Biomedical Informatics

Edward H. Shortliffe • James J. Cimino
Editors

Biomedical Informatics

Computer Applications in Health Care and Biomedicine

Fourth Edition

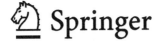 Springer

Editors
Edward H. Shortliffe, MD, PhD
Departments of Biomedical Informatics
at Columbia University
and Arizona State University
New York, NY
USA

James J. Cimino, MD
Bethesda, MD
USA

ISBN 978-1-4471-4473-1   ISBN 978-1-4471-4474-8   (eBook)
DOI 10.1007/978-1-4471-4474-8
Springer London Heidelberg New York Dordrecht

Library of Congress Control Number: 2013955588

Printed on acid-free paper

Springer is part of Springer Science+Business Media (www.springer.com)

Dedicated to Homer R. Warner, MD, PhD, FACMI
   A Principal Founder of the Field of Biomedical Informatics
   1922–2012

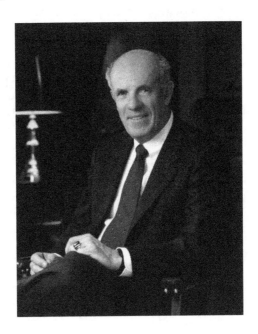

The Fourth Edition of *Biomedical Informatics*: *Computer Applications in Health Care and Biomedicine* is dedicated to the memory and professional contributions of Homer R. Warner. Homer was not only a pioneer in biomedical informatics but a sustained contributor who is truly one of the founders of the field that mourned his loss in November of 2012. Homer's publications on the use of computers in health care span 50 years, from 1963 to 2012, but he can claim an additional decade of informatics research that predated digital computer use, including the use of analog computers and mathematical models ranging from details of cardiac function all the way up to medical diagnosis.[1]

He is best known for his development of the Health Evaluation through Logical Processing (HELP) system, which was revolutionary in its own right as a hospital information system, but was truly visionary in its inclusion of the logical modules for generating alerts and reminders. The HELP system,

---

[1] Warner, H. R., Toronto, A. F., Veasey, L. G., & Stephenson, R. 1961. A mathematical approach to medical diagnosis. Application to congenital heart disease. *JAMA: The Journal of the American Medical Association, 177*, 177–183.

begun in 1968, is still running today at the LDS Hospital in Salt Lake City; innovations are continually added while commercial systems struggle to replicate functions that HELP has had for almost half a century. Homer's other contributions are far too numerous to recount here, but you will find them described in no less than six different chapters of this book.

Homer's contributions go far beyond merely the scientific foundation of biomedical informatics. He also provided extensive leadership to define informatics as a separate academic field. He accomplished this in many settings; locally by founding the first degree-granting informatics department at the University of Utah, nationally as the President of the American College of Medical Informatics, and internationally as the founding editor of the well-known and influential journal *Computers and Biomedical Research* (now the *Journal of Biomedical Informatics*). But perhaps his greatest impact is the generations of researchers and trainees that he personally inspired who have gone on to mentor additional researchers and trainees who together are the life blood of biomedical informatics. Homer's true influence on the field is therefore incalculable. Just consider the convenience sample of this book's 60 chapter co-authors: the following diagram shows his lineage of professional influence on 52 of us.[2]

Both of us were privileged to have many professional and personal interactions with Homer and we were always struck by his enthusiasm, energy, humor, generosity, and integrity. In 1994, Homer received the American College of Medical Informatics' highest honor, the Morris F Collen Award of Excellence. We are proud to have this opportunity to add to the recognition of Homer's life and career with this dedication.

James J. Cimino
Edward H. Shortliffe

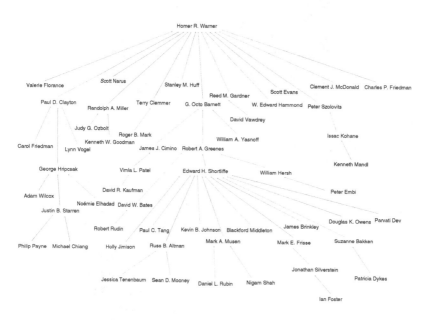

[2] Paul Clayton and Peter Szolovits provide important connections between Homer Warner and ten coauthors but, while they are informatics leaders in their own right, they are not contributors to this edition of this book.

Preface to the Fourth Edition

The world of biomedical research and health care has changed remarkably in the 25 years since the first edition of this book was undertaken. So too has the world of computing and communications and thus the underlying scientific issues that sit at the intersections among biomedical science, patient care, public health, and information technology. It is no longer necessary to argue that it has become impossible to practice modern medicine, or to conduct modern biological research, without information technologies. Since the initiation of the human genome project two decades ago, life scientists have been generating data at a rate that defies traditional methods for information management and data analysis. Health professionals also are constantly reminded that a large percentage of their activities relates to information management—for example, obtaining and recording information about patients, consulting colleagues, reading and assessing the scientific literature, planning diagnostic procedures, devising strategies for patient care, interpreting results of laboratory and radiologic studies, or conducting case-based and population-based research. It is complexity and uncertainty, plus society's overriding concern for patient well-being, and the resulting need for optimal decision making, that set medicine and health apart from many other information-intensive fields. Our desire to provide the best possible health and health care for our society gives a special significance to the effective organization and management of the huge bodies of data with which health professionals and biomedical researchers must deal. It also suggests the need for specialized approaches and for skilled scientists who are knowledgeable about human biology, clinical care, information technologies, and the scientific issues that drive the effective use of such technologies in the biomedical context.

Information Management in Biomedicine

The clinical and research influence of biomedical-computing systems is remarkably broad. Clinical information systems, which provide communication and information-management functions, are now installed in essentially all healthcare institutions. Physicians can search entire drug indexes in a few seconds, using the information provided by a computer program to anticipate harmful side effects or drug interactions. Electrocardiograms (ECGs) are typically analyzed initially by computer programs, and similar techniques are being applied for interpretation of pulmonary-function tests and a variety of laboratory and radiologic abnormalities. Devices with embedded processors routinely monitor patients and provide warnings in critical-care settings, such as the intensive-care unit (ICU) or the operating room. Both biomedical researchers and clinicians regularly use computer programs to search the medical literature, and modern clinical research would be severely hampered without computer-based data-storage techniques and statistical analysis systems. Advanced decision-support tools also are emerging from research laboratories, are being integrated with patient-care systems, and are beginning to have a profound effect on the way medicine is practiced.

Despite this extensive use of computers in healthcare settings and biomedical research, and a resulting expansion of interest in learning more about biomedical computing, many life scientists, health-science students, and professionals have found it difficult to obtain a comprehensive and rigorous, but nontechnical, overview of the field. Both practitioners and basic scientists are recognizing that thorough preparation for their professional futures requires that they gain an understanding of the state of the art in biomedical computing, of the current and future capabilities *and* limitations of the technology, and of the way in which such developments fit within the scientific, social, and financial context of biomedicine and our healthcare system. In turn, the future of the biomedical computing field will be largely determined by how well health professionals and biomedical scientists are prepared to guide and to capitalize upon the discipline's development. This book is intended to meet this growing need for such well-equipped professionals. The first edition appeared in 1990 (published by Addison-Wesley) and was used extensively in courses on medical informatics throughout the world. It was updated with a second edition (published by Springer) in 2000, responding to the remarkable changes that occurred during the 1990s, most notably the introduction of the World Wide Web and its impact on adoption and acceptance of the Internet. The third edition (again published by Springer) appeared in 2006, reflecting the ongoing rapid evolution of both technology and health- and biomedically-related applications, plus the emerging government recognition of the key role that health information technology would need to play in promoting quality, safety, and efficiency in patient care. With that edition the title of the book was changed from *Medical Informatics* to *Biomedical Informatics*, reflecting (as is discussed in Chap. 1) both the increasing breadth of the basic discipline and the evolving new name for academic units, societies, research programs, and publications in the field. Like the first three editions, this new version provides a conceptual framework for learning about the science that underlies applications of computing and communications technology in biomedicine and health care, for understanding the state of the art in computer applications in clinical care and biology, for critiquing existing systems, and for anticipating future directions that the field may take.

In many respects, this new edition is very different from its predecessors, however. Most importantly, it reflects the remarkable changes in computing and communications that continue to occur, most notably in communications, networking, and health information technology policy, and the exploding interest in the role that information technology must play in systems integration and the melding of genomics with innovations in clinical practice and treatment. In addition, new chapters have been introduced, one (healthcare financing) was eliminated, while others have been revamped. We have introduced new chapters on the health information infrastructure, consumer health informatics, telemedicine, translational bioinformatics, clinical research informatics, and health information technology policy. Most of the previous chapters have undergone extensive revisions. Those readers who are familiar with the first three editions will find that the organization and philosophy are unchanged, but the content is either new or extensively updated.[1]

This book differs from other introductions to the field in its broad coverage and in its emphasis on the field's conceptual underpinnings rather than on technical details. Our book presumes no health- or computer-science background, but it does assume that you are interested in a comprehensive summary of the field that stresses the underlying concepts, and that introduces technical details only to the extent that they are necessary to meet the principal goal. It thus differs from an impressive early text in the field (Ledley 1965) that emphasized technical details but did not dwell on the broader social and clinical context in which biomedical computing systems are developed and implemented.

Overview and Guide to Use of This book

This book is written as a text so that it can be used in formal courses, but we have adopted a broad view of the population for whom it is intended. Thus, it may be used not only by students of medicine and of the other health professions, but also as an introductory text by future biomedical informatics professionals, as well as for self-study and for reference by practitioners. The book is probably too detailed for use in a 2- or 3-day continuing-education course, although it could be introduced as a reference for further independent study.

Our principal goal in writing this text is to teach *concepts* in biomedical informatics—the study of biomedical information and its use in decision making—and to illustrate them in the context of descriptions of representative systems that are in use today or that taught us lessons in the past. As you will see, biomedical informatics is more than the study of computers in biomedicine, and we have organized the book to emphasize that point. Chapter 1 first sets the stage for the rest of the book by providing a glimpse of the future, defining important terms and concepts, describing the content of the field, explaining the connections between biomedical informatics and related disciplines, and discussing the forces that have influenced research in biomedical informatics and its integration into clinical practice and biological research.

---

[1] As with the first three editions, this book has tended to draw both its examples and it contributors from North America. There is excellent work in other parts of the world as well, although variations in healthcare systems, and especially financing, do tend to change the way in which systems evolve from one country to the next. The basic concepts are identical, however, so the book is intended to be useful in educational programs in other parts of the world as well.

Broad issues regarding the nature of data, information, and knowledge pervade all areas of application, as do concepts related to optimal decision making. Chapters 2 and 3 focus on these topics but mention computers only in passing. They serve as the foundation for all that follows. Chapter 4 on cognitive science issues enhances the discussions in Chaps. 2 and 3, pointing out that decision making and behavior are deeply rooted in the ways in which information is processed by the human mind. Key concepts underlying system design, human-computer interaction, patient safety, educational technology, and decision making are introduced in this chapter.

Chapters 5 and 6 introduce the central notions of computer architectures and software engineering that are important for understanding the applications described later. Also included is a discussion of computer-system design, with explanations of important issues for you to consider when you read about specific applications and systems throughout the remainder of this book.

Chapter 7 summarizes the issues of standards development, focusing in particular on data exchange and issues related to sharing of clinical data. This important and rapidly evolving topic warrants inclusion given the evolution of the health information exchange, institutional system integration challenges, and the increasingly central role of standards in enabling clinical systems to have their desired influence on healthcare practices.

Chapter 8 addresses a topic of increasing practical relevance in both the clinical and biological worlds: natural language understanding and the processing of biomedical texts. The importance of these methods is clear when one considers the amount of information contained in free-text dictated notes or in the published biomedical literature. Even with efforts to encourage structured data entry in clinical systems, there will likely always be an important role for techniques that allow computer systems to extract meaning from natural language documents.

Chapter 9 is a comprehensive introduction to the conceptual underpinnings of biomedical and clinical image capture, analysis, interpretation and use. This overview of the basic issues and imaging modalities serves as background for Chap. 20, which deals with imaging applications issues, highlighted in the world of radiological imaging and image management (e.g., in picture archiving and communication systems).

Chapter 10 addresses the key legal and ethical issues that have arisen when health information systems are considered. Then, in Chap. 11, the challenges associated with technology assessment and with the evaluation of clinical information systems are introduced.

Chapters 12–26 (which include several new chapters in this edition) survey many of the key biomedical areas in which computers are being used. Each chapter explains the conceptual and organizational issues in building that type of system, reviews the pertinent history, and examines the barriers to successful implementations.

Chapter 27 is a new chapter in the fourth edition, providing a summary of the rapidly evolving policy issues related to health information technology. Although the emphasis is on US government policy, there is some discussion of issues that clearly generalize both to states (in the US) and to other countries. The book concludes in Chap. 28 with a look to the future—a vision of how informatics concepts, computers, and advanced communication devices one day may pervade every aspect of biomedical research and clinical practice.

The Study of Computer Applications in Biomedicine

The actual and potential uses of computers in health care and biomedicine form a remarkably broad and complex topic. However, just as you do not need to understand how a telephone or an ATM machine works to make good use of it and to tell when it is functioning poorly, we believe that technical biomedical-computing skills are not needed by health workers and life scientists who wish simply to become effective users of evolving information technologies. On the other hand, such technical skills are of course necessary for individuals with career commitment to developing information systems for biomedical and health environments. Thus, this book will neither teach you to be a programmer, nor show you how to fix a broken computer (although it might motivate you to learn how to do both). It also will not tell you about every important biomedical-computing system or application; we shall use an extensive bibliography to direct you to a wealth of literature where review articles and individual project reports can be found. We describe specific systems only as examples that can provide you with an understanding of the conceptual and organizational issues to be addressed in building systems for such uses. Examples also help to reveal the remaining barriers to successful implementations. Some of the application systems described in the book are well established, even in the commercial marketplace. Others are just beginning to be used broadly in biomedical settings. Several are still largely confined to the research laboratory.

Because we wish to emphasize the concepts underlying this field, we generally limit the discussion of technical implementation details. The computer-science issues can be learned from other courses and other textbooks. One exception, however, is our emphasis on the details of decision science as they relate to biomedical problem solving (Chaps. 3 and 22). These topics generally are not presented in computer-science courses, yet they play a central role in the intelligent use of biomedical data and knowledge. Sections on medical decision making and computer-assisted decision support accordingly include more technical detail than you will find in other chapters.

All chapters include an annotated list of Suggested Readings to which you can turn if you have a particular interest in a topic, and there is a comprehensive Bibliography, drawn from the individual chapters, at the end of the book. We use **boldface** print to indicate the key terms of each chapter; the definitions of these terms are included in the Glossary at the end of the book. Because many of the issues in biomedical informatics are conceptual, we have included Questions for Discussion at the end of each chapter. You will quickly discover that most of these questions do not have "right" answers. They are intended to illuminate key issues in the field and to motivate you to examine additional readings and new areas of research.

It is inherently limiting to learn about computer applications solely by reading about them. We accordingly encourage you to complement your studies by seeing real systems in use—ideally by using them yourself. Your understanding of system limitations and of what *you* would do to improve a biomedical-computing system will be greatly enhanced if you have had personal experience with representative applications. Be aggressive in seeking opportunities to observe and use working systems.

In a field that is changing as rapidly as biomedical informatics is, it is difficult ever to feel that you have knowledge that is completely current. However, the conceptual basis for study changes much more slowly than do the detailed technological issues. Thus, the lessons you learn from this volume will provide you with a foundation on which you can continue to build in the years ahead.

The Need for a Course in Biomedical Informatics

A suggestion that new courses are needed in the curricula for students of the health professions is generally not met with enthusiasm. If anything, educators and students have been clamoring for *reduced* lecture time, for more emphasis on small group sessions, and for more free time for problem solving and reflection. A 1984 national survey by the Association of American Medical Colleges found that both medical students and their educators severely criticized the traditional emphasis on lectures and memorization. Yet the analysis of a panel on the General Professional Education of the Physician (GPEP) (Association of American Medical Colleges 1984) and several subsequent studies and reports have specifically identified biomedical informatics, including computer applications, as an area in which new educational opportunities need to be developed so that physicians and other health professionals will be better prepared for clinical practice. The AAMC recommended the formation of new academic units in biomedical informatics in our medical schools, and subsequent studies and reports have continued to stress the importance of the field and the need for its inclusion in the educational environments of health professionals.

The reason for this strong recommendation is clear: *The practice of medicine is inextricably entwined with the management of information.* In the past, practitioners handled medical information through resources such as the nearest hospital or medical-school library; personal collections of books, journals, and reprints; files of patient records; consultation with colleagues; manual office bookkeeping; and (all-too-often flawed) memorization. Although these techniques continue to be variably valuable, information technology is offering new methods for finding, filing, and sorting information: online bibliographic-retrieval systems, including full-text publications; personal computers, laptops, tablets, and smart phones, with database software to maintain personal information and commonly used references; office-practice and clinical information systems to capture, communicate, and preserve key elements of the health record; information retrieval and consultation systems to provide assistance when an answer to a question is needed rapidly; practice-management systems to integrate billing and receivable functions with other aspects of office or clinic organization; and other online information resources that help to reduce the pressure to memorize in a field that defies total mastery of all but its narrowest aspects. With such a pervasive and inevitable role for computers in clinical practice, and with a growing failure of traditional techniques to deal with the rapidly increasing information-management needs of practitioners, it has become obvious to many people that an essential topic has emerged for study in schools that train medical and other health professionals.

What is less clear is how the subject should be taught, and to what extent it should be left for postgraduate education. We believe that topics in bio-medical informatics are best taught and learned in the context of health-science training, which allows concepts from both the health sciences and informatics science to be integrated. Biomedical-computing novices are likely to have only limited opportunities for intensive study of the material once their health-professional training has been completed.

The format of biomedical informatics education is certain to evolve as faculty members are hired to develop it at more health-science schools, and as the emphasis on lectures as the primary teaching method continues to diminish. Computers will be used increasingly as teaching tools and as devices for communication, problem solving, and data sharing among students and faculty. In the meantime, key content in biomedical informatics will likely be taught largely in the classroom setting. This book is designed to be used in that kind of traditional course, although the Questions for Discussion also could be used to focus conversation in small seminars and working groups. As resources improve in schools and academic medical centers, integration of biomedical informatics topics into clinical experiences also will become more common. The eventual goal should be to provide instruction in biomedical informatics whenever this field is most relevant to the topic the student is studying. This aim requires educational opportunities throughout the years of formal training, supplemented by continuing-education programs after graduation.

The goal of integrating biomedicine and biomedical informatics is to provide a mechanism for increasing the sophistication of health professionals, so that they know and understand the available resources. They also should be familiar with biomedical computing's successes and failures, its research frontiers and its limitations, so that they can avoid repeating the mistakes of the past. Study of biomedical informatics also should improve their skills in information management and problem solving. With a suitable integration of hands-on computer experience, computer-based learning, courses in clinical problem solving, and study of the material in this volume, health-science students will be well prepared to make effective use of computer-based tools and information management in healthcare delivery.

The Need for Specialists in Biomedical Informatics

As mentioned, this book also is intended to be used as an introductory text in programs of study for people who intend to make their professional careers in biomedical informatics. If we have persuaded you that a course in biomedical informatics is needed, then the requirement for trained faculty to teach the courses will be obvious. Some people might argue, however, that a course on this subject could be taught by a computer scientist who had an interest in biomedical computing, or by a physician or biologist who had taken a few computing courses. Indeed, in the past, most teaching—and research—has been undertaken by faculty trained primarily in one of the fields and later drawn to the other. Today, however, schools have come to realize the need for professionals trained specifically at the interfaces among biomedicine, biomedical informatics, and related disciplines such as computer science, statistics, cognitive science, health economics, and medical ethics. This book outlines a first course for students training for careers in the biomedical informatics field. We specifically address the need for an educational experience in which computing and information-science concepts are synthesized with biomedical issues regarding research, training, and clinical practice. It is the *integration* of the related disciplines that traditionally has been lacking in the educational opportunities available to students with career interests in biomedical informatics. If schools are to establish such courses and training programs (and there are growing numbers of examples of each), they clearly need educators who have a broad familiarity with the field and who can develop curricula for students of the health professions as well as of informatics itself.

The increasing introduction of computing techniques into biomedical environments will require that well-trained individuals be available not only to teach students, but also to design, develop, select, and manage the biomedical-computing systems of tomorrow. There is a wide range of context-dependent computing issues that people can appreciate only by working on problems defined by the healthcare setting and its constraints. The field's development has been hampered because there are relatively few trained personnel to design research programs, to carry out the experimental and developmental activities, and to provide academic leadership in biomedical informatics. A frequently cited problem is the difficulty a health professional (or a biologist) and a technically trained computer scientist experience when they try to communicate with one another. The vocabularies of the two fields are complex and have little overlap, and there is a process of acculturation to biomedicine that is difficult for computer scientists to appreciate through distant observation. Thus, interdisciplinary research and development projects are more likely to be successful when they are led by people who can effectively bridge the biomedical and computing fields. Such professionals often can facilitate sensitive communication among program personnel whose backgrounds and training differ substantially.

It is exciting to be working in a field that is maturing and that is having a beneficial effect on society. There is ample opportunity remaining for innovation as new technologies evolve and fundamental computing problems succumb to the creativity and hard work of our colleagues. In light of the increasing sophistication and specialization required in computer science in general, it is hardly surprising that a new discipline should arise at that field's interface with biomedicine. This book is dedicated to clarifying the definition and to nurturing the effectiveness of that discipline: biomedical informatics.

New York, NY   Edward H. Shortliffe
Bethesda, MD   James J. Cimino
                                                                                                  October 2013

Acknowledgments

In the 1980s, when I was based at Stanford University, I conferred with colleagues Larry Fagan and Gio Wiederhold and we decided to compile the first comprehensive textbook on what was then called medical informatics. As it turned out, none of us predicted the enormity of the task we were about to undertake. Our challenge was to create a multi-authored textbook that captured the collective expertise of leaders in the field yet was cohesive in content and style. The concept for the book first developed in 1982. We had begun to teach a course on computer applications in health care at Stanford's School of Medicine and had quickly determined that there was no comprehensive introductory text on the subject. Despite several published collections of research descriptions and subject reviews, none had been developed with the needs of a rigorous introductory course in mind.

The thought of writing a textbook was daunting due to the diversity of topics. None of us felt that he was sufficiently expert in the full range of important subjects for us to write the book ourselves. Yet we wanted to avoid putting together a collection of disconnected chapters containing assorted subject reviews. Thus, we decided to solicit contributions from leaders in the respective fields to be represented but to provide organizational guidelines in advance for each chapter. We also urged contributors to avoid writing subject reviews but, instead, to focus on the key conceptual topics in their field and to pick a handful of examples to illustrate their didactic points.

As the draft chapters began to come in, we realized that major editing would be required if we were to achieve our goals of cohesiveness and a uniform orientation across all the chapters. We were thus delighted when, in 1987, Leslie Perreault, a graduate of our training program, assumed responsibility for reworking the individual chapters to make an integral whole and for bringing the project to completion. The final product, published in 1990, was the result of many compromises, heavy editing, detailed rewriting, and numerous iterations. We were gratified by the positive response to the book when it finally appeared, and especially by the students of biomedical informatics who have often come to us at scientific meetings and told us about their appreciation of the book.

As the 1990s progressed, however, we began to realize that, despite our emphasis on basic concepts in the field (rather than a survey of existing systems), the volume was beginning to show its age. A great deal had changed since the initial chapters were written, and it became clear that a new edition would be required. The original editors discussed the project and decided that we should redesign the book, solicit updated chapters, and publish a new edition. Leslie Perreault by this time was a busy Director at First Consulting

Group in New York City and would not have as much time to devote to the project as she had when we did the first edition. With trepidation, in light of our knowledge of the work that would be involved, we embarked on the new project.

As before, the chapter authors did a marvelous job, trying to meet our deadlines, putting up with editing changes that were designed to bring a uniform style to the book, and contributing excellent chapters that nicely reflected the changes in the field in the preceding decade.

No sooner had the second edition appeared in print than we started to get inquiries about when the next update would appear. We began to realize that the maintenance of a textbook in a field such as biomedical informatics was nearly a constant, ongoing process. By this time I had moved to Columbia University and the initial group of editors had largely disbanded to take on other responsibilities, with Leslie Perreault no longer available. Accordingly, as plans for a third edition began to take shape, my Columbia colleague Jim Cimino joined me as the new associate editor, whereas Drs. Fagan, Wiederhold, and Perreault continued to be involved as chapter authors. Once again the authors did their best to try to meet our deadlines as the third edition took shape. This time we added several chapters, attempting to cover additional key topics that readers and authors had identified as being necessary enhancements to the earlier editions. We were once again extremely appreciative of all the authors' commitment and for the excellence of their work on behalf of the book and the field.

Predictably, it was only a short time after the publication of the third edition that we began to get queries about a fourth edition. We resisted for a year or two but it became clear that the third edition was becoming rapidly stale in some key areas and that there were new topics that were not in the book and needed to be added. With that in mind we, in consultation with Grant Weston from Springer's offices in London, agreed to embark on a fourth edition. Progress was slowed by my professional moves (to Phoenix, Arizona, then Houston, Texas, and then back to New York) with a very busy three-year stint as President and CEO of the American Medical Informatics Association. Similarly, Jim Cimino left Columbia to assume new responsibilities at the NIH Clinical Center in Bethesda, MD. With several new chapters in mind, and the need to change authors of some of the existing chapters due to retirements (this too will happen, even in a young field like informatics!), we began working on the fourth edition, finally completing the effort in early 2013.

The completed fourth edition reflects the work and support of many people in addition to the editors and chapter authors. Particular gratitude is owed to Maureen Alexander, our developmental editor whose rigorous attention to detail was crucial given the size and the complexity of the undertaking. At Springer we have been delighted to work on this edition with Grant Weston, who has been extremely supportive despite our missed deadlines. And I want to offer my sincere personal thanks to Jim Cimino, who has been a superb and talented collaborator in this effort for the last two editions. Without his hard work and expertise, we would still be struggling to complete the massive editing job associated with this now very long manuscript.

New York, NY   Edward H. Shortliffe

Contents

Part I   Recurrent Themes in Biomedical Informatics

1   **Biomedical Informatics: The Science and the Pragmatics**   3
    Edward H. Shortliffe and Marsden S. Blois

2   **Biomedical Data: Their Acquisition, Storage, and Use**   39
    Edward H. Shortliffe and G. Octo Barnett

3   **Biomedical Decision Making: Probabilistic**
    Clinical Reasoning   67
    Douglas K. Owens and Harold C. Sox

4   **Cognitive Science and Biomedical Informatics** 109
    Vimla L. Patel and David R. Kaufman

5   **Computer Architectures for Health Care and Biomedicine** . . . 149
    Jonathan C. Silverstein and Ian T. Foster

6   **Software Engineering for Health Care and Biomedicine** 185
    Adam B. Wilcox, Scott P. Narus, and David K. Vawdrey

7   **Standards in Biomedical Informatics** 211
    W. Edward Hammond, Charles Jaffe,
    James J. Cimino, and Stanley M. Huff

8   **Natural Language Processing in Health Care**
    and Biomedicine 255
    Carol Friedman and Noémie Elhadad

9   **Biomedical Imaging Informatics** 285
    Daniel L. Rubin, Hayit Greenspan,
    and James F. Brinkley

10 **Ethics in Biomedical and Health Informatics: Users,**
    Standards, and Outcomes 329
    Kenneth W. Goodman, Reid Cushman, and Randolph A. Miller

11 **Evaluation of Biomedical and Health**
    Information Resources 355
    Charles P. Friedman and Jeremy C. Wyatt

Part II   Biomedical Informatics Applications

12   **Electronic Health Record Systems** 391
     Clement J. McDonald, Paul C. Tang, and George Hripcsak

13   **Health Information Infrastructure** 423
     William A. Yasnoff

14   **Management of Information in Health
     Care Organizations**.................................... 443
     Lynn Harold Vogel

15   **Patient-Centered Care Systems**......................... 475
     Judy Ozbolt, Suzanne Bakken, and Patricia C. Dykes

16   **Public Health Informatics** 503
     Martin LaVenture, David A. Ross, and William A. Yasnoff

17   **Consumer Health Informatics and Personal
     Health Records** 517
     Kevin Johnson, Holly Brugge Jimison,
     and Kenneth D. Mandl

18   **Telehealth**.. 541
     Justin B. Starren, Thomas S. Nesbitt, and Michael F. Chiang

19   **Patient Monitoring Systems**............................ 561
     Reed M. Gardner, Terry P. Clemmer, R. Scott Evans,
     and Roger G. Mark

20   **Imaging Systems in Radiology**.......................... 593
     Bradley Erickson and Robert A. Greenes

21   **Information Retrieval and Digital Libraries** 613
     William R. Hersh

22   **Clinical Decision-Support Systems** 643
     Mark A. Musen, Blackford Middleton, and Robert A. Greenes

23   **Computers in Health Care Education**.................... 675
     Parvati Dev and Titus K.L. Schleyer

24   **Bioinformatics**....................................... 695
     Sean D. Mooney, Jessica D. Tenenbaum, and Russ B. Altman

25   **Translational Bioinformatics** 721
     Jessica D. Tenenbaum, Nigam H. Shah, and Russ B. Altman

26   **Clinical Research Informatics** 755
     Philip R.O. Payne, Peter J. Embi, and James J. Cimino

Part III Biomedical Informatics in the Years Ahead

27 Health Information Technology Policy 781
Robert S. Rudin, Paul C. Tang, and David W. Bates

28 The Future of Informatics in Biomedicine 797
Mark E. Frisse, Valerie Florance, Kenneth D. Mandl,
and Isaac S. Kohane

Glossary 813

Bibliography 865

Name Index 927

Subject Index 943

Contributors

Russ B. Altman, MD, PhD, FACMI Departments of Bioengineering, Genetics and Medicine, Stanford University, Stanford, CA, USA

Suzanne Bakken, RN, PhD, FAAN, FACMI Department of Biomedical Informatics, School of Nursing, Columbia University, New York, NY, USA

G. Octo Barnett, MD, FACP, FACMI Laboratory of Computer Science (Harvard Medical School and Massachusetts General Hospital), Boston, MA, USA

David W. Bates, MD, MSc, FACMI Division of General Internal Medicine and Primary Care, Department of Medicine, Brigham and Women's Hospital, Boston, MA, USA

James F. Brinkley, MD, PhD, FACMI Department of Biological Structure, Biomedical Education and Medical Education, Computer Science and Engineering, University of Washington, Seattle, WA, USA

Michael F. Chiang, MD, MA Department of Ophthalmology and Medical Informatics and Clinical Epidemiology, Oregon Health & Science University, Portland, OR, USA

James J. Cimino, MD, FACMI Laboratory for Informatics Development, NIH Clinical Center, Bethesda, MD, USA

Terry P. Clemmer, MD Pulmonary – Critical Care Medicine, LDS Hospital, Salt Lake City, UT, USA

Reid Cushman, PhD Department of Medicine, University of Miami, Miami, FL, USA

Parvati Dev, PhD, FACMI Innovation in Learning Inc., Los Alotos Hills, CA, USA

Patricia C. Dykes, DNSc, MA, FACMI Center for Patient Safety Research and Practice, Brigham and Women's Hospital, Boston, MA, USA

Noémie Elhadad, PhD Department of Biomedical Informatics, Columbia University, New York, NY, USA

Peter J. Embi, MD, MS, FACMI Departments of Biomedical Informatics and Internal Medicine, The Ohio State University Wexner Medical Center, Columbus, OH, USA

Bradley Erickson, MD, PhD Department of Radiology
and Medical Informatics, Mayo Clinic, Rochester, MN, USA

R. Scott Evans, BS, MS, PhD, FACMI Medical Informatics Department,
LDS Hospital, Intermountain Healthcare, Salt Lake City, UT, USA

Valerie Florance, PhD, FACMI Division of Extramural Programs,
National Library of Medicine, National Institutes of Health, DHHS,
Bethesda, MD, USA

Ian T. Foster, PhD Searle Chemistry Laboratory, Computation Institute,
University of Chicago and Argonne National Laboratory, Chicago, IL, USA

Carol Friedman, PhD, FACMI Department of Biomedical Informatics,
Columbia University, New York, NY, USA

Charles P. Friedman, PhD, FACMI Schools of Information and
Public Health, University of Michigan, Ann Arbor, MI, USA

Mark E. Frisse, MD, MS, MBA, FACMI Department of Biomedical
Informatics, Vanderbilt University Medical Center, Nashville, TN, USA

Reed M. Gardner, PhD, FACMI Department of Informatics,
University of Utah, Biomedical Informatics, Salt Lake City, UT, USA

Kenneth W. Goodman, PhD, FACMI University of Miami Bioethics
Program, Miami, FL, USA

Robert A. Greenes, MD, PhD, FACMI Department of Biomedical
Informatics, Arizona State University, Tempe, AZ, USA
Division of Health Sciences Research, College of Medicine,
Mayo Clinic, Scottsdale, AZ, USA

Hayit Greenspan, PhD Department of Biomedical Engineering,
Faculty of Engineering, TelAviv University, Tel Aviv, Israel

W. Edward Hammond, PhD, FACMI Duke Center for Health
Informatics, Duke University Medical Center, Durham, NC, USA

William R. Hersh, MD FACMI, FACP Department of Medical
Informatics and Clinical Epidemiology, Oregon Health and Science
University, Portland, OR, USA

George Hripcsak, MD, MS, FACMI Department of Biomedical
Informatics, Columbia University Medical Center, New York, NY, USA

Stanley M. Huff, MD, FACMI Medical Informatics,
Intermountain Healthcare, Murray, UT, USA

Charles Jaffe, PhD Health Level Seven International,
Del Mar, CA, USA

Holly Brugge Jimison, PhD, FACMI Consortium on Technology for
Proactive Care, Colleges of Computer and Information Sciences and Health
Sciences, Northeastern University, Boston, MA, USA

Kevin Johnson, MD, MS, FACMI Department of Biomedical Informatics, Vanderbilt University School of Medicine, Nashville, TN, USA

David R. Kaufman, PhD Department of Biomedical Informatics, Arizona State University, Scottsdale, AZ, USA

Isaac S. Kohane, MD, PhD, FACMI Harvard Medical School Center for Biomedical Informatics and Children's Hospital Informatics Program, Boston, MA, USA

Martin LaVenture, MPH, PhD, FACMI Minnesota Department of Health, Office of HIT and e-Health, Center for Health Informatics, St. Paul, MN, USA

Kenneth D. Mandl, MD, MPH, FACMI Children's Hospital Informatics Program, Harvard Medical School, Boston Children's Hospital, Boston, MA, USA

Roger G. Mark, MD, PhD Institute of Medical Engineering and Science, Department of Electrical Engineering and Computer Science (EECS), Massachusetts Institute of Technology, Cambridge, MA, USA

Clement J. McDonald, MD, FACMI Office of the Director, Lister Hill National Center for Biomedical Communications, National Library of Medicine, National Institutes of Health, Bethesda, MD, USA

Blackford Middleton, MD, MPH, MSc, FACMI Informatics Center, Vanderbilt University Medical Center, Nashville, TN, USA

Randolph A. Miller, MD, FACMI Department of Biomedical Informatics, Vanderbilt University Medical Center, Nashville, TN, USA

Sean D. Mooney, PhD Buck Institute for Research on Aging, Novato, CA, USA

Mark A. Musen, MD, PhD, FACMI Center for Biomedical Informatics Research, Stanford University School of Medicine, Stanford, CA, USA

Scott P. Narus, PhD Department of Medical Informatics, Intermountain Healthcare, Murray, UT, USA

Thomas S. Nesbitt, MD, MPH Department of Family and Community Medicine, School of Medicine, UC Davis Health System, Sacramento, CA, USA

Douglas K. Owens, MD, MS, VA Palo Alto Health Care System and H.J. Kaiser Center for Primary Care and Outcomes Research/Center for Health Policy, Stanford University, Stanford, CA, USA

Judy Ozbolt, PhD, RN, FAAN, FACMI, FAIMBE Department of Organizational Systems and Adult Health, University of Maryland School of Nursing, Baltimore, MD, USA

Vimla L. Patel, PhD, DSc, FACMI Center for Cognitive Studies in Medicine and Public Health, The New York Academy of Medicine, New York, NY, USA

Philip R.O. Payne, PhD, FACMI Department of Biomedical Informatics, The Ohio State University Wexner Medical Center, Columbus, OH, USA

David A. Ross, D.Sc Public Health Informatics Institute/ The Task Force for Global Health, Decatur, GA, USA

Daniel L. Rubin, MD, MS, FACMI Departments of Radiology and Medicine, Stanford University, Stanford, CA, USA

Robert S. Rudin, BS, SM, PhD Health Unit, Rand Corporation, Boston, MA, USA

Titus K.L. Schleyer, DMD, PhD, FACMI Center for Biomedical Informatics Regenstrief Institute, Inc., Indianapolis, IN

Nigam H. Shah, MBBS, PhD Department of Medicine, Stanford University, Stanford, CA, USA

Edward H. Shortliffe, MD, PhD, MACP, FACMI Departments of Biomedical Informatics, Arizona State University, Columbia University, Weill Cornell Medical College, and the New York Academy of Medicine, New York, NY, USA

Jonathan C. Silverstein, MD, MS, FACMI Research Institute, NorthShore University Health System, Evanston, IL, USA

Harold C. Sox, MD, MACP Dartmouth Institute, Geisel School of Medicine, Dartmouth College, West Lebanon, NH, USA

Justin B. Starren, MD, PhD, FACMI Division of Health and Biomedical Informatics, Department of Preventive Medicine and Medical Social Sciences, Northwestern University Feinberg School of Medicine, Chicago, IL, USA

Paul C. Tang, MD, MS, FACMI David Druker Center for Health Systems Innovation, Palo Alto Medical Foundation, Mountain View, CA, USA

Jessica D. Tenenbaum, PhD Duke Translational Medicine Institute, Duke University, Durham, NC, USA

David K. Vawdrey, PhD Department of Biomedical Informatics, Columbia University, New York, NY, USA

Lynn Harold Vogel, PhD LH Vogel Consulting, LLC, Ridgewood, NJ, USA

Adam B. Wilcox, PhD, FACMI Department of Biomedical Informatics, Intermountain Healthcare, New York, NY, USA

Jeremy C. Wyatt, MB BS, FRCP, FACMI Leeds Institute of Health Sciences, University of Leeds, Leeds, UK

William A. Yasnoff, MD, PhD, FACMI NHII Advisors, Arlington, VA, USA

Part I

Recurrent Themes in Biomedical Informatics

Biomedical Informatics: The Science and the Pragmatics

Edward H. Shortliffe and Marsden S. Blois[†]

After reading this chapter, you should know the answers to these questions:

- Why is information and knowledge management a central issue in biomedical research and clinical practice?
- What are integrated information management environments, and how might we expect them to affect the practice of medicine, the promotion of health, and biomedical research in coming years?
- What do we mean by the terms *biomedical informatics, medical computer science, medical computing, clinical informatics, nursing informatics, bioinformatics, public health informatics,* and *health informatics*?
- Why should health professionals, life scientists, and students of the health professions learn about biomedical informatics concepts and informatics applications?
- How has the development of modern computing technologies and the Internet changed the nature of biomedical computing?
- How is biomedical informatics related to clinical practice, public health, biomedical engineering, molecular biology, decision science, information science, and computer science?

- How does information in clinical medicine and health differ from information in the basic sciences?
- How can changes in computer technology and the way patient care is financed influence the integration of biomedical computing into clinical practice?

1.1 The Information Revolution Comes to Medicine

After scientists had developed the first digital computers in the 1940s, society was told that these new machines would soon be serving routinely as memory devices, assisting with calculations and with information retrieval. Within the next decade, physicians and other health professionals had begun to hear about the dramatic effects that such technology would have

[†]Author was deceased at the time of publication.

E.H. Shortliffe, MD, PhD
Departments of Biomedical Informatics
at Columbia University and Arizona State University,
Weill Cornell Medical College,
and The New York Academy of Medicine,
272 W 107th St #5B, New York 10025, NY, USA
e-mail: ted@shortliffe.net

Dr. Blois coauthored the 1990 (1st edition) version of this chapter shortly before his death in 1988, a year prior to the completion of the full manuscript. Although the chapter has evolved in subsequent editions, we continue to name Dr. Blois as a coauthor because of his seminal contributions to the field as well as to this chapter. Section 1.5 was written by him and, since it is timeless, remains unchanged in each edition of the book. To learn more about this important early leader in the field of informatics, see his classic volume (Blois 1984) and a tribute to him at http://www.amia.org/about-amia/leadership/acmi-fellow/marsden-s-blois-md-facmi (Accessed 3/3/2013).

E.H. Shortliffe, J.J. Cimino (eds.), *Biomedical Informatics*,
DOI 10.1007/978-1-4471-4474-8_1, © Springer-Verlag London 2014

on clinical practice. More than six decades of remarkable progress in computing have followed those early predictions, and many of the original prophesies have come to pass. Stories regarding the "information revolution" and "big data" fill our newspapers and popular magazines, and today's children show an uncanny ability to make use of computers (including their increasingly mobile versions) as routine tools for study and entertainment. Similarly, clinical workstations have been available on hospital wards and in outpatient offices for years, and are being gradually supplanted by mobile devices with wireless connectivity. Yet many observers cite the health care system as being slow to understand information technology, slow to exploit it for its unique practical and strategic functionalities, slow to incorporate it effectively into the work environment, and slow to understand its strategic importance and its resulting need for investment and commitment. Nonetheless, the enormous technological advances of the last three decades—personal computers and graphical interfaces, new methods for human-computer interaction, innovations in mass storage of data (both locally and in the "cloud"), mobile devices, personal health monitoring devices and tools, the Internet, wireless communications, social media, and more—have all combined to make the routine use of computers by all health workers and biomedical scientists inevitable. A new world is already with us, but its greatest influence is yet to come. This book will teach you both about our present resources and accomplishments and about what you can expect in the years ahead.

When one considers the penetration of computers and communication into our daily lives today, it is remarkable that the first personal computers were introduced as recently as the late 1970s; local area networking has been available only since ~1980; the World Wide Web dates only to the early 1990s; and smart phones, social networking, and wireless communication are even more recent. This dizzying rate of change, combined with equally pervasive and revolutionary changes in almost all international health care systems, makes it difficult for public-health planners and health-institutional managers to try to deal with both issues at once. Yet many observers now believe that the two topics are inextricably related and that planning for the new health care environments of the coming decades requires a deep understanding of the role that information technology is likely to play in those environments.

What might that future hold for the typical practicing clinician? As we shall discuss in detail in Chap. 12, no applied clinical computing topic is gaining more attention currently than is the issue of electronic health records (EHRs). Health care organizations have recognized that they do not have systems in place that effectively allow them to answer questions that are crucially important for strategic planning, for their better understanding of how they compare with other provider groups in their local or regional competitive environment, and for reporting to regulatory agencies. In the past, administrative and financial data were the major elements required for such planning, but comprehensive clinical data are now also important for institutional self-analysis and strategic planning. Furthermore, the inefficiencies and frustrations associated with the use of paper-based medical records are now well accepted (Dick and Steen 1991 (Revised 1997)), especially when inadequate access to clinical information is one of the principal barriers that clinicians encounter when trying to increase their efficiency in order to meet productivity goals for their practices.

1.1.1 Integrated Access to Clinical Information: The Future Is Now

Encouraged by **health information technology (HIT)** vendors (and by the US government, as is discussed later), most health care institutions are seeking to develop integrated computer-based information-management environments. These are single-entry points into a clinical world in which computational tools assist not only with patient-care matters (reporting results of tests, allowing direct entry of orders or patient information by clinicians, facilitating access to transcribed reports, and in some cases supporting telemedicine applications or decision-support functions) but also administrative and financial topics (e.g., tracking of patients within the hospital, managing materials and inventory, supporting personnel functions, and managing the payroll), research (e.g., analyzing the outcomes associated with treatments and procedures, performing quality assurance, supporting clinical trials, and implementing various treatment protocols), scholarly information (e.g., accessing digital libraries, supporting bibliographic search, and providing access to drug information databases), and even office automation (e.g., providing access to spreadsheets and document-management software). The key idea, however, is that at the heart of the evolving integrated environments lies an electronic health record that is intended to be accessible, confidential, secure, acceptable to clinicians and patients, and integrated with other types of useful information to assist in planning and problem solving.

1.1.2 Moving Beyond the Paper Record

The traditional paper-based medical record is now recognized as woefully inadequate for meeting the needs of modern medicine. It arose in the nineteenth century as a highly personalized "lab notebook" that clinicians could use to record their observations and plans so that they could be reminded of pertinent details when they next saw the same patient. There were no regulatory requirements, no assumptions that the record would be used to support communication among varied providers of care, and few data or test results to fill up the record's pages. The record that met the needs of clinicians a century ago struggled mightily to adjust over the decades and to accommodate to new requirements as health care and medicine changed. Today the inability of paper charts to serve the best interests of the patient, the clinician, and the health system has become clear (see Chaps. 12 and 14).

Most organizations have found it challenging (and expensive) to move to a paperless, electronic clinical record. This observation forces us to ask the following questions: "What is a health record in the modern world? Are the available products and systems well matched with the modern notions of a comprehensive health record? Do they meet the needs of individual users as well as the health systems themselves?"

The complexity associated with automating clinical-care records is best appreciated if one analyzes the processes associated with the creation and use of such records rather than thinking of the record as a physical object that can be moved around as needed within the institution. For example, on the input side (Fig. 1.1), the EHR requires the integration of processes for data capture and for merging information from diverse sources. The contents of the paper record have traditionally been organized chronologically—often a severe limitation when a clinician seeks to find a specific piece of information that could occur almost anywhere within the chart. To be useful, the record system must make it easy to access and display needed data, to analyze them, and to share them among colleagues and with secondary users of the record who are not involved in direct patient care (Fig. 1.2). Thus, the EHR is best viewed not as an object, or a product, but rather as a set of processes that an organization must put into place, supported by technology (Fig. 1.3). Implementing electronic records is inherently a systems-integration task; it is not possible to buy a medical record system for a complex organization as an off-the-shelf product. Joint development and local adaptation are crucial, which implies that the institutions that purchase such systems must have local expertise that can oversee and facilitate an effective implementation process, including elements of process re-engineering and cultural change that are inevitably involved.

Experience has shown that clinicians are "horizontal" users of information technology (Greenes and Shortliffe 1990). Rather than becoming "power users" of a narrowly defined software package, they tend to seek broad functionality across a wide variety of systems and resources. Thus, routine use of computers, and of EHRs, is most easily achieved when the computing environment offers a critical mass of functionality

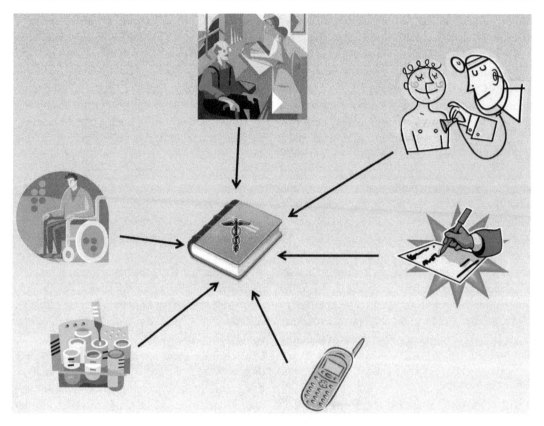

Fig. 1.1 Inputs to the clinical-care record. The traditional paper record is created by a variety of organizational processes that capture varying types of information (notes regarding direct encounters between health professionals and patients, laboratory or radiologic results, reports of telephone calls or prescriptions, and data obtained directly from patients). The record thus becomes a merged collection of such data, generally organized in chronological order

that makes the system both smoothly integrated with workflow and useful for essentially every patient encounter.

The arguments for automating clinical-care records are summarized in Chaps. 2 and 12 and in the now classic Institute of Medicine's report on **computer-based patient records** (**CPRs**) (Dick and Steen 1991 (Revised 1997)). One argument that warrants emphasis is the importance of the EHR in supporting **clinical trials**—experiments in which data from specific patient interactions are pooled and analyzed in order to learn about the safety and efficacy of new treatments or tests and to gain insight into disease processes that are not otherwise well understood. Medical researchers were constrained in the past by clumsy methods for acquiring the data needed for clinical trials, generally relying on manual capture of

information onto datasheets that were later transcribed into computer databases for statistical analysis (Fig. 1.4). The approach was labor-intensive, fraught with opportunities for error, and added to the high costs associated with randomized prospective research protocols.

The use of EHRs has offered many advantages to those carrying out clinical research (see Chap. 26). Most obviously, it helps to eliminate the manual task of extracting data from charts or filling out specialized datasheets. The data needed for a study can often be derived directly from the EHR, thus making much of what is required for research data collection simply a by-product of routine clinical record keeping (Fig. 1.5). Other advantages accrue as well. For example, the record environment can help to ensure compliance with a research protocol, pointing out to a

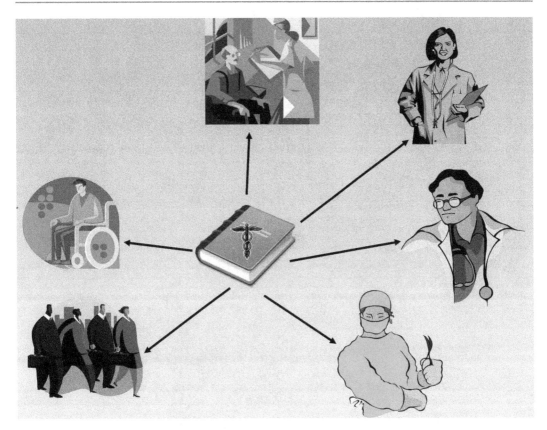

Fig. 1.2 Outputs from the clinical-care record. Once information is collected in the traditional paper chart, it may be provided to a wide variety of potential users of the information that it contains. These users include health professionals and the patients themselves but also a wide variety of "secondary users" (represented here by the individuals in business suits) who have valid reasons for accessing the record but who are not involved with direct patient care. Numerous providers are typically involved in a patient's care, so the chart also serves as a means for communicating among them. The mechanisms for displaying, analyzing, and sharing information from such records results from a set of processes that often varies substantially across several patient-care settings and institutions

clinician when a patient is eligible for a study or when the protocol for a study calls for a specific management plan given the currently available data about that patient. We are also seeing the development of novel authoring environments for clinical trial protocols that can help to ensure that the data elements needed for the trial are compatible with the local EHR's conventions for representing patient descriptors.

Another theme in the changing world of health care is the increasing investment in the creation of **standard order sets**, **clinical guidelines**, and **clinical pathways** (see Chap. 22), generally in an effort to reduce practice variability and to develop consensus approaches to recurring management problems. Several government and professional organizations, as well as individual provider groups, have invested heavily in guideline development, often putting an emphasis on using clear evidence from the literature, rather than expert opinion alone, as the basis for the advice. Despite the success in creating such **evidence-based guidelines**, there is a growing recognition that we need better methods for delivering the decision logic to the point of care. Guidelines that appear in monographs or journal articles tend to sit on shelves, unavailable when the knowledge they contain would be most valuable to practitioners. Computer-based tools for implementing such guidelines, and integrating them with the EHR, present a means for making high-quality advice available in the routine clinical setting.

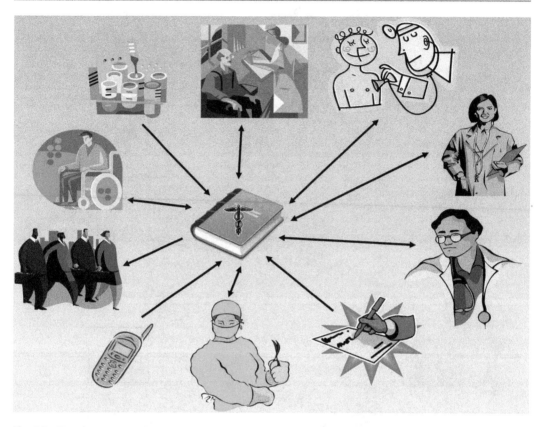

Fig. 1.3 Complex processes demanded of the record. As shown in Figs 1.1 and 1.2, the clinical chart is the incarnation of a complex set of organizational processes, which both gather information to be shared and then distribute that information to those who have valid reasons for accessing it. Paper-based documents are severely limited in meeting the diverse requirements for data collection and information access that are implied by this diagram

Many organizations are accordingly attempting to integrate decision-support tools with their EHR systems, and there are highly visible efforts underway to provide computer-based diagnostic decision support to practitioners.[1]

There are at least four major issues that have consistently constrained our efforts to build effective EHRs: (1) the need for standards in the area of clinical terminology; (2) concerns regarding data privacy, confidentiality, and security; (3) challenges in data entry by physicians; and (4) difficulties associated with the integration of record systems with other information resources in the health care setting. The first of these issues is discussed in detail in Chap. 7, and privacy is one of the central topics in Chap. 10. Issues of direct data entry by clinicians are discussed in Chaps. 2 and 12 and throughout many other chapters as well. Chapter 13 examines the fourth topic, focusing on recent trends in networked data integration, and offers solutions for the ways in which the EHR can be better joined with other relevant information resources and clinical processes, especially within communities where patients may have records with multiple providers and health care systems (Yasnoff et al. 2013).

1.1.3 Anticipating the Future of Electronic Health Records

One of the first instincts of software developers is to create an electronic version of an object or process from the physical world. Some

---

[1] http://www.forbes.com/sites/bruceupbin/2013/02/08/ibms-watson-gets-its-first-piece-of-business-in-healthcare/. (Accessed 4/21/13/).

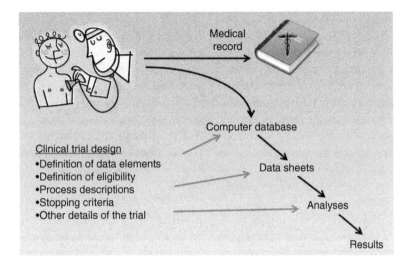

Fig. 1.4 Traditional data collection for clinical trials. Although modern clinical trials routinely use computer systems for data storage and analysis, the gathering of research data is still often a manual task. Physicians who care for patients enrolled in trials, or their research assistants, have traditionally been asked to fill out special data-sheets for later transcription into computer databases. Alternatively, data managers have been hired to abstract the relevant data from the chart. The trials are generally designed to define data elements that are required and the methods for analysis, but it is common for the process of collecting those data in a structured format to be left to manual processes at the point of patient care

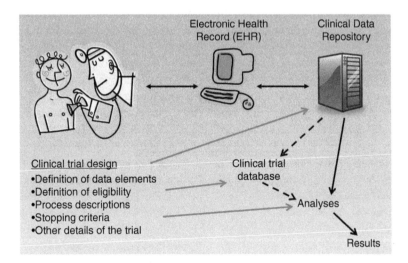

Fig. 1.5 Role of electronic health records (EHRs) in supporting clinical trials. With the introduction of EHR systems, the collection of much of the research data for clinical trials can become a by-product of the routine care of the patients. Research data may be analyzed directly from the clinical data repository, or a secondary research database may be created by downloading information from the online patient records. The manual processes in Fig. 1.4 are thereby largely eliminated. In addition, the interaction of the physician with the EHR permits two-way communication, which can greatly improve the quality and efficiency of the clinical trial. Physicians can be reminded when their patients are eligible for an experimental protocol, and the computer system can also remind the clinicians of the rules that are defined by the research protocol, thereby increasing compliance with the experimental plan

familiar notion provides the inspiration for a new software product. Once the software version has been developed, however, human ingenuity and creativity often lead to an evolution that extends the software version far beyond what was initially contemplated. The computer can thus facilitate paradigm shifts in how we think about such familiar concepts.

Consider, for example, the remarkable difference between today's office automation software and the typewriter, which was the original inspiration for the development of "word processors". Although the early word processors were designed largely to allow users to avoid retyping papers each time a minor change was made to a document, the document-management software of today bears little resemblance to a typewriter. Consider all the powerful desktop-publishing facilities, integration of figures, spelling correction, grammar aids, "publishing" on the Web, use of color, etc. Similarly, today's spreadsheet programs bear little resemblance to the tables of numbers that we once created on graph paper. To take an example from the financial world, consider automatic teller machines (ATMs) and their facilitation of today's worldwide banking in ways that were never contemplated when the industry depended on human bank tellers.

It is accordingly logical to ask what the health record will become after it has been effectively implemented on computer systems and new opportunities for its enhancement become increasingly clear to us. It is clear that EHRs a decade from now will be remarkably different from the antiquated paper folders that until recently dominated most of our health care environments. Note that the state of today's EHR is roughly comparable to the status of commercial aviation in the 1930s. By that time air travel had progressed substantially from the days of the Wright Brothers, and air travel was becoming common. But 1930s air travel seems archaic by modern standards, and it is logical to assume that today's EHRs, albeit much better than both paper records and the early computer-based systems of the 1960s and 1970s, will be greatly improved and further modernized in the decades ahead. If people had failed to use the early airplanes for travel, the quality and

efficiency of airplanes and air travel would not have improved as they have. A similar point can be made about the importance of committing to the use of EHRs today, even though we know that they need to be much better in the future.

1.2   Communications Technology and Health Data Integration

An obvious opportunity for changing the role and functionality of clinical-care records in the digital age is the power and ubiquity of the Internet. The Internet began in 1968 as a U.S. research activity funded by the Advanced Research Projects Agency (ARPA) of the Department of Defense. Initially known as the **ARPANET**, the network began as a novel mechanism for allowing a handful of defense-related mainframe computers, located mostly at academic institutions or in the research facilities of military contractors, to share data files with each other and to provide remote access to computing power at other locations. The notion of electronic mail arose soon thereafter, and machine-to-machine electronic mail exchanges quickly became a major component of the network's traffic. As the technology matured, its value for nonmilitary research activities was recognized, and by 1973 the first medically related research computer had been added to the network (Shortliffe 1998a, 2000).

During the 1980s, the technology began to be developed in other parts of the world, and the National Science Foundation took over the task of running the principal high-speed **backbone network** in the United States. Hospitals, mostly academic centers, began to be connected to what had by then become known as the Internet, and in a major policy move it was decided to allow commercial organizations to join the network as well. By April 1995, the Internet in the United States had become a fully commercialized operation, no longer depending on the U.S. government to support even the major backbone connections. Today, the Internet is ubiquitous, accessible through mobile wireless devices, and has provided the invisible but mandatory infrastructure for social, political, financial, scientific, and entertainment ventures. Many people point to the Internet as a superb example of the facilitating role of federal investment in promoting innovative technologies. The Internet is a major societal force that arguably would never have been created if the research and development, plus the coordinating activities, had been left to the private sector.

The explosive growth of the Internet did not occur until the late 1990s, when the **World Wide Web** (which had been conceived initially by the physics community as a way of using the Internet to share preprints with photographs and diagrams among researchers) was introduced and popularized. Navigating the Web is highly intuitive, requires no special training, and provides a mechanism for access to multimedia information that accounts for its remarkable growth as a worldwide phenomenon.

The societal impact of this communications phenomenon cannot be overstated, especially given the international connectivity that has grown phenomenally in the past two decades. Countries that once were isolated from information that was important to citizens, ranging from consumers to scientists to those interested in political issues, are now finding new options for bringing timely information to the desktop machines and mobile devices of individuals with an Internet connection.

There has in turn been a major upheaval in the telecommunications industry, with companies that used to be in different businesses (e.g., cable television, Internet services, and telephone) now finding that their activities and technologies have merged. In the United States, legislation was passed in 1996 to allow new competition to develop and new industries to emerge. We have subsequently seen the merging of technologies such as cable television, telephone, networking, and satellite communications. High-speed lines into homes and offices are widely available, wireless networking is ubiquitous, and inexpensive mechanisms for connecting to the Internet without using conventional computers (e.g., using cell phones or set-top boxes) have also emerged. The impact on everyone has been great

and hence it is affecting the way that individuals seek health-related information and it is also enhancing how patients can gain access to their health care providers and to their clinical data.

Just as individual hospitals and health care systems have come to appreciate the importance of integrating information from multiple clinical and administrative systems within their organizations (see Chap. 14), health planners and governments now appreciate the need to develop integrated information resources that combine clinical and health data from multiple institutions within regions, and ultimately nationally (see Chaps. 13 and 16). As you will see, the Internet and the role of digital communications has therefore become a major part of modern medicine and health. Although this topic recurs in essentially every chapter in this book, we introduce it in the following sections because of its importance to modern technical issues and policy directions.

1.2.1   A Model of Integrated Disease Surveillance[2]

To emphasize the role that the nation's networking infrastructure is playing in integrating clinical data and enhancing care delivery, consider one example of how disease surveillance, prevention, and care are increasingly being influenced by information and communications technology. The goal is to create an information-management infrastructure that will allow all clinicians, regardless of practice setting (hospitals, emergency rooms, small offices, community clinics, military bases, multispecialty groups, etc.) to use EHRs in their practices both to assist in patient care and to provide patients with counsel on illness prevention. The full impact of this use of electronic resources will occur when data from all such records are pooled in regional and national surveillance databases (Fig. 1.6), mediated through secure connectivity with the Internet. The challenge, of course, is to find a way to integrate data from such diverse practice settings, especially

---

[2] This section is adapted from a discussion that originally appeared in (Shortliffe and Sondik 2004).

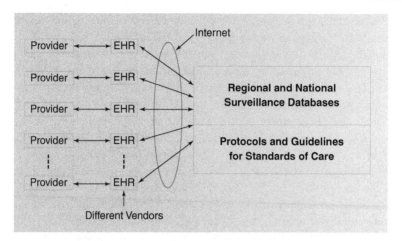

Fig. 1.6 A future vision of surveillance databases, in which clinical data are pooled in regional and national repositories through a process of data submission that occurs over the Internet (with attention to privacy and security concerns as discussed in the text). When information is effectively gathered, pooled, and analyzed, there are significant opportunities for feeding back the results of derived insights to practitioners at the point of care

since there are multiple vendors and system developers active in the marketplace, competing to provide value-added capabilities that will excite and attract the practitioners for whom their EHR product is intended.

The practical need to pool and integrate clinical data from such diverse resources and systems emphasizes the practical issues that need to be addressed in achieving such functionality and resources. Interestingly, most of the barriers are logistical, political, and financial rather than technical in nature:

- *Encryption of data*: Concerns regarding privacy and data protection require that Internet transmission of clinical information occur only if those data are encrypted, with an established mechanism for identifying and authenticating individuals before they are allowed to decrypt the information for surveillance or research use.
- *HIPAA-compliant policies*: The privacy and security rules that resulted from the 1996 **Health Insurance Portability and Accountability Act (HIPAA)** do not prohibit the pooling and use of such data (see Chap. 10), but they do lay down policy rules and technical security practices that must be part of the solution in achieving the vision we are discussing here.

- *Standards for data transmission and sharing*: Sharing data over networks requires that all developers of EHRs and clinical databases adopt a single set of standards for communicating and exchanging information. The de facto standard for such sharing, Health Level 7 (HL7), was introduced decades ago and, after years of work, is beginning to be uniformly adopted, implemented, and utilized (see Chap. 7).
- *Standards for data definitions*: A uniform "envelope" for digital communication, such as HL7, does not assure that the contents of such messages will be understood or standardized. The pooling and integration of data requires the adoption of standards for clinical terminology and potentially for the schemas used to store clinical information in databases (see Chap. 7).
- *Quality control and error checking*: Any system for accumulating, analyzing, and utilizing clinical data from diverse sources must be complemented by a rigorous approach to quality control and error checking. It is crucial that users have faith in the accuracy and comprehensiveness of the data that are collected in such repositories, because policies, guidelines, and a variety of metrics can be derived over time from such information.

- *Regional and national surveillance databases*: Any adoption of the model in Fig. 1.6 will require mechanisms for creating, funding, and maintaining the regional and national databases that are involved (see Chap. 13). The role of state and federal governments will need to be clarified, and the political issues addressed (including the concerns of some members of the populace that any government role in managing or analyzing their health data may have societal repercussions that threaten individual liberties, employability, and the like).

With the establishment of surveillance databases, and a robust system of Internet integration with EHRs, summary information can flow back to providers to enhance their decision making at the point of care (Fig. 1.6). This assumes standards that allow such information to be integrated into the vendor-supplied products that the clinicians use in their practice settings. These may be EHRs or, increasingly, order-entry systems that clinicians use to specify the actions that they want to have taken for the treatment or management of their patients (see Chaps. 12 and 14). Furthermore, as is shown in Fig. 1.6, the databases can help to support the creation of evidence-based guidelines, or clinical research protocols, which can be delivered to practitioners through the feedback process. Thus one should envision a day when clinicians, at the point of care, will receive integrated, non-dogmatic, supportive information regarding:

- Recommended steps for health promotion and disease prevention
- Detection of syndromes or problems, either in their community or more widely
- Trends and patterns of public health importance
- Clinical guidelines, adapted for execution and integration into patient-specific decision support rather than simply provided as text documents
- Opportunities for distributed (community-based) clinical research, whereby patients are enrolled in clinical trials and protocol guidelines are in turn integrated with the clinicians' EHR to support protocol-compliant management of enrolled patients

1.2.2 The Goal: A Learning Health Care System

We have been stressing the cyclical role of information—its capture, organization, interpretation, and ultimate use. You can easily understand the small cycle that is implied: patient-specific data and plans entered into an EHR and subsequently made available to the same practitioner or others who are involved in that patient's care (Fig. 1.7). Although this view is a powerful contributor to improved data management in the care of patients, it fails to include a larger view of the societal value of the information that is contained in clinical-care records. In fact, such straightforward use of EHRs for direct patient care does not meet some of the requirements that the US government has specified when determining eligibility for payment of incentives to clinicians or hospitals who implement EHRs (see the discussion of this government program in Sect. 1.3).

Consider, instead, an expanded view of the health surveillance model introduced in Sect. 1.2.1 (Fig. 1.8). Beginning at the left of the diagram, clinicians caring for patients use electronic health records, both to record their observations and to gain access to information about the patient. Information from these records is then forwarded automatically to

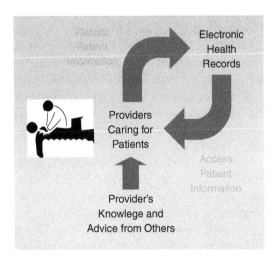

Fig. 1.7 There is a limited view of the role of EHRs that sees them as intended largely to support the ongoing care of the patient whose clinical data are stored in the record

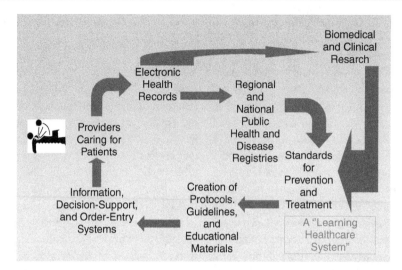

Fig. 1.8 The ultimate goal is to create a cycle of information flow, whereby data from distributed electronic health records (EHRs) are routinely and effortlessly submitted to registries and research databases. The resulting new knowledge then can feed back to practitioners at the point of care, using a variety of computer-supported decision-support delivery mechanisms. This cycle of new knowledge, driven by experience, and fed back to clinicians, has been dubbed a "learning health care system"

regional and national registries as well as to research databases that can support retrospective studies (see Chap. 11) or formal institutional or community-based clinical trials (see Chap. 26). The analyzed information from registries and research studies can in turn be used to develop standards for prevention and treatment, with major guidance from biomedical research. Researchers can draw information either directly from the health records or from the pooled data in registries. The standards for treatment in turn can be translated into protocols, guidelines, and educational materials. This new knowledge and decision-support functionality can then be delivered over the network back to the clinicians so that the information informs patient care, where it is integrated seamlessly with EHRs and order-entry systems.

This notion of a system that allows us to learn from what we do, unlocking the experience that has traditionally been stored in unusable form in paper charts, is gaining wide attention now that we can envision an interconnected community of clinicians and institutions, building digital data resources using EHRs. The concept has been dubbed a **learning health care system** and is an ongoing subject of study by the Institute of Medicine,[3] which has published a series of reports on the topic (IOM 2007; 2011; 2012).

1.2.3 Implications of the Internet for Patients

As the penetration of the Internet continues to grow, it is not surprising that increasing numbers of patients, as well as healthy individuals, are turning to the Internet for health information. It is a rare North American physician who has not encountered a patient who comes to an appointment armed with a question, or a stack of printouts, that arose due to medically related searches on the net. The companies that provide search engines for the Internet report that health-related sites are among the most popular ones being explored by consumers. As a result, physicians and other care providers must be prepared to deal with information that patients discover on the net and bring with them when they seek care from clinicians. Some of the information is timely and excellent; in this sense physicians can often learn

---

[3] http://www.iom.edu/Activities/Quality/LearningHealthCare. aspx (Accessed 3/3/2013).

about innovations from their patients and will need to be increasingly open to the kinds of questions that this enhanced access to information will generate from patients in their practices. On the other hand, much of the health information on the Web lacks peer review or is purely anecdotal. People who lack medical training can be misled by such information, just as they have been poorly served in the past by printed information in books and magazines dealing with fad treatments from anecdotal sources. In addition, some sites provide personalized advice, sometimes for a fee, with all the attendant concerns about the quality of the suggestions and the ability to give valid advice based on an electronic mail or Web-based interaction.

In a positive light, the new communications technologies offer clinicians creative ways to interact with their patients and to provide higher quality care. Years ago medicine adopted the telephone as a standard vehicle for facilitating patient care, and we now take this kind of interaction with patients for granted. If we extend the audio channel to include our visual sense as well, typically relying on the Internet as our communication mechanism, the notion of **telemedicine** emerges (see Chap. 18). This notion of "medicine at a distance" arose early in the twentieth century (see Fig. 1.9), but the technology was too limited for much penetration of the idea beyond telephone conversations until the last 30–40 years. The use of telemedicine has subsequently grown rapidly, and there are specialized settings in which it is already proving to be successful and cost-effective (e.g., rural care, international medicine, **teleradiology**, and video-based care of patients in prisons).

1.2.4   Requirements for Achieving the Vision

Efforts that continue to push the state of the art in Internet technology all have significant implications for the future of health care delivery in general and of EHRs and their integration in particular (Shortliffe 1998b, 2000). But in addition to increasing speed, reliability, security, and availability of the Internet, there are many other areas that need attention if the vision of a learning health care system is to be achieved.

1.2.4.1   Education and Training

There is a difference between computer literacy (familiarity with computers and their routine uses in our society) and knowledge of the role that computing and communications technology can and should play in our health care system. We are generally doing a poor job of training future clinicians in the latter area and are thereby leaving them poorly equipped for the challenges and opportunities they will face in the rapidly changing practice environments that surround them (Shortliffe 2010).

Furthermore, much of the future vision we have proposed here can be achieved only if educational institutions produce a cadre of talented individuals who not only comprehend computing and communications technology but also have a deep understanding of the biomedical milieu and of the needs of practitioners and other health workers. Computer science training alone is not adequate. Fortunately, we have begun to see the creation of formal training programs in what has become known as **biomedical informatics** (see Sect. 1.4) that provide custom-tailored educational opportunities. Many of the trainees are life science researchers, physicians, nurses, pharmacists, and other health professionals who see the career opportunities and challenges at the intersections of biomedicine, information science, computer science, decision science, cognitive science, and communications technologies. As has been clear for over two decades (Greenes and Shortliffe 1990), however, the demand for such individuals far outstrips the supply, both for academic and industrial career pathways.[4,5] We need

---

[4] http://www.healthcare-informatics.com/news-item/survey-strong-demand-health-information-technology-workers (Accessed 3/3/2013); http://www.ehidc.org/about/press/press/803-ehealth-initiative-survey-reveals-high-demand-for-health-information-technology-workers (Accessed 9/11/2013).
[5] http://www.pwc.com/us/HITtalent (Accessed 4/21/13).

Fig. 1.9 "The Radio Doctor": long before television was invented, creative observers were suggesting how doctors and patients could communicate using advanced technologies. This 1924 example is from the cover of a popular magazine and envisions video enhancements to radio (Source: "Radio News" 1924)

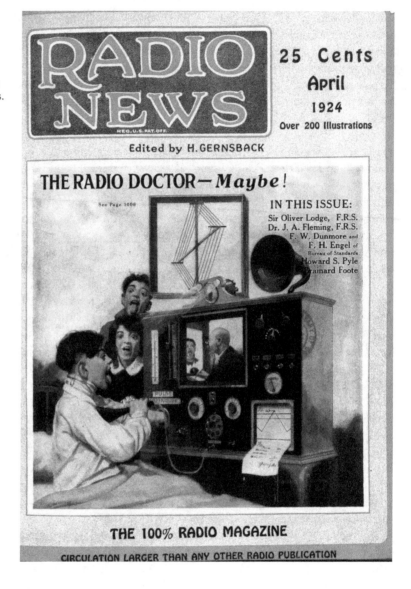

more training programs,[6] expansion of those that already exist, plus support for junior faculty in health science schools who may wish to pursue additional training in this area.

1.2.4.2 Organizational and Management Change

Second, as implied above, there needs to be a greater understanding among health care lead-ers regarding the role of specialized multi-disciplinary expertise in successful clinical systems implementation. The health care system provides some of the most complex organizational structures in society (Begun and Zimmerman 2003), and it is simplistic to assume that off-the-shelf products will be smoothly introduced into a new institution without major analysis, redesign, and cooperative joint-development efforts. Underinvestment and a failure to understand the requirements for process reengineering as part of software implementation, as well as problems with technical leadership and planning, account

---

[6] A directory of some existing training programs is available at http://www.amia.org/education/programs-and-courses (Accessed 3/3/2013).

for many of the frustrating experiences that health care organizations report in their efforts to use computers more effectively in support of patient care and provider productivity.

The notion of a learning health care system described previously is meant to motivate your enthusiasm for what lies ahead and to suggest the topics that need to be addressed in a book such as this one. Essentially all of the following chapters touch on some aspect of the vision of integrated systems that extend beyond single institutions. Before embarking on these topics, however, we must emphasize two points. First, the cyclical creation of new knowledge in a learning health care system will become reality only if individual hospitals, academic medical centers, and national coordinating bodies work together to provide the standards, infrastructure, and resources that are necessary. No individual system developer, vendor, or administrator can mandate the standards for connectivity, data pooling, and data sharing implied by a learning health care system. A national initiative of cooperative planning and implementation for computing and communications resources within and among institutions and clinics is required before practitioners will have routine access to the information that they need (see Chap. 13). A recent federal incentive program for EHR implementation is a first step in this direction (see Sect. 1.3). The criteria that are required for successful EHR implementation are sensitive to the need for data integration, public-health support, and a learning health care system.

Second, although our presentation of the learning health care notion has focused on the clinician's view of integrated information access, other workers in the field have similar needs that can be addressed in similar ways. The academic research community has already developed and made use of much of the technology that needs to be coalesced if the clinical user is to have similar access to data and information. There is also the patient's view, which must be considered in the notion of patient-centered health care that is now broadly accepted and encouraged (Ozkaynak et al. 2013).

1.3 The US Government Steps In

During the early decades of the evolution of clinical information systems for use in hospitals, patient care, and public health, the major role of government was in supporting the research enterprise as new methods were developed, tested, and formally evaluated. The topic was seldom mentioned by the nation's leaders, however, even during the 1990s when the White House was viewed as being especially tech savvy. It was accordingly remarkable when, in the President's State of the Union address in 2004 (and in each of the following years of his administration), President Bush called for universal implementation of electronic health records within 10 years. The Secretary of Health and Human Services, Tommy Thompson, was similarly supportive and, in May 2004, created an entity intended to support the expansion of the use of EHRs—the **Office of the National Coordinator for Health Information Technology** (initially referred to by the full acronym ONCHIT, but later shortened simply to ONC).

There was limited budget for ONC, although the organization served as a convening body for EHR-related planning efforts and the National Health Information Infrastructure (see Chaps. 12, 13, and 27). The topic of EHRs subsequently became a talking point for both major candidates during the Presidential election in 2008, with strong bipartisan support. However, it was the American Recovery and Reinvestment Act (ARRA) in early 2009, also known as the economic "Stimulus Bill", that first provided major funding to provide fiscal incentives for health systems, hospitals, and providers to implement EHRs in their practices. Such payments were made available, however, only when eligible organizations or individual practitioners implemented EHRs that were "certified" as meeting minimal standards and when they could document that they were making "meaningful use" of those systems. You will see references to such certification and **meaningful use** criteria in many chapters in this volume. There is also a discussion of HIT policy and the federal government in Chap. 27. Although the process of EHR implementation is still ongoing at present, the trend is clear: because

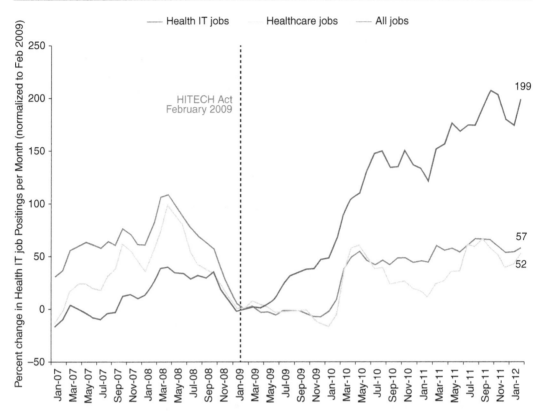

Fig. 1.10 Percent change in online health IT job postings per month, relative to health care jobs and all jobs: normalized to February 2009 when ARRA passed (Source: ONC analysis of data from O'Reilly Job Data Mart, ONC Data Brief, No. 2, May 2012 [http://www.healthit.gov/sites/default/files/pdf/0512_ONCDataBrief2_JobPostings.pdf (Accessed 4/10/13)]

of the federal stimulus package, large numbers of hospitals, systems, and practitioners are investing in EHRs and incorporating them into their practices. Furthermore, the demand for workers skilled in health information technology has grown much more rapidly than has the general job market, even within health care (Fig. 1.10). It is a remarkable example of how government policy and investment can stimulate major transitions in systems such as health care, where many observers had previously felt that progress had been unacceptably slow (Shortliffe 2005).

1.4   Defining Biomedical Informatics and Related Disciplines

With the previous sections of this chapter as background, let us now consider the scientific discipline that is the subject of this volume and

has led to the development of many of the functionalities that need to be brought together in the integrated bio medical-computing environment of the future. The remainder of this chapter deals with biomedical informatics as a field and with biomedical and health information as a subject of study. It provides additional background needed to understand many of the subsequent chapters in this book.

Reference to the use of computers in biomedicine evokes different images depending on the nature of one's involvement in the field. To a hospital administrator, it might suggest the maintenance of clinical-care records using computers; to a decision scientist, it might mean the assistance by computers in disease diagnosis; to a basic scientist, it might mean the use of computers for maintaining, retrieving, and analyzing gene-sequencing information. Many physicians immediately think of office-practice tools for tasks such as patient billing or appointment scheduling. Nurses often think of computer-based tools for charting the care that they deliver, or decision-support tools that assist in applying the most current patient-care guidelines. The field includes study of all these activities and a great many others too. More importantly, it includes the consideration of various external factors that affect the biomedical setting. Unless you keep in mind these surrounding factors, it may be difficult to understand how biomedical computing can help us to tie together the diverse aspects of health care and its delivery.

To achieve a unified perspective, we might consider four related topics: (1) the concept of biomedical information (why it is important in biological research and clinical practice and why we might want to use computers to process it); (2) the structural features of medicine, including all those subtopics to which computers might be applied; (3) the importance of evidence-based knowledge of biomedical and health topics, including its derivation and proper management and use; and (4) the applications of computers and communication methods in biomedicine and the scientific issues that underlie such efforts. We mention the first two topics briefly in this and the next chapter, and we provide references in the Suggested Readings section for those students who wish to learn more. The third topic, knowledge to support effective decision making in support of human health, is intrinsic to this book and occurs in various forms in essentially every chapter. The fourth topic, however, is the principal subject of this book.

Computers have captured the imagination (and attention) of our society. Today's younger individuals have always lived in a world in which computers are ubiquitous and useful. Because the computer as a machine is exciting, people may pay a disproportionate amount of attention to it as such—at the expense of considering what the computer can do given the numbers, concepts, ideas, and cognitive underpinnings of fields such as medicine, health, and biomedical research. Computer scientists, philosophers, psychologists, and other scholars increasingly consider such matters as the nature of information and knowledge and how human beings process such concepts. These investigations have been given a sense of timeliness (if not urgency) by the simple existence of the computer. The cognitive activities of clinicians in practice probably have received more attention over the past three decades than in all previous history (see Chap. 4). Again, the existence of the computer and the possibilities of its extending a clinician's cognitive powers have motivated many of these studies. To develop computer-based tools to assist with decisions, we must understand more clearly such human processes as diagnosis, therapy planning, decision making, and problem solving in medicine. We must also understand how personal and cultural beliefs affect the way in which information is interpreted and decisions are ultimately made.

1.4.1 Terminology

Since the 1960s, by which time a growing number of individuals doing serious biomedical research or clinical practice had access to some kind of computer system, people have been uncertain what name they should use for the biomedical application of computer science concepts. The name computer science was itself new in 1960 and was only vaguely defined. Even today, the term computer science is used more as a matter of convention than as an explanation of the field's scientific content.

In the 1970s we began to use the phrase **medical computer science** to refer to the subdivision of computer science that applies the methods of the larger field to medical topics. As you will see, however, medicine has provided a rich area for computer science research, and several basic computing insights and methodologies have been derived from applied medical-computing research.

The term **information science**, which is occasionally used in conjunction with computer science, originated in the field of library science and is used to refer, somewhat generally, to the broad range of issues related to the management of both paper-based and electronically stored information. Much of what information science originally set out to be is now drawing evolving interest under the name **cognitive science**.

Information theory, in contrast, was first developed by scientists concerned about the physics of communication; it has evolved into what may be viewed as a branch of mathematics. The results scientists have obtained with information theory have illuminated many processes in communications technology, but they have had little effect on our understanding of human information processing.

The terms **biomedical computing** or **biocomputation** have been used for a number of years. They are nondescriptive and neutral, implying only that computers are employed for some purpose in biology or medicine. They are often associated with bioengineering applications of computers, however, in which the devices are viewed more as tools for a bioengineering application than as a primary focus of research.

In the 1970s, inspired by the French term for computer science (*informatique*), the English-speaking community began to use the term **medical informatics**. Those in the field were attracted by the word's emphasis on *information*, which they saw as more central to the field than the computer itself, and it gained momentum as a term for the discipline, especially in Europe, during the 1980s. The term is broader than **medical computing** (it includes such topics as medical statistics, record keeping, and the study of the nature of medical information itself) and deemphasizes the computer while focusing instead on the nature of the field to which computations are applied. Because the term *informatics* became widely accepted in the United States only in the late 1980s, **medical information science** was also used earlier in North America; this term, however, may be confused with library science, and it does not capture the broader implications of the European term. As a result, the name *medical informatics* appeared by the late 1980s to have become the preferred term, even in the United States. Indeed, this is the name of the field that we used in the first two editions of this textbook (from 1990 to 2000), and it is still sometimes used in professional, industrial, and academic settings. However, many observers expressed concern that the adjective "medical" is too focused on physicians and fails to appreciate the relevance of this discipline to other health and life-science professionals. Thus, the term **health informatics**, or health care informatics, gained some popularity, even though it has the disadvantage of tending to exclude applications to biomedical research (Chaps. 24 and 25) and, as we will argue shortly, it tends to focus the field's name on application domains (clinical care, public health, and prevention) rather than the basic discipline and its broad range of applicability.

Applications of informatics methods in biology and genetics exploded during the 1990s due to the human genome project[7] and the growing recognition that modern life-science research was no longer possible without computational support and analysis (see Chaps. 24 and 25). By the late 1990s, the use of informatics methods in such work had become widely known as **bioinformatics** and the director of the National Institutes of Health (NIH) appointed an advisory group called the Working Group on Biomedical Computing. In June 1999, the group provided a report[8] recommending that the NIH undertake an initiative called the **Biomedical Information Science and Technology Initiative** (BISTI). With the subsequent creation of another NIH organization called the Bioinformatics Working Group, the visibility of informatics applications in biology was greatly enhanced. Today bioinformatics is a major area of activity at the NIH[9] and in many universities and biotechnology companies around the world. The explosive growth of this field, however, has added to the confusion regarding the naming conventions we have been discussing. In addition, the relationship between *medical informatics* and *bioinformatics* became unclear. As a result, in an effort to be more inclusive and to embrace the biological applications with which many medical informatics groups had already been involved, the name *medical informatics* gradually gave way to biomedical informatics (BMI). Several academic groups have changed their names, and a major medical informatics journal (*Computers and Biomedical*

---

[7] http://www.ornl.gov/sci/techresources/Human_Genome/home.shtml (Accessed 4/8/2013).
[8] Available at http://www.nih.gov/about/director/060399.html(Accessed 4/8/2013).
[9] See http://www.bisti.nih.gov/. (Accessed 4/8/2013).

Research) was reborn in 2001 as *The Journal of Biomedical Informatics.*[10]

Despite this convoluted naming history, we believe that the broad range of issues in biomedical information management does require an appropriate name and, beginning with the third edition of this book (2006), we used the term biomedical informatics for this purpose. It has become the most widely accepted term for the core discipline and should be viewed as encompassing broadly all areas of application in health, clinical practice, and biomedical research. When we speak specifically about computers and their use within biomedical informatics activities, we use the terms biomedical computer science (for the methodologic issues) or biomedical computing (to describe the activity itself). Note, however, that biomedical informatics has many other component sciences in addition to computer science. These include the decision sciences, statistics, cognitive science, information science, and even management sciences. We return to this point shortly when we discuss the basic versus applied nature of the field when it is viewed as a basic research discipline.

Although labels such as these are arbitrary, they are by no means insignificant. In the case of new fields of endeavor or branches of science, they are important both in designating the field and in defining or restricting its contents. The most distinctive feature of the modern computer is the generality of its application. The nearly unlimited range of computer uses complicates the business of naming the field. As a result, the nature of computer science is perhaps better illustrated by examples than by attempts at formal definition. Much of this book presents examples that do just this for biomedical informatics as well.

The American Medical Informatics Association (AMIA), which was founded in the late 1980s under the former name for the discipline, has recognized the confusion regarding the field and its definition.[11] They accordingly appointed a working group to develop a formal definition of the field and to specify the core competencies that need to be acquired by students seeking graduate training in the discipline. The resulting definition, published in AMIA's journal and approved by the full board of the organization, identifies the focus of the field in a simple sentence and then adds four clarifying corollaries that refine the definition and the field's scope and content (Box 1.1). We adopt this definition, which is very similar to the one we offered in previous editions of this text. It acknowledges that the emergence of biomedical informatics as a new discipline is due in large part to rapid advances in computing and communications technology, to an increasing awareness that the knowledge base of biomedicine is essentially unmanageable by traditional paper-based methods, and to a growing conviction that the process of informed decision making is as important to modern biomedicine as is the collection of facts on which clinical decisions or research plans are made.

Box 1.1: Definition of Biomedical Informatics

Biomedical informatics (BMI) is the interdisciplinary field that studies and pursues the effective uses of biomedical data, information, and knowledge for scientific inquiry, problem solving, and decision making, driven by efforts to improve human health.

Scope and breadth of discipline: BMI investigates and supports reasoning, modeling, simulation, experimentation, and translation across the spectrum from molecules to individuals and to populations, from biological to social systems, bridging basic and clinical research and practice and the health care enterprise.

Theory and methodology: BMI develops, studies, and applies theories, methods, and processes for the generation, storage, retrieval, use, management, and sharing of biomedical data, information, and knowledge.

Technological approach: BMI builds on and contributes to computer, telecommunication, and information sciences and

---

[10] http://www.journals.elsevier.com/journal-of-biomedical-informatics (Accessed 4/8/13).
[11] http://www.amia.org/about-amia/science-informatics (Accessed 4/8/13).

technologies, emphasizing their application in biomedicine.

Human and social context: BMI, recognizing that people are the ultimate users of biomedical information, draws upon the social and behavioral sciences to inform the design and evaluation of technical solutions, policies, and the evolution of economic, ethical, social, educational, and organizational systems.

Reproduced with permission from (Kulikowski et al. 2012)

1.4.2 Historical Perspective

The modern digital computer grew out of developments in the United States and abroad during World War II, and general-purpose computers began to appear in the marketplace by the mid-1950s (Fig. 1.11). Speculation about what might be done with such machines (if they should ever become reliable) had, however, begun much earlier. Scholars, at least as far back as the Middle Ages, often had raised the question of whether human reasoning might be explained in terms of formal or **algorithmic processes**. Gottfried

Wilhelm von Leibnitz, a seventeenth-century German philosopher and mathematician, tried to develop a calculus that could be used to simulate human reasoning. The notion of a "logic engine" was subsequently worked out by Charles Babbage in the mid nineteenth century.

The first practical application of automatic computing relevant to medicine was Herman Hollerith's development of a punched-card data-processing system for the 1890 U.S. census (Fig. 1.12). His methods were soon adapted to **epidemiologic** and public health surveys, initiating the era of electromechanical punched-card data-processing technology, which matured and was widely adopted during the 1920s and 1930s. These techniques were the precursors of the stored program and wholly electronic digital computers, which began to appear in the late 1940s (Collen 1995).

One early activity in biomedical computing was the attempt to construct systems that would assist a physician in decision making (see Chap. 22). Not all biomedical-computing programs pursued this course, however. Many of the early ones instead investigated the notion of a total **hospital information system** (HIS; see Chap. 14). These projects were perhaps less ambitious in that they were more concerned with practical applications in the short term;

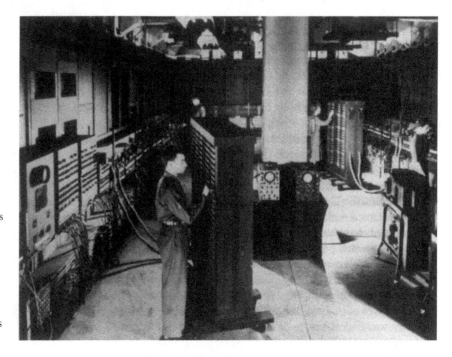

Fig. 1.11 The ENIAC. Early computers, such as the ENIAC, were the precursors of today's personal computers (PCs) and handheld calculators (Photograph courtesy of Unisys Corporation)

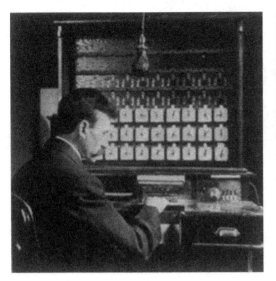

Fig. 1.12 Tabulating machines. The Hollerith Tabulating Machine was an early data-processing system that performed automatic computation using punched cards (Photograph courtesy of the Library of Congress.)

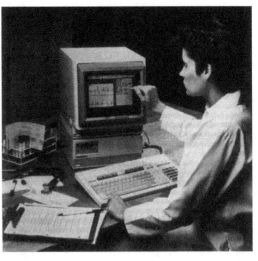

Fig. 1.13 Departmental system. Hospital departments, such as the clinical laboratory, were able to implement their own custom-tailored systems when affordable minicomputers became available. These departments subsequently used microcomputers to support administrative and clinical functions (Copyright 2013 Hewlett-Packard Development Company, LP. Reproduced from ~1985 original with permission)

the difficulties they encountered, however, were still formidable. The earliest work on HISs in the United States was probably that associated with the MEDINET project at General Electric, followed by work at Bolt, Beranek, Newman in Cambridge, Massachusetts, and then at the Massachusetts General Hospital (MGH) in Boston. A number of hospital application programs were developed at MGH by Barnett and his associates over three decades beginning in the early 1960s. Work on similar systems was undertaken by Warner at Latter Day Saints (LDS) Hospital in Salt Lake City, Utah, by Collen at Kaiser Permanente in Oakland, California, by Weiderhold at Stanford University in Stanford, California, and by scientists at Lockheed in Sunnyvale, California.[12]

The course of HIS applications bifurcated in the 1970s. One approach was based on the concept of an integrated or monolithic design in which a single, large, *time-shared computer* would be used to support an entire collection of applications. An alternative was a distributed

design that favored the separate implementation of specific applications on smaller individual computers—minicomputers—thereby permitting the independent evolution of systems in the respective application areas. A common assumption was the existence of a single shared database of patient information. The multi-machine model was not practical, however, until network technologies permitted rapid and reliable communication among distributed and (sometimes) heterogeneous types of machines. Such distributed HISs began to appear in the 1980s (Simborg et al. 1983).

Biomedical-computing activity broadened in scope and accelerated with the appearance of the minicomputer in the early 1970s. These machines made it possible for individual departments or small organizational units to acquire their own dedicated computers and to develop their own application systems (Fig. 1.13). In tandem with the introduction of general-purpose software tools that provided standardized facilities to individuals with limited computer training (such as the UNIX operating system and programming environment), the minicomputer

---

[12] The latter system was later taken over and further developed by the Technicon Corporation (subsequently TDS Healthcare Systems Corporation). Later the system was part of the suite of products available from Eclipsys, Inc. (which in turn was acquired by Allscripts, Inc in 2010).

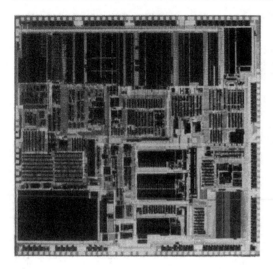

Fig. 1.14 Miniature computer. The microprocessor, or "computer on a chip," revolutionized the computer industry in the 1970s. By installing chips in small boxes and connecting them to a computer terminal, engineers produced the personal computer (PC)—an innovation that made it possible for individual users to purchase their own systems

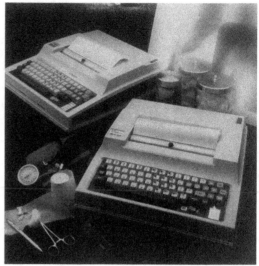

Fig. 1.15 Medical advertising. An early advertisement for a portable computer terminal that appeared in general medical journals in the late 1970s. The development of compact, inexpensive peripheral devices and personal computers (PCs) inspired future experiments in marketing directly to clinicians (Reprinted by permission of copyright holder Texas Instruments Incorporated © 1985)

put more computing power in the hands of more biomedical investigators than did any other single development until the introduction of the microprocessor, a central processing unit (CPU) contained on one or a few chips (Fig. 1.14).

Everything changed radically in the late 1970s and early 1980s, when the microprocessor and the personal computer (PC) or microcomputer became available. Not only could hospital departments afford minicomputers but now individuals also could afford microcomputers. This change enormously broadened the base of computing in our society and gave rise to a new software industry. The first articles on computers in medicine had appeared in clinical journals in the late 1950s, but it was not until the late 1970s that the first use of computers in advertisements dealing with computers and aimed at physicians began to appear (Fig. 1.15). Within a few years, a wide range of computer-based information-management tools were available as commercial products; their descriptions began to appear in journals alongside the traditional advertisements for drugs and other medical products. Today individual physicians find it practical to employ PCs in a variety of settings, including for applications in patient care or clinical investigation.

The stage is now set with a wide range of hardware of various sizes, types, prices, and capabilities, all of which will continue to evolve in the decades ahead. The trend—reductions in size and cost of computers with simultaneous increases in power (Fig. 1.16)—shows no sign of slowing, although scientists foresee the ultimate physical limitations to the miniaturization of computer circuits.[13]

Progress in biomedical-computing research will continue to be tied to the availability of funding from either government or commercial sources. Because most biomedical-computing research is exploratory and is far from ready for commercial application, the federal government has played a key role in funding the work of the last four decades, mainly through the NIH and the Agency for Health Care Research and Quality (AHRQ). The National Library of Medicine (NLM) has assumed a primary role for biomedical informatics, especially with support for basic research in the field (Fig. 1.17). As increasing

---

[13] http://www.sciencedaily.com/releases/2008/01/080112083626.htm (Accessed 4/8/13).

Fig. 1.16 Moore's Law. Former Intel chairman Gordon Moore is credited with popularizing the "law" that the size and cost of microprocessor chips will half every 18 months while they double in computing power. This graph shows the exponential growth in the number of transistors that can be integrated on a single microprocessor by two of the major chip manufacturers (Source: San Jose Mercury News, Dec 2007, used with permission)

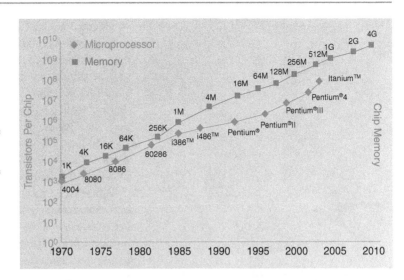

Fig. 1.17 The National Library of Medicine (NLM). The NLM, on the campus of the National Institutes of Health (NIH) in Bethesda, Maryland, is the principal biomedical library for the nation (see Chap. 21). It is also a major source of support for research in biomedical informatics (Photograph courtesy of the National Library of Medicine)

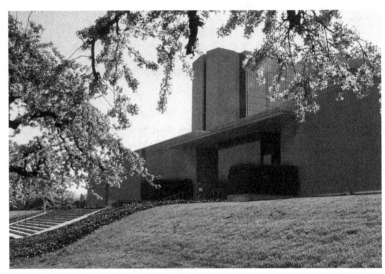

numbers of applications prove to be cost-effective, it is likely that more development work will shift to industrial settings and that university programs will focus increasingly on fundamental research problems viewed as too speculative for short-term commercialization.

1.4.3   Relationship to Biomedical Science and Clinical Practice

The exciting accomplishments of biomedical informatics, and the implied potential for future benefits to medicine, must be viewed in the context of our society and of the existing health care system. As early as 1970, an eminent clinician suggested that computers might in time have a revolutionary influence on medical care, on medical education, and even on the selection criteria for health-science trainees (Schwartz 1970). The subsequent enormous growth in computing activity has been met with some trepidation by health professionals. They ask where it will all end. Will health workers gradually be replaced by computers? Will nurses and physicians need to be highly trained in computer science or informatics before they can practice their professions effectively? Will both patients and health workers eventually revolt rather than accept a trend toward automation that they believe may threaten the traditional

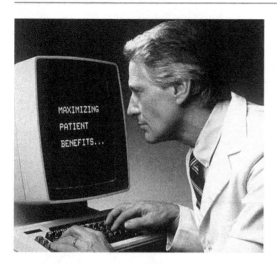

Fig. 1.18 Doctor of the future. By the early 1980s, advertisements in medical journals (such as this one for an antihypertensive agent) began to use computer equipment as props and even portrayed them in a positive light. The suggestion in this photograph seems to be that an up-to-date physician feels comfortable using computer-based tools in his practice (Photograph courtesy of ICI Pharma, Division of ICI Americas, Inc)

humanistic values in health care delivery (see Chap. 10) (Shortliffe 1993)? Will clinicians be viewed as outmoded and backward if they do not turn to computational tools for assistance with information management and decision making (Fig. 1.18)?

Biomedical informatics is intrinsically entwined with the substance of biomedical science. It determines and analyzes the structure of biomedical information and knowledge, whereas biomedical science is constrained by that structure. Biomedical informatics melds the study data, information, knowledge, decision making, and supporting technologies with analyses of biomedical information and knowledge, thereby addressing specifically the interface between the science of information and knowledge management and biomedical science. To illustrate what we mean by the "structural" features of biomedical information and knowledge, we can contrast the properties of the information and knowledge typical of such fields as physics or engineering with the properties of those typical of biomedicine (see Sect. 1.5).

Biomedical informatics is perhaps best viewed as a basic biomedical science, with a wide variety of potential areas of application (Fig. 1.19). The analogy with other **basic sciences** is that biomedical informatics uses the results of past experience to understand, structure, and encode objective and subjective biomedical findings and thus to make them suitable for processing. This approach supports the integration of the findings and their analyses. In turn, the selective distribution of newly created knowledge can aid patient care, health planning, and basic biomedical research.

Biomedical informatics is, by its nature, an **experimental science**, characterized by posing questions, designing experiments, performing analyses, and using the information gained to design new experiments. One goal is simply to search for new knowledge, called **basic research**. A second goal is to use this knowledge for practical ends, called **applications (applied) research**. There is a continuity between these two endeavors (see Fig. 1.19). In biomedical informatics, there is an especially tight coupling between the application areas, broad categories of which are indicated at the bottom of Fig. 1.19, and the identification of basic research tasks that characterize the scientific underpinnings of the field. Research, however, has shown that there can be a very long period of time between the development of new concepts and methods in basic research and their eventual application in the biomedical world (Balas and Boren 2000). Furthermore (see Fig. 1.20), many discoveries are discarded along the way, leaving only a small percentage of basic research discoveries that have a practical influence on the health and care of patients.

Work in biomedical informatics (BMI) is inherently motivated by problems encountered in a set of applied domains in biomedicine. The first of these historically has been clinical care (including medicine, nursing, dentistry, and veterinary care), an area of activity that demands patient-oriented informatics applications. We refer to this area as **clinical informatics**. It includes several subtopics and areas of specialized expertise, including patient-care foci such as **nursing informatics**, **dental informatics**, and even **veterinary informatics**. Furthermore, the former name of the discipline, **medical**

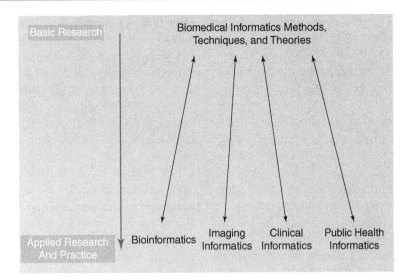

Fig. 1.19 Biomedical informatics as basic science. We view the term biomedical informatics as referring to the basic science discipline in which the development and evaluation of new methods and theories are a primary focus of activity. These core concepts and methods in turn have broad applicability in the health and biomedical sciences. The informatics subfields indicated by the terms across the bottom of this figure are accordingly best viewed as application domains for a common set of concepts and techniques from the field of biomedical informatics. Note that work in biomedical informatics is motivated totally by the application domains that the field is intended to serve (thus the two-headed arrows in the diagram). Therefore the basic research activities in the field generally result from the identification of a problem in the real world of health or biomedicine for which an informatics solution is sought (see text)

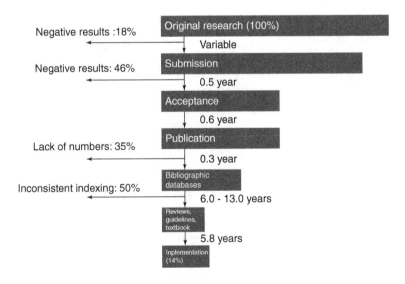

Fig. 1.20 Phases in the transfer of research into clinical practice. A synthesis of studies focusing on various phases of this transfer has indicated that it takes an average of 17 years to make innovation part of routine care (Balas and Boren 2000). Pioneering institutions often apply innovations much sooner, sometimes within a few weeks, but nationwide introduction is usually slow. National utilization rates of specific, well-substantiated procedures also suggests a delay of two decades in reaching the majority of eligible patients (Courtesy of Dr. Andrew Balas)

informatics, is now reserved for those applied research and practice topics that focus on disease and the role of physicians. As was previously discussed, the term "medical informatics" is no longer used to refer to the discipline as a whole.

Closely tied to clinical informatics is **public health informatics** (Fig. 1.19), where similar methods are generalized for application to populations of patients rather than to single individuals (see Chap. 16). Thus clinical informatics and public health informatics share many of the same methods and techniques. Two other large areas of application overlap in some ways with clinical informatics and public health informatics. These include **imaging informatics** (and the set of issues developed around both radiology and other image management and image analysis domains such as pathology, dermatology, and molecular visualization—see Chaps. 9 and 20). Finally, there is the burgeoning area of **bioinformatics**, which at the molecular and cellular levels is offering challenges that draw on many of the same informatics methods as well (see Chap. 24).

As is shown in Fig. 1.21, there is a spectrum as one moves from left to right across these BMI application domains. In bioinformatics, workers

deal with molecular and cellular processes in the application of informatics methods. At the next level, workers focus on tissues and organs, which tend to be the emphasis of imaging informatics work (also called **structural informatics** at some institutions). Progressing to clinical informatics, the focus is on individual patients, and finally to public health, where researchers address problems of populations and of society. The core science of biomedical informatics has important contributions to make across that entire spectrum, and many informatics methods are broadly applicable across the same range of domains.

Note from Fig. 1.19 that biomedical informatics and bioinformatics are not synonyms and it is incorrect to refer to the scientific discipline as bioinformatics, which is, rather, an important area of application of BMI methods and concepts. Similarly, the term health informatics, which refers to applied research and practice in clinical and public-health informatics, is also not an appropriate name for the core discipline, since BMI is applicable to basic human biology as well as to health.

We acknowledge that the four major areas of application shown in Fig. 1.19 have "fuzzy"

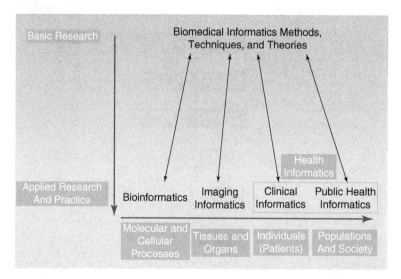

Fig. 1.21 Building on the concepts of Fig. 1.19, this diagram demonstrates the breadth of the biomedical informatics field. The relationship between biomedical informatics as a core scientific discipline and its diverse array of application domains that span biological science, imaging, clinical practice, public health, and others

not illustrated (see text). Note that "health informatics" is the term used to refer to applied research and practice in clinical and public health informatics. It is not a synonym for the underlying discipline, which is "biomedical informatics"

boundaries, and many areas of applied informatics research involve more than one of the categories. For example, **biomolecular imaging** involves both bioinformatics and imaging informatics concepts. Similarly, **consumer health informatics** (see Chap. 17) includes elements of both clinical informatics and public-health informatics. Another important area of BMI research activities is **pharmacogenomics** (see Chap. 25), which is the effort to infer genetic determinants of human drug response. Such work requires the analysis of linked **genotypic** and **phenotypic** databases, and therefore lies at the intersection of bioinformatics and clinical informatics.

In general, BMI researchers derive their inspiration from one of the application areas, identifying fundamental methodologic issues that need to be addressed and testing them in system prototypes or, for more mature methods, in actual systems that are used in clinical or biomedical research settings. One important implication of this viewpoint is that the core discipline is identical, regardless of the area of application that a given individual is motivated to address, although some BMI methods have greater relevance to some domains than to others. This argues for unified BMI educational programs, ones that bring together students with a wide variety of applications interests. Elective courses and internships in areas of specific interest are of course important complements to the core exposures that students should receive, but, given the need for teamwork and understanding in the field, separating trainees based on the application areas that may interest them would be counterproductive and wasteful.[14]

The scientific contributions of BMI also can be appreciated through their potential for benefiting the education of health professionals (Shortliffe 2010). For example, in the education of medical students, the various cognitive activities of physicians traditionally have tended to be considered separately and in isolation—they have been largely treated as though they are independent and distinct modules of performance. One activity attracting increasing interest is that of formal medical decision making (see Chap. 3). The specific content of this area remains to be defined completely, but the discipline's dependence on formal methods and its use of knowledge and information reveal that it is one aspect of biomedical informatics.

A particular topic in the study of medical decision making is **diagnosis**, which is often conceived and taught as though it were a free-standing and independent activity. Medical students may thus be led to view diagnosis as a process that physicians carry out in isolation before choosing therapy for a patient or proceeding to other modular tasks. A number of studies have shown that this model is oversimplified and that such a decomposition of cognitive tasks may be quite misleading (Elstein et al. 1978; Patel and Groen 1986). Physicians seem to deal with several tasks at the same time. Although a diagnosis may be one of the first things physicians think about when they see a new patient, patient assessment (diagnosis, management, analysis of treatment results, monitoring of disease progression, etc.) is a process that never really terminates. A physician must be flexible and open-minded. It is generally appropriate to alter the original diagnosis if it turns out that treatment based on it is unsuccessful or if new information weakens the evidence supporting the diagnosis or suggests a second and concurrent disorder. Chapter 4 discusses these issues in greater detail.

When we speak of making a diagnosis, choosing a treatment, managing therapy, making decisions, monitoring a patient, or preventing disease, we are using labels for different aspects of medical care, an entity that has overall unity. The fabric of medical care is a continuum in which these elements are tightly interwoven. Regardless of whether we view computer and information science as a profession, a technology, or a science, there is no doubt about its importance to biomedicine. We can assume computers will be used

---

[14] Many current biomedical informatics training programs were designed with this perspective in mind. Students with interests in clinical, imaging, public health, and biologic applications are often trained together and are required to learn something about each of the other application areas, even while specializing in one subarea for their own research. Several such programs were described in a series of articles in the *Journal of Biomedical Informatics* in 2007 (Tarczy-Hornoch et al. 2007).

increasingly in clinical practice, biomedical research, and health science education.

1.4.4 Relationship to Computer Science

During its evolution as an academic entity in universities, computer science followed an unsettled course as involved faculty attempted to identify key topics in the field and to find the discipline's organizational place. Many computer science programs were located in departments of electrical engineering, because major concerns of their researchers were computer architecture and design and the development of practical hardware components. At the same time, computer scientists were interested in programming languages and software, undertakings not particularly characteristic of engineering. Furthermore, their work with algorithm design, computability theory,[15] and other theoretical topics seemed more related to mathematics.

Biomedical informatics draws from all of these activities—development of hardware, software, and computer science theory. Biomedical computing generally has not had a large enough market to influence the course of major hardware developments; i.e., computers have not been developed specifically for biomedical applications. Not since the early 1960s (when health-computing experts occasionally talked about and, in a few instances, developed special medical terminals) have people assumed that biomedical applications would use hardware other than that designed for general use.

The question of whether biomedical applications would require specialized programming languages might have been answered affirmatively in the 1970s by anyone examining the MGH Utility Multi-Programming System, known as the MUMPS language (Greenes et al. 1970;

Bowie and Barnett 1976), which was specially developed for use in medical applications. For several years, MUMPS was the most widely used language for medical record processing. Under its new name, M, it is still in widespread use. New implementations have been developed for each generation of computers. M, however, like any programming language, is not equally useful for all computing tasks. In addition, the software requirements of medicine are better understood and no longer appear to be unique; rather, they are specific to the kind of task. A program for scientific computation looks pretty much the same whether it is designed for chemical engineering or for pharmacokinetic calculations.

How, then, does BMI differ from biomedical computer science? Is the new discipline simply the study of computer science with a "biomedical flavor"? If you return to the definition of biomedical informatics that we provided in Sect. 1.4.1, and then refer to Fig.1.19, we believe you will begin to see why biomedical informatics is more than simply the biomedical application of computer science. The issues that it addresses not only have broad relevance to health, medicine, and biology, but the underlying sciences on which BMI professionals draw are inherently interdisciplinary as well (and are not limited to computer science topics). Thus, for example, successful BMI research will often draw on, and contribute to, computer science, but it may also be closely related to the decision sciences (probability theory, decision analysis, or the psychology of human problem solving), cognitive science, information sciences, or the management sciences (Fig. 1.22). Furthermore, a biomedical informatics researcher will be tightly linked to some underlying problem from the real world of health or biomedicine. As Fig. 1.22 illustrates, for example, a biomedical informatics basic researcher or doctoral student will typically be motivated by one of the application areas, such as those shown at the bottom of Fig. 1.21, but a dissertation worthy of a PhD in the field will usually be identified by a generalizable scientific result that also contributes to one of the component disciplines (Fig. 1.22) and on which other scientists can build in the future.

---

[15] Many interesting problems cannot be computed in a reasonable time and require heuristics. Computability theory is the foundation for assessing the feasibility and cost of computation to provide the complete and correct results to a formally stated problem.

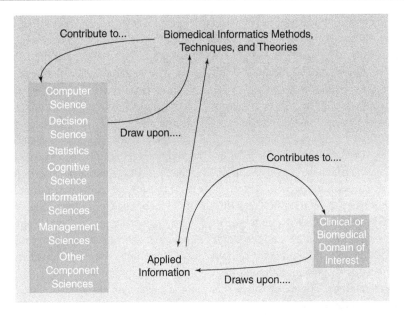

Fig. 1.22 Component sciences in biomedical informatics. An informatics application area is motivated by the needs of its associated biomedical domain, to which it attempts to contribute solutions to problems. Thus any applied informatics work draws upon a biomedical domain for its inspiration, and in turn often leads to the delineation of basic research challenges in biomedical informatics that must be tackled if the applied biomedical domain is ultimately to benefit. At the methodologic level, biomedical informatics draws on, and contributes to, a wide variety of component disciplines, of which computer science is only one. As Figs. 1.19 and 1.21 show explicitly, biomedical informatics is inherently multidisciplinary, both in its areas of application and in the component sciences on which it draws

1.4.5 Relationship to Biomedical Engineering

If BMI is a relatively young discipline, biomedical engineering is an older and more well-established one. Many engineering and medical schools have formal academic programs in the latter subject, often with departmental status and full-time faculty. Only in the last 2 decades or so has this begun to be true of biomedical informatics academic units. How does biomedical informatics relate to biomedical engineering, especially in an era when engineering and computer science are increasingly intertwined?

Biomedical engineering departments emerged 40 years ago, when technology began to play an increasingly prominent role in medical practice.[16] The emphasis in such departments has tended to be research on, and development

of, instrumentation (e.g., as discussed in Chaps. 19 and 20, advanced monitoring systems, specialized transducers for clinical or laboratory use, and image-enhancement techniques for use in radiology), with an orientation toward the development of medical devices, **prostheses**, and specialized research tools. There is also a major emphasis on tissue engineering and related wet-bench research efforts. In recent years, computing techniques have been used both in the design and construction of medical devices and in the medical devices themselves. For example, the "smart" devices increasingly found in most medical specialties are all dependent on computational technology. Intensive care monitors that generate blood pressure records while calculating mean values and hourly summaries are examples of such "intelligent" devices.

---

[16] The Duke University undergraduate major in biomedical engineering was the first department (September 1972) accredited by the Engineering Council for Professional Development.

The overlap between biomedical engineering and BMI suggests that it would be unwise for us to draw compulsively strict boundaries between the two fields. There are ample opportunities for interaction, and there are chapters in this book that clearly overlap with biomedical engineering topics—e.g., Chap. 19 on patient-monitoring systems and Chap. 20 on radiology systems. Even where they meet, however, the fields have differences in emphasis that can help you to understand their different evolutionary histories. In biomedical engineering, the emphasis is on medical devices; in BMI, the emphasis is on biomedical information and knowledge and on their management with the use of computers. In both fields, the computer is secondary, although both use computing technology. The emphasis in this book is on the informatics end of the spectrum of biomedical computer science, so we shall not spend much time examining biomedical engineering topics.

1.5   The Nature of Medical Information

From the previous discussion, you might conclude that biomedical applications do not raise any unique problems or concerns. On the contrary, the biomedical environment raises several issues that, in interesting ways, are quite distinct from those encountered in most other domains of applied computing. Clinical information seems to be systematically different from the information used in physics, engineering, or even clinical chemistry (which more closely resembles chemical applications generally than it does medical ones). Aspects of biomedical information include an essence of uncertainty—we can never know all about a physiological process—and this results in inevitable variability among individuals. These differences raise special problems and some investigators suggest that biomedical computer science differs from conventional computer science in fundamental ways. We shall explore these differences only briefly here; for details, you can consult Blois' book on this subject (see Suggested Readings).

Let us examine an instance of what we will call a low-level (or readily formalized) science. Physics is a natural starting point; in any discussion of the hierarchical relationships among the sciences (from the fourth-century BC Greek philosopher Aristotle to the twentieth-century U.S. librarian Melvil Dewey), physics will be placed near the bottom. Physics characteristically has a certain kind of simplicity, or generality. The concepts and descriptions of the objects and processes of physics, however, are necessarily used in all applied fields, including medicine. The laws of physics and the descriptions of certain kinds of physical processes are essential in representing or explaining functions that we regard as medical in nature. We need to know something about molecular physics, for example, to understand why water is such a good solvent; to explain how nutrient molecules are metabolized, we talk about the role of electron-transfer reactions.

Applying a computer (or any formal computation) to a physical problem in a medical context is no different from doing so in a physics laboratory or for an engineering application. The use of computers in various **low-level processes** (such as those of physics or chemistry) is similar and is independent of the application. If we are talking about the solvent properties of water, it makes no difference whether we happen to be working in geology, engineering, or medicine. Such low-level processes of physics are particularly receptive to mathematical treatment, so using computers for these applications requires only conventional numerical programming.

In biomedicine, however, there are other **higher-level processes** carried out in more complex objects such as organisms (one type of which is patients). Many of the important informational processes are of this kind. When we discuss, describe, or record the properties or behavior of human beings, we are using the descriptions of very high-level objects, the behavior of whom has no counterpart in physics or in engineering. The person using computers to analyze the descriptions of these high-level objects and processes encounters serious difficulties (Blois 1984).

One might object to this line of argument by remarking that, after all, computers are used routinely in commercial applications in which human beings and situations concerning them are involved and that relevant computations are carried out successfully. The explanation is that, in these commercial applications, the descriptions of human beings and their activities have been so highly abstracted that the events or processes have been reduced to low-level objects. In biomedicine, abstractions carried to this degree would be worthless from either a clinical or research perspective.

For example, one instance of a human being in the banking business is the customer, who may deposit, borrow, withdraw, or invest money. To describe commercial activities such as these, we need only a few properties; the customer can remain an abstract entity. In clinical medicine, however, we could not begin to deal with a patient represented with such skimpy abstractions. We must be prepared to analyze most of the complex behaviors that human beings display and to describe patients as completely as possible. We must deal with the rich descriptions occurring at high levels in the hierarchy, and we may be hard pressed to encode and process this information using the tools of mathematics and computer science that work so well at low levels. In light of these remarks, the general enterprise known as **artificial intelligence** (**AI**) can be aptly described as the application of computer science to high-level, real-world problems.

Biomedical informatics thus includes computer applications that range from processing of very low-level descriptions, which are little different from their counterparts in physics, chemistry, or engineering, to processing of extremely high-level ones, which are completely and systematically different. When we study human beings in their entirety (including such aspects as human cognition, self-consciousness, intentionality, and behavior), we must use these high-level descriptions. We will find that they raise complex issues to which conventional logic and mathematics are less readily applicable. In general, the attributes of low-level objects appear sharp, crisp, and unambiguous (e.g., "length," "mass"), whereas those of high-level ones tend to be soft, fuzzy, and inexact (e.g., "unpleasant scent," "good").

Just as we need to develop different methods to describe high-level objects, the inference methods we use with such objects may differ from those we use with low-level ones. In formal logic, we begin with the assumption that a given proposition must be either true or false. This feature is essential because logic is concerned with the preservation of truth value under various formal transformations. It is difficult or impossible, however, to assume that all propositions have truth values when we deal with the many high-level descriptions in medicine or, indeed, in everyday situations. Such questions as "Was Woodrow Wilson a good president?" cannot be answered with a "yes" or "no" (unless we limit the question to specific criteria for determining the goodness of presidents). Many common questions in biomedicine have the same property.

1.6 Integrating Biomedical Informatics and Clinical Practice

It should be clear from the previous discussion that biomedical informatics is a remarkably broad and complex topic. We have argued that information management is intrinsic to clinical practice and that interest in using computers to aid in information management has grown over the last five decades. In this chapter and throughout the book, we emphasize the myriad ways in which computers are used in biomedicine to ease the burdens of information processing and the means by which new technology promises to change the delivery of health care. The degree to which such changes are realized, and their rate of occurrence, will be determined in part by external forces that influence the costs of developing and implementing biomedical applications and the ability of scientists, clinicians, patients, and the health care system to accrue the potential benefits.

We can summarize several global forces that are affecting biomedical computing and that will determine the extent to which computers are assimilated into clinical practice: (1) new developments in computer hardware and software; (2) a gradual increase in the number of individuals who have been trained in both medicine or another health profession and in BMI; and (3) ongoing changes in health care financing designed to control the rate of growth of health-related expenditures. We touched on the first of these factors in Sect. 1.4.2, when we described the historical development of biomedical computing and the trend from mainframe computers, to microcomputers and PCs, and to the mobile devices of today. The future view outlined in Sect. 1.1 similarly builds on the influence that the Internet has provided throughout society during the last decade. The new hardware technologies have made powerful computers inexpensive and thus available to hospitals, to departments within hospitals, and even to individual physicians. The broad selection of computers of all sizes, prices, and capabilities makes computer applications both attractive and accessible. Technological advances in information storage devices,[17] including the movement of files to the "cloud", are facilitating the inexpensive storage of large amounts of data, thus improving the feasibility of data-intensive applications, such as the all-digital radiology department discussed in Chap. 20. Standardization of hardware and advances in network technology are making it easier to share data and to integrate related information-management functions within a hospital or other health care organization.

Computers are increasingly prevalent in all aspects of our lives, whether as an ATM, as the microprocessor in a microwave oven, or as a telephone that takes photographs and shares them wirelessly with others. Physicians trained in recent years may have used computer programs to learn diagnostic techniques or to manage the therapy of simulated patients. They may have learned to use a computer to search the medical literature, either directly or with the assistance of a specially trained librarian. Simple exposure to computers does not, however, guarantee an eagerness to embrace the machine. Clinical personnel will continue to be unwilling to use computer-based systems that are poorly designed, confusing, unduly time-consuming, or lacking in clear benefit (see Chaps. 4 and 6). As they become more sophisticated in the use of computers in other aspects of their lives, their expectations of clinical software will become only more demanding.

The second factor is the increase in the number of professionals who are being trained to understand the biomedical issues as well as the technical and engineering ones. Computer scientists who understand biomedicine are better able to design systems responsive to actual needs and sensitive to workflow and the clinical culture. Health professionals who receive formal training in BMI are likely to build systems using well-established techniques while avoiding the past mistakes of other developers. As more professionals are trained in the special aspects of both fields, and as the programs they develop are introduced, health care professionals are more likely to have useful and usable systems available when they turn to the computer for help with information management tasks.

The third factor affecting the integration of computing technologies into health care settings is managed care and the increasing pressure to control medical spending. The escalating tendency to apply technology to all patient-care tasks is a frequently cited phenomenon in modern medical practice. Mere physical findings no longer are considered adequate for making diagnoses and planning treatments. In fact, medical students who are taught by more experienced physicians to find subtle diagnostic signs by examining various parts of the body nonetheless often choose to bypass or deemphasize physical examinations in favor of ordering one test after another. Sometimes, they do so without paying sufficient attention to the ensuing cost. Some new technologies replace less expensive, but technologically inferior, tests. In such cases, the use of

---

[17] Technological progress in this area is occurring at a dizzying rate. Consider, for example, the announcement that scientists are advancing the notion of "organically-grown" storage and can store as much as 704 terabytes of information in a gram of DNA. http://www.engadget.com/2012/08/19/harvard-stores-704tb-in-a-gram-of-dna/ (Accessed 4/21/13).

the more expensive approach is generally justified. Occasionally, computer-related technologies have allowed us to perform tasks that previously were not possible. For example, the scans produced with computed tomography or magnetic resonance imaging (see Chaps. 9 and 20) have allowed physicians to visualize cross-sectional slices of the body for the first time, and medical instruments in intensive care units perform continuous monitoring of patients' body functions that previously could be checked only episodically (see Chap. 19).

Yet the development of expensive new technologies, and the belief that more technology is better, helped to fuel the rapidly escalating health care costs of the 1970s and 1980s, leading to the introduction of managed care and **capitation**—changes in financing and delivery that were designed to curb spending in the new era of cost consciousness. Integrated computer systems potentially provide the means to capture data for detailed cost accounting, to analyze the relationship of costs of care to the benefits of that care, to evaluate the quality of care provided, and to identify areas of inefficiency. Systems that improve the quality of care while reducing the cost of providing that care clearly will be favored. The effect of cost containment pressures on technologies that increase the cost of care while improving the quality are less clear. Medical technologies, including computers, will be embraced only if they improve the delivery of clinical care while either reducing costs or providing benefits that clearly exceed their costs.

Improvements in hardware and software make computers more suitable for biomedical applications. Designers of medical systems must, however, address satisfactorily many logistical and engineering questions before computers can be fully integrated into medical practice. For example, are computers conveniently located? Should mobile devices replace the tethered workstations of the past? Can users complete their tasks without excessive delays? Is the system reliable enough to avoid loss of data? Can users interact easily and intuitively with the computer? Are patient data secure and appropriately protected from prying eyes? In addition, cost-control pressures produce a growing reluctance to embrace expensive technologies that add to the high cost of health care. The net effect of these opposing trends will in large part determine the degree to which computers continue to be integrated into the health care environment.

In summary, rapid advances in computer hardware and software, coupled with an increasing computer literacy of health care professionals and researchers, favor the implementation of effective computer applications in clinical practice, public health, and life sciences research. Furthermore, in the increasingly competitive health care industry, providers have a greater need for the information management capabilities supplied by computer systems. The challenge is to demonstrate in persuasive and rigorous ways the financial and clinical advantages of these systems (see Chap. 11).

Suggested Readings

Blois, M. S. (1984). *Information and medicine: The nature of medical descriptions*. Berkeley: University of California Press. In this classic volume, the author analyzes the structure of medical knowledge in terms of a hierarchical model of information. He explores the ideas of high- and low-level sciences and suggests that the nature of medical descriptions accounts for difficulties in applying computing technology to medicine.

Coiera E., Magrabi F., Sintchenko V. (2013). *Guide to health informatics* (3rd ed). Boca Raton, FL: CRC Press. This introductory text is a readable summary of clinical and public health informatics, aimed at making the domain accessible and understandable to the non-specialist.

Collen, M. F. (1995). *A history of medical informatics in the United States: 1950 to 1990*. Bethesda: American Medical Informatics Association, Hartman Publishing. This comprehensive book traces the history of the field of medical informatics through 1990, and identifies the origins of the discipline's name (which first appeared in the English-language literature in 1974).

Elstein, A. S., Shulman, L. S., & Sprafka, S. A. (1978). *Medical problem solving: An analysis of clinical reasoning*. Cambridge, MA: Harvard University Press. This classic collection of papers describes detailed studies that have illuminated several aspects of the ways in which expert and novice physicians solve medical problems.

Friedman, C. P., Altman, R. B., Kohane, I. S., McCormick, K. A., Miller, P. L., Ozbolt, J. G., Shortliffe, E. H.,

Stormo, G. D., Szczepaniak, M. C., Tuck, D., & Williamson, J. (2004). Training the next generation of informaticians: The impact of BISTI and bioinformatics. *Journal of American Medical Informatics Association, 11*, 167–172. This important analysis addresses the changing nature of biomedical informatics due to the revolution in bioinformatics and computational biology. Implications for training, as well as organization of academic groups and curriculum development, are discussed.

Hoyt R. E., Bailey N., Yoshihashi A. (2012). *Health informatics: practical guide for healthcare and information technology professionals* (5th ed.). Raleigh, NC: Lulu.com. This introductory volume provides a broad view of informatics and is aimed especially at health professionals in management roles or IT professionals who are entering the clinical world.

Institute of Medicine (1991 [revised 1997]). The Computer-Based Patient Record: An Essential Technology for Health Care. Washington, DC: National Academy Press. National Research Council (1997). For The Record: Protecting Electronic Health Information. Washington, DC: National Academy Press. National Research Council (2000). Networking Health: Prescriptions for the Internet. Washington, DC: National Academy Press. This set of three reports from branches of the US National Academies of Science has had a major influence on health information technology education and policy over the last 25 years.

Institute of Medicine (2000). To Err is Human: Building a Safer Health System. Washington, DC: National Academy Press. Institute of Medicine (2001). Crossing the Quality Chasm: A New Health Systems for the 21st Century. Washington, DC: National Academy Press. Institute of Medicine (2004). Patient Safety: Achieving a New Standard for Care. Washington, DC: National Academy Press. This series of three reports from the Institute of Medicine has outlined the crucial link between heightened use of information technology and the enhancement of quality and reduction in errors in clinical practice. Major programs in patient safety have resulted from these reports, and they have provided motivation for a heightened interest in health care information technology among policy makers, provider organizations, and even patients.

Kalet, I. J. (2008). *Principles of biomedical informatics*. New York: Academic. This volume provides a technical introduction to the core methods in BMI, dealing with storage, retrieval, display, and use of biomedical data for biological problem solving and medical decision making. Application examples are drawn from bioinformatics, clinical informatics, and public health informatics.

Shortliffe, E. (1993). Doctors, patients, and computers: Will information technology dehumanize health care delivery? *Proceedings of the American Philosophical Society, 137*(3), 390–398 In this paper, the author examines the frequently expressed concern that the introduction of computing technology into health care settings will disrupt the development of rapport between clinicians and patients and thereby dehumanize the therapeutic process. He argues, rather, that computers may have precisely the opposite effect on the relationship between clinicians and their patients.

Questions for Discussion

1. How do you interpret the phrase "logical behavior"? Do computers behave logically? Do people behave logically? Explain your answers.

2. What do you think it means to say that a computer program is "effective"? Make a list of a dozen computer applications with which you are familiar. List the applications in decreasing order of effectiveness, as you have explained this concept. Then, for each application, indicate your estimate of how well human beings perform the same tasks (this will require that you determine what it means for a human being to be effective). Do you discern any pattern? If so, how do you interpret it?

3. Discuss three society-wide factors that will determine the extent to which computers are assimilated into clinical practice.

4. Reread the future vision presented in Sect. 1.1. Describe the characteristics of an integrated environment for managing clinical information. Discuss two ways in which such a system could change clinical practice.

5. Do you believe that improving the technical quality of health care entails the risk of dehumanization? If so, is it worth the risk? Explain your reasoning.

6. Consider Fig. 1.19, which shows that bioinformatics, imaging informatics, clinical informatics, and public health informatics are all application domains of the biomedical informatics discipline because they share the same core methods and theories:

    (a) Briefly describe two examples of core biomedical informatics methods and theories that can be applied both to bioinformatics and clinical informatics.

(b) Imagine that you describe Fig. 2.19 to a mathematics faculty member, who responds that "in that case, I'd also argue that statistics, computer science, and physics are all application domains of math because they share the same core mathematical methods and theories." In your opinion, is this a legitimate argument? In what ways is this situation similar to, and different from, the case of biomedical informatics?

(c) Why is biomedical informatics *not* simply computer science applied to biomedicine, or the practice of medicine using computers?

(d) How would you describe the relevance of psychology and cognitive science to the field of biomedical informatics? [Hint: See Fig. 1.22]

7. In 2000, a major report by the Institute of Medicine entitled "To Err is Human: Building a Safer Health System" (see Suggested Readings) stated that up to 98,000 patient deaths are caused by preventable medical errors in American hospitals each year.

(a) It has been suggested that electronic health record (EHR) systems should be used to address this problem. What are three specific ways in which they could reduce the number of adverse events in hospitals?

(b) Are there ways in which computer-based systems could *increase* the incidence of medical errors? Explain.

(c) Describe a practical experiment that could be used to examine the impact of an EHR system on patient safety. In other words, the study design should address whether the computer-based system increases or decreases the incidence of preventable adverse events in hospitals – and by how much.

(d) What are the limitations of the experimental design you proposed in (c)?

8. It has been argued that the ability to capture "nuance" in the description of what a clinician has seen when examining or interviewing a patient may not be as crucial as some people think. The desire to be able to express one's thoughts in an unfettered way (free text) is often used to argue against the use of structured data-entry methods using a controlled vocabulary and picking descriptors from lists.

(a) What is your own view of this argument? Do you believe that it is important to the quality and/or efficiency of care for clinicians to be able to record their observations, at least part of the time, using free text/natural language?

(b) Many clinicians may be unwilling to use an electronic health record (EHR) system requiring structured data entry because of the increased time required for documentation at the point of care. What are two strategies that could be used to address this problem (other than "designing a better user interface for the system")?

Biomedical Data: Their Acquisition, Storage, and Use

2

Edward H. Shortliffe and G. Octo Barnett

After reading this chapter, you should know the answers to these questions:

- What are clinical data?
- How are clinical data used?
- What are the drawbacks of the traditional paper medical record?
- What is the potential role of the computer in data storage, retrieval, and interpretation?
- What distinguishes a database from a knowledge base?
- How are data collection and hypothesis generation intimately linked in clinical diagnosis?
- What are the meanings of the terms *prevalence*, *predictive value*, *sensitivity*, and *specificity*?
- How are the terms related?
- What are the alternatives for entry of data into a clinical database?

E.H. Shortliffe, MD, PhD (✉)
Departments of Biomedical Informatics
at Columbia University and Arizona State University,
Weill Cornell College of Medicine,
and the New York Academy of Medicine,
272 W 107th St #5B, New York 10025, NY, USA
e-mail: ted@shortliffe.net

G.O. Barnett, MD, FACP, FACMI
Laboratory of Computer Science
(Harvard Medical School and Massachusetts
General Hospital),
Boston 02114, MA, USA

2.1 What Are Clinical Data?

From earliest times, the ideas of ill health and its treatment have been wedded to those of the observation and interpretation of data. Whether we consider the disease descriptions and guidelines for management in early Greek literature or the modern physician's use of complex laboratory and X-ray studies, it is clear that gathering data and interpreting their meaning are central to the health care process. With the move toward the use of genomic information in assessing individual patients (their risks, prognosis, and likely responses to therapy), the sheer amounts of data that may be used in patient care have become huge. A textbook on informatics will accordingly refer time and again to issues in data collection, storage, and use. This chapter lays the foundation for this recurring set of issues that is pertinent to all aspects of the use of information, knowledge, and computers in biomedicine, both in the clinical world and in applications related to, public health, biology and human genetics.

If data are central to all health care, it is because they are crucial to the process of decision making (as described in detail in Chaps. 3 and 4 and again in Chap. 22). In fact, simple reflection will reveal that all health care activities involve gathering, analyzing, or using data. Data provide the basis for categorizing the problems a patient may be having or for identifying subgroups within a population of patients. They also help a physician to decide what additional information

E.H. Shortliffe, J.J. Cimino (eds.), *Biomedical Informatics*,
DOI 10.1007/978-1-4471-4474-8_2, © Springer-Verlag London 2014

is needed and what actions should be taken to gain a greater understanding of a patient's problem or most effectively to treat the problem that has been diagnosed.

It is overly simplistic to view data as the columns of numbers or the monitored waveforms that are a product of our increasingly technological health care environment. Although laboratory test results and other numeric data are often invaluable, a variety of more subtle types of data may be just as important to the delivery of optimal care: the awkward glance by a patient who seems to be avoiding a question during the medical interview, information about the details of a patient's symptoms or about his family or economic setting, or the subjective sense of disease severity that an experienced clinician will often have within a few moments of entering a patient's room. No clinician disputes the importance of such observations in decision making during patient assessment and management, yet the precise role of these data and the corresponding decision criteria are so poorly understood that it is difficult to record them in ways that convey their full meaning, even from one clinician to another. Despite these limitations, clinicians need to share descriptive information with others. When they cannot interact directly with one another, they often turn to the chart or electronic health record for communication purposes.

We consider a **clinical datum** to be any single observation of a patient—e.g., a temperature reading, a red blood cell count, a past history of rubella, or a blood pressure reading. As the blood pressure example shows, it is a matter of perspective whether a single observation is in fact more than one datum. A blood pressure of 120/80 might well be recorded as a single element in a setting where knowledge that a patient's blood pressure is normal is all that matters. If the difference between diastolic (while the heart cavities are beginning to fill) and systolic (while they are contracting) blood pressures is important for decision making or for analysis, however, the blood pressure reading is best viewed as two pieces of information (systolic pressure = 120 mmHg, diastolic pressure = 80 mmHg). Human beings can glance at a written blood pressure value

and easily make the transition between its unitary view as a single data point and the decomposed information about systolic and diastolic pressures. Such dual views can be much more difficult for computers, however, unless they are specifically allowed for in the design of the method for data storage and analysis. The idea of a *data model* for computer-stored medical data accordingly becomes an important issue in the design of medical data systems.

If a clinical *datum* is a single observation about a patient, clinical *data* are multiple observations. Such data may involve several different observations made concurrently, the observation of the same patient parameter made at several points in time, or both. Thus, a single datum generally can be viewed as defined by five elements:

1. The *patient* in question
2. The *parameter* being observed (e.g., liver size, urine sugar value, history of rheumatic fever, heart size on chest X-ray film)
3. The *value* of the parameter in question (e.g., weight is 70 kg, temperature is 98.6 °F, profession is steel worker)
4. The *time* of the observation (e.g., 2:30 A.M. on 14FEB2013[1])
5. The method by which the observation was made (e.g., patient report, thermometer, urine dipstick, laboratory instrument).

Time can particularly complicate the assessment and computer-based management of data. In some settings, the date of the observation is adequate—e.g., in outpatient clinics or private offices where a patient generally is seen infrequently and the data collected need to be identified in time with no greater accuracy than a calendar date. In others, minute-to-minute variations may be important—e.g., the frequent blood sugar readings obtained for a patient in diabetic ketoacidosis (acid production due to poorly controlled blood sugar levels) or the continuous measurements of mean arterial blood pressure for a

---

[1] Note that it was the tendency to record such dates in computers as "14FEB12" that led to the end-of-century complexities that we called the *Year 2K problem*. It was shortsighted to think that it was adequate to encode the year of an event with only two digits.

patient in cardiogenic shock (dangerously low blood pressure due to failure of the heart muscle).

It often also is important to keep a record of the circumstances under which a data point was obtained. For example, was the blood pressure taken in the arm or leg? Was the patient lying or standing? Was the pressure obtained just after exercise? During sleep? What kind of recording device was used? Was the observer reliable? Such additional information, sometimes called contexts, methods, or modifiers, can be of crucial importance in the proper interpretation of data. Two patients with the same basic problem or symptom often have markedly different explanations for their problem, revealed by careful assessment of the modifiers of that problem.

A related issue is the uncertainty in the values of data. It is rare that an observation—even one by a skilled clinician—can be accepted with absolute certainty. Consider the following examples:

- An adult patient reports a childhood illness with fevers and a red rash in addition to joint swelling. Could he or she have had scarlet fever? The patient does not know what his or her pediatrician called the disease nor whether anyone thought that he or she had scarlet fever.
- A physician listens to the heart of an asthmatic child and thinks that she hears a heart murmur—but is not certain because of the patient's loud wheezing.
- A radiologist looking at a shadow on a chest X-ray film is not sure whether it represents overlapping blood vessels or a lung tumor.
- A confused patient is able to respond to simple questions about his or her illness, but under the circumstances the physician is uncertain how much of the history being reported is reliable.

As described in Chaps. 3 and 4, there are a variety of possible responses to deal with incomplete data, the uncertainty in them, and in their interpretation. One technique is to collect additional data that will either confirm or eliminate the concern raised by the initial observation. This solution is not always appropriate, however, because the costs of data collection must be considered. The additional observation might be expensive, risky for the patient, or wasteful of time during which treatment could have been instituted. The idea of trade-offs in data collection thus becomes extremely important in guiding health care decision making.

2.1.1 What Are the Types of Clinical Data?

The examples in the previous section suggest that there is a broad range of data types in the practice of medicine and the allied health sciences. They range from narrative, textual data to numerical measurements, genetic information, recorded signals, drawings, and even photographs or other images.

Narrative data account for a large component of the information that is gathered in the care of patients. For example, the patient's description of his or her present illness, including responses to focused questions from the physician, generally is gathered verbally and is recorded as text in the medical record. The same is true of the patient's social and family history, the general review of systems that is part of most evaluations of new patients, and the clinician's report of physical examination findings. Such narrative data were traditionally handwritten by clinicians and then placed in the patient's medical record (Fig. 2.1). Increasingly, however, the narrative summaries are dictated and then transcribed by typists who produce printed summaries or electronic copies for inclusion in paper or electronic medical records. The electronic versions of such reports can easily be integrated into electronic health records (EHRs) and clinical data repositories so that clinicians can access important clinical information even when the paper record is not available.[2] Electronically stored transcriptions of dictated information often include not only patient histories and physical examinations but also other narrative descriptions such as reports of specialty consultations, surgical procedures,

---

[2] As is discussed in Chap. 12, health care organizations are increasingly relying on electronic health records to the exclusion of printed records.

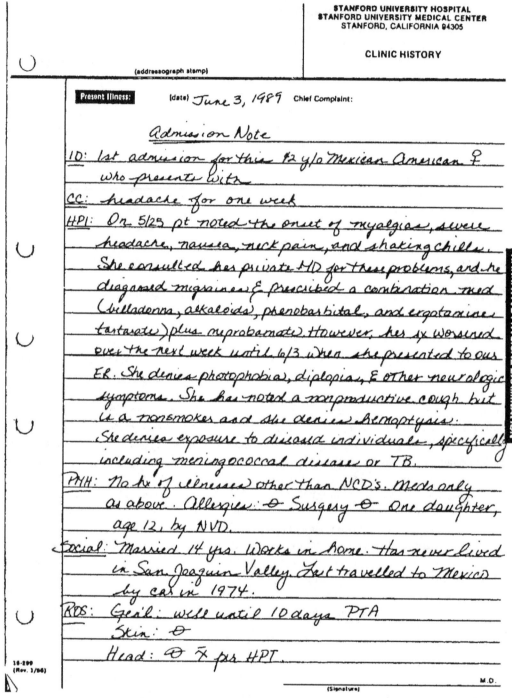

STANFORD UNIVERSITY HOSPITAL
STANFORD UNIVERSITY MEDICAL CENTER
STANFORD, CALIFORNIA 94305

CLINIC HISTORY

(addressograph stamp)

Present Illness: (date) June 3, 1989 Chief Complaint:

Admission Note

ID: 1st admission for this 42 y/o Mexican American ♀ who presents with

CC: headache for one week

HPI: On 5/25 pt noted the onset of myalgias, severe headache, nausea, neck pain, and shaking chills. She consulted her private MD for these problems, and he diagnosed migraines & prescribed a combination med (belladonna, alkaloids, phenobarbital, and ergotamine tartarate) plus meprobamate. However, her sx worsened over the next week until 6/3 when she presented to our ER. She denies photophobia, diplopia, & other neurologic symptoms. She has noted a nonproductive cough but is a nonsmoker and she denies hemoptysis. She denies exposure to diseased individuals, specifically including meningococcal disease or TB.

PMH: No hx of illnesses other than NCD's. Meds only as above. Allergies: ⊖ Surgery ⊖ One daughter, age 12, by NVD.

Social: Married 14 yrs. Works in home. Has never lived in San Joaquin Valley. Last travelled to Mexico by car in 1974.

ROS: Genl: well until 10 days PTA
Skin: ⊖
Head: ⊖ x̄ per HPI.

16-299
(Rev. 1/86)

(Signature) M.D.

NARRATIVE PHYSICAL EXAMINATION

Fig. 2.1 Much of the information gathered during a physician–patient encounter is written in the medical record

pathologic examinations of tissues, and hospitalization summaries when a patient is discharged.

Some narrative data are loosely coded with shorthand conventions known to health personnel,

particularly data collected during the physical examination, in which recorded observations reflect the stereotypic examination process taught to all practitioners. It is common, for example, to find the notation "PERRLA" under the eye examination in a patient's medical record. This encoded form indicates that the patient's "Pupils are Equal (in size), Round, and Reactive to Light and Accommodation (the process of focusing on near objects)."

Note that there are significant problems associated with the use of such abbreviations. Many are not standard and can have different meanings depending on the context in which they are used. For example, "MI" can mean "mitral insufficiency" (leakage in one of the heart's valves) or "myocardial infarction" (the medical term for what is commonly called a heart attack). Many hospitals try to establish a set of "acceptable" abbreviations with meanings, but the enforcement of such standardization is often unsuccessful.

Complete phrases have become loose standards of communication among medical personnel. Examples include "mild dyspnea (shortness of breath) on exertion," "pain relieved by antacids or milk," and "failure to thrive." Such standardized expressions are attempts to use conventional text notation as a form of summarization for otherwise heterogeneous conditions that together characterize a simple concept about a patient.

Many data used in medicine take on discrete numeric values. These include such parameters as laboratory tests, vital signs (such as temperature and pulse rate), and certain measurements taken during the physical examination. When such numerical data are interpreted, however, the issue of precision becomes important. Can physicians distinguish reliably between a 9-cm and a 10-cm liver span when they examine a patient's abdomen? Does it make sense to report a serum sodium level to two-decimal-place accuracy? Is a 1-kg fluctuation in weight from 1 week to the next significant? Was the patient weighed on the same scale both times (i.e., could the different values reflect variation between measurement instruments rather than changes in the patient)?

In some fields of medicine, analog data in the form of continuous signals are particularly important (see Chap. 19). Perhaps the best-known example is an electrocardiogram (ECG), a tracing of the electrical activity from a patient's heart. When such data are stored in medical records, a graphical tracing frequently is included, with a written interpretation of its meaning. There are clear challenges in determining how such data are best managed in computer-based storage systems.

Visual images—acquired from machines or sketched by the physician—are another important category of data. Radiologic images or photographs of skin lesions are obvious examples. It also is common for physicians to draw simple pictures to represent abnormalities that they have observed; such drawings may serve as a basis for comparison when they or another physician next see the patient. For example, a sketch is a concise way of conveying the location and size of a nodule in the prostate gland (Fig. 2.2).

As should be clear from these examples, the idea of data is inextricably bound to the idea of **data recording**. Physicians and other health care personnel are taught from the outset that it is crucial that they do not trust their memory when caring for patients. They must record their observations, as well as the actions they have taken and the rationales for those actions, for later communication to themselves and other people. A glance at a medical record will quickly reveal the wide variety of data-recording techniques that have evolved. The range goes from handwritten text to commonly understood shorthand notation to cryptic symbols that only specialists can understand; few physicians without specialized training know how to interpret the data-recording conventions of an ophthalmologist, for example (Fig. 2.3). The notations may be highly structured records with brief text or numerical information, hand-drawn sketches, machine-generated tracings of analog signals, or photographic images (of the patient or of radiologic or other studies). This range of data-recording conventions presents significant challenges to the person implementing electronic health record systems.

2.1.2 Who Collects the Data?

Health data on patients and populations are gathered by a variety of health professionals. Although conventional ideas of the **health care team** evoke images of coworkers treating ill patients, the team

Fig. 2.2 A physician's hand-drawn sketch of a prostate nodule. A drawing may convey precise information more easily and compactly than a textual description

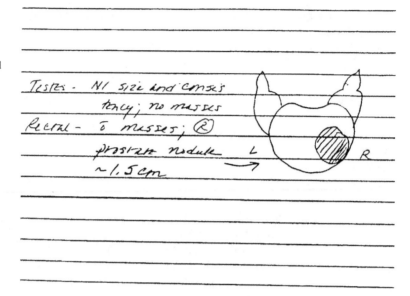

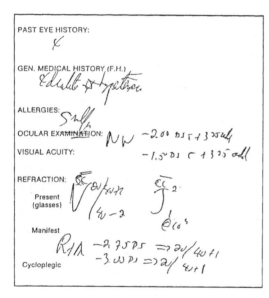

Fig. 2.3 An ophthalmologist's report of an eye examination. Most physicians trained in other specialties would have difficulty deciphering the symbols that the ophthalmologist has used

has much broader responsibilities than treatment per se; data collection and recording are a central part of its task.

Physicians are key players in the process of data collection and interpretation. They converse with a patient to gather narrative descriptive data on the chief complaint, past illnesses, family and social information, and the system review. They examine the patient, collecting pertinent data and recording them during or at the end of the visit. In addition, they generally decide what additional data to collect by ordering laboratory or radiologic studies and by observing the patient's response to therapeutic interventions (yet another form of data that contributes to patient assessment).

In both outpatient and hospital settings, nurses play a central role in making observations and recording them for future reference. The data that they gather contribute to nursing care plans as well as to the assessment of patients by physicians and by other health care staff. Thus, nurses' training includes instruction in careful and accurate observation, history taking, and examination of the patient. Because nurses typically spend more time with patients than physicians do, especially in the hospital setting, nurses often build relationships with patients that uncover information and insights that contribute to proper diagnosis, to understanding of pertinent psychosocial issues, or to proper planning of therapy or discharge management (Fig. 2.4). The role of information systems in contributing to patient care tasks such as care planning by nurses is the subject of Chap. 15.

Various other health care workers contribute to the data-collection process. Office staff and admissions personnel gather demographic and financial information. Physical or respiratory

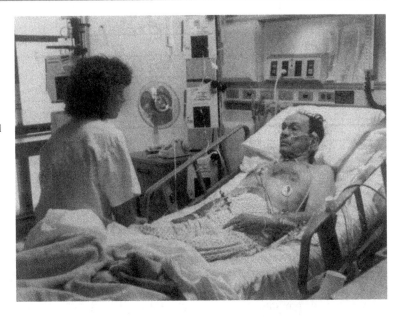

Fig. 2.4 Nurses often develop close relationships with patients. These relationships may allow the nurse to make observations that are missed by other staff. This ability is just one of the ways in which nurses play a key role in data collection and recording (Photograph courtesy of Janice Anne Rohn)

therapists record the results of their treatments and often make suggestions for further management. Laboratory personnel perform tests on biological samples, such as blood or urine, and record the results for later use by physicians and nurses. Radiology technicians perform X-ray examinations; radiologists interpret the resulting data and report their findings to the patients' physicians. Pharmacists may interview patients about their medications or about drug allergies and then monitor the patients' use of prescription drugs. As these examples suggest, many different individuals employed in health care settings gather, record, and make use of patient data in their work.

Finally, there are the technological devices that generate data—laboratory instruments, imaging machines, monitoring equipment in intensive care units, and measurement devices that take a single reading (such as thermometers, ECG machines, sphygmomanometers for taking blood pressure, and spirometers for testing lung function). Sometimes such a device produces a paper report suitable for inclusion in a traditional medical record. Sometimes the device indicates a result on a gauge or traces a result that must be read by an operator and then recorded in the patient's chart. Sometimes a trained specialist must interpret the output. Increasingly, however, the devices feed their results directly into computer equipment so that the data can be analyzed or formatted for electronic storage as well as reported on paper. With the advent of comprehensive EHRs (see Chap. 12), the printing of such data summaries may no longer be required as we move to "paperless" records whereby all access to information is through computer workstations, hand-held tablets, or even smart phones.

2.2 Uses of Health Data

Health data are recorded for a variety of purposes. Clinical data may be needed to support the proper care of the patient from whom they were obtained, but they also may contribute to the good of society through the aggregation and analysis of data regarding populations of individuals (supporting clinical research or public health assessments; see Chaps. 16 and 26). Traditional data-recording techniques and a paper record may have worked reasonably well when care was given by a single physician over the life of a patient. However, given the increased complexity of modern health care, the broadly trained team of individuals who are involved in a patient's care, and the need for multiple providers to access a patient's data and to communicate effectively with one another through the chart, the paper record no longer adequately supports optimal care of individual patients. Another problem occurs because traditional paper-based data-recording techniques have made clinical research across populations of patients extremely cumbersome. Electronic record keeping offers major advantages in this regard, as we discuss in more detail later in this chapter and in Chaps. 12 and 16.

2.2.1 Create the Basis for the Historical Record

Any student of science learns the importance of collecting and recording data meticulously when carrying out an experiment. Just as a laboratory notebook provides a record of precisely what a scientist has done, the experimental data observed, and the rationale for intermediate decision points, medical records are intended to provide a detailed compilation of information about individual patients:

- What is the patient's history (development of a current illness; other diseases that coexist or have resolved; pertinent family, social, and demographic information)?
- What symptoms has the patient reported? When did they begin, what has seemed to aggravate them, and what has provided relief?
- What physical signs have been noted on examination?
- How have signs and symptoms changed over time?
- What laboratory results have been, or are now, available?
- What radiologic and other special studies have been performed?
- What medications are being taken and are there any allergies?
- What other interventions have been undertaken?
- What is the reasoning behind the management decisions?

Each new patient problem and its management can be viewed as a therapeutic experiment, inherently confounded by uncertainty, with the goal of answering three questions when the experiment is over:

1. What was the nature of the disease or symptom?
2. What was the treatment decision?
3. What was the outcome of that treatment?

As is true for all experiments, one purpose is to learn from experience through careful observation and recording of data. The lessons learned in a given encounter may be highly individualized (e.g., the physician may learn how a specific patient tends to respond to pain or how family interactions tend to affect the patient's response to disease). On the other hand, the value of some experiments may be derived only by pooling of data from many patients who have similar problems and through the analysis of the results of various treatment options to determine efficacy.

Although laboratory research has contributed dramatically to our knowledge of human disease and treatment, especially over the last half century, it is careful observation and recording by skilled health care personnel that has always been of fundamental importance in the generation of new knowledge about patient care. We learn from the aggregation of information from large numbers of patients; thus, the historical record for individual patients is of inestimable importance to clinical research.

2.2.2 Support Communication Among Providers

A central function of structured data collection and recording in health care settings is to assist personnel in providing coordinated care to a patient over time. Most patients who have significant medical conditions are seen over months or years on several occasions for one or more problems that require ongoing evaluation and treatment. Given the increasing numbers of elderly patients in many cultures and health care settings, the care given to a patient is less oriented to diagnosis and treatment of a single disease episode and increasingly focused on management of one or more chronic disorders—possibly over many years.

It was once common for patients to receive essentially all their care from a single provider: the family doctor who tended both children and adults, often seeing the patient over many or all the years of that person's life. We tend to picture such physicians as having especially close relationships with their patients—knowing the family and sharing in many of the patient's life events, especially in smaller communities. Such

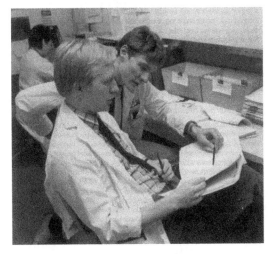

Fig. 2.5 One role of the medical record: a communication mechanism among health professionals who work together to plan patient care (Photograph courtesy of Janice Anne Rohn)

doctors nonetheless kept records of all encounters so that they could refer to data about past illnesses and treatments as a guide to evaluating future care issues.

In the world of modern medicine, the emergence of subspecialization and the increasing provision of care by teams of health professionals have placed new emphasis on the central role of the medical record. Shared access to a paper chart (Fig. 2.5) is now increasingly being replaced by clinicians accessing electronic records, sometimes conferring as they look at the same computer screen (Fig. 2.6). Now the record not only contains observations by a physician for reference on the next visit but also serves as a communication mechanism among physicians and other medical personnel, such as physical or respiratory therapists, nursing staff, radiology technicians, social workers, or discharge planners. In many outpatient settings, patients receive care over time from a variety of physicians—colleagues covering for the primary physician, or specialists to whom the patient has been referred, or a managed care organization's case manager. It is not uncommon to hear complaints from patients who remember the days when it was

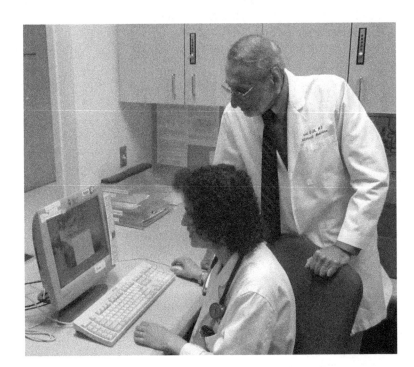

Fig. 2.6 Today similar communication sessions occur around a computer screen rather than a paper chart (see Fig. 2.5) (Photograph courtesy of James J. Cimino)

possible to receive essentially all their care from a single physician whom they had come to trust and who knew them well. Physicians are sensitive to this issue and therefore recognize the importance of the medical record in ensuring quality and **continuity of care** through adequate recording of the details and logic of past interventions and ongoing treatment plans. This idea is of particular importance in a health care system, such as the one in the United States, in which chronic diseases rather than care for trauma or acute infections increasingly dominate the basis for interactions between patients and their doctors.

2.2.3 Anticipate Future Health Problems

Providing high-quality health care involves more than responding to patients' acute or chronic health problems. It also requires educating patients about the ways in which their environment and lifestyles can contribute to, or reduce the risk of, future development of disease. Similarly, data gathered routinely in the ongoing care of a patient may suggest that he or she is at high risk of developing a specific problem even though he or she may feel well and be without symptoms at present. Clinical data therefore are important in screening for risk factors, following patients' risk profiles over time, and providing a basis for specific patient education or preventive interventions, such as diet, medication, or exercise. Perhaps the most common examples of such ongoing risk assessment in our society are routine monitoring for excess weight, high blood pressure, and elevated serum cholesterol levels. In these cases, abnormal data may be predictive of later symptomatic disease; optimal care requires early intervention before the complications have an opportunity to develop fully.

2.2.4 Record Standard Preventive Measures

The medical record also serves as a source of data on interventions that have been performed to prevent common or serious disorders. Sometimes the interventions involve counseling or educational programs (for example, regarding smoking cessation, measures for stopping drug abuse, safe sex practices, and dietary changes to lower cholesterol). Other important preventive interventions include immunizations: the vaccinations that begin in early childhood and continue throughout life, including special treatments administered when a person will be at particularly high risk (e.g., injections of gamma globulin to protect people from hepatitis, administered before travel to areas where hepatitis is endemic). When a patient comes to his local hospital emergency room with a laceration, the physicians routinely check for an indication of when he most recently had a tetanus immunization. When easily accessible in the record (or from the patient), such data can prevent unnecessary treatments (in this case, a repeat injection) that may be associated with risk or significant cost.

2.2.5 Identify Deviations from Expected Trends

Data often are useful in medical care only when viewed as part of a continuum over time. An example is the routine monitoring of children for normal growth and development by pediatricians (Fig. 2.7). Single data points regarding height and weight may have limited use by themselves; it is the trend in such data points observed over months or years that may provide the first clue to a medical problem. It is accordingly common for such parameters to be recorded on special charts or forms that make the trends easy to discern at a glance. Women who want to get pregnant often keep similar records of body temperature. By measuring temperature daily and recording the values on special charts, women can identify the slight increase in temperature that accompanies ovulation and thus may discern the days of maximum fertility. Many physicians will ask a patient to keep such graphical records so that they can later discuss the data with the patient and include the record in the medical chart for ongoing reference. Such graphs are increasingly created and displayed for viewing by clinicians as a feature of a patient's medical record.

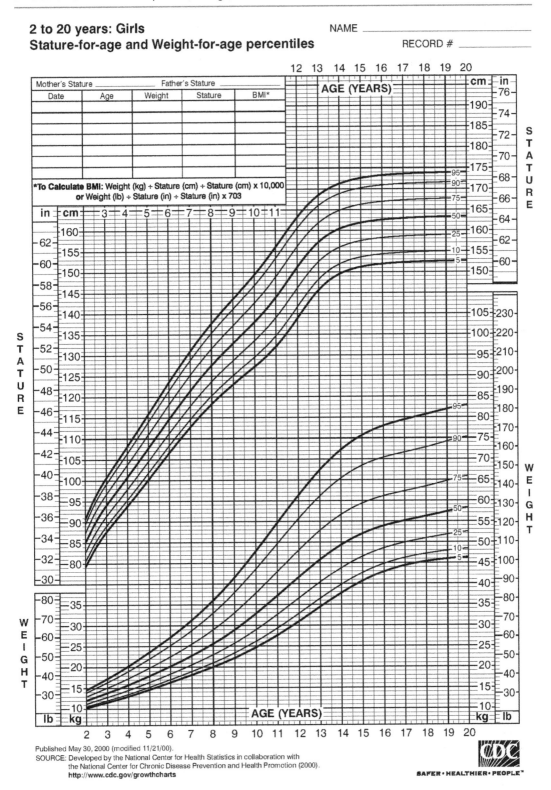

Fig. 2.7 A pediatric growth chart. Single data points would not be useful; it is the changes in values over time that indicate whether development is progressing normally (Source: National Center for Health Statistics in collaboration with the National Center for Chronic Disease Prevention and Health Promotion (2000). http://www.cdc.gov/growthcharts)

2.2.6 Provide a Legal Record

Another use of health data, once they are charted and analyzed, is as the foundation for a legal record to which the courts can refer if necessary. The medical record is a legal document; the responsible individual must sign most of the clinical information that is recorded. In addition, the chart generally should describe and justify both the presumed diagnosis for a patient and the choice of management.

We emphasized earlier the importance of recording data; in fact, data do not exist in a generally useful form unless they are recorded. The legal system stresses this point as well. Providers' unsubstantiated memories of what they observed or why they took some action are of little value in the courtroom. The medical record is the foundation for determining whether proper care was delivered. Thus, a well-maintained record is a source of protection for both patients and their physicians.

2.2.7 Support Clinical Research

Although experience caring for individual patients provides physicians with special skills and enhanced judgment over time, it is only by formally analyzing data collected from large numbers of patients that researchers can develop and validate new clinical knowledge of general applicability. Thus, another use of clinical data is to support research through the aggregation and statistical or other analysis of observations gathered from populations of patients (see Chap. 1).

A **randomized clinical trial** (**RCT**) (see also Chaps. 11 and 26) is a common method by which specific clinical questions are addressed experimentally. RCTs typically involve the random assignment of matched groups of patients to alternate treatments when there is uncertainty about how best to manage the patients' problem. The variables that might affect a patient's course (e.g., age, gender, weight, coexisting medical problems) are measured and recorded. As the study progresses, data are gathered meticulously to provide a record of how each patient fared under

treatment and precisely how the treatment was administered. By pooling such data, sometimes after years of experimentation (depending on the time course of the disease under consideration), researchers may be able to demonstrate a statistical difference among the study groups depending on precise characteristics present when patients entered the study or on the details of how patients were managed. Such results then help investigators to define the standard of care for future patients with the same or similar problems.

Medical knowledge also can be derived from the analysis of large patient data sets even when the patients were not specifically enrolled in an RCT, often referred to as **retrospective studies**. Much of the research in the field of epidemiology involves analysis of population-based data of this type. Our knowledge of the risks associated with cigarette smoking, for example, is based on irrefutable statistics derived from large populations of individuals with and without lung cancer, other pulmonary problems, and heart disease.

2.3 Weaknesses of the Traditional Medical Record System

The preceding description of medical data and their uses emphasizes the positive aspects of information storage and retrieval in the record. All medical personnel, however, quickly learn that use of the traditional paper record is complicated by a bevy of logistical and practical realities that greatly limit the record's effectiveness for its intended uses.

2.3.1 Pragmatic and Logistical Issues

Recall, first, that data cannot effectively serve the delivery of health care unless they are recorded. Their optimal use depends on positive responses to the following questions:

- Can I find the data I need when I need them?
- Can I find the medical record in which they are recorded?

- Can I find the data within the record?
- Can I find what I need quickly?
- Can I read and interpret the data once I find them?
- Can I update the data reliably with new observations in a form consistent with the requirements for future access by me or other people?

All too frequently, the traditional paper record creates situations in which people answer such questions in the negative. For example:

- The patient's paper chart may be unavailable when the health care professional needs it. It may be in use by someone else at another location; it may have been misplaced despite the record-tracking system of the hospital, clinic, or office (Fig. 2.8); or it may have been taken by someone unintentionally and is now buried on a desk.
- Once the chart is in hand, it might still be difficult to find the information required. The data may have been known previously but never recorded due to an oversight by a physician or other health professional. Poor organization in the chart may lead the user to spend an inordinate time searching for the data, especially in the massive paper charts of patients who have long and complicated histories.

- Once the health care professional has located the data, he or she may find them difficult to read. It is not uncommon to hear one physician asking another as they peer together into a chart: "What is that word?" "Is that a two or a five?" "Whose signature is that?" Illegible and sloppy entries can be a major obstruction to effective use of the chart (Fig. 2.9).
- When a chart is unavailable, the health care professional still must provide patient care. Thus, providers make do without past data, basing their decisions instead on what the patient can tell them and on what their examination reveals. They then write a note for inclusion in the chart—when the chart is located. In a large institution with thousands of medical records, it is not surprising that such loose notes often fail to make it to the patient's chart or are filed out of sequence so that the actual chronology of management is disrupted in the record.
- When patients who have chronic or frequent diseases are seen over months or years, their records grow so large that the charts must be broken up into multiple volumes. When a hospital clinic or emergency room orders the patient's chart, only the most recent volume typically is provided. Old but pertinent data

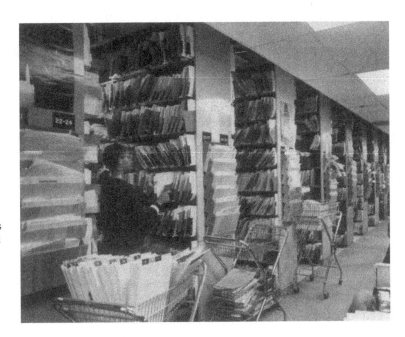

Fig. 2.8 A typical storage room for medical records. It is not surprising that charts sometimes were mislaid, and similarly clear why such paper repositories are being replaced as EHRs increasingly become the standard (Photograph courtesy of Janice Anne Rohn)

Fig. 2.9 Written entries are standard in paper records, yet handwritten notes may be illegible. Notes that cannot be interpreted by other people due to illegibility may cause delays in treatment or inappropriate care—an issue that is largely eliminated when EHRs are used

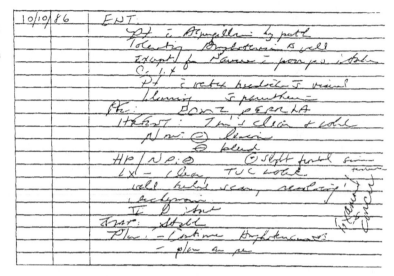

may be in early volumes that are stored offsite or are otherwise unavailable. Alternatively, an early volume may be mistaken for the most recent volume, misleading its users and resulting in documents being inserted out of sequence.

As described in Chap. 12, electronic health record systems offer solutions to all these practical problems in the use of the paper record. It is for this reason that more and more hospitals, health systems, and individual practitioners are implementing EHRs–further encouraged in the US by Federal incentive programs that help to cover the costs of EHR acquisition and maintenance (see Chaps. 1 and 27).

2.3.2 Redundancy and Inefficiency

To be able to find data quickly in the chart, health professionals have developed a variety of techniques that provide redundant recording to match alternate modes of access. For example, the result of a radiologic study typically is entered on a standard radiology reporting form, which is filed in the portion of the chart labeled "X-ray." For complicated procedures, the same data often are summarized in brief notes by radiologists in the narrative part of the chart, which they enter at the time of studies because they know that the formal report will not make it back to the chart for 1 or 2 days. In addition, the study results often are men-

tioned in notes written by the patient's admitting and consulting physicians and by the nursing staff. Although there may be good reasons for recording such information multiple times in different ways and in different locations within the chart, the combined bulk of these notes accelerates the physical growth of the document and, accordingly, complicates the chart's logistical management. Furthermore, it becomes increasingly difficult to locate specific patient data as the chart succumbs to "obesity". The predictable result is that someone writes yet another redundant entry, summarizing information that it took hours to track down.

A similar inefficiency occurs because of a tension between opposing goals in the design of reporting forms used by many laboratories. Most health personnel prefer a consistent, familiar paper form, often with color-coding, because it helps them to find information more quickly (Fig. 2.10). For example, a physician may know that a urinalysis report form is printed on yellow paper and records the bacteria count halfway down the middle column of the form. This knowledge allows the physician to work backward quickly in the laboratory section of the chart to find the most recent urinalysis sheet and to check at a glance the bacterial count. The problem is that such forms typically store only sparse information. It is clearly suboptimal if a rapidly growing physical chart is filled with sheets of paper that report only a single data element.

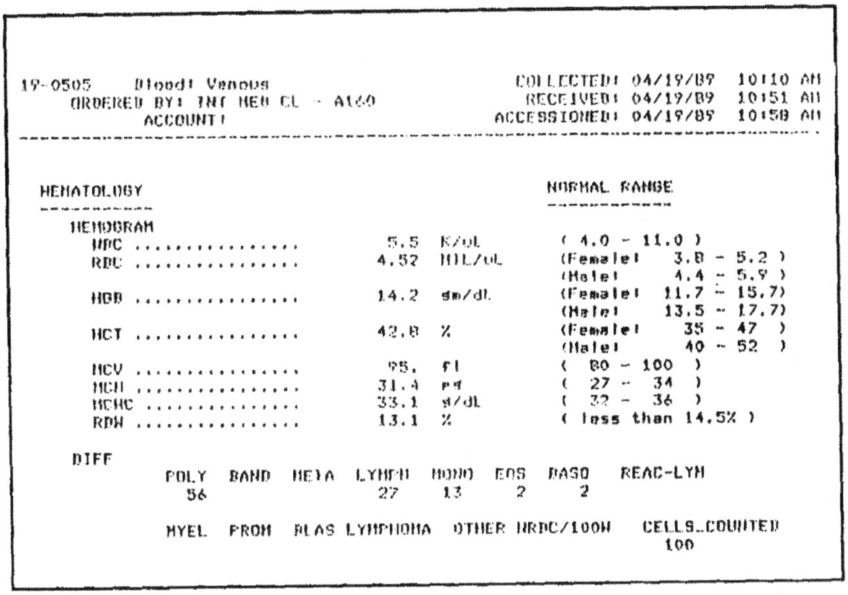

```
19-0505     Blood: Venous                          COLLECTED: 04/19/89   10:10 AM
   ORDERED BY: INT MED CL - A160                    RECEIVED: 04/19/89   10:51 AM
           ACCOUNT:                              ACCESSIONED: 04/19/89   10:58 AM
----------------------------------------------------------------------------------

HEMATOLOGY                                        NORMAL RANGE
----------                                        ------------
   HEMOGRAM
     WBC ................     5.5  K/uL          ( 4.0 - 11.0 )
     RBC ................    4.52  MIL/uL        (Female:   3.8 - 5.2 )
                                                 (Male:     4.4 - 5.9 )
     HGB ................    14.2  gm/dl         (Female:  11.7 - 15.7)
                                                 (Male:    13.5 - 17.7)
     HCT ................    42.8  %             (Female:    35 - 47  )
                                                 (Male:      40 - 52  )
     MCV ................     95.  fl            (  80 - 100  )
     MCH ................    31.4  pg            (  27 -  34  )
     MCHC ...............    33.1  g/dL          (  32 -  36  )
     RDW ................    13.1  %             ( less than 14.5% )

   DIFF
          POLY  BAND  META  LYMPH  MONO  EOS  BASO   REAC-LYM
           56                27     13    2     2

          MYEL  PROM  BLAS LYMPHOMA  OTHER NRBC/100W   CELLS_COUNTED
                                                           100
```

Fig. 2.10 Laboratory reporting forms record medical data in a consistent, familiar format

2.3.3 Influence on Clinical Research

Anyone who has participated in a clinical research project based on chart review can attest to the tediousness of flipping through myriad medical records. For all the reasons described in Chap. 1, it is arduous to sit with stacks of patients' charts, extracting data and formatting them for structured statistical analysis, and the process is vulnerable to transcription errors. Observers often wonder how much medical knowledge is sitting untapped in paper medical records because there is no easy way to analyze experience across large populations of patients without first extracting pertinent data from those charts.

Suppose, for example, that physicians on a medical consultation service notice that patients receiving a certain common oral medication for diabetes (call it drug X) seem to be more likely to have significant postoperative hypotension (low blood pressure) than do surgical patients receiving other medications for diabetes. The doctors have based this hypothesis—that drug X influences postoperative blood pressure—on only a few recent observations, however, so they decide to look into existing hospital records to see whether this correlation has occurred with sufficient frequency to warrant a formal investigation. One efficient way to follow up on their theory from existing medical data would be to examine the hospital records of all patients who have diabetes and also have been admitted for surgery. The task would then be to examine those records (difficult and arduous with paper charts as will be discussed shortly, but subject to automated analysis in the case of EHRs) and to note for all patients (1) whether they were taking drug X when admitted and (2) whether they had postoperative hypotension. If the statistics showed that patients receiving drug X were more likely to have low blood pressure after surgery than were similar diabetic patients receiving alternate treatments, a controlled trial (prospective observation and data gathering) might well be appropriate.

Note the distinction between **retrospective chart review** to investigate a question that was not a subject of study at the time the data were collected and **prospective studies** in which the clinical hypothesis is known in advance and the **research protocol** is designed specifically to collect future data that are relevant to the question under consideration (see also Chaps. 11 and 26). Subjects are assigned **randomly** to different study groups to help prevent researchers—who are bound to be biased, having developed the hypothesis—from unintentionally skewing the results by assigning a specific class of patients all to one group. For the same reason, to the extent possible, the studies are **double blind**; i.e., neither the researchers nor the subjects know which treatment is being administered. Such blinding is of course impractical when it is obvious to patients or physicians what therapy is being given (such as surgical procedures versus drug therapy). Prospective, randomized, double-blind studies are considered the best method for determining optimal management of disease, but it is often impractical to carry out such studies, and then methods such as retrospective chart review are used.

Returning to our example, consider the problems in paper chart review that the researchers would encounter in addressing the postoperative hypotension question retrospectively. First, they would have to identify the charts of interest: the subset of medical records dealing with surgical patients who are also diabetic. In a hospital record room filled with thousands of charts, the task of chart selection can be overwhelming. Medical records departments generally do keep indexes of diagnostic and procedure codes cross-referenced to specific patients (see Sect. 2.5.1). Thus, it might be possible to use such an index to find all charts in which the discharge diagnoses included diabetes and the procedure codes included major surgical procedures. The researcher might compile a list of patient identification numbers and have the individual charts pulled from the file room for review.

The researchers' next task is to examine each chart serially to find out what treatment each patient was receiving for diabetes at the time of the surgery and to determine whether the patient had postoperative hypotension. Finding such information may be extremely time-consuming. Where should the researcher look for it? The admission drug orders might show what the patient received for diabetes control, but it would also be wise to check the medication sheets to see whether the therapy was also administered (as well as ordered) and the admission history to see whether a routine treatment for diabetes, taken right up until the patient entered the hospital, was not administered during the inpatient stay. Information

about hypotensive episodes might be similarly difficult to locate. The researchers might start with nursing notes from the recovery room or with the anesthesiologist's datasheets from the operating room, but the patient might not have been hypotensive until after leaving the recovery room and returning to the ward. So the nursing notes from the ward need to be checked too, as well as vital signs sheets, physicians' progress notes, and the discharge summary.

It should be clear from this example that retrospective paper chart review is a laborious and tedious process and that people performing it are prone to make transcription errors and to overlook key data. One of the great appeals of EHRs (Chap. 12) is their ability to facilitate the chart review process. They obviate the need to retrieve hard copy charts; instead, researchers can use computer-based data retrieval and analysis techniques to do most of the work (finding relevant patients, locating pertinent data, and formatting the information for statistical analyses). Researchers can use similar techniques to harness computer assistance with data management in prospective clinical trials (Chap. 26).

2.3.4 The Passive Nature of Paper Records

The traditional manual system has another limitation that would have been meaningless until the emergence of the computer age. A manual archival system is inherently passive; the charts sit waiting for something to be done with them. They are insensitive to the characteristics of the data recorded within their pages, such as legibility, accuracy, or implications for patient management. They cannot take an active role in responding appropriately to those implications.

Increasingly, EHR systems have changed our perspective on what health professionals can expect from the medical chart. Automated record systems introduce new opportunities for dynamic responses to the data that are recorded in them. As described in many of the chapters to follow, computational techniques for data storage, retrieval, and analysis make it feasible to develop record systems that (1) monitor their contents and generate warnings or advice for providers based on single observations or on logical combinations of data; (2) provide automated quality control, including the flagging of potentially erroneous data; or (3) provide feedback on patient-specific or population-based deviations from desirable standards.

2.4   New Kinds of Data and the Resulting Challenges

The revolution in human genetics that emerged with the **Human Genome Project** in the 1990s is already having a profound effect on the diagnosis, prognosis, and treatment of disease (Palotie et al. 2013). The vast amounts of data that are generated in biomedical research (see Chaps. 24 and 25), and that can be pooled from patient datasets to support clinical research (Chap. 26) and public health (Chap. 16), have created new challenges as well as opportunities. Researchers are finding that the amount of data that they must manage and assess has become so large that they often find that they lack either the capabilities or expertise to handle the analytics that are required. This problem, sometimes dubbed the "big data" problem, has gathered the attention of government funding agencies as well (Mervis 2012; NSF-NIH Interagency Initiative 2012). Some suggest that the genetic material itself will become our next-generation method for storing large amounts of data (Church et al. 2012). Data analytics, and the management of large amounts of genomic/proteomic or clinical/public-health data, have accordingly become major research topics and key opportunities for new methodology development by biomedical informatics scientists (Ohno-Machado 2012).

The issues that arise are practical as well as scientifically interesting. For example, developers of EHRs have begun to grapple with questions regarding how they might be store an individual's personal genome with the electronic health record. New standards will be required,

and tactical questions need answering regarding, for example, whether to store an entire genome or only those components (e.g., genetic markers) that are already understood (Masys et al. 2012). In cancer, for example, where mutations in cell lines can occur, an individual may actually have many genomes represented among his or her cells. These issues will undoubtedly influence the evolution of data systems and EHRs, as well as the growth of **personalized medicine**, in the years ahead.

2.5   The Structure of Clinical Data

Scientific disciplines generally develop a precise terminology or notation that is standardized and accepted by all workers in the field. Consider, for example, the universal language of chemistry embodied in chemical formulae, the precise definitions and mathematical equations used by physicists, the predicate calculus used by logicians, or the conventions for describing circuits used by electrical engineers. Medicine is remarkable for its failure to develop a widely accepted standardized vocabulary and **nomenclature**, and many observers believe that a true scientific basis for the field will be impossible until this problem is addressed (see Chap. 7). Other people argue that common references to the "art of medicine" reflect an important distinction between medicine and the "hard" sciences; these people question whether it is possible to introduce too much standardization into a field that prides itself in humanism.

The debate has been accentuated by the introduction of computers for data management, because such machines tend to demand conformity to data standards and definitions. Otherwise, issues of data retrieval and analysis are confounded by discrepancies between the meanings intended by the observers or recorders and those intended by the individuals retrieving information or doing data analysis. What is an "upper respiratory infection"? Does it include infections of the trachea or of the main stem bronchi? How large does the heart have to be before we can refer to "cardiomegaly"? How should we deal with the plethora of disease names based on eponyms (e.g., Alzheimer's disease, Hodgkin's disease) that are not descriptive of the illness and may not be familiar to all practitioners? What do we mean by an "acute abdomen"? Are the boundaries of the abdomen well agreed on? What are the time constraints that correspond to "acuteness" of abdominal pain? Is an "ache" a pain? What about "occasional" cramping?

Imprecision and the lack of a standardized vocabulary are particularly problematic when we wish to aggregate data recorded by multiple health professionals or to analyze trends over time. Without a controlled, predefined vocabulary, data interpretation is inherently complicated, and the automatic summarization of data may be impossible. For example, one physician might note that a patient has "shortness of breath." Later, another physician might note that she has "dyspnea." Unless these terms are designated as synonyms, an automated program will fail to indicate that the patient had the same problem on both occasions.

Regardless of arguments regarding the "artistic" elements in medicine, the need for health personnel to communicate effectively is clear both in acute care settings and when patients are seen over long periods. Both high-quality care and scientific progress depend on some standardization in terminology. Otherwise, differences in intended meaning or in defining criteria will lead to miscommunication, improper interpretation, and potentially negative consequences for the patients involved.

Given the lack of formal definitions for many medical terms, it is remarkable that medical workers communicate as well as they do. Only occasionally is the care for a patient clearly compromised by miscommunication. If EHRs are to become dynamic and responsive manipulators of patient data, however, their encoded logic must be able to presume a specific meaning for the terms and data elements entered by the observers. This point is discussed in greater detail in Chap. 7, which deals in part with the multiple efforts to develop health care-computing standards, including a shared, controlled terminology for biomedicine.

2.5.1 Coding Systems

We are used to seeing figures regarding the growing incidences of certain types of tumors, deaths from influenza during the winter months, and similar health statistics that we tend to take for granted. How are such data accumulated? Their role in health planning and health care financing is clear, but if their accumulation required chart review through the process described earlier in this chapter, we would know much less about the health status of the populations in various communities (see Chap. 16).

Because of the needs to know about health trends for populations and to recognize epidemics in their early stages, there are various health-reporting requirements for hospitals (as well as other public organizations) and practitioners. For example, cases of gonorrhea, syphilis, and tuberculosis generally must be reported to local public-health organizations, which code the data to allow trend analyses over time. The Centers for Disease Control and Prevention in Atlanta (CDC) then pool regional data and report national as well as local trends in disease incidence, bacterial-resistance patterns, etc.

Another kind of reporting involves the coding of all discharge diagnoses for hospitalized patients, plus coding of certain procedures (e.g., type of surgery) that were performed during the hospital stay. Such codes are reported to state and federal health-planning and analysis agencies and also are used internally at the institution for case-mix analysis (determining the relative frequencies of various disorders in the hospitalized population and the average length of stay for each disease category) and for research. For such data to be useful, the codes must be well defined as well as uniformly applied and accepted.

The World health Organization publishes adiagnostic coding scheme called the International Classification of Disease (ICD). The 10th revision of this standard, ICD10,[3] is currently in use in much of the world, although in the United States a derivative of the previous version, the *International Classification of Diseases, 9th*

---

[3] http://www.icd10data.com/ (Accessed 12/2/2012).

Edition – Clinical Modifications (ICD9-CM), is still transitioning to the new version (see Chap. 7). ICD9-CM is used by all nonmilitary hospitals in the United States for discharge coding, and must be reported on the bills submitted to most insurance companies (Fig. 2.11). Pathologists have developed another widely used diagnostic coding scheme; originally known as Systematized Nomenclature of Pathology (SNOP), it was expanded to the Systematized Nomenclature of Medicine (SNOMED) (Côté and Rothwell 1993; American College of Pathologists 1982) and then merged with the Read Clinical Terms from the Great Britain to become

J45 Asthma
Includes: allergic (predominantly) asthma, allergic bronchitis NOS, allergic rhinitis with asthma, atopic asthma, extrinsic allergic asthma, hay fever with asthma, idiosyncratic asthma, intrinsic nonallergic asthma, nonallergic asthma

Use additional code to identify: exposure to environmental tobacco smoke (Z77.22), exposure to tobacco smoke in the perinatal period (P96.81), history of tobacco use (Z87.891), occupational exposure to environmental tobacco smoke (Z57.31), tobacco dependence (F17.-), tobacco use (Z72.0)

Excludes: detergent asthma (J69.8), eosinophilic asthma (J82), lung diseases due to external agents (J60-J70), miner's asthma (J60), wheezing NOS (R06.2), wood asthma (J67.8), asthma with chronic obstructive pulmonary disease (J44.9), chronic asthmatic (obstructive) bronchitis (J44.9), chronic obstructive asthma (J44.9)

  J45.2 Mild intermittent asthma
    J45.20 Mild intermittent asthma, uncomplicated
          Mild intermittent asthma NOS
    J45.21 Mild intermittent asthma with (acute) exacerbation
    J45.22 Mild intermittent asthma with status asthmaticus
  J45.3 Mild persistent asthma
    J45.30 Mild persistent asthma, uncomplicated
          Mild persistent asthma NOS
    J45.31 Mild persistent asthma with (acute) exacerbation
    J45.32 Mild persistent asthma with status asthmaticus
  J45.4 Moderate persistent asthma
    J45.40 Moderate persistent asthma, uncomplicated
          Moderate persistent asthma NOS
    J45.41 Moderate persistent asthma with (acute) exacerbation
    J45.42 Moderate persistent asthma with status asthmaticus
  J45.5 Severe persistent asthma
    J45.50 Severe persistent asthma, uncomplicated
          Severe persistent asthma NOS
    J45.51 Severe persistent asthma with (acute) exacerbation
    J45.52 Severe persistent asthma with status asthmaticus
  J45.9 Other and unspecified asthma
    J45.90 Unspecified asthma
          Asthmatic bronchitis NOS
          Childhood asthma NOS
          Late onset asthma
    J45.901 Unspecified asthma with (acute) exacerbation
    J45.902 Unspecified asthma with status asthmaticus
    J45.909 Unspecified asthma, uncomplicated
          Asthma NOS
  J45.99 Other asthma
    J45.990 Exercise induced bronchospasm
    J45.991 Cough variant asthma
    J45.998 Other asthma

Fig. 2.11 The subset of disease categories for asthma taken from ICD-10-CM, the new diagnosis coding system that is being developed as a replacement for ICD-9-CM, Volumes 1 and 2 (Source: Centers for Medicare and Medicaid Services, US Department of Health and Human Services, http://www.cms.gov/Medicare/Coding/ICD10/2013-ICD-10-CM-and-GEMs.html, accessed September 11, 2013)

SNOMED-CT (Stearns et al. 2001). In recent years, support for SNOMED-CT, has been assumed by the International Health Terminology Standards Development Organization, based in Copenhagen.[4] Another coding scheme, developed by the American Medical Association, is the Current Procedural Terminology (CPT) (Finkel 1977). It is similarly widely used in producing bills for services rendered to patients. More details on such schemes are provided in Chap. 7. What warrants emphasis here, however, is the motivation for the codes' development: health care personnel need standardized terms that can support pooling of data for analysis and can provide criteria for determining charges for individual patients.

The historical roots of a coding system reveal themselves as limitations or idiosyncrasies when the system is applied in more general clinical settings. For example, ICD9-CM was derived from a classification scheme developed for epidemiologic reporting. Consequently, it has more than 500 separate codes for describing tuberculosis infections. SNOMED versions have long permitted coding of pathologic findings in exquisite detail but only in later years began to introduce codes for expressing the dimensions of a patient's functional status. In a particular clinical setting, none of the common coding schemes is likely to be completely satisfactory. In some cases, the granularity of the code will be too coarse; on the one hand, a hematologist (person who studies blood diseases) may want to distinguish among a variety of hemoglobinopathies (disorders of the structure and function of hemoglobin) lumped under a single code in ICD8-CM. On the other hand, another practitioner may prefer to aggregate many individual codes—e.g., those for active tuberculosis—into a single category to simplify the coding and retrieval of data.

Such schemes cannot be effective unless health care providers accept them. There is an inherent tension between the need for a coding system that is general enough to cover many different patients and the need for precise and unique terms that accurately apply to a specific patient and do not unduly constrain physicians' attempts

to describe what they observe. Yet if physicians view the EHR as a blank sheet of paper on which any unstructured information can be written, the data they record will be unsuitable for dynamic processing, clinical research, and health planning. The challenge is to learn how to meet all these needs. Researchers at many institutions have worked for over two decades to develop a unified medical language system (UMLS), a common structure that ties together the various vocabularies that have been created. At the same time, the developers of specific terminologies are continually working to refine and expand their independent coding schemes (Humphreys et al. 1998) (see Chap. 7).

2.5.2 The Data-to-Knowledge Spectrum

A central focus in bio medical informatics is the information base that constitutes the "substance of medicine." Workers in the field have tried to clarify the distinctions among three terms frequently used to describe the content of computer-based systems: data, information, and knowledge (Blum 1986b; Bernstam et al. 2010). These terms are often used interchangeably. In this volume, we shall refer to a **datum** as a single observational point that characterizes a relationship.[5] It generally can be regarded as the value of a specific parameter for a particular object (e.g., a patient) at a given point in time. The term **information** refers to analyzed data that have been suitably curated and organized so that they have meaning. Data do not constitute information until they have been organized in some way, e.g., for analysis or display. **Knowledge**, then, is derived through the formal or informal analysis (or interpretation) of information that was in turn derived from data. Thus, knowledge includes the results of formal studies and also common sense facts, assumptions, heuristics (strategic rules of thumb), and models—any of which may reflect the expe-

---

[4] http://www.ihtsdo.org/ (Accessed 12/2/2012).

[5] Note that *data* is a plural term, although it is often erroneously used in speech and writing as though it were a collective (singular) noun.

rience or biases of people who interpret the primary data and the resulting information.

The observation that patient Brown has a blood pressure of 180/110 is a *datum*, as is the report that the patient has had a myocardial infarction (heart attack). When researchers pool such data, creating information, subsequent analysis may determine that patients with high blood pressure are more likely to have heart attacks than are patients with normal or low blood pressure. This analysis of organized data (information) has produced a piece of knowledge about the world. A physician's belief that prescribing dietary restriction of salt is unlikely to be effective in controlling high blood pressure in patients of low economic standing (because the latter are less likely to be able to afford special low-salt foods) is an additional personal piece of *knowledge*—a **heuristic** that guides physicians in their decision making. Note that the appropriate interpretation of these definitions depends on the context. Knowledge at one level of abstraction may be considered data at higher levels. A blood pressure of 180/110 mmHg is a raw piece of data; the statement that the patient has hypertension is an interpretation of several such data and thus represents a higher level of information. As input to a diagnostic decision aid, however, the presence or absence of hypertension may be requested, in which case the presence of hypertension is treated as a data item.

A **database** is a collection of individual observations without any summarizing analysis. An EHR system is thus primarily viewed as a database—the place where patient data are stored. When properly collated and pooled with other data, these elements in the EHR provide *information* about the patient. A **knowledge base**, on the other hand, is a collection of facts, heuristics, and models that can be used for problem solving and analysis of organized data (information). If the knowledge base provides sufficient structure, including semantic links among knowledge items, the computer itself may be able to apply that knowledge as an aid to case-based problem solving. Many decision-support systems have been called knowledge-based systems, reflecting this distinction between knowledge bases and databases (see Chap. 22).

2.6 Strategies of Clinical Data Selection and Use

It is illusory to conceive of a "complete clinical data set." All medical databases, and medical records, are necessarily incomplete because they reflect the selective collection and recording of data by the health care personnel responsible for the patient. There can be marked interpersonal differences in both style and problem solving that account for variations in the way practitioners collect and record data for the same patient under the same circumstances. Such variations do not necessarily reflect good practices, however, and much of medical education is directed at helping physicians and other health professionals to learn what observations to make, how to make them (generally an issue of technique), how to interpret them, and how to decide whether they warrant formal recording.

An example of this phenomenon is the difference between the first medical history, physical examination, and summarizing report developed by a medical student and the similar process undertaken by a seasoned clinician examining the same patient. Medical students tend to work from comprehensive mental outlines of questions to ask, physical tests to perform, and additional data to collect. Because they have not developed skills of selectivity, the process of taking a medical history and performing a physical examination may take more than 1 h, after which students develop extensive reports of what they observed and how they have interpreted their observations. It clearly would be impractical, inefficient, and inappropriate for physicians in practice to spend this amount of time assessing every new patient. Thus, part of the challenge for the neophyte is to learn how to ask only the questions that are necessary, to perform only the examination components that are required, and to record only those data that will be pertinent in justifying the ongoing diagnostic approach and in guiding the future management of the patient.

What do we mean by **selectivity** in data collection and recording? It is precisely this process that often is viewed as a central part of the "art of medicine," an element that accounts for individual styles and the sometimes marked distinctions among clinicians. As is discussed with numerous clinical examples in Chaps. 3 and 4, the idea of selectivity implies an ongoing decision-making process that guides data collection and interpretation. Attempts to understand how expert clinicians internalize this process, and to formalize the ideas so that they can better be taught and explained, are central in biomedical informatics research. Improved guidelines for such decision making, derived from research activities in biomedical informatics, not only are enhancing the teaching and practice of medicine (Shortliffe 2010) but also are providing insights that suggest methods for developing computer-based decision-support tools.

2.6.1 The Hypothetico-Deductive Approach

Studies of clinical decision makers have shown that strategies for data collection and interpretation may be imbedded in an iterative process known as the **hypothetico-deductive approach** (Elstein et al. 1978; Kassirer and Gorry 1978). As medical students learn this process, their data collection becomes more focused and efficient, and their medical records become more compact. The central idea is one of sequential, staged data collection, followed by data interpretation and the generation of hypotheses, leading to hypothesis-directed selection of the next most appropriate data to be collected. As data are collected at

each stage, they are added to the growing database of observations and are used to reformulate or refine the active hypotheses. This process is iterated until one hypothesis reaches a threshold level of certainty (e.g., it is proved to be true, or at least the uncertainty is reduced to a satisfactory level). At that point, a management, disposition, or therapeutic decision can be made.

The diagram in Fig. 2.12 clarifies this process. As is shown, data collection begins when the patient presents to the physician with some issue (a symptom or disease, or perhaps the need for routine care). The physician generally responds with a few questions that allow one to focus rapidly on the nature of the problem. In the written report, the data collected with these initial questions typically are recorded as the patient identification, chief complaint, and initial portion of the history of the present illness. Studies have shown that an experienced physician will have an initial set of hypotheses (theories) in mind after hearing the patient's response to the first six or seven questions (Elstein et al. 1978). These hypotheses then serve as the basis for selecting additional questions. As shown in Fig. 2.12, answers to these additional questions allow the physician to refine hypotheses about the source of the patient's problem. Physicians refer to the set of active hypotheses as the **differential diagnosis** for a patient; the differential diagnosis comprises the set of possible diagnoses among which the physician must distinguish to determine how best to administer treatment.

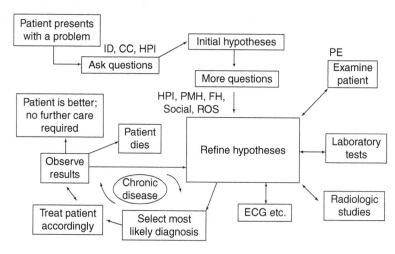

Fig. 2.12 A schematic view of the hypothetico-deductive approach. The process of medical data collection and treatment is intimately tied to an ongoing process of hypothesis generation and refinement. See text for full discussion. *ID* patient identification, *CC* chief complaint, *HPI* history of present illness, *PMH* past medical history, *FH* family history, *Social* social history, *ROS* review of systems, *PE* physical examination

Note that the question selection process is inherently heuristic; e.g., it is personalized and efficient, but it is not guaranteed to collect every piece of information that might be pertinent. Human beings use heuristics all the time in their decision making because it often is impractical or impossible to use an exhaustive problem-solving approach. A common example of heuristic problem solving is the playing of a complex game such as chess. Because it would require an enormous amount of time to define all the possible moves and countermoves that could ensue from a given board position, expert chess players develop personal heuristics for assessing the game at any point and then selecting a strategy for how best to proceed. Differences among such heuristics account in part for variations in observed expertise.

Physicians have developed safety measures, however, to help them to avoid missing important issues that they might not discover when collecting data in a hypothesis-directed fashion when taking the history of a patient's present illness (Pauker et al. 1976). These measures tend to be focused in four general categories of questions that follow the collection of information about the chief complaint: past medical history, family history, social history, and a brief **review of systems** in which the physician asks some general questions about the state of health of each of the major organ systems in the body. Occasionally, the physician discovers entirely new problems or finds important information that modifies the hypothesis list or modulates the treatment options available (e.g., if the patient reports a serious past drug reaction or allergy).

When physicians have finished asking questions, the refined hypothesis list (which may already be narrowed to a single diagnosis) then serves as the basis for a focused physical examination. By this time, physicians may well have expectations of what they will find on examination or may have specific tests in mind that will help them to distinguish among still active hypotheses about diseases based on the questions that they have asked. Once again, as in the question-asking process, focused hypothesis-directed examination is augmented with general

tests that occasionally turn up new abnormalities and generate hypotheses that the physician did not expect on the basis of the medical history alone. In addition, unexplained findings on examination may raise issues that require additional history taking. Thus, the asking of questions generally is partially integrated with the examination process.

When physicians have completed the physical examination, their refined hypothesis list may be narrowed sufficiently for them to undertake specific treatment. Additional data gathering may still be necessary, however. Such testing is once again guided by the current hypotheses. The options available include laboratory tests (of blood, urine, other body fluids, or biopsy specimens), radiologic studies (X-ray examinations, nuclear-imaging scans, computed tomography (CT) studies, magnetic resonance scans, sonograms, or any of a number of other imaging modalities), and other specialized tests (electrocardiograms (ECGs), electroencephalograms, nerve conduction studies, and many others), as well as returning to the patient to ask further questions or perform additional physical examination. As the results of such studies become available, physicians constantly revise and refine their hypothesis list.

Ultimately, physicians are sufficiently certain about the source of a patient's problem to be able to develop a specific management plan. Treatments are administered, and the patient is observed. Note data collected to measure response to treatment may themselves be used to synthesize information that affects the hypotheses about a patient's illness. If patients do not respond to treatment, it may mean that their disease is resistant to that therapy and that their physicians should try an alternate approach, or it may mean that the initial diagnosis was incorrect and that physicians should consider alternate explanations for the patient's problem.

The patient may remain in a cycle of treatment and observation for a long time, as shown in Fig. 2.12. This long cycle reflects the nature of chronic-disease management—an aspect of medical care that is accounting for an increasing proportion of the health care community's work (and an increasing proportion of health care cost).

Alternatively, the patient may recover and no longer need therapy, or he or she may die. Although the process outlined in Fig. 2.12 is oversimplified in many regards, it is generally applicable to the process of data collection, diagnosis, and treatment in most areas of medicine.

Note that the hypothesis-directed process of data collection, diagnosis, and treatment is inherently knowledge-based. It is dependent not only on a significant fact base that permits proper interpretation of data and selection of appropriate follow-up questions and tests but also on the effective use of heuristic techniques that characterize individual expertise.

Another important issue, addressed in Chap. 3, is the need for physicians to balance financial costs and health risks of data collection against the perceived benefits to be gained when those data become available. It costs nothing but time to examine the patient at the bedside or to ask an additional question, but if the data being considered require, for example, X-ray exposure, coronary angiography, or a CT scan of the head (all of which have associated risks and costs), then it may be preferable to proceed with treatment in the absence of full information. Differences in the assessment of cost-benefit trade-offs in data collection, and variations among individuals in their willingness to make decisions under uncertainty, often account for differences of opinion among collaborating physicians.

2.6.2 The Relationship Between Data and Hypotheses

We wrote rather glibly in Sect. 2.6.1 about the "generation of hypotheses from data"; now we need to ask: What precisely is the nature of that process? As is discussed in Chap. 4, researchers with a psychological orientation have spent much time trying to understand how expert problem solvers evoke hypotheses (Pauker et al. 1976; Elstein et al. 1978; Pople 1982) and the traditional probabilistic decision sciences have much to say about that process as well. We provide only a brief introduction to these ideas here; they are discussed in greater detail in Chaps. 3 and 4.

When an observation evokes a hypothesis (e.g., when a clinical finding makes a specific diagnosis come to mind), the observation presumably has some close association with the hypothesis. What might be the characteristics of that association? Perhaps the finding is almost always observed when the hypothesis turns out to be true. Is that enough to explain hypothesis generation? A simple example will show that such a simple relationship is not enough to explain the evocation process. Consider the hypothesis that a patient is pregnant and the observation that the patient is female. Clearly, all pregnant patients are female. When a new patient is observed to be female, however, the possibility that the patient is pregnant is not immediately evoked. Thus, female gender is a highly sensitive indicator of pregnancy (there is a 100 % certainty that a pregnant patient is female), but it is not a good predictor of pregnancy (most females are not pregnant). The idea of **sensitivity**—the likelihood that a given datum will be observed in a patient with a given disease or condition—is an important one, but it will not alone account for the process of hypothesis generation in medical diagnosis.

Perhaps the clinical manifestation seldom occurs unless the hypothesis turns out to be true; is that enough to explain hypothesis generation? This idea seems to be a little closer to the mark. Suppose a given datum is never seen unless a patient has a specific disease. For example, a Pap smear (a smear of cells swabbed from the cervix, at the opening to the uterus, treated with Papanicolaou's stain, and then examined under the microscope) with grossly abnormal cells (called class IV findings) is never seen unless the woman has cancer of the cervix or uterus. Such tests are called **pathognomonic**. Not only do they evoke a specific diagnosis but they also immediately prove it to be true. Unfortunately, there are few pathognomonic tests in medicine and they are often of relatively low sensitivity (that is, although having a particular test result makes the diagnosis, few patients with the condition actually have that finding).

More commonly, a feature is seen in one disease or disease category more frequently than it is in others, but the association is not absolute.

For example, there are few disease entities other than infections that elevate a patient's white blood cell count. Certainly it is true, for example, that leukemia can raise the white blood cell count, as can the use of the drug prednisone, but most patients who do not have infections will have normal white blood cell counts. An elevated white count therefore does not prove that a patient has an infection, but it does tend to evoke or support the hypothesis that an infection is present. The word used to describe this relationship is **specificity**. An observation is highly specific for a disease if it is generally not seen in patients who do not have that disease. A pathognomonic observation is 100% specific for a given disease. When an observation is highly specific for a disease, it tends to evoke that disease during the diagnostic or data-gathering process.

By now, you may have realized that there is a substantial difference between a physician viewing test results that evoke a disease hypothesis and that physician being willing to act on the disease hypothesis. Yet even experienced physicians sometimes fail to recognize that, although they have made an observation that is highly specific for a given disease, it may still be more likely that the patient has other diseases (and does not have the suspected one) unless (1) the finding is pathognomonic or (2) the suspected disease is considerably more common than are the other diseases that can cause the observed abnormality. This mistake is one of the most common errors of intuition that has been identified in the medical decision-making process. To explain the basis for this confusion in more detail, we must introduce two additional terms: prevalence and predictive value.

The **prevalence** of a disease is simply the percentage of a population of interest that has the disease at any given time. A particular disease may have a prevalence of only 5 % in the general population (1 person in 20 will have the disease) but have a higher prevalence in a specially selected subpopulation. For example, black-lung disease has a low prevalence in the general population but has a much higher prevalence among coal miners, who develop black lung from inhaling coal dust. The task of diagnosis therefore involves updating the probability that a patient has a disease from the **baseline rate** (the prevalence in the population from which the patient was selected) to a post-test probability that reflects the test results. For example, the probability that any given person in the United States has lung cancer is low (i.e., the prevalence of the disease is low), but the chance increases if his or her chest X-ray examination shows a possible tumor. If the patient were a member of the population composed of cigarette smokers in the United States, however, the prevalence of lung cancer would be higher. In this case, the identical chest X-ray report would result in an even higher updated probability of lung cancer than it would had the patient been selected from the population of all people in the United States.

The **predictive value (PV)** of a test is simply the post-test (updated) probability that a disease is present based on the results of a test. If an observation supports the presence of a disease, the PV will be greater than the prevalence (also called the pretest risk). If the observation tends to argue against the presence of a disease, the PV will be lower than the prevalence. For any test and disease, then, there is one PV if the test result is positive and another PV if the test result is negative. These values are typically abbreviated PV+ (the PV of a positive test) and PV− (the PV of a negative test).

The process of hypothesis generation in medical diagnosis thus involves both the evocation of hypotheses and the assignment of a likelihood (probability) to the presence of a specific disease or disease category. The PV of a positive test depends on the test's sensitivity and specificity, as well as the prevalence of the disease. The formula that describes the relationship precisely is:

$$PV+ = \frac{(\text{sensitivity})(\text{prevalence})}{(\text{sensitivity})(\text{prevalence}) + (1 - \text{specificity})(1 - \text{prevalence})}$$

There is a similar formula for defining PV− in terms of sensitivity, specificity, and prevalence. Both formulae can be derived from simple probability theory. Note that positive tests with high sensitivity and specificity may still lead to a low post-test probability of the disease (PV+) if the prevalence of that disease is low. You should substitute values in the PV + formula to convince yourself that this assertion is true. It is this relationship that tends to be poorly understood by practitioners and that often is viewed as counterintuitive (which shows that your intuition can misguide you!). Note also (by substitution into the formula) that test sensitivity and disease prevalence can be ignored only when a test is pathognomonic (i.e., when its specificity is 100 %, which mandates that PV+ be 100 %). The PV+ formula is one of many forms of **Bayes' theorem**, a rule for combining probabilistic data that is generally attributed to the work of Reverend Thomas Bayes in the 1700s. Bayes' theorem is discussed in greater detail in Chap. 3.

2.6.3 Methods for Selecting Questions and Comparing Tests

We have described the process of hypothesis-directed sequential data collection and have asked how an observation might evoke or refine the physician's hypotheses about what abnormalities account for the patient's illness. The complementary question is: Given a set of current hypotheses, how does the physician decide what additional data should be collected? This question also has been analyzed at length (Elstein et al. 1978; Pople 1982) and is pertinent for computer programs that gather data efficiently to assist clinicians with diagnosis or with therapeutic decision making (see Chap. 22). Because understanding issues of test selection and data interpretation is crucial to understanding medical data and their uses, we devote Chap. 3 to these and related issues

of medical decision making. In Sect. 3.6, for example, we discuss the use of decision-analytic techniques in deciding whether to treat a patient on the basis of available information or to perform additional diagnostic tests.

2.7 The Computer and Collection of Medical Data

Although this chapter has not directly discussed computer systems, the potential role of the computer in medical data storage, retrieval, and interpretation should be clear. Much of the rest of this book deals with specific applications in which the computer's primary role is data management. One question is pertinent to all such applications: How do you get the data into the computer in the first place?

The need for data entry by physicians has posed a problem for medical-computing systems since the earliest days of the field. Awkward or nonintuitive interactions at computing devices—particularly ones requiring keyboard typing or confusing movement through multiple display screens by the physician—have probably done more to inhibit the clinical use of computers than have any other factor. Doctors, and many other health care staff, sometimes simply refuse to use computers because of the awkward interfaces that are imposed.

A variety of approaches have been used to try to finesse this problem. One is to design systems such that clerical staff can do essentially all the data entry and much of the data retrieval as well. Many clinical research systems (see Chap. 26) have taken this approach. Physicians may be asked to fill out structured paper datasheets, or such sheets may be filled out by data abstractors who review patient charts, but the actual entry of data into the database is done by paid transcriptionists.

In some applications, it is possible for data to be entered automatically into the computer by the device that measures or collects them. For example, monitors in intensive care or coronary care units, pulmonary function or ECG machines, and measurement equipment in the clinical chemistry laboratory can interface directly with a computer in which a database is stored. Certain data can be entered directly by patients; there are systems, for example, that take the patient's history by presenting on a computer screen or tablet multiple-choice questions that follow a branching logic. The patient's responses to the questions are used to generate electronic or hard copy reports for physicians and also may be stored directly in a computer database for subsequent use in other settings.

When physicians or other health personnel do use the machine themselves, specialized devices often allow rapid and intuitive operator–machine interaction. Most of these devices use a variant of the "point-and-select" approach—e.g., touch-sensitive computer screens, mouse-pointing devices, and increasingly the clinician's finger on a mobile tablet or smart phone (see Chap. 5). When conventional computer workstations are used, specialized keypads can be helpful. Designers frequently permit logical selection of items from menus displayed on the screen so that the user does not need to learn a set of specialized commands to enter or review data. There were clear improvements when handheld tablets using pen-based or finger-based mechanisms for data entry were introduced. With ubiquitous wireless data services, such devices are allowing clinicians to maintain normal mobility (in and out of examining rooms or inpatient rooms) while accessing and entering data that are pertinent to a patient's care.

These issues arise in essentially all application areas, and, because they can be crucial to the successful implementation and use of a system, they warrant particular attention in system design. As more physicians are becoming familiar with computers at home, they will find the use of computers in their practice less of a hindrance. We encourage you to consider human–computer interaction, and the cognitive issues that arise in dealing with computer systems (see Chap. 4), as you learn about the application areas and the specific systems described in later chapters.

Suggested Readings

Bernstam, E. V., Smith, J. W., & Johnson, T. R. (2010). What is biomedical informatics? *Journal of Biomedical Informatics, 43*(1), 104–110. The authors discuss the transformation of data into information and knowledge, delineating the ways in which this focus lies at the heart of the field of biomedical informatics.

Klasnja, P., & Pratt, W. (2012). Healthcare in the pocket: mapping the space of mobile-phone health interventions. *Journal of Biomedical Informatics, 45*(1), 184–198. This review article describes the multiple ways in which both patients and providers are being empowered through the introduction of affordable mobile technologies that manage data and apply knowledge to generate advice.

Ohno-Machado, L. (2012). Big science, big data, and a big role for biomedical informatics. *Journal of the American Medical Informatics Association, 19*, e1. This editorial introduces a special online issue of the Journal of the American Medical Informatics Association in which the rapidly evolving world of biomedical and clinical "big data" challenges are the focus. Papers deal with both translational bioinformatics, in which genomic and proteomic data dominate, and clinical research informatics, in which large clinical and public health datasets are prominent.

Patel, V. L., Arocha, J. F., & Kaufman, D. R. (1994). Diagnostic reasoning and medical expertise. *Psychology of Learning and Motivation, 31*, 187–252. This paper illustrates the role of theory-driven psychological research and cognitive evaluation as they relate to medical decision making and the interpretation of clinical data. See also Chap. 4.

Shah, N. H. (2012). Translational bioinformatics embraces big data. *Yearbook of Medical Informatics, 7*(1), 130–134. This article reviews the latest trends and major developments in translational bioinformatics, arguing that the field is ready to revolutionize human health and health care using large-scale measurements on individuals. It discusses data-centric approaches that compute on massive amounts of data ("Big Data") to discover patterns and to make clinically relevant predictions, arguing that research that bridges the latest multimodal measurement technologies with large amounts of electronic health care data is where new medical breakthroughs will occur. See also Chap. 25.

Questions for Discussion

1. You check your pulse and discover that your heart rate is 100 beats per minute. Is this rate normal or abnormal? What additional information would you use in making this judgment? How does the context in which data are collected influence the interpretation of those data?

2. Given the imprecision of many medical terms, why do you think that serious instances of miscommunication among health care professionals are not more common? Why is greater standardization of terminology necessary if computers rather than humans are to manipulate patient data?

3. Based on the discussion of coding schemes for representing clinical information, discuss three challenges you foresee in attempting to construct a standardized terminology to be used in hospitals, physicians' offices, and research institutions.

4. How would medical practice change if nonphysicians were to collect all medical data?

5. Consider what you know about the typical daily schedule of a busy clinician. What are the advantages of wireless devices, connected to the Internet, as tools for such clinicians? Can you think of disadvantages as well? Be sure to consider the safety and protection of information as well as workflow and clinical needs.

6. To decide whether a patient has a significant urinary tract infection, physicians commonly use a calculation of the number of bacterial organisms in a milliliter of the patient's urine. Physicians generally assume that a patient has a urinary tract infection if there are at least 10,000 bacteria per milliliter. Although laboratories can provide such quantification with reasonable accuracy, it is obviously unrealistic for the physician explicitly to count large numbers of bacteria by examining a milliliter of urine under the microscope. As a result, one article offers the following guideline to physicians: "When interpreting ... microscopy of ... stained centrifuged urine, a threshold of one organism per field yields a 95 % sensitivity and five organisms per field a 95 % specificity for bacteriuria [bacteria in the urine] at a level of at least 10,000 organisms per ml." (Senior Medical Review 1987, p. 4)

   (a) Describe an experiment that would have allowed the researchers to determine the sensitivity and specificity of the microscopy.

   (b) How would you expect specificity to change as the number of bacteria per microscopic field increases from one to five?

   (c) How would you expect sensitivity to change as the number of bacteria per microscopic field increases from one to five?

   (d) Why does it take more organisms per microscopic field to obtain a specificity of 95 % than it does to achieve a sensitivity of 95 %?

Biomedical Decision Making: Probabilistic Clinical Reasoning

3

Douglas K. Owens and Harold C. Sox

After reading this chapter, you should know the answers to these questions:

- How is the concept of probability useful for understanding test results and for making medical decisions that involve uncertainty?
- How can we characterize the ability of a test to discriminate between disease and health?
- What information do we need to interpret test results accurately?
- What is expected-value decision making? How can this methodology help us to understand particular medical problems?
- What are utilities, and how can we use them to represent patients' preferences?
- What is a sensitivity analysis? How can we use it to examine the robustness of a decision and to identify the important variables in a decision?
- What are influence diagrams? How do they differ from decision trees?

D.K. Owens, MD, MS (✉)
VA Palo Alto Health Care System,
Palo Alto, CA, USA

Henry J. Kaiser Center for Primary Care
and Outcomes Research/Center for Health Policy,
Stanford University, Stanford, CA, USA
e-mail: owens@stanford.edu

H.C. Sox, MD, MACP
Dartmouth Institute, Geisel School of Medicine at
Dartmouth, Dartmouth College, 31 Faraway Lane,
West Lebanon, NH 03784, USA

3.1 The Nature of Clinical Decisions: Uncertainty and the Process of Diagnosis

Because clinical data are imperfect and outcomes of treatment are uncertain, health professionals often are faced with difficult choices. In this chapter, we introduce probabilistic medical reasoning, an approach that can help health care providers to deal with the uncertainty inherent in many medical decisions. Medical decisions are made by a variety of methods; our approach is neither necessary nor appropriate for all decisions. Throughout the chapter, we provide simple clinical examples that illustrate a broad range of problems for which probabilistic medical reasoning does provide valuable insight.

As discussed in Chap. 2, medical practice is medical decision making. In this chapter, we look at the process of medical decision making. Together, Chaps. 2 and 3 lay the groundwork for the rest of the book. In the remaining chapters, we discuss ways that computers can help clinicians with the decision-making process, and we emphasize the relationship between information needs and system design and implementation.

The material in this chapter is presented in the context of the decisions made by an individual clinician. The concepts, however, are more broadly applicable. Sensitivity and specificity are important parameters of laboratory systems that flag abnormal test results, of patient monitoring systems (Chap. 19), and of information-retrieval systems (Chap. 21). An understanding of what

E.H. Shortliffe, J.J. Cimino (eds.), *Biomedical Informatics*,
DOI 10.1007/978-1-4471-4474-8_3, © Springer-Verlag London 2014

probability is and of how to adjust probabilities after the acquisition of new information is a foundation for our study of clinical decision-support systems (Chap. 22). The importance of probability in medical decision making was noted as long ago as 1922:

> [G]ood medicine does not consist in the indiscriminate application of laboratory examinations to a patient, but rather in having so clear a comprehension of the probabilities and possibilities of a case as to know what tests may be expected to give information of value (Peabody 1922).

Example 1
You are the director of a blood bank. All potential blood donors are tested to ensure that they are not infected with the human immunodeficiency virus (HIV), the causative agent of acquired immunodeficiency syndrome (AIDS). You ask whether use of the polymerase chain reaction (PCR), a gene-amplification technique that can diagnose HIV, would be useful to identify people who have HIV. The PCR test is positive 98 % of the time when antibody is present, and negative 99 % of the time antibody is absent.[1]

---

[1]The test sensitivity and specificity used in Example 1 are consistent with the reported values of the sensitivity and specificity of the PCR test for diagnosis of HIV early in its development (Owens et al. 1996b); the test now has higher sensitivity and specificity.

If the test is positive, what is the likelihood that a donor actually has HIV? If the test is negative, how sure can you be that the person does not have HIV? On an intuitive level, these questions do not seem particularly difficult to answer. The test appears accurate, and we would expect that, if the test is positive, the donated blood specimen is likely to contain the HIV. Thus, we are surprised to find that, if only one in 1,000 donors actually is infected, the test is more often mistaken than it is correct. In fact, of 100 donors with a positive test, fewer than 10 would be infected. There would be ten wrong answers for each correct result. How

are we to understand this result? Before we try to find an answer, let us consider a related example.

Example 2
Mr. James is a 59-year-old man with coronary artery disease (narrowing or blockage of the blood vessels that supply the heart tissue). When the heart muscle does not receive enough oxygen (hypoxia) because blood cannot reach it, the patient often experiences chest pain (angina). Mr. James has twice undergone coronary artery bypass graft (CABG) surgery, a procedure in which new vessels, often taken from the leg, are grafted onto the old ones such that blood is shunted past the blocked region. Unfortunately, he has again begun to have chest pain, which becomes progressively more severe, despite medication. If the heart muscle is deprived of oxygen, the result can be a heart attack (myocardial infarction), in which a section of the muscle dies.

Should Mr. James undergo a third operation? The medications are not working; without surgery, he runs a high risk of suffering a heart attack, which may be fatal. On the other hand, the surgery is hazardous. Not only is the surgical mortality rate for a third operation higher than that for a first or second one but also the chance that surgery will relieve the chest pain is lower than that for a first operation. All choices in Example 2 entail considerable uncertainty. Furthermore, the risks are grave; an incorrect decision may substantially increase the chance that Mr. James will die. The decision will be difficult even for experienced clinicians.

These examples illustrate situations in which intuition is either misleading or inadequate. Although the test results in Example 1 are appropriate for the blood bank, a clinician who uncritically reports these results would erroneously inform many people that they had the AIDS virus—a mistake with profound emotional and social consequences. In Example 2, the decision-making skill of the clinician will affect a patient's quality and length of life. Similar situations are commonplace in medicine. Our goal in this chapter is to show how the use of probability and decision analysis can help to make clear the best course of action.

Decision making is one of the quintessential activities of the healthcare professional. Some decisions are made on the basis of deductive reasoning or of physiological principles. Many decisions, however, are made on the basis of knowledge that has been gained through collective experience: the clinician often must rely on empirical knowledge of associations between symptoms and disease to evaluate a problem. A decision that is based on these usually imperfect associations will be, to some degree, uncertain. In Sects. 3.1.1, 3.1.2 and 3.1.3, we examine decisions made under uncertainty and present an overview of the diagnostic process. As Smith (1985, p. 3) said: "Medical decisions based on probabilities are necessary but also perilous. Even the most astute physician will occasionally be wrong."

3.1.1 Decision Making Under Uncertainty

Example 3
Mr. Kirk, a 33-year-old man with a history of a previous blood clot (thrombus) in a vein in his left leg, presents with the complaint of pain and swelling in that leg for the past 5 days. On physical examination, the leg is tender and swollen to midcalf—signs that suggest the possibility of deep vein thrombosis.[2] A test (ultrasonography) is performed, and the flow of blood in the veins of Mr. Kirk's leg is evaluated. The blood flow is abnormal, but the radiologist cannot tell whether there is a new blood clot.

---

[2]In medicine, a sign is an objective physical finding (something observed by the clinician) such as a temperature of 101.2 °F. A symptom is a subjective experience of the patient, such as feeling hot or feverish. The distinction may be blurred if the patient's experience also can be observed by the clinician.

Should Mr. Kirk be treated for blood clots? The main diagnostic concern is the recurrence of a blood clot in his leg. A clot in the veins of the leg can dislodge, flow with the blood, and cause a blockage in the vessels of the lungs, a potentially fatal event called a pulmonary embolus. Of patients with a swollen leg, about one-half actually have a blood clot; there are numerous other causes of a swollen leg. Given a swollen leg, therefore, a clinician cannot be sure that a clot is the cause. Thus, the physical findings leave considerable uncertainty. Furthermore, in Example 3, the results of the available diagnostic test are equivocal. The treatment for a blood clot is to administer anticoagulants (drugs that inhibit blood clot formation), which pose the risk of excessive bleeding to the patient. Therefore, clinicians do not want to treat the patient unless they are confident that a thrombus is present. But how much confidence should be required before starting treatment? We will learn that it is possible to answer this question by calculating the benefits and harms of treatment.

This example illustrates an important concept: Clinical data are imperfect. The degree of imperfection varies, but all clinical data—including the results of diagnostic tests, the history given by the patient, and the findings on physical examination—are uncertain.

3.1.2 Probability: An Alternative Method of Expressing Uncertainty

The language that clinicians use to describe a patient's condition often is ambiguous—a factor that further complicates the problem of uncertainty in medical decision making. Clinicians use words such as "probable" and "highly likely" to describe their beliefs about the likelihood of disease. These words have strikingly different meanings to different individuals. Because of the widespread disagreement about the meaning of common descriptive terms, there is ample opportunity for miscommunication.

The problem of how to express degrees of uncertainty is not unique to medicine. How is it handled in other contexts? Horse racing has its share of uncertainty. If experienced gamblers are deciding whether to place bets, they will find it unsatisfactory to be told that a given horse has a "high chance" of winning. They will demand to know the odds.

The odds are simply an alternate way to express a probability. The use of probability or odds as an expression of uncertainty avoids the ambiguities inherent in common descriptive terms.

3.1.3 Overview of the Diagnostic Process

In Chap. 2, we described the hypothetico-deductive approach, a diagnostic strategy comprising successive iterations of hypothesis generation, data collection, and interpretation. We discussed how observations may evoke a hypothesis and how new information subsequently may increase or decrease our belief in that hypothesis. Here, we review this process briefly in light of a specific example. For the purpose of our discussion, we separate the diagnostic process into three stages.

The first stage involves making an initial judgment about whether a patient is likely to have a disease. After an interview and physical examination, a clinician intuitively develops a belief about the likelihood of disease. This judgment may be based on previous experience or on knowledge of the medical literature. A clinician's belief about the likelihood of disease usually is implicit; he or she can refine it by making an explicit estimation of the probability of disease. This estimated probability, made before further information is obtained, is the **prior probability** or **pretest probability** of disease.

Example 4

Mr. Smith, a 60-year-old man, complains to his clinician that he has pressure-like chest pain that occurs when he walks quickly. After taking his history and examining him, his clinician believes there is a high enough chance that he has heart disease to warrant ordering an exercise stress test. In the stress test, an electrocardiogram (ECG) is taken while Mr. Smith exercises. Because the heart must pump more blood per stroke and must beat faster (and thus requires more oxygen) during exercise, many heart conditions are evident only when the patient is physically stressed. Mr. Smith's results show abnormal changes in the ECG during exercise—a sign of heart disease.

How would the clinician evaluate this patient? The clinician would first talk to the patient about the quality, duration, and severity of his or her pain. Traditionally, the clinician would then decide what to do next based on his or her intuition about the etiology (cause) of the chest pain. Our approach is to ask the clinician to make his or her initial intuition explicit by estimating the pretest probability of disease. The clinician in this example, based on what he or she knows from talking with the patient, might assess the pretest or prior probability of heart disease as 0.5 (50 % chance or 1:1 odds; see Sect. 3.2). We explore methods used to estimate pretest probability accurately in Sect. 3.2.

After the pretest probability of disease has been estimated, the second stage of the diagnostic process involves gathering more information, often by performing a diagnostic test. The clinician in Example 4 ordered a test to reduce the uncertainty about the diagnosis of heart disease. The positive test result supports the diagnosis of heart disease, and this reduction in uncertainty is shown in Fig. 3.1a. Although the clinician in Example 4 chose the exercise stress test, there are many tests available to diagnose heart disease, and the clinician would like to know which test he or she should order next. Some tests reduce uncertainty more than do others (see Fig. 3.1b), but may cost more. The more a test reduces uncertainty, the more useful it is. In Sect. 3.3, we explore ways to measure how well a test reduces uncertainty, expanding the concepts of test sensitivity and specificity first introduced in Chap. 2.

Fig. 3.1 The effect of test results on the probability of disease. (**a**) A positive test result increases the probability of disease. (**b**) Test 2 reduces uncertainty about presence of disease (increases the probability of disease) more than test 1 does

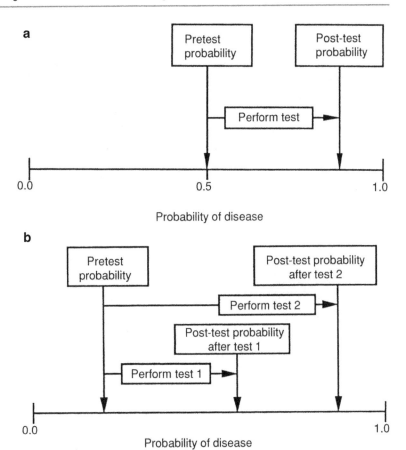

Given new information provided by a test, the third step is to update the initial probability estimate. The clinician in Example 4 must ask: "What is the probability of disease given the abnormal stress test?" The clinician wants to know the **posterior probability**, or **post-test probability**, of disease (see Fig. 3.1a). In Sect. 3.4, we reexamine Bayes' theorem, introduced in Chap. 2, and we discuss its use for calculating the post-test probability of disease. As we noted, to calculate post-test probability, we must know the pretest probability, as well as the sensitivity and specificity, of the test.[3]

3.2   Probability Assessment: Methods to Assess Pretest Probability

In this section, we explore the methods that clinicians can use to make judgments about the probability of disease before they order tests. **Probability** is our preferred means of expressing uncertainty. In this framework, probability (p) expresses a clinician's opinion about the likelihood of an event as a number between 0 and 1. An event that is certain to occur has a probability of 1; an event that is certain not to occur has a probability of 0.[4]

The probability of event A is written p[A]. The sum of the probabilities of all possible, collectively exhaustive outcomes of a chance event must be equal to 1. Thus, in a coin flip,

---

[3]Note that pretest and post-test probabilities correspond to the concepts of prevalence and predictive value. The latter terms were used in Chap. 2 because the discussion was about the use of tests for screening populations of patients; in a population, the pretest probability of disease is simply that disease's prevalence in that population.

[4]We assume a Bayesian interpretation of probability; there are other statistical interpretations of probability.

$$p[heads] + p[tails] = 1.0.$$

The probability of event A and event B occurring together is denoted by p[A&B] or by p[A,B].

Events A and B are considered **independent** if the occurrence of one does not influence the probability of the occurrence of the other. The probability of two independent events A and B both occurring is given by the product of the individual probabilities:

$$p[A,B] = p[A] \times p[B].$$

Thus, the probability of heads on two consecutive coin tosses is $0.5 \times 0.5 = 0.25$. (Regardless of the outcome of the first toss, the probability of heads on the second toss is 0.5.)

The probability that event A will occur given that event B is known to occur is called the **conditional probability** of event A given event B, denoted by p[A|B] and read as "the probability of A given B." Thus a post-test probability is a conditional probability predicated on the test or finding. For example, if 30 % of patients who have a swollen leg have a blood clot, we say the probability of a blood clot given a swollen leg is 0.3, denoted:

$$p[blood\,clot \mid swollen\,leg] = 0.3.$$

Before the swollen leg is noted, the pretest probability is simply the prevalence of blood clots in the leg in the population from which the patient was selected—a number likely to be much smaller than 0.3.

Now that we have decided to use probability to express uncertainty, how can we estimate probability? We can do so by either subjective or objective methods; each approach has advantages and limitations.

3.2.1 Subjective Probability Assessment

Most assessments that clinicians make about probability are based on personal experience. The clinician may compare the current problem to similar problems encountered previously and then ask: "What was the frequency of disease in similar patients whom I have seen?"

To make these subjective assessments of probability, people rely on several discrete, often unconscious mental processes that have been described and studied by cognitive psychologists (Tversky and Kahneman 1974). These processes are termed **cognitive heuristics**.

More specifically, a cognitive heuristic is a mental process by which we learn, recall, or process information; we can think of heuristics as rules of thumb. Knowledge of heuristics is important because it helps us to understand the underpinnings of our intuitive probability assessment. Both naive and sophisticated decision makers (including clinicians and statisticians) misuse heuristics and therefore make systematic—often serious—errors when estimating probability. So, just as we may underestimate distances on a particularly clear day (Tversky and Kahneman 1974), we may make mistakes in estimating probability in deceptive clinical situations. Three heuristics have been identified as important in estimation of probability:

1. Representativeness. One way that people estimate probability is to ask themselves: What is the probability that object A belongs to class B? For instance, what is the probability that this patient who has a swollen leg belongs to the class of patients who have blood clots? To answer, we often rely on the **representativeness** heuristic in which probabilities are judged by the degree to which A is representative of, or similar to, B. The clinician will judge the probability of the development of a blood clot (thrombosis) by the degree to which the patient with a swollen leg resembles the clinician's mental image of patients with a blood clot. If the patient has all the classic findings (signs and symptoms) associated with a blood clot, the clinician judges that the patient is highly likely to have a blood clot. Difficulties occur with the use of this heuristic when the disease is rare (very low prior probability, or prevalence); when the clinician's previous experience with the disease is atypical, thus giving an incorrect mental representation; when the patient's clinical profile is

atypical; and when the probability of certain findings depends on whether other findings are present.

2. Availability. Our estimate of the probability of an event is influenced by the ease with which we remember similar events. Events more easily remembered are judged more probable; this rule is the **availability** heuristic, and it is often misleading. We remember dramatic, atypical, or emotion-laden events more easily and therefore are likely to overestimate their probability. A clinician who had cared for a patient who had a swollen leg and who then died from a blood clot would vividly remember thrombosis as a cause of a swollen leg. The clinician would remember other causes of swollen legs less easily, and he or she would tend to overestimate the probability of a blood clot in patients with a swollen leg.

3. Anchoring and adjustment. Another common heuristic used to judge probability is **anchoring and adjustment**. A clinician makes an initial probability estimate (the anchor) and then adjusts the estimate based on further information. For instance, the clinician in Example 4 makes an initial estimate of the probability of heart disease as 0.5. If he or she then learns that all the patient's brothers had died of heart disease, the clinician should raise the estimate because the patient's strong family history of heart disease increases the probability that he or she has heart disease, a fact the clinician could ascertain from the literature. The usual mistake is to adjust the initial estimate (the anchor) insufficiently in light of the new information. Instead of raising his or her estimate of prior probability to, say, 0.8, the clinician might adjust it to only 0.6.

Heuristics often introduce error into our judgments about prior probability. Errors in our initial estimates of probabilities will be reflected in the posterior probabilities even if we use quantitative methods to derive those posterior probabilities. An understanding of heuristics is thus important for medical decision making. The clinician can avoid some of these difficulties by using published research results to estimate probabilities.

3.2.2 Objective Probability Estimates

Published research results can serve as a guide for more objective estimates of probabilities. We can use the prevalence of disease in the population or in a subgroup of the population, or clinical prediction rules, to estimate the probability of disease.

As we discussed in Chap. 2, the **prevalence** is the frequency of an event in a population; it is a useful starting point for estimating probability. For example, if you wanted to estimate the probability of prostate cancer in a 50-year-old man, the prevalence of prostate cancer in men of that age (5–14 %) would be a useful anchor point from which you could increase or decrease the probability depending on your findings. Estimates of disease prevalence in a defined population often are available in the medical literature.

Symptoms, such as difficulty with urination, or signs, such as a palpable prostate nodule, can be used to place patients into a **clinical subgroup** in which the probability of disease is known. For patients referred to a urologist for evaluation of a prostate nodule, the prevalence of cancer is about 50 %. This approach may be limited by difficulty in placing a patient in the correct clinically defined subgroup, especially if the criteria for classifying patients are ill-defined. A trend has been to develop guidelines, known as clinical prediction rules, to help clinicians assign patients to well-defined subgroups in which the probability of disease is known.

Clinical prediction rules are developed from systematic study of patients who have a particular diagnostic problem; they define how clinicians can use combinations of clinical findings to estimate probability. The symptoms or signs that make an independent contribution to the probability that a patient has a disease are identified and assigned numerical weights based on statistical analysis of the finding's contribution. The result is a list of symptoms and signs for an individual patient, each with a corresponding numerical contribution to a total score. The total score places a patient in a subgroup with a known probability of disease.

Table 3.1 Diagnostic weights for assessing risk of cardiac complications from noncardiac surgery

Clinical finding	Diagnostic weight
Age greater than 70 years	5
Recent documented heart attack	
>6 months previously	5
<6 months previously	10
Severe angina 20	
Pulmonary edema[a]	
Within 1 week	10
Ever	5
Arrhythmia on most recent ECG 5	
>5 PVCs	5
Critical aortic stenosis	20
Poor medical condition	5
Emergency surgery	10

Source: Modified from Palda et al. (1997)
ECG electrocardiogram, *PVCs* premature ventricular contractions on preoperative electrocardiogram
[a]Fluid in the lungs due to reduced heart function

What is the probability that Ms. Troy will suffer a cardiac complication? Clinical prediction rules have been developed to help clinicians to assess this risk (Palda and Detsky 1997). Table 3.1 lists clinical findings and their corresponding diagnostic weights. We add the diagnostic weights for each of the patient's clinical findings to obtain the total score. The total score places the patient in a group with a defined probability of cardiac complications, as shown in Table 3.2. Ms. Troy receives a score of 20; thus, the clinician can estimate that the patient has a 27 % chance of developing a severe cardiac complication.

Objective estimates of pretest probability are subject to error because of bias in the studies on which the estimates are based. For instance, published prevalence data may not apply directly to a

Table 3.2 Clinical prediction rule for diagnostic weights in Table 3.1

Total score	Prevalence (%) of cardiac complications[a]
0–15	5
20–30	27
>30	60

Source: Modified from Palda et al. (1997)
[a]Cardiac complications defined as death, heart attack, or congestive heart failure

particular patient. A clinical illustration is that early studies indicated that a patient found to have microscopic evidence of blood in the urine (microhematuria) should undergo extensive tests because a significant proportion of the patients would be found to have cancer or other serious diseases. The tests involve some risk, discomfort, and expense to the patient. Nonetheless, the approach of ordering tests for any patient with microhematuria was widely practiced for some years. A later study, however, suggested that the probability of serious disease in asymptomatic patients with only microscopic evidence of blood was only about 2 % (Mohr et al. 1986). In the past, many patients may have undergone unnecessary tests, at considerable financial and personal cost.

What explains the discrepancy in the estimates of disease prevalence? The initial studies that showed a high prevalence of disease in patients with microhematuria were performed on patients referred to urologists, who are specialists. The primary care clinician refers patients whom he or she suspects have a disease in the specialist's sphere of expertise. Because of this initial screening by primary care clinicians, the specialists seldom see patients with clinical findings that imply a low probability of disease. Thus, the prevalence of disease in the patient population in a specialist's practice often is much higher than that in a primary care practice; studies performed with the former patients therefore almost always overestimate disease probabilities. This example demonstrates **referral bias**. Referral bias is common because many published studies are performed on patients referred to specialists.

Thus, one may need to adjust published estimates before one uses them to estimate pretest probability in other clinical settings.

We now can use the techniques discussed in this part of the chapter to illustrate how the clinician in Example 4 might estimate the pretest probability of heart disease in his or her patient, Mr. Smith, who has pressure-like chest pain. We begin by using the objective data that are available. The prevalence of heart disease in 60-year-old men could be our starting point. In this case, however, we can obtain a more refined estimate by placing the patient in a clinical subgroup in which the prevalence of disease is known. The prevalence in a clinical subgroup, such as men with symptoms typical of coronary heart disease, will predict the pretest probability more accurately than would the prevalence of heart disease in a group that is heterogeneous with respect to symptoms, such as the population at large. We assume that large studies have shown the prevalence of coronary heart disease in men with typical symptoms of angina pectoris to be about 0.9; this prevalence is useful as an initial estimate that can be adjusted based on information specific to the patient. Although the prevalence of heart disease in men with typical symptoms is high, 10 % of patients with this history do not have heart disease.

The clinician might use subjective methods to adjust his or her estimate further based on other specific information about the patient. For example, the clinician might adjust his or her initial estimate of 0.9 upward to 0.95 or higher based on information about family history of heart disease. The clinician should be careful, however, to avoid the mistakes that can occur when one uses heuristics to make subjective probability estimates. In particular, he or she should be aware of the tendency to stay too close to the initial estimate when adjusting for additional information. By combining subjective and objective methods for assessing pretest probability, the clinician can arrive at a reasonable estimate of the pretest probability of heart disease.

In this section, we summarized subjective and objective methods to determine the pretest probability, and we learned how to adjust the pretest probability after assessing the specific subpopulation of which the patient is representative. The next step in the diagnostic process is to gather further information, usually in the form of formal diagnostic tests (laboratory tests, X-ray studies, etc.). To help you to understand this step more clearly, we discuss in the next two sections how to measure the accuracy of tests and how to use probability to interpret the results of the tests.

3.3   Measurement of the Operating Characteristics of Diagnostic Tests

The first challenge in assessing any test is to determine criteria for deciding whether a result is normal or abnormal. In this section, we present the issues that you need to consider when making such a determination.

3.3.1   Classification of Test Results as Abnormal

Most biological measurements in a population of healthy people are continuous variables that assume different values for different individuals. The distribution of values often is approximated by the normal (gaussian, or bell-shaped) distribution curve (Fig. 3.2). Thus, 95 % of the population will fall within two standard deviations of the mean. About 2.5 % of the population will be more than two standard deviations from the mean at each end of the distribution. The distribution of values for ill individuals may be normally distributed as well. The two distributions usually overlap (see Fig. 3.2).

How is a test result classified as abnormal? Most clinical laboratories report an "upper limit of normal," which usually is defined as two standard deviations above the mean. Thus, a test result greater than two standard deviations above the mean is reported as abnormal (or positive); a test result below that cutoff is reported as normal (or negative). As an example, if the mean cholesterol concentration in the blood is 220 mg/dl, a clinical laboratory might choose as the upper

Fig. 3.2 Distribution of test results in healthy and diseased individuals. Varying the cutoff between "normal" and "abnormal" across the continuous range of possible values changes the relative proportions of false positives (FPs) and false negatives (FNs) for the two populations

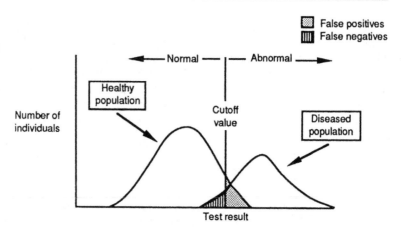

limit of normal 280 mg/dl because it is two standard deviations above the mean. Note that a cutoff that is based on an arbitrary statistical criterion may not have biological significance.

An ideal test would have no values at which the distribution of diseased and nondiseased people overlap. That is, if the cutoff value were set appropriately, the test would be normal in all healthy individuals and abnormal in all individuals with disease. Few tests meet this standard. If a test result is defined as abnormal by the statistical criterion, 2.5 % of healthy individuals will have an abnormal test. If there is an overlap in the distribution of test results in healthy and diseased individuals, some diseased patients will have a normal test (see Fig. 3.2). You should be familiar with the terms used to denote these groups:

- A **true positive** (TP) is a positive test result obtained for a patient in whom the disease is present (the test result correctly classifies the patient as having the disease).
- A **true negative** (TN) is a negative test result obtained for a patient in whom the disease is absent (the test result correctly classifies the patient as not having the disease).
- A **false positive** (FP) is a positive test result obtained for a patient in whom the disease is absent (the test result incorrectly classifies the patient as having the disease).
- A **false negative** (FN) is a negative test result obtained for a patient in whom the disease is present (the test result incorrectly classifies the patient as not having the disease).

Table 3.3 A 2×2 contingency table for test results

Results of test	Disease present	Disease absent	Total
Positive result	TP	FP	TP+FP
Negative result	FN	TN	FN+TN
	TP+FN	FP+TN	

TP true positive, *TN* true negative, *FP* false positive, *FN* false negative

Figure 3.2 shows that varying the cutoff point (moving the vertical line in the figure) for an abnormal test will change the relative proportions of these groups. As the cutoff is moved further up from the mean of the normal values, the number of FNs increases and the number of FPs decreases. Once we have chosen a cutoff point, we can conveniently summarize test performance—the ability to discriminate disease from nondisease—in a 2×2 **contingency table**, as shown in Table 3.3. The table summarizes the number of patients in each group: TP, FP, TN, and FN. Note that the sum of the first column is the total number of diseased patients, TP+FN. The sum of the second column is the total number of nondiseased patients, FP+TN. The sum of the first row, TP+FP, is the total number of patients with a positive test result. Likewise, FN+TN gives the total number of patients with a negative test result.

A perfect test would have no FN or FP results. Erroneous test results do occur, however, and you can use a 2×2 contingency table to define the measures of test performance that reflect these errors.

3.3.2 Measures of Test Performance

Measures of test performance are of two types: measures of agreement between tests or **measures of concordance**, and measures of disagreement or **measures of discordance**. Two types of **concordant test results** occur in the 2×2 table in Table 3.3: TPs and TNs. The relative frequencies of these results form the basis of the measures of concordance. These measures correspond to the ideas of the sensitivity and specificity of a test, which we introduced in Chap. 2. We define each measure in terms of the 2×2 table and in terms of conditional probabilities.

The **true-positive rate** (TPR), or **sensitivity**, is the likelihood that a diseased patient has a positive test. In conditional-probability notation, sensitivity is expressed as the probability of a positive test given that disease is present:

$$p[\text{positive test} \mid \text{disease}].$$

Another way to think of the TPR is as a ratio. The likelihood that a diseased patient has a positive test is given by the ratio of diseased patients with a positive test to all diseased patients:

$$TPR = \left(\frac{\text{number of diseased patients with positive test}}{\text{total number of diseased patients}} \right).$$

We can determine these numbers for our example from the 2×2 table (see Table 3.3). The number of diseased patients with a positive test is TP. The total number of diseased patients is the sum of the first column, TP+FN. So,

$$TPR = \frac{TP}{TP + FN}.$$

The **true-negative** rate (TNR), or **specificity**, is the likelihood that a nondiseased patient has a negative test result. In terms of conditional probability, specificity is the probability of a negative test given that disease is absent:

$$p[\text{negative test} \mid \text{no disease}].$$

Viewed as a ratio, the TNR is the number of nondiseased patients with a negative test divided by the total number of nondiseased patients:

$$TNR = \left(\frac{\begin{array}{c}\text{Number of nondiseased patients}\\\text{with negative test}\end{array}}{\text{Total number of nondiseased patients}} \right).$$

From the 2×2 table (see Table 3.3),

$$TNR = \frac{TN}{TN + FP}$$

The measures of discordance—the **false-positive rate** (FPR) and the **false-negative rate** (FNR)—are defined similarly. The FNR is the likelihood that a diseased patient has a negative test result. As a ratio,

$$FNR = \left(\frac{\begin{array}{c}\text{Number of diseased patients}\\\text{with negative test}\end{array}}{\text{Total number of diseased patients}} \right)$$
$$= \frac{FN}{FN + TP}.$$

The FPR is the likelihood that a nondiseased patient has a positive test result:

$$FPR = \left(\frac{\begin{array}{c}\text{Number of nondiseased patients}\\\text{with positive test}\end{array}}{\text{Total number of nondiseased patients}} \right)$$
$$= \frac{FP}{FP + TN}.$$

Example 6

Consider again the problem of screening blood donors for HIV. One test used to screen blood donors for HIV antibody is an enzyme-linked immunoassay (EIA). So that the performance of the EIA can be measured, the test is performed on 400 patients; the hypothetical results are shown in the 2×2 table in Table 3.4.[5]

---

[5]This example assumes that we have a perfect method (different from EIA) for determining the presence or absence of antibody. We discuss the idea of gold-standard tests in Sect. 3.3.4. We have chosen the numbers in the example to simplify the calculations. In practice, the sensitivity and specificity of the HIV EIAs are greater than 99 %.

Table 3.4 A 2×2 contingency table for HIV anti-body EIA

EIA test result	Antibody present	Antibody absent	Total
Positive EIA	98	3	101
Negative EIA	2	297	299
	100	300	

EIA enzyme-linked immunoassay

To determine test performance, we calculate the TPR (sensitivity) and TNR (specificity) of the EIA antibody test. The TPR, as defined previously, is:

$$\frac{TP}{TP+FN} = \frac{98}{98+2} = 0.98.$$

Thus, the likelihood that a patient with the HIV antibody will have a positive EIA test is 0.98. If the test were performed on 100 patients who truly had the antibody, we would expect the test to be positive in 98 of the patients. Conversely, we would expect two of the patients to receive incorrect, negative results, for an FNR of 2 %. (You should convince yourself that the sum of TPR and FNR by definition must be 1: TPR+FNR=1.)

And the TNR is:

$$\frac{TN}{TN+FP} = \frac{297}{297+3} = 0.99$$

The likelihood that a patient who has no HIV antibody will have a negative test is 0.99. Therefore, if the EIA test were performed on 100 individuals who had not been infected with HIV, it would be negative in 99 and incorrectly positive in 1. (Convince yourself that the sum of TNR and FPR also must be 1: TNR+FPR=1.)

3.3.3 Implications of Sensitivity and Specificity: How to Choose Among Tests

It may be clear to you already that the calculated values of sensitivity and specificity for a continuous-valued test depend on the particular cutoff value chosen to distinguish normal and abnormal results. In Fig. 3.2, note that increasing the cutoff level (moving it to the right) would decrease significantly the number of FP tests but also would increase the number of FN tests. Thus, the test would have become more specific but less sensitive. Similarly, a lower cutoff value would increase the FPs and decrease the FNs, thereby increasing sensitivity while decreasing specificity. Whenever a decision is made about what cutoff to use in calling a test abnormal, an inherent philosophic decision is being made about whether it is better to tolerate FNs (missed cases) or FPs (nondiseased people inappropriately classified as diseased). The choice of cutoff depends on the disease in question and on the purpose of testing. If the disease is serious and if lifesaving therapy is available, we should try to minimize the number of FN results. On the other hand, if the disease in not serious and the therapy is dangerous, we should set the cutoff value to minimize FP results.

We stress the point that sensitivity and specificity are characteristics not of a test per se but rather of the test and a criterion for when to call that test abnormal. Varying the cutoff in Fig. 3.2 has no effect on the test itself (the way it is performed, or the specific values for any particular patient); instead, it trades off specificity for sensitivity. Thus, the best way to characterize a test is by the range of values of sensitivity and specificity that it can take on over a range of possible cutoffs. The typical way to show this relationship is to plot the test's sensitivity against 1 minus specificity (i.e., the TPR against the FPR), as the cutoff is varied and the two test characteristics are traded off against each other (Fig. 3.3). The resulting curve, known as a **receiver-operating characteristic (ROC) curve**, was originally described by researchers investigating methods of electromagnetic-signal detection and was later applied to the field of psychology (Peterson and Birdsall 1953; Swets 1973). Any given point along an ROC curve for a test corresponds to the test sensitivity and specificity for a given threshold of "abnormality." Similar curves can be drawn for any test used to associate observed clinical data with specific diseases or disease categories.

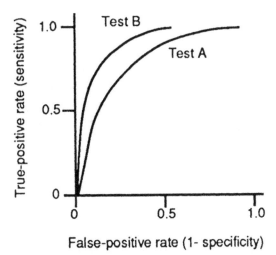

Fig. 3.3 Receiver operating characteristic (ROC) curves for two hypothetical tests. Test B is more discriminative than test A because its curve is higher (e.g., the false-positive rate (FPR) for test B is lower than the FPR for test A at any value of true-positive rate (TPR)). The more discriminative test may not always be preferred in clinical practice, however (see text)

Suppose a new test were introduced that competed with the current way of screening for the presence of a disease. For example, suppose a new radiologic procedure for assessing the presence or absence of pneumonia became available. This new test could be assessed for trade-offs in sensitivity and specificity, and an ROC curve could be drawn. As shown in Fig. 3.3, a test has better discriminating power than a competing test if its ROC curve lies above that of the other test. In other words, test B is more discriminating than test A when its specificity is greater than test A's specificity for any level of sensitivity (and when its sensitivity is greater than test A's sensitivity for any level of specificity).

Understanding ROC curves is important in understanding test selection and data interpretation. Clinicians should not necessarily, however, always choose the test with the most discriminating ROC curve. Matters of cost, risk, discomfort, and delay also are important in the choice about what data to collect and what tests to perform. When you must choose among several available tests, you should select the test that has the highest sensitivity and specificity, provided that other factors, such as cost and risk to the patient, are

equal. The higher the sensitivity and specificity of a test, the more the results of that test will reduce uncertainty about probability of disease.

3.3.4 Design of Studies of Test Performance

In Sect. 3.3.2, we discussed measures of test performance: a test's ability to discriminate disease from no disease. When we classify a test result as TP, TN, FP, or FN, we assume that we know with certainty whether a patient is diseased or healthy. Thus, the validity of any test's results must be measured against a gold standard: a test that reveals the patient's true disease state, such as a biopsy of diseased tissue or a surgical operation. A **gold-standard test** is a procedure that is used to define unequivocally the presence or absence of disease. The test whose discrimination is being measured is called the **index test**. The gold-standard test usually is more expensive, riskier, or more difficult to perform than is the index test (otherwise, the less precise test would not be used at all).

The performance of the index test is measured in a small, select group of patients enrolled in a study. We are interested, however, in how the test performs in the broader group of patients in which it will be used in practice. The test may perform differently in the two groups, so we make the following distinction: the **study population** comprises those patients (usually a subset of the clinically relevant population) in whom test discrimination is measured and reported; the **clinically relevant population** comprises those patients in whom a test typically is used.

3.3.5 Bias in the Measurement of Test Characteristics

We mentioned earlier the problem of referral bias. Published estimates of disease prevalence (derived from a study population) may differ from the prevalence in the clinically relevant population because diseased patients are more likely to be included in studies than are nondiseased patients. Similarly, published values of sensitivity and specificity are derived from study populations that may differ from the clinically relevant populations in terms of average level of health and disease prevalence. These differences may affect test performance, so the reported values may not apply to many patients in whom a test is used in clinical practice.

Example 7

In the early 1970s, a blood test called the carcinoembryonic antigen (CEA) was touted as a screening test for colon cancer. Reports of early investigations, performed in selected patients, indicated that the test had high sensitivity and specificity. Subsequent work, however, proved the CEA to be completely valueless as a screening blood test for colon cancer. Screening tests are used in unselected populations, and the differences between the study and clinically relevant populations were partly responsible for the original miscalculations of the CEA's TPR and TNR (Ransohoff and Feinstein 1978).

The experience with CEA has been repeated with numerous tests. Early measures of test discrimination are overly optimistic, and subsequent test performance is disappointing. Problems arise when the TPR and TNR, as measured in the study population, do not apply to the clinically relevant population. These problems usually are the result of bias in the design of the initial studies— notably spectrum bias, test referral bias, or test interpretation bias.

Spectrum bias occurs when the study population includes only individuals who have advanced disease ("sickest of the sick") and healthy volunteers, as is often the case when a test is first being developed. Advanced disease may be easier to detect than early disease. For example, cancer is easier to detect when it has spread throughout the body (metastasized) than when it is localized to, say, a small portion of the colon. In contrast to the study population, the clinically relevant population will contain more cases of early disease that

are more likely to be missed by the index test (FNs). Thus, the study population will have an artifactually low FNR, which produces an artifactually high TPR (TPR = 1−FNR). In addition, healthy volunteers are less likely than are patients in the clinically relevant population to have other diseases that may cause FP results[6]; the study population will have an artificially low FPR, and therefore the specificity will be overestimated (TNR = 1−FPR). Inaccuracies in early estimates of the TPR and TNR of the CEA were partly due to spectrum bias.

Test-referral bias occurs when a positive index test is a criterion for ordering the gold standard test. In clinical practice, patients with negative index tests are less likely to undergo the gold standard test than are patients with positive tests. In other words, the study population, comprising individuals with positive index–test results, has a higher percentage of patients with disease than does the clinically relevant population. Therefore, both TN and FN tests will be underrepresented in the study population. The result is overestimation of the TPR and underestimation of the TNR in the study population.

Test-interpretation bias develops when the interpretation of the index test affects that of the gold standard test or vice versa. This bias causes an artificial concordance between the tests (the results are more likely to be the same) and spuriously increases measures of concordance—the sensitivity and specificity—in the study population. (Remember, the relative frequencies of TPs and TNs are the basis for measures of concordance). To avoid these problems, the person interpreting the index test should be unaware of the results of the gold standard test.

---

[6]Volunteers are often healthy, whereas patients in the clinically relevant population often have several diseases in addition to the disease for which a test is designed. These other diseases may cause FP test results. For example, patients with benign (rather than malignant) enlargement of their prostate glands are more likely than are healthy volunteers to have FP elevations of prostate-specific antigen (Meigs et al. 1996), a substance in the blood that is elevated in men who have prostate cancer. Measurement of prostate-specific antigen is often used to detect prostate cancer.

To counter these three biases, you may need to adjust the TPR and TNR when they are applied to a new population. All the biases result in a TPR that is higher in the study population than it is in the clinically relevant population. Thus, if you suspect bias, you should adjust the TPR (sensitivity) downward when you apply it to a new population.

Adjustment of the TNR (specificity) depends on which type of bias is present. Spectrum bias and test interpretation bias result in a TNR that is higher in the study population than it will be in the clinically relevant population. Thus, if these biases are present, you should adjust the specificity downward when you apply it to a new population. Test-referral bias, on the other hand, produces a measured specificity in the study population that is lower than it will be in the clinically relevant population. If you suspect test referral bias, you should adjust the specificity upward when you apply it to a new population.

3.3.6 Meta-Analysis of Diagnostic Tests

Often, there are many studies that evaluate the sensitivity and specificity of the same diagnostic test. If the studies come to similar conclusions about the sensitivity and specificity of the test, you can have increased confidence in the results of the studies. But what if the studies disagree? For example, by 1995, over 100 studies had assessed the sensitivity and specificity of the PCR for diagnosis of HIV (Owens et al. 1996a, b); these studies estimated the sensitivity of PCR to be as low as 10 % and to be as high as 100 %, and they assessed the specificity of PCR to be between 40 and 100 %. Which results should you believe? One approach that you can use is to assess the quality of the studies and to use the estimates from the highest-quality studies.

For evaluation of PCR, however, even the high-quality studies did not agree. Another approach is to perform a **meta-analysis**: a study that combines quantitatively the estimates from individual studies to develop a **summary ROC curve** (Moses et al. 1993; Owens et al. 1996a, b;

Hellmich et al. 1999; Leeflang et al. 2008). Investigators develop a summary ROC curve by using estimates from many studies, in contrast to the type of ROC curve discussed in Sect. 3.3.3, which is developed from the data in a single study. Summary ROC curves provide the best available approach to synthesizing data from many studies.

Section 3.3 has dealt with the second step in the diagnostic process: acquisition of further information with diagnostic tests. We have learned how to characterize the performance of a test with sensitivity (TPR) and specificity (TNR). These measures reveal the probability of a test result given the true state of the patient. They do not, however, answer the clinically relevant question posed in the opening example: Given a positive test result, what is the probability that this patient has the disease? To answer this question, we must learn methods to calculate the post-test probability of disease.

3.4 Post-test Probability: Bayes' Theorem and Predictive Value

The third stage of the diagnostic process (see Fig. 3.1a) is to adjust our probability estimate to take into account the new information gained from diagnostic tests by calculating the post-test probability.

3.4.1 Bayes' Theorem

As we noted earlier in this chapter, a clinician can use the disease prevalence in the patient population as an initial estimate of the pretest risk of disease. Once clinicians begin to accumulate information about a patient, however, they revise their estimate of the probability of disease. The revised estimate (rather than the disease prevalence in the general population) becomes the pretest probability for the test that they perform. After they have gathered more information with a diagnostic test, they can calculate the post-test probability of disease with Bayes' theorem.

Bayes' theorem is a quantitative method for calculating post-test probability using the pretest probability and the sensitivity and specificity of the test. The theorem is derived from the definition of conditional probability and from the properties of probability (see the Appendix to this chapter for the derivation).

Recall that a conditional probability is the probability that event A will occur given that event B is known to occur (see Sect. 3.2). In general, we want to know the probability that disease is present (event A), given that the test is known to be positive (event B). We denote the presence of disease as D, its absence as −D, a test result as R, and the pretest probability of disease as p[D]. The probability of disease, given a test result, is written p[D|R]. Bayes' theorem is:

$$p[D \mid R] = \frac{p[D] \times p[R \mid D]}{p[D] \times p[R \mid D] + p[-D] \times p[R \mid -D]}$$

We can reformulate this general equation in terms of a positive test, (+), by substituting p[D|+] for p[D|R], p[+|D] for p[R|D], p[+|−D] for p[R|−D], and 1−p[D] for p[−D]. From Sect. 3.3, recall that p[+|D]=TPR and p[+|−D]=FPR. Substitution provides Bayes' theorem for a positive test:

$$p[D \mid +] = \frac{p[D] \times TPR}{p[D] \times TPR + (1 - p[D]) \times FPR}$$

We can use a similar derivation to develop Bayes' theorem for a negative test:

$$p[D \mid -] = \frac{p[D] \times FNR}{p[D] \times FNR + (1 - p[D]) \times TNR}$$

Example 8
We are now able to calculate the clinically important probability in Example 4: the post-test probability of heart disease after a positive exercise test. At the end of Sect. 3.2.2, we estimated the pretest probability of heart disease as 0.95, based on

the prevalence of heart disease in men who have typical symptoms of heart disease and on the prevalence in people with a family history of heart disease. Assume that the TPR and FPR of the exercise stress test are 0.65 and 0.20, respectively. Substituting in Bayes' formula for a positive test, we obtain the probability of heart disease given a positive test result:

$$p[D \mid +] = \frac{0.95 \times 0.65}{0.95 \times 0.65 + 0.05 \times 0.20} = 0.98$$

Thus, the positive test raised the post-test probability to 0.98 from the pretest probability of 0.95. The change in probability is modest because the pretest probability was high (0.95) and because the FPR also is high (0.20). If we repeat the calculation with a pretest probability of 0.75, the post-test probability is 0.91. If we assume the FPR of the test to be 0.05 instead of 0.20, a pretest probability of 0.95 changes to 0.996.

3.4.2 The Odds-Ratio Form of Bayes' Theorem and Likelihood Ratios

Although the formula for Bayes' theorem is straightforward, it is awkward for mental calculations. We can develop a more convenient form of Bayes' theorem by expressing probability as odds and by using a different measure of test discrimination. Probability and odds are related as follows:

$$odds = \frac{p}{1-p},$$

$$p = \frac{odds}{1 + odds}.$$

Thus, if the probability of rain today is 0.75, the odds are 3:1. Thus, on similar days, we should expect rain to occur three times for each time it does not occur.

A simple relationship exists between pretest odds and post-test odds:

$$\text{post-test odds} = \text{pretest odds} \times \text{likelihood ratio}$$

or

$$\frac{p[D \mid R]}{p[-D \mid R]} = \frac{p[D]}{p[-D]} \times \frac{p[R \mid D]}{p[R \mid -D]}.$$

This equation is the **odds-ratio form** of Bayes' theorem.[7] It can be derived in a straightforward fashion from the definitions of Bayes' theorem and of conditional probability that we provided earlier. Thus, to obtain the post-test odds, we simply multiply the pretest odds by the **likelihood ratio** (LR) for the test in question.

The LR of a test combines the measures of test discrimination discussed earlier to give one number that characterizes the discriminatory power of a test, defined as:

$$\text{LR} = \frac{p[R \mid D]}{p[R \mid -D]}$$

or

$$\text{LR} = \frac{\text{probability of result in diseased people}}{\text{probability of result in nondiseased people}}$$

The LR indicates the amount that the odds of disease change based on the test result. We can use the LR to characterize clinical findings (such as a swollen leg) or a test result. We describe the performance of a test that has only two possible outcomes (e.g., positive or negative) by two LRs: one corresponding to a positive test result and the other corresponding to a negative test. These ratios are abbreviated LR+ and LR−, respectively.

$$\text{LR+} = \left(\frac{\text{probability that test is positive in diseased people}}{\text{probability that test is positive in nondiseased people}} \right) = \frac{\text{TPR}}{\text{FPR}}$$

In a test that discriminates well between disease and nondisease, the TPR will be high, the FPR will be low, and thus LR+ will be much greater than 1. An LR of 1 means that the probability of a test result is the same in diseased and nondiseased individuals; the test has no value. Similarly,

$$\text{LR−} = \left(\frac{\text{probability that test is negative in diseased people}}{\text{probability that test is negative in nondiseased people}} \right) = \frac{\text{FNR}}{\text{TNR}}$$

A desirable test will have a low FNR and a high TNR; therefore, the LR− will be much less than 1.

Example 9

We can calculate the post-test probability for a positive exercise stress test in a 60 year-old man whose pretest probability is 0.75. The pretest odds are:

$$\text{odds} = \frac{p}{1-p} = \frac{0.75}{1-0.75} = \frac{0.75}{0.25} = 3, \text{ or } 3:1$$

The LR for the stress test is:

$$\text{LR+} = \frac{\text{TPR}}{\text{FPR}} = \frac{0.65}{0.20} = 3.25$$

We can calculate the post-test odds of a positive test result using the odds-ratio form of Bayes' theorem:

$$\text{post-test odds} = 3 \times 3.25 = 9.75:1$$

We can then convert the odds to a probability:

$$p = \frac{\text{odds}}{1+\text{odds}} = \frac{9.75}{1+9.75} = 0.91$$

As expected, this result agrees with our earlier answer (see the discussion of Example 8).

The odds-ratio form of Bayes' theorem allows rapid calculation, so you can determine the probability at, for example, your patient's bedside.

---

[7]Some authors refer to this expression as the odds-likelihood form of Bayes' theorem.

The LR is a powerful method for characterizing the operating characteristics of a test: if you know the pretest odds, you can calculate the posttest odds in one step. The LR demonstrates that a useful test is one that changes the odds of disease.

3.4.3 Predictive Value of a Test

An alternative approach for estimation of the probability of disease in a person who has a positive or negative test is to calculate the predictive value of the test. The **positive predictive value** (PV+) of a test is the likelihood that a patient who has a positive test result also has disease. Thus, PV + can be calculated directly from a 2×2 contingency table:

$$PV+ = \frac{\text{number of diseased patients with positive test}}{\text{total number of patients with a positive test}}$$

From the 2×2 contingency table in Table 3.3,

$$PV+ = \frac{TP}{TP + FP}$$

The **negative predictive value** (PV−) is the likelihood that a patient with a negative test does not have disease:

$$PV- = \frac{\text{number of nondiseased patients with negative test}}{\text{Total number of patients with a negative test}}$$

From the 2×2 contingency table in Table 3.3,

$$PV- = \frac{TN}{TN + FN}$$

Example 10

We can calculate the PV of the EIA test from the 2×2 table that we constructed in Example 6 (see Table 3.4) as follows:

$$PV+ = \frac{98}{98 + 3} = 0.97$$

$$PV- = \frac{297}{297 + 2} = 0.99$$

The probability that antibody is present in a patient who has a positive index test (EIA) in this study is 0.97; about 97 of 100 patients with a positive test will have antibody. The likelihood that a patient with a negative index test does not have antibody is about 0.99.

It is worth reemphasizing the difference between PV and sensitivity and specificity, given that both are calculated from the 2×2 table and they often are confused. The sensitivity and specificity give the probability of a particular test result in a patient who has a particular disease state. The PV gives the probability of true disease state once the patient's test result is known.

The PV + calculated from Table 3.4 is 0.97, so we expect 97 of 100 patients with a positive index test actually to have antibody. Yet, in Example 1, we found that fewer than one of ten patients with a positive test were expected to have antibody. What explains the discrepancy in these examples? The sensitivity and specificity (and, therefore, the LRs) in the two examples are identical. The discrepancy is due to an extremely important and often overlooked characteristic of PV: the PV of a test depends on the prevalence of disease in the study population (the prevalence can be calculated as TP + FN divided by the total number of patients in the 2×2 table). The PV cannot be generalized to a new population because the prevalence of disease may differ between the two populations.

The difference in PV of the EIA in Example 1 and in Example 6 is due to a difference in the prevalence of disease in the examples. The prevalence of antibody was given as 0.001 in Example 1 and as 0.25 in Example 6. These examples should remind us that the PV + is not an intrinsic property of a test. Rather, it represents the posttest probability of disease only when the prevalence is identical to that in the 2×2 contingency table from which the PV + was calculated. Bayes' theorem provides a method for calculation of the post-test probability of disease for any prior probability. For that reason, we prefer the use of Bayes' theorem to calculate the post-test probability of disease.

3.4.4 Implications of Bayes' Theorem

In this section, we explore the implications of Bayes' theorem for test interpretation. These ideas are extremely important, yet they often are misunderstood.

Figure 3.4 illustrates one of the most essential concepts in this chapter: The post-test probability of disease increases as the pretest probability of disease increases. We produced Fig. 3.4a by calculating the post-test probability after a positive test result for all possible pretest probabilities of disease. We similarly derived Fig. 3.4b for a negative test result.

The 45-degree line in each figure denotes a test in which the pretest and post-test probability are equal (LR = 1), indicating a test that is useless. The curve in Fig. 3.4a relates pretest and post-test probabilities in a test with a sensitivity and specificity of 0.9. Note that, at low pretest probabilities, the post-test probability after a positive test result is much higher than is the pretest probability. At high pretest probabilities, the post-test probability is only slightly higher than the pretest probability.

Figure 3.4b shows the relationship between the pretest and post-test probabilities after a negative test result. At high pretest probabilities, the post-test probability after a negative test result is much lower than is the pretest probability. A negative test, however, has little effect on the post-test probability if the pretest probability is low.

This discussion emphasizes a key idea of this chapter: the interpretation of a test result depends on the pretest probability of disease. If the pretest probability is low, a positive test result has a large effect, and a negative test result has a small effect. If the pretest probability is high, a positive test result has a small effect, and a negative test result has a large effect. In other words, when the clinician is almost certain of the diagnosis before testing (pretest probability nearly 0 or nearly 1), a confirmatory test has little effect on the posterior probability (see Example 8). If the pretest probability is

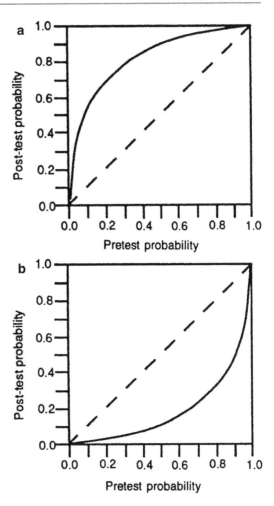

Fig. 3.4 Relationship between pretest probability and post-test probability of disease. The *dashed lines* correspond to a test that has no effect on the probability of disease. Sensitivity and specificity of the test were assumed to be 0.90 for the two examples. (**a**) The post-test probability of disease corresponding to a positive test result (*solid curve*) was calculated with Bayes' theorem for all values of pretest probability. (**b**) The post-test probability of disease corresponding to a negative test result (*solid curve*) was calculated with Bayes' theorem for all values of pretest probability (Source: Adapted from Sox, H.C. (1987). Probability theory in the use of diagnostic tests: Application to critical study of the literature. In: Sox H.C. (Ed.), *Common diagnostic tests: Use and interpretation* (pp. 1–17). American College of Physicians, with permission)

intermediate or if the result contradicts a strongly held clinical impression, the test result will have a large effect on the post-test probability.

Note from Fig. 3.4a that, if the pretest probability is very low, a positive test result can raise the post-test probability into only the intermediate range. Assume that Fig. 3.4a represents the relationship between the pretest and post-test probabilities for the exercise stress test. If the clinician believes the pretest probability of coronary artery disease is 0.1, the post-test probability will be about 0.5. Although there has been a large change in the probability, the post-test probability is in an intermediate range, which leaves considerable uncertainty about the diagnosis. Thus, if the pretest probability is low, it is unlikely that a positive test result will raise the probability of disease sufficiently for the clinician to make that diagnosis with confidence. An exception to this statement occurs when a test has a very high specificity (or a large LR+); e.g., HIV antibody tests have a specificity greater than 0.99, and therefore a positive test is convincing. Similarly, if the pretest probability is very high, it is unlikely that a negative test result will lower the post-test probability sufficiently to exclude a diagnosis.

Figure 3.5 illustrates another important concept: test specificity affects primarily the interpretation of a positive test; test sensitivity affects primarily the interpretation of a negative test. In both parts (a) and (b) of Fig. 3.5, the top family of curves corresponds to positive test results and the bottom family to negative test results. Figure 3.5a shows the post-test probabilities for tests with varying specificities (TNR). Note that changes in the specificity produce large changes in the top family of curves (positive test results) but have little effect on the lower family of curves (negative test results). That is, an increase in the specificity of a test markedly changes the post-test probability if the test is positive but has relatively little effect on the post-test probability if the test is negative. Thus, if you are trying to rule in a diagnosis,[8] you should choose a test with high

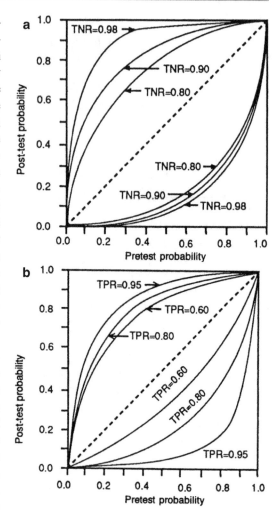

Fig. 3.5 Effects of test sensitivity and specificity on post-test probability. The *curves* are similar to those shown in Fig. 3.4 except that the calculations have been repeated for several values of the sensitivity (*TPR* true-positive rate) and specificity (*TNR* true-negative rate) of the test. (**a**) The sensitivity of the test was assumed to be 0.90, and the calculations were repeated for several values of test specificity. (**b**) The specificity of the test was assumed to be 0.90, and the calculations were repeated for several values of the sensitivity of the test. In both panels, the top family of curves corresponds to positive test results, and the bottom family of curves corresponds to negative test results (Source: Adapted from Sox (1987). Probability theory in the use of diagnostic tests: Application to critical study of the literature. In: Sox (Ed.), *Common diagnostic tests: Use and interpretation* (pp. 1–17), American College of Physicians, with permission)

---

[8]In medicine, to *rule in* a disease is to confirm that the patient *does* have the disease; to *rule out* a disease is to confirm that the patient *does not* have the disease. A doctor who strongly suspects that his or her patient has a bacterial infection orders a culture to *rule in* his or her diagnosis. Another doctor is almost certain that his or her patient has a simple sore throat but orders a culture to rule out streptococcal infection (strep throat). This terminology oversimplifies a diagnostic process that is probabilistic. Diagnostic tests rarely, if ever, rule in or rule out a disease; rather, the tests raise or lower the probability of disease.

specificity or a high LR+. Figure 3.5b shows the post-test probabilities for tests with varying sensitivities. Note that changes in sensitivity produce large changes in the bottom family of curves (negative test results) but have little effect on the top family of curves. Thus, if you are trying to exclude a disease, choose a test with a high sensitivity or a high LR−.

3.4.5 Cautions in the Application of Bayes' Theorem

Bayes' theorem provides a powerful method for calculating post-test probability. You should be aware, however, of the possible errors you can make when you use it. Common problems are inaccurate estimation of pretest probability, faulty application of test-performance measures, and violation of the assumptions of conditional independence and of mutual exclusivity.

Bayes' theorem provides a means to adjust an estimate of pretest probability to take into account new information. The accuracy of the calculated post-test probability is limited, however, by the accuracy of the estimated pretest probability. Accuracy of estimated prior probability is increased by proper use of published prevalence rates, heuristics, and clinical prediction rules. In a decision analysis, as we shall see, a range of prior probability often is sufficient. Nonetheless, if the pretest probability assessment is unreliable, Bayes' theorem will be of little value.

A second potential mistake that you can make when using Bayes' theorem is to apply published values for the test sensitivity and specificity, or LRs, without paying attention to the possible effects of bias in the studies in which the test performance was measured (see Sect. 3.3.5). With certain tests, the LRs may differ depending on the pretest odds in part because differences in pretest odds may reflect differences in the spectrum of disease in the population.

A third potential problem arises when you use Bayes' theorem to interpret a sequence of tests. If a patient undergoes two tests in sequence, you can use the post-test probability after the first test result, calculated with Bayes' theorem, as the pretest probability for the second test. Then, you use Bayes' theorem a second time to calculate the post-test probability after the second test. This approach is valid, however, only if the two tests

are conditionally independent. Tests for the same disease are **conditionally independent** when the probability of a particular result on the second test does not depend on the result of the first test, given (conditioned on) the disease state. Expressed in conditional probability notation for the case in which the disease is present,

$$p \begin{bmatrix} \text{second test positive} \mid \text{first test positive} \\ \text{and disease present} \end{bmatrix}$$
$$= p \begin{bmatrix} \text{second test positive} \mid \text{first test negative} \\ \text{and disease present} \end{bmatrix}$$
$$= p \begin{bmatrix} \text{second test positive} \mid \text{disease present} \end{bmatrix}.$$

If the conditional independence assumption is satisfied, the post-test odds = pretest odds × LR1 × LR2. If you apply Bayes' theorem sequentially in situations in which conditional independence is violated, you will obtain inaccurate post-test probabilities (Gould 2003).

The fourth common problem arises when you assume that all test abnormalities result from one (and only one) disease process. The Bayesian approach, as we have described it, generally presumes that the diseases under consideration are **mutually exclusive**. If they are not, Bayesian updating must be applied with great care.

We have shown how to calculate post-test probability. In Sect. 3.5, we turn to the problem of decision making when the outcomes of a clinician's actions (e.g., of treatments) are uncertain.

3.5 Expected-Value Decision Making

Medical decision-making problems often cannot be solved by reasoning based on pathophysiology. For example, clinicians need a method for choosing among treatments when the outcome of the treatments is uncertain, as are the results of a surgical operation. You can use the ideas developed in the preceding sections to solve such difficult decision problems. Here we discuss two methods: the decision tree, a method for representing and comparing the expected outcomes of each decision alternative; and the threshold probability, a method for deciding whether new information can change a management decision.

These techniques help you to clarify the decision problem and thus to choose the alternative that is most likely to help the patient.

3.5.1 Comparison of Uncertain Prospects

Like those of most biological events, the outcome of an individual's illness is unpredictable.

How can a clinician determine which course of action has the greatest chance of success?

Which of the two therapies is preferable? Example 11 demonstrates a significant fact: a choice among therapies is a choice among gambles (i.e., situations in which chance determines the outcomes). How do we usually choose among gambles? More often than not, we rely on hunches or on a sixth sense. How should we choose among gambles? We propose a method

---

Example 11
There are two available therapies for a fatal illness. The length of a patient's life after either therapy is unpredictable, as illustrated by the frequency distribution shown in Fig. 3.6 and summarized in Table 3.5. Each therapy is associated with uncertainty: regardless of which therapy a patient receives, he will die by the end of the fourth year, but there is no way to know which year will be the patient's last. Figure 3.6 shows that survival until the fourth year is more likely with therapy B, but the patient might die in the first year with

Table 3.5 Distribution of probabilities for the two therapies in Fig. 3.7

Years after therapy	Probability of death	
	Therapy A	Therapy B
1	0.20	0.05
2	0.40	0.15
3	0.30	0.45
4	0.10	0.35

therapy B or might survive to the fourth year with therapy A.

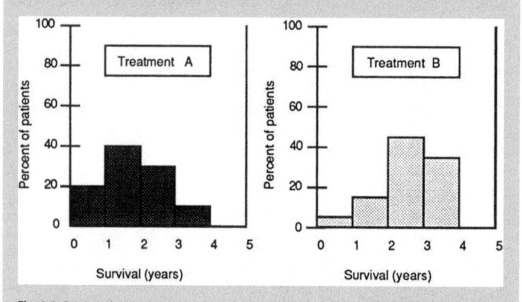

Fig. 3.6 Survival after therapy for a fatal disease. Two therapies are available; the results of either are unpredictable

for choosing called expected-value decision making: we characterize each gamble by a number, and we use that number to compare the gambles.[9] In Example 11, therapy A and therapy B are both gambles with respect to duration of life after therapy. We want to assign a measure (or number) to each therapy that summarizes the outcomes such that we can decide which therapy is preferable.

The ideal criterion for choosing a gamble should be a number that reflects preferences (in medicine, often the patient's preferences) for the outcomes of the gamble. **Utility** is the name given to a measure of preference that has a desirable property for decision making: the gamble with the highest utility should be preferred. We shall discuss utility briefly (Sect. 3.5.4), but you can pursue this topic and the details of decision analysis in other textbooks (see Suggested Readings at the end of this chapter).[10] We use the average duration of life after therapy (survival) as a criterion for choosing among therapies; remember that this model is oversimplified, used here for discussion only. Later, we consider other factors, such as the quality of life.

Because we cannot be sure of the duration of survival for any given patient, we characterize a therapy by the mean survival (average length of life) that would be observed in a large number of patients after they were given the therapy. The first step we take in calculating the mean survival for a therapy is to divide the population receiving the therapy into groups of patients who have similar survival rates. Then, we multiply the survival time in each group[11] by the fraction of the total population in that group. Finally, we sum these products over all possible survival values.

We can perform this calculation for the therapies in Example 11. Mean survival for therapy $A = (0.2 \times 1.0) + (0.4 \times 2.0) + (0.3 \times 3.0) + (0.1 \times 4.0)$

$= 2.3$ years. Mean survival for therapy $B = (0.05 \times 1.0) + (0.15 \times 2.0) + (0.45 \times 3.0) + (0.35 \times 4.0)$ $= 3.1$ years.

Survival after a therapy is under the control of chance. Therapy A is a gamble characterized by an average survival equal to 2.3 years. Therapy B is a gamble characterized by an average survival of 3.1 years. If length of life is our criterion for choosing, we should select therapy B.

3.5.2 Representation of Choices with Decision Trees

The choice between therapies A and B is represented diagrammatically in Fig. 3.7. Events that are under the control of chance can be represented by a **chance node**. By convention, a chance node is shown as a circle from which several lines emanate. Each line represents one of the possible outcomes. Associated with each line is the probability of the outcome occurring. For a single patient, only one outcome can occur. Some physicians object to using probability for just this reason: "You cannot rely on population data, because each patient is an individual." In fact, we often must use the frequency of the outcomes of many patients experiencing the same event to inform our opinion about what might happen to an individual. From these frequencies, we can make patient-specific adjustments and thus estimate the probability of each outcome at a chance node.

A chance node can represent more than just an event governed by chance. The outcome of a chance event, unknowable for the individual, can be represented by the **expected value** at the chance node. The concept of expected value is important and is easy to understand. We can calculate the mean survival that would be expected based on the probabilities depicted by the chance node in Fig. 3.7. This average length of life is called the expected survival or, more generally, the expected value of the chance node. We calculate the expected value at a chance node by the process just described: we multiply the survival value associated with each possible outcome by

---

[9]Expected-value decision making had been used in many fields before it was first applied to medicine.

[10]A more general term for expected-value decision making is expected utility decision making. Because a full treatment of utility is beyond the scope of this chapter, we have chosen to use the term expected value.

[11]For this simple example, death during an interval is assumed to occur at the end of the year.

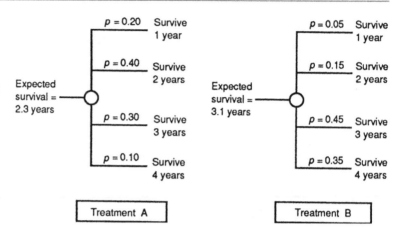

Fig. 3.7 A chance-node representation of survival after the two therapies in Fig. 3.6. The probabilities times the corresponding years of survival are summed to obtain the total expected survival

the probability that that outcome will occur. We then sum the product of probability times survival over all outcomes. Thus, if several hundred patients were assigned to receive either therapy A or therapy B, the expected survival would be 2.3 years for therapy A and 3.1 years for therapy B.

We have just described the basis of expected-value decision making. The term expected value is used to characterize a chance event, such as the outcome of a therapy. If the outcomes of a therapy are measured in units of duration of survival, units of sense of well-being, or dollars, the therapy is characterized by the expected duration of survival, expected sense of well-being, or expected monetary cost that it will confer on, or incur for, the patient, respectively.

To use expected-value decision making, we follow this strategy when there are therapy choices with uncertain outcomes: (1) calculate the expected value of each decision alternative and then (2) pick the alternative with the highest expected value.

3.5.3 Performance of a Decision Analysis

We clarify the concepts of expected-value decision making by discussing an example. There are four steps in decision analysis:
1. Create a decision tree; this step is the most difficult, because it requires formulating the decision problem, assigning probabilities, and measuring outcomes.
2. Calculate the expected value of each decision alternative.

3. Choose the decision alternative with the highest expected value.
4. Use sensitivity analysis to test the conclusions of the analysis.

Many health professionals hesitate when they first learn about the technique of decision analysis, because they recognize the opportunity for error in assigning values to both the probabilities and the utilities in a decision tree. They reason that the technique encourages decision making based on small differences in expected values that are estimates at best. The defense against this concern, which also has been recognized by decision analysts, is the technique known as sensitivity analysis. We discuss this important fourth step in decision analysis in Sect. 3.5.5.

The first step in decision analysis is to create a **decision tree** that represents the decision problem. Consider the following clinical problem.

Example 12
The patient is Mr. Danby, a 66-year-old man who has been crippled with arthritis of both knees so severely that, while he can get about the house with the aid of two canes, he must otherwise use a wheelchair. His other major health problem is emphysema, a disease in which the lungs lose their ability to exchange oxygen and carbon dioxide between blood and air, which in turn causes shortness of breath (dyspnea). He is able to breathe comfortably

when he is in a wheelchair, but the effort of walking with canes makes him breathe heavily and feel uncomfortable. Several years ago, he seriously considered knee replacement surgery but decided against it, largely because his internist told him that there was a serious risk that he would not survive the operation because of his lung disease. Recently, however, Mr. Danby's wife had a stroke and was partially paralyzed; she now requires a degree of assistance that the patient cannot supply given his present state of mobility. He tells his doctor that he is reconsidering knee replacement surgery.

Mr. Danby's internist is familiar with decision analysis. She recognizes that this problem is filled with uncertainty: Mr. Danby's ability to survive the operation is in doubt, and the surgery sometimes does not restore mobility to the degree required by such a patient. Furthermore, there is a small chance that the prosthesis (the artificial knee) will become infected, and Mr. Danby then would have to undergo a second risky operation to remove it. After removal of the prosthesis, Mr. Danby would never again be able to walk, even with canes. The possible outcomes of knee replacement include death from the first procedure and death from a second mandatory procedure if the prosthesis becomes infected (which we will assume occurs in the immediate postoperative period, if it occurs at all). Possible functional outcomes include recovery of full mobility or continued, and unchanged, poor mobility. Should Mr. Danby choose to undergo knee replacement surgery, or should he accept the status quo?

Using the conventions of decision analysis, the internist sketches the decision tree shown in Fig. 3.8. According to these conventions, a square box denotes a **decision node**, and each line emanating from a decision node represents an action that could be taken.

According to the methods of expected-value decision making, the internist first must assign a probability to each branch of each chance node. To accomplish this task, the internist asks several orthopedic surgeons for their estimates of the chance of recovering full function after surgery (p[full recovery] = 0.60) and the chance of developing infection in the prosthetic joint (p[infection] = 0.05). She uses her subjective estimate of the probability that the patient will die during or immediately after knee surgery (p[operative death] = 0.05).

Next, she must assign a value to each outcome. To accomplish this task, she first lists the outcomes. As you can see from Table 3.6, the outcomes differ in two dimensions: length of life (survival) and quality of life (functional status). To characterize each outcome accurately, the internist must develop a measure that takes into account these two dimensions. Simply using duration of survival is inadequate because Mr. Danby values 5 years of good health more than he values 10 years of poor health. The internist can account for this trade-off factor by converting outcomes with two dimensions into outcomes with a single dimension: duration of survival in good health. The resulting measure is called a **quality-adjusted life year** (QALY).[12]

She can convert years in poor health into years in good health by asking Mr. Danby to indicate the shortest period in good health (full mobility) that he would accept in return for his full expected lifetime (10 years) in a state of poor health (status quo). Thus, she asks Mr. Danby: "Many people say they would be willing to accept a shorter life in excellent health in preference to a longer life with significant disability. In your case, how many years with normal mobility do you feel is equivalent in value to 10 years in your current state of disability?" She asks him this question for each outcome. The patient's responses are shown in the third column of Table 3.6. The patient decides that 10 years of limited mobility are equivalent to 6 years of normal mobility,

---

[12]QALYs commonly are used as measures of utility (value) in medical decision analysis and in health policy analysis.

Fig. 3.8 Decision tree for knee replacement surgery. The *box* represents the decision node (whether to have surgery); the *circles* represent chance nodes

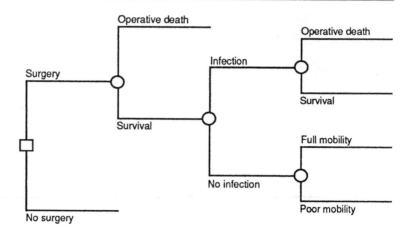

Table 3.6 Outcomes for Example 12

Survival (years)	Functional status	Years of full function equivalent to outcome
10	Full mobility (successful surgery)	10
10	Poor mobility (status quo or unsuccessful surgery)	6
10	Wheelchair-bound (the outcome if a second surgery is necessary)	3
0	Death	0

whereas 10 years of wheelchair confinement are equivalent to only 3 years of full function. Figure 3.9 shows the final decision tree—complete with probability estimates and utility values for each outcome.[13]

The second task that the internist must undertake is to calculate the expected value, in healthy years, of surgery and of no surgery. She calculates the expected value at each chance node, moving from right (the tips of the tree) to left (the root of the tree). Let us consider, for example, the expected value at the chance node representing the outcome of surgery to remove an infected prosthesis (Node A in Fig. 3.9). The calculation requires three steps:

1. Calculate the expected value of operative death after surgery to remove an infected prosthesis. Multiply the probability of operative death (0.05) by the QALY of the outcome—death (0 years): $0.05 \times 0 = 0$ QALY.
2. Calculate the expected value of surviving surgery to remove an infected knee prosthesis. Multiply the probability of surviving the operation (0.95) by the number of healthy years equivalent to 10 years of being wheelchair-bound (3 years): $0.95 \times 3 = 2.85$ QALYs.
3. Add the expected values calculated in step 1 (0 QALY) and step 2 (2.85 QALYs) to obtain the expected value of developing an infected prosthesis: $0 + 2.85 = 2.85$ QALYs.

Similarly, the expected value at chance node B is calculated: $(0.6 \times 10) + (0.4 \times 6) = 8.4$ QALYs. To obtain the expected value of surviving knee replacement surgery (Node C), she proceeds as follows:

1. Multiply the expected value of an infected prosthesis (already calculated as 2.85 QALYs) by the probability that the prosthesis will become infected (0.05): $2.85 \times 0.05 = 0.143$ QALYs.
2. Multiply the expected value of never developing an infected prosthesis (already calculated as 8.4 QALYs) by the probability that the prosthesis will not become infected (0.95): $8.4 \times 0.95 = 7.98$ QALYs.
3. Add the expected values calculated in step 1 (0.143 QALY) and step 2 (7.98 QALYs) to get the expected value of surviving knee replacement surgery: $0.143 + 7.98 = 8.123$ QALYs.

---

[13]In a more sophisticated decision analysis, the clinician also would adjust the utility values of outcomes that require surgery to account for the pain and inconvenience associated with surgery and rehabilitation.

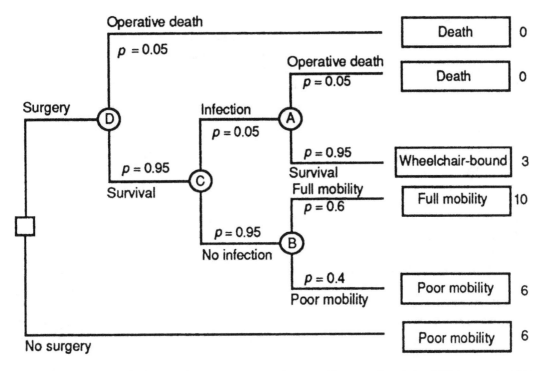

Fig. 3.9 Decision tree for knee-replacement surgery. Probabilities have been assigned to each branch of each chance node. The patient's valuations of outcomes (measured in years of perfect mobility) are assigned to the tips of each branch of the tree

The clinician performs this process, called **averaging out at chance nodes**, for node D as well, working back to the root of the tree, until the expected value of surgery has been calculated. The outcome of the analysis is as follows. For surgery, Mr. Danby's average life expectancy, measured in years of normal mobility, is 7.7. What does this value mean? It does not mean that, by accepting surgery, Mr. Danby is guaranteed 7.7 years of mobile life. One look at the decision tree will show that some patients die in surgery, some develop infection, and some do not gain any improvement in mobility after surgery. Thus, an individual patient has no guarantees. If the clinician had 100 similar patients who underwent the surgery, however, the average number of mobile years would be 7.7. We can understand what this value means for Mr. Danby only by examining the alternative: no surgery.

In the analysis for no surgery, the average length of life, measured in years of normal mobility, is 6.0, which Mr. Danby considered equivalent to 10 years of continued poor mobility. Not all patients will experience this outcome; some who have poor mobility will live longer than, and some will live less than, 10 years. The average length of life, however, expressed in years of normal mobility, will be 6. Because 6.0 is less than 7.7, on average the surgery will provide an outcome with higher value to the patient. Thus, the internist recommends performing the surgery.

The key insight of expected-value decision making should be clear from this example: given the unpredictable outcome in an individual, the best choice for the individual is the alternative that gives the best result on the average in similar patients. Decision analysis can help the clinician to identify the therapy that will give the best results when averaged over many similar patients. The decision analysis is tailored to a specific patient in that both the utility functions and the probability estimates are adjusted to the individual. Nonetheless, the results of the analysis represent the outcomes that would occur on average in a population of patients who have similar utilities and for whom uncertain events have similar probabilities.

3.5.4 Representation of Patients' Preferences with Utilities

In Sect. 3.5.3, we introduced the concept of QALYs, because length of life is not the only outcome about which patients care. Patients' preferences for a health outcome may depend on the length of life with the outcome, on the quality of life with the outcome, and on the risk involved in achieving the outcome (e.g., a cure for cancer might require a risky surgical operation). How can we incorporate these elements into a decision analysis? To do so, we can represent patients' preferences with utilities. The utility of a health state is a quantitative measure of the desirability of a health state from the patient's perspective. Utilities are typically expressed on a 0 to 1 scale, where 0 represents death and 1 represents ideal health. For example, a study of patients who had chest pain (angina) with exercise rated the utility of mild, moderate, and severe angina as 0.95, 0.92, and 0.82 (Nease et al. 1995), respectively. There are several methods for assessing utilities.

The **standard-gamble** technique has the strongest theoretical basis of the various approaches to utility assessment, as shown by Von Neumann and Morgenstern and described by Sox et al. (1988). To illustrate use of the standard gamble, suppose we seek to assess a person's utility for the health state of asymptomatic HIV infection. To use the standard gamble, we ask our subject to compare the desirability of asymptomatic HIV infection to those of two other health states whose utility we know or can assign. Often, we use ideal health (assigned a utility of 1) and immediate death (assigned a utility of 0) for the comparison of health states. We then ask our subject to choose between asymptomatic HIV infection and a gamble with a chance of ideal health or immediate death. We vary the probability of ideal health and immediate death systematically until the subject is indifferent between asymptomatic HIV infection and the gamble. For example, a subject might be indifferent when the probability of ideal health is 0.8 and the probability of death is 0.2. At this point of indifference, the utility of the gamble and that of asymptomatic HIV infection are equal. We calculate the utility of the gamble

as the weighted average of the utilities of each outcome of the gamble $[(1 \times 0.8) + (0 \times 0.2)] = 0.8$. Thus in this example, the utility of asymptomatic HIV infection is 0.8. Use of the standard gamble enables an analyst to assess the utility of outcomes that differ in length or quality of life. Because the standard gamble involves chance events, it also assesses a person's willingness to take risks—called the person's **risk attitude**.

A second common approach to utility assessment is the **time-trade-off** technique (Sox et al. 1988; Torrance and Feeny 1989). To assess the utility of asymptomatic HIV infection using the time-trade-off technique, we ask a person to determine the length of time in a better state of health (usually ideal health or best attainable health) that he or she would find equivalent to a longer period of time with asymptomatic HIV infection. For example, if our subject says that 8 months of life with ideal health was equivalent to 12 months of life with asymptomatic HIV infection, then we calculate the utility of asymptomatic HIV infection as $8 \div 12 = 0.67$. The time-trade-off technique provides a convenient method for valuing outcomes that accounts for gains (or losses) in both length and quality of life. Because the time trade-off does not include gambles, however, it does not assess a person's risk attitude. Perhaps the strongest assumption underlying the use of the time trade-off as a measure of utility is that people are risk neutral. A **risk-neutral** decision maker is indifferent between the expected value of a gamble and the gamble itself. For example, a risk-neutral decision maker would be indifferent between the choice of living 20 years (for certain) and that of taking a gamble with a 50 % chance of living 40 years and a 50 % chance of immediate death (which has an expected value of 20 years). In practice, of course, few people are risk-neutral. Nonetheless, the time-trade-off technique is used frequently to value health outcomes because it is relatively easy to understand.

Several other approaches are available to value health outcomes. To use the **visual analog scale**, a person simply rates the quality of life with a health outcome (e.g., asymptomatic HIV infection) on a scale from 0 to 100. Although the visual analog scale is easy to explain and use, it has no theoretical justification as a valid measure of utility. Ratings with the visual analog scale, however, correlate modestly well with utilities assessed by the standard gamble and time trade-off. For a demonstration of the use of standard gambles, time trade-offs, and the visual analog scale to assess utilities in patients with angina, see Nease et al. (1995); in patient living with HIV, see Joyce et al. (2009) and (2012). Other approaches to valuing health outcomes include the Quality of Well-Being Scale, the Health Utilities Index, and the EuroQoL (see Gold et al. 1996, ch. 4). Each of these instruments assesses how people value health outcomes and therefore may be appropriate for use in decision analyses or cost-effectiveness analyses.

In summary, we can use utilities to represent how patients value complicated health outcomes that differ in length and quality of life and in riskiness. Computer-based tools with an interactive format have been developed for assessing utilities; they often include text and multimedia presentations that enhance patients' understanding of the assessment tasks and of the health outcomes (Sumner et al. 1991; Nease and Owens 1994; Lenert et al. 1995).

3.5.5 Performance of Sensitivity Analysis

Sensitivity analysis is a test of the validity of the conclusions of an analysis over a wide range of assumptions about the probabilities and the values, or utilities. The probability of an outcome at a chance node may be the best estimate that is available, but there often is a wide range of reasonable probabilities that a clinician could use with nearly equal confidence. We use sensitivity analysis to answer this question: Do my conclusions regarding the preferred choice change when the probability and outcome estimates are assigned values that lie within a reasonable range?

The knee-replacement decision in Example 12 illustrates the power of sensitivity analysis. If the conclusions of the analysis (surgery is preferable

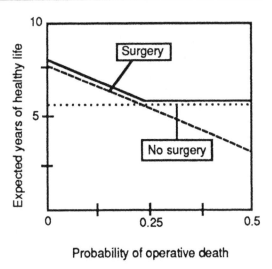

Fig. 3.10 Sensitivity analysis of the effect of operative mortality on length of healthy life (Example 12). As the probability of operative death increases, the relative values of surgery versus no surgery change. The point at which the two lines cross represents the probability of operative death at which no surgery becomes preferable. The *solid line* represents the preferred option at a given probability

to no surgery) remain the same despite a wide range of assumed values for the probabilities and outcome measures, the recommendation is trustworthy. Figures 3.10 and 3.11 show the expected survival in healthy years with surgery and without surgery under varying assumptions of the probability of operative death and the probability of attaining perfect mobility, respectively. Each point (value) on these lines represents one calculation of expected survival using the tree in Fig. 3.8. Figure 3.10 shows that expected survival is higher with surgery over a wide range of operative mortality rates. Expected survival is lower with surgery, however, when the operative mortality rate exceeds 25 %. Figure 3.11 shows the effect of varying the probability that the operation will lead to perfect mobility. The expected survival, in healthy years, is higher for surgery as long as the probability of perfect mobility exceeds 20 %, a much lower figure than is expected from previous experience with the operation. (In Example 12, the consulting orthopedic surgeons estimated the chance of full recovery at 60 %.) Thus, the internist can proceed with confidence

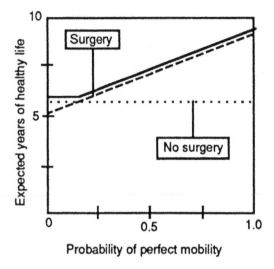

Fig. 3.11 Sensitivity analysis of the effect of a successful operative result on length of healthy life (Example 12). As the probability of a successful surgical result increases, the relative values of surgery versus no surgery change. The point at which the two lines cross represents the probability of a successful result at which surgery becomes preferable. The *solid line* represents the preferred option at a given probability

to recommend surgery. Mr. Danby cannot be sure of a good outcome, but he has valid reasons for thinking that he is more likely to do well with surgery than he is without it.

Another way to state the conclusions of a sensitivity analysis is to indicate the range of probabilities over which the conclusions apply. The point at which the two lines in Fig. 3.10 cross is the probability of operative death at which the two therapy options have the same expected survival. If expected survival is to be the basis for choosing therapy, the internist and the patient should be indifferent between surgery and no surgery when the probability of operative death is 25 %.[14] When the probability is lower, they should select surgery. When it is higher, they should select no surgery.

---

[14]An operative mortality rate of 25 % may seem high; however, this value is correct when we use QALYs as the basis for choosing treatment. A decision maker performing a more sophisticated analysis could use a utility function that reflects the patient's aversion to risking death.

The approach to sensitivity analyses we have described enables the analyst to understand how uncertainty in one, two, or three parameters affects the conclusions of an analysis. But in a complex problem, a decision tree or decision model may have a 100 or more parameters. The analyst may have uncertainty about many parameters in a model. **Probabilistic sensitivity analysis** is an approach for understanding how the uncertainty in all (or a large number of) model parameters affects the conclusion of a decision analysis. To perform a probabilistic sensitivity analysis, the analyst must specify a probability distribution for each model parameter. The analytic software then chooses a value for each model parameter randomly from the parameter's probability distribution. The software then uses this set of parameter values and calculates the outcomes for each alternative. For each evaluation of the model, the software will determine which alternative is preferred. The process is usually repeated 1,000–10,000 times. From the probabilistic sensitivity analysis, the analyst can determine the proportion of times an alternative is preferred, accounting for all uncertainty in model parameters simultaneously. For more information on this advanced topic, see the article by Briggs and colleagues referenced at the end of the chapter.

3.5.6 Representation of Long-Term Outcomes with Markov Models

In Example 12, we evaluated Mr. Danby's decision to have surgery to improve his mobility, which was compromised by arthritis. We assumed that each of the possible outcomes (full mobility, poor mobility, death, etc.) would occur shortly after Mr. Danby took action on his decision. But what if we want to model events that might occur in the distant future? For example, a patient with HIV infection might develop AIDS 10–15 years after infection; thus, a therapy to prevent or delay the development of AIDS could affect events that occur 10–15 years, or more, in the future. A similar

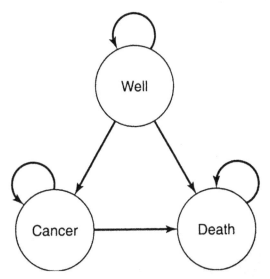

Fig. 3.12 A simple Markov model. The states of health that a person can experience are indicated by the *circles*; *arrows* represent allowed transitions between health states

Table 3.7 Transition probabilities for the Markov model in Fig. 3.13

Health state transition	Annual probability
Well to well	0.9
Well to cancer	0.06
Well to death	0.04
Cancer to well	0.0
Cancer to cancer	0.4
Cancer to death	0.6
Death to well	0.0
Death to cancer	0.0
Death to death	1.0

problem arises in analyses of decisions regarding many chronic diseases: we must model events that occur over the lifetime of the patient. The decision tree representation is convenient for decisions for which all outcomes occur during a short time horizon, but it is not always sufficient for problems that include events that could occur in the future. How can we include such events in a decision analysis? The answer is to use Markov models (Beck and Pauker 1983; Sonnenberg and Beck 1993; Siebert et al. 2012).

To build a **Markov model**, we first specify the set of health states that a person could experience (e.g., Well, Cancer, and Death in Fig. 3.12). We then specify the **transition probabilities**, which are the probabilities that a person will transit from one of these health states to another during a specified time period. This period—often 1 month or 1 year—is the length of the **Markov cycle**. The Markov model then simulates the transitions among health states for a person (or for a hypothetical cohort of people) for a specified number of cycles; by using a Markov model, we can calculate the probability that a person will be in each of the health states at any time in the future. As an illustration, consider a simple

Markov model that has three health states: Well, Cancer, and Death (see Fig. 3.12). We have specified each of the transition probabilities in Table 3.7 for the cycle length of 1 year. Thus, we note from Table 3.7 that a person who is in the well state will remain well with probability 0.9, will develop cancer with probability 0.06, and will die from non-cancer causes with probability 0.04 during 1 year. The calculations for a Markov model are performed by computer software. Based on the transition probabilities in Table 3.7, the probabilities that a person remains well, develops cancer, or dies from non-cancer causes over time is shown in Table 3.8. We can also determine from a Markov model the expected length of time that a person spends in each health state. Therefore, we can determine life expectancy, or quality-adjusted life expectancy, for any alternative represented by a Markov model.

In decision analyses that represent long-term outcomes, the analysts will often use a Markov model in conjunction with a decision tree to model the decision (Owens et al. 1995; Salpeter et al. 1997; Sanders et al. 2005). The analyst models the effect of an intervention as a change in the probability of going from one state to another. For example, we could model a cancer-prevention intervention (such as screening for breast cancer with mammography) as a reduction in the transition probability from Well to Cancer in Fig. 3.12. (See the articles by Beck and Pauker (1983) and Sonnenberg and Beck (1993) for further explanation of the use of Markov models.)

Table 3.8 Probability of future health states for the Markov model in Fig. 3.12

Health state	Probability of health state at end of year						
	Year 1	Year 2	Year 3	Year 4	Year 5	Year 6	Year 7
Well	0.9000	0.8100	0.7290	0.6561	0.5905	0.5314	0.4783
Cancer	0.0600	0.0780	0.0798	0.0757	0.0696	0.0633	0.0572
Death	0.0400	0.1120	0.1912	0.2682	0.3399	0.4053	0.4645

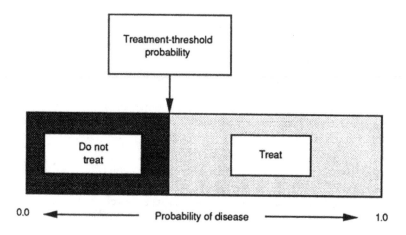

Fig. 3.13 Depiction of the treatment threshold probability. At probabilities of disease that are less than the treatment threshold probability, the preferred action is to withhold therapy. At probabilities of disease that are greater than the treatment threshold probability, the preferred action is to treat

3.6 The Decision Whether to Treat, Test, or Do Nothing

The clinician who is evaluating a patient's symptoms and suspects a disease must choose among the following actions:

1. Do nothing further (neither perform additional tests nor treat the patient).
2. Obtain additional diagnostic information (test) before choosing whether to treat or do nothing.
3. Treat without obtaining more information.

When the clinician knows the patient's true state, testing is unnecessary, and the doctor needs only to assess the trade-offs among therapeutic options (as in Example 12). Learning the patient's true state, however, may require costly, time-consuming, and often risky diagnostic procedures that may give misleading FP or FN results. Therefore, clinicians often are willing to treat a patient even when they are not absolutely certain about a patient's true state. There are risks in this course: the clinician may withhold therapy from a person who has the disease of concern, or he may administer therapy to someone who does not have the disease yet may suffer undesirable side effects of therapy.

Deciding among treating, testing, and doing nothing sounds difficult, but you have already learned all the principles that you need to solve this kind of problem. There are three steps:

1. Determine the treatment threshold probability of disease.
2. Determine the pretest probability of disease.
3. Decide whether a test result could affect your decision to treat.

The **treatment threshold probability** of disease is the probability of disease at which you should be indifferent between treating and not treating (Pauker and Kassirer 1980). Below the treatment threshold, you should not treat. Above the treatment threshold, you should treat (Fig. 3.13). Whether to treat when the diagnosis is not certain is a problem that you can solve with a decision tree, such as the one shown in Fig. 3.14.

You can use this tree to learn the treatment threshold probability of disease by leaving the probability of disease as an unknown, setting the expected value of surgery equal to the expected value for medical (i.e., nonsurgical, such as drugs or physical therapy) treatment, and solving for the probability of disease. (In this example, surgery corresponds to the "treat" branch of the tree

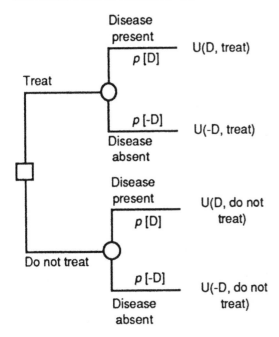

Disease
present
$U(D, treat)$
$p[D]$

Treat

$p[-D]$
$U(-D, treat)$
Disease
absent

Disease
present
$U(D, do\ not$
$treat)$
$p[D]$

Do not treat

$p[-D]$
$U(-D, do\ not$
$treat)$
Disease
absent

Fig. 3.14 Decision tree with which to calculate the treatment threshold probability of disease. By setting the utilities of the treat and do not treat choices to be equal, we can compute the probability at which the clinician and patient should be indifferent to the choice. Recall that $p[-D] = 1 - p[D]$

in Fig. 3.14, and nonsurgical intervention corresponds to the "do not treat" branch.) Because you are indifferent between medical treatment and surgery at this probability, it is the treatment threshold probability. Using the tree completes step 1. In practice, people often determine the treatment threshold intuitively rather than analytically.

An alternative approach to determination of the treatment threshold probability is to use the equation:

$$p^* = \frac{H}{H + B},$$

where p^* = the treatment threshold probability, H = the harm associated with treatment of a nondiseased patient, and B = the benefit associated with treatment of a diseased patient (Pauker and Kassirer 1980; Sox et al. 1988). We define B as the difference between the utility (U) of diseased patients who are treated and diseased patients who are not treated (U[D, treat] − U[D, do not

treat], as shown in Fig. 3.14). The utility of diseased patients who are treated should be greater than that of diseased patients who are not treated; therefore, B is positive. We define H as the difference in utility of nondiseased patients who are not treated and nondiseased patients who are treated (U[−D, do not treat] − U[−D, treat], as shown in Fig. 3.14). The utility of nondiseased patients who are not treated should be greater than that of nondiseased patients who are treated; therefore, H is positive. The equation for the treatment threshold probability fits with our intuition: if the benefit of treatment is small and the harm of treatment is large, the treatment threshold probability will be high. In contrast, if the benefit of treatment is large and the harm of treatment is small, the treatment threshold probability will be low.

Once you know the pretest probability, you know what to do in the absence of further information about the patient. If the pretest probability is below the treatment threshold, you should not treat the patient. If the pretest probability is above the threshold, you should treat the patient. Thus you have completed step 2.

One of the guiding principles of medical decision making is this: do not order a test unless it could change your management of the patient. In our framework for decision making, this principle means that you should order a test only if the test result could cause the probability of disease to cross the treatment threshold. Thus, if the pretest probability is above the treatment threshold, a negative test result must lead to a post-test probability that is below the threshold. Conversely, if the pretest probability is below the threshold probability, a positive result must lead to a post-test probability that is above the threshold. In either case, the test result would alter your decision of whether to treat the patient. This analysis completes step 3.

To decide whether a test could alter management, we simply use Bayes' theorem. We calculate the post-test probability after a test result that would move the probability of disease toward the treatment threshold. If the pretest probability is above the treatment threshold, we calculate the probability of disease if the test result is negative.

If the pretest probability is below the treatment threshold, we calculate the probability of disease if the test result is positive.

Example 13

You are a pulmonary medicine specialist. You suspect that a patient of yours has a pulmonary embolus (blood clot lodged in the vessels of the lungs). One approach is to do a computed tomography angiography (CTA) scan, a test in which a computed tomography (CT) of the lung is done after a radiopaque dye is injected into a vein. The dye flows into the vessels of the lung. The CT scan can then assess whether the blood vessels are blocked. If the scan is negative, you do no further tests and do not treat the patient.

To decide whether this strategy is correct, you take the following steps:
1. Determine the treatment threshold probability of pulmonary embolus.
2. Estimate the pretest probability of pulmonary embolus.
3. Decide whether a test result could affect your decision to treat for an embolus.

First, assume you decide that the treatment threshold should be 0.10 in this patient. What does it mean to have a treatment threshold probability equal to 0.10? If you could obtain no further information, you would treat for pulmonary embolus if the pretest probability was above 0.10 (i.e., if you believed that there was greater than a 1 in 10 chance that the patient had an embolus), and would withhold therapy if the pretest probability was below 0.10. A decision to treat when the pretest probability is at the treatment threshold means that you are willing to treat nine patients without pulmonary embolus to be sure of treating one patient who has pulmonary embolus. A relatively low treatment threshold is justifiable because treatment of a pulmonary embolism with blood-thinning medication substantially reduces the high mortality of pulmonary embolism, whereas there is only a relatively small danger

(mortality of less than 1 %) in treating someone who does not have pulmonary embolus. Because the benefit of treatment is high and the harm of treatment is low, the treatment threshold probability will be low, as discussed earlier. You have completed step 1.

You estimate the pretest probability of pulmonary embolus to be 0.05, which is equal to a pretest odds of 0.053. Because the pretest probability is lower than the treatment threshold, you should do nothing unless a positive CTA scan result could raise the probability of pulmonary embolus to above 0.10. You have completed step 2.

To decide whether a test result could affect your decision to treat, you must decide whether a positive CTA scan result would raise the probability of pulmonary embolism to more than 0.10, the treatment threshold. You review the literature and learn that the LR for a positive CTA scan is approximately 21 (Stein et al. 2006).

A negative CTA scan result will move the probability of disease away from the treatment threshold and will be of no help in deciding what to do. A positive result will move the probability of disease toward the treatment threshold and could alter your management decision if the post-test probability were above the treatment threshold. You therefore use the odds-ratio form of Bayes' theorem to calculate the post-test probability of disease if the lung scan result is reported as high probability.

$$\text{Post-test odds} = \text{pretest odds} \times \text{LR}$$
$$= 0.053 \times 21 = 1.11.$$

A post-test odds of 1.1 is equivalent to a probability of disease of 0.53. Because the post-test probability of pulmonary embolus is higher than the treatment threshold, a positive CTA scan result would change your management of the patient, and you should order the lung scan. You have completed step 3.

This example is especially useful for two reasons: first, it demonstrates one method for making decisions and second, it shows how the concepts that were introduced in this chapter all fit together in a clinical example of medical decision making.

3.7 Alternative Graphical Representations for Decision Models: Influence Diagrams and Belief Networks

In Sects. 3.5 and 3.6, we used decision trees to represent decision problems. Although decision trees are the most common graphical representation for decision problems, **influence diagrams** are an important alternative representation for such problems (Nease and Owens 1997; Owens et al. 1997).

As shown in Fig. 3.15, influence diagrams have certain features that are similar to decision trees, but they also have additional graphical elements. Influence diagrams represent decision nodes as squares and chance nodes as circles. In contrast to decision trees, however, the influence diagram also has arcs between nodes and a diamond-shaped value node. An arc between two chance nodes indicates that a probabilistic relationship may exist between the chance nodes (Owens et al. 1997). A **probabilistic relationship** exists when the occurrence of one chance event affects the probability of the occurrence of another chance event. For example, in Fig. 3.15, the probability of a positive or negative PCR test result (PCR result) depends on whether a person has HIV infection (HIV status); thus, these nodes have a probabilistic relationship, as indicated by the arc. The arc points from the **conditioning event** to the **conditioned event** (PCR test result is conditioned on HIV status in Fig. 3.15). The absence of an arc between two chance nodes, however, always indicates that the nodes are independent or conditionally independent. Two events are conditionally independent, given a third event, if the occurrence of one of the events does not affect the probability of the other event conditioned on the occurrence of the third event.

Unlike a decision tree, in which the events usually are represented from left to right in the order in which the events are observed, influence diagrams use arcs to indicate the timing of events. An arc from a chance node to a decision node indicates that the chance event has been observed at the time the decision is made. Thus, the arc from PCR result to Treat? in Fig. 3.15 indicates

that the decision maker knows the PCR test result (positive, negative, or not obtained) when he or she decides whether to treat. Arcs between decision nodes indicate the timing of decisions: the arc points from an initial decision to subsequent decisions. Thus, in Fig. 3.15, the decision maker must decide whether to obtain a PCR test before deciding whether to treat, as indicated by the arc from Obtain PCR? to Treat?

The probabilities and utilities that we need to determine the alternative with the highest expected value are contained in tables associated with chance nodes and the value node (Fig. 3.16). These tables contain the same information that we would use in a decision tree. With a decision tree, we can determine the expected value of each alternative by averaging out at chance nodes and folding back the tree (Sect. 3.5.3). For influence diagrams, the calculation of expected value is more complex (Owens et al. 1997), and generally must be performed with computer software. With the appropriate software, we can use influence diagrams to perform the same analyses that we would perform with a decision tree. Diagrams that have only chance nodes are called **belief networks**; we use them to perform probabilistic inference.

Why use an influence diagram instead of a decision tree? Influence diagrams have both advantages and limitations relative to decision trees. Influence diagrams represent graphically the probabilistic relationships among variables (Owens et al. 1997). Such representation is advantageous for problems in which probabilistic conditioning is complex or in which communication of such conditioning is important (such as may occur in large models). In an influence diagram, probabilistic conditioning is indicated by the arcs, and thus the conditioning is apparent immediately by inspection. In a decision tree, probabilistic conditioning is revealed by the probabilities in the branches of the tree. To determine whether events are conditionally independent in a decision tree requires that the analyst compare probabilities of events between branches of the tree. Influence diagrams also are particularly useful for discussion with content experts who can help to structure a problem but who are not familiar with decision analysis. In contrast, problems that have decision

Fig. 3.15 A decision tree
(*top*) and an influence
diagram (*bottom*) that
represent the decisions to test
for, and to treat, HIV
infection. The structural
asymmetry of the alternatives
is explicit in the decision
tree. The influence diagram
highlights probabilistic
relationships. *HIV* human
immunodeficiency virus,
HIV+ HIV infected,
HIV− not infected with HIV,
QALE quality-adjusted life
expectancy, *PCR* polymerase
chain reaction. Test results
are shown in quotation marks
("HIV+"), whereas the true
disease state is shown
without quotation marks
(HIV+) (Source: Owens
et al. (1997). Reproduced
with permission)

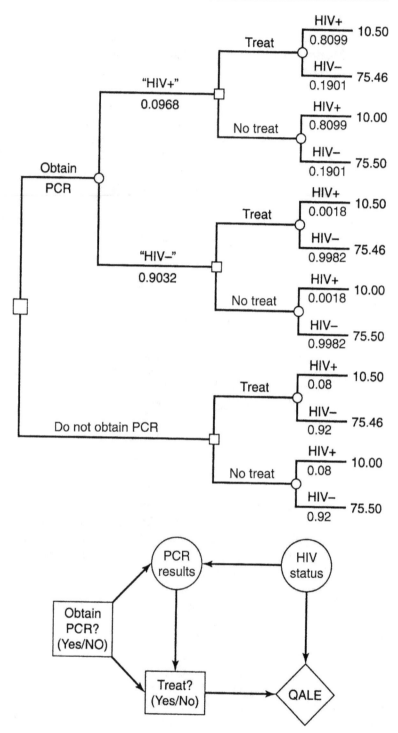

alternatives that are structurally different may be easier for people to understand when represented with a decision tree, because the tree shows the structural differences explicitly, whereas the influence diagram does not. The choice of whether to use a decision tree or an influence diagram depends

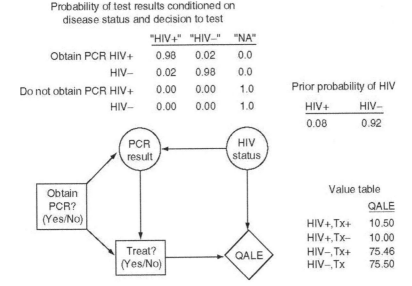

Probability of test results conditioned on disease status and decision to test

	"HIV+"	"HIV−"	"NA"
Obtain PCR HIV+	0.98	0.02	0.0
HIV−	0.02	0.98	0.0
Do not obtain PCR HIV+	0.00	0.00	1.0
HIV−	0.00	0.00	1.0

Prior probability of HIV

HIV+	HIV−
0.08	0.92

Value table

	QALE
HIV+,Tx+	10.50
HIV+,Tx−	10.00
HIV−,Tx+	75.46
HIV−,Tx	75.50

Fig. 3.16 The influence diagram from Fig. 3.15, with the probability and value tables associated with the nodes. The information in these tables is the same as that associated with the branches and endpoints of the decision tree in Fig. 3.15. *HIV* human immunodeficiency virus, *HIV+* HIV infected, *HIV−* not infected with HIV, *QALE* quality-adjusted life expectancy, *PCR* polymerase chain reaction, *NA* not applicable, *TX+* treated, *TX−* not treated. Test results are shown in quotation marks ("HIV+"), and the true disease state is shown without quotation marks (HIV+) (Source: Owens et al.. (1997). Reproduced with permission)

on the problem being analyzed, the experience of the analyst, the availability of software, and the purpose of the analysis. For selected problems, influence diagrams provide a powerful graphical alternative to decision trees.

3.8 Other Modeling Approaches

We have described decision trees, Markov models and influence diagrams. An analyst also can choose several other approaches to modeling. The choice of modeling approach depends on the problem and the objectives of the analysis. Although how to choose and design such models is beyond our scope, we note other type of models that analysts use commonly for medical decision making. **Microsimulation models** are individual-level health state transition models, similar to Markov models, that provide a means to model very complex events flexibly over time. They are useful when the clinical history of a problem is complex, such as might occur with cancer, heart disease, and other chronic diseases. **Dynamic transmission models** are particularly well-suited for assessing the outcomes of infectious diseases. These models divide a population into compartments (for example, uninfected, infected, recovered, dead), and transitions between compartments are governed by differential or difference equations. The rate of transition between compartments depends in part on the number of individuals in the compartment, an important feature for infectious diseases in which the transmission may depend on the number of infected or susceptible individuals. **Discrete event simulation models** also are often used to model interactions between people. These models are composed of entities (a patient) that have attributes (clinical history), and that experience events (a heart attack). An entity can interact with other entities and use resources. For more information on these types of models, we suggest a recent series of papers on best modeling practices; the paper by Caro and colleagues noted in the suggested readings at the end of the chapter is an overview of this series of papers.

3.9 The Role of Probability and Decision Analysis in Medicine

You may be wondering how probability and decision analysis might be integrated smoothly into medical practice. An understanding of probability and measures of test performance will prevent any number of misadventures. In Example 1, we discussed a hypothetical test that, on casual inspection, appeared to be an accurate way to screen blood donors for previous exposure to the AIDS virus. Our quantitative analysis, however, revealed that the hypothetical test results were misleading more often than they were helpful because of the low prevalence of HIV in the clinically relevant population. Fortunately, in actual practice, much more accurate tests are used to screen for HIV.

The need for knowledgeable interpretation of test results is widespread. The federal government screens civil employees in "sensitive" positions for drug use, as do many companies. If the drug test used by an employer had a sensitivity and specificity of 0.95, and if 10 % of the employees used drugs, one-third of the positive tests would be FPs. An understanding of these issues should be of great interest to the public, and health professionals should be prepared to answer the questions of their patients.

Although we should try to interpret every kind of test result accurately, decision analysis has a more selective role in medicine. Not all clinical decisions require decision analysis. Some decisions depend on physiologic principles or on deductive reasoning. Other decisions involve little uncertainty. Nonetheless, many decisions must be based on imperfect data, and they will have outcomes that cannot be known with certainty at the time that the decision is made. Decision analysis provides a technique for managing these situations.

For many problems, simply drawing a tree that denotes the possible outcomes explicitly will clarify the question sufficiently to allow you to make a decision. When time is limited, even a "quick and dirty" analysis may be helpful. By using expert clinicians' subjective probability estimates and asking what the patient's utilities

might be, you can perform an analysis quickly and learn which probabilities and utilities are the important determinants of the decision.

Health care professionals sometimes express reservations about decision analysis because the analysis may depend on probabilities that must be estimated, such as the pretest probability. A thoughtful decision maker will be concerned that the estimate may be in error, particularly because the information needed to make the estimate often is difficult to obtain from the medical literature. We argue, however, that uncertainty in the clinical data is a problem for any decision-making method and that the effect of this uncertainty is explicit with decision analysis. The method for evaluating uncertainty is sensitivity analysis: we can examine any variable to see whether its value is critical to the final recommended decision. Thus, we can determine, for example, whether a change in pretest probability from 0.6 to 0.8 makes a difference in the final decision. In so doing, we often discover that it is necessary to estimate only a range of probabilities for a particular variable rather than a precise value. Thus, with a sensitivity analysis, we can decide whether uncertainty about a particular variable should concern us.

The growing complexity of medical decisions, coupled with the need to control costs, has led to major programs to develop clinical practice guidelines. Decision models have many advantages as aids to guideline development (Eddy 1992): they make explicit the alternative interventions, associated uncertainties, and utilities of potential outcomes. Decision models can help guideline developers to structure guideline-development problems (Owens and Nease 1993), to incorporate patients' preferences (Nease and Owens 1994; Owens 1998), and to tailor guidelines for specific clinical populations (Owens and Nease 1997). In addition, Web-based interfaces for decision models can provide distributed decision support for guideline developers and users by making the decision model available for analysis to anyone who has access to the Web (Sanders et al. 1999).

We have not emphasized computers in this chapter, although they can simplify many aspects of decision analysis (see Chap. 22). MEDLINE and other bibliographic retrieval systems (see Chap. 21) make it easier to obtain published estimates of disease prevalence and test performance. Computer programs for performing statistical analyses can be used on data collected by hospital information systems. Decision analysis software, available for personal computers, can help clinicians to structure decision trees, to calculate expected values, and to perform sensitivity analyses. Researchers continue to explore methods for computer-based automated development of practice guidelines from decision models and use of computer-based systems to implement guidelines (Musen et al. 1996). With the growing maturity of this field, there are now companies that offer formal analytical tools to assist with clinical outcome assessment and interpretation of population datasets.[15]

Medical decision making often involves uncertainty for the clinician and risk for the patient. Most health care professionals would welcome tools that help them make decisions when they are confronted with complex clinical problems with uncertain outcomes. There are important medical problems for which decision analysis offers such aid.

Suggested Readings

Briggs, A., Weinstein, M., Fenwick, E., Karnon, J., Sculpher, M., & Paltiel, A. (2012). Model parameter estimation and uncertainty analysis: A report of the ISPOR-SMDM modeling good research practices task force-6. *Medical Decision Making, 32*(5), 722–732. This article describes best practices for estimating model parameters and for performing sensitivity analyses, including probabilistic sensitivity analysis.

Caro, J., Briggs, A., Siebert, U., & Kuntz, K. (2012). Modeling good research practices – overview: A report of the ISPOR-SMDM modeling good research practices task force-1. *Value in Health, 15,* 796–803. This paper is an introduction to a series of papers that describe best modeling practices.

Gold, M. R., Siegel, J. E., Russell, L. B., & Weinstein, M. C. (1996). *Cost effectiveness in health and medicine.* New York: Oxford University Press. This book provides authoritative guidelines for the conduct of cost-effectiveness analyses. Chapter 4 discusses approaches for valuing health outcomes.

Hunink, M., Glasziou, P., Siegel, J., Weeks, J., Pliskin, J., Einstein, A., & Weinstein, M. (2001). *Decision making in health and medicine.* Cambridge: Cambridge University Press. This textbook addresses in detail most of the topics introduced in this chapter.

Nease, R. F., Jr., & Owens, D. K. (1997). Use of influence diagrams to structure medical decisions. *Medical Decision Making, 17*(13), 263–275. This article provides a comprehensive introduction to the use of influence diagrams.

Owens, D. K., Schacter, R. D., & Nease, R. F., Jr. (1997). Representation and analysis of medical decision problems with influence diagrams. *Medical Decision Making, 17*(3), 241–262. This article provides a comprehensive introduction to the use of influence diagrams.

Raiffa, H. (1970). *Decision analysis: Introductory lectures on choices under uncertainty.* Reading: Addison-Wesley. This now classic book provides an advanced, nonmedical introduction to decision analysis, utility theory, and decision trees.

Sox, H. C. (1986). Probability theory in the use of diagnostic tests. *Annals of Internal Medicine, 104*(1), 60–66. This article is written for clinicians; it contains a summary of the concepts of probability and test interpretation.

Sox, H. C., Higgins, M. C., & Owens, D. K. (2013). *Medical decision making.* Chichester: Wiley-Blackwell. This introductory textbook covers the subject matter of this chapter in greater detail, as well as discussing many other topics.

Tversky, A., & Kahneman, D. (1974). Judgment under uncertainty: Heuristics and biases. *Science, 185,* 1124. This now classic article provides a clear and interesting discussion of the experimental evidence for the use and misuse of heuristics in situations of uncertainty.

Questions for Discussion

1. Calculate the following probabilities for a patient about to undergo CABG surgery (see Example 2):

   (a) The only possible, mutually exclusive outcomes of surgery are death, relief of symptoms (angina and dyspnea), and continuation of symptoms. The probability of death is 0.02, and the probability of relief of symptoms is 0.80. What is the probability that the patient will continue to have symptoms?

   (b) Two known complications of heart surgery are stroke and heart attack, with probabilities of 0.02 and 0.05, respectively. The patient asks what chance he or she has of having both

---

[15]See, for example, the Archimedes tools described at http://archimedesmodel.com/.

Table 3.9 A 2×2 contingency table for the hypothetical study in problem 2

PCR test result	Gold standard test positive	Gold standard test negative	Total
Positive PCR	48	8	56
Negative PCR	2	47	49
Total	50	55	105

PCR polymerase chain reaction

Table 3.10 A 2×2 contingency table to complete for problem 2b

PCR test result	Gold standard test positive	Gold standard test negative	Total
Positive PCR	x	x	x
Negative PCR	100	99,900	x
Total	x	x	x

PCR polymerase chain reaction
x quantities that the question ask students to calculate

complications. Assume that the complications are conditionally independent, and calculate your answer.

(c) The patient wants to know the probability that he or she will have a stroke given that he or she has a heart attack as a complication of the surgery. Assume that 1 in 500 patients has both complications, that the probability of heart attack is 0.05, and that the events are independent. Calculate your answer.

2. The results of a hypothetical study to measure test performance of a diagnostic test for HIV are shown in the 2×2 table in Table 3.9.

(a) Calculate the sensitivity, specificity, disease prevalence, PV+, and PV−.

(b) Use the TPR and TNR calculated in part (a) to fill in the 2×2 table in Table 3.10. Calculate the disease prevalence, PV+, and PV−.

3. You are asked to interpret the results from a diagnostic test for HIV in an asymptomatic man whose test was positive when he volunteered to donate blood. After taking his history, you learn that he has a history of intravenous-drug use. You know that the overall prevalence of HIV infection in your community is 1 in 500 and that the prevalence in people who have injected drugs is 20 times as high as in the community at large.

(a) Estimate the pretest probability that this man is infected with HIV.

(b) The man tells you that two people with whom he shared needles subsequently died of AIDS. Which heuristic will be useful in making a subjective adjustment to the pretest probability in part (a)?

(c) Use the sensitivity and specificity that you worked out in 2(a) to calculate the post-test probability of the patient having HIV after a positive and negative test. Assume that the pretest probability is 0.10.

(d) If you wanted to increase the post-test probability of disease given a positive test result, would you change the TPR or TNR of the test?

4. You have a patient with cancer who has a choice between surgery or chemotherapy. If the patient chooses surgery, he or she has a 2 % chance of dying from the operation (life expectancy=0), a 50 % chance of being cured (life expectancy=15 years), and a 48 % chance of not being cured (life expectancy=1 year). If the patient chooses chemotherapy, he or she has a 5 % chance of death (life expectancy=0), a 65 % chance of cure (life expectancy=15 years), and a 30 % chance that the cancer will be slowed but not cured (life expectancy=2 years). Create a decision tree.

Calculate the expected value of each option in terms of life expectancy.

5. You are concerned that a patient with a sore throat has a bacterial infection that would require antibiotic therapy (as opposed to a viral infection, for which no treatment is available). Your treatment threshold is 0.4, and based on the examination you estimate the probability of bacterial infection as 0.8. A test is available (TPR=0.75, TNR=0.85) that indicates the presence or absence of bacterial infection. Should you perform the test? Explain your reasoning. How would your analysis change if the test were extremely costly or involved a significant risk to the patient?

6. What are the three kinds of bias that can influence measurement of test performance? Explain what each one is, and state how you would adjust the post-test probability to compensate for each.

7. How could a computer system ease the task of performing a complex decision analysis?

8. When you search the medical literature to find probabilities for patients similar to one you are treating, what is the most important question to consider? How should you adjust probabilities in light of the answer to this question?

9. Why do you think clinicians sometimes order tests even if the results will not affect their management of the patient? Do you think the reasons that you identify are valid? Are they valid in only certain situations? Explain your answers. See the January 1998 issue of Medical Decision Making for articles that discuss this question.

10. Explain the differences in three approaches to assessing patients' preferences for health states: the standard gamble, the time trade-off, and the visual analog scale.

Appendix: Derivation of Bayes' Theorem

Bayes' theorem is derived as follows. We denote the conditional probability of disease, D, given a test result, R, p[D|R]. The prior (pretest) probability of D is p[D]. The definition of conditional probability is:

$$p[D \mid R] = \frac{p[R,D]}{p[R]} \qquad (3.1)$$

The probability of a test result (p[R]) is the sum of its probability in diseased patients and its probability in nondiseased patients:

$$p[R] = p[R,D] + p[R,-D].$$

Substituting into Equation 3.1, we obtain:

$$p[D \mid R] = \frac{p[R,D]}{p[R,D] + p[R-D]} \qquad (3.2)$$

Again, from the definition of conditional probability,

$$p[R|D] = \frac{p[R,D]}{p[D]} \text{ and } p[R \mid -D] = \frac{p[R,-D]}{p[-D]}$$

These expressions can be rearranged:

$$p[R,D] = p[D] \times p[R \mid D], \qquad (3.3)$$

$$p[R,-D] = p[-D] \times p[R \mid -D]. \qquad (3.4)$$

Substituting Eqs. 3.3 and 3.4 into Eq. 3.2, we obtain Bayes' theorem:

$$p[D \mid R] = \frac{p[D] \times p[R \mid D]}{p[D] \times p[R \mid D] + p[-D] \times p[R \mid -D]}$$

Cognitive Science and Biomedical Informatics

4

Vimla L. Patel and David R. Kaufman

After reading this chapter, you should know the answers to these questions:

- How can cognitive science theory meaningfully inform and shape design, development and assessment of healthcare information systems?
- What are some of the ways in which cognitive science differs from behavioral science?
- What are some of the ways in which we can characterize the structure of knowledge?
- What are the basic HCI and cognitive science methods that are useful for healthcare information system evaluation and design?
- What are some of the dimensions of difference between experts and novices?
- What are the attributes of system usability?
- What are the gulfs of execution and evaluation? What role do these considerations play in system design?
- Why is it important to consider cognition and human factors in dealing with issues of patient safety?

V.L. Patel, PhD, DSc (✉)
Department of Center for Cognitive Studies in Medicine and Public Health, The New York Academy of Medicine, 1216 Fifth Avenue,
New York, NY 10029, USA
e-mail: vpatel@nyam.org, vimla.patel@uth.tmc.edu

D.R. Kaufman, PhD
Biomedical Informatics, Arizona State University,
13212 East Shea Blvd., Scottsdale, AZ 85259
e-mail: kaufman@dbmi.columbia.edu

4.1 Introduction

Enormous advances in health information technologies and more generally, in computing over the course of the past two decades have begun to permeate diverse facets of clinical practice. The rapid pace of technological developments such as the Internet, wireless technologies, and hand-held devices, in the last decade affords significant opportunities for supporting, enhancing and extending user experiences, interactions and communications (Rogers 2004). These advances coupled with a growing computer literacy among healthcare professionals afford the potential for great improvement in healthcare. Yet many observers note that the healthcare system is slow to understand information technology and effectively incorporate it into the work environment (Shortliffe and Blois 2001). Innovative technologies often produce profound cultural, social, and cognitive changes. These transformations necessitate adaptation at many different levels of aggregation from the individual to the larger institution, sometimes causing disruptions of workflow and user dissatisfaction.

Similar to other complex domains, biomedical information systems embody ideals in design that often do not readily yield practical solutions in implementation. As computer-based systems infiltrate clinical practice and settings, the consequences often can be felt through all levels of the organization. This impact can have deleterious effects resulting in systemic inefficiencies and suboptimal practice, which can lead to frustrated

E.H. Shortliffe, J.J. Cimino (eds.), *Biomedical Informatics*,
DOI 10.1007/978-1-4471-4474-8_4, © Springer-Verlag London 2014

healthcare practitioners, unnecessary delays in healthcare delivery, and even adverse events (Lin et al. 1998; Weinger and Slagle 2001). In the best-case scenario, mastery of the system necessitates an individual and collective learning curve yielding incremental improvements in performance and satisfaction. In the worst-case scenario, clinicians may revolt and the hospital may be forced to pull the plug on an expensive new technology. How can we manage change? How can we introduce systems that are designed to be more intuitive and also implemented to be coherent with everyday practice?

4.1.1 Introducing Cognitive Science

Cognitive science is a multidisciplinary domain of inquiry devoted to the study of cognition and its role in intelligent agency. The primary disciplines include cognitive psychology, artificial intelligence, neuroscience, linguistics, anthropology, and philosophy. From the perspective of informatics, cognitive science can provide a framework for the analysis and modeling of complex human performance in technology-mediated settings. Cognitive science incorporates basic science research focusing on fundamental aspects of cognition (e.g., attention, memory, reasoning, early language acquisition) as well as applied research. Applied cognitive research is focally concerned with the development and evaluation of useful and usable cognitive artifacts. **Cognitive artifacts** are human-made materials, devices, and systems that extend people's abilities in perceiving objects, encoding and retrieving information from memory, and problem-solving (Gillan and Schvaneveldt 1999). In this regard, applied cognitive research is closely aligned with the disciplines of **human-computer interaction** (HCI) and **human factors**. It also has a close affiliation with educational research. In everyday life, we interact with cognitive artifacts to receive and/or manipulate information so as to alter our thinking processes and offload effort-intensive cognitive activity to the external world, thereby reducing mental workload.

The past couple of decades have produced a cumulative body of experiential and practical knowledge about system design and implementation that can guide future initiatives. This practical knowledge embodies the need for sensible and intuitive user interfaces, an understanding of workflow, and the ways in which systems impact individual and team performance. However, experiential knowledge in the form of anecdotes and case studies is inadequate for producing robust generalizations or sound design and implementation principles. There is a need for a theoretical foundation. Biomedical informatics is more than the thin intersection of biomedicine and computing (Patel and Kaufman 1998). There is a growing role for the social sciences, including the cognitive and behavioral sciences, in biomedical informatics, particularly as they pertain to human-computer interaction and other areas such as **information retrieval** and **decision support**. In this chapter, we focus on the foundational role of cognitive science in biomedical informatics research and practice. Theories and methods from the cognitive sciences can illuminate different facets of design and implementation of information and knowledge-based systems. They can also play a larger role in characterizing and enhancing human performance on a wide range of tasks involving clinicians, patients and healthy consumers of biomedical information. These tasks may include developing training programs and devising measures to reduce errors or increase efficiency. In this respect, cognitive science represents one of the component basic sciences of biomedical informatics (Shortliffe and Blois 2001).

4.1.2 Cognitive Science and Biomedical Informatics

How can cognitive science theory meaningfully inform and shape design, development and assessment of health-care information systems? Cognitive science provides insight into principles of system usability and *learnability*, the mediating role of technology in clinical performance, the process of medical judgment and decision-making, the training of healthcare professionals, patients and health consumers, and

Table 4.1 Correspondences between cognitive science, medical cognition and applied cognitive research in medical informatics

Cognitive Science	Medical Cognition	Biomedical Informatics
Knowledge organization and human memory	Organization of clinical and basic science knowledge	Development and use of medical knowledge bases
Problem solving, Heuristics/ reasoning strategies	Medical problem solving and decision making	Medical artificial intelligence/decision support systems/medical errors
Perception/attention	Radiologic and dermatologic diagnosis	Medical imaging systems
Text comprehension	Learning from medical texts	Information retrieval/digital libraries/ health literacy
Conversational analysis	Medical discourse	Medical natural language processing
Distributed cognition	Collaborative practice and research in health care	Computer-based provider order entry systems
Coordination of theory and evidence	Diagnostic and therapeutic reasoning	Evidence-based clinical guidelines
Diagrammatic reasoning	Perceptual processing of patient data displays	Biomedical information visualization

the design of a safer workplace. The central argument is that it can inform our understanding of human performance in technology-rich healthcare environments (Carayon 2007).

Precisely how will cognitive science theory and methods make such a significant contribution towards these important objectives? The translation of research findings from one discipline into practical concerns that can be applied to another is rarely a straight-forward process (Rogers 2004). Furthermore, even when scientific knowledge is highly relevant in principle, making that knowledge effective in a design context can be a significant challenge. In this chapter, we discuss (a) basic cognitive science research and theories that provide a foundation for understanding the underlying mechanisms guiding human performance (e.g., findings pertaining to the structure of human memory), and (b) research in the areas of **medical errors** and **patient safety** as they interact with health information technology),

As illustrated in Table 4.1, there are correspondences between basic cognitive science research, medical cognition and cognitive research in biomedical informatics along several dimensions. For example, theories of human memory and knowledge organization lend themselves to characterizations of expert clinical knowledge that can then be contrasted with representation

of such knowledge in clinical systems. Similarly, research in text comprehension has provided a theoretical framework for research in understanding biomedical texts. This in turn has influenced applied cognitive research on information retrieval (Chap. 21) from biomedical knowledge sources and research on **health literacy**. Similarly, theories of problem solving and reasoning can be used to understand the processes and knowledge associated with diagnostic and therapeutic reasoning. This understanding provides a basis for developing biomedical artificial intelligence and decision support systems.

In this chapter, we demonstrate that cognitive research, theories and methods can contribute to applications in informatics in a number of ways including: (1) seed *basic research findings* that can illuminate dimensions of design (e.g., attention and memory, aspects of the visual system), (2) provide an *explanatory vocabulary* for characterizing how individuals process and communicate health information (e.g., various studies of medical cognition pertaining to doctor-patient interaction), (3) present an *analytic framework* for identifying problems and modeling certain kinds of user interactions, (4) characterize the relationship between health information technology, human factors and patient safety, (5) provide *rich descriptive accounts* of clinicians employing technologies in the context of work, and (6) furnish a generative approach for novel designs and productive applied research programs in informatics (e.g., intervention strategies for supporting low literacy populations in health information seeking).

Since the last edition of this text, there has been a significant growth in cognitive research in biomedical informatics. We conducted an informal comparison of studies across three leading informatics journals, Journal of Biomedical Informatics, Journal of the American Medical Informatics Association and the International Journal of Medical Informatics of two time periods over the last decade, the first being 2001–2005 and the second 2006–2010. A keyword search of ten common terms (e.g., cognition, usability testing and human factors) found an increase of almost 70 % in the last 5 years over the previous 5 years. Although this doesn't constitute a rigorous systematic analysis, it is suggestive of a strong growth of cognitive research in informatics.

The social sciences are constituted by multiple frameworks and approaches. **Behaviorism** constitutes a framework for analyzing and modifying behavior. It is an approach that has had an enormous influence on the social sciences for most of the twentieth Century. Cognitive science partially emerged as a response to the limitations of behaviorism. The next section of the chapter contains a brief history of the cognitive and behavioral sciences that emphasizes the points of difference between the two approaches. It also serves to introduce basic concepts in the study of cognition.

4.2 Cognitive Science: The Emergence of an Explanatory Framework

Cognitive science is, of course, not really a new discipline, but recognition of a fundamental set of common concerns shared by the disciplines of psychology, computer science, linguistics, economics, epistemology, and the social sciences generally. All of these disciplines are concerned with information processing systems, and all of them

are concerned with systems that are adaptive-that are what they are from being ground between the nether millstone of their physiology or hardware, as the case may be, and the upper millstone of a complex environment in which they exist. Herbert A. Simon (1980. P 33) (H. A. Simon 1980)

In this section, we sketch a brief history of the emergence of cognitive science in view to differentiate it with competing theoretical frameworks in the social sciences. The section also serves to introduce core concepts that constitute an explanatory framework for cognitive science.

Behaviorism is the conceptual framework underlying a particular science of behavior (Zuriff 1985). This framework dominated experimental and applied psychology as well as the social sciences for the better part of the twentieth century (Bechtel et al. 1998). Behaviorism represented an attempt to develop an objective, empirically based science of behavior and more specifically, learning. Empiricism is the view that experience is the only source of knowledge (Hilgard and Bower 1975). Behaviorism endeavored to build a comprehensive framework of scientific inquiry around the experimental analysis of observable behavior. Behaviorists eschewed the study of thinking as an unacceptable psychological method because it was inherently subjective, error prone, and could not be subjected to empirical validation. Similarly, hypothetical constructs (e.g., mental processes as mechanisms in a theory) were discouraged. All constructs had to be specified in terms of operational definitions so they could be manipulated, measured and quantified for empirical investigation (Weinger and Slagle 2001). Radical behaviorism as espoused by B.F. Skinner proposed that behavioral events may be understood and analyzed entirely in relation to past and present environment and evolutionary history without any reference to internal states (Baum 2011).

Behavioral theories of learning emphasized the correspondence between environmental stimuli and the responses emitted. These studies generally attempted to characterize the changing relationship between stimulus and response under different reinforcement and punishment contingencies. For example, a behavior that was followed by a satisfying state of affairs is more likely to increase the frequency of the act. According to behavior theories, knowledge is nothing more than sum of an individual's learning history and transformations of mental states play no part in the learning process.

For reasons that go beyond the scope of this chapter, classical behavioral theories have been largely discredited as a comprehensive unifying theory of behavior. However, behaviorism continues to provide a theoretical and methodological foundation in a wide range of social science disciplines. For example, behaviorist tenets continue to play a central role in public health research. In particular, health behavior research places an emphasis on antecedent variables and environmental contingencies that serve to sustain unhealthy behaviors such as smoking (Sussman 2001). Around 1950, there was an increasing dissatisfaction with the limitations and methodological constraints (e.g., the disavowal of the unobserved such as mental states) of behaviorism. In addition, developments in logic, information theory, cybernetics, and perhaps most importantly the advent of the digital computer, aroused substantial interest in "information processing (Gardner 1985).

Newell and Simon (1972) date the beginning of the "cognitive revolution" to the year 1956. They cite Bruner, Goodnow and Austin's "Study of Thinking," George Miller's influential journal publication "The magic number seven" in psychology, Noam Chomsky's writings on syntactic grammars in linguistics (see Chap. 8), and their own logic theorist program in computer science as the pivotal works. Cognitive scientists placed "thought" and "mental processes" at the center of their explanatory framework.

The "computer metaphor" provided a framework for the study of human cognition as the manipulation of "symbolic structures." It also provided the foundation for a model of memory, which was a prerequisite for an information processing theory (Atkinson and Shiffrin 1968). The implementation of models of human performance as computer programs provided a measure of objectivity and a *sufficiency test* of a theory and also serves to increase the objectivity of the study of mental processes (Estes 1975).

Arguably, the most significant landmark publication in the nascent field of cognitive science is Newell and Simon's "Human Problem Solving" (Newell and Simon 1972). This was the culmination of more than 15 years of work on problem solving and research in artificial intelligence. It was a mature thesis that described a theoretical framework, extended a language for the study of cognition, and introduced protocol-analytic methods that have become ubiquitous in the study of high-level cognition. It laid the foundation for the formal investigation of symbolic-information processing (more specifically, problem solving). The development of models of human information processing also provided a foundation for the discipline of human-computer interaction and the first formal methods of analysis (Card et al. 1983).

The early investigations of problem solving focused primarily on investigations of experimentally contrived or toy-world tasks such as elementary deductive logic, the Tower of Hanoi, illustrated in Fig. 4.1, and mathematical word problems (Greeno and Simon 1988). These tasks required very little background knowledge and were well structured, in the sense that all the variables necessary for solving the problem were present in the problem statement. These tasks allowed for a complete description of the task environment; a step-by-step description of the sequential behavior of the subjects' performance; and the modeling of subjects' cognitive and overt behavior in the form of a computer simulation. The Tower of Hanoi, in particular, served as an important test bed for the development of an explanatory vocabulary and framework for analyzing problem solving behavior.

The Tower of Hanoi (TOH) is a relatively straight-forward task that consists of three pegs (A, B, and C) and three or more disks that vary in size. The goal is to move the three disks from peg A to peg C one at a time with the constraint that a larger disk can never rest on a smaller one. Problem solving can be construed as *search* in a **problem space**. A problem space has an *initial state*, a *goal state*, and a *set of operators*. Operators are any moves that transform a given state to a successor state. For example, the first

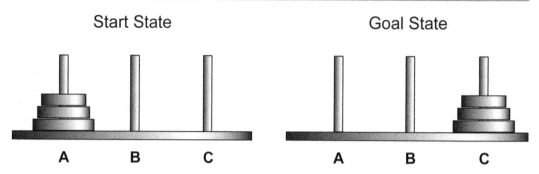

Fig. 4.1 Tower of Hanoi task illustrating a start state and a goal state

move could be to move the small disk to peg B or peg C. In a three-disk TOH, there are a total of 27 possible states representing the complete problem space. TOH has 3^n states where n is the number of disks. The minimum number of moves necessary to solve a TOH is 2^{n-1}. Problem solvers will typically maintain only a small set of states at a time.

The search process involves finding a solution strategy that will minimize the number of steps. The metaphor of movement through a problem space provides a means for understanding how an individual can sequentially address the challenges they confront at each stage of a problem and the actions that ensue. We can characterize the problem-solving behavior of the subject at a local level in terms of state transitions or at a more global level in terms of *strategies*. For example, *means ends analysis* is a commonly used strategy for reducing the difference between the start state and goal state. For instance, moving all but the largest disk from peg A to peg B is an interim goal associated with such a strategy. Although TOH bears little resemblance to the tasks performed by either clinicians or patients, the example illustrates the process of analyzing task demands and task performance in human subjects.

The most common method of data analysis is known as **protocol analysis**[1] (Newell and Simon 1972). Protocol analysis refers to a class of

techniques for representing verbal **think-aloud protocols** (Greeno and Simon 1988). Think aloud protocols are the most common source of data used in studies of problem solving. In these studies, subjects are instructed to verbalize their thoughts as they perform a particular experimental task. Ericsson and Simon (1993) specify the conditions under which verbal reports are acceptable as legitimate data. For example, retrospective think-aloud protocols are viewed as somewhat suspect because the subject has had the opportunity to reconstruct the information in memory and the verbal reports are inevitably distorted. Think aloud protocols recorded in concert with observable behavioral data such as a subject's actions provide a rich source of evidence to characterize cognitive processes.

Cognitive psychologists and linguists have investigated the processes and properties of language and memory in adults and children for many decades. Early research focused on basic laboratory studies of list learning or processing of words and sentences (as in a sentence completion task) (Anderson 1983). Beginning in the early 1970s, van Dijk and Kintsch (1983) developed an influential method of analyzing the process of **text comprehension** based on the realization that text can be described at multiple levels of realization from surface codes (e.g., words and syntax) to deeper level of semantics. Comprehension refers to cognitive processes associated with understanding or deriving meaning from text, conversation, or other informational resources. It involves the processes that people use when trying to make sense of a piece of text, such as a sentence, a book, or a verbal utterance. It also involves the final product of

---

[1] The term protocol refers to that which is produced by a subject during testing (e.g., a verbal record). It differs from the more common use of protocol as defining a code or set of procedures governing behavior or a situation.

such processes, which is, the mental representation of the text, essentially what people have understood.

Comprehension often precedes problem solving and decision making, but is also dependent on perceptual processes that focus attention, the availability of relevant knowledge, and the ability to deploy knowledge in a given context. In fact, some of the more important differences in medical problem solving and decision making arise from differences in knowledge and comprehension. Furthermore, many of the problems associated with decision making are the result of either lack of knowledge or failure to understand the information appropriately.

The early investigations provided a well-constrained artificial environment for the development of the basic methods and principles of problem solving. They also provide a rich explanatory vocabulary (e.g., problem space), but were not fully adequate in accounting for cognition in knowledge-rich domains of greater complexity and involving uncertainty. In the mid to late 1970s, there was a shift in research to complex "real-life" knowledge-based domains of enquiry (Greeno and Simon 1988). Problem-solving research was studying performance in domains such as physics (1980), medical diagnoses (Elstein et al. 1978) and architecture (Akin 1982). Similarly the study of text comprehension shifted from research on simple stories to technical and scientific texts in a range of domains including medicine. This paralleled a similar change in artificial intelligence research from "toy programs" to addressing "real-world" problems and the development of expert systems (Clancey and Shortliffe 1984). The shift to real-world problems in cognitive science was spearheaded by research exploring the nature of expertise. Most of the early investigations on expertise involved laboratory experiments. However, the shift to knowledge-intensive domains provided a theoretical and methodological foundation to conduct both basic and applied research in real-world settings such as the workplace (Vicente 1999) and the classroom (Bruer 1993). These areas of application provided a fertile test bed for assessing and extending the cognitive science framework.

In recent years, the conventional information-processing approach has come under criticism for its narrow focus on the rational/cognitive processes of the solitary individual. One of the most compelling proposals has to do with a shift from viewing cognition as a property of the solitary individual to viewing cognition as distributed across groups, cultures, and artifacts. This claim has significant implications for the study of collaborative endeavors and human-computer interaction. We explore the concepts underlying *distributed cognition* in greater detail in a subsequent section.

4.3 Human Information Processing

It is well known that product design often fails to adequately consider cognitive and physiological constraints and imposes an unnecessary burden on task performance (Preece et al. 2007). Fortunately, advances in theory and methods provide us with greater insight into designing systems for the human condition.

Cognitive science serves as a basic science and provides a framework for the analysis and modeling of complex human performance. A computational theory of mind provides the fundamental underpinning for most contemporary theories of cognitive science. The basic premise is that much of human cognition can be characterized as a series of operations or computations on mental representations. **Mental representations** are internal cognitive states that have a certain correspondence with the external world. For example, they may reflect a clinician's hypothesis about a patient's condition after noticing an abnormal gait as he entered the clinic. These are likely to elicit further inferences about the patient's underlying condition and may direct the physician's information-gathering strategies and contribute to an evolving problem representation.

Two interdependent dimensions by which we can characterize cognitive systems are: (1) architectural theories that endeavor to provide a unified theory for all aspects of cognition and

(2) distinction the different kinds of knowledge necessary to attain competency in a given domain. Individuals differ substantially in terms of their knowledge, experiences, and endowed capabilities. The architectural approach capitalizes on the fact that we can characterize certain regularities of the human information processing system. These can be either structural regularities—such as the existence of and the relations between perceptual, attentional, and memory systems and memory capacity limitations— or processing regularities, such as processing speed, selective attention, or problem solving strategies. Cognitive systems are characterized functionally in terms of the capabilities they enable (e.g., focused attention on selective visual features), the way they constrain human cognitive performance (e.g. limitations on memory), and their development during the lifespan. In regards to the lifespan issue, there is a growing body of literature on cognitive aging and how aspects of the cognitive system such as attention, memory, vision and motor skills change as a function of aging (Fisk et al. 2009). This basic science research is of growing importance to informatics as we seek to develop e-health applications for seniors, many of whom suffer from chronic health conditions such as arthritis and diabetes. A graphical user interface or more generally, a website designed for younger adults may not be suitable for older adults.

Differences in knowledge organization are a central focus of research into the nature of expertise. In medicine, the expert-novice paradigm has contributed to our understanding of the nature of medical expertise and skilled clinical performance.

4.3.1 Cognitive Architectures and Human Memory Systems

Fundamental research in perception, cognition, and psychomotor skills over the course of the last 50 years has provided a foundation for design principles in human factors and human-computer interaction. Although cognitive guidelines have made significant inroads in the design community, there remains a significant gap in applying basic cognitive research (Gillan and Schvaneveldt 1999). Designers routinely violate basic assumptions about the human cognitive system. There are invariably challenges in applying basic research and theory to applications. A more human-centered design and cognitive research can instrumentally contribute to such an endeavor (Zhang et al. 2004).

Over the course of the last 25 years, there have been several attempts to develop a unified theory of cognition. The goal of such a theory is to provide a single set of mechanisms for all cognitive behaviors from motor skills, language, memory, to decision making, problem solving and comprehension (Newell 1990). Such a theory provides a means to put together a voluminous and seemingly disparate body of human experimental data into a coherent form. Cognitive architecture represents unifying theories of cognition that are embodied in large-scale computer simulation programs. Although there is much plasticity evidenced in human behavior, cognitive processes are bound by biological and physical constraints. Cognitive architectures specify functional rather than biological constraints on human behavior (e.g., limitations on working memory). These constraints reflect the information-processing capacities and limitations of the human cognitive system. Architectural systems embody a relatively fixed permanent structure that is (more or less) characteristic of all humans and doesn't substantially vary over an individual's lifetime. It represents a scientific hypothesis about those aspects of human cognition that are relatively constant over time and independent of task (Carroll 2003). Cognitive architectures also play a role in providing blueprints for building future intelligent systems that embody a broad range of capabilities similar to those of humans (Duch et al. 2008).

Cognitive architectures include short-term and long-term memories that store content about an individual's beliefs, goals, and knowledge, the representation of elements that are contained in these memories as well as their organization into larger-scale structures (Langley et al. 2009). An extended discussion of architectural theories and systems is beyond the scope of this chapter. However, we employ the architectural frame of reference to introduce some basic distinctions in memory systems. Human memory is typically divided into at least two structures: **long-term memory** and **short-term/working memory**. Working memory is an emergent property of interaction with the environment. Long-term memory (LTM) can be thought of as a repository of all knowledge, whereas working memory (WM) refers to the resources needed to maintain information active during cognitive activity (e.g., text comprehension). The information maintained in working memory includes stimuli from the environment (e.g., words on a display) and knowledge activated from long-term memory. In theory, LTM is infinite, whereas WM is limited to five to ten "chunks" of information. A chunk is any stimulus or patterns of stimuli that has become familiar from repeated exposure and is subsequently stored in memory as a single unit (Larkin et al. 1980). Problems impose a varying **cognitive load** on working memory. This refers to an excess of information that competes for few cognitive resources, creating a burden on working memory (Chandler and Sweller 1991). For example, maintaining a seven-digit phone number in WM is not very difficult. However, to maintain a phone number while engaging in conversation is nearly impossible for most people. Multi-tasking is one factor that contributes to cognitive load. The structure of the task environment, for example, a crowded computer display is another contributor. High velocity/high workload clinical environments such as intensive care units also impose cognitive loads on clinicians carrying out task.

4.3.2 The Organization of Knowledge

Architectural theories specify the structure and mechanisms of memory systems, whereas theories of knowledge organization focus on the content. There are several ways to characterize the kinds of knowledge that reside in LTM and that support decisions and actions. Cognitive

psychology has furnished a range of domain-independent constructs that account for the variability of mental representations needed to engage the external world.

A central tenet of cognitive science is that humans actively construct and interpret information from their environment. Given that environmental stimuli can take a multitude of forms (e.g., written text, speech, music, images, etc.), the cognitive system needs to be attuned to different representational types to capture the essence of these inputs. For example, we process written text differently than we do mathematical equations. The power of cognition is reflected in the ability to form abstractions - to represent perceptions, experiences and thoughts in some medium other than that in which they have occurred without extraneous or irrelevant information (Norman 1993). Representations enable us to remember, reconstruct, and transform events, objects, images, and conversations absent in space and time from our initial experience of the phenomena. Representations reflect states of knowledge.

Propositions are a form of natural language representation that captures the essence of an idea (i.e., semantics) or concept without explicit reference to linguistic content. For example, "hello", "hey", and "what's happening" can typically be interpreted as a greeting containing identical propositional content even though the literal semantics of the phrases may differ. These ideas are expressed as language and translated into speech or text when we talk or write. Similarly, we recover the propositional structure when we read or listen to verbal information. Numerous psychological experiments have demonstrated that people recover the gist of a text or spoken communication (i.e., propositional structure) not the specific words (Anderson 1985; van Dijk and Kintsch 1983). Studies have also shown the individuals at different levels of expertise will differentially represent a text (Patel and Kaufman 1998). For example, experts are more likely to selectively encode relevant propositional information that will inform a decision. On the other hand, non-experts will often remember more information, but much of the recalled information may not be relevant to the decision (Patel

Fig. 4.2 Propositional analysis of a think-aloud protocol of a primary care physician

1. 43-year-old white female who developed diarrhea after a brief period of 2 days of GI upset.

1.1	female	ATT: Age (old); DEG: 43 year; ATT: white
1.2	develop	PAT: [she]; THM: diarrhea; TNS: past
1.3	period	ATT: brief; DUR: 2 days; THM: 1.4
1.4	upset	LOC: GI
1.5	TEM:ORD	[1.3], [1.2]

and Groen 1991a, b). Propositional representations constitute an important construct in theories of comprehension and are discussed later in this chapter.

Propositional knowledge can be expressed using a predicate calculus formalism or as a semantic network. The predicate calculus representation is illustrated below. A subject's response, as given on Fig. 4.2, is divided into sentences or segments and sequentially analyzed. The formalism includes a head element of a segment and a series of arguments. For example in proposition 1.1, the focus is on a female who has the attributes of being 43 years of age and white. The TEM:ORD or temporal order relation indicates that the events of 1.3 (GI upset) precede the event of 1.2 (diarrhea). The formalism is informed by an elaborate propositional language (Frederiksen 1975) and was first applied to the medical domain by Patel and her colleagues (Patel et al. 1986). The method provides us with a detailed way to characterize the information subjects understood from reading a text, based on their summary or explanations.

Kintsch (1998) theorized that comprehension involves an interaction between what the text conveys and the schemata in long-term memory. Comprehension occurs when the reader uses prior knowledge to process the incoming information presented in the text. The text information is called the *textbase* (the propositional content of the text). For instance, in medicine the textbase could consist of the representation of a patient problem as written in a patient chart. The situation model is constituted by the textbase representation plus the domain-specific and everyday knowledge that the reader uses to derive a broader meaning from the text. In medicine, the situation model would enable a physician to draw inferences from a patient's history leading to a diagnosis, therapeutic plan or prognosis (Patel

and Groen 1991a, b). This situation model is typically derived from the general knowledge and specific knowledge acquired through medical teaching, readings (e.g., theories and findings from biomedical research), clinical practice (e.g., knowledge of associations between clinical findings and specific diseases, knowledge of medications or treatment procedures that have worked in the past) and the textbase representation. Like other forms of knowledge representation, the situation model is used to "fit in" the incoming information (e.g., text, perception of the patient). Since the knowledge in LTM differs among physicians, the resulting situation model generated by any two physicians is likely to differ as well. Theories and methods of text comprehension have been widely used in the study of medical cognition and have been instrumental in characterizing the process of guideline development and interpretation (Arocha et al. 2005).

Schemata represent higher-level knowledge structures. They can be construed as data structures for representing categories of concepts stored in memory (e.g., fruits, chairs, geometric shapes, and thyroid conditions). There are schemata for concepts underlying situations, events, sequences of actions and so forth. To process information with the use of a schema is to determine which model best fits the incoming information. Schemata have constants (all birds have wings) and variables (chairs can have between one and four legs). The variables may have associated default values (e.g., birds fly) that represent the prototypical circumstance.

When a person interprets information, the schema serves as a "filter" for distinguishing relevant and irrelevant information. Schemata can be considered as generic knowledge structures that contain slots for particular kinds of propositions. For instance, a schema for myocardial infarction may contain the findings of "chest pain," "sweating," "shortness of breath," but not the finding of "goiter," which is part of the schema for thyroid disease.

The schematic and propositional representations reflect abstractions and don't necessarily preserve literal information about the external world. Imagine that you are having a conversation at the office about how to rearrange the furniture in your living room. To engage in such a conversation, one needs to be able to construct images of the objects and their spatial arrangement in the room. **Mental images** are a form of internal representation that captures perceptual information recovered from the environment. There is compelling psychological and neuropsychological evidence to suggest that mental images constitute a distinct form of mental representation (Bartolomeo 2008) Images play a particularly important role in domains of visual diagnosis such as dermatology and radiology.

Mental models are an analogue-based construct for describing how individuals form internal models of systems. Mental models are designed to answer questions such as "how does it work?" or "what will happen if I take the following action?" "Analogy" suggests that the representation explicitly shares the structure of the world it represents (e.g., a set of connected visual images of a partial road map from your home to your work destination). This is in contrast to an abstraction-based form such as propositions or schemas in which the mental structure consists of either the gist, an abstraction, or summary representation. However, like other forms of mental representation, mental models are always incomplete, imperfect and subject to the processing limitations of the cognitive system. Mental models can be derived from perception, language or from one's imagination (Payne 2003). *Running* of a model corresponds to a process of mental simulation to generate possible future states of a system from observed or hypothetical state. For example, when one initiates a Google Search, one may reasonably anticipate that system will return a list of relevant (and less than relevant) websites that correspond to the query. Mental models are a particularly useful construct in understanding human-computer interaction.

An individual's mental models provide predictive and explanatory capabilities of the function of a physical system. More often the construct has been used to characterize models that have a spatial and temporal context, as is the case in reasoning about the behavior of electrical circuits (White and Frederiksen 1990). The model can be used to simulate a process (e.g., predict the effects of network interruptions on getting cash from an ATM machine). Kaufman, Patel and Magder (1996) characterized clinicians' mental models of the cardiovascular system (specifically, cardiac output). The study characterized the development of understanding of the system as a function of expertise. The research also documented various conceptual flaws in subjects' models and how these flaws impacted subjects' predictions and explanations of physiological manifestations. Figure 4.3 illustrates the four chambers of the heart and blood flow in the pulmonary and cardiovascular systems. The claim is that clinicians and medical students have variably robust representations of the structure and function of the system. This model enables prediction and explanation of the effects of perturbations in the system on blood flow and on various clinical measures such as left ventricular ejection fraction.

Conceptual and *procedural* knowledge provide another useful way of distinguishing the functions of different forms of representation. **Conceptual knowledge** refers to one's understanding of domain-specific concepts. **Procedural knowledge** is a kind of knowing related to how to perform various activities. There are numerous technical skills in medical contexts that necessitate the acquisition of procedural knowledge. Conceptual knowledge and procedural knowledge are acquired through different learning mechanisms. Conceptual knowledge is acquired through mindful engagement with materials in a range of contexts (from reading texts to conversing with colleagues). Procedural knowledge is developed as a function of deliberate practice that results in a learning process known as *knowledge compilation* (Anderson 1983). However, the development of skills may involve a transition from a declarative or interpretive stage

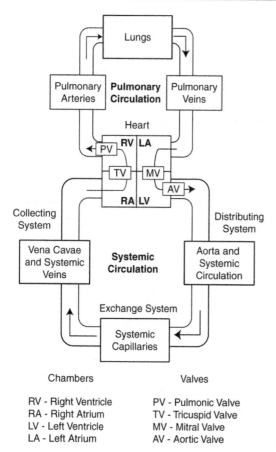

Chambers

RV - Right Ventricle
RA - Right Atrium
LV - Left Ventricle
LA - Left Atrium

Valves

PV - Pulmonic Valve
TV - Tricuspid Valve
MV - Mitral Valve
AV - Aortic Valve

Fig. 4.3 Schematic model of circulatory and cardiovascular physiology. The diagram illustrates various structures of the pulmonary and systemic circulation system and the process of blood flow. The illustration is used to exemplify the concept of mental model and how it could be applied to explaining and predicting physiologic behavior

toward increasingly proceduralized stages. For example, in learning to use an electronic health record (EHR) system designed to be used as part of a consultation, a less experienced user will need to attend carefully to every action and input, whereas, a more experienced user of this system can more effortlessly interview a patient and simultaneously record patient data (Kushniruk et al. 1996; Patel et al. 2000b). Procedural knowledge supports more efficient and automated action, but is often used without conscious awareness.

Procedural knowledge is often modeled in cognitive science and in artificial intelligence as a production *rule*, which is a condition-action rule that states "if the conditions are satisfied,

then execute the specified action" (either an inference or overt behavior). Production rules are a common method for representing knowledge in medical expert systems such as MYCIN (Davis et al. 1977).

In addition to differentiating between procedural and conceptual knowledge, one can differentiate **factual knowledge** from conceptual knowledge. Factual knowledge involves merely knowing a fact or set of facts (e.g., risk factors for heart disease) without any in-depth understanding. Facts are routinely disseminated through a range of sources such as pamphlets and websites. The acquisition of factual knowledge alone is not likely to lead to any increase in understanding or behavioral change (Bransford et al. (1999). The acquisition of conceptual knowledge involves the integration of new information with prior knowledge and necessitates a deeper level of understanding. For example, risk factors may be associated in the physician's mind with biochemical mechanisms and typical patient manifestations. This is contrast to a new medical student who may have largely factual knowledge.

Thus far, we have only considered domain-general ways of characterizing the organization of knowledge. In view to understand the nature of medical cognition, it is necessary to characterize the domain-specific nature of knowledge organization in medicine. Given the vastness and complexity of the domain of medicine, this can be a rather daunting task. Clearly, there is no single way to represent all biomedical (or even clinical) knowledge, but it is an issue of considerable importance for research in biomedical informatics. Much research has been conducted in biomedical artificial intelligence with the aim of developing biomedical ontologies for use in knowledge-based systems. Patel et al. (1997) address this issue in the context of using empirical evidence from psychological experiments on medical expertise to test the validity of the AI systems. **Biomedical taxonomies**, **nomenclatures** and **vocabulary** systems such as UMLS or SNOMED (see Chap. 7) are engaged in a similar pursuit.

We have employed an epistemological framework developed by Evans and Gadd (1989). They

Fig. 4.4 Epistemological frameworks representing the structure of medical knowledge for problem solving

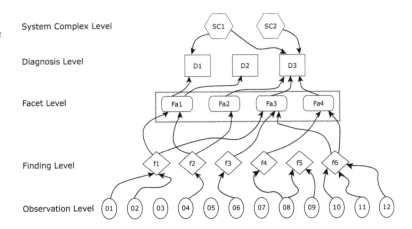

proposed a framework that serves to characterize the knowledge used for medical understanding and problem solving, and also for differentiating the levels at which biomedical knowledge may be organized. This framework represents a formalization of biomedical knowledge as realized in textbooks and journals, and can be used to provide us with insight into the organization of clinical practitioners' knowledge (see Fig. 4.4).

The framework consists of a hierarchical structure of concepts formed by *clinical observations* at the lowest level, followed by *findings*, *facets*, and *diagnoses*. Clinical observations are units of information that are recognized as potentially relevant in the problem-solving context. However, they do not constitute clinically useful facts. Findings are composed of observations that have potential clinical significance. Establishing a finding reflects a decision made by a physician that an array of data contains a significant cue or cues that need to be taken into account. Facets consist of clusters of findings that indicate an underlying medical problem or class of problems. They reflect general pathological descriptions such as left-ventricular failure or thyroid condition. Facets resemble the kinds of constructs used by researchers in medical artificial intelligence to describe the partitioning of a problem space. They are interim hypotheses that serve to divide the information in the problem into sets of manageable sub-problems and to suggest possible solutions. Facets also vary in terms of their levels of abstraction. Diagnosis is the level of classification that subsumes and explains all levels beneath it. Finally, the systems level consists of information that serves to contextualize a particular problem, such as the ethnic background of a patient.

4.4   Medical Cognition

The study of expertise is one of the principal paradigms in problem-solving research. Comparing experts to novices provides us with the opportunity to explore the aspects of performance that undergo change and result in increased problem-solving skill (Lesgold 1984; Glaser 2000). It also permits investigators to develop domain-specific models of competence that can be used for assessment and training purposes.

A goal of this approach has been to characterize expert performance in terms of the knowledge and cognitive processes used in comprehension, problem solving, and decision making, using carefully developed laboratory tasks (Chi and Glaser 1981), (Lesgold et al. 1988). deGroot's (1965) pioneering research in chess represents one of the earliest characterizations of expert-novice differences. In one of his experiments, subjects were allowed to view a chess board for 5–10 seconds and were then required to reproduce the position of the chess pieces from memory. The grandmaster chess players were able to reconstruct the mid-game positions with better than 90 % accuracy, while novice chess players could only reproduce approximately 20 % of the correct positions. When the chess pieces were placed on the board in a random configuration, not encountered in the course of a normal chess match, expert chess masters' recognition ability fell to that of novices. This result suggests that superior recognition ability is not a function of superior memory, but is a result of an enhanced ability to recognize typical situations (Chase and Simon 1973). This phenomenon is accounted for by a process known as "chunking." It is the most general representational construct that makes the fewest assumptions about cognitive processing.

It is well known that knowledge-based differences impact the problem representation and determine the strategies a subject uses to solve a problem. Simon and Simon (1978) compared a novice subject with an expert subject in solving textbook physics problems. The results indicated that the expert solved the problems in one quarter of the time required by the novice with fewer errors. The novice solved most of the problems by working *backward* from the unknown problem solution to the givens of the problem statement. The expert worked *forward* from the givens to solve the necessary equations and determine the particular quantities they are asked to solve for. Differences in the directionality of reasoning by levels of expertise has been demonstrated in diverse domains from computer programming (Perkins et al. 1990) to medical diagnoses (Patel and Groen 1986).

The expertise paradigm spans the range of content domains including physics (Larkin et al. 1980), sports (Allard and Starkes 1991), music (Sloboda 1991), and medicine (Patel et al. 1994). Edited volumes (Ericsson 2006; Chi et al. 1988 Ericsson and Smith 1991; Hoffman 1992) provide an informative general overview of the area. This research has focused on differences between subjects varying in levels of expertise in terms of memory, reasoning strategies, and in particular the role of domain specific knowledge. Among the expert's characteristics uncovered by this research are the following: (1) experts are capable of perceiving large patterns of meaningful information in their domain, which novices cannot perceive; (2) they are fast at processing and at deployment of different skills required for problem solving; (3) they have superior short-term and long-term memories for materials (e.g., clinical findings in medicine) within their domain of expertise, but not outside of it; (4) they typically represent problems in their domain at deeper, more principled levels whereas novices show a superficial level of representation; (5) they spend more time assessing the problem prior to solving it, while novices tend to spend more time working on the solution itself and little time in problem assessment; (6) individual experts may differ substantially in terms of exhibiting these kinds of performance characteristics (e.g., superior memory for domain materials).

Usually, someone is designated as an expert based on a certain level of performance, as exemplified by Elo ratings in chess; by virtue of being certified by a professional licensing body, as in medicine, law, or engineering; on the basis of academic criteria, such as graduate degrees; or simply based on years of experience or peer evaluation (Hoffman et al. 1995). The concept of an expert, however, refers to an individual who surpasses competency in a domain (Sternberg and Horvath 1999). Although competent performers, for instance, may be able to encode relevant information and generate effective plans of action in a specific domain, they often lack the speed and the flexibility that we see in an expert. A domain expert (e.g., a medical practitioner) possesses an extensive, accessible knowledge base that is organized for use in practice and is tuned to the particular problems at hand. In the study of medical expertise, it has been useful to distinguish different types of expertise.

Patel and Groen (1991a, b) distinguished between general and specific expertise, a distinction supported by research indicating differences between subexperts (i.e., experts physicians who solve a case outside their field of specialization) and experts (i.e., domain specialist) in terms of reasoning strategies and organization of knowledge. General expertise corresponds to expertise that cuts across medical subdisciplines (e.g., general medicine). Specific expertise results from detailed experience within a medical subdomain, such as cardiology or endocrinology. An individual may possess both, or only generic expertise.

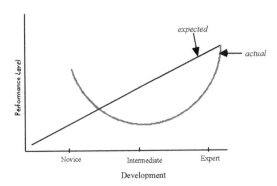

Fig. 4.5 Schematic representation of intermediate effect. The straight line gives a commonly assumed representation of performance development by level of expertise. The curved line represents the actual development from novice to expert. The Y-axis may represent any of a number of performance variables such as the number of errors made, number of concepts recalled, number of conceptual elaborations, or number of hypotheses generated in a variety of tasks

The development of expertise can follow a somewhat unusual trajectory. It is often assumed that the path from novice to expert goes through a steady process of gradual accumulation of knowledge and fine-tuning of skills. That is, as a person becomes more familiar with a domain, his or her level of performance (e.g., accuracy, quality) gradually increases. However, research has shown that this assumption is often incorrect (Lesgold et al. 1988; Patel et al. 1994). Cross-sectional studies of experts, intermediates, and novices have shown that people at intermediate levels of expertise may perform more poorly than those at lower level of expertise on some tasks. Furthermore, there is a longstanding body of research on learning that has suggested that the learning process involves phases of error-filled performance followed by periods of stable, relatively error-free performance. In other words, human learning does not consist of the gradually increasing accumulation of knowledge and fine-tuning of skills. Rather, it requires the arduous process of continually learning, re-learning, and exercising new knowledge, punctuated by periods of apparent decrease in mastery and declines in performance, which may be necessary for learning to take place. Figure 4.5 presents an illustration of this learning and developmental phenomenon known as the **intermediate effect**.

The intermediate effect has been found in a variety of tasks and with a great number of performance indicators. The tasks used include comprehension and explanation of clinical problems, doctor-patient communication, recall and explanation of laboratory data, generation of diagnostic hypotheses, and problem solving (Patel and Groen 1991a, b). The performance indicators used have included recall and inference of medical-text information, recall and inference of diagnostic hypotheses, generation of clinical findings from a patient in doctor-patient interaction, and requests for laboratory data, among others. The research has also identified developmental levels at which the intermediate phenomenon occurs, including senior medical students and residents. It is important to note, however, that in some tasks, the development is **monotonic**. For instance, in diagnostic accuracy, there is a gradual increase, with an intermediate exhibiting higher degree of accuracy than the novice and the expert demonstrating a still higher degree than the intermediate. Furthermore, when relevancy of the stimuli to a problem is taken into account, an appreciable monotonic phenomenon appears. For instance, in recall studies, novices, intermediates, and experts are assessed in terms of the total number of propositions recalled showing the typical non-monotonic effect. However, when propositions are divided in terms of their relevance to the problem (e.g., a clinical case), experts recall more relevant propositions than intermediates and novices, suggesting that intermediates have difficulty separating what is relevant from what is not.

During the periods when the intermediate effect occurs, a reorganization of knowledge and skills takes place, characterized by shifts in perspectives or a realignment or creation of goals. The intermediate effect is also partly due to the unintended changes that take place as the person reorganizes for intended changes. People at intermediate levels typically generate a great deal of irrelevant information and seem incapable of discriminating what is relevant from what is not. As compared to a novice student (Fig. 4.6), the reasoning pattern of an intermediate student shows the generation of long chains of discussion

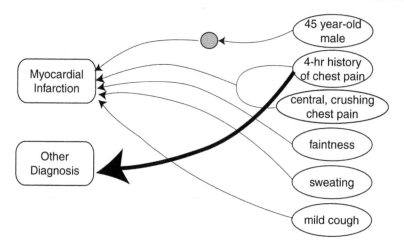

Fig. 4.6 Problem interpretations by a novice medical student. The given information from patient problem is represented on the *right side of the figure* and the new generated information is given on the *left side*, information in the box represents diagnostic hypothesis. Intermediate hypothesis are represented as *solid dark* circles (*filled*). Forward driven or data driven inference *arrows* are shown from left to right (*solid dark line*). Backward or hypothesis driven inference *arrows* are shown from right to left (*solid light line*). *Thick solid dark line* represents rule out strategy

Fig. 4.7 Problem interpretations by an intermediate medical student

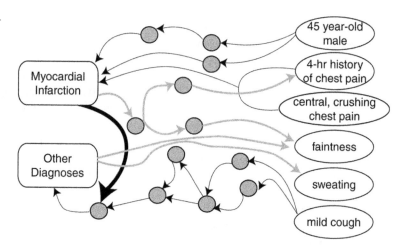

evaluating multiple hypotheses and reasoning in haphazard direction (Fig. 4.7). A well-structured knowledge structure of a senior level student leads him more directly to a solution (Fig. 4.8). Thus, the intermediate effect can be explained as a function of the learning process, maybe as a necessary phase of learning. Identifying the factors involved in the intermediate effect may help in improving performance during learning (e.g., by designing decision-support systems or intelligent tutoring systems that help the user in focusing on relevant information).

There are situations, however, in which the intermediate effect disappears. Schmidt reported that the intermediate recall phenomenon disappears when short text-reading times are used. Novices, intermediates, and experts given only a short time to read a clinical case (about thirty seconds) recalled the case with increasing accuracy. This suggests that under time-restricted

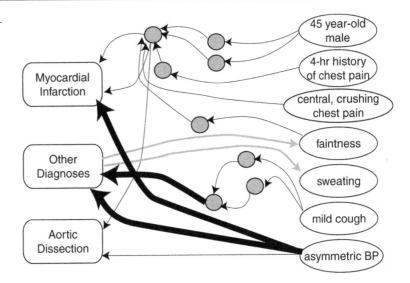

Fig. 4.8 Problem interpretations by a senior medical student

conditions, intermediates cannot engage in extraneous search. In other words, intermediates that are not under time pressure process too much irrelevant information whereas experts do not. On the other hand, novices lack the knowledge to do much searching. Although intermediates may have most of the pieces of knowledge in place, this knowledge is not sufficiently well organized to be efficiently used. Until this knowledge becomes further organized, the intermediate is more likely to engage in unnecessary search.

The intermediate effect is not a one-time phenomenon. Rather, it occurs repeatedly at strategic points in a student or physician's training and follow periods in which large bodies of new knowledge or complex skills are acquired. These periods are followed by intervals in which there is a decrement in performance until a new level of mastery is achieved.

4.4.1 Expertise in Medicine

The systematic investigation of medical expertise began more than 50 years ago with research by Ledley and Lusted (1959) into the nature of clinical inquiry. They proposed a two-stage model of clinical reasoning involving a hypothesis generation stage followed by a hypothesis evaluation stage. This latter stage is most amenable to

formal decision analytic techniques. The earliest empirical studies of medical expertise can be traced to the works of Rimoldi (1961) and Kleinmuntz (1968) who conducted experimental studies of diagnostic reasoning by contrasting students with medical experts in simulated problem-solving tasks. The results emphasized the greater ability of expert physicians to selectively attend to relevant information and narrow the set of diagnostic possibilities (i.e., consider fewer hypotheses).

The origin of contemporary research on medical thinking is associated with the seminal work of Elstein, Shulman, and Sprafka (1978) who studied the problem solving processes of physicians by drawing on then contemporary methods and theories of cognition. This model of problem solving has had a substantial influence both on studies of medical cognition and medical education. They were the first to use experimental methods and theories of cognitive science to investigate clinical competency.

Their research findings led to the development of an elaborated model of **hypothetico-deductive reasoning**, which proposed that physicians reasoned by first generating and then testing a set of hypotheses to account for clinical data (i.e., reasoning from hypothesis to data). First, physicians generated a small set of hypotheses very early in the case, as soon as the first pieces of data became available. Second, physicians were selective in the data they collected, focusing only on the relevant data. Third, physicians made use of a hypothetico-deductive method of diagnostic reasoning. The hypothetico-deductive process was viewed as consisting of four stages: cue acquisition, hypothesis generation, cue interpretation, and hypothesis evaluation. Attention to initial cues led to the rapid generation of a few select hypotheses. According to the authors, each cue was interpreted as positive, negative or non-contributory to each hypothesis generated. They were unable to find differences their diagnostic reasoning strategies between superior physicians (as judged by their peers) and other physicians (Elstein et al. 1978).

The previous research was largely modeled after early problem-solving studies in knowledge-lean tasks. Medicine is clearly a knowledge-rich domain and a different approach was needed. Feltovich, Johnson, Moller, and Swanson (1984), drawing on models of knowledge representation from medical artificial intelligence, characterized fine-grained differences in knowledge organization between subjects of different levels of expertise in the domain of pediatric cardiology. For example, novice's knowledge was described as "classically-centered", built around the prototypical instances of a disease category. The disease models were described as sparse and lacking cross-referencing between shared features of disease categories in memory. In contrast, experts' memory store of disease models was found to be extensively cross-referenced with a rich network of connections among diseases that can present with similar symptoms. These differences accounted for subjects' inferences about diagnostic cues and evaluation of competing hypotheses.

Patel and colleagues studied the knowledge-based solution strategies of expert cardiologists as evidenced by their pathophysiological explanations of a complex clinical problem (Patel and Groen 1986). The results indicated that subjects who accurately diagnosed the problem, employed a forward-oriented (data-driven) reasoning strategy—using patient data to lead toward a complete diagnosis (i.e., reasoning from data to hypothesis).

This is in contrast to subjects who misdiagnosed or partially diagnosed the patient problem. They tended to use a backward or hypothesis-driven reasoning strategy. The results of this study presented a challenge to the hypothetico-deductive model of reasoning as espoused by Elstein, Shulman, and Sprafka (1978), which did not differentiate expert from non-expert reasoning strategies.

Patel and Groen (1991a, b) investigated the nature and directionality of clinical reasoning in a range of contexts of varying complexity. The objectives of this research program were both to advance our understanding of medical expertise and to devise more effective ways of teaching clinical problem solving. It has been established that the patterns of data-driven and hypothesis-driven reasoning are used differentially by novices and experts. Experts tend to use data-driven reasoning, which depends on the physician possessing a highly organized knowledge base about the patient's disease (including sets of signs and symptoms). Because of their lack of substantive knowledge or their inability to distinguish relevant from irrelevant knowledge, novices and intermediates use more hypothesis-driven reasoning resulting often in very complex reasoning patterns. The fact that experts and novices reason differently suggests that they might reach different conclusions (e.g., decisions or understandings) when solving medical problems. Similar patterns of reasoning have been found in other domains (Larkin et al. 1980). Due to their extensive knowledge base and the high level inferences they make, experts typically skip steps in their reasoning.

Although experts typically use data-driven reasoning during clinical performance, this type of reasoning sometimes breaks down and the expert has to resort to hypothesis-driven reasoning. Although data-driven reasoning is highly efficient, it is often error prone in the absence of adequate domain knowledge, since there are no built-in checks on the legitimacy of the inferences that a person makes. Pure data-driven reasoning is only successful in constrained situations, where one's knowledge of a problem can result in a complete chain of inferences from

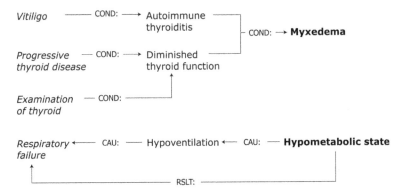

Fig. 4.9 Diagrammatic representation of data-driven (*top down*) and hypothesis-driven (*bottom-up*) reasoning. From the presence of vitiligo, a prior history of progressive thyroid disease, and examination of the thyroid (clinical findings on the *left side of figure*), the physician reasons forward to conclude the diagnosis of Myxedema (*right of figure*). However, the anomalous finding of respiratory failure, which is inconsistent with the main diagnosis, is accounted for as a result of a hypometabolic state of the patient, in a backward-directed fashion. *COND* refers to a conditional relation, *CAU* indicates a causal relation, and *RSLT* identifies a resultive relation

the initial problem statement to the problem solution, as illustrated in Fig. 4.9. In contrast, hypothesis-driven reasoning is slower and may make heavy demands on working memory, because one has to keep track of such things as goals and hypotheses. It is, therefore, most likely to be used when domain knowledge is inadequate or the problem is complex. Hypothesis-driven reasoning is usually exemplary of a *weak method* of problem solving in the sense that is used in the absence of relevant prior knowledge and when there is uncertainty about problem solution. In problem-solving terms, strong methods engage knowledge whereas weak methods refer to general strategies. Weak does not necessarily imply ineffectual in this context.

Studies have shown that the pattern of data-driven reasoning breaks down in conditions of case complexity, unfamiliarity with the problem, and uncertainty (Patel et al. 1990). These conditions include the presence of "loose ends" in explanations, where some particular piece of information remains unaccounted for and isolated from the overall explanation. Loose ends trigger explanatory processes that work by hypothesizing a disease, for instance, and trying to fit the loose ends within it, in a hypothesis-driven reasoning fashion. The presence of loose ends may foster learning, as the person searches for an explanation for them. For instance, a medical student or

a physician may encounter a sign or a symptom in a patient problem and look for information that may account for the finding by searching for similar cases seen in the past, reading a specialized medical book, or consulting a domain expert.

However, in some circumstances, the use of data-driven reasoning may lead to a heavy cognitive load. For instance, when students are given problems to solve while training in the use of problem solving strategies, the situation produces a heavy load on cognitive resources and may diminish students' ability to focus on the task. The reason is that students have to share cognitive resources (e.g., attention, memory) between learning to solve the problem-solving method and learning the content of the material. It has been found that when subjects used a strategy based on the use of data-driven reasoning, they were more able to acquire a schema for the problem. In addition, other characteristics associated with expert performance were observed, such as a reduced number of moves to the solution. However, when subjects used a hypothesis-driven reasoning strategy, their problem solving performance suffered (Patel et al. 1990).

Visual diagnosis has also been an active area of inquiry in medical cognition. Studies have investigated clinicians at varying levels of expertise in their ability to diagnose skin lesions presented on a slide. The results revealed a monotonic increase in accuracy as a function of expertise. In a classification task, novices categorized lesions by their surface features (e.g., "scaly lesions"), intermediates grouped the slides according to diagnosis and expert dermatologists organized the slides according to superordinate categories, such as viral infections, that reflected the underlying pathophysiological structure.

The ability to abstract the underlying principles of a problem is considered to be one of the hallmarks of expertise, both in medical problem solving and in other domains (Chi and Glaser 1981). Lesgold et al. (1988) investigated the abilities of radiologists at different levels of expertise, in the interpretation of chest x-ray pictures. The results revealed that the experts were able to rapidly invoke the appropriate schema and initially detect a general pattern of disease, which resulted in a gross anatomical localization and served to constrain the possible interpretations. Novices experienced greater difficulty focusing in on the important structures and were more likely to maintain inappropriate interpretations despite discrepant findings in the patient history.

Crowley, Naus, Stewart, and Friedman (2003) employed a similar protocol-analytic approach to the Lesgold study to examine differences in expertise in breast pathology. The results suggests systematic differences between subjects at varying levels of expertise corresponding to accuracy of diagnosis, and all aspects of task performance including microscopic search, feature detection, feature identification and data interpretation. The authors propose a model of visual diagnostic competence that involves development of effective search strategies, fast and accurate recognition of anatomic location, acquisition of visual data interpretation skills and explicit feature identification strategies that results from a well-organized knowledge base.

The study of medical cognition has been summarized in a series of articles (Patel et al. 1994) and edited volumes (e.g., Evans and Patel 1989). Other active areas of research include medical text comprehension, therapeutic reasoning and mental models of physiological systems. Medical cognition remains an active area of research and continues to inform debates regarding medical curricula and approaches to learning (Patel et al. 2005; Schmidt and Rikers 2007).

4.5 Human Computer Interaction

Human computer interaction (HCI) is a multifaceted discipline devoted to the study and practice of design and usability (Carroll 2003). The history of computing and more generally, the history of artifacts design, are rife with stories of dazzlingly powerful devices with remarkable capabilities that are thoroughly unusable by anyone except for the team of designers and their immediate families. In the Psychology of Everyday Things, Norman (1988) describes a litany of poorly designed artifacts ranging from programmable VCRs to answering machines and water faucets that are inherently non-intuitive and very difficult to use. Similarly, there have been numerous innovative and promising medical information technologies that have yielded decidedly suboptimal results and deep user dissatisfaction when implemented in practice. At minimum, difficult interfaces result in steep learning curves and structural inefficiencies in task performance. At worst, problematic interfaces can have serious consequences for patient safety (Lin et al. 1998; Zhang et al. 2004; Koppel et al. 2005) (see Chap. 11).

Twenty years ago, Nielsen (1993) reported that around 50 % of software code was devoted to the user interface and a survey of developers indicated that, on average, 6 % of their project budgets were spent on usability evaluation. Given the ubiquitous presence of graphical user interfaces (GUI), it is likely that more than 50 % of code is now devoted to the GUI. On the other hand, usability evaluations have greatly increased over the course of the last 10 years (Jaspers 2009). There have been numerous texts devoted to promoting effective user interface design (Preece et al. 2007; Shneiderman 1998) and the importance of enhancing the user experience has been widely acknowledged by both consumers and producers of information technology (see Chap. 11). Part of the impetus is that usability has been demonstrated to be highly cost effective. Karat (1994) reported that for every dollar a company invests in the usability of a product, it receives between $10 and $100 in benefits. Although much has changed in the world of computing since Karat's estimate (e.g., the flourishing of the World Wide Web), it is very clear that investments in usability still yield substantial rates of return (Nielsen et al. 2008). It remains far more costly to fix a problem after product release than in an early design phase. In our view, usability evaluation of medical information technologies has grown substantially in prominence. The concept of usability as well as the methods and tools to measure and promote it are now "touchstones in the culture of computing" (Carroll 2003).

Usability methods have been used to evaluate a wide range of medical information technologies including infusion pumps (Dansky et al. 2001), ventilator management systems, physician order entry (Ash et al. 2003a; Koppel et al. 2005), pulmonary graph displays (Wachter et al. 2003), information retrieval systems, and research web environments for clinicians (Elkin et al. 2002). In addition, usability techniques are increasingly used to assess patient-centered environments (Cimino et al. 2000; Kaufman et al. 2003; Chan and Kaufman 2011). The methods include observations, focus groups, surveys and experiments. Collectively, these studies make a compelling case for the instrumental value of such research to improve efficiency, user acceptance and relatively seamless integration with current workflow and practices.

What do we mean by usability? Nielsen (1993) suggests that usability includes the following five attributes: (1) *learnability*: system should be relatively easy to learn, (2) *efficiency*: an experienced user can attain a high level of productivity, (3) *memorability*: features supported by the system should be easy to retain once learned, (4) *errors*: system should be designed to minimize errors and support error detection and recovery, and (5) *satisfaction*: the user experience should be subjectively satisfying.

Even with growth of usability research, there remain formidable challenges to designing and developing usable systems. This is exemplified by the events at Cedar Sinai Medical Center in which a decision was made to suspend use of a computer-based physician order entry system just a few months after implementation. Physicians complained that the system, which was designed to reduce medical errors, compromised patient safety, took too much time and was difficult to use (Benko 2003). To provide another example, we have been working with a mental health computer-based patient record system that is rather comprehensive and supports a wide range of functions and user populations (e.g., physicians, nurses, and administrative staff). However, clinicians find it exceptionally difficult and time-consuming to use. The interface is based on a form (or template) metaphor and is neither user- nor task-centered. The interface emphasizes completeness of data entry for administrative purposes rather than the facilitation of clinical communication and is not optimally designed to support patient care (e.g., efficient information retrieval and useful summary reports). In general, the capabilities of this system are not readily usefully deployed to improve human performance. We further discuss issues of EHRs in a subsequent section.

Innovations in technology guarantee that usability and interface design will be a perpetually moving target. In addition, as health information technology reaches out to populations across the digital divide (e.g., seniors and low literacy patient populations), there is a need to consider new interface requirements. Although evaluation methodologies and guidelines for design yield significant contributions, there is a need for a scientific framework to understand the nature of user interactions. **Human computer interaction** (HCI) is a multifaceted discipline devoted to the study and practice of usability. HCI has emerged as a central area of both computer science, development and applied social science research (Carroll 2003).

HCI has spawned a professional orientation that focuses on practical matters concerning the integration and evaluation of applications of technology to support human activities. There are also active academic HCI communities that have contributed significant advances to the science of computing. HCI researchers have been devoted to the development of innovative design concepts such as **virtual reality, ubiquitous computing, multimodal interfaces, collaborative workspaces**, and **immersive environments**. HCI research has been instrumental in transforming the software engineering process towards a more user-centered iterative system development (e.g., rapid prototyping). HCI research has also been focally concerned with the cognitive, social, and cultural dimensions of the computing experience. In this regard, it is concerned with developing analytic frameworks for characterizing how technologies can be used more productively across a range of tasks, settings, and user populations.

Carroll (1997) traces the history of HCI back to the 1970s with the advent of **software psychology**, a behavioral approach to understanding and furthering software design. Human factors, ergonomics, and industrial engineering research were pursuing some of the same goals along parallel tracks. In the early 1980s, Card et al. (1983) envisioned HCI as a test bed for applying cognitive science research and also furthering theoretical development in cognitive science. The Goals, Operators, Methods, and Selection Rules (GOMS) approach to modeling was a direct outgrowth of this initiative. GOMS is a powerful predictive tool, but it is limited in scope to the analysis of routine skills and expert performance. Most medical information technologies such as provider-order entry systems, engage complex cognitive skills.

HCI research has embraced a diversity of approaches with an abundance of new theoretical frameworks, design concepts, and analytical foci (Rogers 2004). Although we view this as an exciting development, it has also contributed to a certain scientific fragmentation (Carroll 2003). Our own research is grounded in a cognitive engineering framework, which is an interdisciplinary approach to the development of principles, methods and tools to assess and guide the design of computerized systems to support human performance (Roth et al. 2002). In supporting performance, the focus is on cognitive functions such as attention, perception, memory, comprehension, problem solving, and decision making. The approach is centrally concerned with the analysis of cognitive tasks and

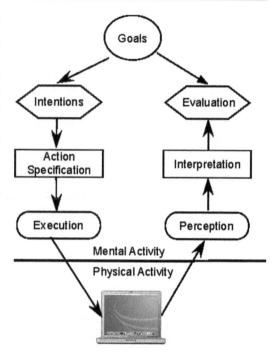

Fig. 4.10 Norman's seven stage model of action

the processing constraints imposed by the human cognitive system.

Models of **cognitive engineering** are typically predicated on a cyclical pattern of interaction with a system. This pattern is embodied in Norman's (1986) seven stage model of action, illustrated in Fig. 4.10. The action cycle begins with a *goal*, for example, retrieving a patient's medical record. The goal is abstract and independent of any system. In this context, let's presuppose that the clinician has access to both a paper record and an electronic record. The second stage involves the formation of an *intention*, which in this case might be to retrieve the record online. The intention leads to the *specification of an action* sequence, which may include logging onto the system (which in itself may necessitate several actions), engaging a search facility to retrieve information, and entering the patient's medical record number or some other identifying information. The specification results in *executing an action*, which may necessitate several behaviors. The system responds in some fashion (or doesn't respond at all). The user may or may not perceive a change in system state (e.g., system provides no indicators of a wait state). The perceived system response must then be *interpreted* and *evaluated* to determine whether the goal has been achieved. This will then determine whether the user has been successful or whether an alternative course of action is necessary.

A complex task will involve substantial nesting of subgoals, involving a series of actions that are necessary before the primary goal can be achieved. To an experienced user, the action cycle may appear to be completely seamless. However to a novice user, the process may break down at any of the seven stages. There are two primary means in which the action cycle can break down. The *gulf of execution* reflects the difference between the goals and intentions of the user and the kinds of actions enabled by the system. A user may not know the appropriate action sequence or the interface may not provide the prerequisite features to make such sequences transparent. For example, many systems require a goal completion action, such as pressing "Enter", after the primary selection had been made. This is a source of confusion, especially for novice users. The *gulf of evaluation* reflects the degree to which the user can interpret the state of the system and determine how well their expectations have been met. For example, it is sometimes difficult to interpret a state transition and determine whether one has arrived at the right place. Goals that necessitate multiple state or screen transitions are more likely to present difficulties for users, especially as they learn the system. Bridging gulfs involves both bringing about changes to the system design and educating users to foster competencies that can be used to make better use of system resources.

Gulfs are partially attributable to differences in the designer's model and the users' mental models. The designer's model is the conceptual model of intent of the system, partially based on an estimation of the user population and task requirements (Norman 1986). The users' mental models of system behavior are developed through interacting with similar systems and gaining an understanding of how actions (e.g., clicking on a link) will produce predictable and desired outcomes. Graphical user interfaces that involve direct manipulation of screen objects represent an attempt to reduce the distance between a designer's and users' model. The distance is more difficult to close in a system of greater complexity that incorporates a wide range of functions, like many medical information technologies.

Norman's theory of action has given rise to (or in some case reinforced) the need for sound design principles. For example, the state of a system should be plainly *visible* to the user. There is a need to provide good mappings between the actions (e.g., clicking on a button) and the results of the actions as reflected in the state of the system (e.g., screen transitions). Similarly, a well-designed system will provide full and continuous feedback so that the user can understand whether one's expectations have been met.

The model has also informed a range of cognitive task-analytic usability evaluation methods such as the cognitive walkthrough (Polson et al. 1992), described below. The study of human performance is predicated on an analysis of both the information-processing demands of a task and the kinds of domain-specific knowledge required performing it. This analysis is often referred to as **cognitive task analysis**. The principles and methods that inform this approach can be applied to a wide range of tasks, from the analysis of written guidelines to the investigation of EHR systems. Generic tasks necessitate similar cognitive demands and have a common underlying structure that involves similar kinds of reasoning and patterns of inference. For example, clinical tasks in medicine include diagnostic reasoning, therapeutic reasoning, and patient monitoring and management. Similarly, an admission order-entry task can be completed using written orders or one of many diverse computer-based order-entry systems. The underlying task of communicating orders in view to admit a patient remains the same. However, the particular implementation will greatly impact the performance of the task. For example, a system may eliminate the need for redundant entries and greatly facilitate the process. On the other hand, it may introduce unnecessary complexity leading to suboptimal performance.

These are a class of usability evaluation methods performed by expert analysts or reviewers and unlike usability testing, don't typically involve the use of subjects (Nielsen 1994)). The **cognitive walkthrough** (CW) and the heuristic evaluation are the most commonly used inspection methods. **Heuristic evaluation** (HE) is a method by which an application is evaluated on the basis of a small set of well-tested design principles such as visibility of system status, user control and freedom, consistency and standards, flexibility and efficiency of use (Nielsen 1993). We illustrate HE in the context of a human factors study later in the chapter. The CW is a cognitive task analytic method that has been applied to the study of usability and learnability of several distinct medical information technologies (Kushniruk et al. 1996). The purpose of a CW is to characterize the cognitive processes of users performing a task. The method involves identifying sequences of actions and goals needed to accomplish a given task. The specific aims of the procedure are to determine whether the typical user's background knowledge and the cues generated by the interface are likely to be sufficient to produce the correct goal-action sequence required to perform a task. The method is intended to identify potential usability problems that may impede the successful completion of a task or introduce complexity in a way that may frustrate real users. The method is performed by an analyst or group of analysts 'walking through' the sequence of actions necessary to achieve a goal. Both behavioral or physical actions such as mouse clicks and cognitive actions (e.g., inference needed to carry out a physical action) are coded. The principal assumption underlying this method is that a given task has a specifiable goal-action structure (i.e., the ways in which a user's objectives can be translated into specific actions). As in Norman's model, each action results in a system response (or absence of one), which is duly noted.

The CW method assumes a cyclical pattern of interaction as described previously. The codes for analysis include *goals,* which can be decomposed into a series of *subgoals* and *actions.* For example, opening an Excel spreadsheet (goal) may involve locating an icon or shortcut on one's desktop (subgoal) and double clicking on the application (action). The system response (e.g.,

change in screen, update of values) is also characterized and an attempt is made to discern potential problems. This is illustrated below in a partial walkthrough of an individual obtaining money from an automated teller system.

Goal: Obtain $80 Cash from Checking Account

1. **Action:** Enter Card (Screen 1)

System response: Enter PIN > (Screen 2)

2. **Subgoal:** Interpret prompt and provide input
3. **Action:** Enter "Pin" on Numeric keypad
4. **Action:** Hit Enter (press lower white button next to screen)

System response: "Do you Want a Printed Transaction Record".

Binary Option: Yes or No (Screen 3)

5. **Subgoal:** Decide whether a printed record is necessary
6. **Action:** Press Button Next to No Response

System response: Select Transaction-8 Choices (Screen 4)

7. **Subgoal:** Choose Between Quick Cash and Cash Withdrawal
8. **Action:** Press Button Next to Cash Withdrawal

System response: Select Account (Screen 5)

9. **Action:** Press Button Next to Checking

System response: Enter Dollar Amounts in Multiples of 20 (Screen 6)

10. **Action:** Enter $80 on Numeric Key Pad
11. **Action:** Select Correct

The walkthrough of the ATM reveals that process of obtaining money from the ATM necessitated a minimum of eight actions, five goals and subgoals, and six screen transitions. In general, it is desirable to minimize the number of actions necessary to complete a task. In addition, multiple screen transitions are more likely to confuse the user. We have employed a similar approach to analyze the complexity of a range of medical information technologies including EHRs, a home telecare system, and infusion pumps used in intensive care settings. The CW process emphasizes the sequential process, not unlike problem solving, involved in completing a computer-based task. The focus is more on the process rather than the content of the displays.

Usability testing represents the gold standard in usability evaluation methods. It refers to a class of methods for collecting empirical data of representative users performing representative tasks. It is known to capture a higher percentage of the more serious usability problems and provides a greater depth of understanding into the nature of the interaction (Jaspers 2009). Usability testing commonly employs video capture of users performing the tasks as well as video-analytic methods of analysis (Kaufman et al. 2003; Kaufman et al. 2009). It involves in-depth testing of a small number of subjects. The assumption is that a test can be perfectly valid with as few as five or six subjects. In addition, five or six subjects may find upwards of 80 % of the usability problems. A typical usability testing study will involve five to ten subjects who are asked to think aloud as they perform the task.

It's not uncommon to employ multiple methods such as the cognitive walkthrough and usability testing (Beuscart-Zephir et al. 2005a, b). The methods are complementary and serve as a means to triangulate significant findings. Kaufman et al. (2003) conducted a cognitive evaluation of the IDEATel home telemedicine system (Shea et al. 2002; 2009); Starren et al. 2002; Weinstock et al. 2010) with a particular focus on a) system usability and learnability, and b) the core competencies, skills and knowledge necessary to productively use the system. The study employed both a cognitive walkthrough and in-depth usability testing. The focal point of the intervention was the home telemedicine unit (HTU), which provided the following functions: (1) synchronous video-conferencing with a nurse case manager, (2) electronic transmission of fingerstick glucose and blood pressure readings, (3) email to a physician and nurse case manager, (4) review of one's clinical data and (5) access to Web-based educational materials (see Chap. 18 for more details on IDEATel). The usability study revealed dimensions of the interface that impeded optimal access to system resources. In addition, significant obstacles corresponding to perceptual-motor skills, mental models of the system, and health literacy were documented.

4.6 Human Factors Research and Patient Safety

Human error in medicine, and the adverse events which may follow, are problems of psychology and engineering not of medicine "(Senders, 1993)" (cited in (Woods et al. 2007).

Human factors research is a discipline devoted to the study of technology systems and how people work with them or are impacted by these technologies (Henriksen 2010). Human factors research discovers and applies information about human behavior, abilities, limitations, and other characteristics to the design of tools, machines, systems, tasks, and jobs, and environments for productive, safe, comfortable, and effective human use (Chapanis 1996). In the context of healthcare, human factors is concerned with the full complement of technologies and systems used by a diverse range of individuals including clinicians, hospital administrators, health consumers and patients (Flin and Patey 2009). Human factors work approaches the study of health practices from several perspectives or levels of analysis. The focus is on the ways in which organizational, cultural, and policy issues inform and shape healthcare processes. A full exposition of human factors in medicine is beyond the scope of this chapter. For a detailed treatment of these issues, the reader is referred to the Handbook of Human Factors and Ergonomics in Health Care and Patient Safety (Carayon 2007). The focus in this chapter is on cognitive work in human factors and healthcare, particularly in relation to issues having to do with patient safety. We recognize that patient safety is a systemic challenge at a multiple levels of aggregation beyond the individual. It is clear that understanding, predicting and transforming human performance in any complex setting requires a detailed understanding of both the setting and the factors that influence performance (Woods et al. 2007).

Our objective in this section is to introduce a theoretical foundation, establish important concepts and discuss illustrative research in **patient safety**. Human factors and human computer

interaction are different disciplines with different histories and different professional and
academic societies. HCI is more focused on computing and cutting-edge design and technology,
whereas human factors focus on a broad range
of systems that include, but are not restricted to
computing technologies (Carayon 2007). Patient
safety is one of the central issues in human factors research and we address this issue in greater
detail in a subsequent section. Both human factors and HCI employ many of the same methods
of evaluation and both strongly emphasize a
user-centered approach to design and a systems-
centered approach to the study of technology use.
Researchers and professionals in both domains
draw on certain theories including cognitive
engineering. The categorization of information
technology-based work as either human factors
or HCI is sometimes capricious.

The field of human factors is guided by principles of engineering and applied cognitive psychology (Chapanis 1996). Human factors analysis
applies knowledge about the strengths and limitations of humans to the design of interactive
systems, equipment, and their environment. The
objective is to ensure their effectiveness, safety,
and ease of use. Mental models and issues of
decision making are central to human factors
analysis. Any system will be easier and less burdensome to use to the extent that that it is co-
extensive with users' mental models. Human
factors focus on different dimensions of cognitive capacity, including memory, attention, and
workload. Our perceptual system inundates us
with more stimuli than our cognitive systems can
possibly process. Attentional mechanisms enable
us to selectively prioritize and attend to certain
stimuli and attenuate other ones. They also have
the property of being sharable, which enables us
to multitask by dividing our attention between
two activities. For example, if we are driving on a
highway, we can easily have a conversation with
a passenger at the same time. However, as the
skies get dark or the weather changes or suddenly
you find yourself driving through winding moun-
tainous roads, you will have to allocate more of
your attentional resources to driving and less to
the conversation.

Human factors research leverages theories and
methods from cognitive engineering to characterize human performance in complex settings and
challenging situations in aviation, industrial process control, military command control and space
operations (Woods et al. 2007). The research has
elucidated empirical regularities and provides
explanatory concepts and models of human performance. This enables us to discern common
underlying patterns in seemingly disparate
settings (Woods et al. 2007).

4.6.1 Patient Safety

When human error is viewed as a cause rather than
a consequence, it serves as a cloak for our ignorance. By serving as an end point rather than a
starting point, it retards further understanding.
(Henriksen 2008)

Patient safety refers to the prevention of healthcare errors, and the elimination or mitigation of
patient injury caused by healthcare errors (Patel
and Zhang 2007). It has been an issue of considerable concern for the past quarter century, but
the greater community was galvanized by the
Institute of Medicine Report, "To Err is Human,"
released in 1999. This report communicated the
surprising fact that 98,000 preventable deaths
every single year in the United States are attributable to human error, which makes it the 8th leading cause of death in this country. Although one
may argue over the specific numbers, there is no
disputing that too many patients are harmed or
die every year as a result of human actions or
absence of action.

The Harvard Medical Practice Study was published several years prior to the IOM report and
was a landmark study at the time. Based on an
extensive review of patient charts in New York
State, they were able to determine that an adverse
event occurred in almost 4 % of the cases (Leape
et al. 1991). An adverse event refers to any unfavorable change in health or side effect that occurs
in a patient who is receiving the treatment. They
further determined that almost 70 % of these
adverse events were caused by errors and 25 % of
all errors were due to negligence.

We can only analyze errors after they happened and they often seem to be glaring blunders after the fact. This leads to assignment of blame or search for a single cause of the error. However, in hindsight, it is exceedingly difficult to recreate the situational context, stress, shifting attention demands and competing goals that characterized a situation prior to the occurrence of an error. This sort of retrospective analysis is subject to hindsight bias. **Hindsight bias** masks the dilemmas, uncertainties, demands and other latent conditions that were operative prior to the mishap. Too often the term 'human error' connotes blame and a search for the guilty culprits, suggesting some sort of human deficiency or irresponsible behavior. Human factors researchers recognized that this approach error is inherently incomplete and potentially misleading. They argue for the need for a more comprehensive systems-centered approach that recognizes that error could be attributed to a multitude of factors as well as the interaction of these factors. Error is the failure of a planned sequence of mental or physical activities to achieve its intended outcome when these failures cannot be attributed to chance (Arocha et al. 2005; Reason 1990). Reason (1990) introduced an important distinction between **latent** and **active failures**. Active failure represents the face of error. The effects of active failure are immediately felt. In healthcare, active errors are committed by providers such as nurses, physicians, or pharmacists who are actively responding to patient needs at the "sharp end". The latent conditions are less visible, but equally important. Latent conditions are enduring systemic problems that may not be evident for some time, combine with other system problems to weaken the system's defenses and make errors possible. There is a lengthy list of potential latent conditions including poor interface design of important technologies, communication breakdown between key actors, gaps in supervision, inadequate training, and absence of a safety culture in the workplace—a culture that emphasizes safe practices and the reporting of any conditions that are potentially dangerous.

Zhang, Patel, Johnson, and Shortliffe (2004) have developed a taxonomy of errors partially based on the distinctions proposed by Reason (1990). We can further classify errors in terms of **slips** and **mistakes** (Reason 1990). A slip occurs when the actor selected the appropriate course of action, but it was executed inappropriately. A mistake involves an inappropriate course of action reflecting an erroneous judgment or inference (e.g., a wrong diagnosis or misreading of an x-ray). Mistakes may either be knowledge-based owing to factors such as incorrect knowledge or they may be rule-based, in which case the correct knowledge was available, but there was a problem in applying the rules or guidelines. They further characterize medical errors as a progression of events. There is a period of time when everything is operating smoothly. Then an unsafe practice unfolds resulting in a kind of error, but not necessarily leading to an adverse event. For example, if there is a system of checks and balances that is part of routine practice or if there is systematic supervisory process in place, the vast majority of errors will be trapped and defused in this middle zone. If these measures or practices are not in place, an error can propagate and cross the boundary to become an adverse event. At this point, the patient has been harmed. In addition, if an individual is subject to a heavy workload or intense time pressure, then that will increase the potential for an error, resulting in an adverse event.

The notion that human error should not be tolerated is prevalent in both the public and personal perception of the performance of most clinicians. However, researchers in other safety-critical domains have long since abandoned the quest for zero defect, citing it as an impractical goal, and choosing to focus instead on the development of strategies to enhance the ability to recover from error (Morel et al. 2008). Patel and her colleagues conducted empirical investigations into error detection and recovery by experts (attending physicians) and non-experts (resident trainees) in the critical care domain, using both laboratory-based and naturalistic approaches (Patel et al. 2011). These studies show that expertise is more closely tied to ability to detect and recover from errors and not so much to the ability not to make errors. The study results show that both the experts and non-experts are prone to commit and recover from errors, but experts' ability to detect and recover from knowledge based errors is better than that of trainees. Error detection and correction in complex real-time critical care situations appears to induce certain urgency for quick action in a high alert condition, resulting in rapid detection and correction. Studies on expertise and understanding of the limits and failures of human decision-making are important if we are to build robust decision-support systems to manage the boundaries of risk of error in decision making (Patel and Cohen 2008).

There has been a wealth of studies regarding patient safety and medical errors in a range of contexts. Holden and Karsh (2007) argue that much of the work is atheoretical in nature and that this diminishes the potential generalizability of the lessons learned. They propose a multifaceted theoretical framework incorporating theories from different spheres of research including motivation, decision-making, and social-cognition. They also draw on a sociotechnical approach, which is a perspective that interweaves technology, people, and the social context of interaction for the design of systems. The end result is a model that can be applied to health information technology usage behavior and that guides a set of principles for design and implementation. The authors propose that through iterative testing of the model, the efforts of researchers and practitioners will yield greater success in the understanding, design, and implementation of health information technology.

4.6.2 Unintended Consequences

It is widely believed that health information technologies have the potential to transform healthcare in a multitude of ways including the reduction of errors. However, it is increasingly apparent that technology-induced errors are deeply consequential and have had deleterious consequences for patient safety. Ash, Stavri, and Kuperman (2003b) were among the first to give voice to this problem in the informatics community. They also endeavored to describe and enumerate the primary kinds of errors caused by health information systems, those related to entering and retrieving information and those related to communication and coordination. The authors characterize several problems that are not typically found in usability studies. For example, many interfaces are not suitable for settings that are highly interruptive (e.g., a cluttered display with too many options). They also characterize a problem in which an information entry screen that is highly structured and requires completeness of entry can cause cognitive overload.

Medical devices include any healthcare product, excluding drugs, that are used for the purpose of prevention, diagnosis, monitoring, treatment or alleviation of an illness (Ward and Clarkson 2007). There is considerable evidence that suggests that medical devices can also cause substantial harm (Jha et al. 2010). It has been reported that more than one million adverse medical device events occur annually in the United States (Bright and Brown 2007). Although medical devices are an integral part of medical care in hospital settings, they are complex in nature and clinicians often do not receive adequate training (Woods et al. 2007). In addition, many medical devices such as such as smart infusion pumps, patient controlled analgesia (PCA) devices, and bar coded medication administration systems have been partially automated and offer a complex programmable interface (Beuscart-Zephir et al. 2005a, 2007). Although this affords opportunities to facilitate clinical care and medical decision making, it may add layers of complexity and uncertainty.

There is evidence to suggest that a poorly designed user interface can present substantial challenges even for the well-trained and highly skilled user (Zhang et al. 2003). Lin and colleagues (1998) conducted a series of studies on a patient controlled analgesic or PCA device, a method of pain relief that uses disposable or electronic infusion devices and allows patients to self-administer analgesic drugs as required. The device is programmed by a nurse or technician and this limits the maximum level of drug administration to keep the dose within safe levels. Lin and colleagues investigated the effects of two interfaces to a commonly used PCA device including the original interface. Based on a **cognitive task analysis**, they redesigned the original interface so that it was more in line with sound human factors principles. As described previously, cognitive task analysis is a method that breaks a task into sets of subtasks or steps (e.g., a single action), the system responses (e.g., changes in the display as a result of an action) and inferences that are needed to interpret the state of the system. It is an effective gauge of the complexity of a system. For example, a simple task that necessitates 25 steps or more to complete using a given system is likely to be unnecessarily complex. On the basis of the cognitive task analysis, they found the existing PCA interface to be problematic in several different ways. For example, the structure of many subtasks in the programming sequence was unnecessarily complex. There was a lack of information available on the screen to provide meaningful feedback and to structure the user experience (e.g., negotiating the next steps). For example, a nurse would not know that he or she was on the third of five screens or when they were half way through the task.

On the basis of the CTA analysis, Lin and colleagues (1998) also redesigned the interface according to sound human factors principles. The new system was designed to simplify the entire process and provide more consistent feedback. It's important to note that the revised screen was a computer simulation and was not actually implemented in the physical device. They conducted a cognitive study with 12 nurses comparing simulations of the old and new interface. They found that programming the new interface was 15 % faster. The average workload rating for the old interface was twice as high. The new interface led to 10 errors as compared to 20 for the old one. This is a compelling demonstration that medical equipment can be made safer and more efficient by adopting sound human factors design principles.

This methodology embodies a particular philosophy that emphasizes simplicity and functionality over intricacy of design and presentation.

Zhang and colleagues employed a modified heuristic evaluation method (see section 4.5, above) to test the safety of two infusion pumps (Zhang et al. 2003). On the basis of an analysis by 4 evaluators, a total of 192 violations with the user interface design were documented. Consistency and visibility (the ease in which a user can discern the system state) were the most widely documented violations. Several of the violations were classified as problems of substantial severity. Their results suggested that one of the two pumps was likely to induce more medical errors than the other ones.

It is clear that usability problems are consequential and have the potential to impact patient safety. Kushniruk et al. (2005) examined the relationship between particular kinds of usability problems and errors in a handheld prescription writing application. They found that particular usability problems were associated with the occurrence of error in entering medication. For example, the problem of inappropriate default values automatically populating the screen was found to be correlated with errors in entering wrong dosages of medications. In addition, certain types of errors were associated with mistakes (not detected by users) while others were associated with slips pertaining to unintentional errors. Horsky et al. (2005) analyzed a problematic medication order placed using a CPOE system that resulted in an overdose of potassium chloride being administered to an actual patient. The authors used a range of investigative methods including inspection of system logs, semi-structured interviews, examination of the electronic health record, and cognitive evaluation of the order entry system involved. They found that the error was due to a confluence of factors including problems associated with the display, the labeling of functions and ambiguous dating of the dates in which a medication was administered. The poor interface design did not provide assistance with the decision-making process, and in fact, its design served as a hindrance, where the interface was a poor fit for the *conceptual operators* utilized by clinicians when calculating medication dosage (i.e., based on volume not duration).

Koppel and colleagues (2005) published an influential study examining the ways in which computer-provider order-entry systems (CPOE) facilitated medical errors. The study, which was published in JAMA (Journal of the American Medical Association), used a series of methods including interviews with clinicians, observations and a survey to document the range of errors. According to the authors, the system facilitated 22 types of medication error and many of them occurred with some frequency. The errors were classified into two broad categories: (1) information errors generated by fragmentation of data and failure to integrate the hospital's information systems and (2) human-machine interface flaws reflecting machine rules that do not correspond to work organization or usual behaviors.

It is a well-known phenomenon that users come to rely on technology and often treat it as an authoritative source that can be implicitly trusted. This can result in information/fragmentation errors. In this case, clinicians relied on CPOE displays to determine the minimum effective dose or a routine dose for a particular kind of patient. However, there was a discrepancy between their expectations and the dose listing. The dosages listed on the display were based on the pharmacy's warehousing and not on clinical guidelines. For example, although normal dosages are 20 or 30 mg, the pharmacy might stock only 10-mg doses, so 10-mg units are displayed on the CPOE screen. Clinicians mistakenly assumed that this was the minimal dose. Medication discontinuation failures are a commonly documented problem with CPOE systems. The system expects a clinician to (1) order new medications and (2) cancel existing orders that are no longer operative. Frequently, clinicians fail to cancel the existing orders leading to duplicative medication orders and thereby increasing the possibility of medical errors. Perhaps, a reminder that prior orders exist and may need to be canceled may serve to mitigate this problem.

As is the case with other clinical information systems, CPOE systems suffer from a range of usability problems. The study describes three kinds of problems. When selecting a patient, it is relatively easy to select the wrong patient because names and drugs are close together, the font is small, and, patients' names do not appear on all screens. On a similar note, physicians can order medications at computer terminals not yet "logged out" by the previous physician. This can result in either unintended patients receiving medication or patients not receiving the intended medication. When patients undergo surgery, the CPOE system cancels their previous medications. Physicians must reenter CPOE and reactivate each previously ordered medication. Once again, a reminder to do so may serve to reduce the frequency of such mistakes.

The growing body of research on unintended consequences spurred the American Medical Informatics Association to devote a policy meeting to consider ways to understand and diminish their impact (Bloomrosen et al. 2011). The matter is especially pressing given the increased implementation of health information technologies nationwide including ambulatory care practices that have little experience with health information technologies. The authors outline a series of recommendations, including a need for more cognitively-oriented research to guide study of the causes and mitigation of unintended consequences resulting from health information technology implementations. These changes could facilitate improved management of those consequences, resulting in enhanced performance, patient safety as well as greater user acceptance.

4.6.3 External Representations and Information Visualization

To reiterate, internal representations reflect mental states that correspond to the external world. The term external representation refers to any object in the external world which has the potential to be internalized. External representations such as images, graphs, icons, audible sounds, texts with symbols (e.g., letters and numbers), shapes and textures are vital sources of knowledge, means of communication and cultural transmission. The classical model of information-processing cognition viewed external representations as mere inputs to the mind (Zhang 1997). For example, the visual system would process the information in a display that would serve as input to the cognitive system for further processing (e.g., classifying dermatological lesions), leading to knowledge being retrieved from memory and resulting in a decision or action. These external representations served as a stimulus to be internalized (e.g., memorized) by the system. The hard work is then done by the machinery of the mind, which develops an internal copy of a slice of the external world and stores it as a mental representation. The appropriate internal representation is then retrieved when needed.

This view has changed considerably. Norman (1993) argues that external representations play a critical role in enhancing cognition and intelligent behavior. These durable representations (at least those that are visible) persist in the external world and are continuously available to augment memory, reasoning, and computation. Consider a simple illustration involving multi-digit multiplication with a pencil and paper. First, imagine calculating 37×93 without any external aids. Unless you are unusually skilled in such computations, they will exert a reasonably heavy load on working memory in relatively short order. One may have to engage in a serial process of calculation and maintain partial products in working memory (e.g., $3 \times 37 = 111$). Now consider the use of pencil and paper as illustrated below.

			3	7
		x	9	3
		1	1	1
3		3	3	
3		4	4	1

The individual brings to the task knowledge of the meaning of the symbols (i.e., digits and their place value), arithmetic operators, and addition and multiplication tables (that enable a look-up from memory). The external representations include the positions of the symbols, the partial products of interim calculations and their spatial relations (i.e., rows and columns). The visual representation, by holding partial results outside the mind, extends a person's working

memory (Card et al. 1999). Calculations can rapidly become computationally prohibitive without recourse to cognitive aids. The offloading of computations is a central argument in support of distributed cognition, which is the subject of the next section.

It is widely understood that not all representations are equal for a given task and individual. The representational effect is a well-documented phenomenon in which different representations of a common abstract structure can have a significant effect on reasoning and decision making (Zhang and Norman 1994). For example, different forms of graphical displays can be more or less efficient for certain tasks. A simple example is that Arabic numerals are more efficient for arithmetic (e.g., 37×93) than Roman numerals ($XXXVII \times XCIII$) even though the representations or symbols are identical in meaning. Similarly, a digital clock provides an easy readout for precisely determining the time (Norman 1993). On the other hand, an analog clock provides an interface that enables one to more readily determine time intervals (e.g., elapsed or remaining time) without recourse to calculations. Larkin and Simon (1987) argued that effective displays facilitate problem-solving by allowing users to substitute perceptual operations (i.e., recognition processes) for effortful symbolic operations (e.g., memory retrieval and computationally intensive reasoning) and that displays can reduce the amount of time spent searching for critical information. Research has demonstrated that different forms of graphical representations such as graphs, tables and lists can dramatically change decision-making strategies (Kleinmuntz and Schkade 1993; Scaife and Rogers 1996).

Medical prescriptions are an interesting case in point. Chronic illness affects over 100 million individuals in the United States, many of whom suffer from multiple of these individuals suffer from multiple afflictions and must adhere to complex medication regimens. There are various pill organizers and mnemonic devices designed to promote patient compliance. Although these are helpful, prescriptions written by clinicians are inherently hard for patients to follow. The following prescriptions were given to a patient following a mild stroke (Day, 1988 reported in Norman 1993).

Inderal	–1 tablet 3 times a day
Lanoxin	–1 tablet every AM
Carafate	–1 tablet before meals and at bedtime
Zantac	–1 tablet every 12 h (twice a day)
Quinaglute	–1 tablet 4 times a day
Coumadin	–1 tablet a day

The physician's list is concise and presented in a format whereby a pharmacist can readily fill the prescription. However, the organization by medication does not facilitate a patient's decision of what medications to take at a given time of day. Some computation, memory retrieval (e.g., I took my last dose of Lanoxin 6 h ago) and inference (what medications to bring when leaving one's home for some duration of hours) are necessary to make such a decision. Day proposed an alternative tabular representation (Table 4.2).

In this matrix representation in Table 4.2, the items can be organized by time of day (columns) and by medication (rows). The patient can simply scan the list by either time of day or medication. This simple change in representation can transform a cognitively taxing task

Table 4.2 Tabular representation of medications

	Breakfast	Lunch	Dinner	Bedtime
Lanoxin	X			
Inderal	X	X	X	
Quinaglute	X	X	X	X
Carafate	X	X	X	X
Zantac		X		X
Coumadin				X

Adapted from Norman (1988)

into a simpler one that facilitates search (e.g., when do I take Zantac) and computation (e.g., how many pills are taken at dinner time). Tables can support quick and easy lookup and embody a compact and efficient representational device. However, a particular external representation is likely to be effective for some populations of users and not others (Ancker and Kaufman 2007). For example, reading a table requires a certain level of numeracy that is beyond the abilities of certain patients with very basic education. Kaufman and colleagues (2003) characterized the difficulties some older adult patients experienced in dealing with numeric data, especially when represented in tabular form. For example, when reviewing their blood glucose or blood pressure values, several patients appeared to lack an abstract understanding of covariation and how it can be expressed as a functional relationship in a tabular format (i.e., cells and rows) as illustrated in Fig. 4.11. Others had difficulty establishing the correspondence between the values expressed on the interface of their blood pressure monitoring device and mathematical representation in tabular format (systolic/diastolic). The familiar monitoring device provided an easy readout and patients could readily make appropriate inferences (e.g., systolic value is higher than usual) and take appropriate measures. However, when interpreting the same values in a table, certain patients had difficulty recognizing anomalous or abnormal results even when these values were rendered as salient by a color–coding scheme.

The results suggest that even the more literate patients were challenged when drawing inferences over bounded periods of time. They tended to focus on discrete values (i.e., a single reading)

Date	Time	Glucose	Blood Pressure
7/23/02	7:20 AM	135	144/82
7/23/02	6:52 PM	163	154/100
7/24/02	6:30 AM	145	161/134
7/24/02	7:08 PM	166	152/88

Fig. 4.11 Mapping values between blood pressure monitor and IDEATel Table

in noting whether it was within their normal or expected range. In at least one case, the problems with the representation seemed to be related to the medium of representation rather than the form of representation. One patient experienced considerable difficulty reading the table on the computer display, but maintained a daily diary with very similar representational properties.

Instructions can be embodied in a range of external representations from text to list of procedures to diagrams exemplifying the steps. Everyday nonexperts are called upon to follow instructions in a variety of application domains (e.g., completing income-tax forms, configuring and using a digital video recorder (DVR), cooking something for the first time, or interpreting medication instructions), where correct processing of information is necessary for proper functioning. The comprehension of written information in such cases frequently involves both quantitative and qualitative reasoning, as well as a minimal familiarity with the application domain. This is nowhere more apparent, and critical, than in the case of over-the-counter pharmaceutical labels, the correct understanding of which often demands that the user translate minimal, quantitative formulas into qualitative, and frequently complex, procedures. Medical errors involving the use of therapeutic drugs are amongst the most frequent.

The calculation of dosages for pharmaceutical instructions can be remarkably complex. Consider the following instructions for an over-the-counter cough syrup.

Each teaspoonful (5 mL) contains 15 mg of dextromethorphan hydrobromide U.S.P., in a palatable yellow, lemon flavored syrup. DOSAGE ADULTS: 1 or 2 teaspoonfuls three or four times daily. DOSAGE CHILDREN: 1 mg/kg of body weight daily in 3 or 4 divided doses.

If you wish to administer medication to a 22 lb child three times a day and wish to determine the dosage, the calculations are as follows:

$$22\text{lbs} / 2.2\text{lbs} / \text{kg} \times 1\text{mg} / \text{kg} / \text{day} / 15\text{mg} / \text{tsp} / 3\text{doses} / \text{day} = 2 / 9\text{tsp} / \text{dose}$$

Patel, Branch, and Arocha (2002a) studied 48 lay subjects' responses to this problem. The majority of participants (66.5 %) were unable to correctly calculate the appropriate dosage of cough syrup. Even when calculations were correct, they were unable to estimate the actual amount to administer. There were no significant differences based on cultural or educational background. One of the central problems is that there is a significant mismatch between the designer's conceptual model of the pharmaceutical text and procedures to be followed and the user's mental model of the situation.

Diagrams are tools that we use daily in communication, information storage, planning, and problem-solving. Diagrammatic representations are not new devices for communicating ideas. They of course have a long history as tools of science and cultural inventions that augment thinking. For example, the earliest maps, a graphical representation of regions of geographical space, date back thousands of years. The phrase "a picture is worth 10,000 words" is believed to be an ancient Chinese proverb (Larkin and Simon 1987). External representations have always been a vital means for storing, aggregating and communicating patient data. The psychological study of information displays similarly has a long history dating back to Gestalt psychologists beginning around the turn of the twentieth century. They produced a set of laws of pattern perception for describing how we see patterns in visual images (Ware 2003). For example, the **law of proximity** states that visual entities that are close together are perceptually grouped. The **law of symmetry** indicates that symmetric objects are more readily perceived.

Advances in graphical user interfaces afford a wide range of novel external representations. Card and colleagues (1999) define **information visualization** as "the use of computer-supported, interactive, visual representations of abstract data to amplify cognition". Information visualization of medical data is a vigorous area of research and application (Kosara and Miksch 2002; Starren and Johnson 2000). Medical data can include single data elements or more complex data structures. Representations can also be characterized as either numeric (e.g., laboratory data) or non-numeric information such as symptoms and diseases. Visual representations may be either static or dynamic (changing as additional temporal data become available). EHRs need to include a wide range of data representation types, including both numeric and nonnumeric (Tang and McDonald 2001). EHR data representations are employed in a wide range of clinical, research and administrative tasks by different kinds of users. Medical imaging systems are used for a range of purposes including visual diagnosis (e.g., radiology), assessment and planning, communication, and education and training (Greenes and Brinkley 2001). The purposes of these representations are to display and manipulate digital images to reveal different facets of anatomical structures in either two or three dimensions.

Patient monitoring systems employ static and dynamic representations (e.g., continuously updated observations) for the presentation of the presentation of physiological parameters such as heart rate, respiratory rate, and blood pressure (Gardner and Shabot 2001) (see Chap. 19). As discussed previously, Lin et al. found that that the original display of a PCA device introduced substantial cognitive complexity into the task and impacted performance (Lin et al. 1998). They also demonstrated that redesigning interface in a manner consistent with human factors principles could lead to significantly faster, easier, and more reliable performance.

Information visualization is an area of great importance in bioinformatics research, particularly in relation to genetic sequencing and alignment. The tools and applications are being produced at a very fast pace. Although there is tremendous promise in such modeling systems, we know very little about what constitutes a usable interface for particular tasks. What sorts of competencies or prerequisite skills are necessary to use such representations effectively? There is a significant opportunity for cognitive methods and theories to play an instrumental role in this area.

In general, there have been relatively few cognitive studies characterizing how different kinds of medical data displays impact performance. However, there have been several efforts to develop a typology of medical data representations. Starren and Johnson (2000) proposed a taxonomy of data representations. They characterized five major classes of representation types including list, table, graph, icon, and generated text. Each of these data types has distinct measurement properties (e.g., ordinal scales are useful for categorical data) and they are variably suited for different kinds of data, tasks and users. The authors propose some criteria for evaluating the efficacy of a representation including: (1) latency (the amount of time it takes a user to answer a question based on information in the representation), (2) accuracy, and (3) compactness (the relative amount of display space required for the representation). Further research is needed to explore the cognitive consequences of different forms of external medical data representations. For example, what inferences can be more readily gleaned from a tabular representation versus a line chart? How does configuration of objects in a representation affect latency?

At present, computational advances in information visualization have outstripped our understanding of how these resources can be most effectively deployed for particular tasks. However, we are gaining a better understanding of the ways in which external representations can amplify cognition. Card et al. (1999) propose six major ways: (1) by increasing the memory and processing resources available to the users (offloading cognitive work to a display), (2) by reducing the search for information (grouping data strategically), (3) by using visual presentations to enhance the detection of patterns, (4) by using perceptual attention mechanisms for monitoring (e.g., drawing attention to events that require immediate attention), and (5) by encoding information in a manipulable medium (e.g., the user can select different possible views to highlight variables of interest).

4.6.4 Distributed Cognition and Electronic Health Records

In this chapter, we have considered a classical model of information-processing cognition in which mental representations mediate all activity and constitute the central units of analysis. The analysis emphasizes how an individual formulates internal representations of the external world. To illustrate the point, imagine an expert user of a word processor who can effortlessly negotiate tasks through a combination of key commands and menu selections. The traditional cognitive analysis might account for this skill by suggesting that the user has formed an image or schema of the layout structure of each of eight menus, and retrieves this information from memory each time an action is to be performed. For example, if the goal is to "insert a clip art icon", the user would simply recall that this is subsumed under pictures that are the ninth item on the "Insert" menu and then execute the action, thereby achieving the goal. However, there are some problems with this model. Mayes, Draper, McGregor, and Koatley (1988) demonstrated that even highly skilled users could not recall the names of menu headers, yet they could routinely make fast and accurate menu selections. The results indicate that many or even most users relied on cues in the display to trigger the right menu selections. This suggests that the display can have a central role in controlling interaction in graphical user interfaces.

As discussed, the conventional information-processing approach has come under criticism for its narrow focus on the rational/cognitive processes of the solitary individual. In the previous section, we consider the relevance of external representations to cognitive activity. The emerging perspective of **distributed cognition** offers a more far-reaching alternative. The distributed view of cognition represents a shift in the study of cognition from being the sole property of the individual to being "stretched" across groups, material artifacts and cultures (Hutchins 1995; Suchman 1987). This viewpoint is increasingly gaining acceptance in cognitive science and human-computer interaction research. In the distributed approach to HCI research, cognition is viewed as a process of coordinating distributed internal (i.e., knowledge) and external representations (e.g., visual displays, manuals). Distributed cognition has two central points of inquiry, one that emphasizes the inherently social and collaborative nature of cognition (e.g., doctors, nurses and technical support staff in neonatal care unit jointly contributing to a decision process), and one that characterizes the mediating effects of technology or other artifacts on cognition.

The distributed cognition perspective reflects a spectrum of viewpoints on what constitutes the appropriate unit of analysis for the study of cognition. Let us first consider a more radical departure from the classical model of information-processing. Cole and Engestrom (1997) suggest that the natural unit of analysis for the study of human behavior is an activity system, comprising relations among individuals and their proximal, "culturally-organized environments". A system consisting of individuals, groups of individuals, and technologies can be construed as a single indivisible unit of analysis. Berg is a leading proponent of the sociotechnical point of view within the world of medical informatics. He argues that "work practices are conceptualized as networks of people, tools, organizational routines, documents and so forth" (Berg 1999). An emergency ward, outpatient clinic or obstetrics and gynecology department is seen as an interrelated assembly of things (including humans) whose functioning is primarily geared to the delivery of patient care. Berg (1999) goes on to emphasize that the "elements that constitute these networks should then not be seen as discrete, well-circumscribed entities with pre-fixed characteristics (p 89).

In Berg's view, the study of information systems must reject an approach that segregates individual and collective, human and machine, as well as the social and technical dimensions of IT. Although there are compelling reasons for adapting a strong socially-distributed approach, an individual's mental representations and external representations are both instrumental tools in cognition (Park et al. 2001; Patel et al. 2002b). This is consistent with a distributed cognition framework that embraces the centrality of external representations as mediators of cognition, but also considers the importance of an individual's internal representations (Perry 2003).

The mediating role of technology can be evaluated at several levels of analysis from the individual to the organization. Technologies, whether they be computer-based or an artifact in another medium, transform the ways individuals and groups think. They do not merely augment, enhance or expedite performance, although a given technology may do all of these things. The difference is not merely one of quantitative change, but one that is qualitative in nature.

In a distributed world, what becomes of the individual? We believe it is important to understand how technologies promote enduring changes in individuals Salomon et al. (1991) introduce an important distinction in considering the mediating role of technology on individual performance, the effects with technology and the effects of technology. The former is concerned with the changes in performance displayed by users while equipped with the technology. For example, when using an effective medical information system, physicians should be able to gather information more systematically and efficiently. In this capacity, medical information technologies may alleviate some of the cognitive load associated with a given task and permit physicians to focus on higher-order thinking skills, such as diagnostic hypothesis generation and evaluation. The effects of technology refer to enduring changes in general cognitive capacities (knowledge and skills) as a consequence of interaction with a technology. This effect is illustrated subsequently in the context of the enduring effects of an EHR (see Chap. 12).

We employed a pen-based EHR system, DCI (Dossier of Clinical Information), in several of our studies (see Kushniruk et al. 1996). Using the pen or computer keyboard, physicians can directly enter information into the EHR, such as the patient's chief complaint, past history, history of present illness, laboratory tests, and differential diagnoses. Physicians were encouraged to use the system while collecting data from patients (e.g., during the interview). The DCI system incorporates an extended version of the ICD-9 vocabulary standard (see Chap. 7). The system allows the physician to record information about the patient's differential diagnosis, the ordering of tests, and the prescription of medication. The system also provides supporting reference information in the form of an integrated electronic version of the Merck Manual, drug monographs for medications, and information on laboratory tests. The graphical interface provides a highly structured set of resources for representing a clinical problem as illustrated in Fig. 4.12.

We have studied the use of this EHR in both laboratory-based research (Kushniruk et al. 1996) and in actual clinical settings using cognitive methods (Patel et al. 2000). The laboratory research included a simulated doctor-patient

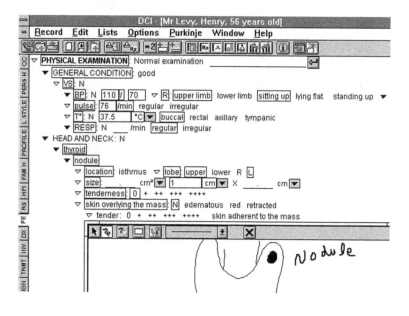

Fig. 4.12 Display of a structured electronic medical record with graphical capabilities

interview. We have observed two distinct patterns of EHR usage in the interactive condition, one in which the subject pursues information from the patient predicated on a hypothesis; the second strategy involves the use of the EHR display to provide guidance for asking the patient questions. In the screen-driven strategy, the clinician is using the structured list of findings in the order in which they appear on the display to elicit information. All experienced users of this system appear to have both strategies in their repertoire.

In general, a screen-driven strategy can enhance performance by reducing the cognitive load imposed by information-gathering goals and allow the physician to allocate more cognitive resources toward testing hypotheses and rendering decisions. On the other hand, this strategy can encourage a certain sense of complacency. We observed both effective as well as counter-productive uses of this screen-driven strategy. A more experienced user consciously used the strategy to structure the information-gathering process, whereas a novice user used it less discriminately. In employing this screen-driven strategy, the novice elicited almost all of the relevant findings in a simulated patient encounter. However, she also elicited numerous irrelevant findings and pursued incorrect hypotheses. In this particular case, the subject became too reliant on the technology and had difficulty imposing her own set of working hypotheses to guide the information-gathering and diagnostic-reasoning processes.

The use of a screen-driven strategy is evidence of the ways in which technology transforms clinical cognition, as evidenced in clinicians' patterns of reasoning. Patel and colleagues (2000) extended this line of research to study the cognitive consequences of using the same EHR system in a diabetes clinic. The study considered the following questions (1) How do physicians manage information flow when using an EHR system? (2) What are the differences in the way physicians organize and represent this information using paper-based and EHR systems, and (3) Are there long-term, enduring effects of the use of EHR systems on knowledge representations and clinical reasoning? One study focused on an in-depth characterization of changes in knowledge organi-

zation in a single subject as a function of using the system. The study first compared the contents and structure of patient records produced by the physician using the EHR system and paper-based patient records, using ten pairs of records matched for variables such as patient age and problem type. After having used the system for 6 months, the physician was asked to conduct his next five patient interviews using only hand-written paper records.

The results indicated that the EHRs contained more information relevant to the diagnostic hypotheses. In addition, the structure and content of information was found to correspond to the structured representation of the particular medium. For example, EHRs were found to contain more information about the patient's past medical history, reflecting the query structure of the interface. The paper-based records appear to better preserve the integrity of the time course of the evolution of the patient problem, whereas, this is notably absent from the EHR. Perhaps, the most striking finding is that, after having used the system for 6 months, the structure and content of the physician's paper-based records bore a closer resemblance to the organization of information in the EHR than the paper-based records produced by the physician prior to exposure to the system. This finding is consistent with the enduring *effects of* technology even in absence of the particular system.

Patel et al. (2000) conducted a series of related studies with physicians in the same diabetes clinic. The results of one study replicated and extended the results of the single subject study (reported above) regarding the differential effects of EHRs on paper-based records on represented (recorded) patient information. For example, physicians entered significantly more information about the patient's chief complaint using the EHR. Similarly, physicians represented significantly more information about the history of present illness and review of systems using paper-based records. It's reasonable to assert that such differences are likely to have an impact on clinical decision making. The authors also video-recorded and analyzed 20 doctor-patient computer interactions by 2 physicians with varying levels of expertise.

One of the physicians was an intermediate-level user of the EHR and the other was an expert user. The analysis of the physician-patient interactions revealed that the less expert subject was more strongly influenced by the structure and content of the interface. In particular, he was guided by the order of information on the screen when asking the patient questions and recording the responses. This screen-driven strategy is similar to what we documented in a previous study (Kushniruk et al. 1996). Although the expert user similarly used the EHR system to structure his questions, he was much less bound to the order and sequence of presented information on the EHR screen. This body of research documented both *effects with* and *effects of* technology in the context of EHR use (Salomon et al. 1991). These include effects on knowledge-organization and information-gathering strategies. The authors conclude that given these potentially enduring effects, the use of a particular EHR will almost certainly have a direct effect on medical decision making.

The previously discussed research demonstrates the ways in which information technologies can mediate cognition and even produce enduring changes in how one performs a task. What dimensions of an interface contribute to such changes? What aspects of a display are more likely to facilitate efficient task performance and what aspects are more likely to impede it? Norman (1986) argued that well-designed artifacts could reduce the need for users to remember large amounts of information, whereas poorly designed artifacts increased the knowledge demands on the user and the burden of working memory. In the distributed approach to HCI research, cognition is viewed as a process of coordinating distributed internal and external representations and this in effect constitutes an indivisible information-processing system.

How do artifacts in the external world "participate" in the process of cognition? The ecological approach of perceptual psychologist Gibson was based on the analysis of invariant structures in the environment in relation to perception and action. The concept of *affordance* has gained substantial currency in human computer interaction. It has been used to refer to attributes of objects that enable individuals to know how to use them (Rogers 2004). When the affordances of an object are perceptually obvious, they render humans interactions with objects as effortless. For example, one can often perceive the affordances of a door handle (e.g., afford turning or pushing downwards to open the door) or a water faucet. One the other hand, there are numerous artifacts in which the affordances are less transparent (e.g., door handles that appear to suggest a pulling motion but actually need to be pushed to open the door). External representations constitute affordances in that they can be picked up, analyzed, and processed by perceptual systems alone. According to theories of distributed cognition, most cognitive tasks have an internal and external component (Hutchins 1995), and as a consequence, the problem-solving process involves coordinating information from these representations to produce new information.

One of the appealing features of the distributed cognition paradigm is that it can be used to understand how properties of objects on the screen (e.g., links, buttons) can serve as external representations and reduce cognitive load. The distributed resource model proposed by Wright, Fields, & Harrison (2000) addresses the question of "what information is required to carry out some task and where should it be located: as an interface object or as something that is mentally represented to the user." The relative difference in the distribution of representations (internal and external) is central to determining the efficacy of a system designed to support a complex task. Wright, Fields, and Harrison (2000) were among the first to develop an explicit model for coding the kinds of resources available in the environment and the ways in which they are embodied on an interface.

Horsky, Kaufman and Patel (2003a) applied the distributed resource model and analysis to a provider order entry system. The goal was to analyze specific order entry tasks such as those involved in admitting a patient to a hospital and then to identify areas of complexity that may impede optimal recorded entries. The research consisted of two component analyses: a cognitive walkthrough evaluation that was modified based on the distributed resource model and a simulated clinical ordering task performed by seven physicians. The CW analysis revealed that the configuration of resources (e.g., very long menus, complexly configured displays) placed unnecessarily heavy cognitive demands on users, especially those who were new to the system. The resources model was also used to account for patterns of errors produced by clinicians. The authors concluded that the redistribution and reconfiguration of resources may yield guiding principles and design solutions in the development of complex interactive systems.

The distributed cognition framework has proved to be particularly useful in understanding the performance of teams or groups of individuals in a particular work setting (Hutchins 1995). Hazlehurst and colleagues (Hazlehurst et al. 2003, 2007) have drawn on this framework to illuminate the ways in which work in healthcare settings is constituted using shared resources and representations. The *activity system* is the primary explanatory construct. It is comprises actors and tools, together with shared understandings among actors that structure interactions in a work setting. The "propagation of representational states through activity systems" is used to explain cognitive behavior and investigate the organization of system and human performance. Following Hazlehurst et al. (2007, p. 540), "a **representational state** is a particular configuration of an information-bearing structure, such as a monitor display, a verbal utterance, or a printed label, that plays some functional role in a process within the system." The author has used the concept to explain the process of medication ordering in an intensive care unit and the coordinated communications of a surgical team in a heart room.

Kaufman and colleagues (2009) employed the concept of representational states to understand nursing workflow in a complex technology-mediated telehealth setting. They extended the construct by introducing the concept of the "state of the patient" as a kind of representational state that reflects the knowledge about the patient embodied in different individuals and inscribed in different media (e.g., EHRs, displays, paper documents and blood pressure monitors) at a given point in time. The authors conducted a qualitative study of the ways in different media and communication practices shaped nursing workflow and patient-centered decision making. The study revealed barriers to the productive use of system technology as well as adaptations that circumvented such limitations. Technologies can be deployed more effectively to establish common ground in clinical communication and can serve to update the state of the patient in a more timely and accurate way.

The framework for distributed cognition is still an emerging one in human-computer interaction. It offers a novel and potentially powerful approach for illuminating the kinds of difficulties users encounter and finding ways to better structure the interaction by redistributing the resources. Distributed cognition analyses may also provide a window into why technologies sometimes fail to reduce errors or even contribute to them.

4.7 Conclusion

Theories and methods from the cognitive sciences can shed light on a range of issues pertaining to the design and implementation of health information technologies. They can also serve an instrumental role in understanding and enhancing the performance of clinicians and patients as they engage in a range of cognitive tasks related to health. The potential scope of applied cognitive research in biomedical informatics is very broad. Significant inroads have been made in areas such as EHRs and patient safety. However, there are promising areas of future cognitive research that remain largely uncharted. These include understanding how to capitalize on health information technology without compromising patient safety (particularly in providing adequate decision support), understanding how various visual representations/graphical forms mediate reasoning in biomedical informatics and how these representations can be used by patients and health consumers with varying degrees of literacy. These are only a few of the cognitive challenges related to harnessing the potential of cutting-edge technologies in order to improve patient safety.

Suggested Readings

Carayon, P. (Ed.). (2007). *Handbook of human factors and ergonomics in health care and patient safety.* Mahwah: Lawrence Erlbaum Associates. A multifaceted introduction to many of the issues related to human factors, healthcare and patient safety.

Carroll, J. M. (2003). *HCI models, theories, and frameworks: toward a multidisciplinary science.* San Francisco: Morgan Kaufmann. An edited volume on cognitive approaches to HCI.

Evans, D. A., & Patel, V. L. (1989). *Cognitive science in medicine.* Cambridge, MA: MIT Press. The first (and only) book devoted to cognitive issues in medicine. This multidisciplinary volume contains chapters by many of the leading figures in the field.

Norman, D. A. (1993). *Things that make us smart: defending human attributes in the age of the machine.* Reading: Addison-Wesley Pub. Co.. This book addresses significant issues in human-computer interaction in a very readable and entertaining fashion.

Patel, V. L., Kaufman, D. R., & Arocha, J. F. (2002). Emerging paradigms of cognition in medical decision-making. *Journal of Biomedical Informatics, 35,* 52–75. This relatively recent article summarizes new directions in decision-making research. The authors articulate a need for alternative paradigms for the study of medical decision making.

Patel, V. L., Yoskowitz, N. A., Arocha, J. F., & Shortliffe, E. H. (2009). Cognitive and learning sciences in biomedical and health instructional design: a review with lessons for biomedical informatics education. *Journal of Biomedical Informatics, 42*(1), 176–97. A review of learning and cognition with a particular focus on biomedical informatics.

Preece, J., Rogers, Y., & Sharp, H. (2007). *Interaction design: beyond human-computer interaction* (2nd ed.). West Sussex: Wiley. A very readable and relatively comprehensive introduction to human-computer interaction.

Questions for Discussion

1. What are some of the assumptions of the distribute cognition framework? What implications does this approach have for the evaluation of electronic health records?

2. Explain the difference between the *effects of technology* and the *effects with technology.* How can each of these effects contribute to improving patient safety and reducing medical errors?

3. Although diagrams and graphical materials can be extremely useful to illustrate quantitative information, they also present challenges for low numeracy patients. Discuss the various considerations that need to be taken into account in the development of effective quantitative representations for lower literacy populations.

4. The use of electronic health records (EHR) has been shown to differentially affect clinical reasoning relative to paper charts. Briefly characterize the effects they have on reasoning, including those that persist after the clinician ceases to use the system. Speculate about the potential impact of EMRs on patient care.

5. A large urban hospital is planning to implement a provider order entry system. You have been asked to advise them on system usability and to study the cognitive effects of the system on performance. Discuss the issues involved and suggests some of the steps you would take to study system usability.

6. Discuss some of the ways in which external representations can amplify cognition. How can the study of information visualization impact the development of representations and tools for biomedical informatics.

7. "When human error is viewed as a cause rather than a consequence, it serves as a cloak for our ignorance" (Henriksen 2008). Discuss the meaning of this quote in the context of studies of patient safety.

8. Koppel and colleagues (2005) documented two categories of errors in clinicians' use of CPOE systems: 1) Information errors generated by fragmentation of data and 2) human-machine interface flaws. What are the implications of these error types for system design?

Computer Architectures for Health Care and Biomedicine

Jonathan C. Silverstein and Ian T. Foster

After reading this chapter, you should know the answers to these questions:

- What are the components of computer architectures?
- How are medical data stored and manipulated in a computer?
- How can information be displayed clearly?
- What are the functions of a computer's operating system?
- What is the technical basis and business model of cloud computing?
- What advantages does using a database management system provide over storing and manipulating your own data directly?
- How do local area networks facilitate data sharing and communication within health care institutions?
- What are the maintenance advantages of Software-as-a-Service?
- How can the confidentiality of data stored in distributed computer systems be protected?
- How is the Internet used for medical applications today?

- How are wireless, mobile devices, federated and hosted systems changing the way the Internet will be used for biomedical applications?

5.1 Computer Architectures

Architectures are the designs or plans of systems. Architectures have both physical and conceptual aspects. Computer architectures for health care and biomedicine are the physical designs and conceptual plans of computers and information systems that are used in biomedical applications.

Health professionals and the general public encounter computers constantly. As electronic health records are increasingly deployed, clinicians use information systems to record medical observations, order drugs and laboratory tests, and review test results. Physicians and patients use personal computing environments such as desktop computers, laptops, and mobile devices to access the Internet, to search the medical literature, to communicate with colleagues and friends, and to do their clinical and administrative work. In fact, computers are ubiquitous, touching every aspect of human life, and increasingly image-intense, interactive, and collaborative.

This chapter is adapted from an earlier version in the third edition authored by GioWiederhold and Thomas C. Rindfleisch.

J.C. Silverstein, MD, MS (✉)
Research Institute, NorthShore University HealthSystem, 1001 University Place, Evanston 60201, IL, USA
e-mail: jcs@uchicago.edu

I.T. Foster, PhD
Searle Chemistry Laboratory, Computation Institute, University of Chicago and Argonne National Laboratory, 5735 South Ellis Avenue, Chicago 60637, IL, USA
e-mail: foster@uchicago.edu

Individual computers differ in speed, storage capacity, and cost; in the number of users that they can support; in the ways that they are interconnected; in the types of applications that they can run; in the way they are managed and shared; in the way they are secured; and in the way people interact with them. On the surface, the differences among computers can be bewildering, but the selection of appropriate hardware, software, and the architecture under which they are assembled is crucial to the success of computer applications. Despite these differences, however, computers use the same basic mechanisms to store and process information and to communicate with the outside world whether desktop, laptop, mobile device, gaming system, digital video recorder, or massive computer cluster. At the conceptual level, the similarities among all these computers greatly outweigh the differences.

In this chapter, we will cover fundamental concepts related to computer hardware, software, and distributed systems (multiple computers working together), including data acquisition, processing, communications, security, and sharing. We assume that you use computers but have not been concerned with their internal workings or how computers work together across the global Internet. Our aim is to give you the background necessary for understanding the underpinning technical architecture of the applications discussed in later chapters. We will describe the component parts that make up computers and their assembly into complex distributed systems that enable biomedical applications.

5.2 Hardware

Early computers were expensive to purchase and operate. Only large institutions could afford to acquire a computer and to develop its software. In the 1960s, the development of integrated circuits on silicon chips resulted in dramatic increases in computing power per dollar. Since that time, computer hardware has become dramatically smaller, faster, more reliable and personal. As computation, storage, and communication capabilities have increased so have data

volumes, particularly genomic and imaging data. At the same time, software packages have been developed that remove much of the burden of writing the infrastructure of applications via encapsulation or abstraction of underlying software to "higher level" commands. The result is that computers are increasingly complex in their layered hardware and software architectures, but simpler for individuals to program and to use.

Essentially all modern general-purpose computers have similar base hardware (physical equipment) architectures. This is generally true whether they are large systems supporting many users, such as hospital information systems, individual personal computers, laptops, mobile devices, or even whole computers on one silicon "chip" embedded in medical devices. The scale of computing, memory, display and style of usage largely distinguish different individual hardware devices. Later we will discuss assemblies of computers for complex applications.

General computer architectures follow principles expressed by John von Neumann in 1945. Figure 5.1 illustrates the configuration of a simple **von Neumann machine**. Extending this to modern computers, they are composed of one or more

- **Central processing units** (**CPUs**) that perform general computation
- **Computer memories** that store programs and data that are being used actively by a CPU
- **Storage devices**, such as **magnetic disks** and tapes, **optical disks**, and **solid state drives**, that provide long-term storage for programs and data
- **Graphics processing units** (**GPUs**) that perform graphic displays and other highly parallel computations
- **Input** and **output** (I/O) devices, such as keyboards, pointing devices, touch screens, controllers, video displays, and printers, that facilitate user interaction and storage
- **Communication** equipment, such as network interfaces, that connect computers to networks of computers
- **Data buses**, electrical pathways that transport encoded information between these subsystems

Most computers are now manufactured with multiple CPUs on a single chip, and in some

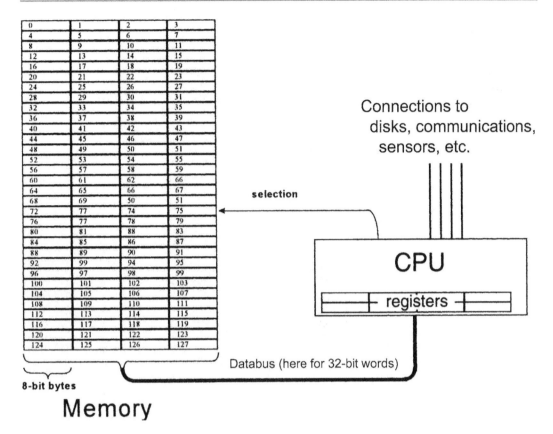

0	1	2	3
4	5	6	7
8	9	10	11
12	13	14	15
16	17	18	19
20	21	22	23
24	25	26	27
28	29	30	31
32	33	34	35
36	37	38	39
40	41	42	43
44	45	46	47
48	49	50	51
52	53	54	55
56	57	58	59
60	61	62	66
64	65	66	67
68	69	50	51
72	77	74	75
76	77	78	79
80	81	88	83
84	85	86	87
88	89	90	91
92	99	94	95
96	97	98	99
100	101	102	103
104	105	106	107
108	109	110	111
112	113	114	115
116	117	118	119
120	121	122	123
124	125	126	127

Connections to disks, communications, sensors, etc.

selection

CPU

registers

Databus (here for 32-bit words)

8-bit bytes

Memory

Fig. 5.1 The von Neumann model: the basic architecture of most modern computers. The computer comprises a single central processing unit (CPU), an area for memory, and a data bus for transferring data between the two

cases multiple GPUs, as well as multiple layers of memory, storage, I/O devices and communication interfaces. Multiple interconnected CPUs with shared memory layers further enable **parallel processing** (performing multiple computations simultaneously). The challenge then is for the software to distribute the computation across these units to gain a proportionate benefit.

5.2.1 Central Processing Unit

Although complete computer systems appear to be complex, the underlying principles are simple. A prime example is a processing unit itself. Here simple components can be carefully combined to create systems with impressive capabilities. The structuring principle is that of hierarchical organization: primitive units (electronic switches) are combined to form basic units that can store letters

and numbers, add digits, and compare values with one another. The basic units are assembled into **registers** capable of storing and manipulating text and large numbers. These registers in turn are assembled into the larger functional units that make up the central component of a computer: the CPU.

The logical atomic element for all digital computers is the *binary digit* or **bit**. Each bit can assume one of two values: 0 or 1. An electronic switch that can be set to either of two states stores a single bit value. (Think of a light switch that can be either on or off.) These primitive units are the building blocks of computer systems. Sequences of bits (implemented as sequences of switches) are used to represent larger numbers and other kinds of information. For example, four switches can store 2^4, or 16, different combination of values: 0000, 0001, 0010, 0011, 0100, 0101, 0110, and so on, up to 1111. Thus, 4 bits

Fig. 5.2 The American Standard Code for Information Interchange (ASCII) is a standard scheme for representing alphanumeric characters using 7 bits. The upper-case and lower-case alphabet, the decimal digits, and common punctuation characters are shown here with their ASCII representations

Character	Binary code	Character	Binary code	Character	Binary code
blank	010 0000	@	100 0000	`	110 0000
!	010 0001	A	100 0001	a	110 0001
"	010 0010	B	100 0010	b	110 0010
#	010 0011	C	100 0011	c	110 0011
$	010 0100	D	100 0100	d	110 0100
%	010 0101	E	100 0101	e	110 0101
&	010 0110	F	100 0110	f	110 0110
'	010 0111	G	100 0111	g	110 0111
(	010 1000	H	100 1000	h	110 1000
)	010 1001	I	100 1001	i	110 1001
*	010 1010	J	100 1010	j	110 1010
+	010 1011	K	100 1011	k	110 1011
,	010 1100	L	100 1100	l	110 1100
-	010 1101	M	100 1101	m	110 1101
.	010 1110	N	100 1110	n	110 1110
/	010 1111	O	100 1111	o	110 1111
0	011 0000	P	101 0000	p	111 0000
1	011 0001	Q	101 0001	q	111 0001
2	011 0010	R	101 0010	r	111 0010
3	011 0011	S	101 0011	s	111 0011
4	011 0100	T	101 0100	t	111 0100
5	011 0101	U	101 0101	u	111 0101
6	011 0110	V	101 0110	v	111 0110
7	011 0111	W	101 0111	w	111 0111
8	011 1000	X	101 1000	x	111 1000
9	011 1001	Y	101 1001	y	111 1001
:	011 1010	Z	101 1010	z	111 1010
;	011 1011	[	101 1011	{	111 1011
<	011 1100	\	101 1100	|	111 1100
=	011 1101	]	101 1101	}	111 1101
>	011 1110	^	101 1110	~	111 1110
?	011 1111	_	101 1111	null	111 1111

can represent any decimal value from 0 to 15; e.g., the sequence 0101 is the **binary** (base 2) representation of the decimal number 5—namely, $0 \times 2^3 + 1 \times 2^2 + 0 \times 2^1 + 1 \times 2^0 = 5$. A byte is a sequence of 8 bits; it can take on 2^8 or 256 values (0–255).

Groups of bits and bytes can represent not only decimal integers but also fractional numbers, general characters (upper-case and lower-case letters, digits, and punctuation marks), instructions to the CPU, and more complex data types such as pictures, spoken language, and the content of a medical record. Figure 5.2 shows the **American Standard Code for Information Interchange** (**ASCII**), a convention for representing 95 common characters using 7 bits. These 7 bits are commonly placed into an 8-bit unit, a byte, which is the common way of transmitting and storing these characters. The eighth bit may be used for formatting information (as in a word processor) or for additional special characters (such as currency and mathematical symbols or characters with diacritic marks), but the ASCII base standard does not cover its use. Not all characters seen on a keyboard can be encoded and stored as ASCII. The Delete and Arrow keys are often dedicated to edit functions, and the Control, Escape, and Function keys are used to modify other keys or to interact directly with programs. A standard called **Unicode** represents characters needed for foreign languages using up to 16 bits; ASCII is a small subset of Unicode.

The CPU works on data that it retrieves from memory, placing them in working registers. By manipulating the contents of its registers, the CPU performs the mathematical and logical functions that are basic to information processing: addition, subtraction, and comparison ("is greater than," "is equal to," "is less than"). In addition to registers that perform computation, the CPU also has registers that it uses to store instructions—a computer program is a set of such instructions—and to control processing. In essence, a computer is an instruction follower: it fetches an instruction from memory and then executes the instruction, which usually is an operation that requires the retrieval, manipulation, and storage of data into memory or registers. The processor often performs a simple loop, fetching and executing each instruction of a program in sequence. Some instructions can direct the processor to begin fetching instructions from a different place in memory or point in the program. Such a transfer of flow control provides flexibility in program execution. Parallel flows may also be invoked.

5.2.2 Memory

The computer's working memory stores the programs and data currently being used by the CPU. Working memory has two parts: **read-only memory (ROM)** and **random-access memory (RAM)**.

ROM, or fixed memory, is permanent and unchanging. It can be read, but it cannot be altered or erased. It is used to store a few crucial programs that do not change and that must be available at all times. One such predefined program is the **bootstrap** sequence, a set of initial instructions that is executed each time the computer is started. ROM also is used to store programs that must run quickly—e.g., the base graphics that run the Macintosh computer interface.

More familiar to computer programmers is RAM, often just called **memory**. RAM can be both read and written into. It is used to store the programs, control values, and data that are in current use. It also holds the intermediate results of computations and the images to be displayed on the screen. RAM is much larger than ROM. For example, we might speak of a 2 gigabyte memory chip. A **kilobyte** is 2^{10}, or 10^3, or 1,024 bytes; a **megabyte** is 2^{20}, or 10^6, or 1,048,576 bytes; and a

gigabyte is 2^{30}, or 10^9, or 1,073,741,824 bytes. Increasing powers of 2^{10}, or 10^3, are **terabytes**, **petabytes**, and **exabytes** (10^{18}).

A sequence of bits that can be accessed by the CPU as a unit is called a **word**. The **word size** is a function of the computer's design. Early computers had word sizes of 8 or 16 bits; newer, faster computers had 32-bit and now 64-bit word sizes that allow processing of larger chunks of information at a time. The bytes of memory are numbered in sequence. The CPU accesses each word in memory by specifying the sequence number, or **address**, of its starting byte.

5.2.3 Long-Term Storage

The computer's memory is relatively expensive, being specialized for fast read–write access; therefore, it is limited in size. It is also **volatile**: its contents are changed when the next program runs, and memory contents are not retained when power is turned off. For many medical applications we need to store more information than can be held in memory, and we want to save all that information for a long time. To save valuable programs, data, or results we place them into **long-term storage**.

Programs and data that must persist over longer periods than in volatile memory are stored on long-term storage devices, such as hard disks, flash memory or solid state disks, optical disks, or magnetic tape, each of which provide persistent storage for less cost per byte than memory and are widely available. The needed information is loaded from such storage into working memory whenever it is used. Conceptually, long-term storage can be divided into two types: (1) **active storage** is used to store data that may need to be retrieved with little delay, e.g., the medical record of a patient who currently is being treated within the hospital; and (2) **archival storage** is used to store data for documentary or legal purposes, e.g., the medical record of a patient who is deceased.

Computer storage also provides a basis for the sharing of information. Whereas memory is dedicated to an executing program, data written on storage in **file systems** or in **databases** is available to other users or processes that can access the computer's storage devices. Files and databases complement direct communication among computer users and have the advantage that the writers and readers need not be present at the same time in order to share information.

5.2.4 Graphics Processing Unit

Graphics processing units are specialized for handling computation over many bytes simultaneously. They can be thought of as enabling of simultaneous processing of many data elements with tight coupling to their memory, or frame buffers, but with limited instruction sets. This allows rapid manipulation of many memory locations simultaneously, essential to their power for computer graphics, but leaves less flexibility in general. For example, GPUs are much more efficient than CPUs for video display, the primary purpose for which they were invented, or for highly parallel computation on a single machine, such as comparing genomic sequences or image processing. However, GPUs generally require different, less mature, programming languages and software architectures than CPUs making them harder to use to date. Newer languages, such as Open CL, enable some computer codes to run over either CPUs or GPUs. When GPUs are used for general computation, rather than for video or graphics display, they are referred to as general purpose GPUs or **GPGPUs**.

5.2.5 Input Devices

Data and user-command entry remain the most costly and awkward aspects of medical data processing. Certain data can be acquired automatically; e.g., many laboratory instruments provide electronic signals that can be transmitted to computers directly, and many diagnostic radiology instruments produce output in digital form. Furthermore, redundant data entry can be minimized if data are shared among computers over networks or across direct interfaces. The most common instrument for data entry is the **keyboard** on which the user types. A **cursor** indicates the current position on the screen. Most programs allow the cursor to be moved with a **pointing device**, such as a **mouse, track pad, or touch screen**, so that making insertions and corrections is convenient. Systems developers continue to experiment with a variety of alternative input devices that minimize or eliminate the need to type.

There are also three-dimensional pointing devices, where an indicator, or just the user's own body, using optical capture, is positioned in front of the screen, and a three-dimensional display may provide feedback to the user. Some three-dimensional pointing devices used in medical virtual-reality environments also provide computer-controlled force or **tactile feedback**, so that a user can experience the resistance, for example, of a simulated needle being inserted for venipuncture or a simulated scalpel making a surgical incision.

In automatic speech recognition, digitized voice signals captured through a microphone are matched to the patterns of a vocabulary of known words, and use grammar rules to allow recognition of sentence structures. The speech input is then stored as ASCII-coded text. This technology is improving in flexibility and reliability, but error rates remain sufficiently high that manual review of the resulting text is needed. This is easier for some users than typing.

5.2.6 Output Devices

The presentation of results, or of the **output**, is the complementary step in the processing of medical data. Many systems compute information that is transmitted to health care providers and is displayed immediately on local personal computers or printed so that action can be taken. Most immediate output appears at its destination on a display screen, such as the flat-panel **liquid crystal display** (**LCD**) or **light-emitting diode** (**LED**) based displays of a personal computer (PC). The near-realistic quality of computer displays enables unlimited interaction with text, images, video, and interactive graphical elements. Graphical output is essential for summarizing and presenting the information derived from voluminous data.

A graphics screen is divided into a grid of picture elements called **pixels**. One or more bits in memory represent the output for each pixel. In a black-and-white monitor, the value of each pixel on the screen is associated with the level of intensity, or gray scale. For example, 2 bits can distinguish 2^2 or 4 display values per pixel: black, white, and two intermediate shades of gray. For color displays, the number of bits per pixel, or **bit depth**, determines the **contrast** and **color resolution** of an image. Three sets of multiple bits are necessary to specify the color of pixels on LCDs, giving the intensity for red, green, and blue components of each pixel color, respectively. For instance, three sets of 8 bits per pixel provide 2^{24} or 16,777,216 colors. The number of pixels per square inch determines the **spatial resolution** of the image (Fig. 5.3). Both parameters determine the size requirements for storing images. LCD color projectors are readily available so that the output of a workstation can also be projected onto a screen for group presentations. Multiple standard hardware interfaces, such as VGA and HDMI also enable computers to easily display to high definition and even stereoscopic televisions (3DTVs). Much diagnostic information is produced in image formats that can be shown on graphics terminals. Examples are ultrasound observations, magnetic resonance images (MRIs), and computed tomography (CT) scans.

For portability and traditional filing, output is printed on paper. Printing information is slower than displaying it on a screen, so printing is best done in advance of need. In a clinic, relevant portions of various patient records may be printed on high-volume printers the night before scheduled visits. **Laser printers** use an electromechanically controlled laser beam to generate an image on a xerographic surface, which is then used to produce paper copies, just as is done in a copier. Their spatial resolution is often better than that of displays, allowing 600 dots (pixels) per inch (commercial typesetting equipment may have a resolution of several thousand dots per inch).

Color **ink-jet printers** are inexpensive, but the ink cartridges raise the cost under high use. Liquid ink is sprayed on paper by a head that moves back and forth for each line of pixels. Ink-jet printers have lower resolution than laser printers and are relatively slow, especially at high resolution. Ink-jet printers that produce images of photographic quality are also readily available. Here the base colors are merged while being sprayed so that true color mixes are placed on the paper.

Other output mechanisms are available to computer systems and may be used in medical applications, particularly sound, for alerts, feedback and instruction, such as for Automatic External Defibrillators (AEDs). A computer can produce sound via digital-to-analog conversion (see Sect. 5.3). There are also 3D printers which create objects.

5.2.7 Local Data Communications

Information can be shared most effectively by allowing access for all authorized participants whenever and wherever they need it. Transmitting data electronically among applications and computer systems facilitates such sharing by minimizing delays and by supporting interactive collaborations. Videoconferencing is also supported on PCs. Transmitting paper results in a much more passive type of information sharing. Data communication and integration are critical functions of health care information systems. Modern computing and communications are deeply intertwined.

Computer systems used in health care are specialized to fulfill the diverse needs of health professionals in various areas, such as physicians' offices, laboratories, pharmacies, intensive care units, and business offices. Even if their hardware is identical, their content will differ, and some of that content must be shared with other applications in the health care organization. Over time, the hardware in the various areas will also diverge—e.g., imaging departments will require more capable displays and larger storage, other areas will use more processor power. Demand for growth and funding to accommodate change

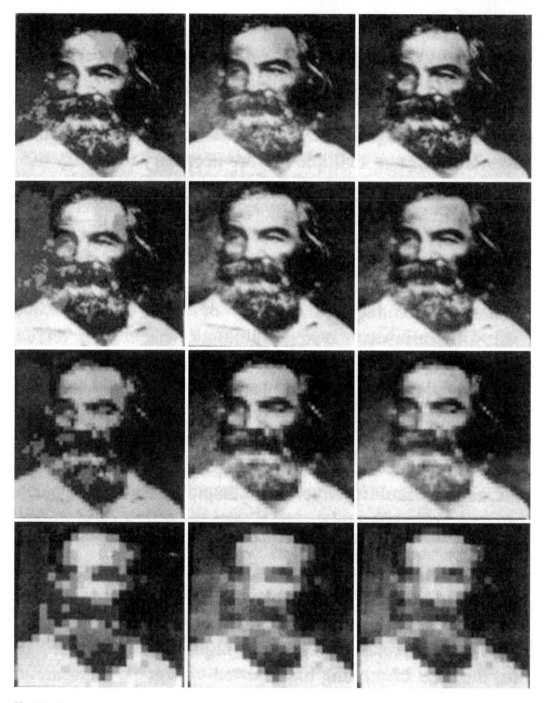

Fig. 5.3 Demonstration of how varying the number of pixels and the number of bits per pixel affects the spatial and contract resolution of a digital image. The image in the upper right corner was displayed using a 256 x 256 array of pixels, 8 bits per pixel; the subject (Walt Whitman) is easily discernible (Source: Reproduced with permission from Price R.R., & James A.E. (1982). Basic principles and instrumentation of digital radiography. In: Price R.R., et al. (Eds.). *Digital radiography: A focus on clinical utility*. Orlando: WB Saunders)

occurs at different times. Communication among diverse systems bridges the differences in computing environments.

Communication can occur via telephone lines, dedicated or shared wires, fiber-optic cables, infrared, or radio waves (wireless). In each case different communication interfaces must be enabled with the computer, different conventions or communication protocols must be obeyed, and a different balance of performance and reliability can be expected. For example, wired connections are typically higher volume communication channels and more reliable. However, communication paths can reach capacity; so for example, a wired computer in a busy hotel where the network is overloaded may communicate less reliably than a wireless smart phone with a strong wireless signal. Thus, specific communication needs and network capabilities and loads must always be considered when designing applications and implementing them.

The overall **bit rate** of a digital communication link is a combination of the rate at which symbols can be transmitted and the efficiency with which digital information (in the form of bits) is encoded in the symbols. There are many available data transmission options for connecting local networks (such as in the home). **Integrated services digital network** (**ISDN**) and, later, **digital subscriber line** (**DSL**) technologies allow network communications using conventional telephone wiring (twisted pairs). These allow sharing of data and voice transmission ranging from 1 to 10 **megabits** per second (Mbps), depending on the distance from the distribution center.

In areas remote to wired lines, these digital services may be unavailable, but the communications industry is broadening access to digital services over wireless channels. In fact, in many countries, usable wireless bandwidth exceeds wired bandwidth in many areas. Transmission for rapid distribution of information can occur via cable modems using coaxial cable (up to 30 Mbps) or direct satellite broadcast. These alternatives have a very high capacity, but all subscribers then share that capacity. Also for DSL, digital cable services and wireless services, transmission

speeds are often asymmetrical, with relatively low-speed service used to communicate back to the data source. This design choice is rationalized by the assumption that most users receive more data than they send, for example, in downloading and displaying graphics, images, and video, while typing relatively compact commands to make this happen. This assumption breaks down if users generate large data objects on their personal machine that then have to be sent to other users. In this case it may be more cost-effective in terms of user time to purchase a symmetric communication service. Home networking has been further expanded with the use of WiFi (IEEE 802.11 standard for wireless communications). Computers, cell phones, and many personal health and fitness devices with embedded computers now support WiFi to establish access to other computers and the Internet, while Bluetooth is another wireless protocol generally used for communicating among computer components (such as wireless headsets to cell phones and wireless keyboards to computers).

Frame Relay is a network protocol designed for sending digital information over shared, **wide-area networks** (**WANs**). It transmits variable-length messages or packets of information efficiently and inexpensively over dedicated lines that may handle aggregate speeds up to 45 Mbps. **Asynchronous Transfer Mode** (**ATM**) is a protocol designed for sending streams of small, fixed-length cells of information over very high-speed dedicated connections—most often digital optical circuits. The underlying optical transmission circuit sends cells synchronously and supports multiple ATM circuits. The cells associated with a given ATM circuit are queued and processed asynchronously with respect to each other in gaining access to the multiplexed (optical) transport medium. Because ATM is designed to be implemented by hardware switches, information bit rates over 10 gigabits per second (Gbps) are typical.

For communication needs within an office, a building, or a campus, installation of a **local-area network** (**LAN**) allows local data communication without involving the telephone company or **network access provider**. Such a network is dedicated to linking multiple computer nodes together at high speeds to facilitate the sharing of resources—data, software, and equipment—among multiple users. Users working at individual workstations can retrieve data and programs from network **file servers**: computers dedicated to storing local files, both shared and private. The users can process information locally and then save the results over the network to the file server or send output to a shared printer.

There are a variety of **protocols** and technologies for implementing LANs, although the differences should not be apparent to the user. Typically data are transmitted as messages or **packets** of data; each packet contains the data to be sent, the network addresses of the sending and receiving nodes, and other control information. LANs are limited to operating within a geographical area of at most a few miles and often are restricted to a specific building or a single department. Separate remote LANs may be connected by **bridges**, routers, or switches (see below), providing convenient communication between machines on different networks. The information technology department of a health care organization typically takes responsibility for implementing and linking multiple LANs to form an enterprise network. Important services provided by such network administrators include integrated access to WANs, specifically to the Internet (see later discussion on Internet communication), service reliability, and security.

Early LANs used coaxial cables as the communication medium because they could deliver reliable, high-speed communications. With improved communication signal–processing technologies, however, **twisted-pair wires** (Cat-5 and better quality) have become the standard. Twisted-pair wiring is inexpensive and has a high **bandwidth** (capacity for information transmission) of at least 100 Mbps. An alternate medium, **fiber-optic cable**, offers the highest bandwidth (over 1 billion bps or 1 Gbps) and a high degree of reliability because it uses light waves to transmit information signals and is not susceptible to electrical interference. Fiber-optic cable is used in LANs to increase transmission speeds and distances by at least one order of magnitude over twisted-pair

wire. Splicing and connecting into optical cable is more difficult than into twisted-pair wire, however, so in-house delivery of networking services to the desktop is still easier using twisted-pair wires. Fiber-optic cable, twisted-pair wires, and WiFi are often used in a complementary fashion—fiber-optic cable for the high-speed, shared backbone of an enterprise network or LAN and twisted-pair wires extending out from side-branch hubs to bring service to small areas and twisted-pair wires or WiFi to the individual workstation.

Rapid data transmission is supported by LANs. Many LANs still operate at 10 Mbps, but 100-Mbps networks are now cost-effective. Even at 10 Mbps, the entire contents of this book could be transmitted in a few seconds. Multiple users and high-volume data transmissions such as video may congest a LAN and its servers, however, so the effective transmission speed seen by each user may be much lower. When demand is high, LANs can be duplicated in parallel. Gateways, routers, and switches shuttle packets among these networks to allow sharing of data between computers as though the machines were on the same LAN. A **router** or a **switch** is a special device that is connected to more than one network and is equipped to forward packets that originate on one network segment to machines on another network. **Gateways** perform routing and can also translate packet formats if the two connected networks run different communication protocols.

Messages also can be transmitted through the air by radio, microwave, infrared, satellite signal, or line-of-sight laser-beam transmission. Application of these have many special trade-offs and considerations. **Broadband** has a specific technical meaning related to parallelization of signal transmission, but has been used more recently as a term to refer to any relatively high bandwidth network connection, such as cable service or third generation (3G) or fourth generation (4G) wireless cellular telephone services, which are now widespread means of broadband Internet access and communication.

Wireless users of a hospital or clinic can use these radio signals from portable devices to communicate with the Internet and, when authorized, to servers that contain clinical data and thus can gain entry to the LANs and associated services. Hospitals have many instruments that generate electronic interference, and often have reinforced concrete walls, so that radio transmission may not be reliable internally over long distances. In fact, in many medical settings the use of cellular or similar radio technologies was also prohibited for a time for perhaps justified fear of electromagnetic interference with telemetry or other delicate instruments. You experience electromagnetic interference when proximity of a cell phone causes public address speakers to make chattering sounds. These features and short battery life had made portable wireless devices weakly fit computers in medical applications until recently. Now, with: (1) better battery life due to improvements in battery technology; (2) smarter wireless radio use by the portable devices (e.g. cellular phones, tablet computers), which decrease the radio transmission power when they have stronger wireless signals (also reducing the risk for electromagnetic interference); (3) more reliable hospital wireless networks; and (4) better applications; portable wireless devices (e.g. tablet computers) are exploding in use in hospital environments.

5.3 Data Acquisition and Signal Processing Considerations

A prominent theme of this book is that capturing and entering data into a computer manually is difficult, time-consuming, error-prone, and expensive. **Real-time acquisition** of data from the actual source by direct electrical connections to instruments can overcome these problems. Direct acquisition of data avoids the need for people to measure, encode, and enter the data manually. Sensors attached to a patient convert biological signals—such as blood pressure, pulse rate, mechanical movement, and electrocardiogram (ECG)—into electrical signals, which are transmitted to the computer. The signals are sampled periodically and are converted to digital representation for storage and processing. Automated

data-acquisition and signal-processing techniques are particularly important in patient-monitoring settings (see Chap. 19). Similar techniques also apply to the acquisition and processing of human voice input.

Most naturally occurring signals are **analog signals**—signals that vary continuously. The first bedside monitors, for example, were wholly analog devices. Typically, they acquired an analog signal (such as that measured by the ECG) and displayed its level on a dial or other continuous display (see, for example, the continuous signal recorded on the ECG strip shown in Fig. 19.4).

The computers with which we work are **digital computers**. A digital computer stores and processes values in discrete values collected at discrete points and at discrete times. Before computer processing is possible, analog signals must be converted to digital units. The conversion process is called **analog-to-digital conversion** (**ADC**). You can think of ADC as sampling and rounding—the continuous value is observed (sampled) at some instant and is rounded to the nearest discrete unit (Fig. 5.4). You need one bit to distinguish between two levels (e.g., on or off); if you wish to discriminate among four levels, you need two bits (because $2^2 = 4$), and so on.

Two parameters determine how closely the digital data represent the original analog signal:

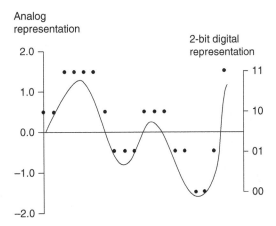

Fig. 5.4 Analog-to-digital conversion (ADC). ADC is a technique for transforming continuous-valued signals to discrete values. In this example, each sampled value is converted to one of four discrete levels (represented by 2 bits)

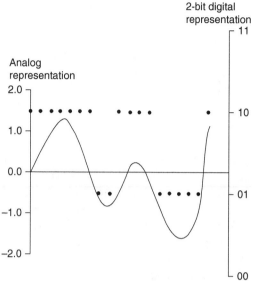

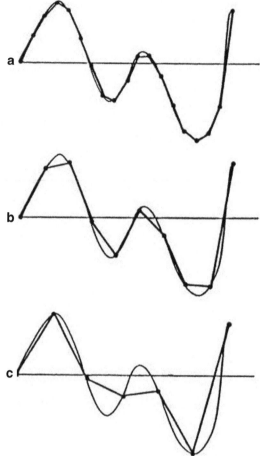

Fig. 5.5 Effect on precision of ranging. The amplitude of signals from sensors must be ranged to account, for example, for individual patient variation. As illustrated here, the details of the signal may be lost if the signal is insufficiently amplified. On the other hand, over amplification will produce clipped peaks and troughs

Fig. 5.6 The greater the sampling rate is, the more closely the sampled observations will correspond to the underlying analog signal. The sampling rate in (**a**) is highest; that in (**b**) is lower; and that in (**c**) is the lowest. When the sampling rate is very low (as in **c**), the results of the analog-to-digital conversion (ADC) can be misleading. Note the degradation of the quality of the signal from (**a**) to (**c**)

the precision with which the signal is recorded and the frequency with which the signal is sampled. The **precision** is the degree to which a digital estimate of a signal matches the actual analog value. The number of bits used to encode the digital estimate and their correctness determines precision; the more bits, the greater the number of levels that can be distinguished. Precision also is limited by the accuracy of the equipment that converts and transmits the signal. Ranging and calibration of the instruments, either manually or automatically, is necessary for signals to be represented with as much accuracy as possible. Improper ranging will result in loss of information. For example, a change in a signal that varies between 0.1 and 0.2 V will be undetectable if the instrument has been set to record changes between −2.0 and 2.0 in 0.5 V increments. Figure 5.5 shows another example of improper ranging.

The **sampling rate** is the second parameter that affects the correspondence between an analog signal and its digital representation. A sampling rate that is too low relative to the rate with which a signal changes value will produce a poor representation (Fig. 5.6). On the other hand, oversampling increases the expense of processing and storing the data. As a general rule, you need to sample at least twice as frequently as the highest-frequency component that you need to observe in a signal. For instance, looking at an ECG, we find that the basic contraction repetition frequency is at most a few per second, but that the **QRS wave** within each beat (see Sect. 17.5) contains useful frequency components on the order of 150 cycles per second, i.e., the QRS signal rises and falls within a much shorter interval than the basic heart beat. Thus, the ECG data-sampling rate should be at least 300 measurements per second. The rate calculated by doubling the highest frequency is called the **Nyquist frequency**. The ideas of sampling and signal estimation apply just as well to spatially varying signals (like images) with the temporal dimension replaced by one or more spatial dimensions.

Another aspect of signal quality is the amount of **noise** in the signal—the component of the acquired data that is not due to the specific phenomenon being measured. Primary sources of noise include random fluctuations in a signal detector or electrical or magnetic signals picked up from nearby devices and power lines. Once the signal has been obtained from a sensor, it must be transmitted to the computer. Often, the signal is sent through lines that pass near other equipment. En route, the analog signals are susceptible to electromagnetic interference. Inaccuracies in the sensors, poor contact between sensor and source (e.g., the patient), and disturbances from signals produced by processes other than the one being studied (e.g., respiration interferes with the ECG) are other common sources of noise.

Three techniques, often used in combination, minimize the amount of noise in a signal before its arrival in the computer:

1. **Shielding**, isolation, and grounding of cables and instruments carrying analog signals all reduce electrical interference. Often, two twisted wires are used to transmit the signal—one to carry the actual signal and the other to transmit the ground voltage at the sensor. At the destination, a differential amplifier measures the difference. Most types of interference affect both wires equally; thus, the difference should reflect the true signal. The use of glass fiber-optic cables, instead of copper wires, for signal transmission eliminates interference from electrical machinery, because optical signals are not affected by relatively slow electrical or magnetic fields.

2. For robust transmission over long distances, analog signals can be converted into a frequency-modulated representation. An FM signal represents changes of the signal as changes of frequency rather than of amplitude. **Frequency modulation** (**FM**) reduces noise greatly, because interference directly disturbs only the amplitude of the signal. As long as the interference does not create amplitude changes near the high carrier frequency, no loss of data will occur during transmission.

Conversion of analog signals to digital form provides the most robust transmission. The closer to the source the conversion occurs, the more reliable the data become. Digital transmission of signals is inherently less noise-sensitive than is analog transmission: interference rarely is great enough to change a 1 value to a 0 value or vice versa. Furthermore, digital signals can be coded, permitting detection and correction of transmission errors. Placing a microprocessor near the signal source is now the most common way to achieve such a conversion. The development of **digital signal processing** (**DSP**) chips—also used for computer voice mail and other applications—facilitates such applications.

3. **Filtering algorithms** can be used to reduce the effect of noise. Usually, these algorithms are applied to the data once they have been stored in memory. A characteristic of noise is its relatively random pattern. Repetitive signals, such as an ECG, can be integrated over several cycles, thus reducing the effects of random noise. When the noise pattern differs from the signal pattern, Fourier analysis can be used to filter the signal; a signal is decomposed into its individual components, each with a distinct period and amplitude. (The article by Wiederhold and Clayton (1985) in the Suggested Readings explains Fourier analysis in greater detail.) Unwanted components of the signal are assumed to be noise and are eliminated. Some noise (such as the 60-cycle interference caused by a building's electrical circuitry) has a regular pattern. In this case, the portion of the signal that is known to be caused by interference can be filtered out.

Once the data have been acquired and cleaned up, they typically are processed to reduce their volume and to abstract information for use by interpretation programs. Often, the data are analyzed to extract important parameters, or features, of the signal—e.g., the duration or intensity of the ST segment of an ECG. The computer also can analyze the shape of the waveform by comparing one part of a repetitive signal to another, e.g., to detect ECG beat irregularities, or by comparing a waveform to models of known patterns, or templates. In **speech recognition**, the voice signals can be compared with stored profiles of spoken words. Further analysis is necessary to determine the meaning or importance of the signals— e.g., to allow automated ECG-based cardiac diagnosis or to respond properly to the words recognized in a spoken input.

5.4   Internet Communication

External routers link the users on a LAN to a **regional network** and then to the **Internet**. The Internet is a WAN that is composed of many regional and local networks interconnected by long-range **backbone links**, including international links. The Internet was begun by the National Science Foundation in the 1980s, a period in which various networking approaches were overtaken by a common protocol designed and inspired by military considerations to enable scalability and robustness to failure of individual links in the network.

All Internet participants agree on many standards. The most fundamental is the protocol suite referred to as the **Transmission Control Protocol/Internet Protocol (TCP/IP)**. Data transmission is always by structured packets, and all machines are identified by a standard for IP addresses. An **Internet address** consist of a sequence of four 8-bit numbers, each ranging from 0 to 255— most often written as a dotted sequence of numbers: a.b.c.d. Although IP addresses are not assigned geographically (the way ZIP codes are), they are organized hierarchically, with a first component identifying a network, a second identifying a subnet, and a third identifying a specific computer. Computers that

are permanently linked into the Internet may have a fixed IP address assigned, whereas users whose machines reach the Internet by making a wireless connection only when needed, may be assigned a temporary address that persists just during a connected session. The Internet is in the process of changing to a protocol (IPv6) that supports 64-bit IP addresses, because the worldwide expansion of the Internet, the block address assignment process, and proliferation of networked individual computer devices are exhausting the old 32-bit address space. While the changeover is complex and has been moving slowly for more than a decade, much work has gone into making this transition transparent to the user.

Because 32-bit (and 64-bit) numbers are difficult to remember, computers on the Internet also have names assigned. Multiple names may be used for a given computer that performs distinct services. The names can be translated to IP addresses—e.g., when they are used to designate a remote machine—by means of a hierarchical name management system called the **Domain Name System** (DNS). Designated computers, called **name-servers**, convert a name into an IP address before the message is placed on the network; routing takes place based on only the numeric IP address. Names are also most often expressed as dotted sequences of name segments, but there is no correspondence between the four numbers of an IP address and the parts of a name. The Internet is growing rapidly; therefore, periodic reorganizations of parts of the network are common. Numeric IP addresses may have to change, but the logical name for a resource can stay the same and the (updated) DNS can take care of keeping the translation up to date. This overall process is governed today by **the Internet Corporation for Assigned Names and Numbers (ICANN)**. Three conventions are in use for composing Internet names from segments:

1. Functional convention: Under the most common convention for the United States, names are composed of hierarchical segments increasing in specificity from right to left, beginning with one of the top-level domain-class identifiers—e.g., computer.institution.class (ci.uchicago.edu) or institution.class (whitehouse.gov).

Initially the defined top-level domain classes were .com, .edu, .gov, .int, .mil, .org, and .net (for commercial, educational, government, international organizations, military, non-profit, and ISP organizations, respectively). As Internet use has grown, many more classes have been added. Other conventions have evolved as well: www was often used as a prefix to name the **World Wide Web** (**WWW**) services on a computer (e.g., www.nlm.nih. gov).

2. Geographic convention: Names are composed of hierarchical segments increasing in specificity from right to left and beginning with a two-character top-level country domain identifier—e.g., institution.town.state.country (cnri.reston.va.us or city.paloalto.ca.us). Many countries outside of the United States use a combination of these conventions, such as csd.abdn.ac.uk, for the Computer Science Department at the University of Aberdeen (an academic institution in the United Kingdom). Note that domain names are **case-insensitive**, although additional fields in a URL, such as file names used to locate content resources, may be **case-sensitive**.

3. Attribute list address (X.400) convention: Names are composed of a sequence of attribute-value pairs that specifies the components needed to resolve the address— e.g.,/C = GB/ ADMD = BT/PRMD = AC/O = Abdn/ OU = csd/, which is equivalent to the address csd.abdn.ac.uk. This convention derives from the X.400 address standard that is used mainly in Europe. It has the advantage that the address elements (e.g., /C for Country name, /ADMD for Administrative Management Domain name, and /PRMD for Private Management Domain name) are explicitly labeled and may come in any order. Country designations differ as well. However, this type of address is generally more difficult for humans to understand and has not been adopted broadly in the Internet community.

An institution that has many computers may provide a service whereby all communications (e.g., incoming e-mails) go to a single address (e.g., uchicago.edu or apple.com), and then local tables are used to direct each message to the right computer or individual. Such a scheme insulates outside users from internal naming conventions and changes, and can allow dynamic machine selection for the service in order to distribute loading. Such a central site can also provide a firewall—a means to attempt to keep viruses and unsolicited and unwanted connections or messages (spam) out. The nature of attacks on networks and their users is such that constant vigilance is needed at these service sites to prevent system and individual intrusions.

The routing of packets of information between computers on the Internet is the basis for a rich array of information services. Each such service— be it resource naming, electronic mail, file transfer, remote computer log in, World Wide Web, or another service— is defined in terms of sets of protocols that govern how computers speak to each other. These worldwide inter-computer linkage conventions allow global sharing of information resources, as well as personal and group communications. The Web's popularity and growing services continues to change how we deal with people, form communities, make purchases, entertain ourselves, and perform research. The scope of all these activities is more than we can cover in this book, so we restrict ourselves to topics important to health care. Even with this limitation, we can only scratch the surface of many topics.

Regional and national networking services are now provided by myriad commercial communications companies, and users get access to the regional networks through their institutions or privately by paying an **Internet service provider** (**ISP**), who in turn gets WAN access through a **network access provider** (NAP). There are other WANs besides the Internet, some operated by demanding commercial users, and others by parts of the federal government, such as the Department of Defense, the National Aeronautics and Space Administration, and the Department of Energy. Nearly all countries have their own networks connected to the Internet so that information can be transmitted to most computers in the world. Gateways of various types connect all these networks, whose capabilities may differ. It is no longer possible to show the Internet map on a single diagram.

5.5   Software

All the functions performed by the hardware of a computer system are directed by computer programs, or software (e.g. data acquisition from input devices, transfer of data and programs to and from working memory, computation and information processing by the CPU, formatting and presentation of results via the GPU, exchange of data across networks).

5.5.1   Programming Languages

In our discussion of the CPU in Sect. 5.2, we explained that a computer processes information by manipulating words of information in registers. Instructions that tell the processor which operations to perform also are sequences of 0's and 1's, a binary representation called **machine language** or **machine code** or just **code**. Machine-code instructions are the only instructions that a computer can process directly. These binary patterns, however, are difficult for people to understand and manipulate. People think best symbolically. Thus, a first step toward making programming easier and less error prone was the creation of an assembly language. **Assembly language** replaces the sequences of bits of machine-language programs with words and abbreviations meaningful to humans; a programmer instructs the computer to LOAD a word from memory, ADD an amount to the contents of a register, STORE it back into memory, and so on. A program called an **assembler** translates these instructions into binary machine-language representation before execution of the code. There is a one-to-one correspondence between instructions in assembly and machine languages. To increase efficiency, we can combine sets of assembly instructions into **macros** and thus reuse them. An assembly-language programmer must consider problems on a hardware-specific level, instructing the computer to transfer data between regis-

Assembly-language program:

```
        ORG  0        /Origin of program is location 0
        LDA A         /Load operand from location A
        ADD B         /Add operand from location B
        STA C         /Store sum in location C
        HLT           /Halt
   A,   DEC  3        /Location A contains decimal 3
   B,   DEC  15       /Location B contains decimal 15
   C,   DEC  0        /Location C contains decimal 0
        END           /End of program
```

Machine-language program:

Location	Instruction code
0	0010 0000 0000 0100
1	0001 0000 0000 0101
10	0011 0000 0000 0110
11	0111 0000 0000 0001
100	0000 0000 0000 0011
101	0000 0000 0000 1111
110	0000 0000 0000 0000

Fig. 5.7 An assembly-language program and a corresponding machine-language program to add two numbers and to store the result.

ters and memory and to perform primitive operations, such as incrementing registers, comparing characters, and handling all processor exceptions (Fig. 5.7).

On the other hand, the problems that the users of a computer wish to solve are real-world problems on a higher conceptual level. They want to be able to instruct the computer to perform tasks such as to retrieve the latest trends of their test results, to monitor the status of hypertensive patients, or to order new medications. To make communication with computers more understandable and less tedious, computer scientists developed higher-level, user-oriented **symbolic-programming languages**.

Using a higher-level language, such as one of those listed in Table 5.1, a programmer defines variables to represent higher-level entities and specifies arithmetic and symbolic operations without worrying about the details of how the hardware performs these operations. The details

Table 5.1 Distinguishing features of 17 common programming languages

Programming language	First year	Primary application domain	Type	Operation	Type checks	Procedure call method	Data management method
FORTRAN	1957	Mathematics	Procedural	Compiled	Weak	By reference	Simple files
COBOL	1962	Business	Procedural	Compiled	Yes	By name	Formatted files
Pascal	1978	Education	Procedural	Compiled	Strong	By name	Record files
Smalltalk	1976	Education	Object	Interpreted	Yes	By defined methods	Object persistence
PL/1	1965	Math, business	Procedural	Compiled	Coercion	By reference	Formatted files
Ada	1980	Math, business	Procedural	Compiled	Strong	By name	Formatted files
Standard ML	1989	Logic, math	Functional	Compiled	Yes	By value	Stream files
MUMPS (M)	1962	Data handling	Procedural	Interpreted	No	By reference	Hierarchical files
LISP	1964	Logic	Functional	Either	No	By value	Data persistence
C	1976	Data handling	Procedural	Compiled	Weak	By reference	Stream files
C++	1986	Data handling	Hybrid	Compiled	Strong	By reference	Object files
Java	1995	Data display	Object	Either	Strong	By value	Object classes
JavaScript	1995	Interactive Web	Object	Interpreted	Weak	By value or reference	Context-specific object classes
Perl	1987	Text processing	Hybrid	Interpreted	Dynamic	By reference	Stream files
Python	1990	Scripting	Hybrid	Interpreted	Dynamic	By reference	Stream files
Erlang	1986	Real-time systems	Functional; concurrent	Compiled	Dynamic	By reference	Stream files

of managing the hardware are hidden from the programmer, who can specify with a single statement an operation that may translate to thousands of machine instructions. A compiler is used to translate automatically a high-level program into machine code. Some languages are interpreted instead of compiled. An **interpreter** converts and executes each statement before moving to the next statement, whereas a compiler translates all the statements at one time, creating a binary program, which can subsequently be executed many times. MUMPS (M) is an interpreted language, LISP may either be interpreted or compiled, and FORTRAN routinely is compiled before execution. Hundreds of languages have been developed—here we touch on only a few that are important from a practical or conceptual level.

Each statement of a language is characterized by syntax and semantics. The syntactic rules describe how the statements, declarations, and other language constructs are written—they define the language's grammatical structure. Semantics is the meaning given to the various syntactic constructs. The following sets of statements (written in Pascal, FORTRAN, COBOL, and LISP) all have the same semantics:

```
C := A + B              C := A + B            LN IS "The value        (SETQ C
PRINTF(C)               WRITE 10,              is NNN.FFF"             (PLUS A B))
no layout               6 c 10               ADD A TO B, GIVING C     (format file
choice                  FORMAT                MOVE C TO LN            6 "The value
                        ("The value is" F5.2)  WRITE LN                is ~ 5, 2F" C)
```

Each set of statements instructs the computer to add the values of variables A and B, to assign the result to variable C, and to write the result onto a file. Each language has a distinct syntax for indicating which operations to perform. Regardless of the particular language in which a program is written, in the end, the computer executes similar (perhaps exactly the same) instructions to manipulate sequences of 0's and 1's within its registers.

Computer languages are tailored to handle specific types of computing problems, as shown in Table 5.1, although all these languages are sufficiently flexible to deal with nearly any type of problem. Languages that focus on a flexible, general computational infrastructure, such as C or Java have to be augmented with large collections of libraries of procedures, and learning the specific libraries takes more time than does learning the language itself. Languages also differ in usability. A language meant for education and highly reliable programs will include features to make it foolproof, by way of checking that the types of values, such as integers, decimal numbers, and strings of characters, match throughout their use—this is called **type checking**. Such features may cause programs to be slower in execution, but more reliable. Without type checking, smart programmers can instruct the computers to perform some operations more efficiently than is possible in a more constraining language.

Sequences of statements are grouped into *procedures*. Procedures enhance the clarity of larger programs and also provide a basis for reuse of the work by other programmers. Large programs are in turn mainly sequences of invocations of such procedures, some coming from libraries (such as format in LISP) and others written for the specific application. These procedures are called with *arguments*—e.g., the medical record number of a patient—so that a procedure to retrieve a value, such as the patient's age might be: age (medical record number). An important distinction among languages is how those arguments are transmitted. Just giving the value in response to a request is the safest method. Giving the name provides the most information to the procedure, and giving the reference (a pointer to where the value is stored) allows the procedure to go back to the source, which can be efficient but also allows changes that may not be

wanted. Discussions about languages often emphasize these various features, but the underlying concern is nearly always the trade-off of protection versus power.

Programmers work in successively higher levels of abstraction by writing, and later invoking, standard procedures in the form of functions and subroutines. Within these they may also have routines that spawn other routines, called **threads**. Threads allow multiple execution units, or concurrency, in programming, and as systems scale they become increasingly important, particularly as multiple functions are being run over the same data simultaneously. Built-in functions and subroutines create an environment in which users can perform complex operations by specifying single commands. Tools exist to combine related functions for specific tasks—e.g., to build a forms interface that displays retrieved data in a certain presentation format.

Specialized languages can be used directly by nonprogrammers for well-understood tasks, because such languages define additional procedures for specialized tasks and hide yet more detail. For example, users can search for, and retrieve data from, large databases using the Structured Query Language (SQL) of database management systems (discussed later in this section). With the help of statistical languages, such as SAS or R, users can perform extensive statistical calculations, such as regression analysis and correlation. Other users may use a spreadsheet program, such as Excel, to record and manipulate data with formulas in the cells of a spreadsheet matrix. In each case, the physical details of the data storage structures and the access mechanisms are hidden from the user.

The end users of a computer may not even be aware that they are programming per se, if the language is so natural that it matches their needs in an intuitive manner. Moving icons on a screen and dragging and dropping them into boxes or onto other icons is a form of programming supported by many layers of interpreters and compiler-generated code. If the user saves a **script** (a keystroke-by-keystroke record) of the actions performed for later reuse, then he or she has created a program. Some systems allow such scripts to be viewed and edited for later updates and changes; e.g., there is a macro function available in the Microsoft Excel spreadsheet and on Macintosh computers via AppleScript.

Even though many powerful languages and packages handle these diverse tasks, we still face the challenge of incorporating multiple functions into a larger system. It is easy to envision a system where a Web browser provides access to statistical results of data collected from two related databases. Such interoperation is not simple; however, modern layers of software coupled with programming expertise now make such complex interactions routine in health information systems and our everyday lives.

5.5.2 Data Management

Data provide the infrastructure for recording and sharing information. Data become information when they are organized to affect decisions, actions, and learning (see Chap. 2). Accessing and moving data from the points of collection to the points of use are among the primary functions of computing in medicine. These applications must deal with large volumes of varied data and manage them, for persistence, on external storage. The mathematical facilities of computer languages are based on common principles and are, strictly speaking, equivalent. The same conceptual basis is not available for data management facilities. Some languages allow only internal structures to be made persistent; in that case, external library programs are used for handling storage.

Handling data is made easier if the language supports moving structured data from internal memory to external, persistent storage. Data can, for instance, be viewed as a stream, a model that matches

Table 5.2 A simple patient data file containing records for four pediatric patients

Record number	Name	Sex	Date of Birth
22-546-998	Adams, Clare	F	11 Nov 1998
62-847-991	Barnes, Tanner	F	07 Dec 1997
47-882-365	Clark, Laurel	F	10 May 1998
55-202-187	Davidson, Travis	M	10 Apr 2000

Note: The key field of each record contains the medical record number that uniquely identifies the patient. The other fields of the record contain demographic information

well with data produced by some instruments, by TCP connections over the Internet, or by a ticker tape. Data can also be viewed as records, matching well with the rows of a table (Table 5.2); or data can be viewed as a hierarchy, matching well with the structure of a medical record, including patients, their visits, and their findings during a visit.

If the language does not directly support the best data structure to deal with an application, additional programming must be done to construct the desired structure out of the available facilities. The resulting extra layer, however, typically costs effort (and therefore money) and introduces inconsistencies among applications trying to share information.

5.5.3 Operating Systems

Users ultimately interact with the computer through an **operating system (OS)**: a program that supervises and controls the execution of all other programs and that directs the operation of the hardware. The OS is software that is typically included with a computer system and it manages the resources, such as memory, storage, and devices for the user. Once started, the **kernel** of the OS resides in memory at all times and runs in the background. It assigns the CPU to specific tasks, supervises other programs running in the computer, controls communication among hardware components, manages the transfer of data from input devices to output devices, and handles the details of file management such as the creation, opening, reading, writing, and closing of data files. In shared systems, it allocates the resources of the system among the competing users. The OS insulates users from much of the complexity of handling these processes. Thus, users are able to concentrate on higher-level problems of information management. They do get involved in specifying which programs to run and in giving names to the directory structures and files that are to be made persistent. These names provide the links to the user's work from one session to another. Deleting files that are no longer needed and archiving those that should be kept securely are other interactions that users have with the OS.

Programmers can write **application programs** to automate routine operations that store and organize data, to perform analyses, to facilitate the integration and communication of information, to perform bookkeeping functions, to monitor patient status, to aid in education—in short, to perform all the functions provided by medical computing systems. These programs are then filed by the OS and are available to its users when needed.

PCs typically operate as **single-user systems**, whereas servers are **multiuser systems**. In a multiuser system, all users have simultaneous access to their **jobs**; users interact through the OS, which switches resources rapidly among all the jobs that are running. Because people work slowly compared with CPUs, the computer can respond to multiple users, seemingly at the same time. Thus, all users have the illusion that they have the full attention of the machine, as long as they do not make very heavy demands. Such shared resource access is important where databases must be shared, as we discuss below in Database Management Systems. When it is managing sharing, the OS spends resources for queuing, switching, and re-queuing jobs. If the total demand is too high, the overhead increases disproportionately and slows the service for everyone. High individual demands are best allocated to distributed systems (discussed in Sect. 5.6), or to dedicated machines where all resources are prioritized to a primary user.

Because computers need to perform a variety of services, several application programs reside in main memory simultaneously. **Multiprogramming** permits the effective use of multiple devices; while the CPU is executing one program, another program may be receiving input from external storage, and another may be generating results on a printer. With the use of multiple simultaneous programs executing in one system it becomes important to ensure one program does not interfere with another or with the OS. Thus, **protected memory** comes in to play. Protected memory is only available to the program that allocated it. Web browsers and the Apple iOS (operating system for smart phones and tablets) similarly protect one process from another for security (unless authorized by the user). In **multiprocessing** systems, several processors (CPUs) are used by the OS within a single computer system, thus increasing the overall processing power. Note, however, that multiprogramming does not necessarily imply having multiple processors.

Memory may still be a scarce resource, especially under multiprogramming. When many programs and their data are active simultaneously, they may not all fit in the physical memory on the machine at the same time. To solve this problem, the OS will partition users' programs and data into **pages**, which can be kept in tempo-

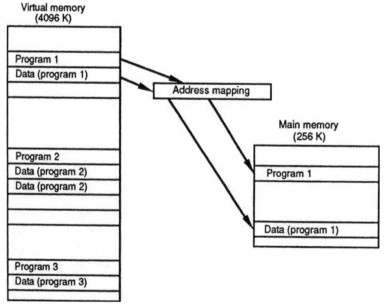

Fig. 5.8 Virtual-memory system. Virtual memory provides users with the illusion that they have many more addressable memory locations than there are in real memory—in this case, more than five times as much. Programs and data stored on peripheral disks are swapped into main memory when they are referenced; logical addresses are translated automatically to physical addresses by the hardware

rary storage on disk and are brought into main memory as needed. Such a storage allocation is called **virtual memory**. Virtual memory can be many times the size of real memory, so users can allocate many more pages than main memory can hold. Also individual programs and their data can use more memory than is available on a specific computer. Under virtual memory management, each address referenced by the CPU goes through an address mapping from the **virtual address** of the program to a physical address in main memory (Fig. 5.8). When a memory page is referenced that is not in physical storage, the CPU creates space for it by swapping out a little-used page to secondary storage and bringing in the needed page from storage. This mapping is handled automatically by the hardware on most machines but still creates significant delays, so the total use of virtual memory must be limited to a level that permits the system to run efficiently.

A large collection of **system programs** are generally associated with the **kernel** of an OS. These programs include utility programs, such as **graphical user interface** (**GUI**) routines; security management; compilers to handle programs written in higher-level languages; **debuggers** for newly created programs; communication software; diagnostic programs to help maintain the computer system; and substantial libraries of standard routines (such as for listing and viewing files, starting and stopping programs, and checking on system status). Modern software libraries include tools such as sorting programs and programs to perform complex mathematical functions and routines to present and manipulate graphical displays that access a variety of application programs, handle their point-and-click functions, allow a variety of fonts, and the like.

5.5.4 Database Management Systems

Throughout this book, we emphasize the importance to good medical decision making of timely access to relevant and complete data from diverse sources. Computers provide the primary means for organizing and accessing these data; however, the programs to manage the data are complex and

are difficult to write. Database technology supports the integration and organization of data and assists users with data entry, long-term storage, and retrieval. Programming data management software is particularly difficult when multiple users share data (and thus may try to access data simultaneously), when they must search through voluminous data rapidly and at unpredictable times, and when the relationships among data elements are complex. For health care applications, it is important that the data be complete and virtually error-free. Furthermore, the need for long-term reliability makes it risky to entrust a medical database to locally written programs. The programmers tend to move from project to project, computers will be replaced, and the organizational units that maintain the data may be reorganized.

Not only the individual data values but also their meanings and their relationships to other data must be stored. For example, an isolated data element (e.g., the number 99.7) is useless unless we know that that number represents a human's body temperature in degrees Fahrenheit and is linked to other data necessary to interpret its value—the value pertains to a particular patient who is identified by a unique medical record number, the observation was taken at a certain time (02:35, 7 Feb 2000) in a certain way (orally), and so on. To avoid loss of descriptive information, we must keep together clusters of related data throughout processing. These relationships can be complex; e.g., an observation must be linked not only to the patient but also to the person recording the observation, to the instrument that he used to acquire the values, and to the physical state of the patient.

The meaning of data elements and the relationships among those elements are captured in the structure of the database. **Databases** are collections of data, typically organized into fields, records, and files (see Table 5.2), as well as descriptive metadata. The **field** is the most primitive building block; each field represents one data element. For example, the database of a hospital's registration system typically has fields such as the patient's identification number, name, date of birth, gender, admission date, and admitting diagnosis. Fields are usually grouped together to form **records**. A record is uniquely identified by one or more **key fields**—e.g., patient identification number and observation time. Records that contain similar information are grouped in **files**. In addition to files about patients and their diagnoses, treatments, and drug therapies, the database of a health care information system will have separate files containing information about charges and payments, personnel and payroll, inventory, and many other topics. All these files relate to one another: they may refer to the same patients, to the same personnel, to the same services, to the same set of accounts, and so on.

Metadata describes where in the record specific data are stored, and how the right record can be located. For instance, a record may be located by searching and matching patient ID in the record. The metadata also specifies where in the record the digits representing the birth date are located and how to convert the data to the current age. When the structure of the database changes—e.g., because new fields are added to a record—the metadata must be changed as well. When data are to be shared, there will be continuing requirements for additions and reorganizations to the files and hence the metadata. The desire for **data independence**—i.e., keeping the applications of one set of users independent from changes made to applications by another group—is the key reason for using a database management system for shared data.

A **database management system (DBMS)** is an integrated set of programs that helps users to store and manipulate data easily and efficiently. The conceptual (logical) view of a database provided by a DBMS allows users to specify what the results should be without worrying too much about how they will be obtained; the DBMS handles the details of managing and accessing data. A crucial part of a database kept in a DBMS is the **schema**, containing the needed metadata. A schema is the machine-readable definition of the contents and organization of the records of all the data files. Programs are insulated by the DBMS from changes in the way that data are stored, because the programs access data by field name rather than by address. A DBMS also provides facilities for entering, editing, and retrieving data. Often, fields are associated with lists or ranges of valid values; thus, the DBMS can detect

SELECT	Patient ID, Name, Age, Systolic
FROM	Patients
WHERE	Sex = 'M' and
	Age >= 45 and
	Age <= 64 and
	Systolic > 140

Fig. 5.9 An example of a simple database query written in Structured Query Language (SQL). The program will retrieve the records of males whose age is between 45 and 64 years and whose systolic blood pressure is greater than 140 mmHg

and request correction of some data-entry errors, thereby improving database integrity.

Users retrieve data from a database in either of two ways. Users can query the database directly using a query language to extract information in an ad hoc fashion—e.g., to retrieve the records of all male hypertensive patients aged 45–64 years for inclusion in a retrospective study. Figure 5.9 shows the syntax for such a query using SQL. Query formulation can be difficult, however; users must understand the contents and underlying structure of the database to construct a query correctly. Often, database programmers formulate the requests for health professionals.

To support occasional use, **front-end applications** to database systems can help a user retrieve information using a menu based on the schema. More often, transactional applications, such as a drug order–entry system, will use a database system without the pharmacist or ordering physician being aware of the other's presence. The medication-order records placed in the database by the physician create communication transactions with the pharmacy; then, the pharmacy application creates the daily drug lists for the patient care units.

Some database queries are routine requests—e.g., the resource utilization reports used by health care administrators and the end-of-month financial reports generated for business offices. Thus, DBMSs often also provide an alternative, simpler means for formulating such queries, called **report generation**. Users specify their data requests on the input screen of the report-generator program. The report generator then produces the actual query program using information stored in the schema, often at predetermined intervals. The reports are formatted such that they can be distributed without modification. The report-generation programs can extract header information from the schema. Routine report generation should, however, be periodically reviewed in terms of its costs and benefits. Reports that are not read are a waste of computer, natural, and people resources. A reliable database will be able to provide needed and up-to-date information when that information is required.

Many DBMSs support multiple **views**, or models, of the data. The data stored in a database have a single physical organization, yet different user groups can have different perspectives on the contents and structure of a database. For example, the clinical laboratory and the finance department might use the same underlying database, but only the data relevant to the individual application area are available to each group. Basic patient information will be shared; the existence of other data is hidden from groups that do not need them. Application-specific descriptions of a database are stored in such **view schemas**. Through the views, a DBMS controls access to data. Thus, a DBMS facilitates the integration of data from multiple sources and avoids the expense of creating and maintaining multiple files containing redundant information. At the same time, it accommodates the differing needs of multiple users. The use of database technology, combined with communications technology (see the following discussion on Software for Network Communications), will enable health care institutions to attain the benefits both of independent, specialized applications and of large integrated databases.

Database design and implementation has become a highly specialized field. An introduction to the topic is provided by Garcia-Molina et al. (2002). Wiederhold's book (1981) discusses the organization and use of databases in health care settings. Most medical applications use standard products from established vendors. However, these databases and application architectures are inherently oriented toward the transactions needed for the workflows of the applications, one patient at a time. Thus, these are called **on line transaction processing** (**OLTP**) systems, typically designed for use by thousands of simultaneous

users doing simple repetitive queries. Data warehousing or **on line analytic processing** (**OLAP**) systems focus on use of DBMS differently, for querying across multiple patients simultaneously, typically by few users for infrequent, but complex queries, often for research. To achieve both of these architectural goals, hospital information systems will duplicate the data in two separate DBMS with different data architectures. Thus computer architectures may require the coordination of multiple individual computer systems, especially when both systems use data derived from a single source.

5.5.5 Software for Network Communications

The ability of computers to communicate with each other over local and remote networks brings tremendous power to computer users. Internet communications make it possible to share data and resources among diverse users and institutions around the world. Network users can access shared patient data (such as a hospital's medical records) or international databases (such as bibliographic databases of scientific literature or genomics databases describing what is known about the biomolecular basis of life and disease). Networks make it possible for remote users to communicate with one another and to collaborate. In this section, we introduce the important concepts that will allow you to understand network technology.

5.5.5.1 The Network Stack

Network power is realized by means of a large body of communications software. This software handles the physical connection of each computer to the network, the internal preparation of data to be sent or received over the network, and the interfaces between the network data flow and applications programs. There are now tens of millions of computers of different kinds on the Internet and hundreds of programs in each machine that service network communications. Two key ideas make it possible to manage the complexity of network software: network service stacks and network protocols. These strategies

ISO Level	TCP/IP Service Level
5–7	Applications: SMTP, FPT, TELNET, DNS, ...
4	Transport: TCP and UDP
3	Network: IP (including ICMP, ARP, and RARP)
1–2	Data link and Physical transport: (Ethernet, Token Rings, Wireless, ...)

Fig. 5.10 TCP/IP network service level stack and corresponding levels of the Open Systems Interconnection (OSI) Reference model developed by the International Standards Organization (ISO). Each level of the stack specifies a progressively higher level of abstraction. Each level serves the level above and expects particular functions or services from the level below it. *SMTP* Simple Mail Transport Protocol, *FTP* File Transfer Protocol, *DNS* Domain Name System, *TCP* Transmission Control Protocol, *UDP* User Datagram Protocol, *IP* Internet Protocol, *ICMP* Internet Control Message Protocol, *ARP* Address Resolution Protocol, *RARP* Reverse Address Resolution Protocol

allow communication to take place between any two machines on the Internet, ensure that application programs are insulated from changes in the network infrastructure, and make it possible for users to take advantage easily of the rapidly growing set of information resources and services. The **network stack** serves to organize communications software within a machine. Network software is made modular by dividing the responsibilities for network communications into different levels, with clear interfaces between the levels. The four-level network stack for TCP/IP is shown in Fig. 5.10, which also compares that stack to the seven-level stack defined by the International Standards Organization.

At the lowest level—the Data Link and Physical Transport level—programs manage the physical connection of the machine to the network, the physical-medium packet formats, and the means for detecting and correcting errors. The Network level implements the IP method of addressing packets, routing packets, and controlling the timing and sequencing of transmissions. The Transport level converts packet-level communications into several services for the Application level, including a reliable serial byte stream (TCP), a transaction-oriented User Datagram Protocol (UDP), and newer services such as real-time video.

The Application level is where programs run that support electronic mail, file sharing and transfer, Web posting, downloading, browsing, and many other services. Each layer communicates with only the layers directly above and below it and does so through specific interface conventions. The network stack is machine- and OS-dependent—because it has to run on particular hardware and to deal with the OS on that machine (filing, input–output, memory access, etc.). But its layered design serves the function of modularization. Applications see a standard set of data-communication services and do not each have to worry about details such as how to form proper packets of an acceptable size for the network, how to route packets to the desired machine, how to detect and correct errors, or how to manage the particular network hardware on the computer. If a computer changes its network connection from a wired to a wireless network, or if the **topology** of the network changes, the applications are unaffected. Only the lower level Data Link and Network layers need to be updated.

Internet protocols(see Sect. 5.3) are shared conventions that serve to standardize communications among machines—much as, for two people to communicate effectively, they must agree on the syntax and meaning of the words they are using, the style of the interaction (lecture versus conversation), a procedure for handling interruptions, and so on. Protocols are defined for every Internet service (such as routing, electronic mail, and Web access) and establish the conventions for representing data, for requesting an action, and for replying to a requested action. For example, protocols define the format conventions for e-mail addresses and text messages (RFC822), the attachment of multimedia content (Multipurpose Internet Mail Extensions (MIME)), the delivery of e-mail messages (Simple Mail Transport Protocol (SMTP)), the transfer of files (File Transfer Protocol (FTP)), connections to remote computers (SSH), the formatting of Web pages (Hypertext Markup Language (HTML)), the exchange of routing information, and many more. By observing these protocols, machines of different types can communicate openly and can interoperate with each other. When requesting a Web page from a server using the Hypertext Transfer Protocol (HTTP), the client does not have to know whether the server is a UNIX machine, a Windows machine, or a mainframe running VMS—they all appear the same over the network if they adhere to the HTTP protocol. The layering of the network stack is also supported by protocols. As we said, within a machine, each layer communicates with only the layer directly above or below. Between machines, each layer communicates with only its peer layer on the other machine, using a defined protocol. For example, the SMTP application on one machine communicates with only an SMTP application on a remote machine. Similarly, the Network layer communicates with only peer Network layers, for example, to exchange routing information or control information using the Internet Control Message Protocol (ICMP).

We briefly describe four of the basic services available on the Internet: electronic mail, FTP, SSH, and access to the World Wide Web.

5.5.5.2 Electronic Mail

Users send to and receive messages from other users via electronic mail, mimicking use of the postal service. The messages travel rapidly: except for queuing delays at gateways and receiving computers, their transmission is nearly instantaneous. Electronic mail was one of the first protocols invented for the Internet (around 1970, when what was to become the Internet was still called the **ARPANET**). A simple e-mail message consists of a **header** and a **body**. The header contains information formatted according to the RFC822 protocol, which controls the appearance of the date and time of the message, the address of the sender, addresses of the recipients, the subject line, and other optional header lines. The body of the message contains free text. The user addresses the e-mail directly to the intended reader by giving the reader's account name or a personal alias followed by the IP address or domain name of the machine on which the reader receives mail—e.g., JohnSmith@ domain.name. If the body of the e-mail message is encoded according to the MIME standard it may also contain arbitrary multimedia information, such as drawings, pictures, sound, or video. Mail is sent to the recipient using the SMTP standard. It may either be read on the machine holding the addressee's account or it may be downloaded to the addressee's local computer for reading.

It is easy to broadcast electronic mail by sending it to a **mailing list** or a specific **list-server**, but electronic mail etiquette conventions dictate that such communications be focused and relevant. **Spamming**, which is sending e-mail solicitations or announcements to broad lists, is annoying to recipients, but is difficult to prevent. Conventional e-mail is sent in clear text over the network so that anyone observing network traffic can read its contents. Protocols for encrypted e-mail, such as Privacy-Enhanced Mail (PEM) or encrypting attachments, are also available, but are not yet widely deployed. They ensure that the contents are readable by only the intended recipients. Because secure email is generally not in use, communication of protected health information from providers to patients is potentially in violation of the HIPAA regulations in that the information is not secure in transit. It remains less clear, however, if it is appropriate for physicians to answer direct questions from patients in email, given that the patient has begun the insecure communication. Large health systems have generally deployed secure communication portals over the Web (where both participants must authenticate to the same system) to overcome this.

5.5.5.3 File Transfer Protocol (FTP)

FTP facilitates sending and retrieving large amounts of information—of a size that is uncomfortably large for electronic mail. For instance, programs and updates to programs, complete medical records, papers with many figures or images for review, and the like could be transferred via FTP. FTP access requires several steps: (1) accessing the remote computer using the IP address or domain name; (2) providing user identification to authorize access; (3) specifying the name of a file to be sent or fetched using the file-naming convention at the destination site; and (4) transferring the data. For open sharing of information by means of FTP sites, the user identification is by convention "anonymous" and the requestor's e-mail address is used as the password. **Secure FTP (SFTP)** uses the same robust security mechanism as SSH (below), but provides poor performance. **Globus Online** is a SaaS data movement solution (see Sect. 5.7.4) that provides both security and high performance.

5.5.5.4 SSH

Secure Shell allows a user to log in on a remote computer securely over unsecured networks using public-key encryption (discussed in next section). If the log-in is successful, the user becomes a fully qualified user of the remote system, and the user's own machine becomes a relatively passive terminal in this context. The smoothness of such a terminal emulation varies depending on the differences between the local and remote computers. Secure Shell replaced Telnet which was used for terminal emulation until network security became important. Secure Shell enables complete command line control of the remote system to the extent the user's account is authorized.

5.5.5.5 World Wide Web (WWW)

Web **browsing** facilitates user access to remote information resources made available by Web servers. The user interface is typically a **Web browser** that understands the World Wide Web protocols. The **Universal Resource Locator (URL)** is used to specify where a resource is located in terms of the protocol to be used, the domain name of the machine it is on, and the name of the information resource within the remote machine. The **Hyper Text Markup Language (HTML)** describes what the information should look like when displayed. HTML supports conventional text, font settings, headings, lists, tables, and other display specifications. Within HTML documents, highlighted **buttons** can be defined that point to other HTML documents or services. This **hypertext** facility makes it possible to create a web of cross-referenced works that can be navigated by the user. HTML can also refer to subsidiary documents that contain other types of information—e.g., graphics, equations, images, video, speech— that can be seen or heard if the browser has been augmented with **helpers** or **plug-ins** for the particular format used. The **Hyper Text Transfer Protocol (HTTP)** is used to communicate between browser clients and servers and to retrieve HTML documents. Such communications can be **encrypted** to protect sensitive contents (e.g., credit card information or patient information) from external view using protocols such as **Secure Sockets Layer (SSL:** recently renamed to **Transport Level Security, TLS)** which is used by the HTTPS protocol (and generally shows a "lock" icon when the browser is securely communicating with the host in the URL).

HTML documents can also include small programs written in the Java language, called **applets**, which will execute on the user's computer when referenced. Applets can provide animations and also can compute summaries, merge information, and interact with selected files on the user's computer. The Java language is designed such that operations that might be destructive to the user's machine environment are blocked, but downloading remote and untested software still represents a substantial security risk (see Sect. 5.3). The JavaScript language, distinct from the Java language (unfortunately similarly named) runs in the browser itself (much like protected memory), thus reducing this security risk, and is becoming increasingly powerful, enhancing substantially the capabilities and capacity of the Web browser as a computer platform.

HTML captures many aspects of document description from predefined markup related to the appearance of the document on a display to markup related to internal links, scripts, and other semantic features. To separate appearance-related issues from other types of markup, to provide more flexibility in terms of markup types, and to work toward more open, self-defining document descriptions, a more powerful markup framework, called **eXtensible Markup Language** (XML), has emerged. Coupled with JavaScript, XML further enhances the capabilities of the Web browser itself as a computer platform.

5.5.5.6 Client-Server Interactions

A client–server interaction is a generalization of the four interactions we have just discussed, involving interactions between a client (requesting) machine and a server (responding) machine. A **client–server** interaction, in general, supports collaboration between the user of a local machine and a remote computer. The server provides information and computational services according to some protocol, and the user's computer—the client—generates requests and does complementary processing (such as displaying HTML documents and images). A common function provided by servers is database access. Retrieved information is transferred to the client in response to requests, and then the client may perform specialized analyses on the data. The final results can be stored locally, printed, or mailed to other users.

5.6   Data and System Security

Medical records contain much information about us. These documents and databases include data ranging from height and weight measurements, blood pressures, and notes regarding bouts with the flu, cuts, or broken bones to information about topics such as fertility and abortions, emotional problems and psychiatric care, sexual behaviors, sexually transmitted diseases, human

immunodeficiency virus (HIV) status, substance abuse, physical abuse, and genetic predisposition to diseases. Some data are generally considered to be mundane, others highly sensitive. Within the medical record, there is much information about which any given person may feel sensitive. As discussed in Chap. 10, health information is confidential, and access to such information must be controlled because disclosure could harm us, for example, by causing social embarrassment or prejudice, by affecting our insurability, or by limiting our ability to get and hold a job. Medical data also must be protected against loss. If we are to depend on electronic medical records for care, they must be available whenever and wherever we need care, and the information that they contain must be accurate and up to date. Orders for tests or treatments must be validated to ensure that they are issued by authorized providers. The records must also support administrative review and provide a basis for legal accountability. These requirements touch on three separate concepts involved in protecting health care information.

Privacy refers to the desire of a person to control disclosure of personal health and other information. **Confidentiality** applies to information—in this context, the ability of a person to control the release of his or her personal health information to a care provider or information custodian under an agreement that limits the further release or use of that information. **Security** is the protection of privacy and confidentiality through a collection of policies, procedures, and safeguards. Security measures enable an organization to maintain the integrity and availability of information systems and to control access to these systems' contents. Health privacy and confidentiality are discussed further in Chap. 10.

Concerns about, and methods to provide, security are part of most computer systems, but health care systems are distinguished by having especially complex considerations for the use and release of information. In general, the security steps taken in a health care information system serve five key functions (National Research Council, 1997), namely availability, accountability, perimeter control, role-limited access, and comprehensibility and control. We discuss each of these functions in turn.

5.6.1 Availability

Availability ensures that accurate and up-to-date information is available when needed at appropriate places. It is primarily achieved to protect against loss of data by ensuring redundancy—performing regular system backups. Because hardware and software systems will never be perfectly reliable, information of long-term value is copied onto archival storage, and copies are kept at remote sites to protect the data in case of disaster. For short-term protection, data can be written on duplicate storage devices. Critical medical systems must be prepared to operate even during environmental disasters. If one of the storage devices is attached to a remote processor, additional protection is conferred. Therefore, it is also important to provide secure housing and alternative power sources for CPUs, storage devices, network equipment, etc. It is also essential to maintain the integrity of the information system software to ensure availability. Backup copies provide a degree of protection against software failures; if a new version of a program damages the system's database, the backups allow operators to roll back to the earlier version of the software and database contents.

Unauthorized software changes—e.g., in the form of **viruses** or **worms**—are also a threat. A virus may be attached to an innocuous program or data file, and, when that program is executed or data file is opened, several actions take place:

1. The viral code copies itself into other files residing in the computer.
2. It attaches these files to outgoing messages, to spread itself to other computers.
3. The virus may collect email addresses to further distribute its copies.
4. The virus may install other programs to destroy or modify other files, often to escape detection.
5. A program installed by a virus may record keystrokes with passwords or other sensitive information, or perform other deleterious actions.

A software virus causes havoc with computer operations, even if it does not do disabling damage, by disturbing operations and system access and by producing large amounts of Internet traffic as it repeatedly distributes itself (what is called a denial of service attack). To protect against viruses, all programs loaded onto the system should be checked against known viral codes and for unexpected changes in size or configuration. It is not always obvious that a virus program has been imported. For example, a word-processing document may include macros that help in formatting the document. Such a macro can also include viral codes, however, so the document can be infected. Spreadsheets, graphical presentations, and so on are also subject to infection by viruses.

5.6.2 Accountability

Accountability for use of medical data can be promoted both by surveillance and by technical controls. It helps to ensure that users are responsible for their access to, and use of, information based on a documented need and right to know. Most people working in a medical environment are highly ethical. In addition, knowledge that access to, and use of, data records are being watched, through scanning of access **audit trails**, serves as a strong impediment to abuse. Technical means to ensure accountability include two additional functions: authentication and authorization.

1. The user is **authenticated** through a positive and unique identification process, such as name and password combination.
2. The authenticated user is **authorized** within the system to perform only certain actions appropriate to his or her role in the health care system—e.g., to search through certain medical records of only patients under his or her care.

Authentication and authorization can be performed most easily within an individual computer system, but, because most institutions operate multiple computers, it is necessary to coordinate these access controls consistently across all the systems. Enterprise-wide and remote access-control standards and systems are available and are being deployed extensively.

5.6.3 Perimeter Definition

Perimeter definition requires that you know who your users are and how they are accessing the information system. It allows the system to control the boundaries of trusted access to an information system, both physically and logically. For health care providers within a small physician practice, physical access can be provided with a minimum of hassle using simple name and password combinations. If a clinician is traveling or at home and needs remote access to a medical record, however, greater care must be taken to ensure that the person is who he or she claims to be and that communications containing sensitive information are not observed inappropriately. But where is the boundary for being considered a trusted insider? Careful control of where the network runs and how users get outside access is necessary. Most organizations install a **firewall** to define the boundary: all sharable computers of the institution are located within the firewall. Anyone who attempts to access a shared system from the outside must first pass through the firewall, where strong authentication and protocol access controls are in place. Having passed this authentication step, the user can then access enabled services within the firewall (still limited by the applicable authorization controls). Even with a firewall in place, it is important for enterprise system administrators to monitor and ensure that the firewall is not bypassed. For example, a malicious intruder could install a new virus within the perimeter, install or use surreptitiously a wireless base station, or load unauthorized software.

Virtual Private Network (**VPN**) technologies offer a powerful way to let bona fide users access information resources remotely. Using a client–server approach, an encrypted communication link is negotiated between the user's client machine and an enterprise server. This approach protects all communications and uses strong authentication to identify the user. No matter how secure the connection is, however, sound security ultimately depends on responsible users and care that increasingly portable computers (laptops, tablets, or handheld devices) are not lost or stolen

so that their contents are accessible by unauthorized people. This is the single most common mechanism by which HIPAA violations occur. Health systems are therefore requiring whole machine encryption on portable devices.

Strong authentication and authorization controls depend on cryptographic technologies. **Cryptographic encoding** is a primary tool for protecting data that are stored or are transmitted over communication lines. Two kinds of cryptography are in common use— secret-key cryptography and public-key cryptography. In **secret-key cryptography**, the same key is used to encrypt and to decrypt information. Thus, the key must be kept secret, known to only the sender and intended receiver of information. In **public-key cryptography**, two keys are used, one to encrypt the information and a second to decrypt it. One is kept secret. The other one can be made publicly available. It is thus asymmetric and one end of the transaction can be proven to have been done by a specific entity. By using this twice (four keys), one can certify both the sender and receiver. This arrangement leads to important services in addition to the exchange of sensitive information, such as digital signatures (to certify authorship), content validation (to prove that the contents of a message have not been changed), and nonrepudiation (to ensure that an action cannot be denied as having been done by the actor). Under either scheme, once data are encrypted, a key is needed to decode and make the information legible and suitable for processing.

Keys of longer length provide more security, because they are harder to guess. Because powerful computers can help intruders to test millions of candidate keys rapidly, single-layer encryption with keys of 56-bit length (the length prescribed by the 1975 **Data Encryption Standard** (**DES**)) are no longer considered secure, and keys of 128 and even 256 bits are routine. If a key is lost, the information encrypted with the key is effectively lost as well. If a key is stolen, or if too many copies of the key exist for them to be tracked, unauthorized people may gain access to information. Holding the keys in **escrow** by a trusted party can provide some protection against loss.

Cryptographic tools can be used to control authorization as well. The authorization information may be encoded as digital **certificates**, which then can be validated with a certification authority and checked by the services so that the services do not need to check the authorizations themselves. Centralizing authentication and authorization functions simplifies the coordination of access control, allows for rapid revocation of privileges as needed, and reduces the possibility of an intruder finding holes in the system. A central authentication or authorization server must itself be guarded and managed with extreme care, however, so that the chain of access-control information is not broken. Modern browsers contain the public certificates for major certificate authorities thus enabling them to check the veracity of Web sites using HTTPS (enabling the locked browser icon discussed earlier).

5.6.4 Role-Limited Access

Role-limited access control is based on extensions of authorization schemes. It allows access for personnel to only that information essential to the performance of their jobs and limits the real or perceived temptation to access information beyond a legitimate need. Even when overall system access has been authorized and is protected, further checks must be made to control access to specific data within the record. A medical record is partitioned according to access criteria based upon use privileges; the many different collaborators in health care all have diverse needs for the information collected in the medical record. Examples of valid access privileges include the following:

- Patients: the contents of their own medical records
- Community physicians: records of their patients
- Specialty physicians: records of patients referred for consultations
- Public health agencies: incidences of communicable diseases
- Medical researchers: consented data, or by waiver of authorization for patient groups approved by an **Institutional Review Board (IRB)**

- Billing clerks: records of services, with supporting clinical documentation as required by insurance companies
- Insurance payers: justifications of charges

Different types of information kept in medical records have different rules for release, as determined by state and federal law such as provisions of the Health Insurance Portability and Accountability Act (HIPAA) and as set by institutional policy following legal and ethical considerations and the IRB.

5.6.5 Comprehensibility and Control

Comprehensibility and Control ensures that record owners, data stewards, and patients can understand and have effective control over appropriate aspects of information confidentiality and access. From a technological perspective, while authentication and access control are important control mechanisms, audit trails are perhaps the most important means for allowing record owners and data stewards to understand whether data is being accessed correctly or incorrectly. Many hospitals also allow employees to review who has accessed their personal records. This ability both reassures employees and builds awareness of the importance of patient privacy.

An audit trail contains records indicating what data was accessed, when, by who, from where, and if possible some indication of the reason for the access. If backed by strong authentication and protected against improper deletion, such records can both provide a strong disincentive for improper access (because individuals will know that accesses will be recorded) and allow responsible parties to detect inadequate controls.

5.7 Distributed System Architectures

As noted in Sect. 5.5.5, computer networks have become fundamental to both health care and biomedical research, allowing for quasi-instantaneous information sharing and communication within and between clinical and research institutions. Applications such as the Web, email, videoconferencing, and SSH for remote access to computers are all widely used to reduce barriers associated with physical separation.

As health care becomes more information driven, we see increased interest in not just enabling ad hoc access to remote data, but in linking diverse information systems into **distributed systems**. A distributed system links multiple computer systems in such a way that they can function, to some extent at least, as a single information system. The systems to be linked may live within a single institution (e.g., an electronic medical record system operated by a hospital's information technology services organization, a pathology database operated by the Department of Pathology, and a medical PACS system operated by the Department of Radiology); within multiple institutions of similar type (e.g., electronic medical record systems operated by different hospitals); or within institutions of quite different types (e.g., a hospital and a third-party cloud (see Sect. 5.7.5) service provider). They may be linked for a range of reasons: for example, to federate database systems, so as to permit federated queries (see Sect. 5.7.2) across different databases—e.g., to find records corresponding to multiple admissions for a single patient at different hospitals, or to identify potential participants in a clinical trial; to enable cross-institutional workflows, such as routing of infectious disease data to a public health organization; or to outsource expensive tasks to third-party providers, as when a medical center maintains an off-site backup of its databases in a cloud provider.

Distributed systems can be challenging to construct and operate. They are, first of all, networked systems, and thus are inevitably subject to a wide range of failures. Yet more seriously, they commonly span administrative boundaries, and in the absence of strong external control and/or incentives, different administrative units tend to adopt distinct and incompatible technical solutions, information representations, policies, and governance structures. These problems seem to be particularly prevalent within health care, which despite much effort towards standardization over many decades, remains dominated by non-standards-based products. This situation can make even point-to-point integration of two systems within a single hospital challenging; the creation of large-scale distributed systems that span many institutions remains difficult.

To illustrate the types of problems that may exist, consider a distributed system that is intended to provide a unified view of electronic medical records maintained in databases D_A and D_B at two hospitals, H_A and H_B. We may find that:

- Databases D_A and D_B use different database management systems (see Sect. 5.4), with different access protocols and query languages
- Databases D_A and D_B use different schemas and vocabularies to represent patient information
- Hospitals H_A and H_B assign different identifiers to the same patient
- Hospital H_A does not allow remote access to its electronic medical record system, restricting access to computers located within its firewall (see Sect. 5.4)
- Hospital H_B interprets HIPAA rules as preventing information about its patients to be shared with personnel who are not H_B employees
- Hospitals H_A and H_B both have a governance structure that reviews proposed changes to computer and data systems ahead of implementation, but neither includes representation from the developers of the distributed system.

As this brief and partial list shows, the development of a successful distributed system can require solutions to a wide range of heterogeneity problems, including syntactic (e.g., different formats used to represent data in databases), semantic (e.g., different meanings assigned to a clinical diagnosis), policy, and governance. The use of appropriate distributed system technologies can assist with overcoming these problems, but any effective and robust solution must take into account all aspects of the problem.

5.7.1 Distributed System Programming

To build a distributed system, it must be possible for a program running on one computer to issue a request that results in a program being run in another computer. Various approaches have been pursued over the years to this **distributed system programming** problem. All seek to hide heterogeneity across different platforms via the introduction of a standardized remote procedure call mechanism. Under the covers, communication typically occurs via the Internet protocols described in Sect. 5.5.5; distributed system programming methods build on that base to allow a programmer to name a remote procedure that is to be called (e.g., "query database"), specify arguments to that procedure (e.g., "find patients with influenza"), specify how results are to be returned, provide required security credentials, and so forth—all without the programmer needing to know anything about how the remote program is implemented. Other related methods may allow a programmer to discover what procedures are supported by a particular remote system, or alternatively what remote system should be contacted for a particular purpose.

One distributed system programming approach on which much effort has been spent is **CORBA**, the Common Object Request Broker Architecture. Starting in the mid 1990s, numerous technology providers and adopters formed the Object Management Group (OMG) to define standards for describing remotely accessible procedures (an Interface Definition Language: **IDL**) and for invoking those procedures over a network. Building on that base, a wide range of other standards have been developed defining interaction patterns important for different fields. In the field of health care, the CORBAmed activity defined a range of specifications for such things as personal identification and medical image access. Unfortunately, while CORBA has had some success in certain industries (e.g., manufacturing), a combination of technical limitations in its specifications and inter-company conflict (e.g., Microsoft never adopted CORBA) had prevented it from having broad impact as a distributed system programming technology.

In the mid 2000s, a new technology called **Web Services** emerged that implemented simi-lar concepts to those found in CORBA, but in a simpler and more flexible form. Web Services uses XML (Sect. 5.5.5.5) to encode remote procedure calls and HTTP (Sect. 5.5.5.5) to communicate them, and defines an IDL called Web Services Description Language (**WSDL**). These technologies have seen wide use in many areas, including biomedical research, with many research datasets and analytic procedures being made accessible over the network via Web Service interfaces. However, adoption within clinical systems remains modest for reasons listed above.

Over the past 5 years, the commercial and consumer Web/Cloud market — as typified, for example, by the likes of Google, Facebook, Twitter, and Amazon — has largely converged on a yet simpler architectural approach for defining interfaces to services. This approach is based on a small set of protocol standards and methodologies, namely REST and HTTP, JSON and XML, TLS, and O Auth 2.0. These same methods are seeing increasingly widespread use in health care as well, due to their simplicity and the substantial investment in relevant technologies occurring within industry. At the core of this approach is **REpresentational State Transfer** (**REST**), an HTTP-based approach to distributed system architecture in which components are modeled as *resources* that are named by URLs and with which interaction occurs through standard HTTP actions (POST, GET, PUT, DELETE). For example, Table 5.3 illustrates a simple REST encoding of an interface to a medical record system. This interface models patients as resources with the following form, where {patient-id} is the patient identifier:

/patients/{patient-id}

Table 5.3 Example REST representation of a patient record interface. On the left, the format of each request; on the right, a brief description

Request	Description
GET/patients	Retrieve list of patients
GET or POST/patients/{patient-id}	Get/put profile for a specific patient
GET/patients/{patient-id}/lab results	Request lab results for a specific patient

Thus, to request all patients that we have permission to see we send the following HTTP request:
GET/patients/
while to obtain the profile for a specific patient named NAME we send this request:
GET/patients/NAME
and to update that profile we send the request:
POST/patients/NAME

REST and HTTP define how to name resources (URLs) and messaging semantics, but not how to encode message contents. Two primary message encoding schemes are used: **Java Script Object Notation** (**JSON**) and XML. The following is a potential JSON encoding of a response to a GET/patients/request. The response provides a list of patient identifiers plus (because there may be many more patients that can fit in a single response) information regarding the number of patients included in this response (X), an offset that can be provided in a subsequent request to get new patients (Y), and the number of patients remaining (Z):

```
{"patients":
{"list":[list of patients],
"count":X,
"offset":Y,
"remain":Z}
}
```

5.7.2   Distributed Databases

Distributed databases are a special case of a distributed system. The problem here is to enable queries against data located in multiple databases. Two different methods are commonly used. In a **data warehouse** approach, an **extract-transform-load** (**ETL**) process is used to extract data from the various sources, transform it as required to fit the schema and semantics used by the data warehouse, and then load the transformed data into the data warehouse. In a **federated query** approach, a query is dispatched to the different databases, applied to each of them independently, and then the results combined to get the complete answer. Intermediate components called **mediators** may be used to convert between different syntaxes and semantics used in different systems.

These two approaches have various advantages and disadvantages. The data warehouse requires a potentially expensive ETL process, requires storage for a separate copy of all relevant data, and may not be up to date with all source databases. However, it can permit highly efficient queries against the entirety of the data. The federated query approach can provide access to the latest data from each source database, but requires potentially complex mediator technology.

5.7.3   Parallel Computing

Parallel computers combine many microprocessors and/or GPUs (see Sect. 5.2) to provide an aggregate computing capacity greater than that of a single workstation. The largest such systems available today have more than one million processing cores. While systems of that scale are not used in medicine, parallel computers are becoming more commonly used in biomedical computing as a means of performing large-scale computational simulations and/or analyzing large quantities of data. In basic research, parallel computers are used for such purposes as mining clinical records, genome sequence analysis, protein folding, simulation studies of cell membranes, and modeling of blood flow. In translational research, parallel computers are commonly used to compute parameters for computer programs that are then used in clinical settings, for example, for computed aided diagnosis of mammograms.

When computing over large quantities of data, it is often useful to employ a **parallel database management system**. These systems support the same SQL query language as sequential database management systems (see Sect. 5.5.4.) but can run queries faster when using multiple processors. Another increasingly popular approach to parallel data analysis is to use the **MapReduce** model, popularized by Google and widely available via the free **Hadoop** software. MapReduce programs may be less efficient than equivalent SQL programs but do not require that data be loaded into a database prior to processing.

5.7.4 Grid Computing

Grid computing technologies allow for the federation of many computers and/or data resources in such a way that they can be used in an integrated manner. Grid computing is the foundation, for example, for the worldwide distributed system that analyzes data from the Large Hadron Collider (LHC) in Geneva, Switzerland. The 10 or more petabytes (10×10^{15} bytes) produced per year at the LHC is distributed to several hundred institutions worldwide for analysis. Each institution that participates in this worldwide system has its own local computer system administration team, user authentication system, accounting system, and so forth. Grid technologies bridge these institutional barriers, allowing a user to authenticate once (to "the grid"), and then submit jobs for execution at any or all computers in the grid.

Grid computing is used in many academic campuses to link small and large computer clusters and even idle desktop computers for parallel computing applications. But its biggest use in research is to enable sharing of large quantities of data across institutional boundaries. By addressing the challenges of authentication, access control, and high-speed data movement, grid computing technologies make it possible, for example, to acquire genome sequence from a commercial sequencing provider, transport that data over the network to a cloud computing provider (see Sect. 5.7.5), perform analysis there, and then load results into a database at a researcher's home institution.

5.7.5 Cloud Computing

The late 2000s saw the emergence of successful commercial providers of on-demand computing and software services. This concept is certainly not new: for example, McCarthy first referred to "utility computing" in 1961, various time sharing services provided computing over the network in the 1970s and 1980s, and grid computing provided such services in the 1990s and 2000s. However, it is clear that—perhaps driven by a combination of quasi-ubiquitous high-speed Internet, vastly increased demand from e-commerce, powerful lightweight Web protocols, and an effective business model— cloud computing has achieved large-scale adoption in ways that previous efforts had not. The implications of these developments for medical informatics will surely be profound.

The **National Institutes of Standards and Technology** (NIST) defines cloud computing as "a model for enabling ubiquitous, convenient, on-demand network access to a shared pool of configurable computing resources (e.g., networks, servers, storage, applications, and services) that can be rapidly provisioned and released with minimal management effort or service provider interaction" (Mell and Grance, 2011). They distinguish between three distinct types of cloud service (see Fig. 5.11):

- *Software as a Service* (*SaaS*) allows the consumer to use the provider's applications running on a cloud infrastructure. Examples include Google mail, Google Docs, Salesforce.com customer relationship management, and a growing number of electronic medical record and practice management systems.
- *Platform as a Service* (*PaaS*) allows the consumer to deploy consumer-created or acquired applications onto the cloud infrastructure, created using programming languages, libraries, services, and tools supported by the provider. Google's App Engine and Salesforce's Force.com are examples of such platforms.
- *Infrastructure as a Service* (*IaaS*) allows the consumer to provision processing, storage, networks, and other fundamental computing resources on which the consumer is able to deploy and run arbitrary software. Amazon Web Services and Microsoft Azure are popular IaaS providers.

Each level of the stack can, and often does, build on services provided by the level below. For example, Google Mail is a SaaS service that runs on compute and storage infrastructure services operated by Google; Globus Online is a SaaS research data management service that runs on infrastructure services operated by Amazon Web Services.

NIST further distinguishes between public cloud providers, which deliver such capabilities

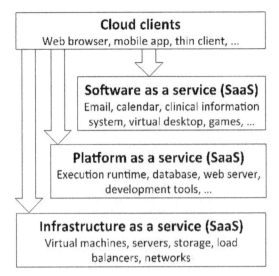

Fig. 5.11 The NIST taxonomy of cloud providers. SaaS, PaaS, and IaaS providers each offer different types of services to their clients. Cloud services are distinguished by their Web 2.0 interfaces, which can be accessed either via Web browsers or (for access from other programs or scripts) via simple APIs

to anyone, and private cloud providers, which provide such on-demand services for consumers within an organization.

Benefits claimed for cloud computing include increased reliability, higher usability, and reduced cost relative to equivalent software deployed and operated within the consumer's organization, due to expert operations and economies of scale. (IaaS providers such as Amazon charge for computing and storage on a per-usage basis.) Potential drawbacks include security challenges associated with remote operations, lock-in to a remote cloud provider, and potentially higher costs if usage becomes large.

Outside health care, cloud computing has proven particularly popular among smaller businesses, who find that they can outsource essentially all routine information technology functions (e.g., email, Web presence, accounting, billing, customer relationship management) to SaaS providers. Many companies also make considerable use of IaaS from the likes of Amazon Web Services and Microsoft Azure for compute- and data-intensive computations that exceed local capacity. In research, we see the emergence of a

growing number of both commercial and non-profit SaaS offerings designed to accelerate common research tasks. For example, Mendeley organizes bibliographic information, while Globus Online provides research data management services.

Similarly, in health care, we see many independent physicians and smaller practices adopting SaaS electronic medical record systems. The relatively high costs and specialized expertise required to operate in-house systems, plus a perception that SaaS providers do a good job of addressing usability and security concerns, seem to be major drivers of adoption. Similarly, a growing number of biomedical researchers are using IaaS for data- and compute-intensive research. Meanwhile, some cloud providers (e.g., Microsoft) are prepared to adhere to security and privacy provisions defined in HIPAA and the HITECH act. Nevertheless, while some hospitals are using IaaS for remote backup (e.g., by storing encrypted database dumps), there is not yet any significant move to outsource major hospital information systems.

5.8   Summary

As we have discussed in this chapter, the synthesis of large-scale information systems is accomplished through the careful construction of hierarchies of hardware and software. Each successive layer is more abstract and hides many of the details of the preceding layer. Simple methods for storing and manipulating data ultimately produce complex information systems that have powerful capabilities. Communication links that connect local and remote computers in arbitrary configurations, and the security mechanisms that span these systems, transcend the basic hardware and software hierarchies. Thus, without worrying about the technical details, users can access a wealth of computational resources and can perform complex information management tasks, such as storing and retrieving, communicating, authorizing, and processing information. As the technology landscape evolves and computer architectures continuously increase in complexity, they will also increasingly, necessarily, hide that complexity from the user. Therefore, it is paramount that systems designers, planners, and implementers remain sufficiently knowledgeable about the underlying mechanisms and distinguishing features of computing architectures so as to make optimal technology choices.

Suggested Readings

Council, N.R. (1997). *For the record: Protecting electronic health information*. Washington, DC: National Academy Press. This report documents an extensive study of current security practices in US health care settings and recommends significant changes. It sets guidelines for policies, technical protections, and legal standards for acceptable access to, and use of, health care information. It is well suited for lay, medical, and technical readers who are interested in an overview of this complex topic.

Garcia-Molina, H., Ullman, J.D., & Widom, J.D. (2008). *Database systems: The complete book* (2nd ed.). Englewood Cliffs: Prentice-Hall. The first half of the book provides in-depth coverage of databases from the point of view of the database designer, user, and application programmer. It covers the latest database standards SQL:1999, SQL/PSM, SQL/CLI, JDBC, ODL, and XML, with broader coverage of SQL than most other texts. The second half of the book provides in-depth coverage of databases from the point of view of the DBMS implementer. It focuses on storage structures, query processing, and transaction management. The book covers the main techniques in these areas with broader coverage of query optimization than most other texts, along with advanced topics including multidimensional and bitmap indexes, distributed transactions, and information-integration techniques.

Hennessy, J.L., & Patterson, D.A. (2011). *Computer architecture: a quantitative approach* (5th ed.). San Francisco: Morgan Kaufmann. This technical book provides an in-depth explanation of the physical and conceptual underpinnings of computer hardware and its operation. It is suitable for technically oriented readers who want to understand the details of computer architecture.

Mell, P. and Grance, T. (2011). *The NIST definition of cloud computing*. NIST Special Publication 800–145, National Institute of Standards and Technology. This brief document provides a concise and clear definition of cloud computing.

Tanenbaum, A., & Wetherall, D. (2010). *Computer networks* (5th ed.). Englewood Cliffs: Prentice-Hall. The heavily revised edition of a classic textbook on computer communications, this book is well organized, clearly written, and easy to understand. It first describes the physical layer of networking and then works up to network applications, using real-world example networks to illustrate key principles. Covers applications and services such as email, the domain name system, the World Wide Web, voice over IP, and video conferencing.

Teorey, T., Lightstone, S., Nadeau, T., & Jagadish, H. (2011). *Database modeling and design: Logical design* (5th ed.). San Francisco: Elsevier. This text provides and excellent and compact coverage of multiple topics regarding database architectures, including core concepts, universal modeling language, normalization, entity-relationship diagrams, SQL, and data warehousing.

Wiederhold, G., & Clayton, P.D. (1985). Processing biological data in real time. M.D. *Computing, 2*(6), 16–25. This article discusses the principles and problems of acquiring and processing biological data in real time. It covers much of the material discussed in the signal-processing section of this chapter and it provides more detailed explanations of analog-to-digital conversion and Fourier analysis.

Questions for Discussion

1. What are four considerations in deciding whether to keep data in active versus archival storage?
2. Explain how operating systems and cloud architectures insulate users from hardware changes.
3. Discuss what characteristics determine whether computer clusters or cloud architectures are better for scaling a given computational problem.
4. Explain how grid computing facilitates federation of resources.
5. Describe the architectural advantages and disadvantages of different computing environments.
6. Explain how REST and XML enable flexibility, modularity, and scale.
7. How can you prevent inappropriate access to electronic medical record information? How can you detect that such inappropriate access might have occurred?
8. You are asked whether a medical practice should outsource its information technology functions to third party cloud providers. What factors would enter into your recommendation?

Software Engineering for Health Care and Biomedicine

6

Adam B. Wilcox, Scott P. Narus,
and David K. Vawdrey

After reading this chapter, you should know the answers to these questions:

- What key functions do software applications perform in health care?
- How are the components of the software development life cycle applied to health care?
- What are the trade-offs between purchasing commercial, off-the-shelf systems and developing custom applications?
- What are important considerations in comparing commercial software products?
- Why do systems in health care, both internally-developed and commercially-purchased, require continued software development?

6.1 How Can a Computer System Help in Health Care?

Chapter 5 discusses basic concepts related to computer and communications hardware and software. In this chapter, we focus on the software

applications and components of health care information systems, and describe how they are used and applied to support health care delivery. We give examples of some basic functions that may be performed by health information systems, and discuss important considerations in how the software may be acquired, implemented and used. This understanding of how a system gets put to use in health care settings will help as you read about the various specific applications in the chapters that follow.

Health care is an information-intensive field. Clinicians are constantly collecting, gathering, reviewing, analyzing and communicating information from many sources to make decisions. Humans are complex, and individuals have many different characteristics that are relevant to health care and that need to be considered in decision-making. Health care is complex, with a huge body of existing knowledge that is expanding at ever-increasing rates. Health care information software is intended to facilitate the use of this information at various points in the delivery process. Software defines how data are obtained, organized and processed to yield information. Software, in terms of design, development, acquisition, configuration and maintenance, is therefore a major component of the field. Here we

A.B. Wilcox, PhD (⌧) • S.P. Narus, PhD
Department of Medical Informatics,
Intermountain Healthcare,
5171 South Cottonwood St,
Murray, UT 84107, USA
e-mail: aw115@columbia.edu; scott.narus@hsc.utah.edu

D.K. Vawdrey, PhD
Department of Biomedical Informatics,
Columbia University, 622 W. 168th Street, VC-5,
New York, NY10032, USA
e-mail: david.vawdrey@dbmi.columbia.edu

The authors gratefully acknowledge the co-authors of the previous chapter edition titled "System Design and Engineering in Health Care," GioWiederhold and Edward H. Shortliffe.

E.H. Shortliffe, J.J. Cimino (eds.), *Biomedical Informatics*,
DOI 10.1007/978-1-4471-4474-8_6, © Springer-Verlag London 2014

provide an introduction to the practical considerations regarding health information software. This includes both understanding of general software engineering principles, and then specifically how these principles are applied to health care settings.

To this aim, we first describe the major software functions within a health care environment or health information system. While not all functions can be covered in detail, some specific examples are given to indicate the breadth of software applications as well as to provide an understanding of their relevance. We also describe the software development life cycle, with specific applications to health care. We then describe important considerations and strategies for acquiring and implementing software in health care settings. Finally, we discuss emerging software engineering influences and issues and their impact on health information systems. Each system can be considered in regard to what it would take to make it functional in a health care system, and what advantages and disadvantage the software may have, based on how it was created and implemented. Understanding this will help you identify the risks and benefits of various applications, so that you can identify how to optimize the positive impact of health information systems.

6.2 Software Functions in Health Care

6.2.1 Cases Study of Health Care Software

The following case study illustrates many important functions of health care software.

James Johnson is a 42-year old man living in a medium-sized western U.S. city. He is married and has two children. He has Type-II diabetes, but it is currently well-controlled and he has no other health concerns. There is some history of cardiovascular disease in

his family. James has a primary care physician, Linda Stark, who practices at a clinic that is part of a larger health delivery network, Generation Healthcare System (GHS). GHS includes a physician group, primary and specialty care clinics, a tertiary care hospital and an affiliated health insurance plan.

*James needs to make an appointment with Dr. Stark. He logs into the GHS **patient portal** and uses an online scheduling application to request an appointment. While in the patient portal, James also reviews results from his most recent visit and prints a copy of his current medication list in order to discuss the addition of an over-the-counter supplement he recently started taking.*

*Before James arrives for his visit, the clinic's scheduling system has already alerted the staff of James's appointment and the need to collect information related to his diabetes. Upon his arrival, Dr. Stark's nurse gathers the requested diabetes information and other vital signs data and enters these into the **electronic health record** (EHR). In the exam room, Dr. Stark reviews James's history, the new information gathered today, and recommendations and reminders provided by the EHR on a report tailored to her patient's medical history. They both go over James's medication list and Dr. Stark notes that, according to the EHR's drug interaction tool, the supplement he is taking may have an interaction with one of his diabetes medications. One of the reminders suggests that James is due for an HbA1c test and Dr. Stark orders this in the EHR. Dr. Stark's nurse, who has been alerted to the lab test order, draws a blood sample from James. Before the appointment ends, Dr. Stark completes and signs his progress note and forwards a visit summary for James to review on the patient portal.*

A few days after his appointment, James receives an email from GHS that alerts him to an important piece of new information in his patient record. Logging into the patient portal application, James sees that his HbA1c test is back. The test indicates that the result is elevated. Dr. Stark has added a note to the result saying that she has reviewed the lab and would like to refer James to the GHS Diabetes Specialty Clinic for additional follow-up. James uses the messaging feature in the patient portal to respond to Dr. Stark and arrange for an appointment. James also clicks on an **infobutton** next to the lab result to obtain more information about the abnormal value. He is linked to patient-focused material about HbA1c testing, common causes for high results, and common ways this might be addressed. Lastly, James reviews the visit summary note from his appointment with Dr. Stark to remind him about suggestions she had for replacing his supplement.

At his appointment with the Diabetes Specialty Clinic, James notes that they have access to all the information in his record. A diabetes care manager reviews the important aspects of James's medical history. She suggests more frequent monitoring of his laboratory test results to see if he is able to control his diabetes without changes to his medications. She highlights diet and exercise suggestions in his patient portal record that have been shown to help. The care manager sends a summary of the visit to Dr. Stark so that Dr. Stark knows that James did follow-up with the Clinic.

A year later, James is experiencing greater difficulty controlling his diabetes. Dr. Stark and the Diabetes Care Manager have continued to actively monitor his HbA1c and other laboratory test results, and occasionally make changes to his treatment regimen. They are able to use the EHR to track and graph laboratory test results and correlate them with changes in medications. Due to family problems, James struggles with adherence to his medication regimen, and he is not maintaining a healthy diet. As a result, his blood sugar has become seriously unstable and he is taken to the GHS hospital emergency department. Doctors in the ED are able to access his electronic record through a Web-based interface to the clinic EHR. His medication and lab history, as well as notes from Dr. Stark and the care manager, help them quickly assess his condition and develop a plan. James is admitted as an inpatient for overnight observation and, again, doctors and nurses on the ward are able to access his full record and record new observations and treatments, which are automatically shared with the outpatient EHR. They are also able to reconcile his outpatient prescriptions with his inpatient medications to ensure continuity. James is stabilized by the next day. He receives new discharge medications, which simultaneously discontinue his existing orders.

Because Dr. Stark is listed as James's primary care physician, she is notified both at admission and discharge of his current status. She is able to review his discharge summary in the EHR. She instructs her staff to send a message through the patient portal to James to let him know she had reviewed his inpatient record and to schedule a follow-up appointment.

The GMS EHR is also part of a statewide **health information exchange** (HIE), which allows medical records to be easily shared with health care providers outside a patient's primary care provider. This means that if James should need to visit a hospital, emergency department or specialty care clinic outside the GMS network, his record would be available for review and any information entered by these outside providers would be available to Dr. Stark and the rest of the GMS network. In James's state, the local and state health departments are also linked to the HIE. This allows clinics, hospitals and labs to electronically submit information to the health departments for disease surveillance and case reporting purposes.

Back at home, James's wife, Gina, is able to view his record on the GHS patient portal because he has granted her proxy access to his account. This allows her to see the note from Dr. Stark and schedule the follow-up appointment. Gina also views the discharge *instructions that were electronically sent to James's patient record. As she looks deeper into information about diabetes that GHS had automatically linked to James's record, Gina sees a note about a research study into genetic links with diabetes. Concerned about their two children, Gina discusses the study with James, and he reviews the on-line material about the study. Growing interested in the possible benefits of the research, James enrolls electronically in the study and is later contacted by a study coordinator. Because GHS researchers are conducting the study, relevant parts of James's EHR can be easily shared with the research data tracking system.*

This fictional case study highlights many of the current goals for improving health care delivery, including: improved access to care, increased patient engagement, shared patient-provider decision-making, better care management, medication reconciliation, improved transitions of care, and research recruitment. In the case study, each of these goals required software to make health information accessible to the correct individuals at the proper time.

In today's health care system, few individuals enjoy the interaction with software depicted in the case study with James Johnson. Although the functions described in the scenario exist at varying levels of maturity, most health care delivery institutions have not connected all the functions together as described. The current role of software engineering in health care is therefore twofold: to design and implement software applications that provide required functions, and to connect these functions in a seamless experience for both the clinicians and the patients.

The case study also highlights the usefulness of several functions provided by health care software applications for clinicians, patients, and administrators. Some of these functions include:
1. Acquiring and storing data
2. Summarizing and displaying data
3. Facilitating communication and information exchange
4. Generating alerts, reminders, and other forms of decision support
5. Supporting educational, research, and public health initiatives

6.2.2 Acquiring and Storing Data

The amount of data needed to describe the state of even a single person is huge. Health professionals require assistance with data acquisition to deal with the data that must be collected and processed. One of the first uses of computers in a medical setting was the automatic analysis of specimens of blood and other body fluids by instruments that measure chemical concentrations or that count cells and organisms. These systems generated printed or electronic results to health care workers and identified values that were outside normal limits. Computer-based patient monitoring that collected physiological data directly from patients were another early application of computing technology (see Chap. 19). These systems provided frequent, consistent collection of vital signs, electrocardiograms (ECGs), and other indicators of patient status. More recently, researchers have developed medical imaging applications as described in Chaps. 9 and 20, including computed tomography (CT), magnetic resonance imaging (MRI), and digital subtraction angiography. The calculations for these computationally intensive applications cannot be performed manually; computers are required to collect and manipulate millions of individual observations.

Early computer-based medical instruments and measurement devices provided results only to human beings. Today, most instruments can transmit data directly into the EHR, although the interfaces are still awkward and poorly standardized (see Chaps. 4 and 7). Computer-based systems that acquire information, such as one's health history, from patients are also data-acquisition systems; they free health professionals from the need to collect and enter routine demographic and history information.

Various departments within a hospital use computer systems to store clinical data. For instance, clinical laboratories use information systems to keep track of orders and specimens and to report test results; most pharmacy and radiology departments use computers to perform analogous functions. Their systems may connect to outside services (e.g., pharmacy systems are typically connected to one or more drug distributors so that ordering and delivery are rapid and local inventories can be kept small). By automating processing in areas such as these, health care facilities are able to speed up services, reduce direct labor costs, and minimize the number of errors.

6.2.3 Summarizing and Displaying Data

Computers are well suited to performing tedious and repetitive data-processing tasks, such as collecting and tabulating data, combining related data, and formatting and producing reports. They are particularly useful for processing large volumes of data.

Raw data as acquired by computer systems are detailed and voluminous. Data analysis systems must aid decision makers by reducing and presenting the intrinsic information in a clear and understandable form. Presentations should use graphs to facilitate trend analysis and compute secondary parameters (means, standard deviations, rates of change, etc.) to help spot abnormalities. Clinical research systems have modules for performing powerful statistical analyses over large sets of patient data. The researcher, however, should have insight into the methods being used. For clinicians, graphical displays are useful for interpreting data and identifying trends.

Fast retrieval of information is essential to all computer systems. Data must be well organized and indexed so that information recorded in an EHR system can be easily retrieved. Here the variety of users must be considered. Getting cogent recent information about a patient entering the office differs from the needs that a researcher will have in accessing the same data. The query interfaces provided by EHRs and clinical research systems assist researchers in retrieving pertinent records from the huge volume of patient information. As discussed in Chap. 21, bibliographic retrieval systems are an essential component of health information services.

6.2.4 Facilitating Communication and Information Exchange

In hospitals and other large-scale health care institutions, myriad data are collected by multiple health professionals who work in a variety of settings; each patient receives care from a host of providers—nurses, physicians, technicians, pharmacists, and so on. Communication among the members of the team is essential for effective health care delivery. Data must be available to decision makers when and where they are needed, independent of when and where they were obtained. Computers help by storing, transmitting, sharing, and displaying those data. As described in Chaps. 2 and 12, the patient record is the primary vehicle for communication of clinical information. The limitation of the traditional paper-based patient record is the concentration of information in a single location, which prohibits simultaneous entry and access by multiple people. Hospital information systems (HISs; see Chap. 13) and EHR systems (Chap. 12) allow distribution of many activities, such as admission, appointment, and resource scheduling; review of laboratory test results; and inspection of patient records to the appropriate sites.

Information necessary for specific decision-making tasks is rarely available within a single computer system. Clinical systems are installed and updated when needed, available, and affordable. Furthermore, in many institutions, inpatient, outpatient, and financial activities are supported by separate organizational units.

Patient treatment decisions require inpatient and outpatient information. Hospital administrators must integrate clinical and financial information to analyze costs and to evaluate the efficiency of health care delivery. Similarly, clinicians may need to review data collected at other health care institutions, or they may wish to consult published biomedical information. Communication networks that permit sharing of information among independent computers and geographically distributed sites are now widely available. Actual integration of the information they contain requires additional software, adherence to standards, and operational staff to keep it all working as technology and systems evolve.

6.2.5   Generating Alerts, Reminders, and Other Forms of Decision Support

In the end, all the functions of storing, displaying and transmitting data support decision making by health professionals, patients, and their caregivers. The distinction between decision-support systems and systems that monitor events and issue alerts is not clear-cut; the two differ primarily in the degree to which they interpret data and recommend patient-specific action. Perhaps the best-known examples of decision-support systems are the clinical consultation systems or event-monitoring systems that use population statistics or encode expert knowledge to assist physicians in diagnosis and treatment planning (see Chap. 22). Similarly, some nursing information systems help nurses to evaluate the needs of individual patients and thus assist their users in allocating nursing resources. Chapter 22 discusses systems that use algorithmic, statistical, or artificial-intelligence (AI) techniques to provide advice about patient care.

Timely reactions to data are crucial for quality in health care, especially when a patient has unexpected problems. Data overload, created by the ubiquity of information technology, is as detrimental to good decision making as is data insufficiency. Data indicating a need for action

may be available but are easily overlooked by overloaded health professionals. Surveillance and monitoring systems can help people cope with all the data relevant to patient management by calling attention to significant events or situations, for example, by reminding doctors of the need to order screening tests and other preventive measures (see Chaps. 12 and 22) or by warning them when a dangerous event or constellation of events has occurred.

Laboratory systems routinely identify and flag abnormal test results. Similarly, when patient-monitoring systems in intensive care units detect abnormalities in patient status, they sound alarms to alert nurses and physicians to potentially dangerous changes. A pharmacy system that maintains computer-based drug-profile records for patients can screen incoming drug orders and warn physicians who order a drug that interacts with another drug that the patient is receiving or a drug to which the patient has a known allergy or sensitivity. By correlating data from multiple sources, an integrated clinical information system can monitor for complex events, such as interactions among patient diagnosis, drug regimen, and physiological status (indicated by laboratory test results). For instance, a change in cholesterol level can be due to prednisone given to an arthritic patient and may not indicate a dietary problem.

6.2.6   Supporting Educational, Research, and Public Health Initiatives

Rapid growth in biomedical knowledge and in the complexity of therapy management has produced an environment in which students cannot learn all they need to know during training—they must learn how to learn and must make a lifelong educational commitment. Today, physicians and nurses have available a broad selection of computer programs designed to help them to acquire and maintain the knowledge and skills they need to care for their patients. The simplest programs are of the drill-and-practice variety; more sophisticated programs can help students to learn complex problem-solving skills, such as diagnosis and therapy management (see Chap. 21). Computer-aided instruction provides a valuable means by which health professionals can gain experience and learn from mistakes without endangering actual patients. Clinical decision-support systems and other systems that can explain their recommendations also perform an educational function. In the context of real patient cases, they can suggest actions and explain the reasons for those actions.

Surveillance also extends beyond the health care setting. Appearances of new infectious diseases, unexpected reactions to new medications, and environmental effects should be monitored. Thus the issue of data integration has a national or global scope (see the discussion of the National Health Information Infrastructure in Chaps. 1 and 16 that deals with public health informatics).

6.3   Software Development and Engineering

Clearly, software can be used in many different ways to manage and manipulate health information to facilitate health care delivery. However, just using a computer or a software program does not improve care. If critical information is unavailable, or if processes are not organized to operate smoothly, a computer program will only expose challenges and waste time of clinical staff that could be better applied in delivering care. To be useful, software must be developed with an understanding of its role in the care setting, be geared to the specific functions that are required, and it must be developed correctly. To be used, software must be integrated to support the users' workflow. We will discuss both aspects of software engineering – development and integration.

6.3.1   Software Development

Software development can be a complex, resource-intensive undertaking, particularly in environments like health care where safety and security provide added risk. The **software**

development life cycle (SDLC) is a framework imposed over software development in order to better ensure a repeatable, predictable process that controls cost and improves quality of the software product (usually an application). SDLC is a subset of the systems development life cycle, focusing on the software component of a larger system. In practice, and particularly in heath care, software development encompasses more than just the software, often stretching into areas such as process re-engineering in order to maximize the benefits of the software product. Although SDLC most literally applies to an in-house development project, all or most of the life cycle framework is also relevant to shared development and even purchase of commercial off-the-shelf (COTS) software. The following is an overview of the phases of the SDLC.

6.3.1.1 Planning/Analysis

The software development life cycle begins with the formation of a project goal during the planning phase. This goal typically derives from an organization's or department's mission/vision, focusing on a particularly need or outcome. This is sometimes called project conceptualization. Planning includes some initial scoping of the project as well as resource identification (including funding). It is important that the project's scope also addresses what is not in the project in order to create appropriate expectations for the final product. A detailed analysis of current processes and needs of the target users is often done. As part of the analysis, specific user requirements are gathered. Depending on the development process, this might include either detailed instructions on specific functions and operating parameters or more general user stories that explain in simple narrative the needs, expected workflow and outcomes for the software. It is important that real users of the system are consulted, as well as those in the organization who will implement and maintain the software. The decision of whether to develop the software in-house, partner with a developer, or purchase a vendor system will likely determine the level of detail needed in the requirements. Vendors will want very specific requirements that allow them to properly scope and price their work. The requirements document will usually become part of a contract with a vendor and will be used to determine if the final product meets the agreed specification for the software. In-house development can have less detailed requirements, as the contract to build the software is with the organization itself, and can allow some evolution of the requirements as the project progresses. However, the more flexibility that is allowed and the longer changes or enhancements are permitted, the higher the likelihood of "scope creep" and schedule and cost overruns.

Other tasks performed during analysis include an examination of existing products and potential alternative solutions, and, particularly for large projects, a cost/benefit analysis. A significant and frequently overlooked aspect of the planning and analysis phase is to determine outcome measures that can be used during the life cycle to demonstrate progress and success or failure of the project. These measures can be refined and details added as the project progresses. The planning and analysis phase typically ends when a decision to proceed is made, along with at least a rough plan of how to implement the next steps in the SDLC. If the organization decides to purchase a solution, a request for proposals (RFP) that contains the requirements document is released to the vendor community.

The planning and analysis stage of software development is perhaps both the most difficult and the most important stage in the development lifecycle as it is applied to health care. Requirements for software in health care are inherently difficult to define for many reasons. Health care practice is constantly changing, and as new therapies or approaches are discovered and validated, these new advancements can change how care is practiced. In addition, the end users of health care software are comparatively advanced relative to other industries. Unlike industries where front-line workers may be directed by supervisors with more advanced training and greater flexibility in decision making, in health care the front-line workers are often physicians, who are the most advance-trained workers in the system (although not necessarily the most advanced with respect to computer

literacy) and require the greatest flexibility for decisions. This flexibility makes it difficult to define workflows or even get indications of the workflows being followed, since physicians will not always make explicit what actions or plans are being pursued. This flexibility is important for patient care, because it allows front-line clinicians to adapt appropriately to different settings, staffing levels, and specialties. The need for flexibility is such that defining requirements for software that could reduce flexibility is criticized as "cookbook" medicine, and a common reason for resistance to software adoption. However, this resistance is not just characteristic of software – clinical guidelines and other approaches to structured or formalized care processes are also criticized, and the challenge of applying discovered knowledge to clinical care processes remains difficult.

Over time, however, there have been some successful efforts that have defined standard requirements for health information software. Among the most notable efforts have been in the EHRs, where groups have created lists of requirements and certified systems that match those requirements. The Certification Commission for Health Information Technology (CCHIT) began in 2004 and has emerged as perhaps the most notable of these efforts. CCHIT defines criteria for electronic health records' functionality, interoperability and security (Leavitt and Gallagher 2006). In addition, because CCHIT released criteria in different stages, it gave a preliminary prioritization of EHR functions. Later, the certification approach was adopted by the Office of the National Coordinator of Health Information Technology (ONC) in 2010, when they created a list of EHR functions that were most related to "meaningful use" of EHRs (Blumenthal and Tavenner 2010). These efforts have been significant in creating a consistent set of functions that have been subsequently incorporated into software products (Mostashari 2011).

6.3.1.2 Design

During the Design phase, potential software solutions are explored. System architectures are examined for their abilities to meet the needs stated in the requirements. Data storage and interface technologies are researched for appropriate fit. User front-end solutions are investigated to assess capabilities for required user input and data display functions. Other details, such as security, performance, internationalization, etc., are also addressed during design. Analysts with domain knowledge in the target environment are often employed during this phase in order to translate user requirements into suitable proposals. Simple mock-ups of the proposed system may be developed, particularly for user-facing components, in order to validate the design and identify potential problems and missing information. Closely related to this, an integrated, automated testing architecture, with appropriate testing scripts/procedures, may be designed in this phase in order to ensure the software being developed is both high quality and responsive to the requirements. The depth and completeness of the design is contingent on the software development process, as well as other factors. In some cases, the entire design is completed before moving on to software coding. In other development strategies, a high-level system architecture is designed but the details of the software components are delayed until each component or component feature is being programmed. The pros and cons of these approaches are discussed later in this chapter. For vendor-developed systems, the purchasing organization will often hold design reviews and demonstrations of mock-ups or prototypes with the vendor to assess the solutions. In the case of pre-built COTS software, the purchasing organization relies on the vendor's system description and reviews from third parties, supplemented by system demonstrations, to determine the appropriateness of the design. As with the Analysis phase, it is important to include the target users and IT operations personnel in the design reviews.

Ideally, the software could be designed solely around the care requirements and the use of information. However, rarely are the clinical requirements of the use case the only consideration. In the design phase, other requirements are considered, such as the software cost and how it integrates with an existing health IT strategy of an organization. Resources applied to a development project are not available for other potential projects, so costs are always influential. The design phase must consider various alternatives to meet the most important requirements, recognizing trade-offs and contingency approaches. Additional considerations are how the software will support long-term factors, not just the immediate requirements that have been identified. Clinicians and clinical workflow analysts are often the primary participants in the requirements analysis stage, whereas informaticians are more prominent in the design phase. This is because during this latter phase the clinical goals and strategies are considered together with what can be vastly different design approaches, and the ability to consider the various strengths and weaknesses of these different approaches is critical. Often, design considerations are between custom development, purchasing niche applications, or purchasing components of a monolithic EHR. The considerations of development versus COTS software is discussed in more detail in the Acquisition Strategy Sect. 6.3.3.1 below.

6.3.1.3 Development

Coding of the software is done during the Development phase of the SDLC. The software engineers use the requirements and system designs as they program the code. Analysts help resolve questions about requirements and designs for the programmers when it is unclear how software might address a particular feature. The software process defines the pace and granularity of the development. In some cases, an entire software component or system is developed at once by the team. In other cases, the software is broken down into logical pieces and the programmers only work on the features that are relevant to the piece they are currently working on. As software components are completed, unit tests are run to confirm the component is free of known bugs and produces expected outputs or results.

In health care, development includes coding of custom software as well as configuration of COTS software. Health care practices across institutions (and even within larger organizations) are so variable that all software requires some level –often substantial – of configuration. Configuration can range from assigning local values to generic variables within the software, to complete development of documentation templates, reports, and terminology. In fact, configuration can be so considerable that institutions name the software separately as their own configuration, with all the content that the users interact with being defined locally. This configuration is often done using tools built specifically for the commercial software, which facilitate the integration of the configuration products into the software infrastructure. The tools can be complex, requiring significant training for developers. Typically, tools work well for basic configuration and may also have advanced functionality that can configure more complicated templates or reports. The most intensive time investment for configuration is typically when the tools do not directly support certain configurations, and developers must find approaches to creatively adapt the development "around the tools."

6.3.1.4 Integration and Test

For complex software projects consisting of several components and/or interfaces with outside systems, an Integration phase in the SDLC is employed to tie together the various pieces. Some aspects of the integration software are likely done during the Development phase by simulating or mocking the outputs to, and inputs from, other systems. During Integration, these connections are finalized. Simulations are run to demonstrate functional integration of the various system components. Once the various components are integrated, a thorough testing regimen is conducted in order to prove the end-to-end operation of the entire software system. Specific test scenarios are run with known inputs and expected outputs. This is typically done in a safe, non-operational environment in order to avoid conflicts or issues with real-world people (e.g., patients and clinicians) and environments, although some inbound information from live systems may be used to verify scenarios that are difficult to simulate.

Testing and integration in health care are similar to other complex environments, in that it can be difficult to create a testing environment that matches the dynamics of the real-world setting.

Generally, testing is done around multiple use cases or case studies, using data to support the cases. In the real world, however, there may be data and information that don't match the case studies, since both people and health care are complex. As a result, internally-developed applications are often provisionally used in a "pilot" phase as part of testing. For COTS software, companies may use simulation laboratories that try to mimic the clinical environment, or work with specific health care organizations as development and testing partners. Later, however, this can lead to challenges if data representing the dynamics of one organization are not easily transferrable, and software must be further tested with new environments. Issues with software transferability between institutions have been demonstrated in studies, even for specific applications (Hripcsak et al. 1998). Another challenge is that with current privacy laws, organizations are more reluctant to release data to vendors for testing.

6.3.1.5 Implementation

Once the software passes integration testing it moves to the implementation phase. In this phase, the software is installed in the live environment. In preparation for installation, server hardware, user devices, network infrastructure, facilities changes, etc., may need to be implemented and tested, too. In addition, user training will be performed in the weeks before the software goes live. Any changes to policies and procedures required by the software will also be implemented in the build-up to installation.

Health care presents interesting considerations in each phase of the software development cycle, but the challenges have been more visible in implementation than any other phase. This may be because health IT, while intended to facilitate more efficient workflows with information, is still disruptive. Disruption happens most during implementation, when clinicians actually begin using the software, and studies have shown that during this time clinical productivity does decline (Shekelle et al. 2006). If users do not perceive that the benefits are sufficient to justify this disruption, or if the efficiency does not improve quickly enough after the initial implementation, they may choose to disregard the software or even revolt against its implementation. There have been prominent examples in biomedical informatics of software implementations failing during implementation (Bates 2006; Smelcer et al. 2009), and even studies demonstrating harm (Han et al. 2005). Because of these risks, health IT professionals need to be flexible in implementation, and adapt the implementation strategies to how the system is adopted. Users have been shown to use health IT software in different ways for different benefits, and may need incentives or prodding to advance to different levels of use.

6.3.1.6 Verification and Validation

To ensure that the software satisfies the original requirements for the system and meets the need of the organization, a formal verification and validation of the software is performed. The implementing organization will *verify* that the software has the features and performs all the functions specified in the requirements document. The software is also *validated* to show that it performs according to specified operational requirements, that it produces valid outputs, and that it can be operated in a safe manner. For purchased software, the verification and validation phase is used by the purchasing organization in order to officially accept the software.

Since clinicians often use software at different levels or in different ways, tracking patterns of use can be an important approach for verification and validation of software in health care. Additionally, because they have experience working in complicated environments, users can be good at identifying inconsistencies in data or software functions. Two approaches that have been used and can be successful for validation are monitoring use, and facilitating user feedback.

6.3.1.7 Operations and Maintenance

Software eventually enters an operations and maintenance (O&M) phase where it is being regularly used to support the operational needs of the organization. During this phase, an O&M team will ensure that the software is operating as desired and will be fielding the support needs of the users. Updates may need to be installed as new versions of the software are released. This may require new integration and testing, implementation, and verification and validation steps. Ongoing training will be required for new users and system updates. The O&M team may conduct regular security reviews of the system and its use. Data repositories and software interfaces will be monitored for proper operation and continued information validity. Software bugs and feature enhancement requests will be collected. These may drive an entire new development life cycle as new requirements persuade an organization to explore significant upgrades to its current software or even an entirely new system.

Maintenance is a demanding task in health information software. It involves correcting errors; adapting configurations and software to growth, new standards, and new regulations; and linking to other information sources. Maintenance tasks can exceed by more than double the initial acquisition costs, making it a substantial consideration that should affect software design. COTS suppliers often provide maintenance services for 15–30 % of the purchase price annually, but custom development or configuration maintenance must be supported by the purchasing organization. If the software is not maintained, it can quickly become unusable in a health care setting.

6.3.1.8 Evaluation

An important enhancement to the SDLC suggested by Thompson et al. (1999) is the inclusion of an evaluation process during each of the phases of the life cycle. The evaluation is influenced by risk factors that may affect a particular SDLC segment. An organization might perform formative evaluations during each phase, depending on specific needs, in order to assess the inputs, processes and resources employed during development. During Verification and Validation or O&M, a summative evaluation may be performed to assess the outcome effects, organizational impact, and cost-benefit of the software solution.

Health IT is considered an intervention into the health care delivery system, so evaluations have been done and published as comparative studies in clinical literature (Bates et al. 1998; Evans et al. 1998; Hunt et al. 1998). These evaluations and syntheses of multiple studies have identified areas of impact and areas where the effect of health IT software is inconsistent. Researchers have also noted that most of these studies have occurred in institutions where software was developed internally, with disproportionate under-representation of COTS software systems in evaluations, especially considering that most health care institutions use COTS rather than internal development (Chaudhry et al. 2006). It is hoped that the existing evaluations can be a model for software evaluations of COTS, to clarify their impact on care.

6.3.2 Software Development Models

Different software development processes or methods can be used in an SDLC. The **software development process** describes the day-to-day methodology followed by the development team, while the life cycle describes a higher-level view that encompasses aspects that take place well before code is ever written and after an application is in use. The following are two of the most common examples of different development processes in clinical information systems development.

6.3.2.1 Waterfall Model

The Waterfall model of software development suggests that each step in the process happens sequentially, as shown in Fig. 6.1. The term "Waterfall" refers to the analogy of water cascading downward in stages. A central concept of the Waterfall methodology is to solidify all of the requirements, establish complete functional specifications, and create the final software design prior to performing programming tasks. This concept is referred to as "Big Design Up Front," and reflects the thinking that time spent early-on making sure requirements and design are correct saves considerable time and effort later. Steve McConnell, an expert in software development, estimated that "… a requirements defect that is left undetected until construction or

maintenance will cost 50–200 times as much to fix as it would have cost to fix at requirements time" (McConnell 1996).

The waterfall model provides a structured, linear approach that is easy to understand. Application of the model is best suited to software projects with stable requirements that can be completely designed in advance. In practice, it may not be possible to create a complete design for software a priori. Requirements and design specifications can change even late in the development process. Clients may not know exactly what requirements they need before reviewing a working prototype. In other cases, software developers may identify problems during the implementation that necessitate reworking the design or modifying the requirements.

6.3.2.2 Agile Models

In contrast to the Waterfall model, modern software development approaches have attempted to provide more flexibility, particularly in terms of involving the customer throughout the process. In 2001, a group of software developers published the Manifesto for Agile Software Development, which emphasizes iterative, incremental development and welcomes changes to software requirements even late in the development process (Beck et al. 2001).

Agile development eschews long-term planning in favor of short iterations that usually last from 1 to 4 weeks. During each iteration, a small collaborative team (typically five to ten people) conducts planning, requirements analysis, design, coding, unit testing, and acceptance testing activities with direct involvement of a customer representative. Multiple iterations are required to release a product, and larger development efforts involve several small teams working toward a common goal. The agile method is value-driven, meaning that customers set priorities at the beginning of each iteration based on perceived business value.

Agile methods emphasize face-to-face communication over written documents. Frequent communication exposes problems as they arise during the development process. Typically, a

Fig. 6.1 The Waterfall model of software development

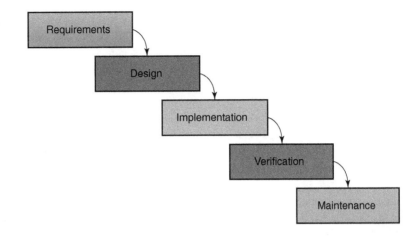

formal meeting is held each morning during which team members report to each other what they did the previous day, what they intend to do today, and what their roadblocks are. The brief meeting, sometimes called a "stand-up," "scrum," or "huddle," usually lasts 5–15 minutes, and includes the development team, customer representatives and other stakeholders. A common implementation of agile development is Extreme Programming.

6.3.3   Software Engineering

The software development life cycle can be used to actually create the software, and understanding it is critical for those developing software in biomedical informatics. However, as the field has expanded, software has matured to the point that it is developed by and available from commercial companies, so that software development has become less of a concern for most of the field. A more important consideration in biomedical informatics has been the strategy of whether to develop and how to develop. Software vendors can spread development costs over multiple organizations, rather than one organization having to fund the full development, which can make purchasing software economically advantageous. On the other hand, as biomedical informatics remains an emerging field, the core requirements for the software continue to change, and

sometimes organizations need specific capabilities that are not met by existing vendor software options. In addition to software development, informaticians often need to participate in software acquisition, and subsequent enhancements to the acquired software.

6.3.3.1 Software Acquisition

In health care information technology applications, the next significant question is whether to develop the software internally, or purchase an existing system from a vendor. As illustrated above, this "build vs. buy" is a core decision in design, and influences most of the other considerations about software.

Considerations for purchasing software begin with how the software will be selected. Software can be a component of a monolithic vendor system, be a secondary application sold by the same vendor as the EHR, or be "best-of-breed," meaning the software that meets the requirements best, independent of its architecture or source. Another consideration is whether the software needs to integrate with other applications. Some specialty applications are sufficient with minimal data sharing with other software, while other applications must be tightly integrated with existing systems to achieve a benefit. Two examples are a picture archiving and communications system (PACS) and a laboratory information system (LIS). The most important requirement for the PACS may be allowing access to images for a radiologist, who can then separately document a report. On the other hand, the LIS may need greater integration if the users require lab data to be stored in the EHR. Another consideration, related to integration, is the storage mechanism. A stand-alone system will likely have a separate database, while an integrated system may be able to store and retrieve data using a data repository. User interface deployment is also important, and possibilities include Web-based clients, **thin clients** (e.g., Citrix), and locally-installed **thick-client** applications. Functionality may be more available with a thick client, but Web-based and thin clients are easier to update and distribute to users. Finally, security and privacy considerations are critical in health care, and can influence both the requirements and design of software. Security considerations can include whether **user authentication** is shared with other applications, or what data access events are audited for identifying potential security threats.

With some notable exceptions, most health care delivery organizations today use commercial – as opposed to locally developed – EHRs. But in reality, there is a mix between building and buying. As mentioned, organizations using commercial systems still require substantial local configuration that ranges from application-specific parameter configuration to arranging multiple software applications to link together. There is no single solution, commercial or internally-developed, that meets all the health information needs of most health care organizations, and most implementations involve a mixture of software from multiple vendors. While there can be advantages to allowing best-of-breed, recently we have observed a trend among organizations to consolidate as much functionality as possible with one vendor. Another observed trend is for organizations that build systems to consider purchasing COTS, due to the substantial maintenance costs and increased functionality of the vendor solutions. Over time, organizations are expected to move from internally-developed to COTS as functionality of commercial software becomes more advanced.

Usually, if vendor software exists that meets the requirements, it is more cost-efficient to purchase the software than build it internally. This is because the vendor can spread development costs over multiple organizations, rather than one organization having to fund the full development. In fact, few organizations have the existing infrastructure and personnel to consider internal development for anything other than small applications. However, those few institutions with developed EHRs and health information systems are notable for the success of their software. So while the costs may be higher for internal development, the benefits may also be higher. Still, these institutions have invested decades in building an infrastructure that makes these benefits possible, and it is unlikely that other organizations can afford the time investment to follow the same model. Even within historically internally-developing organizations, buying systems that can integrate with the existing system is more efficient than development. An appropriate guide is therefore, "Buy where you can, build where you can't."

Once an organization decides to acquire a health information system, there are many other decisions beyond whether to build or buy. (In fact, since the costs in time and money are prohibitive for internal development, the decision to buy is typically the easiest decision to make.) The next decision is what commercial system to purchase. There is a wide variation in the functionalities between different EHR systems, even though certification efforts have defined basic functions that each system should have. Even systems with the same certified functions may approach the functions so differently that some implementations will be incongruent to an organization. The main factors an organization should consider when choosing which system are (a) the core functionality of the software, including integration with other systems, (b) total system cost, (c) the service experience of other customers, and (d) the system's certification status. Some organizations have performed systematic reviews of different commercial software offerings that can be a helpful start to identify possible vendors and understand variations between systems. For example, KLAS Research publishes periodic assessments of both software functions and vendor performance that can be used to identify potential software products. However, since systems are complex, it is important to meet with and discuss experiences with actual organizations that have used the software. This is typically done through site visits to existing customer organizations. It is also common for organizations to make a broad request of vendors for proposals to address a specific software need, especially when the needs are not standard components of EHR software.

After a commercial product is selected, an organization must then choose how extensive the software will be. EHR companies typically have a core EHR system, with additional modules that have either been developed or acquired and integrated into their system. The set of modules used by each institution varies. One organization may use the core EHR system and accompanying modules for certain specialties, such as internal medicine and family practice, while choosing to purchase separate best-of breed software for other specialties, like obstetrics/gynecology and emergency medicine, even when the core EHR vendor has functional modules for those areas. Another organization may choose to purchase and implement all specialty systems offered from the core EHR vendor, and only purchase other software if a similar module is not available from the vendor. These decisions also must be made for all ancillary systems, including laboratory, pharmacy, radiology, etc. This is both a pre-implementation decision and a long-term strategy. Once the EHR is implemented, many specialties that were not included in the initial implementation plan may request software and data integration, depending on the success of the EHR implementation.

For organizations that choose components of multiple vendor offerings to any degree, they will need to also address how to integrate the components together so that they are not disruptive to the users' workflow. There are various strategies that can be pursued to integrate modules, either at the user context (user authentication credentials are maintained), the application view (one application is viewable as a component within another application), or at the data (data are exchanged between the applications). If components are not integrated, a user must access each application separately, by opening the software application, logging into each separately, and selecting the patient within each. When data are integrated at the user context, a user moves between both applications, but the user and patient context are shared. This "single sign-on" approach alleviates one of the main barriers to the user, by facilitating the login and patient selection, while retaining all the functionality of each system. The **Clinical Context Object Workgroup** (CCOW) is a common protocol for single sign-on implementations in health care.

A deeper level of integration is at the application view. In this case, one application will have an integrated viewer to another application, that shares user and patient context, but is accessible through the user's main workflow system. The integrated viewer functions within the primary application, but acts as a portal to the data in the secondary application. With this approach, the user workflow is retained in one system, but some of the functionality in the secondary system may be reduced because the integrated viewers are not full applications.

The deepest level of integration is at the data, where actual data elements from one system are also stored in the other system. With this approach, one system is determined to be the main repository, and data from the other systems are automatically stored into the repository. This approach has the advantage of the most complete use of data, e.g., decision support logic can use data from multiple systems, which can be more accurate. The disadvantage is that the integration can be expensive, requiring new interfaces for each integrated system.

Another and often overlooked consideration of EHR software modules is the data analytics module, usually in conjunction with a data warehouse. EHR systems generally include a reporting function, where specific reports can be configured to extract data stored in the system. However, these systems often don't facilitate ad hoc reports that are commonly needed for more complicated data analysis. Additionally, if modules from multiple software vendors are used, the data reporting functions will not work unless data are fully integrated. A solution is to use a separate data warehouse and analysis system, with functions to create ad hoc reports, that can integrate data from multiple systems. Data integration with warehouses is less expensive than with repositories, because the data do not need to be synchronized. Instead, data can be extracted in batches from source systems, transformed to the warehouse data model, and then loaded into the warehouse at periodic intervals. The greatest cost of the integration is the data transformation, but this transformation is similar to what is required when receiving data through a real-time interface.

The incentives for **Meaningful Use** have important influences on the systems that are installed by an institution. As mentioned above, the ONC created a list of important EHR functions. They also created a requirement that an organization must use a "certified" system – i.e., one that has demonstrated it provides those functions – to receive the incentives, and other criteria that the functions must be used in clinical care. As a result, health care organizations are now more likely to choose among those that are certified, and are also more likely to implement functions that support the Meaningful Use measures.

6.3.3.2 Case Studies of EHR Adoption

Consider the following case studies of institutions adopting EHR systems. All examples are fictional, but reflect the reality of the issues with EHR software.

Hospital A had been using information systems for many years, dating back to when some researchers in the cardiology department built a small system to integrate data from the purchased laboratory and pharmacy information systems. Over time, the infection control group for the hospital began using the system, and contributed efforts to expand its functionality. Other departments began developing decision support rules, and the system continued to grow. Eventually, the institution made a

commitment to redevelop the infrastructure to support a much larger group of users and functions, and named it A-Chart. Satisfaction with the system was high where it had been initially developed, and with other related specialties. However, over time there was disproportionate development in these areas, and clinicians in other specialties complained about the rudimentary functions, especially when compared to existing vendor systems for their specialty. As a result, the organization decided to purchase a new vendor system. This made the other specialties happy, but was a big concern to the groups that had been using A-Chart for years. These clinicians feared that they would have to reconfigure their complicated decision support rules with a new system, or worse, that functionality would no longer be supported. To alleviate concerns, representatives from each department were asked to participate in both drafting a Request for Proposals and then reviewing the proposals from four different vendors. Many clinicians liked System X, but in the end the hospital chose System Y, which seemed to have most of the same functions but was more affordable. However, System Y did not include a laboratory system, so the hospital purchased a separate laboratory system and built interfaces to connect it with the core EHR.

Integrated Delivery System (IDS) B had a different history of its EHRs. Years ago, it existed as a separate system of hospitals and clinics. Shortly after the merger of these institutions, both the hospitals and clinics purchased separate EHRs, InPatSys and CliniCare. At the time, the institution felt that each would be best off with a best-of-breed system, to support the different workflows, and there was no system that both sides of the organization could tolerate. Years later, as IDS B began to integrate care between the hospitals and clinics, the clinicians and administrators became increasingly frustrated at how different the InPatSys and CliniCare systems were, and that they had to use two separate systems to care for the same patients. A team was formed to evaluate the options, and the CliniCare system was eventually replaced by OutPatSys, the outpatient version of InPatSys. To prevent losing data as they moved from one system to the other, the IDS IT department prepared the OutPatSys system by loading existing laboratory results and vital sign measurements from CliniCare. Then they purchased CCOW software to allow single sign-on between systems during the first 6 months of OutPatSys implementation, while they transformed the other data from CliniCare.

Community Hospital C (CHC) had various niche information systems throughout its organization, but no EHR to organize it all together. With the availability of Meaningful Use incentives, the hospital determined it needed to finally acquire a commercial EHR. A leadership team of four people visited six different hospitals to look at how various EHRs were used. Finally, the hospital made a decision to purchase eCompuChart, because it was among the best systems and seemed best adapted to their community size. CHC hired a new chief information officer who had recently implemented eCompuChart at a community hospital in a neighboring state. They also promoted Dr. Jones, who had recently moved from another hospital that had also used eCompuChart, to chief medical information officer (CMIO). Then they contracted with DigiHealth, a consulting company with experience in implementing EHRs, to plan and coordinate the implementation with the new CMIO and CIO. Based on DigiHealth's recommendations, all existing overlapping systems were replaced with modules from eCompuChart, to simplify maintenance.

In practice, organizations rarely adopt a complete "build" or a complete "buy" strategy. EHR vendors have come a long way in the last 5–10 years in creating systems that meet the standard and even non-standard needs in health care. Still, no system exists to date that can fully address all information needs for an organization, in part because the information needs expand as more data are stored and are available. Additionally, EHR strategies become malleable over time, as commercial software capabilities increase and data become more consistent. As indicated through some of the examples above, organizational strategies may change over time to adapt to these capabilities and needs.

One consideration that is not always stated in the software selection process, but is significant in its influence over the decision, is how the organization will pay for the application. In organizations where software purchases are requested from the information technology department and budget, overall maintenance costs are considered more prominently, and software that integrates with and is a component of the overall EHR vendor offering is often selected. However, if a clinical department has direct control over their spending for the software, functionality becomes a greater concern. An additional case study illustrates this situation.

Hospital D has recently decided to purchase eCompuChart as an overall clinical information system strategy. eCompuChart has award-winning software for the emergency department and intensive care units. However, there were strong complaints about its capabilities for labor and delivery management and radiology. After considering capabilities of best-of-breed options and their ability to integrate with eCompuChart, Hospital D eventually made a split decision. The labor and delivery module for eCompuChart was purchased because other systems with more elaborate functionality could not integrate data as well with the overall EHR. On the other hand, a separate best-of-breed system was purchased for radiology, because interfaces between the systems were seen as an acceptable solution for integrating data.

6.3.3.3 Enhancing Acquired Software

Although most institutions will choose to acquire a system rather than building it from scratch, software engineering is still required to make the systems function effectively. This involves more than just installing and configuring the software to the local environment. There is still a significant need for software development in implementing COTS, because (1) applications must be integrated with existing systems, and (2) health care institutions increasingly develop custom applications that supplement commercial systems.

6.3.3.4 Integration with existing systems

In all but the most basic health care information technology environments, multiple software applications are used for treatment, payment, and operations purposes. A partial list of applications that might be used in a hospital environment is shown in Table 6.1.

To facilitate the sharing of information among various software applications, standards have emerged for exchanging messages and defining clinical terminology (see Chap. 7). Message exchange between different software applications enables the following scenario:

1. A patient is admitted to the hospital. A registration clerk uses the bed management system to assign the patient's location and attending physician of record.
2. The physician orders a set of routine blood tests for the patient in the inpatient EHR computerized order entry module.
3. The request for blood work is sent electronically to the laboratory information system, where the blood specimen is matched to the patient using a bar code.

Table 6.1 Partial list of software applications that may be used in a hospital setting

System	Primary users
Inpatient EHR (results review, order entry, documentation)	Physicians, nurses, allied health professionals
Pharmacy information system	Pharmacists, pharmacy technicians
Laboratory information system	Laboratory technicians, phlebotomists
Radiology information system	Radiologists, radiology technicians
Pathology information system	Pathologists
Registration/bed management	Registration staff
Hospital billing system	Medical coders
Professional services billing system	Physicians, medical coders

4. The results of the laboratory tests are sent to the results review module of the EHR

Message exchange is an effective means of integrating disparate software applications in health care when the users rely primarily on a single "workflow system" (e.g., physician uses the inpatient EHR and the laboratory technician uses the LIS). Because message exchange is handled by a sophisticated "interface engine" (see Chap. 7), little software development in the traditional sense is typically required. When a user accesses multiple workflow systems to perform a task, message exchange may not be sufficient and a deeper level of integration may be required. For example, consider the following addition to the previously described scenario:

5. The physician reviews the patient's blood work and notes that the patient may be suffering from renal insufficiency as evidenced by his elevated creatinine level.
6. The physician would like to review a trend of the patient's creatinine over the past 3 years. Because the hospital installed their commercial EHR less than a year ago, data from prior to that time are available in a legacy results review system that was developed locally. The physician logs into the legacy application (entering her username and password), searches for the correct patient, and reviews the patient's creatinine history.

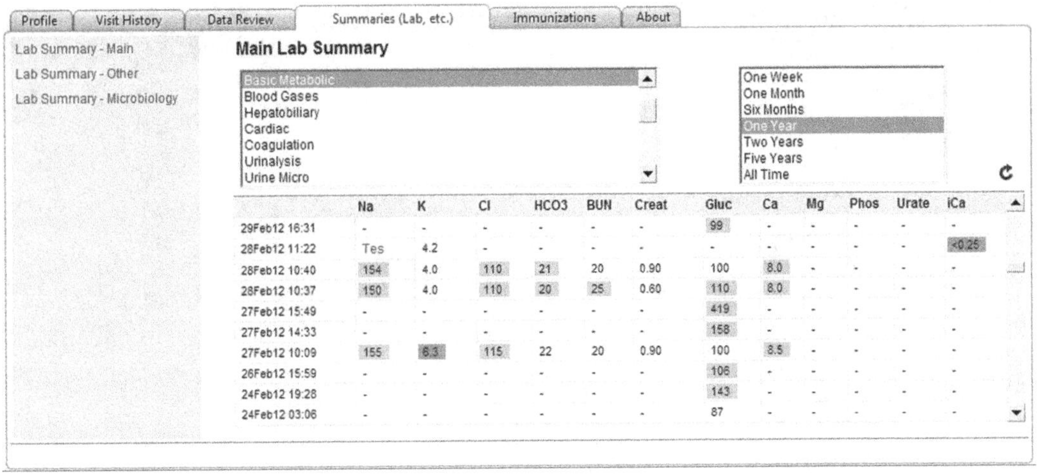

| Profile | Visit History | Data Review | Summaries (Lab, etc.) | Immunizations | About |

Lab Summary - Main
Lab Summary - Other
Lab Summary - Microbiology

Main Lab Summary

	Basic Metabolic ▲	One Week
	Blood Gases	One Month
	Hepatobiliary	Six Months
	Cardiac	One Year
	Coagulation	Two Years
	Urinalysis	Five Years
	Urine Micro ▼	All Time

	Na	K	Cl	HCO3	BUN	Creat	Gluc	Ca	Mg	Phos	Urate	iCa	▲
29Feb12 16:31	-	-	-	-	-	-	99	-	-	-	-	-	
28Feb12 11:22	Tes	4.2	-	-	-	-	-	-	-	-	-	<0.25	
28Feb12 10:40	154	4.0	110	21	20	0.90	100	8.0	-	-	-	-	
28Feb12 10:37	150	4.0	110	20	25	0.60	110	8.0	-	-	-	-	
27Feb12 15:49	-	-	-	-	-	-	419	-	-	-	-	-	
27Feb12 14:33	-	-	-	-	-	-	158	-	-	-	-	-	
27Feb12 10:09	155	6.3	115	22	20	0.90	100	8.5	-	-	-	-	
26Feb12 15:59	-	-	-	-	-	-	106	-	-	-	-	-	
24Feb12 19:28	-	-	-	-	-	-	143	-	-	-	-	-	
24Feb12 03:06	-	-	-	-	-	-	87	-	-	-	-	-	▼

Fig. 6.2 Example screen from a custom lab summary display application integrated into a commercial EHR. The application shows a longitudinal view of laboratory results that can span multiple patient encounters

While it may seem preferable in this scenario to load all data from the legacy system into the new EHR, commercial applications may not support importing such data for various reasons. To simplify and improve the user experience for reviewing information from a legacy application within a commercial EHR, one group of informaticians created the custom application shown in Fig. 6.2. The application is accessed by clicking a link within the commercial EHR and does not require login or patient look-up.

In an example of a more sophisticated level of "workflow integration" is shown in Fig. 6.3. In this example, informaticians developed a custom billing application within an inpatient commercial EHR. Users of the application were part of a physician practice that used a different outpatient EHR with a professional billing module with which they were already familiar. When the physicians in the practice rounded on their patients who were admitted to the hospital, they documented their work by writing notes within the inpatient EHR, and then used their outpatient EHR to submit their professional service charges. This practice not only required a separate login to submit a bill, but also required duplicate patient lists to be maintained in each application, as well as a duplicate problem list for each patient to be managed in each application. The integrated charge application was accessed from the inpatient EHR but provided the same look-and-feel as

the outpatient EHR billing module. Charges were submitted through the outpatient EHR infrastructure and would appear as normal charges in the outpatient system, with the substantial improvement of displaying the information (note name, author, and time) for the documentation that supported the charge.

6.3.3.5 Development of Custom Applications That Supplement or Enhance Commercial Systems

Commercial EHRs frequently provide customers with the ability to develop custom software modules. Some EHRs provide a flexible clinical decision support infrastructure that allows customers to develop modules that execute medical logic to generate alerts, reminders, corollary orders, and so on. Vendors may also provide customers with tools to access the EHR database, which allows development of stand-alone applications that make use of EHR data. Additionally, vendors may foster development of custom user interfaces within the EHR by providing an application programming interface through which developers can obtain information on user and patient context.

The ability to provide patient-specific clinical decision support is one of the key benefits of EHRs. Many commercial EHRs either directly support or have been influenced by the **Arden Syntax for Medical Logic Modules** (Pryor and

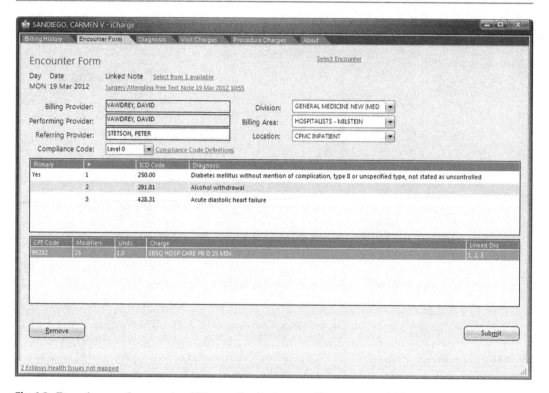

Fig. 6.3 Example screen from a custom billing application integrated into a commercial EHR. This replaced a separate application that was not integrated into the clinicians' workflow

Hripcsak 1993). The Arden Syntax is part of the **Health Level Seven** (HL7) family of standards. It encodes medical knowledge as **Medical Logic Modules** (MLMs), which can be triggered by various events within the EHR (e.g., the placing of a medication order) and execute serially as a sequence of instructions to access and manipulate data and generate output. MLMs have been used to generate clinical alerts and reminders, to screen for eligibility in clinical research studies, to perform quality assurance functions, and to provide administrative support (Dupuits 1994; Ohno-Machado et al. 1999; Jenders and Shah 2001; Jenders 2008). Although one goal of the Arden Syntax was to make knowledge portable, MLMs developed for one environment are not easily transferrable to another. Developers of clinical decision support logic require skills in both computer programming as well as medical knowledge representation.

An example of a standalone, locally developed software application that relies on EHR data is shown in Fig. 6.4. The Web-based application, EpiPortal™, provides a comprehensive, electronic hospital epidemiology decision support system. The application can be accessed from a Web browser or directly from within the EHR. It relies on EHR data such as microbiology results, clinician orders, and bed tracking information to provide users with timely information related to infection control and prevention.

In some cases, it is desirable to develop custom applications to address specific clinical needs that are not met by a commercial EHR. For example, most commercial EHRs lack dedicated tools to support patient handoff activities. For hospitalized patients, handoffs between providers affect continuity of care and increase the risk of medical errors. Informaticians at one academic medical center developed a collaborative application supporting patient handoff that is fully integrated with a commercial EHR (Fred et al. 2009). An example screen from the application is shown in

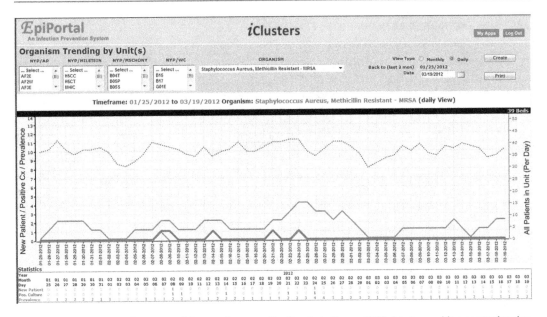

Fig. 6.4 Example screen from a standalone, software application thatrelies on EHR data to provide a comprehensive, electronic hospital epidemiology decision support system (Courtesy of New York-Presbyterian Hospital)

Fig. 6.5. The application creates user-customizable printed reports with automatic inclusion of patient allergies, active medications, 24-hour vital signs, recent common laboratory test results, isolation requirements, code status, and other EHR data. The application is currently used extensively at several academic medical centers by thousands of physicians, nurses, medical students, pharmacists, social workers, and others.

6.4   Emerging Influences and Issues

Several trends in software engineering are beginning to significantly influence biomedical information systems. While many of the trends may not be considered new to software engineering in general, they are more novel to the biomedical environment because of the less rapid and less broad adoption of information technology in this field. One area in particular that has received growing attention is **service oriented architectures** (SOA). Sometimes called "software as a service", SOA is a software design framework that allows specific processing or information functions (services) to run on an independent

computing platform that can be called by simple messages from another computer application. For example, an EHR application might have native functionality to maintain a patient's medication list, but might call a drug-drug interaction program running on a third party system to check the patient's medications for potential interactions. This allows the EHR provider to off-load developing this functionality, while the drug-drug interaction service provider can concentrate efforts on this focused task, and in particular on ensuring that the drug interaction database is kept up-to-date for all users of the service. Since the service is independent of any EHR application, many different EHR providers can call the same service, as can other applications such as patient health record (PHR) applications that are focused on consumer functionality. (SOA might also be grouped with the more recent computer phrase "cloud computing", which includes providing functional services to other applications, but also encompasses running entire applications and storing data in offsite or disconnected locations.)

The important property of SOA that makes this paradigm appealing to software designers is the use of open, discoverable message formats. These message formats describe the published

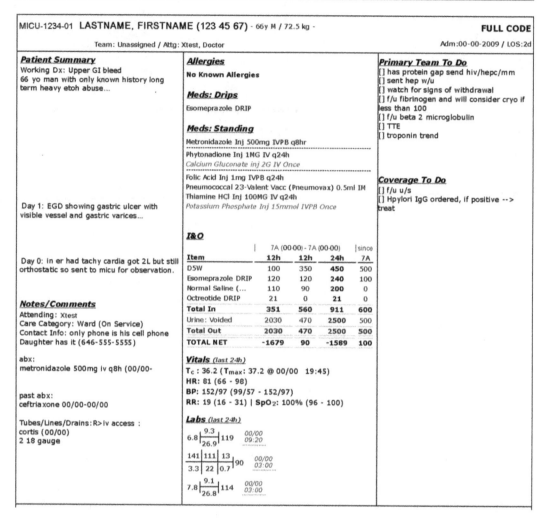

| MICU-1234-01 **LASTNAME, FIRSTNAME (123 45 67)** - 66y M / 72.5 kg - |||| **FULL CODE** |

Fig. 6.5 Example screen from a custom patient handoff application integrated into a commercial EHR. The application creates user-customizable printed reports with automatic inclusion of patient allergies, active medications, 24-h vital signs, recent common laboratory test results, isolation requirements, code status, and other EHR data

name of the service (e.g., "Get Drug Interactions") as well as the service inputs and outputs. In the case of our drug interaction service example, the input would be the medications of interest and the output would be the interacting drugs and a description of the interaction(s). Although the services might be designed according to a proprietary **application programming interface** (API), modern implementations of SOA make use of open internet standards, particularly the **Hypertext Transfer Protocol** (HTTP), so that service providers can offer their services to a wider audience of consumers. One of the more widely used SOA protocols for the World-Wide Web is the **Simple Object Access Protocol** (SOAP), which uses HTTP and the **Extensible Markup Language** (XML) to describe the message format. SOAP also uses a simple mechanism, **Web Services Discovery Language** (WSDL), to allow service consumers to discover the format and functionality of a service. It is easy to imagine how an EHR or other biomedical application might be designed to allow use of SOA services to provide significant additional functionality, and how an application developer might allow an application user to configure a personal version of the program to call "favorite" or custom services to support specific needs.

Another important trend in clinical information systems is the development of local, regional and statewide **health information exchanges** (HIE). The HIE allows health organizations to share information about patients through a common electronic framework. The HIE is typically an independent or co-owned entity that provides the exchange service to the partner organizations. The HIE can support a query interface so that a provider can use a local EHR to search for patient data across the partner network. A subscription model can also be used to deliver relevant data as it is produced (e.g., lab results, consultation reports, etc.) to a provider on the exchange network with a need to receive that information. The HIE will often publish APIs for accessing the exchange, which could be Web-based SOA services, for example. The HIE makes it much more efficient to share patient information between organizations versus trying to create point-to-point interfaces between all the clinical information systems a particular provider might need to communicate with. Often, a large health organization will have an interface engine to link together the many disparate information systems that support clinical operations. Interfaces from the engine can be developed to support the incoming and outgoing messages from the local organization to the HIE. An important aspect of the HIE is its ability to transform or map a message from one organization's internal format and content to a representation that can be consumed by other organizations. The HIE might require that each data provider on the exchange use standard message formats and terminologies before sending information, or the HIE might handle the data translations using a central terminology and data model mapping capability.

Software engineering is an ever-evolving discipline, and new ideas are emerging rapidly in this field. It is less than 20 years since the first graphical browser (**Mosaic**) was used to access the World Wide Web, but today Web-based applications are ubiquitous. Access to information through search engines like Google has changed the way that people find and evaluate information. Social networking applications like Facebook have altered our views on privacy and personal interaction. All of these developments have shaped the development of health care software, too. Today it is unimaginable that an EHR would not support a Web interface. Clinicians and consumers use the Web to search for health-related information in growing numbers and with growing expectations. It is not atypical for patients to discuss health issues in online forums and share intimate details on sites like PatientsLikeMe. Two other emerging developments in software engineering are also driving clinical software development: **applets** and **open source**.

Applets, or "apps", are small programs that are designed to accomplish very focused tasks. They are also designed to run in low resource environments like smart phones and tablets. The growth of the iPhone and iPad from Apple has accelerated the growth in app development, although some may argue that it is the boom in app development by a wide variety of programmers and small software companies that has fed the growth of smart phones and other smaller computer devices. Other companies, like Google and its Android operating system, have joined in the app development frenzy. One of the appeals of apps is that they are easily available: users can find apps in "app stores" and can download them effortlessly, sometimes for free but often at very low prices. This also makes apps very democratic because many potential users can try a variety of apps with very little investment and "vote" for winners through online reviews, which encourages additional downloads by new users. In the health software environment, many apps have been developed for efficient access to medical information, such as drug indexes and anatomical viewers. Vendors are beginning to offer apps that allow views into their EHR products. EHR apps are also being written to reside entirely on mobile devices like smart phones and tablets. The question is whether the democratic nature of apps that allows users to choose the solution that best fits their personal needs fits the model of a health care organization that needs to standardize on solutions in order to share information accurately, safely and appropriately and have common training and support models. An effort by researchers at Harvard, called SMArt (Substitutable Medical Applications, reusable technologies), is seeking to build a platform and interface that allows software developers to develop medical apps that can be easily plugged together to support health care environments (Kohane and Mandl 2011).

Although the concept of open source software development, or free sharing of intellectual ideas and source code, has been around for many years, and has led to many software advances, such as **Linux** and **Apache**, its use in the medical field has been more limited. Research communities, particularly at universities, have been more supportive of open source software in support of biomedical research. But software to support medical operations has been largely dominated by commercial systems that are closed and proprietary. A notable exception is the open source version of the Veterans Affairs EHR software, VistA (Brown et al. 2003). Others have collaborated on developing open source standards for EHR components, interfaces and messaging standards. Federal efforts to push interoperability standards in health care IT are forcing vendors, independent developers, and public researchers to look to open source development. Other "special needs" areas that aren't supported widely by software vendors are also potential areas of growth for open source development.

6.5 Summary

The goal of software engineering in health care is to create a system that facilitates delivery of care. Much has changed in the past decade with EHRs, and today most institutions will purchase rather than build an EHR. But engineering these systems to facilitate care is still challenging, and following appropriate software development practices is increasingly important. The success of a system depends on interaction among designers of health care software applications and those that use the systems. Communication among the participants is very difficult when it comes to commercial applications. Informaticians have an important role to play in bridging the gaps among designers and users that result from the wide variety in background, education, experience, and styles of interaction. They can improve the process of software development by specifying accurately and realistically the need for a system and of designing workable solutions to satisfy those needs.

Suggested Readings

Carter, J. H. (2008). *Electronic health records* (2nd ed.). Philadelphia: ACP Press. Written by a clinician and for clinicians, this is a practical guide for the planning, selection, and implementation of an electronic health record. It first describes the basic infrastructure of an EHR, and then how they can be used effectively in health care. The second half of the book is written more as a workbook for someone participating in the selection and implementation of an EHR.

KLAS Reports. http://www.klasresearch.com/reports. These reports are necessary tools for a project manager who needs to know the latest industry and customer information about vendor health information technology products. The reports include information on functionality available from vendors as well as customer opinions about how vendors are meeting the needs of organizations and whose products are the best in a particular user environment.

McConnell, S. (1996). *Rapid development: Taming wild software schedules*. Redmond: Microsoft Press. For those who would like a deeper understanding of software development and project methodologies like Agile, this is an excellent source. It is targeted to code developers, system architects, and project managers.

President's Council of Advisors on Science and Technology (2010 December). Report to the President Realizing the Full Potential of Health Information Technology to Improve Healthcare for Americans: the Path Forward. http://www.whitehouse.gov/sites/default/files/microsites/ostp/pcast-health-it-report.pdf. This PCAST report focuses on what changes could be made in the field of electronic health records to make them more useful and transformational in the future. It gives a good summary of the current state of EHRs in general, and compares the barriers to those faced in adopting information technology in other fields. Time will tell if the suggestions really become the solution.

Stead, W. W., & Lin, H. S. (Eds.). (2009). *Computational technology for effective health care: Immediate steps and strategic directions*. Washington, DC: National Academies Press. This is a recent National Research Council report about the current state of health information technology and the vision of the Institute of Medicine about how such technology could be used. It can help give a good understanding of how health IT could be used in health care, especially to technology professionals without a health care background.

Tang (Chair), P. C. (2003). *Key capabilities of an electronic health record system*. Washington, DC: National Academies Press. This is a short, letter report from an Institute of Medicine committee that briefly describes the core functionalities of an electronic health record system. Much of the report is tables that list specific capabilities of EHRs in some core functional areas, and indicate their maturity in hospitals, ambulatory care, nursing homes, and personal health records.

Questions for Discussion

1. Reread the hypothetical case study in Sect. 6.2.1.
   (a) What are three primary benefits of the software used in James's care?
   (b) How many different ways is James's information used to help manage his care?
   (c) Without the software and information, how might his care be different?
   (d) How has health care that you have experienced similar or different to this example?

2. For what types of software development projects would an agile development approach be better than a waterfall approach? For what types of development would waterfall be preferred?

3. What are reasons an institution would choose to develop software instead of purchase it from a vendor?

4. How is would various stages in the software development life cycle be different when developing software versus configuring or adding enhancements to an existing software program?

5. Reread the case studies in Sect. 6.3.3.2.
   (a) What are the benefits and advantages of the different approaches to development and acquisition among the scenarios?
   (b) What were the initial costs for each institution for the software? Where will most of the long-term costs be?

6. In what ways might new trends in software (small "apps" that accomplish focused tasks) change long-term strategies for electronic health record architectures?

Standards in Biomedical Informatics

7

W. Edward Hammond, Charles Jaffe, James J. Cimino, and Stanley M. Huff

After reading this chapter, you should know the answers to these questions:

- Why are standards important in biomedical informatics?
- What data standards are necessary to be able to exchange data seamlessly among systems?
- What organizations are active in standards development?
- What aspects of biomedical information management are supported today by standards?
- What is the process for creating consensus standards?
- What factors and organizations influence the creation of standards?

W.E. Hammond (✉)
Duke Center for Health Informatics, Duke University Medical Center, Room 12053, Hock Plaza,
2424 Erwin Road, Durham, NC 27705, USA
e-mail: william.hammond@duke.edu

C. Jaffe, PhD
Health Level Seven International, 122 15th Street,
#2250, Del Mar, CA 92014, USA

J.J. Cimino, MD
Laboratory for Informatics Development,
NIH Clinical Center, 10 Center Drive,
Room 6-2551, Bethesda, MD 20892, USA
e-mail: ciminoj@mail.nih.gov

S.M. Huff, MD
Medical Informatics, Intermountain Healthcare,
South Office Building, Suite 600,
5171 Cottonwood Street, Murray, UT 84107, USA
e-mail: stan.huff@imail.org, coshuff@ihc.com

7.1 The Idea of Standards

Ever since Eli Whitney developed interchangeable parts for rifle assembly, standards have been created and used to make things or processes work more easily and economically—or, sometimes, to work at all. A standard can be defined in many physical forms, but essentially it comprises a set of rules and definitions that specify how to carry out a process or produce a product. Sometimes, a standard is useful because it provides a way to solve a problem that other people can use without having to start from scratch. Generally, though, a standard is useful because it permits two or more disassociated people to work in some cooperative way. Every time you screw in a light bulb or play a music CD, you are taking advantage of a standard. Some standards make things work more easily. Some standards evolve over time,[1] others are developed deliberately.

The first computers were built without standards, but hardware and software standards quickly became a necessity. Although computers work with values such as 1 or 0, and with "words" such as 10101100, humans need a more readable language (see Chap. 5). Thus, standard

---

[1] The current standard for railroad-track gauge originated with Roman chariot builders, who set the axle length based on the width of two horses. This axle length became a standard as road ruts developed, requiring that the wheels of chariots—and all subsequent carriages—be the right distance apart to drive in the ruts. When carriage makers were called on to develop railway rolling stock, they continued to use the same axle standard.

E.H. Shortliffe, J.J. Cimino (eds.), *Biomedical Informatics*,
DOI 10.1007/978-1-4471-4474-8_7, © Springer-Verlag London 2014

character sets, such as ASCII and EBCDIC, were developed. The first standard computer language, COBOL, was written originally to simplify program development but was soon adopted as a way to allow sharing of code and development of software components that could be integrated. As a result, COBOL was given official standard status by the American National Standards Institute (ANSI).[2] In like manner, hardware components depend on standards for exchanging information to make them as interchangeable as were Whitney's gun barrels.

A 1987 technical report from the International Standards Organization (ISO) states that "any meaningful exchange of utterances depends upon the prior existence of an agreed upon set of semantic and syntactic rules" (International Standards Organization 1987). In biomedical informatics, where the emphasis is on collection, manipulation, and transmission of information, standards are greatly needed but have only recently begun to be available. At present, the standards scene is evolving so rapidly that any description is inevitably outdated within a few months. This chapter emphasizes the need for standards in general, standards development processes, current active areas of standards development, and key participating organizations that are making progress in the development of usable standards.

7.2 The Need for Health Informatics Standards

Standards are generally required when excessive diversity creates inefficiencies or impedes effectiveness. The health care environment has traditionally consisted of a set of loosely connected, organizationally independent units. Patients receive care across primary, secondary, and tertiary care settings, with little bidirectional communication and coordination among the services. Patients are cared for by one or more primary physicians, as well as by specialists. There is little coordination and sharing of data between

inpatient care and outpatient care. Both the system and patients, by choice, create this diversity in care. Within the inpatient setting, the clinical environment is divided into clinical specialties that frequently treat the patient without regard to what other specialties have done. Ancillary departments function as detached units, performing their tasks as separate service units, reporting results without follow-up about how those results are used or whether they are even seen by the ordering physician. Reimbursement requires patient information that is often derived through a totally separate process, based on the fragmented data collected in the patient's medical record and abstracted specifically for billing purposes. The resulting set of diagnosis and procedure codes often correlates poorly with the patient's original information (Jollis et al. 1993).

7.2.1 Early Standards to Support the Use of IT in Health Care

Early interest in the development of standards was driven by the need to exchange data between clinical laboratories and clinical systems, and then between independent units within a hospital. Therefore, the first standards were for data exchange and were referred to as messaging standards. Early systems were developed within independent service units, functional applications such as ADT (admission-discharge-transfer) and billing, and within primary care and specialty units. The first uses of computers in hospitals were for billing and accounting purposes and were developed on large, monolithic mainframe computers (see Chap. 13). Initially the cost of computers restricted expansion into clinical areas. But in the 1960s, hospital information systems (HISs) were developed to support service operations within a hospital. These systems followed a pattern of diversity similar to that seen in the health care system itself. As new functions were added in the 1970s, they were implemented on mainframe computers and were managed by a data processing staff that usually was independent of the clinical and even of the administrative staff. The advent of the minicomputer supported the development of departmental systems, such as those for the

---

[2] Interestingly, medical informaticians were responsible for the second ANSI standard language: MUMPS (now known as M).

clinical laboratory, radiology department, or pharmacy. With the advent of minicomputers, departmental systems were introduced but connectivity to other parts of the hospital was either by paper or independent electronic systems. It was common to see two terminals sitting side-by-side with an operator typing data from one system to another. Clinical systems, as they developed, continued to focus on dedicated departmental operations and clinical-specialty systems and thus did not permit the practicing physician to see a unified view of the patient. Most HISs were either supported entirely by a single vendor or were still functionally independent and unconnected.

In the 1980s, the need to move laboratory data directly into developing electronic health records systems (although this term was not used then), early standards were created in ASTM (formerly, the American Society for Testing and Materials, see Sect. 7.3.2) for the transfer of laboratory data from local and commercial laboratories (American Society for Testing and Materials 1999). In the late 1980s, Simborg and others developed an HIS by interfacing independent systems using a "Best of Breed" approach to create an integrated HIS (Simborg et al. 1983) Unfortunately, the cost of developing and maintaining those interfaces was prohibitive, and the need for a broader set of standards was realized. This effort resulted in the creation of the **standards development organization** (SDO) Health Level Seven (**HL7**) in 1987. Other SDOs were created in this same time frame: EDIFACT by the United Nations and ASC X12N by ANSI to address standards for claims and billing, IEEE for device standards, ACR/NEMA (later DICOM) for imaging standards, and NCPDP for prescription standards. Internationally, the 1990s saw the creation of the European Normalization Committee (CEN) and ISO Technical Committee 215 for Health Informatics (TC251). These organizations are described in more detail in Sect. 7.3.2.

7.2.2 Transitioning Standards to Meet Present Needs

Early standards were usually applied within a single unit or department in which the standards addressed mainly local requirements. Even then, data acquired locally came from another source introducing the need for additional standards. These many pressures caused health care information systems to change the status quo such that data collected for a primary purpose could be reused in a multitude of ways. Newer models for health care delivery, such as integrated delivery networks, health maintenance organizations (HMOs), preferred provider organizations (PPOs), and now accountable care organizations (ACOs) have increased the need for coordinated, integrated, and consolidated information (see Chap. 11), even though the information comes from disparate departments and institutions. Various management techniques, such as continuous quality improvement and case management, require up-to-date, accurate abstracts of patient data. Post hoc analyses for clinical and outcomes research require comprehensive summaries across patient populations. Advanced tools, such as clinical workstations (Chap. 5) and decision-support systems (Chap. 3), require ways to translate raw patient data into generic forms for tasks as simple as summary reporting and as complex as automated medical diagnosis. All these needs must be met in the existing setting of diverse, interconnected information systems—an environment that cries out for implementation of standards.

One obvious need is for standardized identifiers for individuals, health care providers, health plans, and employers so that such participants can be recognized across systems. Choosing such an identifier is much more complicated than simply deciding how many digits the identifier should have. Ideal attributes for these sets of identifiers have been described in a publication from the ASTM (1999). The identifier must include a check digit to ensure accuracy when the identifier is entered by a human being into a system. A standardized solution must also determine mechanisms for issuing identifiers to individuals, facilities, and organizations; for maintaining databases of identifying information; and for authorizing access to such information (also see Chap. 5).

The Centers for Medicare and Medicaid Services (CMS), has defined a National Provider

Identifier (NPI) as a national standard. This number is a seven-character alphanumeric base identifier plus a one-character check digit. No meaning is built into the number, each number is unique, it is never reissued, and alpha characters that might be confused with numeric characters have been eliminated (e.g., 0, 1, 2, 4, and 5 can be confused with O, I or L, Z, Y, and S). CMS was tasked to define a Payer ID for identifying health care plans. The Internal Revenue Service's employer identification number has been adopted as the Employer Identifier.

The most controversial issue is identifying each individual or patient. Many people consider assignment and use of such a number to be an invasion of privacy and are concerned that it could be easily linked to other databases. Public Law 104–191, passed in August 1996 (see Sect. 7.3.2), required that Congress formally define suitable identifiers. Pushback by privacy advocates and negative publicity in the media resulted in Congress declaring that this issue would not be moved forward until privacy legislation was in place and implemented (see Chap. 10). The Department of Health and Human Services has recommended the identifiers discussed above, except for the person identifier. This problem has still not been resolved, although the momentum for creating such a unique personal identified seems to be increasing. The United States is one of the few developed countries without such an identifier.

7.2.3   Settings Where Standards Are Needed

A hospital admissions system records that a patient has the diagnosis of diabetes mellitus, a pharmacy system records that the patient has been given gentamicin, a laboratory system records that the patient had certain results on kidney function tests, and a radiology system records that a doctor has ordered an X-ray examination for the patient that requires intravenous iodine dye. Other systems need ways to store these data, to present the data to clinical users, to send warnings about possible drug-drug

interactions, to recommend dosage changes, and to follow the patient's outcome. A standard for coding patient data is nontrivial when one considers the need for agreed-on definitions, use of qualifiers, differing (application-specific) levels of granularity in the data, and synonymy, not to mention the breadth and depth that such a standard would need to have.

The inclusion of medical knowledge in clinical systems is becoming increasingly important and commonplace. Sometimes, the knowledge is in the form of simple facts such as the maximum safe dose of a medication or the normal range of results for a laboratory test. Much medical knowledge is more complex, however. It is challenging to encode such knowledge in ways that computer systems can use (see Chap. 22), especially if one needs to avoid ambiguity and to express logical relations consistently. Thus the encoding of clinical knowledge using an accepted standard would allow many people and institutions to share the work done by others. One standard designed for this purpose is the Arden Syntax, discussed in Chap. 3.

Because the tasks we have described require coordination of systems, methods are needed for transferring information from one system to another. Such transfers were traditionally accomplished through custom-tailored point-to-point interfaces, but this technique has become unworkable as the number of systems and the resulting permutations of necessary connections have grown. A current approach to solving the multiple-interface problem is through the development of messaging standards. Such messages must depend on the preexistence of standards for patient identification and data encoding.

Although the technical challenges are daunting, methods for encoding patient data and shipping those data from system to system are not sufficient for developing practical systems. Security must also be addressed before such exchanges can be allowed to take place. Before a system can divulge patient information, it must ensure that requesters are who they say they are and that they are permitted access to the requested information (see Chap. 5). Although each clinical system can have its own security features, system builders would rather draw on available standards and avoid reinventing the wheel. Besides, the secure exchange of information requires that interacting systems use standard technologies. Fortunately, many researchers are busy developing such standards.

7.3 Standards Undertakings and Organizations

It is helpful to separate our discussion of the general process by which standards are created from our discussion of the specific organizations and the standards that they produce. The process is relatively constant, whereas the organizations form, evolve, merge, and are disbanded. This section will discuss how standards are created then identify the many SDOs and an overview of the types of standards they create. This section will also identify other groups and organizations that contribute or relate to standards activities.

7.3.1 The Standards Development Process

The process of creating standards is biased and highly competitive. Most standards are created by volunteers who represent multiple, disparate stakeholders. They are influenced by direct or indirect self-interest rather than judgment about what is best or required. The process is generally slow and inefficient; multiple international groups create competitive standards; and new groups continue to be formed as they become aware of the need for standards and do not look to see what standards exist. Yet, the process of creating standards largely works, and effective standards are created.

There are four ways in which a standard can be produced:

1. Ad hoc method: A group of interested people and organizations (e.g., laboratory-system and hospital-system vendors) agree on a standard specification. These specifications are informal and are accepted as standards through mutual agreement of the participating groups.

A standard example produced by this method is the DICOM standard for medical imaging.

2. De facto method: A single vendor controls a large enough portion of the market to make its product the market standard. An example is Microsoft's Windows.

3. Government-mandate method: A government agency, such as CMS or the National Institute for Standards and Technology (NIST) creates a standard and legislates its use. An example is the HIPPA standard.

4. Consensus method: A group of volunteers representing interested parties works in an open process to create a standard. Most health care standards are produced by this method. An example is the Health Level 7 (HL7) standard for clinical-data interchange (Fig. 7.1).

The process of creating a standard proceeds through several stages (Libicki 1995). It begins with an identification stage, during which someone becomes aware that there exists a need for a standard in some area and that technology has reached a level that can support such a standard. For example, suppose there are several laboratory systems sending data to several central hospital systems—a standard message format would allow each laboratory system to talk to all the hospital systems without specific point-to-point interface programs being developed for each possible laboratory-to-laboratory or laboratory-to-hospital combination. If the time for a standard is ripe, then several individuals can be identified and organized to help with the conceptualization stage, in which the characteristics of the standard are defined. What must the standard do? What is the scope of the standard? What will be its format? In the early years of standards development, this approach led the development of standards, and the process was supported by vendors and providers. As those early standards have become successful, the need for "gap-standards" has arisen. These gap-standards have no champion but are necessary for completeness of an interoperable data exchange network. The need for these standards is not as obvious as for the primary standards, people are less likely to volunteer to do work, putting stress on the voluntary approach.

Fig. 7.1 Standards development meetings. The development of effective standards often requires the efforts of dedicated volunteers, working over many years. Work is often done in small committee meetings and then presented to a large group to achieve consensus. Here we see meetings of the HL7. Vocabulary Technical Committee (*top*) and an HL7 plenary meeting (*bottom*). See Sect. 7.5.2 for a discussion on HL7

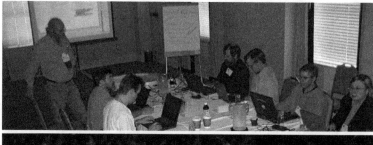
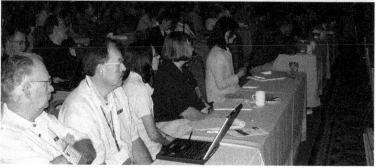

In such cases, the need of such standards must be sold to the volunteers or developed by paid professionals.

Let us consider, for purposes of illustration, how a standard might be developed for sending laboratory data in electronic form from one computer system to another in the form of a message. The volunteers for the development might include laboratory system vendors, clinical users, and consultants. One key discussion would be on the scope of the standard. Should the standard deal only with the exchange of laboratory data, or should the scope be expanded to include other types of data exchange? Should the data elements being exchanged be sent with a XML tag identifying the data element, or should the data be defined positionally? In the ensuing discussion stage, the participants will begin to create an outline that defines content, identifies critical issues, and produces a time line. In the discussion, the pros and cons of the various concepts are discussed. What will be the specific form for the standard? For example, will it be message based or document based? Will the data exchange be based on a query or on a trigger event? Will the standard define the message content, the message syntax, the terminology, the network protocol, or a subset of these issues? How will a data model or information model be incorporated?

The participants are generally well informed in the domain of the standard, so they appreciate the needs and problems that the standard must address. Basic concepts are usually topics for heated discussion; subsequent details may follow at an accelerated pace. Many of the participants will have experience in solving problems to be addressed by the standard and will protect their own approaches. The meanings of words are often debated. Compromises and loosely defined terms are often accepted to permit the process to move forward. For example, the likely participants would be vendors of competing laboratory systems and vendors of competing HISs. All participants would be familiar with the general problems but would have their own proprietary approach to solving them. Definitions of basic concepts normally taken for granted, such as what constitutes a test or a result, would need to be clearly stated and agreed on.

The writing of the draft standard is usually the work of a few dedicated individuals—typically people who represent the vendors in the field. Other people then review that draft; controversial points are discussed in detail and solutions are proposed and finally accepted. Writing and refining the standard is further complicated by the introduction of people new to the process who have not been privy to the original discussions and who want to revisit points that have been resolved earlier. The balance between moving forward and being open is a delicate one. Most standards-writing groups have adopted an **open standards development policy**: Anyone can join the process and can be heard. Most standards development organizations—certainly those by accredited groups— support an open balloting process. A draft standard is made available to all interested parties, inviting comments and recommendations. All comments are considered. Negative ballots must be addressed specifically. If the negative comments are persuasive, the standard is modified. If they are not, the issues are discussed with the submitter in an attempt to convince the person to remove the negative ballot. If neither of these efforts is successful, the comments are sent to the entire balloting group to see whether the group is persuaded to change its vote. The resulting vote then determines the content of the standard. Issues might be general, such as deciding what types of laboratory data to include (pathology? blood bank?), or specific, such as deciding the specific meanings of specific fields (do we include the time the test was ordered? specimen drawn? test performed?).

A standard will generally go through several versions on its path to maturity. The first attempts at implementation are frequently met with frustration as participating vendors interpret the standard differently and as areas not addressed by the standard are encountered. These problems may be dealt with in subsequent versions of the standard. Backward compatibility is a major concern as the standard evolves. How can the standard evolve, over time, and still be economically responsible to both vendors and users? An implementation guide is usually produced to help new vendors profit from the experience of the early implementers.

A critical stage in the life of a standard is early implementation, when acceptance and rate of implementation are important to success. This process is influenced by accredited standards bodies, by the federal government, by major vendors, and the marketplace. The maintenance and promulgation of the standard are also important to ensure widespread availability and continued value of the standard. Some form of conformance testing is ultimately necessary to ensure that vendors adhere to the standard and to protect its integrity.

Producing a standard is an expensive process in terms of both time and money. Vendors and users must be willing to support the many hours of work, usually on company time; the travel expense; and the costs of documentation and distribution. In the United States, the production of a consensus standard is voluntary, in contrast to in Europe and elsewhere, where most standards development is funded by governments.

An important aspect of standards is conformance, a concept that covers compliance with the standard and also usually includes specific agreements among users of the standard who affirm that specific rules will be followed. A conformance document identifies specifically what data elements will be sent, when, and in what form. Even with a perfect standard, a conformance document is necessary to define business relationships between two or more partners.

The creation of the standard is only the first step. Ideally the first standard would be a Draft Standard for Trial Use (DSTU), and two or more vendors would implement and test the standard to identify problems and issues. Those items would be corrected, and in a short period of time (usually 1 year) the standards would be advanced to a normative stage.

Even then, the process is only beginning. Implementation that conforms to the standard is essential if the true value of the standard is to be realized. The use of most standards is enhanced by a certification process in which a neutral body certifies that a vendor's product, in fact, does comply and conform to the standard.

There is currently no body that certifies conformance of specific standards from a vendor. There is, however, the certification of an application that uses standards. In 2010, the Office of the National Coordinator (ONC)[3] engaged with the CCHIT to certify EHR products. That certification process evolved in 2011 to include

---

[3] http://www.healthit.gov/newsroom/about-onc (accessed 4/26/13)

eight groups that could certify EHR products, and to date over 500 EHR products have been certified. The certification process is still undergoing change.

7.3.2 Data Standards Organizations

Sometimes, standards are developed by organizations that need the standard to carry out their principal functions; in other cases, coalitions are formed for the express purpose of developing a particular standard. The latter organizations are discussed later, when we examine the particular standards developed in this way. There are also standards organizations that exist for the sole purpose of fostering and promulgating standards. In some cases, they include a membership with expertise in the area where the standard is needed. In other cases, the organization provides the rules and framework for standard development but does not offer the expertise needed to make specific decisions for specific standards, relying instead on participation by knowledgeable experts when a new standard is being studied.

This section describes in some detail several of the best known SDOs. Our goal has been to familiarize you with the names or organizational and historical aspects of the most influential health-related standards groups. Additional organizations are listed in Table 7.1. In Sect. 7.5 we describe many of the most important standards. For a detailed understanding of an organization or the standards it has developed, you will need to refer to current primary resources. Many of the organizations maintain Web sites with excellent current information on their status.

7.3.2.1 ISO Technical Committee 215—Health Informatics

In 1989, interests in the European Committee for Standardization (CEN) and the United States led to the creation of Technical Committee (TC) 215 for Health Information within ISO.

TC 215 meets once in a year as a TC and once as a Joint Working Group. TC 215 follows rather rigid procedures to create ISO standards. Thirty-five countries are active participants in the TC

with another 23 countries acting as observers. While the actual work is done in the working groups, the balloting process is very formalized— one vote for each participating country. For most work there are a defined series of steps, beginning with a New Work Item Proposal and getting five countries to participate; a Working Document, a Committee Document; a Draft International Standard, a Final Draft International Standard (FDIS); and finally an International Standard. This process, if fully followed, takes several years to produce an International Standard. Under certain conditions, a fast track to FDIS is permitted. Technical Reports and Technical Specifications are also permitted.

The United States has been assigned the duties of Secretariat, and that function is carried out by ANSI. Currently, AHIMA acts for ANSI as Secretariat. AHIMA also serves as the U.S. Technical Advisory Group Administrator, which represents the U.S. position in ISO.

A recent change in ISO policy is permitting standards developed by other bodies to move directly to become ISO standards. Originally, CEN and ISO developed an agreement, called the Vienna Agreement, which permits CEN standards to move into ISO for parallel development and be balloted in each organization. In 2000, a new process was added with the Institute of Electrical and Electronics Engineers (IEEE) called the ISO/IEEE Standards partners in which IEEE standards could be moved directly to ISO for approval as ISO standards. HL7 also has an agreement with ISO which permits HL7 standards to be submitted to TC 215 for approval to become ISO standards.

7.3.2.2 European Committee for Standardization Technical Committee 251

The European Committee for Standardization (CEN) established, in 1991, Technical Committee 251 (TC 251—not to be confused with ISO TC 215 described below) for the development of standards for health care informatics. The major goal of TC 251 is to develop standards for communication among independent medical information systems so that clinical and management

Table 7.1 List of health-related standards groups

Organization	Description
Accredited Standards Organization X12 (ASC X12)	ASC X12 was charted by the American National Standards Institute (ANSI) to develop and maintain several data interchange standards.
American National Standards Institute	ANSI is a private, nonprofit membership organization responsible for approving official American National Standards. ANSI assists standards developers and users from the private sector and from government to reach consensus on the need for standards.
ASTM	ASTM (formerly known as the American Society for Testing and Materials) develops standard test methods for materials, products, systems, and services.
Clinical Data Interchange Standards Consortium (CDISC)	CDISC creates standards in support of the clinical research community. Its membership includes pharma, academic researchers, vendors and others.
European Committee for Standardization Technical Committee 251	The European Committee for Standardization (CEN) established Technical Committee 251 in 1991. The major goal of TC 251 is to develop standards for communication among independent medical information systems so that clinical and management data produced by one system could be transmitted to another system.
GS1	GS1 is a global standards organization with over one million members world-wide. It has a presence in over 100 countries. Its primary standards relate to the supply chain and for assigning object identifiers and standards for bar codes.
Health Level Seven International (HL7)	HL7 was founded in 1987 to create standards for the exchange of clinical data. HL7 is ANSI accredited, and many of the HL7 standards have been designed for required use by the U.S. government as part of Meaningful Use.
Institution of Electrical and Electronic Engineering (IEEE)	The IEEE is an international SDO that has developed standards in many areas. In the health care area, the applicable standards are for the interfacing of instruments and mobile devices.
Integrating the Health care Enterprise	The goal of the Integrating the Health care Enterprise (IHE) initiative is to stimulate integration of health care information resources. IHE enables vendors to direct product development resources toward building increased functionality rather than redundant interfaces.
International Health Terminology Standards Organization (IHTSDO)	The primary purpose of IHTSDO is the continued development and maintenance of SNOMED-CT. Member countries make SNOMED-CT freely available to its citizens. IHTSDO has a number of Special Interest Groups, including Anesthesia, Concept Model, Education, Implementation, International Pathology & Laboratory Medicine, Mapping, Nursing, Pharmacy, and Translation.
ISO Technical Committee 215—Health Informatics	Formed by the European Committee for Standardization (CEN) and the United States in 1989 to create ISO standards in health informatics.
Joint Initiative Council (JIC)	The Joint Initiative Council was formed to enable the creation of common, timely health information standards by addressing gaps, overlaps, and competitive standards efforts by jointly creating, as equal partners, health IT standards. Current members of JIC include ISO, CEN, HL7, CDISC, IHTSDO, and GS1. Ownership of standards created by this group is shared among the participating partners.
National Council for Prescription Drug Programs (NCPDP)	NCPDP creates data interchange standards for the pharmacy services, most specifically for the prescribing process (ePrescribing) and reimbursement for medications.
National Institute of Standards and Technology	Non-regulatory federal agency within the U.S. Department of Commerce whose mission is to develop and promote measurement, standards, and technology to enhance productivity, facilitate trade, and improve the quality of life. In health care, NIST is providing measurement tools, manufacturing assistance, research and development support and quality guidelines as an effort to contain health care costs without compromising quality.

(continued)

Table 7.1 (continued)

Organization	Description
National Quality Forum	Private, not for profit, whose purpose is to develop and implement a national strategy for health care quality measurement and reporting.
openEHR	International organization that develops standards loosely based on ISO 13606. Key work is the development of archetypes.
Standards Development Organizations Charter Committee (SCO)	The SCO was created through an initiative of NCPDP to harmonize the efforts of U.S. SDOs. Membership is limited to SDOs, but associate membership is award to other organizations with an interest in U.S. Health Data Standards.
The Digital Imaging and Communications in Medicine (DICOM)	DICOM was created through a joint effort by the American College of Radiology and NEMA (and was thus initially known as the ACR/NEMA) to develop standards for imaging and waveforms.
U.S. Technical Advisory Group	Represents the U.S. interests in ISO.
Workgroup for Electronic Data Interchange	Broad health care coalition to promote greater health care electronic commerce and connectivity; one of the four organizations named specifically in HIPAA to be consulted in the development of health care standards that would be selected to meet HIPAA requirements.

data produced by one system could be transmitted to another system. The organization of TC 251 parallels efforts in the United States through various working groups. These groups similarly deal with data interchange standard, medical record standards, code and terminology standards, imaging standards, and security, privacy and confidentiality. Both Europe and the United States are making much effort toward coordination in all areas of standardization. Draft standards are being shared. Common solutions are being accepted as desirable. Groups are working together at various levels toward a common goal.

CEN has made major contributions to data standards in health care. One important CEN prestandard ENV 13606 on the electronic health record (EHR) is being advanced by CEN as well as significant input from Australia and the OpenEHR Foundation. There is an increasing cooperation among the CEN participants and several of the U.S. standards bodies. CEN standards may be published through the ISO as part of the Vienna Agreement.

7.3.2.3 Health Level Seven International (HL7)

Health Level 7 was founded as an ad hoc standards group in March 1987 to create standards for the exchange of clinical data, adopting the name "HL7" to reflect the application (seventh) level

of the OSI (see Sect. 7.5.1) reference model. The primary motivation was the creation of a Hospital Information System from "Best of Breed" components. The HL7 data interchange standard (version 2.n series) reduced the cost of interfacing between disparate systems to an affordable cost. Today HL7 is one of the premier SDOs in the world. It has become an international standards body with approximately 40 Affiliates, over 500 organizational members and over 2,200 individual members. HL7 is ANSI accredited, and many of the HL7 standards are required by the U.S. government as part of the certification requirements of Meaningful Use (see Chap. 13). The HL7 standards are described in Sect. 7.5.2.3, below.

7.3.2.4 Integrating the Health Care Enterprise

The goal of the Integrating the Health care Enterprise (IHE) initiative is to stimulate integration of health care information resources. While information systems are essential to the modern health care enterprise, they cannot deliver full benefits if they operate using proprietary protocols or incompatible standards. Decision makers need to encourage comprehensive integration among the full array of imaging and information systems.

IHE is sponsored jointly by the Radiological Society of North America (RSNA) and the

HIMSS. Using established standards and working with direction from medical and information technology professionals, industry leaders in health care information and imaging systems cooperate under IHE to agree upon implementation profiles for the transactions used to communicate images and patient data within the enterprise. Their incentive for participation is the opportunity to demonstrate that their systems can operate efficiently in standards-based, multi-vendor environments with the functionality of real HISs. Moreover, IHE enables vendors to direct product development resources toward building increased functionality rather than redundant interfaces.

7.3.2.5 International Health Terminology Standards Organization (IHTSDO)

IHTSDO was founded in 2007 with nine charter members. Currently 19 countries, including the United States, are members. The primary purpose of IHTSDO is the continued development and maintenance of the Systematized Nomenclature of Medicine – Clinical Terms (SNOMED-CT). Member countries make SNOMED-CT freely available to its citizens. SNOMED has a number of Special Interest Groups: Anesthesia, Concept Model, Education, Implementation, International Pathology & Laboratory Medicine, Mapping, Nursing, Pharmacy, and Translation. SNOMED-CT is described in Sect. 7.4.4.7, below.

7.3.2.6 American National Standards Institute

ANSI is a private, nonprofit membership organization founded in 1918. It originally served to coordinate the U.S. voluntary census standards systems. Today, it is responsible for approving official American National Standards. ANSI membership includes over 1,100 companies; 30 government agencies; and 250 professional, technical, trade, labor, and consumer organizations.

ANSI does not write standards; rather, it assists standards developers and users from the private sector and from government to reach consensus on the need for standards. It helps them to avoid duplication of work, and it provides a forum for

resolution of differences. ANSI administers the only government-recognized system for establishing American National Standards. ANSI also represents U.S. interests in international standardization. ANSI is the U.S. voting representative in the ISO and the International Electrotechnical Commission (IEC). There are three routes for a standards development body to become ANSI approved so as to produce an American National Standard: Accredited Organization; Accredited Standards Committee (ASCs); and Accredited Canvass.

An organization that has existing organizational structure and procedures for standards development may be directly accredited by ANSI to publish American National Standards, provided that it can meet the requirements for due process, openness, and consensus. HL7 (discussed in Sect. 7.5.2) is an example of an ANSI Accredited Organization.

ANSI may also create internal ASCs to meet a need not filled by an existing Accredited Organization. ASC X12 is an example of such a committee.

The final route, Accredited Canvass, is available when an organization does not have the formal structure required by ANSI. Through a canvass method that meets the criterion of balanced representation of all interested parties, a standard may be approved as an American National Standard. ASTM (discussed below) creates its ANSI standards using this method.

7.3.2.7 ASTM

ASTM (formerly known as the American Society for Testing and Materials) was founded in 1898 and chartered in 1902 as a scientific and technical organization for the development of standards for characteristics and performance of materials. The original focus of ASTM was development of standard test methods. The charter was subsequently broadened in 1961 to include products, systems, and services, as well as materials. ASTM is the largest nongovernment source of standards in the United States. It has over 30,000 members who reside in over 90 different countries. ASTM is a charter member of ANSI. ASTM Committee E31 on

Table 7.2 ASTM E31 subcommittees

Subcommittee	Medical information standard
E31.01	Controlled Vocabularies for Health Care Informatics
E31.10	Pharmaco-Informatics Standards
E31.11	Electronic Health Record Portability
E31.13	Clinical Laboratory Information Management Systems
E31.14	Clinical Laboratory Instrument Interface
E31.16	Interchange of Electrophysiological Waveforms and Signals
E31.17	Access, Privacy, and Confidentiality of Medical Records
E31.19	Electronic Health Record Content and Structure
E31.20	Data and System Security for Health Information
E31.21	Health Information Networks
E31.22	Health Information Transcription and Documentation
E31.23	Modeling for Health Informatics
E31.24	Electronic Health Record System Functionality
E31.25	XML for Document Type Definitions in Health care
E31.26	Personal (Consumer) Health Records
E31.28	Electronic Health Records

Computerized Systems is responsible for the development of the medical information standards. Table 7.2 shows the domains of its various subcommittees.

7.4 Detailed Clinical Models, Coded Terminologies, Nomenclatures, and Ontologies

As discussed in Chap. 2, the capture, storage, and use of clinical data in computer systems is complicated by lack of agreement on terms and meanings. In recent years there has also been a growing recognition that just standardizing the terms and codes used in medicine is not sufficient to enable interoperability. The structure or form of medical data provides important context for computable understanding of the data. Terms and codes need to be interpreted in the context of clinical information models. The many terminologies and detailed clinical modeling activities discussed in this section have been developed to ease the communication of coded medical information.

7.4.1 Motivation for Structured and Coded Data

The structuring and encoding of medical information is a basic function of most clinical systems. Standards for such structuring and encoding can serve two purposes. First, they can save system developers from reinventing the wheel. For example, if an application allows caregivers to compile problem lists about their patients, using a standard structure and terminology saves developers from having to create their own. Second, using commonly accepted standards can facilitate exchange of data, applications, and clinical decision support logic among systems. For example, if a central database is accepting clinical data from many sources, the task is greatly simplified if each source is using the same logical data structure and coding scheme to represent the data. System developers often ignore available standards and continue to develop their own solutions. It is easy to believe that the developers have resisted adoption of standards because it is too much work to understand and adapt to any system that was "not invented here." The reality, however, is that the available standards are often inadequate for the needs of the users (in this case, system developers). As a result, no standard terminology enjoys the wide acceptance sufficient to facilitate the second function: exchange of coded clinical information.

The need for detailed clinical models is directly related to the second goal discussed above, that of creating interoperability between systems. The subtle relationship between terminologies and models is best understood using a couple of examples. If a physician wants to record the idea that a patient had "chest pain that radiated to the back", the following coded terms could be used from SNOMED-CT (see Sect. 7.4.4, below):

51185008	Chest (Thoracic structure)
22253000	Pain
8754004	Radiating to
302552004	Back (Entire back)

However, by just reordering the codes, as shown below, one could use the same codes to represent the idea of "back pain radiating to the chest."

302552004	Back (Entire back)
22253000	Pain
8754004	Radiating to
51185008	Chest (Thoracic structure)

In this simple example, changing the order of the codes changes the implied meaning. Creating an ordering of the codes is one way of imposing structure. The need for structure is often overlooked because people can make sense of the set of codes because of medical context and knowledge. Chest pain radiating to the back is much more common than back pain that radiates to the chest, so most clinicians seeing the data would not be confused. However, computer systems do not have the same kind of intuition. To render the representation so that it is unambiguous even to a computer one can make an explicit structure that includes the elements of *finding*, *finding location*, *radiates to location*:

Finding: PainFinding

Location: Chest

Radiates to location: Back

Using the SNOMED-CT codes as values in a data structure removes the ambiguity that exists if just the list of codes is used as a representation of finding.

A second example of why detailed clinical models are needed is closely related to the idea of **pre-coordination** and **post-coordination**. In this example, we are trying to represent the measurement of a patient's dry weight. Two different sites could choose two different ways of representing the measurement:

Site#1: Dry   70 ●kg ○lbs
         weight:

Site #2: Weight: 70 ●kg ○lbs ○Wet ●Dry ○Ideal

At the first site, they have chosen a single concept or label to represent the idea of *dry weight*. The second site decided to use one concept for the generic idea of a *weight measurement*, and to couple that measurement, with a second piece of information indicating the *kind of weight* (dry, wet, or ideal). The first site is using a precoordinated approach, while the second site is using a postcoordinated approach. If you put the measurements from these two different sites into spreadsheets or databases, the information might be structured as shown below:

Site #1:	Patient ID	Date	Observation	Value	Unit
	12345678	10/20/2012	Dry weight	70	kg
	12345678	10/26/2012	Current weight	72	kg

Site #2:	Patient ID	Date	Observation	Type	Value	Unit
	12345678	10/20/2012	Weight	Dry	70	kg
	12345678	10/26/2012	Weight	Current	72	kg

It is intuitively clear that the information content of both the pre- and post-coordination representations is identical. However, if data from both sites were being combined to support a clinical study, it is equally clear that the data from the two sites cannot be referenced or manipulated in exactly the same way. The information that is in the *Observation Type* column in the first site is being represented by information in two columns (*Observation Type* and *Weight type*) in the second site. The logic to query and then calculate the desired weight loss for a patient is different for data from the two sites. Even though the information content is equivalent in the two cases, a computer would need models to know how to transform data from one site into data that could be used interoperably with data from the second site.

The weight example is a very simple case. Problem list data, family history data, complex physical exam observations, and the use of negation all have much greater complexity and degrees of freedom in how the data could be represented, and the need for models to formally represent the explicit structure is even more evident. Because of this interdependence of structure with terms and codes, we will discuss terminologies and detailed clinical models together in this section. We will first discuss detailed clinical models, and then discuss how terminologies relate to the models.

7.4.2   Detailed Clinical Models

The creation of unambiguous data representation is a combination of creating appropriate structures (models) for representing the form of the data and then linking or "binding" specific sets of codes to the coded elements in the structures. Several modeling languages or formalisms have been found to be useful in describing the structure of the data. They include:

- UML – the Unified Modeling Language, Object Management Group
- ADL – Archetype Definition Language, OpenEHR Foundation
- CDL – Constraint Definition Language, General Electric and Intermountain Health care
- MIF – Model Interchange Format, Health Level Seven International Inc.
- OWL – Web Ontology Language, World Wide Web Consortium

All languages used for clinical modeling need to accomplish at least two major things: they need to show the "logical" structure of the data, and they need to show how sets of codes from standard terminologies participate in the logical structure. Defining the logical structure is simply showing how the named parts of a model relate to one another. Model elements can be contained in other elements, creating hierarchies of elements. It is also import to specify which elements of the model can occur more than once (cardinality), which elements are required, and which are optional. Terminology binding is the act of creating connections between the elements in a model and concepts in a coded terminology. For each coded element in a model, the set of allowed values for the coded element are specified. The HL7 Vocabulary Working Group has created a comprehensive discussion of how value sets can be

defined and used with information models [HL7 Core Vocabulary Foundation].

There are many clinical information modeling activities worldwide. Some of the most important activities are briefly listed below.

- HL7 Activities
  - HL7 Detailed Clinical Models – This group has developed a method for specifying clinical models based on the HL7 Reference Information Model (RIM) that guarantees that data that conforms to the model could be sent in HL7 Version 3 messages.
  - HL7 Clinical Document Architecture (CDA) Templates – This group has defined a standard way of specifying the structure of data to be sent in XML documents that conform to the CDA standard.
  - HL7 TermInfo – This Workgroup of HL7 has specified a set of guidelines for how SNOMED-CT codes and concepts should be used in conjunction with the HL7 RIM to represent data sent in HL7 Version 3 messages.
- The openEHR Foundation is developing models based on a core reference model and the Archetype Definition Language. This approach has been adopted by several national health information programs.
- EN 13606 is developing models based on the ISO/CEN 13606 standard and core reference model.
- Tolven is an open source initiative that creates models as part of an overall architecture to support open Electronic Health Record implementation.
- The US Veterans Administration (VA) is creating models for integrating data across all VA facilities and for integration with military hospitals that are part of the US Department of Defense. The modeling is done primarily using Unified Modeling Language.
- US Department of Defense is creating models for integrating data across all DoD facilities and for integration with VA facilities. The modeling is done primarily using Unified Modeling Language.
- The National Health Service in the United Kingdom (UK) is developing the Logical

Fig. 7.2 Terminologic terms, adapted from ISO Standard 1087. Terms not defined here—such as definition, lexical unit, and linguistic expression—are assumed by the Standard to have common meanings

- **Object:** Any part of the perceivable or conceivable world
- **Name:** Designation of an object by a linguistic expression
- **Concept:** A unit of thought constituted through abstraction on the basis of properties common to a set of objects
- **Term:** Designation of a defined concept in a special language by a linguistic expression
- **Terminology:** Set of terms representing the system of concepts of a particular subject field
- **Nomenclature:** System of terms that is elaborated according to preestablished naming rules
- **Dictionary:** Structured collection of lexical units, with linguistic information about each of them
- **Vocabulary:** Dictionary containing the terminology of a subject field

Record Architecture to provide models for interoperability across all health care facilities in the UK. The modeling is done primarily using UML.

- Clinical Element Models - Intermountain Health care and General Electric have created a set of detailed clinical models using a core reference model and Constraint Definition Language. The models are free-for-use and are available for download from the Internet.
- SHARE Models – CDISC is creating models to integrate data collected as part of clinical trials.
- SMArt Team – This group at Boston Children's Hospital is defining standard application programming interfaces (APIs) for services that store and retrieve medical data.
- Clinical Information Modeling Initiative (CIMI) – This is an international consortium that has the goal of establishing a free-for-use repository of detailed clinical models, where the models are expressed in a single common modeling language with explicit bindings to standard terminologies.

7.4.3 Vocabularies, Terminologies, and Nomenclatures

In discussing coding systems, the first step is to clarify the differences among a **terminology**, a **vocabulary**, and a **nomenclature**. These terms are often used interchangeably by creators of coding systems and by authors discussing the subject. Fortunately, although there are few accepted standard terminologies, there is a generally accepted standard about terminology: ISO Standard 1087 (Terminology—Vocabulary). Figure 7.2 lists the various definitions for these terms. For our purposes, we consider the currently available standards from the viewpoint of their being terminologies.

The next step in the discussion is to determine the basic use of the terminology. In general, there are two different levels relevant to medical data encoding: abstraction and representation. **Abstraction and classification** entail examination of the recorded data and then selection of items from a terminology with which to label the data. For example, a patient might be admitted to the hospital and have a long and complex course; for the purposes of billing, however, it might be relevant that the patient was diagnosed only as having had a myocardial infarction. Someone charged with abstracting the record to generate a bill might then reduce the entire set of information to a single code. **Representation**, on the other hand, is the process by which as much detail as possible is coded. Thus, for the medical record example, the representation might include codes for each physical finding noted, laboratory test performed and its result, and medication administered.

When we discuss a controlled terminology, we should consider the domain of discourse. Virtually any subject matter can be coded, but there must be a good match with any standard selected for the purpose. For example, a terminology that only included diseases might be a poor choice for coding entries on a problem list because it might lack items such as "abdominal pain," "cigarette smoker," or "health maintenance."

The next consideration is the content of the standard itself. There are many issues, including the degree to which the standard covers the terminology of the intended domain; the degree to which data are coded by assembly of terms into descriptive phrases (post-coordination) versus selection of a single, precoordinated term; and the overall structure of the terminology (list, strict hierarchy, multiple hierarchy, semantic network, and so on). There are also many qualitative issues to consider, including the availability of synonyms and the possibility of redundant terms (i.e., more than one way to encode the same information).

Finally, we should consider the methods by which the terminology is maintained. Every standard terminology must have an ongoing maintenance process, or it will rapidly become obsolete. The process must be timely and must not be too disruptive to people using an older version of the terminology. For example, if the creators of the terminology choose to rename a code, what happens to the data previously recorded with that code?

7.4.4 Specific Terminologies

With these considerations in mind, let us survey some of the available controlled terminologies. People often say, tongue in cheek, that the best thing about standards is that there are so many from which to choose. We give introductory descriptions of a few current and common terminologies. New terminologies appear annually, and existing proprietary terminologies often become publicly available. When reviewing the following descriptions, try to keep in mind the background motivation for a development effort. All these standards are evolving rapidly, and one should consult the Web sites or other primary sources for the most recent information.

7.4.4.1 International Classification of Diseases and Its Clinical Modifications

One of the best known terminologies is the International Classification of Diseases (ICD).

First published in 1893, it has been revised at roughly 10-year intervals, first by the Statistical International Institute and later by the World Health Organization (WHO). The Ninth Edition (ICD-9) was published in 1977 (World Health Organization, 1977) and the Tenth Edition (ICD-10) in 1992 (World Health Organization 1992). The ICD-9 coding system consists of a core classification of three-digit codes that are the minimum required for reporting mortality statistics to WHO. A fourth digit (in the first decimal place) provides an additional level of detail; usually .0 to .7 are used for more specific forms of the core term, .8 is usually "other," and .9 is "unspecified." Codes in the ICD-10 coding system start with an alpha character and consist of three to seven characters. In both systems, terms are arranged in a strict hierarchy, based on the digits in the code. For example, bacterial pneumonias are classified as shown in Figs. 7.3 and 7.4. In addition to diseases, ICD includes several "families" of terms for medical-specialty diagnoses, health status, disease-related events, procedures, and reasons for contact with health care providers.

ICD-9 has generally been perceived as inadequate for the level of detail desired for statistical reporting in the United States (Kurtzke 1979). In response, the U.S. National Center for Health Statistics published a set of **clinical modifications** (CM) (Commission on Professional and Hospital Activities 1978). **ICD-9-CM**, as it is known, is compatible with ICD-9 and provides extra levels of detail in many places by adding fourth-digit and fifth-digit codes. Figure 7.3 shows a sample of additional material. Most of the diagnoses assigned in the United States are coded in ICD-9-CM, allowing compliance with international treaty (by conversion to ICD-9) and supporting billing requirements (by conversion to diagnosis-related groups or DRGs). A clinical modification for ICD-10 has also been created; examples are shown in Fig. 7.4.

7.4.4.2 Diagnosis-Related Groups

Another U.S. creation for the purpose of abstracting medical records is the DRGs, developed initially at Yale University for use in

Fig. 7.3 Examples of codes in ICD-9 and ICD-9-CM (*) showing how bacterial pneumonia terms are coded. Tuberculosis terms, pneumonias for which the etiologic agent is not specified, and other intervening terms are not shown. Note that some terms, such as "Salmonella Pneumonia" were introduced in ICD-9-CM as a children of organism-specific terms, rather than under 482 (other bacterial pneumonia)

```
003 Other salmonella infections
    003.2 Localized salmonella infections
        003.22 Salmonella pneumonia *
020 Plague
    020.3 Primary pneumonic plague
    020.4 Secondary pneumonic plague
    020.5 Pneumonic plague, unspecified
021 Tularemia
    021.2 Pulmonary tularemia *
022 Anthrax
    022.1 Pulmonary anthrax
481 Pneumococcal pneumonia
482 Other bacterial pneumonia
    482.0 Pneumonia due to Klebsiella pneumoniae
    482.1 Pneumonia due to Pseudomonas
    482.2 Pneumonia due to Hemophilus influenzae
    482.3 Pneumonia due to Streptococcus
        482.30 Pneumonia due to Streptococcus, unspecified *
        482.31 Pneumonia due to Group A Streptococcus *
        482.32 Pneumonia due to Group B Streptococcus *
        482.39 Other streptococcal pneumonia *
    482.4 Pneumonia due to Staphylococcus
        482.40 Pneumonia due to Staphylococcus, unspecified *
        482.41 Pneumonia due to Staphylococcus aureus *
        482.49 Other Staphylococcus pneumonia *
    482.8 Pneumonia due to other specified bacteria
        482.81 Pneumonia due to anaerobes *
        482.82 Pneumonia due to Escherichia coli *
        482.83 Pneumonia due to other Gram-negative bacteria *
        482.84 Legionnaires' disease *
        482.89 Pneumonia due to other specified bacteria *
    482.9 Bacterial pneumonia, unspecified
483 Pneumonia due to other specified organism
    483.0 Mycoplasma pneumoniae *
484 Pneumonia in infectious diseases classified elsewhere *
    484.3 Pneumonia in whooping cough *
    484.5 Pneumonia in anthrax *
```

prospective payment in the Medicare program (3M Health Information System, updated annually). In this case, the coding system is an abstraction of an abstraction; it is applied to lists of ICD-9-CM codes that are themselves derived from medical records. The purpose of DRG coding is to provide a relatively small number of codes for classifying patient hospitalizations while also providing some separation of cases based on severity of illness. The principal bases for the groupings are factors that affect cost and length of stay. Thus, a medical record containing the ICD-9-CM primary diagnosis of pneumococcal pneumonia (481) might be coded with one of 18 codes (Fig. 7.5), depending on associated conditions and procedures; additional codes are possible if the pneumonia is a secondary diagnosis.

Fig. 7.4 Examples of codes in ICD-10 and ICD-10-CM (*) showing how bacterial pneumonia terms are coded. Tuberculosis terms, pneumonias for which the etiologic agent is not specified, and other intervening terms are not shown. Note that ICD-10 classifies Mycoplasma pneumoniae as a bacterium, while ICD-9 does not. Also, neither ICD-10 nor ICD-10-CM have a code for "Melioidosis Pneumonia," but ICD-10-CM specifies that the code A24.1 Acute and fulminating melioidosis (not shown) should be used

A01 Typhoid and paratyphoid fevers
  A01.0 Typhoid Fever
    A01.03 Typhoid Pneumonia *
A02 Other salmonella infection
  A02.2 Localized salmonella infections
    A02.22 Salmonella pneumonia *
A20 Plague
  A20.2 Pneumonic plague
A22 Anthrax
  A22.1 Pulmonary anthrax
A37 Whooping cough
  A37.0 Whooping cough due to *Bordetella pertussis*
    A37.01 Whooping cough due to *Bordetella pertussis* with pneumonia *
  A37.1 Whooping cough due to *Bordetella parapertussis*
    A37.11 Whooping cough due to *Bordetella parapertussis* with pneumonia *
  A37.8 Whooping cough due to other Bordetella species
    A37.81 Whooping cough due to other Bordetella species with pneumonia *
  A37.9 Whooping cough, unspecified
    A37.91 Whooping cough, unspecified species with pneumonia *
A50 Congenital syphilis
  A50.0 Early congenital syphilis, symptomatic
    A50.04 Early congenital syphilitic pneumonia *
A54 Gonococcal infection
  A54.8 Other gonococcal infection
    A54.84 Gonococcal pneumonia *
J13 Pneumonia due to *Streptococcus pneumoniae*
J14 Pneumonia due to *Hemophilus influenzae*
J15 Bacterial pneumonia, not elsewhere classified
  J15.0 Pneumonia due to *Klebsiella pneumoniae*
  J15.1 Pneumonia due to Pseudomonas
  J15.2 Pneumonia due to staphylococcus
    J15.20 Pneumonia due to staphylococcus, unspecified *
    J15.21 Pneumonia due to *Staphylococcus aureus* *
    J15.29 Pneumonia due to other staphylococcus *
  J15.3 Pneumonia due to streptococcus, group B
  J15.4 Pneumonia due to other streptococci
  J15.5 Pneumonia due to *Escherichia coli*
  J15.6 Pneumonia due to other aerobic Gram-negative bacteria
  J15.7 Pneumonia due to *Mycoplasma pneumoniae*
  J15.8 Other bacterial pneumonia
  J15.9 Bacterial pneumonia, unspecified
P23 Congenital pneumonia
  P23.2 Congenital pneumonia due to staphylococcus
  P23.3 Congenital pneumonia due to streptococcus, group B
  P23.4 Congenital pneumonia due to *Escherichia coli*
  P23.5 Congenital pneumonia due to Pseudomonas
  P23.6 Congenital pneumonia due to other bacterial agents

7.4.4.3 International Classification of Primary Care

The World Organization of National Colleges, Academies and Academic Associations of General Practitioners/Family Physicians (WONCA) publishes the International Classification of Primary Care (ICPC) with the WHO, the latest version of which is ICPC-2, published in 1998. ICPC-2 is a classification of some 1,400 diagnostic concepts that are partially mapped into ICD-9 and ICD-10. ICPC-2 contains all 380 concepts of the International Classification of Health Problems in Primary Care (ICHPPC), Third Edition, including reasons for an encounter. ICPC provides seven axes of terms and a structure to combine them to represent clinical encounters. Although the granularity of the terms is generally larger than that of other classification schemes (e.g.,

Respiratory disease w/ major chest operating room procedure, no major complication or comorbidity	75
Respiratory disease w/ major chest operating room procedure, minor complication or comorbidity	76
Respiratory disease w/ other respiratory system operating procedure, no complication or comorbidity	77
Respiratory infection w/ minor complication, age greater than 17	79
Respiratory infection w/ no minor complication, age greater than 17	80
Simple Pneumonia w/ minor complication, age greater than 17	89
Simple Pneumonia w/ no minor complication, age greater than 17	90
Respiratory disease w/ ventilator support	475
Respiratory disease w/ major chest operating room procedure and major complication or comorbidity	538
Respiratory disease, other respiratory system operating procedure and major complication	539
Respiratory infection w/ major complication or comorbidity	540
Respiratory infection w/ secondary diagnosis of bronchopulmonary dysplasia	631
Respiratory infection w/ secondary diagnosis of cystic fibrosis	740
Respiratory infection w/ minor complication, age not greater than 17	770
Respiratory infection w/ no minor complication, age not greater than 17	771
Simple Pneumonia w/ minor complication, age not greater than 17	772
Simple Pneumonia w/ no minor complication, age not greater than 17	773
Respiratory infection w/ primary diagnosis of tuberculosis	798

Fig. 7.5 Diagnosis-related group codes assigned to cases of bacterial pneumonia depending on co-occurring conditions or procedures (mycobacterial disease is not shown here except as a cooccurring condition). "Simple Pneumonia" codes are used when the primary bacterial pneumonia corresponds to ICD-9 code 481, 482.2, 482.3, or 482.9, and when there are only minor or no complica- tions. The remaining ICD-9 bacterial pneumonias (482.0, 482.1, 482.2, 482.4, 482.8, 484, and various other codes such as 003.22) are coded as "Respiratory Disease" or "Respiratory Infection." Cases in which pneumonia is a secondary diagnosis may also be assigned other codes (such as 798), depending on the primary condition

all pneumonias are coded as R81), the ability to represent the interactions of the concepts found in a medical record is much greater through the **post-coordination** of atomic terms. In post-coor- dination, the coding is accomplished through the use of multiple codes as needed to describe the data. Thus, for example, a case of bacterial pneu- monia would be coded in ICPC as a combination of the code R81 and the code for the particular test result that identifies the causative agent. This method is in contrast to the **pre-coordination** approach in which every type of pneumonia is assigned its own code.

7.4.4.4 Current Procedural Terminology

The American Medical Association developed the Current Procedural Terminology (CPT) in 1966 (American Medical Association, updated annually) to provide a precoordinated coding scheme for diagnostic and therapeutic procedures that has since been adopted in the United States for billing and reimbursement. Like the DRG codes, CPT codes specify information that dif- ferentiates the codes based on cost. For example, there are different codes for pacemaker inser- tions, depending on whether the leads are "epi- cardial, by thoracotomy" (33200), "epicardial, by xiphoid approach" (33201), "transvenous, atrial" (33206), "transvenous, ventricular" (33207), or "transvenous, atrioventricular (AV) sequential" (33208). CPT also provides information about the reasons for a procedure. For example, there are codes for arterial punctures for "withdrawal of blood for diagnosis" (36600), "monitoring" (36620), "infusion therapy" (36640), and "occlu- sion therapy" (75894). Although limited in scope and depth (despite containing over 8,000 terms), CPT-4 is the most widely accepted nomenclature in the United States for reporting physician pro- cedures and services for federal and private insurance third-party reimbursement.

7.4.4.5 Diagnostic and Statistical Manual of Mental Disorders

The American Psychiatric Association published the Fifth Edition of the Diagnostic and Statistical Manual of Mental Disorders (DSM-5) in May 2013. DSM-5 is the standard classification of mental disorders used by mental health professionals in the U.S. and contains a listing of diagnostic criteria for every psychiatric disorder recognized by the U.S. healthcare system. The previous edition, DSM-IV, was originally published in 1994 and revised in 2000 as DSM-IV-TR. DSM-5 is coordinated with ICD-10.

7.4.4.6 Read Clinical Codes

The Read Clinical Codes comprise a set of terms designed specifically for use in coding electronic medical records. Developed by James Read in the 1980s (Read and Benson 1986; Read 1990), the first version was adopted by the British National Health Service (NHS) in 1990. Version 2.0 was developed to meet the needs of hospitals for cross-mapping their data to ICD-9. Version 3.0 (NHS Centre for Coding and Classification 1994) was developed to support not only medical record summarization but also patient-care applications directly. Whereas previous versions of the Read Codes were organized in a strict hierarchy, Version 3.0 took an important step by allowing terms to have multiple parents in the hierarchy, i.e., the hierarchy became that of a directed acyclic graph. Version 3.1 added the ability to make use of term modifiers through a set of templates for combining terms in specific, controlled ways so that both pre-coordination and post-coordination are used. Finally, the NHS undertook a series of "clinical terms" projects that expanded the content of the Read Codes to ensure that the terms needed by practitioners are represented in the Codes (NHS Centre for Coding and Classification 1994). Clinical Terms version 3 was merged with SNOMED in 2001 to create the first version of SNOMED-CT (see next section).

7.4.4.7 SNOMED Clinical Terms and Its Predecessors

Drawing from the New York Academy of Medicine's Standard Nomenclature of Diseases and Operations (SNDO) (Plunkett 1952; Thompson and Hayden 1961) (New York Academy of Medicine 1961), the College of American Pathologists (CAP) developed the Standard Nomenclature of Pathology (SNOP) as a multiaxial system for describing pathologic findings (College of American Pathologists, 1971) through post-coordination of topographic (anatomic), morphologic, etiologic, and functional terms. SNOP has been used widely in pathology systems in the United States; its successor, the Systematized Nomenclature of Medicine (SNOMED) has evolved beyond an abstracting scheme to become a comprehensive coding system.

Largely the work of Roger Côté and David Rothwell, SNOMED was first published in 1975, was revised as SNOMED II in 1979, and then greatly expanded in 1993 as the Systematized Nomenclature of Human and Veterinary Medicine—SNOMED.

International (Côté and Rothwell 1993). Each of these versions was **multi-axial**; coding of patient information was accomplished through the post-coordination of terms from multiple axes to represent complex terms that did not exist as single codes in SNOMED. In 1996, SNOMED changed from a multi-axial structure to a more logic-based structure called a Reference Terminology (Spackman et al. 1997a, b; Campbell et al. 1998), intended to support more sophisticated data encoding processes and resolve some of the problems with earlier versions of SNOMED (see Fig. 7.6). In 1999, CAP and the NHS announced an agreement to merge their products into a single terminology called SNOMED Clinical Terms (SNOMED-CT) (Spackman 2000), containing terms for over 344,000 concepts (see Fig. 7.7). SNOMED-CT is currently maintained by a not-for-profit association called the International Health Terminology Standards Development Organization (IHTSDO).

Despite the broad coverage of SNOMED-CT, it continues to allow users to create new, ad hoc terms through post-coordination of existing terms. While this increases the expressivity, users must be careful not to be too expressive because there are few rules about how the post-coordination coding should be done, the same expression might end up being represented differently by different coders. For example,

```
Concept: Bacterial pneumonia
    Concept Status Current
    Fully defined by ...
        Is a
            Infectious disease of lung
            Inflammatory disorder of lower respiratory tract
            Infective pneumonia
            Inflammation of specific body organs
            Inflammation of specific body systems
            Bacterial infectious disease
        Causative agent:
            Bacterium
        Pathological process:
            Infectious disease
        Associated morphology:
            Inflammation
        Finding site:
            Lung structure
        Onset:
            Subacute onset
            Acute onset
            Insidious onset
            Sudden onset
        Severity:
            Severities
        Episodicity:
            Episodicities
        Course:
            Courses
    Descriptions:
        Bacterial pneumonia (disorder)
        Bacterial pneumonia
    Legacy codes:
        SNOMED: DE-10100
        CTV3ID: X100H
```

Fig. 7.6 Description-logic representation of the SNOMED-CT term "Bacterial Pneumonia." The "Is a" attributes define bacterial pneumonia's position in SNOMED-CT's multiple hierarchy, while attributes such as "Causative Agent" and "Finding Site" provide definitional information. Other attributes such as "Onset" and "Severities" indicate ways in which bacterial pneumonia can be postcoordinated with others terms, such as "Acute Onset" or any of the descendants of the term "Severities." "Descriptions" refers to various text strings that serve as names for the term, while "Legacy Codes" provide backward compatibility to SNOMED and Read Clinical Terms

```
Pneumonia
    Bacterial pneumonia
        Proteus pneumonia
        Legionella pneumonia
        Anthrax pneumonia
        Actinomycotic pneumonia
        Nocardial pneumonia
        Meningococcal pneumonia
        Chlamydial pneumonia
            Neonatal chlamydial pneumonia
            Ornithosis
                Ornithosis with complication
                Ornithosis with pneumonia
        Congenital bacterial pneumonia
            Congenital staphylococcal pneumonia
            Congenital group A hemolytic streptococcal pneumonia
            Congenital group B hemolytic streptococcal pneumonia
            Congenital Escherichia coli pneumonia
            Congenital pseudomonal pneumonia
        Chlamydial pneumonitis in all species except pig
            Feline pneumonitis
        Staphylococcal pneumonia
        Pulmonary actinobacillosis
        Pneumonia in Q fever
        Pneumonia due to Streptococcus
            Group B streptococcal pneumonia
            Congenital group A hemolytic streptococcal pneumonia
            Congenital group B hemolytic streptococcal pneumonia
            Pneumococcal pneumonia
                Pneumococcal lobar pneumonia
                AIDS with pneumococcal pneumonia
        Pneumonia due to Pseudomonas
            Congenital pseudomonal pneumonia
        Pulmonary tularemia
        Enzootic pneumonia of calves
        Pneumonia in pertussis
        AIDS with bacterial pneumonia
        Enzootic pneumonia of sheep
        Pneumonia due to Klebsiella pneumoniae
        Hemophilus influenzae pneumonia
        Porcine contagious pleuropneumonia
        Pneumonia due to pleuropneumonia-like organism
        Secondary bacterial pneumonia
    Pneumonic plague
        Primary pneumonic plague
        Secondary pneumonic plague
    Salmonella pneumonia
        Pneumonia in typhoid fever
    Infective pneumonia
        Mycoplasma pneumonia
            Enzootic mycoplasmal pneumonia of swine
    Achromobacter pneumonia
    Bovine pneumonic pasteurellosis
    Corynebacterial pneumonia of foals
    Pneumonia due to Escherichia coli
    Pneumonia due to Proteus mirabilis
```

Fig. 7.7 Examples of codes in SNOMED-CT, showing some of the hierarchical relationships among bacterial pneumonia terms. Tuberculosis terms and certain terms that are included in SNOMED-CT for compatability with other terminologies are not shown. Note that some terms such as "Congenital group A hemolytic streptococcal pneumonia" appear under multiple parent terms, while other terms, such as "Congenital staphylococcal pneumonia" are not listed under all possible parent terms (e.g., it is under "Congenital pneumonia" but not under "Staphylococcal pneumonia"). Some terms, such as "Pneumonic plague" and "Mycoplasma pneumonia" are not classified under Bacterial Pneumonia, althogh the causative agents in their descriptions ("Yersinia pestis" and "Myocplasma pneumioniae", respectively) are classified under "Bacterium", the causative agent of Bacterial pneumonia

"acute appendicitis" can be coded as a single disease term, as a combination of a modifier ("acute") and a disease term ("appendicitis"), or as a combination of a modifier ("acute"), a morphology term ("inflammation") and a topography term ("vermiform appendix"). Users must therefore be careful when post-coordinating terms, not to recreate a meaning that is satisfied by an already existing single code. SNOMED-CT's description logic, such as the example in Fig. 7.6, can help guide users when selecting modifiers.

7.4.4.8 Galen

In Europe, a consortium of universities, agencies, and vendors, with funding from the Advanced Informatics in Medicine initiative (AIM), has formed the GALEN project to develop standards for representing coded patient information (Rector et al. 1995). GALEN developed a reference model for medical concepts using a formalism called Structured Meta Knowledge (SMK) and a formal representation language called GALEN Representation and Integration Language (GRAIL). Using GRAIL, terms are defined through relationships to other terms, and grammars are provided to allow combinations of terms into sensible phrases. The reference model is intended to allow representation of patient information in a way that is independent of the language being recorded and of the data model used by an electronic medical record system. The GALEN developers are working closely with CEN TC 251 (see Sect. 7.3.2) to develop the content that will populate the reference model with actual terms. In 2000, an open source foundation called OpenGALEN[4] was developed. Active development of OpenGALEN has since ceased. However, the website is still active and all of the GALEN content and educational materials are available for download and use free of charge.

7.4.4.9 Logical Observations, Identifiers, Names, and Codes

An independent consortium, led by Clement J. McDonald and Stanley M. Huff, has created a naming system for tests and observations. The system is called Logical Observation Identifiers Names and Codes (LOINC).[5] The coding system contains names and codes for laboratory tests, patient measurements, assessment instruments, document and section names, and radiology exams. Figure 7.8 shows some typical fully specified names for common laboratory tests.

The standard specifies structured coded semantic information about each test, such as the substance measured and the analytical method used.

7.4.4.10 Nursing Terminologies

Nursing organizations and research teams have been extremely active in the development of standard coding systems for documenting and evaluating nursing care. One review counted a total of 12 separate projects active worldwide (Coenen et al. 2001), including coordination with SNOMED and LOINC. These projects have arisen because general medical terminologies fail to represent the kind of clinical concepts needed in nursing care. For example, the kinds of problems that appear in a physician's problem list (such as "myocardial infarction" and "diabetes mellitus") are relatively well represented in many of the terminologies that we have described, but the kinds of problems that appear in a nurse's assessment (such as "activity intolerance" and "knowledge deficit related to myocardial infarction") are not. Preeminent nursing terminologies include the North American Nursing Diagnosis Association (NANDA) codes, the Nursing Interventions Classification (NIC), the Nursing Outcomes Classification (NOC), the Georgetown Home Health Care Classification (HHCC), and the Omaha System (which covers problems, interventions, and outcomes).

Despite the proliferation of standards for nursing terminologies, gaps remain in the coverage of this domain (Henry and Mead 1997). The International Council of Nurses and the International Medical Informatics Association Nursing Informatics Special Interest Group have worked together to produce the International Classification for Nursing Practice (ICNP®). This system uses a post-coordinated approach for describing nursing diagnoses, actions, and outcomes.

7.4.4.11 Drug Codes

A variety of public and commercial terminologies have been developed to represent terms used for prescribing, dispensing and administering drugs. The WHO Drug Dictionary is an international classification of drugs that provides proprietary drug names used in different countries, as

---

[4] www.opengalen.org (accessed 4/26/13)

[5] loinc.org (accessed 4/26/13)

```
Blood glucose              GLUCOSE:MCNC:PT:BLD:QN:
Plasma glucose             GLUCOSE:MCNC:PT:PLAS:QN:
Serum glucose              GLUCOSE:MCNC:PT:SER:QN:
Urine glucose concentration GLUCOSE:MCNC:PT:UR:QN:
Urine glucose by dip stick  GLUCOSE:MCNC:PT:UR:SQ:TEST STRIP
Glucose tolerance test at   GLUCOSE"2H POST 100 G GLUCOSE PO:
   2 hours                    MCNC:PT:PLAS:QN:
Ionized whole blood calcium CALCIUM.FREE:SCNC:PT:BLD:QN:
Serum or plasma            CALCIUM.FREE:SCNC:PT:SER/PLAS:QN:
   ionized calcium
24-hour calcium excretion   CALCIUM.TOTAL:MRAT:24H:UR:QN:
Whole blood total calcium   CALCIUM.TOTAL:SCNC:PT:BLD:QN:
Serum or plasma total       CALCIUM.TOTAL:SCNC:PT:SER/PLAS:QN:
   calcium
Automated hematocrit        HEMATOCRIT:NFR:PT:BLD:QN:  AUTOMATED COUNT
Manual spun hematocrit      HEMATOCRIT:NFR:PT:BLD:QN:SPUN
Urine erythrocyte casts     ERYTHROCYTE CASTS:ACNC:PT:URNS:SQ:
                              MICROSCOPY.LIGHT
Erythrocyte MCHC            ERYTHROCYTE MEAN CORPUSCULAR HEMOGLOBIN
                              CONCENTRATION:MCNC:PT:RBC:QN:AUTOMATED
                              COUNT
Erythrocyte MCH            ERYTHROCYTE MEAN CORPUSCULAR
                              HEMOGLOBIN:MCNC:PT:RBC:QN: AUTOMATED
                              COUNT
Erythrocyte MCV            ERYTHROCYTE MEAN CORPUSCULAR
                              VOLUME:ENTVOL:PT:RBC:QN:AUTOMATED COUNT
Automated Blood RBC         ERYTHROCYTES:NCNC:PT:BLD:QN: AUTOMATED
                              COUNT
Manual blood RBC           ERYTHROCYTES:NCNC:PT:BLD:QN: MANUAL
                              COUNT
ESR by Westergren method   ERYTHROCYTE SEDIMENTATION
                              RATE:VEL:PT:BLD:QN:WESTERGREN
ESR by Wintrobe method     ERYTHROCYTE SEDIMENTATION
                              RATE:VEL:PT:BLD:QN:WINTROBE
```

Fig. 7.8 Examples of common laboratory test terms as they are encoded in LOINC. The major components of the fully specified name are in separate columns and consist of the analyte, the property (e.g., *Mcnc* mass concentration, *Scnc* substance concentration, *Acnc* arbitrary concentration, *Vfr* volume fraction, *EntMass* entitic mass, *EntVol* entitic volume, *Vel* velocity, and *Ncnc* number concentration), the timing (*Pt* point in time), the system (specimen), and the method (*Ord* ordinal, *Qn* quantitative)

well as all active ingredients and the chemical substances, with Chemical Abstract numbers. Drugs are classified according to the Anatomical-Therapeutic-Chemical (ATC) classification, with cross-references to manufacturers and reference sources. The current dictionary contains 25,000 proprietary drug names, 15,000 single ingredient drugs, 10,000 multiple ingredient drugs, and 7,000 chemical substances. The dictionary now covers drugs from 34 countries and grows at a rate of about 2,000 new entries per year.

The National Drug Codes (NDC), produced by the U.S. Food and Drug Administration (FDA), is applied to all drug packages. It is widely used in the United States, but it is not as comprehensive as the WHO codes. The FDA designates part of the code based on drug manufacturer, and each manufacturer defines the specific codes for their own products. As a result, there is no uniform class hierarchy for the codes, and codes may be reused at the manufacturer's discretion. Due in part to the inadequacies of the NDC codes, pharmacy information systems typically purchase proprietary terminologies from knowledge base vendors. These terminologies map to NDC, but provide additional information about therapeutic classes, allergies, ingredients, and forms.

The need for standards for drug terminologies led to a collaboration between the FDA, the U.S. National Library of Medicine (NLM), the Veterans Administration (VA), and the pharmacy knowledge base vendors that has produced a representational model for drug terms called RxNorm. The NLM provides RxNorm to the

Respiratory Tract Diseases
    Lung Diseases
        Pneumonia
            Bronchopneumonia
            Pneumonia, Aspiration
                Pneumonia, Lipid
            Pneumonia, Lobar
            Pneumonia, Mycoplasma
            Pneumonia, *Pneumocystis carinii*
            Pneumonia, Rickettsial
            Pneumonia, Staphylococcal
            Pneumonia, Viral
        Lung Diseases, Fungal
            Pneumonia, *Pneumocystis carinii*
Respiratory Tract Infections
    Pneumonia
            Pneumonia, Lobar
            Pneumonia, Mycoplasma
            Pneumonia, *Pneumocystis carinii*
            Pneumonia, Rickettsial
            Pneumonia, Staphylococcal
            Pneumonia, Viral
        Lung Diseases, Fungal
            Pneumonia, *Pneumocystis carinii*

Fig. 7.9 Partial tree structure for the Medical Subject Headings showing pneumonia terms. Note that terms can appear in multiple locations, although they may not always have the same children, implying that they have somewhat different meanings in different contexts. For example, Pneumonia means "lung inflammation" in one context (line 3) and "lung infection" in another (line 16)

public as part of the Unified Medical Language System (UMLS) (see below) to support mapping between NDC codes, the VA's National Drug File (VANDF) and various proprietary drug terminologies (Nelson et al. 2002). RxNorm currently contains 14,000 terms.

7.4.4.12 Medical Subject Headings

The Medical Subject Headings (MeSH), maintained by the NLM (updated annually), is the terminology by which the world medical literature is indexed. MeSH arranges terms in a structure that breaks from the strict hierarchy used by most other coding schemes. Terms are organized into hierarchies and may appear in multiple places in the hierarchy (Fig. 7.9). Although it is not generally used as a direct coding scheme for patient information, it plays a central role in the UMLS.

7.4.4.13 RadLex

RadLex is a terminology produced by the Radiology Society of North America (RSNA). With more than 30,000 terms, RadLex is intended to be a unified language of radiology terms for standardized indexing and retrieval of radiology information resources. RadLex includes the names of anatomic parts, radiology devices, imaging exams and procedure steps performed in radiology. Given the scope of the radiology domain, many RadLex terms overlap with SNOMED-CT, and LOINC.

7.4.4.14 Bioinformatics Terminologies

For the most part, the terminologies discussed above fail to represent the levels of detail needed by biomolecular researchers. This has become a more acute problem with the advent of bioinformatics and the sequencing of organism genomes (see Chap. 24). As in other domains, researchers have been forced to develop their own terminologies. As these researchers have begun to exchange information, they have recognized the need for standard naming conventions as well as standard ways of representing their data with terminologies. Prominent efforts to unify naming systems include the Gene Ontology (GO) (Harris et al. 2004) from the Gene Ontology Consortium and the gene naming database of the HUGO Gene Nomenclature Committee (HGNC). A related resource is the RefSeq database of the National Center for Biotechnology Information (NCBI) which contains identifiers for reference sequences.

7.4.4.15 Unified Medical Language System

In 1986, Donald Lindberg and Betsy Humphreys, at the NLM, began working with several academic centers to identify ways to construct a resource that would bring together and disseminate controlled medical terminologies. An experimental version of the UMLS was first published in 1989 (Humphreys 1990); the UMLS has been updated annually since then. Its principal component is the Metathesaurus, which contains over 8.9 million terms collected from over 160 different sources (including many of those that we

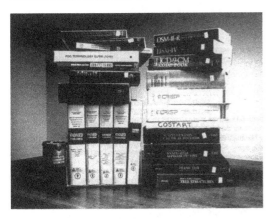

Fig. 7.10 Growth of the UMLS. The UMLS Metathesaurus contains over 8.9 million terms collected from over 160 different sources and attempts to relate synonymous and similar terms from across the different sources into over 2.6 million concepts. The content continues to grow dynamically in response to user needs (Source: U.S. National Library of Medicine)

have discussed), and attempts to relate synonymous and similar terms from across the different sources into over 2.6 million concepts (Fig. 7.10). Figure 7.11 lists the preferred names for many of the pneumonia concepts in the Metathesaurus; Fig. 7.12 shows how like terms are grouped into concepts and are tied to other concepts through semantic relationships.

7.5   Data Interchange Standards

The recognition of the need to interconnect health care applications led to the development and enforcement of **data interchange standards**. The conceptualization stage began in 1980 with discussions among individuals in an organization called the American Association for Medical Systems and Informatics (AAMSI). In 1983, an AAMSI task force was established to pursue those interests in developing standards. The discussions were far ranging in topics and focus. Some members wanted to write standards for everything, including a standard medical terminology, standards for HISs, standards for the computer-based patient record, and standards for data interchange. Citing the need for data interchange between commercial

laboratories and health care providers, the task force agreed to focus on data-interchange standards for clinical laboratory data. Early activities were directed mainly toward increasing interest of AAMSI members in working to create health care standards.

The development phase was multifaceted. The AAMSI task force became subcommittee E31.11 of the ASTM and developed and published ASTM standard 1238 for the exchange of clinical-laboratory data. Two other groups—many members of which had participated in the earlier AAMSI task force—were formed to develop standards, each with a slightly different emphasis: HL7 and Institute of Electrical and Electronics Engineering (IEEE) Medical Data Interchange Standard. The American College of Radiology (ACR) joined with the National Electronic Manufacturers Association (NEMA) to develop a standard for the transfer of image data. Two other groups developed related standards independent of the biomedical informatics community: (1) ANSI X12 for the transmission of commonly used business transactions, including health care claims and benefit data, and (2) National Council for Prescription Drug Programs (NCPDP) for the transmission of third-party drug claims. Development was further complicated by the independent creation of standards by several groups in Europe, including EDIFACT United Nations/Electronic Data Interchange For Administration, Commerce and Transport which is the EDI standard developed under the United Nations. The adoption of EDIFACT has been hampered by competing standards that are based upon XML.

7.5.1   General Concepts and Requirements

The purpose of a data-interchange standard is to permit one system, the **sender**, to transmit to another system, the **receiver**, all the data required to accomplish a specific communication, or **transaction set**, in a precise, unambiguous fashion. To complete this task successfully, both systems must know what format and content is being

Fig. 7.11 Some of the bacterial pneumonia concepts in the Unified Medical Language System Metathesaurus

```
C0004626: Pneumonia, Bacterial
C0023241: Legionnaires' Disease
C0032286: Pneumonia due to other specified bacteria
C0032308: Pneumonia, Staphylococcal
C0152489: Salmonella pneumonia
C0155858: Other bacterial pneumonia
C0155859: Pneumonia due to Klebsiella pneumoniae
C0155860: Pneumonia due to Pseudomonas
C0155862: Pneumonia due to Streptococcus
C0155865: Pneumonia in pertussis
C0155866: Pneumonia in anthrax
C0238380: PNEUMONIA, KLEBSIELLA AND OTHER GRAM NEGATIVE BACILLI
C0238381: PNEUMONIA, TULAREMIC
C0242056: PNEUMONIA, CLASSIC PNEUMOCOCCAL LOBAR
C0242057: PNEUMONIA, FRIEDLAENDER BACILLUS
C0275977: Pneumonia in typhoid fever
C0276026: Hemophilus influenzae pneumonia
C0276039: Pittsburgh pneumonia
C0276071: Achromobacter pneumonia
C0276080: Pneumonia due to Proteus mirabilis
C0276089: Pneumonia due to Escherichia coli
C0276523: AIDS with bacterial pneumonia
C0276524: AIDS with pneumococcal pneumonia
C0339946: Pneumonia with tularemia
C0339947: Pneumonia with anthrax
C0339952: Secondary bacterial pneumonia
C0339953: Pneumonia due to Escherichia coli
C0339954: Pneumonia due to proteus
C0339956: Typhoid pneumonia
C0339957: Meningococcal pneumonia
C0343320: Congenital pneumonia due to staphylococcus
C0343321: Congenital pneumonia due to group A hemolytic streptococcus
C0343322: Congenital pneumonia due to group B hemolytic streptococcus
C0343323: Congenital pneumonia due to Escherichia coli
C0343324: Congenital pneumonia due to pseudomonas
C0348678: Pneumonia due to other aerobic Gram-negative bacteria
C0348680: Pneumonia in bacterial diseases classified elsewhere
C0348801: Pneumonia due to streptococcus, group B
C0349495: Congenital bacterial pneumonia
C0349692: Lobar (pneumococcal) pneumonia
C0375322: Pneumococcal pneumonia {Streptococcus pneumoniae pneumonia}
C0375323: Pneumonia due to Streptococcus, unspecified
C0375324: Pneumonia due to Streptococcus Group A
C0375326: Pneumonia due to other Streptococcus
C0375327: Pneumonia due to anaerobes
C0375328: Pneumonia due to Escherichia coli
C0375329: Pneumonia due to other Gram-negative bacteria
C0375330: Bacterial pneumonia, unspecified
```

sent and must understand the words or terminology, as well as the delivery mode. When you order merchandise, you fill out a form that includes your name and address, desired items, quantities, colors, sizes, and so on. You might put the order form in an envelope and mail it to the supplier at a specified address. There are standard requirements, such as where and how to write the receiver's (supplier's) address, your (the sender's) address, and the payment for delivery (the postage stamp). The receiver must have a mailroom, a post office box, or a mailbox to receive the mail.

A communications model, called the Open Systems Interconnection (OSI) reference model (ISO 7498–1), has been defined by the ISO (see Chap. 5 and the discussion of software for network communications). It describes seven levels

Fig. 7.12 Some of the information available in the Unified Medical Language System about selected pneumonia concepts. Concept's preferred names are shown in italics. Sources are identifiers for the concept in other terminologies. Synonyms are names other than the preferred name. ATX is an associated Medical Subject Heading expression that can be used for Medline searches. The remaining fields (Parent, Child, Broader, Narrower, Other, and Semantic) show relationships among concepts in the Metathesaurus. Note that concepts may or may not have hierarchical relations to each other through Parent–Child, Broader–Narrower, and Semantic (is-a and inverseis-a) relations. Note also that Pneumonia, Streptococcal and Pneumonia due to Streptococcus are treated as separate concepts, as are Pneumonia in Anthrax and Pneumonia, Anthrax

Bacterial pneumonia
    Source: CSP93/PT/2596-5280; DOR27/DT/U000523;
                ICD91/PT/482.9; ICD91/IT/482.9
    Parent: Bacterial Infections; Pneumonia; Influenza with Pneumonia
    Child: Pneumonia, Mycoplasma
    Narrower: Pneumonia, Lobar; Pneumonia, Rickettsial; Pneumonia,
                Staphylococcal; Pneumonia due to *Klebsiella pneumoniae*;
                Pneumonia due to Pseudomonas; Pneumonia due to *Hemophilus
                influenzae*
    Other: *Klebsiella pneumoniae, Streptococcus pneumoniae*

Pneumonia, Lobar
    Source: ICD91/IT/481; MSH94/PM/D011018; MSH94/MH/D011018;
                SNM2/RT/M-40000; ICD91/PT/481; SNM2/PT/D-0164;
                DXP92/PT/U000473; MSH94/EP/D011018;
                INS94/MH/D011018;INS94/SY/D011018
    Synonym: Pneumonia, diplococcal
    Parent: Bacterial Infections; Influenza with Pneumonia
    Broader: Bacterial Pneumonia; Inflammation
    Other: *Streptococcus pneumoniae*
    Semantic: inverse-is-a: *Pneumonia*
                has-result: *Pneumococcal Infections*

Pneumonia, Staphylococcal
    Source: ICD91/PT/482.4; ICD91/IT/482.4; MSH94/MH/D011023;
                MSH94/PM/D011023; MSH94/EP/D011023; SNM2/PT/D-017X;
                INS94/MH/D011023; INS94/SY/D011023
    Parent: Bacterial Infections; Influenza with Pneumonia
    Broader: Bacterial Pneumonia
    Semantic   inverse-is-a: Pneumonia; Staphylococcal Infections

Pneumonia, Streptococcal
    Source: ICD91/IT/482.3
    Other: *Streptococcus pneumoniae*

Pneumonia due to Streptococcus
    Source: ICD91/PT/482.3
    ATX: Pneumonia AND Streptococcal Infections AND NOT Pneumonia, Lobar
    Parent: Influenza with Pneumonia

Pneumonia in Anthrax
    Source: ICD91/PT/484.5; ICD91/IT/022.1; ICD91/IT/484.5
    Parent: Influenza with Pneumonia
    Broader: Pneumonia in other infectious diseases classified elsewhere
    Other: Pneumonia, Anthrax

Pneumonia, Anthrax
    Source: ICD91/IT/022.1; ICD91/IT/484.5
    Other: Pneumonia in Anthrax

of requirements or specifications for a communications exchange: physical, data link, network, transport, session, presentation, and application (Stallings 1987a; Tanenbaum 1987; Rose 1989). Level 7, the application level, deals primarily with the semantics or data-content specification of the transaction set or message. For the data-interchange standard, HL7 requires the definition of all the data elements to be sent in response to a specific task, such as the admission of a patient to a hospital. In many cases, the data content requires a specific terminology that can be understood by both sender and receiver. For example,

if a physician orders a laboratory test that is to be processed by a commercial laboratory, the ordering system must ensure that the name of the test on the order is the same as the name that the laboratory uses. When a panel of tests is ordered, both systems must share a common understanding of the panel composition. This terminology understanding is best ensured through use of a terminology table that contains both the test name and a unique code. Unfortunately, several code sets exist for each data group, and none are complete. An immediate challenge to the medical-informatics community is to generate one complete set. In other cases, the terminology requires a definition of the domain of the set, such as what are the possible answers to the data parameter "ethnic origin."

The sixth level, presentation, deals with what the syntax of the message is, or how the data are formatted. There are both similarities and differences at this level across the various standards bodies. Two philosophies are used for defining syntax: one proposes a position-dependent format; the other uses a tagged-field format. In the position-dependent format, the data content is specified and defined by position. For example, the sixth field, delimited by "|," is the gender of the patient and contains an M, F, or U or is empty. A tagged-field representation is "SEX = M."

The remaining OSI levels—session, transport, network, data link, and physical—govern the communications and networking protocols and the physical connections made to the system. Obviously, some understanding at these lower levels is necessary before a linkage between two systems can be successful. Increasingly, standards groups are defining scenarios and rules for using various protocols at these levels, such as TCP/IP (see Chap. 5). Much of the labor in making existing standards work lies in these lower levels.

Typically, a transaction set or message is defined for a particular event, called a **trigger event**. This trigger event, such as a hospital admission, then initiates an exchange of messages. The message is composed of several data segments; each data segment consists of one or more data fields. Data fields, in turn, consist of data elements that may be one of several data types. The message must identify the sender and the receiver, the message number for subsequent referral, the type of message, special rules or flags, and any security requirements. If a patient is involved, a data segment must identify the patient, the circumstances of the encounter, and additional information as required. A reply from the receiving system to the sending system is mandatory in most circumstances and completes the communications set.

It is important to understand that the sole purpose of the data-interchange standard is to allow data to be sent from the sending system to the receiving system; the standard is not intended to constrain the application system that uses those data. Application independence permits the data-interchange standard to be used for a wide variety of applications. However, the standard must ensure that it accommodates all data elements required by the complete application set.

7.5.2 Specific Data Interchange Standards

As health care increasingly depends on the connectivity within an institution, an enterprise, an integrated delivery system, a geographic system, or even a national integrated system, the ability to interchange data in a seamless manner becomes critically important. The economic benefits of data-interchange standards are immediate and obvious. Consequently, it is in this area of health care standards that most effort has been expended. All of the SDOs in health care have some development activity in data-interchange standards.

In the following sections we summarize many of the current standards for data-interchange. Examples are provided to give you a sense of the technical issues that arise in defining a data-exchange standard, but details are beyond the scope of this book. For more information, consult the primary resources or the Web sites for the relevant organizations.

7.5.2.1 Digital Imaging and Communications in Medicine (DICOM) Standards

With the introduction of computed tomography and other digital diagnostic imaging modalities, people needed a standard method for transferring images and associated information between devices, manufactured by different vendors, that display a variety of digital image formats. ACR formed a relationship with the NEMA in 1983 to develop such a standard for exchanging radiographic images, creating a unique professional/vendor group. The purposes of the ACR/NEMA standard were to promote a generic digital-image communication format, to facilitate the development and expansion of picture-archiving and communication systems (PACSs; see Chap. 18), to allow the creation of diagnostic databases for remote access and to enhance the ability to integrate new equipment with existing systems. Later the group became an international organization with ACR becoming just a member organization. NEMA still manages the organization in the United States.

Version 1.0 of the DICOM standard, published in 1985, specified a hardware interface, a data dictionary, and a set of commands. This standard supported only point-to-point communications. Version 2.0, published in 1988, introduced a message structure that consisted of a command segment for display devices, a new hierarchy scheme to identify an image, and a data segment for increased specificity in the description of an image (e.g., the details of how the image was made and of the settings).

In the DICOM standard, individual units of information, called data elements, are organized within the data dictionary into related groups. Groups and elements are numbered. Each individual data element, as contained within a message, consists of its group-element tag, its length, and its value. Groups include command, identifying, patient, acquisition, relationship, image presentation, text, overlay, and pixel data.

The latest version of DICOM is Version 3.0, which incorporates an object-oriented data model and adds support for ISO standard communications. DICOM provides full networking capability and specifies levels of conformance. The standard itself is structured as a nine-part document to accommodate evolution of the standard. In addition, DICOM introduces explicit information objects for images, graphics, and text reports; introduces service classes to specify well-defined operations across the network, and specifies an established technique for identifying uniquely any information object. DICOM also specifies image-related management information exchange, with the potential to interface to HISs and radiology information systems. An updated Version 3.0 is published annually.

The general syntax used by DICOM in representing data elements includes a data tag, a data length specification, and the data value. That syntax is preserved over a hierarchical nested data structure of items, elements, and groups. Data elements are defined in a data dictionary and are organized into groups. A data set consists of the structured set of attributes or data elements and the values related to an information object. Data-set types include images, graphics, and text

The protocol architecture for DICOM Version 3.0 is shown in Fig. 7.13, which illustrates the communication services for a point-to-point environment and for a networked environment, identifies the communication services and the upper-level protocols necessary to support communication between DICOM Application Entities. The upper-layer service supports the use of a fully conformant stack of OSI protocols to achieve effective communication. It supports a wide variety of international standards-based network technologies using a choice of physical networks such as Ethernet, FDDI, ISDN, X.25, dedicated digital circuits, and other local area network (LAN) and wide area network (WAN) technologies. In addition, the same upper-layer service can be used in conjunction with TCP/IP transport protocols. DICOM is now producing a number of standards including structured reports and Web access to, and presentation of, DICOM persistent objects.

7.5.2.2 ASTM International Standards

In 1984, the first ASTM health care data-interchange standard was published: E1238, Standard Specification for Transferring Clinical Observations Between Independent Systems. This standard is used in large commercial and reference clinical laboratories in the United States and has been adopted by a consortium of French laboratory system vendors who serve 95 % of the laboratory volume in France. The ASTM E1238 standard is message based; it uses position-defined syntax and is similar to the HL7 standard (see next section). An example of the ASTM 1238 standard describing a message transmitted between a clinic and a commercial clinical laboratory is shown in Fig. 7.14. Related data-interchange standards include E1467 (from Subcommittee E31.16), Specification for Transferring Digital

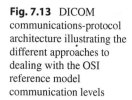

Fig. 7.13 DICOM communications-protocol architecture illustrating the different approaches to dealing with the OSI reference model communication levels

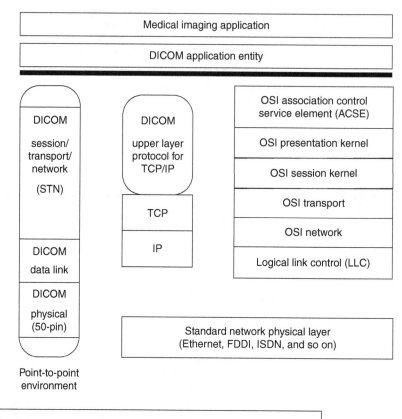

Fig. 7.14 An example of a message in the ASTM 1238 format. The message consists of the header segment, H, the patient segment, P, and general order segments, OBR. Primary delimiters are the vertical bars (|); secondary delimiters are the carets (^). Note the similarities of this message to the HL7 message in Fig. 7.3

Neurophysiological Data Between Independent Computer Systems. Another important ASTM standard is E1460, Defining and Sharing Modular Health Knowledge Bases (Arden Syntax for Medical Logic Modules; see Chap. 20). In 1998, ownership of the Arden Syntax was transferred to HL7, where it will be developed by the Arden Syntax and Clinical Decision Support Technical Committee.

In 2005, ASTM developed an electronic format for a paper-based record, initially created by the Massachusetts Medical Society to improve data exchange when transferring patients. This standard became known as the Continuity of Care Record (CCR), and embodies a core data set, represented in XML. The published format of the CCR was jointly developed by ASTM International, the Massachusetts Medical Society[1] (MMS), the Health Care Information and Management Systems Society (HIMSS), the American Academy of Family Physicians (AAFP), the American Academy of Pediatrics, and other health informatics vendors. The CCR represents a summary of the patient record, rather than clinical encounter. The CCR is both machine- and human-readable, which accelerated its adoption. In the delineation of the Meaningful Use requirements from the US Department of Health and Human Services, the CCR data set provided a constraint on the HL7 Clinical Document Architecture (CDA) specification (see below), now referred to as the Continuity of Care Document (CCD).

7.5.2.3 Health Level 7 Standards

The initial HL7 (see Sect. 7.3.2.3) standard was built on existing production protocols—particularly ASTM 1238. The HL7 standard is message based and uses an event trigger model that causes the sending system to transmit a specified message to the receiving unit, with a subsequent response by the receiving unit. Messages are defined for various trigger events. Version 1.0 was published in September 1987 and served mainly to define the scope and format of standards. Version 2.0, September 1988, was the basis for several data-interchange demonstrations involving more than ten vendors. Version 2.1, June 1990, was widely implemented in the United States and abroad. In 1991, HL7 became a charter member of ANSI; on June 12, 1994, it became an ANSI-accredited Standard Developers Organization (SDO). Version 2.2 was published in December 1994 and on February 8, 1996, it was approved by ANSI as the first health care data-interchange American National Standard. Version 2.3, March 1997, considerably expanded the scope by providing standards for the interchange of data relating to patient administration (admission, discharge, transfer, and outpatient registration), patient accounting (billing), order entry, clinical-observation data, medical information management, patient and resource scheduling, patient-referral messages, patient-care messages that support communication for problem-oriented records, adverse-event reporting, immunization reporting, and clinical trials, as well as a generalized interface for synchronizing common reference files.

Version 2.4, which became an ANSI standard in October 2000 introduced conformance query profiles and added messages for laboratory automation, application management, and personnel management. ANSI recently approved the HL7 Version 2.0 Extensible Markup Language (XML) Encoding Syntax. The XML capability of HL7 v2.xml makes messages Web-enabled. Version 2.5, which is more consistent and supports more functionality than any other previous version, became an ANSI standard in 2003. Figure 7.15 illustrates the exchange that occurs when a patient is transferred from the operating room (which uses a system called DHIS) to the surgical intensive-care unit (which uses a system called TMR). Note the similarity between these messages and the ASTM example.

Version 3.0 of the standard (currently in the ballot process) is object oriented and based on a **Reference Information Model** (**RIM**) being developed by HL7. The RIM has evolved from a number of commercial and academic health care data models, and it accommodates the data elements defined in the current Version 2.x HL7 standard.

The RIM is a collection of subject areas, scenarios, classes, attributes, use cases, actors, trigger events, interactions, and so on that depict the information needed to specify HL7 messages. In this sense it is more than a data-interchange standard, seeking to merge standards notions that include terminology and representation as well as data exchange. The stated purpose of the RIM is to provide a model for the creation of message specifications and messages for HL7. The RIM was approved as an ANSI standard in 2003, and has been introduced as an ISO standard. HL7 has also introduced a V3 suite of standards including V3 Abstract Data Types; Clinical Data Architecture, Release 2; and Context Management Standard (CCOW). In some health information system architectures, notably those of UK and Canada, there has been a successful blending of messaging specifications, incorporating those from both V2 and V3.

Since its initial development in 2001, the Clinical Document Architecture (CDA) standard has become globally adopted for a broad range of use. Now an ISO standard and advanced to Release 2, CDA is a document mark-up standard

Fig. 7.15 An example of
an HL7 ADT transaction
message. This message
includes the Message
Heading segment, the EVN
trigger definition segment,
the PID patient-identification
segment, the PV1 patient-
visit segment, the OBR
general-order segment,
and several OBX results
segments

```
MSH|^~&\|DHIS|OR|TMR|SICU|199212071425|password|ADT|16603529|P|2.1<cr>

EVN|A02|199212071425||<cr>

PID|||Z99999^5^M11||GUNCH^MODINE^SUE|RILEY|19430704 |F||C|RT. 1, BOX
97^ZIRCONIA^NC^27401 |HEND|(704)982-1234|(704)983-1822||S|C||245-33-
9999<cr>

PV1|1|I|N22^2204|||OR^03|0940^DOCTOR^HOSPITAL^A||| SUR|||||A3<cr>

OBR|7|||93000^EKG REPORT|R|199401111000|199401111330|||RMT||||19940111
11330|?|P030|||||199401120930||||||88-126666|A111|VIRANYI^ANDREW<cr>

OBX|1|ST|93000.1^VENTRICULAR RATE(EKG)||91|/MIN|60-100<cr>

OBX|2|ST|93000.2^ATRIAL RATE(EKG)||150|/MIN|60-100<cr>

. . .

OBX|8|ST|93000&IMP^EKG DIAGNOSIS|1|^ATRIAL FIBRILATION<cr>
```

for the structure and semantics of an exchanged "clinical document." CDA is built upon the RIM and relies upon reusable templates for its ease of implementation. A CDA document is a defined and complete information object that can exist outside of a message and can include text, images, sounds, and other multimedia content. CDA supports the following features: persistence, stewardship, potential for authentication, context, wholeness, and human-readability. In the US, CDA is one of the core components of data exchange for Meaningful Use. The competing implementation processes for CCD profile development were successfully harmonized into a broadly adopted *Consolidated* Continuity of Care Document (CCCD).

In order to ease the path to implementation of CDA, HL7 has developed a more narrowly defined specification called greenCDA, which limits the requirements of the RIM, provides greater ease of template composition, and consumes much less bandwidth for transmission. An additional effort to promote CDA adoption was achieved with the release of the CDA Trifolia repository, which, in addition to offering a library of templates, includes tooling for template modification as well as a template-authoring language. This has enabled the adoption of native CDA for exchange of laboratory data, clinical summaries, and electronic prescriptions and well as for clinical decision support.

Fast Health care Interoperability Resources (FHIR, pronounced "Fire") is a new highly innovative approach to standards development, first introduced by HL7in 2011. FHIR was created in order to overcome the complexity of development based upon the HL7 Reference Information Model (RIM), without losing the successful interoperability that model-driven data interchange demands. At the same time, FHIR delivers greater ease of implementation than other high-level development processes. It is designed to be compatible with legacy systems that conform to V2 and/or V3 messaging, and it supports system-development utilizing broadly deployed Clinical Document Architecture (CDA) platforms and ubiquitous templated CDA implementations, such as *Consolidated CDA*.

Although FHIR is built upon more than a decade of the development and refinement of the RIM, FHIR utilizes unique methodologies, artifacts, tooling, and publishing approach. While FHIR is based upon the RIM, it does not require implementers to know the RIM or know the modeling language upon which it was built. FHIR defines a limited set of data elements (or *resources*) as XML objects, but provides extension mechanisms for creating any elements which are incomplete or missing. The resulting structures are native XLM objects which do not require knowledge of the

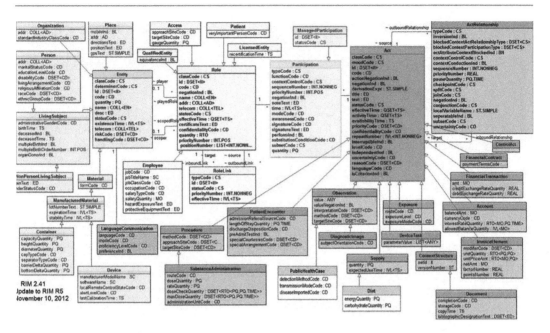

Fig. 7.16   Current version of the HL7 Reference Information Model. Most newer standards from HL7 are based on this model. The model is under constant revision

RIM abstraction in order to be implemented. Fundamentally, each clinical concept is created as a single resource, which need not change over time. The resources remain as the smallest unit of abstraction, and the creation of each resource is based upon *RESTful* design principles.

Inherently, development can precede around a *services* (SOA) model, which will support cloud-based applications. While a RESTful framework is enabled, it is not required. In addition, a well-defined ontology persists in the background, but knowledge of the vocabulary is not necessary for implementation. Fundamental to FHIR, all resources, as well as all resource attributes have a free-text expression, an encoded expression or both. Thus, FHIR supports a human-readable format, which is so valuable to the implementations supported by CDA.

Finally, FHIR is built with new *datatypes*, conformant with the familiar ISO 21090 format. As such, these datatypes are far simpler to use, with much of the complexity captured in the *extensions*. This allows mapping to other models, including those developed using *archetypes*, upon which the CEN format for electronic medical

records is predicated. This allows an inherently much smaller library of resources, all mapped to the HL7 RIM, and which can be maintained in perpetuity. FHIR developers have estimated that fewer than 150 such resources will define all of health care. Other concepts can be described as extensions.

As it is now envisioned, legacy systems will not map their interfaces to FHIR. Instead, FHIR will most likely serve in those environments or applications in which classical V2 messaging and/or CDA do not currently exist. This provides a unique opportunity for creation of both new applications in mature computing environments and for low and medium resource countries without legacy implementations. Nonetheless, migrations from V2 or V3 environments to FHIR implementations are achievable through native tooling.

Most often, HL7 is recognized for its messaging standards, but there is a large contribution to technical specifications that support the development and implementation of these messaging standards. These standards are also based on the RIM. A copy of the current version of the RIM is shown in Fig. 7.16.

Other HL7 standards that may be of interest the reader include:

- Clinical Decision Support (CDS) Standards
  - Arden Syntax – Begun at Columbia University, migrated to ASTM, and currently resides in HL7; syntax for CDS
  - GELLO – common expression language for clinical guidelines
- Functional Requirements for Electronic Health Records
  - Electronic Health Record – System Functional Model (EHR-S FM)
  - Personal Health Record (PHR FM)
- Functional Profiles – defines function and conformances
  - Behavioral Health
  - Child Health
  - Clinical Research
  - Records Management and Evidentiary Support
  - Long Term Care
  - Vital Records
  - Pharmacist/Pharmacy Provider
  - Public Health
- Domain Analysis Models – an informative document that defines work and data flow; actors and entities, and data elements
  - Immunization
  - Cardiology; Acute Coronary Syndrome
  - Clinical Trials Registration and Results
  - Tuberculosis Surveillance, Diagnosis, Treatment and Research
  - Virtual Medical Record for Clinical Decision Support
  - Vital Records
- Implementation Guides
  - Orders and Observations Ambulatory Lab Result (v2.5.1)
  - CDA R2: Quality Reporting Document Architecture
  - S&I Framework Lab Results Interface (v2.5.1)
  - Clinical Genomics; Fully LOINC-Qualified Genetic Variation Model
  - CDA R2: IHE Health Story Consolidation
  - URL-Based Implementations of Context-Aware Information Retrieval (Infobutton)
  - Virtual Medical Record for Clinical Decision Support for GELLO

- Electronic Laboratory Reporting to Public Health
- Interoperable Laboratory Result Reporting to EHR
- Infobutton Service Oriented Architecture
- Continuity of Care Document
- Laboratory Test Compendium Framework
- Blood Bank Donation Services
- Emergency Medical Services Run Report
- CDA R2: Consent Directives
- Unique Object Identifiers
- CDA R2: Level 1 and 2 Care Record Summary
- CDA R2: Personal Health care Monitoring Report
- CDA R2: History and Physical Notes
- CDA R2: Patient Assessments
- CDA R2: Procedure Note
- CDA R2: Unstructured Documents
- Imaging Integration; Basic Imaging Reports in CDA and DICOM
- CDA R2: Neonatal Care Reports
- CDA R2: Care Record Summary Discharge Summary
- CDA R2: Consult Notes
- CDA R2: Operative Notes
- CDA R@: Plan-to-plan Personal Health Record Data Transfer
- CDA R2: greenCDA Modules for CCD
- HL7-NCPDP Prescribing Coordination Mapping Document
- CDA R2: Health care Associated Infection
- CDA R2: Public Health Case Reports
- Vital Records Death Reporting
- Structured Product Labeling
- Annotated ECG
- Drug Stability Reporting
- Regulated Product Submission
- Genomics
  - Family History/Pedigree
- Regulatory Standards
  - Structured Product Labeling
  - Individual Case Safety Report (ICSR)
- Common Terminology Services
- Claims Attachment
- Data Types
- HL7 Vocabulary Tables

7.5.2.4 Institute of Electrical and Electronics Engineers Standards

IEEE is an international organization that is a member of both ANSI and ISO. Through IEEE, many of the world's standards in telecommunications, electronics, electrical applications, and computers have been developed. There were two major IEEE standards projects in health care.

IEEE 1073, Standard for Medical Device Communications, has produced a family of documents that defines the entire seven-layer communications requirements for the **Medical Information Bus** (MIB). The MIB is a robust, reliable communication service designed for bedside devices in the intensive care unit, operating room, and emergency room (see Chap. 19 for further discussion of the MIB in patient-monitoring settings). These standards have been harmonized with work in CEN, and the results are being released as ISO standards. IEEE and HL7 have collaborated on several key standards, including those for mobile medical devices.

7.5.2.5 National Council for Prescription Drug Programs (NCPDP) Standards

NCPDP is an ANSI-accredited SDO and is a trade organization. Its mission is to create and promote data-interchange standards for the pharmacy services sector of the health care industry and to provide information and resources that educate the industry. Currently, NCPDP has developed three ANSI-approved standards: a telecommunication standard (Version 3.2 and Version 7.0), a SCRIPT standard (Version 5.0), and a manufacturer rebate standard (Version 3.01). The telecommunication standard provides a standard format for the electronic submission of third-party drug claims. The standard was developed to accommodate the eligibility verification process at the point of sale and to provide a consistent format for electronic claims processing. Primarily pharmacy providers, insurance carriers, third-party administrators, and other responsible parties use the standard. This standard addresses the data format and content, transmission protocol, and other appropriate telecommunication requirements. Version 5.1 (September, 1999) of this standard is one of the transactions standards required for use by HIPAA.

Version 1.0, released in 1988, used formats that were limited to only fixed fields.. Version 2.0 added only typographic corrections to the Version 1.0 standard. The major thrust of the changes in Versions 3.0 and 3.1, in 1989, was the change from fixed-field transactions to a hybrid or variable format in which the fields can be tailored to the required content of the message. The current release is Version 3.2 (February, 1992). It introduces the fixed-length Recommended Transaction Data Sets (RTDS), which define three different message types, and a separate Data Dictionary format. The Data Dictionary defines permissible values and default values for fields contained in the specification. An online, real-time version was developed in 1996.

The standard uses defined separator characters at a group and a field level. The telecommunications specifications for sending two or more prescriptions include three required sections (Transaction Header; Group Separator, First-Claim Information; and Group Separator, Second-Claim Information [R]) and three optional sections (Header Information, First-Claim Information, and Second-Claim Information [O]). The NCPDP communication standard is used in more than 60 % of the nation's total prescription volume.

The SCRIPT Standard and Implementation Guide was developed for transmitting prescription information electronically between prescribers and providers. The standard, which adheres to EDIFACT syntax requirements and utilizes ASC X12 data types where possible, addresses the electronic transmission of new prescriptions, prescription refill requests, prescription fill status notifications, and cancellation notifications.

7.5.2.6 Accredited Standards Committee X12 (ASC X12) Standards

ASC X12, an independent organization accredited by ANSI, has developed message standards for purchase-order data, invoice data, and other commonly used business documents. The subcommittee X12N has developed a group of standards related to providing claim, benefits, and claim payment or advice. The specific standards that strongly relate to the health care industry are shown in Table 7.3.

The X12 standards define commonly used business transactions in a formal, structured manner called transaction sets. A transaction set is composed of a transaction-set header control segment, one or more data segments, and a transaction-set trailer control segment. Each segment is composed of a unique segment ID; one or more logically related simple data elements or composite data structures, each preceded by a data element separator; and a segment terminator. Data segments are defined in a data segment directory; data elements are defined in a data element directory; composite data structures are defined in a composite data structure directory; control segments and the binary segment are defined in a data segment directory.

A sample 835 Interchange Document is shown in Fig. 7.17. This standard is similar to ASTM and HL7 in that it uses labeled segments with positionally defined components.

There are several additional organizations that either create standards related to health care or have influence on the creation of standards.

7.5.2.7 American Dental Association Standards

In 1983, the American Dental Association (ADA) committee MD 156 became an ANSI-accredited committee responsible for all specifications for dental materials, instruments, and equipment. In 1992, a Task Group of the ASC MD 156 was established to initiate the development of technical reports, guidelines, and standards on electronic technologies used in dental practice. These include digital radiography, digital intraoral video cameras, digital voice-text-image transfer, periodontal probing devices, and CAD/CAM. Proposed standards include Digital Image Capture in Dentistry,

Table 7.3 ANSI X12N standards

Code	Title	Purpose
148	First Report of Injury, Illness or Incident	Facilitates the first report of an injury, incident, or illness
270	Health-Care Eligibility/Benefit Inquiry	Provide for the exchange of eligibility information and for response to individuals in a health care plan
271	Health-Care Eligibility/Benefit Information	
275	Patient Information	Supports the exchange of demographic, clinical, and other patient information to support administrative reimbursement processing as it relates to the submission of health-care claims for both health-care products and services reports the status of a submitted claim
276	Health-Care Claim Status Request	Queries the status of a submitted claim and reports the status of a submitted claim
277	Health-Care Claim Status Notification	
278	Health-Care Service Review Information	Provides referral certification and authorization
811	Consolidated Service Invoice/Statement	Facilitate health-plan premium billing and payment
820	Payment Order/Remittance Advice	
IHCLME Interactive Health-Care Claim/Encounter		Supports administrative reimbursement processing as it relates to the submission of health-care claims for both health-care products and services in an interactive environment
IHCE/BI Interactive Health-Care Eligibility/ Benefit Inquiry		Provide for the exchange of eligibility information and for response to individuals within a health plan
IHCE/BR Interactive Health-Care Eligibility/ Benefit Response		

```
ST*835*0001<n/l>
BPR*X*3685*C*ACH*CTX*01*122000065*DA*296006596*IDNUMBER*
SUPPLECODE*01*134999883*DA*867869899*940116<n/l>
TRN*1*45166*IDNUMBER<n/l>
DTM*009*940104<n/l>
N1*PR*HEALTHY INSURANCE COMPANY<n/l>
N3*1002 WEST MAIN STREET<n/l>
N4*DURHAM*NC*27001<n/l>
N1*PE*DUKE MEDICAL CENTER<n/l>
N3*2001 ERWIN ROAD<n/l>
N4*DURHAM*NC*27710<n/l>
CLP*078189203*1*6530*4895*CIN<n/l>
CAS*PR*1*150<n/l>
CAS*PR*2*550<n/l>
NM1*15*IAM*A*PATIENT<n/l>
REF*1K*942238493<n/l>
DTM*232*940101<n/l>
DTM*233*940131<n/l>
SE*22*0001<n/l>
```

Fig. 7.17 An example of ANSI X12 Interchange Document (Standard 835). This message is derived from a batch process, business-document orientation to a data-interchange model. The example does not include the control header or the functional-group header. The first line identifies the segment as a transaction-set header (ST). The last line is the transaction-set trailer (SE). The leading alphanumeric characters are tags that identify data content. For example, DTM is a date/time reference; N3 is address information; and BPR is the beginning segment for payment order/remittance advice

Infection Control in Dental Informatics, Digital Data Formats for Dentistry, Construction and Safety for Dental Informatics, Periodontal Probe Standard Interface, Computer Oral Health Record, and Specification for the Structure and Content of electronic medical record integration.

7.5.2.8 Uniform Code Council Standards

The Uniform Code Council (UCC) is an ANSI-approved organization that defines the universal product code. Standards include specifications for the printing of machine-readable representations (bar codes).

7.5.2.9 Health Industry Business Communications Council Standards

The Health Industry Business Communications Council (HIBCC) has developed the Health Industry Bar Code (HIBC) Standard, composed of two parts. The HIBC Supplier Labeling Standard describes the data structures and bar code symbols for bar coding of health care products. The HIBCC Provider Applications Standard describes data structures and bar code symbols for bar coding of identification data in a health care provider setting. HIBCC also issues and maintains Labeler Identification Codes that identify individual manufacturers. The HIBCC administers the Health Industry Number System, which provides a unique identifier number and location information for every health care facility and provider in the United States The HIBCC also administers the Universal Product Number Repository, which identifies specific products and is recognized internationally.

7.5.2.10 The Electronic Data Interchange for Administration, Commerce, and Transport Standard

The EDI for Administration, Commerce, and Transport (EDIFACT) is a set of international standards, projects, and guidelines for the electronic interchange of structured data related to trade in goods and services between independent computer-based information systems (National Council for Prescription Drug Programs Data Dictionary, 1994). The standard includes application-level syntax rules, message design guidelines, syntax implementation guidelines, data element dictionary, code list, composite data-elements dictionary, standard message dictionary, uniform rules of conduct for the interchange of trade data by transmission, and explanatory material.

The basic EDIFACT (ISO 9735) syntax standard was formally adopted in September 1987 and has undergone several updates. In addition to the common syntax, EDIFACT specifies standard messages (identified and structured sets of statements covering the requirements of specific transactions), segments (the groupings of functionally related data elements), data elements (the smallest items in a message that can convey data), and code sets (lists of codes for data elements). The ANSI ASC X12 standard is similar in purpose to EDIFACT, and work is underway to coordinate and merge the two standards.

EDIFACT is concerned not with the actual communications protocol but rather with the structuring of the data that are sent. EDIFACT is independent of the machine, media, system, and application and can be used with any communications protocol or with physical magnetic tape.

7.5.2.11 Clinical Data Interchange Standards Consortium

The Clinical Data Interchange Standards Consortium (CDISC) was founded in 1997 in order to facilitate electronic regulatory submission of clinical trial data. The current standards include a study data model, a data analysis model, a lab data model and an operational data model that supports audit trails and metadata. In 2007, CDISC began a collaborative project with HL7, the National Institutes of Health and the USFDA to link research data with data derived from clinical care. This modeling effort, BRIDG (Biomedical Research Integrated Domain Group), has created a domain analysis model of clinical research based upon the HL7 Reference Information Model (RIM).

7.6 Today's Reality and Tomorrow's Directions

7.6.1 The Interface: Standards and Systems

Historically, interchange standards evolved to support sharing of information over complex networks of distributed systems. This served a simple business model in which data was pushed from disparate repositories with inconsistent architectures and data structures. This permitted the exchange of data for both business needs and patient care.

In today's medical environment, there are several competing forces that place a burden on standards requirements. The traditional scope of data sources included business level information, principally for payment needs. These were developed utilizing coding methodologies and business architecture that did not rely upon inclusion of primary clinical data into the reimbursement decision. With the advent of statutory requirements that demand justification of insurance claims and reimbursement, additional data forms and formats became essential. This lead to the development of claims attachment standards (see X12, above) that enabled more complex adjudication, comparative effectiveness, and accountable care. These standards will most certainly require structured, coded data rather than free-text and unstructured narrative.

Complexity of data requirements is constantly growing to better support evidence-based medicine, clinical decision support, personalized medicine, and accountable care. Each of these has overlapping, but fundamentally unique data streams. Moreover, the data provided at the point of care, if unfiltered, is likely to overwhelm the clinical decision making process. Elements of clinical data, such as events in pediatric years, must not compete for the attention of the caregiver. To an extent, this was solved with specifications, such as CCOW (see Sect. 7.5.2.3), which were developed to provide context aware data to that process. There are growing demands for increasing the depth and breadth of data delivered to that clinical environment. In addition, these standards must support the implicit policy decisions about the nature of this data.

To date, clinical and pre-clinical information populates many of the alerts that clinicians receive at the point of care. Typically, these range from information supporting complex decision trees to the selection of testing and interventions. This has been abetted by increasing knowledge of genomic data and implication for therapeutic decisions. Although this has had its greatest impact on the chemotherapy of cancer, the importance in many other clinical domains, for more common conditions (including the treatment of diabetes, hypertension, and arthritis) is now recognized. Current architectural systems are ill-prepared to manage this process. Moreover, data formats for genomic and genetic information are disparate and often incompatible.

Data privacy requirements, and the variability of these requirements among legal entities, currently pose a different set of demands for information access technologies. For example, some states permit line-item exclusion of clinical data that is transferred between providers, based on the primacy of the information and the role of the caregiver. Other jurisdictions allow participation of health information exchanges to those individuals who agree only to dissemination of data from complete sources.

Existing data architectures enable a constant stream of data to be passed in an untended and unmonitored fashion. In evolving models, data request and acknowledgement require a more complex query and response logic. In fact, most inquiries demand the validation of the provider system and privileges that are afforded to both the caregiver and the primary data repository. This places another component of interface design between the respective systems, and necessitated the development of analogous provider indices and provider repositories. Concerns of both privacy and security must be met by these specifications. The system effectively asks not only who you are but why you want the information.

Much of this process overhead has been addressed by the design and architecture of health information exchanges. Often the business case supersedes the demand for clinical knowledge.

At the same time, these exchanges are designed to behave in an entirely agnostic fashion, placing no demand on either the sender or recipient for data quality, but only for source identification. In fact, the metadata, so responsible for the value of the information, is often capable of specifying only its origin and value sets.

In today's clinical environment, there has been very little attention paid to the capture and validation of patient-initiated data. While so very critical to diagnosis and ongoing management, only scant standards exist for embedding patient derived information into the clinical record without intermediate human interaction and adjudication. When allowed by current systems, data provided by patients often lies within the audit trail, as a comment, rather than in the record as source data. Steps are sorely needed to define and attribute such data since it is so critical to many aspects of accountable care. Data obtained directly from patient sources is often attributed to "subjective" status, but it is no less objective that many clinician observations. Perhaps justification for that lies in the fact that this patient derived data is neither quantifiable nor codeable. This is supported by valid concerns about the patient's health care literacy, or lack thereof, but is no less required than validated decision support for caregivers.

Data obtained from clinical research and clinical data provided to inform clinical studies suffer from other concerns of failed interoperability. This is attributed, and rightfully so, to disparities of vocabularies utilized for patient care and those used in clinical research. This is most dramatically highlighted in the terminology deployed by regulation for adverse event reporting (MedDRA; Medical Dictionary of Regulatory Affairs). Mapping between the MedDRA dictionary and other clinical terminologies (SNOMED-CT, LOINC, ICD, and CPT) has not proven successful. Moreover, many aspects pertaining to study subject inquiries in clinical research are often designed to elicit yes-no responses (Have you smoked in the last 5 years), rather than data that many caregivers deem relevant. Yet, today, it is more critical than ever to enable clinical research to inform patient care and care derived data to enable clinical trials. The business model of developing drugs for billon dollar markets ("blockbuster drugs") has proven itself to be unsustainable, as the cost of developing a new drug entity has now exceeded a billion dollars. From the clinical perspective, current estimates suggest that information from basic science research experiences delays of nearly 17 years before that knowledge can be incorporated into clinical care.

Semantic interoperability of clinical data inherently requires *data reuse*. It is not sufficient for systems to unambiguously exchange machine readable data. Data, once required only for third party payment, must be shared by other partners in the wellness and health care delivery ecosystems. Certainly, these data must be presented to research systems, as noted above. The data must also be available for public health reporting and analysis, for comparative effectiveness research, for accountable care measurement and for enhancement of decision support systems (including those for patients and their families). The immediate beneficiaries have been systems developed to support biosurveillance and pharmacovigilance. In practical terms, the business practices that govern our delivery systems (and the government policies and regulations that enable them) must enable these data streams to both enhance care and control costs.

7.6.2   Future Directions

The new models for health care require a very different approach. The concept of a patient-centric EHR (Chap. 15) requires the aggregation of any and all data created from, for, and about a patient into a single real or virtual record that provides access to the required data for effective care at the place and time of care. Health information exchange (HIE; see Chap. 12) at regional, state, national, and potentially at a global level is now the goal. This goal can only be reached through the effective use of information technology, and that use can only be accomplished through the use of common global standards that are ubiquitously implemented across all sites of care.

Three other future trends influence the need for new and different standards. The first is secondary use of data by multiple stakeholders. This requirement can only be met through semantic interoperability – a universal ontology that covers all aspects of health, health care, clinical research, management, and evaluation. Standards for expressing what is to be exchanged and under what circumstances are important as well as standards for the exchange of data. Included in multiple uses of data is reporting to other organizations such as immunization and infectious disease reports to the **Centers for Disease Control and Prevention** (CDC), performance reports to the **National Quality Forum** (NQF) and audit reports to **The Joint Commission** (TJC). Such systems as described also enable population health studies and health surveillance for natural and bioterrorism outbreaks.

The second trend area is the expansion of the types of data that are to be included in the EHR. The new emphasis on translational informatics will require new standards for the transport, inclusion into the EHR, and use of genetic information including genes, biomarkers, and phenotypic data. Imaging, videos, waveforms, audio, and consumer-generated data will require new types of standards. Effective use of these new types of data as well as exponential increases in the volume of data will require standards for decision support, standards for creating effective filters for presentation and data exchange, and new forms of presentation including visualization. New sources of data will include geospatial coding, health environmental data, social and community data, financial data, and cultural data. Queries and navigation of very large databases will require new standards. Establishing quality measures and trust will require new standards. Ensuring integrity and trust as data is shared and used by other than the source of data will require new standards addressing provenance and responsibility.

The third trend area is the use of mobile devices, smart devices, and personal health devices. How, when and where such devices should be used is still being explored. Standards will be required for safe design, presentation, interface, integrity, and protection from interference.

True global interoperability will require a suite of standards starting with the planning of systems, the definition and packaging of the data, collection of the data including usability standards, the exchange of data, the storage and use of data, and a wealth of applications that enable the EHR for better care. IT systems must turn data collected into information for use – a process that will require the use of knowledge in real time with data to produce information for patient care. Selecting the correct knowledge from literature, clinical trials, and other forms of documentation will require standards. Knowledge representation, indexing, and linkages will require standards.

A major, and challenging, requirement to address these new types and use of data will be effective standards for privacy and security. These standards must protect, but not restrict the use of data and access to that data for determining and giving the best care possible. The aggregation of data requires an error-free way for patient identification that will permit merger of data across disparate sources. Sharing data also requires standards for the de-identification of patient data.

The effective management of all of these resources will require additional output from the standards communities. Standards for defining the required functionality of systems and ways for certifying adherence to required functionality is essential for connecting a seamless network of heterogeneous EHRs from multiple vendors. Testing of standards, including IHE Connectathons before wide-spread dissemination and perhaps mandated use of standards is critical to use and acceptance. Standards for registries, standards for the rules that govern the sharing of research data, standards for patient consent, and standards for identification of people, clinical trials, collaboration, and other similar areas are necessary. Profiles for use and application from the suite of standards are a necessity. Detailed implementation guides are key to use and implementation of standards. Tools that enable content population and use of standards are mandatory for easy use of standards.

Standards for these new and evolving business and social needs must be supported by changes in the standards development methodologies and harmonization. Legacy systems are not easily discarded. Recommendations for complete replacement of existing standards are neither politically expedient nor fiscally supportable. Currently, there is increasing attention to new approaches to standards development that speeds the creation process and improves the quality of standards that are developed. These evolving development platforms pay appropriate homage to existing standards and leverage previously developed models of development and analysis.

The use of the FHIR, which leverages the HL7 Reference Information Model, may provide a much needed solution While relying upon historically developed and refined interoperability specifications, it hides the complexity of authoring messages within the FHIR development process. This leads to more usable specifications, created in a dramatically abbreviated time frame. Other approaches to standards development, such as those focused upon services, are rapidly evolving. These services-aware architectures are governed by strict development principles that help ensure both interoperability and the ability of components to be reused.

Increasingly large data stores ("big data") have demanded some of these changes. These data have emanated from a highly diverse universe of scientific development. In fact, some of the new bio-analytic platforms for *in vitro* cellular research are generating data at a rate, which by some estimates, is faster than the data can be analyzed. Medical images, for which storage requirements are growing, must now be principally evaluated by human inspection. Newly evolving algorithms and the technologies to support them, initially developed for star wars-type image analysis, are replacing radiologist and pathologists for the establishment of diagnoses. These machines have proven to be faster and more accurate than their human counterparts. In the very near future, such instrumentation will supplant medical scientists the same way that comparable technologies replaced human inspection in the estimation of cell differentials for blood counts. These new technologies are demanding the development of specifications and the terminologies to support them.

Tomorrow's technologies will transition from early vision through prototyping to commercial products in a more compressed life cycle. A model for this process in biomedical science was established with the emergence of the Human Genome Project (see Chap. 24). Within the next decade, routine genome determination and archiving, as well as their application to disease management, will require greatly enhanced solutions for data management and analysis. Innovative strategies for recognizing and validating biomarkers will grow exponentially from the current stable of imaging and cell surface determinants. These data streams will require adaption of existing decision support systems and comparative effectiveness paradigms. Lastly, scientific evidence supporting the diagnosis and management with the field of behavioral medicine will change the entire clinical spectrum and approach to evaluation and care. As we emerge from the dark ages of behavioral medicine, we will certainly require new systems for recognizing, diagnosing, naming and intervening on behalf of our patients.

In some sense, the development of standards is just beginning. The immediate future years will be important to create effective organizations that include the right experts in the right setting to produce standards that are in themselves interoperable. That goal still remains in the future.

Suggested Readings

Abbey, L. M., & Zimmerman, J. (Eds.). (1991). Dental informatics: integrating technology into the dental environment. New York: Springer. This text demonstrates that the issues of standards extend throughout the areas of application of biomedical informatics. The standards issues discussed in this chapter for clinical medicine are shown to be equally pertinent for dentistry.

American Psychiatric Association Committee on Nomenclature and Statistics (1994). *Diagnostic and Statistical Manual of Mental Disorders.* (4th ed.). Washington, D.C.: The American Psychiatric Association.

Benson, T. (2012). *Principles of health interoperability HL7 and SNOMED* (2nd ed.). London: Springer. This book presents a detail discussion of the HL7 version 2 messaging standard and a detail presentation of SNOMED-CT.

Boone, K. W. (2012). *The CDA™ book.* London: Springer. This book provides an excellent presentation of the HL7 Clinical Document Architecture and related topics.

Chute, C. G. (2000). Clinical classification and terminology: some history and current observations. Journal of the American Medical Informatics Association, 7(3), 298–303. This article reviews the history and current status of controlled terminologies in health care.

Cimino, J. J. (1998). Desiderata for controlled medical vocabularies in the twenty-first century. Methods of Information in Medicine, 37(4–5), 394–403. This article enumerates a set of desirable characteristics for controlled terminologies in health care.

Executive Office of the President; President's Council of Advisors on Science and Technology (2010). *Report to the President realizing the full potential of health information technology to Improve healthcare for Americans: the path forward.*

Henderson, M. (2003). *HL7 messaging.* Silver Spring: OTech Inc.. Description of HL7 V2 with examples. Available from HL7.

Institute of Medicine. (2003). *Patient safety: achieving a new standard for care.* Washington, D.C.: National Academy Press. Discusses approaches to the standardization of collection and reporting of patient data.

New York Academy of Medicine (1961). *Standard Nomenclature of Diseases and Operations.* (5th ed.). New York: McGraw-Hill.

Richesson, R. L., & Andrews, J. E. (2012). *Clinical research informatics.* London: Springer. This book includes a discussion of standards and applications from the clinical research perspectives.

Stallings, W. (1987). *Handbook of computer-communications standards.* New York: Macmillan. This text provides excellent details on the Open Systems Interconnection model of the International Standards Organization.

Stallings, W. (1997). *Data and computer communications.* Englewood Cliffs: Prentice-Hall. This text provides details on communications architecture and protocols and on local and wide area networks.

Questions for Discussion

1. Who should be interested in interoperability and health data standards?

2. What are the five possible approaches to accelerating the creation of standards?

3. Define five health care standards, not mentioned in the chapter, which might also be needed?

4. What role should the government play in the creation of standards?

5. At what level might a standard interfere with a vendor's ability to produce a unique product?

6. Define a hypothetical standard for one of the areas mentioned in the text for which no current standard exists. Include the conceptualization and discussion points. Specifically state the scope of the standard.

Natural Language Processing in Health Care and Biomedicine

8

Carol Friedman and Noémie Elhadad

After reading this chapter, you should know the answers to these questions:

- Why is natural language processing important?
- What are the potential uses for natural language processing (NLP) in the biomedical and health domains?
- What forms of knowledge are used in NLP?
- What are the principal techniques of NLP?
- What are challenges for NLP in the clinical, biological, and health consumer domains?

8.1 Motivation for Natural Language Processing

Natural language is the primary means of human communication. In biomedical and health areas,[1] knowledge and data are disseminated in textual form as articles in the scientific literature, as technical and administrative reports on the Web, and as textual fields databases. In health care facilities, patient information mainly occurs in narrative notes and reports. Because of the growing adoption of electronic health records and the promise of health information exchange, it is common for a patient to have records at multiple facilities, and for a chart of a single patient at one institution to comprise several hundred notes. Because of the explosion of online textual information available, it is difficult for scientists and health care professionals to keep up with the latest discoveries, and they need help to find, manage, and analyze the enormous amounts of online knowledge and data. On the Web, individuals exchange and look for health-related information, and health consumers and patients are often overwhelmed by the amount of the information available to them, whether in traditional websites or through online health communities. There is also much information disseminated verbally through scientific interactions in conferences, in care teams at hospitals, and in patient-doctor encounters. In this chapter however, we focus on the written form.

While there is valuable information conveyed in text, it is not in a format amenable to further computer processing. Texts are difficult to process reliably because of the inherent characteristics and variability of language. Since structured standardized data are more useful for most automated applications, a significant amount of manual work is currently devoted to mapping textual information into a structured or coded representation: in the clinical realm, for instance, professional

---

[1] Unless stated otherwise, the general domain and the topics of text materials discussed in this chapter refer to biomedicine and health.

C. Friedman, PhD (✉) • N. Elhadad, PhD
Department of Biomedical Informatics,
Columbia University, 622 West 168th Street,
VC Bldg 5, New York 10032, NY, USA
e-mail: friedman@dbmi.columbia.edu;
noemie@dbmi.columbia.edu

This chapter is adapted from an earlier version in the third edition authored by Carol Friedman and Stephen B. Johnson.

coders assign billing codes corresponding to diagnoses and procedures to hospital admissions; indexers at the National Library of Medicine assign MeSH terms to represent the main topics of scientific articles; and database curators extract genomic and phenotypic information on organisms from the literature. Because of the overwhelmingly large amount of textual information, manual work is very costly, time-consuming, and impossible to keep up to date. One aim of **natural language processing** (NLP) is to facilitate these tasks by enabling use of automated methods that represent the relevant information in the text with high validity and reliability.

Another aim of NLP is to help advance many of the fundamental aims of biomedical informatics, which include the discovery and validation of scientific knowledge, improvement in the quality and cost of health care, and support to patients and health consumers.

The massive amounts of texts amassed through clinical care or published in the scientific literature or on the Web can be leveraged to acquire and organize knowledge from the information conveyed in text, and to promote discovery of new phenomena. For instance, the information in patient notes, while not originally entered for discovery purposes, but rather for the care of individual patients, can be processed, aggregated and mined to discover patterns across patients. This process, commonly referred to as secondary use of data, shows much promise for some of the current challenges of informatics, such as **comparative effectiveness research**, **phenotype definition**, **hypothesis generation** for clinical research and understanding of disease, and **pharmacovigilance**. For the literature, NLP can speed up the high throughput access needed for scientific discoveries and their meta-analysis across individual articles, by identifying similar results across articles (i.e. recent treatments for diseases, reports of adverse drug events), and by connecting pieces of information among articles (i.e. constructing biomolecular pathways).

For clinicians interacting with an electronic health record and treating a particular patient, NLP can support several points in a clinician workflow: when reviewing the patient chart, NLP can be leveraged to aggregate and consolidate information spread across many notes and reports, and to highlight relevant facts about the patient. During the decision-making and actual care phase, information extracted through NLP from the notes can contribute to the decision support systems in the EHR. Finally, when health care professionals are documenting patient information, higher quality notes can be generated with the help of NLP-based methods.

For quality and administrative purposes, NLP can signal potential errors, conflicting information, or missing documentation in the chart. For public health administrators, EHR patient information can be monitored for **syndromic surveillance** through the analysis of ambulatory notes or chief complaints in the emergency room.

Finally, NLP can support health consumers and patients looking for information about a particular disease or treatment, through automated **question understanding** which can then facilitate better access to relevant information, targeted to their information needs, and to their health literacy levels through the analysis of the topics conveyed in a document as well as the vocabulary used in the document.

Across all these use cases of NLP, the techniques of natural language processing provide the means to bridge the gap between unstructured text and data by transforming the text to data in a computable format, allowing humans to interact using familiar natural language, while enabling computer applications to process data effectively and to provide users with easy access and synthesis of the raw textual information. The next section gives a more in-depth definition of NLP and a quick history of NLP in biomedicine and health. Section 8.3 presents some of the well-studied applications of NLP. Sections 8.4 and 8.5 introduce linguistic background and ways in which linguistic knowledge is leveraged to build NLP tools. Section 8.5 also focuses on evaluation methodology for NLP-based systems. Section 8.6 provides a discussion of the challenges entailed in processing texts in the biological, clinical and general health domains, which are currently active areas of research in the NLP community. Finally Sect. 8.7 provides pointers to useful resources for NLP research and development.

8.2 What Is NLP

Natural language processing is currently a very active and exciting research area in informatics. The term NLP is often used to include a group of methods that involve the processing of unstructured text, although the methods themselves range widely in their use of knowledge of language. Some methods use minimal linguistic knowledge, and are based solely on the presence of words in text. For these methods, the only linguistic knowledge needed is the knowledge of what constitutes a word; these methods often depend on a **keyword** or **bag-of-words** approach. One example of a method that uses only words is a search engine that retrieves documents containing the presence of a combination of words in a collection, although these words may have no relation to each other in the retrieved documents. Another example is a **machine learning** method that uses words independently of each other as features when building a statistical model. Other NLP methods contain more advanced knowledge of language, and these are the methods that are the focus of this chapter. Generally, these more advanced linguistic methods aim to determine some or all of the syntactic or semantic structure in text and to interpret some of the meaning of relevant information in text.

The reason why it is possible to process natural language using computational methods is that language is formulaic: it consists of discrete symbols (words), and rules (a grammar) specifying how different linguistic elements can be combined to create a sequence of words that represents a well-formed sentence or phrase that conveys a particular meaning. According to Harris (1982), it is possible to represent the content of a sentence in an operator argument structure, similar to formulations in **predicate logic**. The formulaic aspect of language can also explain why machine-learning approaches have been

successful at some NLP tasks. In particular, patterns, when present in large amounts of text can be detected automatically.

Early work in NLP began in the 1950s. In the 1960s and 1970s, some successful general language NLP systems were developed that involved a very limited domain along with highly specific tasks, such as Eliza (Weizenbaum 1966), SHRDLU (Winograd 1972), and LUNAR (Woods 1973). In the 1970s, the Linguistic String Project (LSP) under the leadership of Dr. Naomi Sager, a pioneer in NLP, developed a comprehensive computer grammar and parser of English (Grishman et al. 1973; Sager 1981), and also began work in NLP of clinical reports (Sager 1972, 1978; Sager et al. 1987) that continued into the 1990s. A number of other clinical NLP systems were developed starting in the late 1980s and early 1990s, and are discussed in more detail by Spyns (Spyns 1996). Some clinical NLP systems that were associated with numerous publications in that period include SPRUS (which evolved into Symtext and then MPLUS) (Haug et al. 1990, 1994; Christensen et al. 2002), MedLEE (Friedman et al. 1994; Hripcsak et al. 1995), the Geneva System (Baud et al. 1992, 1998), MeneLAS (Zweigenbaum and Courtois 1998), and MEDSYNDIKATE (Hahn et al. 2002). NLP processing of the literature started to take hold in the late 1990s with the large increase in publications concerning biomolecular discoveries and the need to facilitate access to the information. Early work in the biomolecular NLP area involved identification of biomolecular entities in text (Fukuda et al. 1998; Jenssen and Vinterbo 2000), and then extraction of certain relations between the entities (Sekimizu et al. 1998; Rindflesch et al. 2000; Humphreys et al. 2000; Park et al. 2001; Yakushiji et al. 2001; Friedman et al. 2001). Meanwhile, in the clinical literature, similar work was carried out to recognize mentions of disorders, findings, and treatments (Aronson 2001) as well as certain relationships, such as diseases and their corresponding treatments in order to mine results conveyed across clinical studies (Srinivasan and Rindflesch 2002).

The assumption concerning much of the early NLP work was that successful NLP systems required substantial knowledge of language integrated with real-world knowledge in order to process text and solve real-world problems. Thus, the primary focus of much of the early work concerned representation of syntactic and semantic knowledge, which was a complex task generally requiring linguistic expertise (Sager 1981; Grishman and Kittredge 1986) along with development of rule-based systems that used the knowledge to parse and interpret the text. The trend started to shift in the biomedical domain from rule-based systems to probabilistic NLP systems in the early 2000s, likely due to the availability of large collections of annotated textual material in the general language domain (Marcus et al. 1993; Palmer et al. 2005) and in the biomolecular domain (Kim et al. 2003), to the rise of machine learning approaches that use the text collections to uncover patterns in text (Manning and Schütze 1999; Bishop 2007).

NLP is multi-disciplinary at its core, weaving together theories of linguistics, computation, representation, and knowledge of biology, medicine and health. Within the computational field itself, NLP intersects with many fields of research, including computational linguistics, knowledge representation and reasoning, knowledge and information management, and machine and statistical learning. Furthermore, because NLP tools are often part of systems targeted at end-users, NLP also intersects with the field of human-computer interaction and cognitive science. The inter-disciplinary nature of NLP has important implications for the design, development and evaluation of NLP-based systems. For instance, it would be impossible to perform a proper error analysis of an NLP tool without expertise in the domain, whether biological or clinical.

8.3   Applications of NLP

Natural language processing has a wide range of potential applications. The following are important applications of NLP technology for biomedicine and health:

- **Information extraction**, the most common application of NLP in biomedicine, locates and structures specific information in text, usually without performing a complete linguistic analysis of the text, but rather by looking for patterns in the text. Once textual information is extracted and structured it can be used for a number of different tasks. In **biosurveillance**, for instance, one can extract symptoms from a chief complaint field in a note written for a patient admitted to the emergency department of a hospital (Chapman et al. 2004) or from ambulatory electronic health records (Hripcsak et al. 2009). The extracted data, when collected across many patients, can help understand the prevalence as well as the progression of a particular epidemic. In biology, biomolecular interactions extracted from one article or from different articles can be merged to construct biomolecular pathways. Figure 8.1 shows a pathway in the form of a graph that was created by extracting interactions from one article published in the journal Cell (Maroto et al. 1997). In the clinical domain, pharmacovigilance systems can use structured data obtained by means of NLP on huge numbers of patient records to discover adverse drug events (Wang et al. 2009a).
- The techniques for information extraction may be limited to the identification of names of people or places, dates, and numerical expressions, or to certain types of terms in text (e.g.

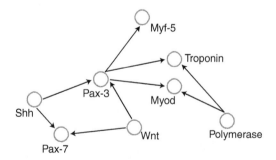

Fig. 8.1 A graph showing interactions that were extracted from an article. A vertex represents a gene or protein, and an edge represents the interaction. The *arrow* represents the direction of the interaction so that the agent is represented by the outgoing end of the arrow and the target by the incoming end

mentions of medications or proteins), which can then be mapped to canonical or standardized forms. This is referred as **named-entity recognition** or **named-entity normalization**. More sophisticated techniques identify and represent the modifiers attached to a named entity. Such advanced methods are necessary for reliable retrieval of information because the correct interpretation of a term typically depends on its relation with other terms in a given sentence. For example, the term *fever* has different interpretations in *no fever, high fever, fever lasted 2 days*, and *check for fever*. Defining the types of **modifiers of interest** (e.g. *no* is a negation modifier, while *lasted 2 days* is a temporal modifier), as well as techniques to recognize them in text, is an active topic of research. Identifying **relations among named entities** is another important information extraction method. For example, when extracting adverse events associated with a medication, the sentences "*the patient developed a rash from amoxicillin*" and "*the patient came in with a rash and was given benadryl*" must be distinguished. In both sentences, there is a relation between a rash and a drug, but the first sentence conveys a potential adverse drug event whereas the second sentence conveys a treatment for an adverse event. As entities are extracted within one document or across documents, one important step consists of **reference resolution**, that is, recognizing that two mentions in two different textual locations refer to the same entity. In some cases, resolving the references is very challenging. For instance, mentions of *stroke* in two different notes associated with the same patient could refer to the same stroke or two different strokes; additional contextual information and domain knowledge is often needed to resolve this problem.

- **Information retrieval** (IR) and NLP overlap in some of the methods that are used. IR is discussed in Chap. 21, but here we discuss basic differences between IR and NLP. IR methods are generally geared to help users access documents in large collections, such as electronic health records, the scientific literature, or the Web in general . This is a crucial application in biomedicine and health, due to the explosion of information available in electronic form. The essential goal of information retrieval is to match a user's query against a document collection and return a ranked list of relevant documents. A search is performed on an **index** of the document collection. The most basic form of indexing isolates simple words and terms, and therefore, uses minimal linguistic knowledge. More advanced approaches use NLP-based methods similar to those employed in information extraction, identifying complex named entities and determining their relationships in order to improve the accuracy of retrieval. For instance, one could search for *hypertension* and have the search operate at the concept level, returning documents that mention the phrase *high blood pressure* in addition to the ones mentioning *hypertension* only. In addition, one could search for *hypertension* in a specific context, such as treatment or etiology.

- **Question answering** (QA) involves a process whereby a user submits a natural language question that is then automatically answered by a QA system. The availability of information in journal articles and on the Web makes this type of application increasingly important as health care consumers, health care professionals, and biomedical researchers frequently search the Web to obtain information about a disease, a medication, or a medical procedure. A QA system can be very useful for obtaining the answers to factual questions, like "*In children with an acute febrile illness, what is the efficacy of single-medication therapy with acetaminophen or ibuprofen in reducing fever?*" (Demner-Fushman and Lin 2007). QA systems provide additional functionalities to an IR system. In an IR system, the user has to translate a question into a list of keywords and generate a query, but this step is carried out automatically by a QA system. Furthermore, a QA system presents the user with an actual answer (often one or several passages extracted from the source documents), rather than a list of relevant source documents. QA has focused on the literature thus far (Demner-Fushman and Lin 2007; Cao et al. 2011).

- **Text summarization** takes one or several documents as input and produces a single, coherent text that synthesizes the main points of the input documents. Summarization helps users make sense of a large amount of data, by identifying and presenting the salient points in texts automatically. Summarization can be generic or query-focused (i.e. taking a particular information need into account when selecting important content of input documents). Query-focused summarization can be viewed as a post-processing of IR and QA: the relevant passages corresponding to an input question are further processed into a single, coherent text. Several steps are involved in the summarization process: content selection (identifying salient pieces of information in the input document(s)), content organization (identifying redundancy and contradictions among the selected pieces of information, and ordering them so the resulting summary is coherent), and content re-generation (producing natural language from the organized pieces of information). Like question answering, text summarization has also focused on the literature (Elhadad et al. 2005; Zhang et al. 2011).
- Other tasks: **Text generation** formulates natural language sentences from a given source of information that is not directly readable by humans. Generation can be used to create a text from a structured database, such as summarizing trends and patterns in laboratory data (Jordan et al. 2001). **Machine translation** converts text in one language (e.g. English) into another (e.g. Spanish). These applications are important in multilingual environments in which human translation is too expensive or time consuming (Deleger et al. 2009). **Text readability assessment and simplification** is becoming relevant to the health domain, as patients and health consumers access more and more medical information on the Web, but need support because their health literacy levels do not match the ones of the documents they read (Elhadad 2006; Keselman et al. 2007). Finally, **sentiment analysis and emotion detection** are slightly more recent

applications of NLP and belong to the general task of automated content analysis. There are promising research results showing that patients' discourse can be analyzed automatically to help detect their mental states (Pestian and Matykiewicz 2008).

8.4 Linguistic Levels of Knowledge and Their Representations

While current linguistic theories differ in certain details, there is broad consensus that linguistic knowledge consists of multiple levels: **morphology** (words and meaningful parts of words), **syntax** (structure of phrases and sentences), **semantics** (meaning of words, phrases, and sentences), **pragmatics** (impact of context and of intent of the speaker on meaning), and **discourse** (paragraphs and documents). Human language processing may appear deceptively simple, because we are not conscious of the effort involved in learning and using language. However, a long process of acculturation is necessary to attain proficiency in speaking, reading, writing, and understanding with further intensive study to master a different language or the specialized languages of biological science and medicine. This section introduces the types of knowledge entailed in each of the levels as well as their representations. Traditionally, lexicography (the study of the morphology, syntax and semantics of words), the development of rules, or grammars, and the acquisition of linguistic knowledge in general was performed by trained linguists through the careful, manual analysis of texts. This process is extremely time intensive and requires expertise. Therefore, more recent methods have leveraged machine-learning (ML) techniques to acquire linguistic knowledge, with the hope of reducing manual effort and dependence on linguistic expertise.

8.4.1 Morphology

Morphology concerns the combination of **morphemes** (roots, prefixes, suffixes) to produce words or lexemes, where a lexeme generally constitutes several forms of the same word (e.g. *activate, activates, activating, activated, activation*). **Free morphemes** can occur as separate words, while **bound morphemes** cannot (e.g. *de-* in *detoxify*, *-tion* in *creation*, *-s* in *dogs*). **Inflectional morphemes** express grammatically required features or indicate relations between different words in the sentence, but do not change the basic syntactic category; for example, *big, bigg-er, biggest* are all adjectives. **Derivational morphemes** change the part of speech or the basic meaning of a word: thus *-ation* added to a verb may form a noun (*activ-ation*) and *re-activate* means activate again. Biomedical language has a very rich morphological structure especially for chemicals (e.g. *Hydr-oxy-nitro-di-hydro-thym-ine*) and procedures (*hepatico-cholangio-jejuno-stom-y*), but recognizing morphemes is complex. In the previous chemical example, the first split must be made after *hydr-* (because the *-o-* is part of *–oxy*), while the fifth split occurs after *hydro-*. In the procedure example, an automated morphological analyzer would have to distinguish *stom* (mouth) from *tom* (cut) in *-stom*. NLP systems in the biomedical domain do not generally incorporate morphological knowledge. Instead many systems use **regular expressions** to represent what textual words consist of, and a **lexicon** to specify the words or lexemes in the domain and their linguistic characteristics.

Patterns are conveniently represented by the formalism known as a regular expression or equivalently, **finite state automata** (Jurafsky and Martin 2009, pp. 17–42). For example, the following simple regular expression represents what patterns are to be recognized as morphemes.

$$[\,a-z]+\,|\,[\,0-9]+$$

The vertical bar (|) separates alternative expressions, which in this case specify two different kinds of **tokens** (alphabetic and numeric). Expressions in square brackets represent a range or choice of characters. The expression [a-z] indicates a lower case letter, while [0–9] indicates a digit. The plus sign denotes one or more occurrences of an expression. According to this regular expression, the sentence "*patient's wbc dropped to 12.*" contains six morphemes, and the string *patient's* would contain two morphemes,

patient and *s*; in this case, the *s* is a morpheme denoting a possessive construct. This regular expression is very limited, and would not represent a comprehensive set of tokens found in text. For example, it does not represent other morphological variations, such as negation (*n't*) or numbers with a decimal point (*3.4*).

More complex regular expressions can handle many of the morphological phenomena described above. However, situations that are locally ambiguous are more challenging, and representations that can encode more knowledge are preferable. For instance, **Markov processes** (see Chap. 3) that encode some level of context by assigning probabilities to the presence of individual morphemes and to possible combinations of morphemes, can help characterize morphological knowledge. While an important field of study, there has been little work concerning morphology in the field of NLP in the biomedicine and health domains, especially for the English language. Encoding morphological knowledge is necessary in languages that are morphologically rich (e.g. Turkish, German, and Hebrew).

8.4.2 Syntax

Syntax concerns the categorization of the words in the language, and the structure of the phrases and sentences. Each word belongs to one or more **parts of speech** in the language, such as noun (e.g. *chest*), adjective (e.g. *mild*), or tensed verb (e.g. *improves*), which are the elementary components of the grammar and are generally specified in a **lexicon**. Words may also have subcategories, depending on the corresponding basic part of speech, which are usually expressed by inflectional morphemes. For example, nouns have number (e.g. plural or singular as in *legs, leg*), person (e.g. first, second, third as in *I, you, he*, respectively), and case (e.g. subjective, objective, possessive as in *I, me, my*, respectively). **Lexemes** can consist of more than one word as in foreign phrases (*ad hoc*), prepositions (*along with*), and idioms (*follow up, on and off*). Biomedical lexicons tend to contain many multi-word lexemes, e.g. lexemes in the clinical domain include multiword terms such as *congestive heart* *failure* and *diabetes mellitus*, and in the biomolecular domain include the gene named *ALL1-fused gene from chromosome 1q*.

Lexemes combine (according to their parts of speech) in well-defined ways to form sequences of words or phrases, such as noun phrases (e.g. *severe chest pain*), adjectival phrases (e.g. *painful to touch*), or verb phrases (e.g. *has increased*). Each phrase generally consists of a main part of speech and modifiers, e.g. nouns are frequently modified by adjectives, while verbs are frequently modified by adverbs. The phrases then combine in well-defined ways to form sentences (e.g. *"he complained of severe chest pain" is a well-formed sentence, but "he severe complained chest pain of" is not*). General English imposes many restrictions on the formation of sentences, e.g. every sentence requires a verb, and count nouns (like *cough*) require an article (e.g., *a* or *the*). Clinical language, in contrast, is often **telegraphic**, relaxing many of these restrictions of the general language to achieve a highly compact form. For example, clinical language allows all of the following as sentences: *"the cough worsened," "cough worsening,"* and *"cough."* Because the community widely uses and accepts these alternate forms, they are not considered ungrammatical, but constitute a **sublanguage** (Grishman and Kittredge 1986; Kittredge and Lehrberger 1982; Friedman 2002). There are a wide variety of sublanguages in the biomedical domain, each exhibiting specialized content and linguistic forms.

8.4.2.1 Representation of Syntactic Knowledge

Syntactic knowledge can be represented by means of a lexicon and a grammar. Representing such knowledge in a computable fashion is important, as it enables the creation of tools that parse the syntax of any given sentence, by matching the sentence against the lexicon and the grammar. A **lexicon** is used to delineate the lexemes along with their corresponding parts of speech and canonical forms so that each lexical entry assigns a word to one or more parts of speech, and also to a canonical form or lemma. For example, *abdominal* is an adjective where the canonical form is *abdomen*, and *activation* is a noun that is the nominal

form of the verb *activate*. A **grammar** specifies the structure of the phrases and sentences in the language. It specifies how the words combine into well-formed structures through use of rules where categories combine with other categories or structures to produce a well-formed structure with underlying relations. A lexicon and grammar should be compatible with each other in that the parts of speech or categories specified in the lexicon should be the same as those specified in the rules of the grammar. In many systems, the parts of speech are typically standard and are based on the parts of speech specified by the Penn Treebank Project (Marcus et al. 1993). Table 8.1 provides some examples of Penn Treebank parts of speech, also called tags.

Generally, words combine to form phrases consisting of a **head word** and modifiers, and phrases combine to form sentences or clauses. For example, in English, there are noun phrases (NP) that contain a noun and optionally left and right modifiers, such as definite articles, adjectives, or prepositional phrases (i.e. *the patient, lower extremities, pain in lower extremities, chest pain*), and verb phrases (VP), such as *had pain, will be discharged*, and *denies smoking*. Phrases and sentences can be represented as a sequence where each word is followed by its corresponding part of speech. For example, *Severe joint pain* can be represented as *Severe/JJ joint/NN pain/NN*.

The field of computer science provides a number of formalisms that can be used to represent syntactic linguistic knowledge. These include symbolic or logical formalisms (e.g. **regular expressions** and **context free grammars**) and statistical formalisms (e.g. **probabilistic context free grammars**). Simple phrases, which are phrases that do not contain right modifiers, can be represented using **regular expressions**. When using regular expressions to represent the syntax of simple phrases, syntactic categories are used in the expression. An example of a regular expression (using the Penn Treebank parts of speech defined in Table 8.1) for a simple noun phrase is:

$$\textbf{DT?JJ*NN*(NN|NNS)}$$

Table 8.1 Description of some part-of-speech tags from the Penn Treebank

Tag	Meaning (example)
CC	Conjunction (*and*)
CD	Cardinal number (*2*)
DT	Article (*the*)
IN	Preposition (*of*)
JJ	Adjective (*big*)
NN	Singular noun (*pain*)
NNS	Plural noun (*arms*)
PP$	Possessive pronoun (*her*)
PRP	Personal pronoun (*she*)
VB	Infinitive verb (*fall*)
VBD	Past-tense verb (*fell*)
VBG	Progressive verb form (*falling*)
VBN	Past participle (*fallen*)
VBZ	Present-tense verb (*falls*)

```
S       → NP VP .
NP      → DT? JJ* (NN | NNS) CONJN* PP* | NP and NP
VP      → (VBZ | VBP) NP? PP*
PP      → IN NP
CONJN   → and (NN | NNS)
```

Fig. 8.2 A simple syntactic context-free grammar of English. A sentence is represented by the rule S, a noun phrase by the rule NP, a verb phrase by VP, and a prepositional phrase by PP. Terminal symbols in the grammar that correspond to syntactic parts of speech, are underlined in the figure

This structure specifies a simple noun phrase as consisting of an optional determiner (i.e. *a*, *the*, *some*, *no*), followed by zero or more adjectives, followed by zero or more singular nouns, and terminated by a singular or plural noun. For example, the above regular expression would match the noun phrase "*no/DT usual/JJ congestive/JJ heart/NN failure/NN symptoms/NNS*" but would not match "*heart/NN the/DT unusual/JJ*" because in the above regular expression *the* cannot occur in the middle of a noun phrase. In addition, the above regular expression does not cover many legitimate simple noun phrases, such as "*3/CD days/NNS*", "*her/PRP$ arm/NN*", and "*pain/NN and/CC fever/NN*".

A complex noun phrase with right modifiers, however, cannot be handled using a regular expression because a right modifier may contain **nested structures**, such as nested prepositional phrases or nested relative clauses. More complex language structures, like phrases with right modifiers, can be represented by a **context-free grammar** (CFG) or by equivalent formalisms (Jurafsky and Martin 2009, pp 386–421). A CFG is concerned with how sequences of words combine to form phrases or constituents. A very simple grammar of English is shown in Fig. 8.2. Context-free rules use **part-of-speech tags** (see Table 8.1) and

the operators found in regular expressions. The difference is that each rule has a non-terminal symbol on the left side (S, NP, VP, PP) that represents a syntactic structure, and consists of a rule that specifies a sequence of grammar symbols (non-terminal and terminal) on the right side. Thus, in Fig. 8.2, the S (sentence) rule contains a sequence consisting of the symbols NP, followed by VP, which in turn are followed by a literal that is a '.'. Additionally, other rules may refer to these symbols or to the atomic parts of speech. In the NP rule there is an optional determiner DT as well as an optional prepositional phrase PP, which in turn contains an embedded NP to define noun phrases such as "*the pain*", "*pain*", "*pain in arm*", and "*pain in elbow of left arm*".

CFG grammar rules generally give rise to many possible structures for a parse tree, which represent sequences of alternative choices of rules in the grammar, but some choices are more likely than others. For example, in the sentence "*she experienced pain in chest*", it is more likely that *in chest* modifies *pain* and not *experienced*. The preferences can be represented using a **probabilistic context free grammar** that associates a probability with each choice in a rule (Jurafsky and Martin 2009, pp 459–479). The grammar shown in Fig. 8.2 can be augmented with probabilities for each rule (see Fig. 8.3). The number indicates the probability of including the given category in the parse tree. For example, the probability assigned to having a determiner (DT) in a NP can be 0.9 (and conversely not having a DT at the beginning of a NP has a probability of 0.1). The probability of a present tense verb (VBZ) is 0.4, while a past tense verb (VBD) is 0.6. The

S	→	NP VP .
NP	→	DT?$^{.9}$ JJ*$^{.8}$ (NN │ $^{.6}$NNS) PP*$^{.8}$
VP	→	(VBZ │ $^{.4}$VBD) NP?$^{.9}$ PP*$^{.7}$
PP	→	<u>IN</u> NP

Fig. 8.3 A simple probabilistic context-free grammar of English. Probabilities for each rule are part of the grammar and are derived from a large corpus annotated with syntactic information

probabilities are usually estimated from a large corpus of text that has been annotated with the correct syntactic structures.

Recently, there has been increased interest in the **dependency grammar** formalism (Jurafsky and Martin 2009, 414–416), which focuses on how words relate to other words, although there are many different theories and forms of dependency grammars. Dependency is a binary asymmetrical relation between a head and its dependents or modifiers. The head of a sentence is usually a tensed verb. Thus, unlike CFGs, dependency structures do not contain phrasal structures but are basically directed relations between words. For example, in the sentence, *The patient had pain in lower extremities*, the head of the sentence is the verb *had*, which has two arguments, a subject noun *patient* and an object noun *extremities*, *the* modifies or is dependent on *patient*, and *in* is dependent on *pain*, *extremities* is dependent on *in*, and *lower* is dependent on *extremities*. As such, in a dependency grammar, the relations among words and the concept of head in particular (e.g. *extremities* is the head of *lower*) is closer to the semantics of a sentence. We introduce the concept of semantics next.

8.4.3   Semantics

Semantics concerns the meaning or interpretation of words, phrases and sentences, generally associated with real-world applications. There are many different theories for representation of meaning, such as **logic-based**, **frame-based**, or **conceptual graph** formalisms. In this section, we discuss semantics involved in interpretation of the text in order to accomplish practical tasks, and do not aim to discuss representation of complete

meaning. Each word has one or more meanings or **word senses** (e.g. *capsule*, as in *renal capsule*, *vitamin B12 capsule*, or *shoulder capsule*), and other terms may modify the senses (e.g. *no*, as in *no fever*, or *last week* as in *fever last week*). Additionally, the meanings of the words combine to form a meaningful sentence, as in *there was thickening in the renal capsule*). Representation of the semantics of general language is extremely important, but the underlying concepts are not as clear or uniform as those concerning syntax. Interpreting the meaning of words and text for general language is very challenging, but interpreting the meaning of text within a sublanguage is more feasible. More specifically, biomedical sublanguages are easier to interpret than general languages because they exhibit more restrictive semantic patterns that can be represented more easily (Harris et al. 1989; Harris 1991; Sager et al. 1987). Sublanguages tend to have a relatively small number of well-defined **semantic types** (e.g. medication, gene, disease, body part, or organism) and a small number of **semantic patterns** (e.g. medication-treats-disease, gene-interacts with-gene).

8.4.3.1   Representation of Semantic Knowledge

Semantic interpretations must be assigned to individual terms (e.g. single words or multi-word terms that function as single words) that are then combined into larger semantic structures (Jurafsky and Martin 2009, pp 545–580). The notion of what constitutes an individual term is not straightforward, particularly in the biomedical domain where there are many multi-word terms that have specific meanings that are different from the combined meanings of the parts. For example, *burn* in *heart burn* has a different meaning than in *finger burn*. Semantic information about words can be maintained in a lexicon or a domain-specific dictionary. A **semantic type or class** is usually a broad class that is associated with a specific domain and includes many instances, while a **semantic sense** distinguishes individual word meanings (Jurafsky and Martin 2009, pp 611–617). For example, *heart attack*, *myocardial infarct*, and *systemic lupus* *eryhtematosus* (*SLE*) all have the same semantic type (disease); *heart attack* and *myocardial infarct* share the same semantic sense (they are synonymous) that is distinct from the sense of *SLE* (a different condition).

A lexicon containing semantic knowledge may be created manually by a linguist, or be derived from external knowledge sources. Examples of semantic knowledge sources are the **Unified Medical Language System** (UMLS) (Lindberg et al. 1993), which assigns semantic types to terms, such as **disease**, **procedure**, or **medication**, and also specifies the sense of the concept through a unique concept identifier (CUI), and GenBank (Benson et al. 2003), which lists the names of genes and also specifies a unique identifier for each gene concept. While external sources can save a substantial effort, the types and senses provided may not be the appropriate granularity for the text being analyzed. Narrow categories may be too restrictive, and broad categories may introduce ambiguities. Morphological knowledge can be helpful in determining semantic types in the absence of lexical information. For example, in the clinical domain, suffixes like *–itis* and *-osis* indicate diseases, while *-otomy* and *ectomy* indicate procedures. However, such techniques cannot determine the specific sense of a word.

Semantic structures consisting of **semantic relations** can be identified using regular expressions, which specify patterns of semantic types that are relevant in a specific domain, and that are associated with a real-word interpretation. The expressions may be semantic and look only at the semantic categories of the words in the sentence. For example, this method may be applied in the biomolecular domain to identify interactions between genes or proteins. For example, the regular expression

$$[\text{GENE} \mid \text{PROT}]\text{MFUN}[\text{GENE} \mid \text{PROT}]$$

will match sentences consisting of very simple gene or protein interactions (e.g. *Pax-3/GENE activated/MFUN Myod/GENE*). In this case, the elements of the pattern consist of semantic classes: gene (GENE), molecular function (MFUN), and protein (PROT). This pattern is

very restrictive, and regular expressions that skip over parts of the sentence can be written to detect relevant patterns for a broader variety of text, although it will incur some loss of specificity and precision while achieving increased sensitivity. For example, the regular expression

$$[\text{GENE} \mid \text{PROT}].*\text{MFUN}.*[\text{GENE} \mid \text{PROT}]$$

specifies a pattern that provides for skipping over terms in the text. The dot (.) matches any tag, and the asterisk (*) allows for an arbitrary number of occurrences. Using the above expression, the interpretation of the interaction, *Pax-3 activated Myod* would be obtained for the sentence "*Pax-3/GENE, only when activated/MFUN by Myod/GENE, inhibited/MFUN phosphorylation/MFUN*". In this example, the match does not capture the information correctly because "*only when*" was skipped. The correct interpretation of the individual interactions in this sentence should be "*Myod activated Pax-3*", and "*Pax-3 inhibited phosphorylation*". Note that the simple regular expression shown above does not provide for the latter pattern (i.e. GENE-MFUN-MFUN), for the connective relation *only when*, or for the passive structure *activated by*.

Frequently, simple semantic relations are not represented using regular expressions. Instead, relations and the roles of the elements in the relation are specified by manual or semi-automated annotation so that machine-learning methods could be leveraged to develop models that detect the relations. For example, interaction type relations could be annotated so that it has an element that is an agent, and an element that is a target. Therefore, the above sentence would be annotated as consisting of two relations: an interaction relation *inhibit* where the agent is *Pax-3* and the target is *phosphorylation*, and an interaction relation *activate* where the agent is *Myod* and the target is *Pax-3*.

More complex semantic structures containing nesting can be represented using a **semantic grammar**, which is a context free grammar based on semantic categories. As shown in Fig. 8.4, a simple semantic grammar for clinical texts might define a clinical sentence as a Finding, which

```
S            → Finding .
Finding      → DegreePhrase? ChangePhrase? SYMP
ChangePhrase → NEG? CHNG
DegreePhrase → DEGR | NEG
```

Fig. 8.4 A simple semantic context-free grammar for the English clinical domain. A sentence S consists of a Finding that consists of an optional DegreePhrase, an optional ChangePhrase and a Symptom. The DegreePhrase consists of a degree type word or a negation type word; the ChangePhrase consists of an optional negation type word followed by a change type word. The terminal symbols in the grammar correspond to semantic parts of speech and are underlined

consists of optional degree information and optional change information followed by a symptom. Such a semantic grammar can parse the sentence "increased/CHNG tenderness/SYMP", a typical sentence in the clinical domain, which often omits subjects and verbs.

NLP systems can represent more complex language structures by integrating syntactic and semantic structures into the grammar (Friedman et al. 1994). In this case, the grammar would be similar to that shown in Fig. 8.4, but the rules would also include syntactic structures. Additionally, the grammar rule may also specify the representational output form that represents the underlying interpretation of the relations. For example, in Fig. 8.4, the rule for Finding would specify an output form denoting that SYMP is the primary finding and the other elements are the modifiers.

More comprehensive syntactic structures can be recognized using a broad-coverage CFG of English that is subsequently combined with a semantic component (Sager et al. 1987). After the syntactic structures are recognized, they are followed by syntactic rules that regularize the structures. For example, passive sentences, such as "*the chest x-ray was interpreted by a radiologist*", would be transformed to the active form (e.g. "*a radiologist interpreted the chest x-ray*"). Another set of semantic rules would then operate on the regularized syntactic structures to interpret their semantic relations.

The representation of a probabilistic CFG that contains semantic information would be similar to that of a CFG for syntax, but it would require a large corpus that has been annotated with both syntactic and semantic information. Since a semantic grammar is domain and/or application specific, annotation involving the phrase structure would be costly and not portable, and therefore is not generally done.

8.4.4 Pragmatics and Discourse

Pragmatics concerns how knowledge concerning the intent of the author of the text, or more generally the context in which the text is written, influences the meaning of a sentence or a text. For example, in a mammography report *mass* generally denotes *breast mass*, whereas a radiological report of the chest denotes *mass in lung*. In yet a different genre of texts, like a religious journal, it is likely to denote a ceremony. Similarly, in a health care setting, *he drinks heavily*, is assumed to be referring to alcohol and not water. In these two examples, pragmatics influences the meaning of individual words. It can also influence the meaning of larger linguistic units. For instance, when physicians document the chief-complaint section of a note, they list symptoms and signs, as reported by the patient. The presence of a particular symptom, however, does not imply that the patient actually has the symptom. Rather, it is understood implicitly by both the author of the note and its reader that this is the patient's impression rather than the truth. Thus, the meaning of the chief-complaint section of a note is quite different from the assessment and plan, for instance. Another pragmatic consideration is the interpretation of pronouns and other referential expressions (*there, tomorrow*). For example, in the two following sentences "*An infiltrate was noted in right upper lobe. It was patchy*", the pronoun *it* refers to *infiltrate* and not *lobe*. In a sentence containing the term *tomorrow*, it would be necessary to know when the note was written in order to interpret the actual date denoted by *tomorrow*.

In the biomedical domain, pragmatics is taken into account, but knowledge about the pragmatics of the domain is not modeled explicitly. In NLP applications limited to a specific subdomain, it can be encoded through the semantic lexicon (like the one described in Sect. 8.4.3) and rules about the discourse of a text.

While sentences in isolation convey individual pieces of information, sentences together combine to form a text, obeying a **discourse** structure (e.g. a group of sentences about the same topic can be grouped into coherent paragraphs, whereas a dialogue between a physician and a patient can be structured as a sequence of conversation turns). Complete analysis of a text requires analysis of relationships between sentences and larger units of discourse, such as paragraphs and sections (Jurafsky and Martin 2009, pp 681–723).

There has been much work regarding discourse in computational linguistics and in NLP in the general domain. One of the most important mechanisms in language for creating linkages between sentences is the use of **referential expressions**, which include pronouns (*he, she, her, himself*), proper nouns (*Dr. Smith, Atlantic Hospital*) and noun phrases modified by the definite article or a demonstrative (*the left breast, this medication, that day, these findings*). **Coreference chains** provide a compact representation for encoding the words and phrases in a text that all refer to the same entity. Figure 8.5 shows a text and the coreference chains corresponding to two entities in the discourse. Each referential expression has a unique referent that must be identified in order to make sense of the text. In the figure, the proper noun *Dr. Smith* refers to the physician who is treating the patient. In the first two sentences, *his* and *he* refer to the patient, while *he* refers to the physician in the fourth sentence. In that figure, there also are several definite noun phrases (e.g. *the epithelium, the trachea,* and *the lumen*) that have to be resolved. In this case, the referents are parts of the patient's body and are not mentioned previously in the text.

[Mr. Jones's$_1$] laboratory values on admission were notable for a chest x-ray showing a right upper lobe pneumonia. [He$_1$] underwent upper endoscopy with dilatation. It was noted that [his$_1$] respiratory function became compromised each time the balloon was dilated. Subsequently, [Dr. Smith$_2$] saw [him$_1$] in consultation. [He$_2$] performed a bronchoscopy and verified that there was an area of tumor. It had not invaded the epithelium or the trachea. But it did partially occlude the lumen.

Fig. 8.5 A text and two coreference chains, one about the patient and one about the clinician. *Brackets* denotes the span of the reference, and the indices inside the *brackets* refer to the entity. Note that even though we show two chains only, there are many other entities in the text (such as "laboratory values," "chest x-ray, and "tumor")

8.5 NLP Techniques

Most NLP systems are designed with separate modules that handle different functions. The modules typically roughly coincide with the linguistic levels described in Sect. 8.4. In general, the output from each lower level serves as input to the next higher level. For example, the output of **tokenization** transforms a textual string into tokens that will undergo lexical analysis to determine their parts of speech and possibly other properties as specified in a lexicon; the parts of speech along with the corresponding lexical definitions will then be the input to syntactic analysis that will determine the structure of the sentence; the structure will be the input to semantic analysis that will interpret the meaning. Each system packages these processing steps somewhat differently. At each stage of processing, the module for that stage aims to regularize the data in some aspect to reduce variety while preserving the informational content as much as possible.

8.5.1 Low-Level Text Processing

In addition to different linguistic levels introduced in the previous section, there is an additional practical level involved in NLP that pertains to the low-level processing of an input file. **Text processing**, as it is commonly referred to, is a sometimes-tedious part of developing an NLP system, but it is a critical one, as it impacts the processing at all the subsequent linguistic levels. Below, we review a few of the characteristics of low-level text that need to be considered when implementing an NLP system or when preparing input for an off-the-shelf NLP system.

8.5.1.1 File Formats

Documents in a corpus (a collection of documents, plural: corpora) can be stored using different formats. In some EHRs, for instance, it is not uncommon to have patient notes stored in **Rich Text Format** (RTF). PubMed citations can be downloaded from the Web in an **Extensible Markup Language** (XML) format, whereas full-text articles from PubMed can be **Hypertext Markup Language** (HTML) files, and Twitter feeds can come in the XML-based **Really Simple Syndication** (RSS) format. While there is no established way to convert one format into another or to clean up HTML tags, there are several packages available in many programming languages that can help deal with different file formats.

8.5.1.2 Character Sets and Encodings

Characters can be encoded in different ways in a computer (e.g. ASCII, which contains 128 characters, or Unicode, which contains over 100,000 characters). Knowing the character encoding used in a document is essential to recognize the characters and process the text further.

8.5.2   Document Structure

Journal articles generally have well-defined section headers, associated with the informational content (e.g. Introduction, Background, Methods, Results) and other information, such as references and data about the authors and their affiliations. In clinical reports, there often are well-defined sections (e.g. History of Present Illness, Past Medical History, Family History, Allergies, Medications, Assessment and Plan) that would be important for an NLP system to recognize. For example, medications mentioned in the Medication Section have been prescribed to patients whereas medications mentioned in the Allergy Section should not be. Within sections, other document-level constructs must be identified, such as paragraphs, tables in various formats, and (often nested) list items. In many cases however, a text comes "raw," that is, without any formatting information, or with some idiosyncratic formatting. In the clinical domain, for instance, there is evidence that many typed notes have no explicit section headers.

Tokens. The next step in processing generally consists of separating the cleaned up ASCII text, which is usually one large string at this stage, into individual units called tokens (a process called tokenization), which include morphemes, words (often morpheme sequences), numbers, symbols (e.g. mathematical operators), and punctuation. The notion of what constitutes a token is far from trivial. The primary indication of a token

in general English is the occurrence of white space before and after it; however there are many exceptions: a token may be followed by certain punctuation marks without an intervening space, such as by a period, comma, semicolon, or question mark, or may have a '-'in the middle. In biomedicine, periods and other punctuation marks can be part of words (e.g. *q.d.* meaning *every day* in the clinical domain or *M03F4.2A*, a gene name that includes a period), and are used inconsistently, thereby complicating the tokenization process. For instance, in the string "*5 mg. given*" the tokenization process determines whether to keep the string "*mg.*" as one token or two ("*mg*" and "*.*"). In addition, chemical and biological names often include parentheses, commas and hyphens (for example, "*(w)adh-2*") that also complicate the tokenization process.

Symbolic approaches to tokenization are generally based on pattern matching using regular expressions, but most current approaches use statistical methods. One method consists of comparing which alternatives are most frequent in a correctly-tokenized corpus (e.g. is the token *M03F4.2A* more frequent than the two tokens *M03F4* and *2A* one next to another, but separated by a white space).

8.5.2.1 Sentence Boundaries

Detecting the beginning and end of a sentence may seem like an easy task, but is a highly domain-dependent one. Not all sentences end with a punctuation mark (this is especially true in texts with minimal editing, such as online patient posts and clinical notes entered by physicians). Conversely, the presence of a period does not necessarily mean the end of a sentence (as discussed in tokenization). While there are statistically trained models available for general NLP, they are based on an annotated corpus of general language text, and do not perform as well on biomedical and health-related text. Therefore, many NLP systems rely on hand-built rules to detect an end of sentence.

8.5.2.2 Case

Most NLP techniques operate on words as their smallest unit of processing. The definition of a word is not trivial, however. One question is whether to consider strings with different cases the same. In some situations, it makes sense to keep all tokens in lowercase, as it reduces variations in vocabulary. But in others, it might hinder further NLP: there are many acronyms that, when lowercased, might be confused with regular words, such as *TEN*, which is an abbreviation for *toxic epidermal necrosis*.

8.5.3 Syntax

There are generally two tasks involved in syntactic analysis: one involves determining the syntactic categories or parts of speech of the words, and the other involves determining and representing the structures of the sentences.

8.5.3.1 Output of Syntactic Parse

Applying grammar rules to a given sentence is called parsing, and if the grammar rules can be satisfied, the grammar yields a nested structure that can be represented graphically as a **parse tree**. For example, based on the CFG shown in Fig. 8.2, the sentence "*the patient had pain in lower extremities*" would be parsed successfully and would be assigned the parse tree shown in Fig. 8.6. Alternatively, brackets can be used to

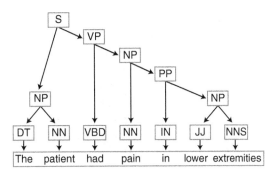

Fig. 8.6 A parse tree for the sentence *the patient had pain in lower extremities* according to the context-free grammar shown in Fig. 8.2. Notice that the terminal nodes in the tree correspond to the syntactic categories of the words in the sentence

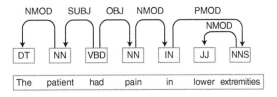

Fig. 8.7 A parse tree for the sentence *the patient had pain in lower extremities* in a dependency grammar framework

represent the nesting of phrases instead of a parse tree. Subscripts on the brackets specify the type of phrase or tag:

$$[_S [_{NP} [_{DT} \text{the}] [_{NN} \text{patient}]] [_{VP} [_{VBD} \text{had}]$$
$$[_{NP} [_{NN} \text{pain}] [_{PP} [_{IN} \text{in}] [_{NP} [_{JJ} \text{lower}] [_{NNS} \text{extremities}]]]]]]]$$

The following shows an example of a parse in the biomolecular domain for the sentence *Activation of Pax-3 blocks Myod phosphorylation*:

$$[_S [_{NP} [_{NN} \text{Activation}] [_{PP} [_{IN} \text{of}] [_{NP} [_{NN} \text{Pax-3}]]]]$$
$$[_{VP} [_{VBZ} \text{blocks}] [_{NP} [_{JJ} \text{Myod}] [_{NN} \text{phosphorylation}]]]]$$

When a dependency grammar is used, the representation of the parsed structure would be different from the structure generated by a CFG, and would reflect relations between words instead of structures. Figure 8.7 shows a representation of a dependency structure for the same sentence as the one illustrated in Fig. 8.6. In this example, the noun *patient* and the noun *pain* are the subject and object arguments of the verb *had*, and thus

are both dependent on the verb. Similarly, the determiner *the* modifies (i.e. is dependent on) *patient*, and the preposition *in* modifies *pain*.

8.5.3.2 Part-of-Speech Tagging and Lexical Lookup

Once text is tokenized, an NLP system needs to identify the words or multi-word terms known to the system, and determine their categories and canonical forms. Many systems carry out tokenization on complete words and perform **part-of-speech tagging**, and then some form of lexical look up immediately afterwards. This requires that the tagger and lexicon contain all the possible combinations of morphemes. A few systems perform morphological analysis during tokenization. In that case, the lexicon only needs entries for roots, prefixes, and suffixes, with additional entries for irregular forms. For example, the lexicon would contain entries for the roots *abdomen* (with variant *abdomin-*) and *activat-*, the adjective suffix *-al*, verb suffix *-e*, and noun suffix *-ion*.

Part-of-speech tagging is not straightforward because a word may be associated with more than one part of speech. For example, *stay* may be a noun (as in *her hospital stay*) or a verb (as in *refused to stay*). Without resolution, such ambiguities can lead to creating different structures for the sentence causing inaccuracies in parsing and interpretation, resulting in a substantial decrease in performance. For example, when *eating* occurs before a noun, it can be an adjective (JJ) that modifies the noun, or it can be a verb form (VBG) with the noun as object:

She/PRP denied/VBD eating/JJ difficulties/NN
She/PRP denied/VBD eating/VBG food/NN

In the first example, the patient is having a difficulty associated with eating, whereas in the second the patient is denying the act of eating food. Various methods for part-of-speech tagging may be used to resolve ambiguities by considering the surrounding words. A rule-based approach generally consists of rules based on the word that precedes or follows the current word. For example, if *stay* follows *the* or *her*, a rule may specify that it should be tagged as a noun, but if it follows *to* it should be tagged as a verb.

Currently, the most widely used approaches are statistically based part-of-speech taggers. One type of approach is based on Markov models (as described above for morphology). In this case, the **transition matrix** specifies the probability of one part of speech following another (see Table 8.2):

The following sentence shows the correct assignment of part-of-speech tags: *Rheumatology/NN consult/NN continued/VBD to/TO follow/VB patient/NN.*

Table 8.2 Transition probabilities for part-of-speech tags

	NN	VB	VBD	VBN	TO	IN
NN	0.34	0.00	0.22	0.02	0.01	0.40
VB	0.28	0.01	0.02	0.27	0.04	0.39
VBD	0.12	0.01	0.01	0.62	0.05	0.19
VBN	0.21	0.00	0.00	0.03	0.11	0.65
TO	0.02	0.98	0.00	0.00	0.00	0.00
IN	0.85	0.00	0.02	0.05	0.00	0.08

Table 8.3 Probabilities of alternative part-of-speech tag sequences

Part of speech tag sequence	Probability
NN NN VBD TO VB NN	0.001149434
NN NN VBN TO VB NN	0.000187779
NN VB VBN TO VB NN	0.000014194
NN NN VBD IN VB NN	0.000005510
NN NN VBN IN VB NN	0.000001619
NN VB VBD TO VB NN	0.000000453
NN VB VBN IN VB NN	0.000000122
NN VB VBD IN VB NN	0.000000002

This assignment is challenging for a computer, because *consult* can be tagged VB (*Orthopedics asked to consult*), *continued* can be tagged VBN (*penicillin was continued*), and *to* can be tagged IN. However, probabilities can be calculated for these sequences using the matrix in Table 8.2 (these were estimated from a large corpus of clinical text). By multiplying the transitions together, a probability for each sequence can be obtained (as described above for morphology), and is shown in Table 8.3. Note that the correct assignment has the highest probability.

8.5.3.3 Parsing

Many NLP systems perform some type of syntactic parsing to determine the structure of the sentence. Some systems perform **partial parsing** or **shallow parsing**, and are based on a number of different methods (Jurafsky and Martin 2009; pp 450–458). Partial parsing systems determine the structure of local phrases, such as simple noun phrases (i.e. noun phrases without right adjuncts) and simple adjectival phrases but do not determine relations among the phrases. Determining non-recursive phrases where each phrase corresponds to a specific part of speech is also called

chunking. These systems tend to be robust because it is easier to recognize isolated phrases than it is to recognize complete sentences, but typically they lose some information. For example, in *amputation below knee*, the two noun phrases *amputation* and *knee* would be extracted, but the relation *below* might not be. Rule-based methods use regular expressions that are manually created, while statistical models are developed based on an annotated corpus.

Complete syntactic parsing recognizes and determines the structure of a complete sentence. A system based on a CFG tries to find a match between the sentence and the grammar rules. Therefore, parsing can be thought of as a search problem that tries to fit the sequence of part-of-speech tags associated with the sentence to all possible combinations of grammar rules. There are a number of different approaches to parsing, such as searching through the rules in a **top-down** or **bottom-up** fashion, or using dynamic programming methods for efficiency, as in the **Cocke–Younger–Kasami** (CYK), **Earley**, or **chart parsing** methods (Jurafsky and Martin 2009; pp 427–450).

Additionally, grammar rules generally give rise to many possible structures for a parse tree (structural ambiguity) because the sequence of alternative choices of rules in the grammar can yield different groupings of phrases based on syntax alone. For example, sentence 1a below corresponds to a parse based on the grammar rules shown in Fig. 8.2 where the VP rule contains a PP (e.g. *denied in the ER*) and the NP rule contains only a noun (e.g. *pain*). Sentence 1b corresponds to the same atomic sequence of syntactic categories but the parse is different because the VP rule contains only a verb (e.g. *denied*) and the NP contains a noun followed by a PP (e.g. *pain in the abdomen*). Prepositions

and conjunctions are also a frequent cause of ambiguity. In 2a, the NP consists of a conjunction of the head nouns so that the left adjunct (e.g. *pulmonary*) is distributed across both nouns (i.e. this is equivalent to an interpretation *pulmonary edema* and *pulmonary effusion*), whereas in 2b, the left adjunct *pulmonary* is attached only to *edema* and is not related to *anemia*. In 3a the NP in the prepositional phrase PP contains a conjunction (i.e. this is equivalent to *pain in hands* and *pain in feet*) whereas in 3b two NPs are also conjoined but the first NP consists of *pain in hands* and the second consists of *fever*.

1a. *Denied* [*pain*] [*in the ER*]
1b. *Denied* [*pain* [*in the abdomen*]]
2a. *Pulmonary* [*edema and effusion*]
2b. [*Pulmonary edema*] *and anemia*
3a. *Pain in* [*hands and feet*]
3b. [*Pain in hands*] *and fever*

More complex forms of ambiguity do not exhibit differences in parts of speech or in grouping, but require determining deeper syntactic relationships. For example, when a verb ending in *–ing* is followed by *of*, the following noun can be either the subject or object of the verb.

Feeling of lightheadedness improved.
Feeling of patient improved.

Statistical approaches provide one method of addressing parsing ambiguity, and provide a mechanism where it is possible to prefer the more likely parses over less likely ones based on the probability of a parse tree that is the product of the probabilities of each grammar rule used to make it. For example, there are two ways to parse *x-ray shows patches in lung* using this grammar (shown below). The first interpretation in which *shows* is modified by *lung* has probability 3.48×10^{-8}, while the second interpretation in which *patches* is modified by *lung* has probability 5.97×10^{-8}.

$$[_S [_{NP} NN\ 0.1 \times 0.2 \times 0.6 \times 0.2] [_{VP} VBZ [_{NP} NN\ 0.1 \times 0.2 \times 0.6 \times 0.2]$$
$$[_{PP} IN [_{NP} NN\ 0.1 \times 0.2 \times 0.6 \times 0.2]]\ 0.4 \times .9 \times .7]]$$

$$[_S [_{NP} NN\ 0.1 \times 0.2 \times 0.6 \times 0.2]$$
$$[_{VP} VBZ [_{NP} [_{PP} IN [_{NP} NN\ 0.1 \times 0.2 \times 0.6 \times 0.2] NN\ 0.1 \times 0.2 \times 0.6 \times 0.8]\ 0.4 \times 0.9 \times 0.3]]$$

The probabilities are generally established based on a large corpus that has been parsed and annotated correctly. Therefore, it is critical that the corpus be of a genre similar to the text to be parsed; otherwise, performance will likely deteriorate.

8.5.4 Semantics

Semantic analysis involves steps analogous to those described above for syntax. First, semantic interpretations must be assigned to individual words, and then, these are combined into larger semantic structures, including modifications and relations. There are a number of formalisms for representing information in language (see Jurafsky and Martin 2009; pp 545–580), such as database tables, XML, **frames**, **conceptual graphs**, or **predicate logic**. Below, we discuss a few general approaches within this domain.

NLP systems may capture the clinical information at many different levels of granularity. One level of coarse granularity consists of classification of reports. For example, several systems (Aronow et al. 1995; Aronow et al. 1999) classified reports as positive or negative for specific clinical conditions, such as breast cancer. Another level of granularity that is useful for information retrieval and indexing, captures relevant terms by mapping the information to a controlled vocabulary, such as the UMLS (Aronson 2001; Nadkarni et al. 2001), but modifier relations are not captured. A more specific level of granularity also captures positive and negative modification (Mutalik et al. 2001; Chapman et al. 2001) or temporal status (Harkema et al. 2009). An even more specific level of granularity captures a comprehensive set of modifiers associated with the term, facilitating reliable information extraction (Friedman et al. 2004).

8.5.4.1 Output of Semantic Interpretation

Typically within a specific domain, semantic interpretation is limited in the sense that NLP systems in that domain do not attempt to capture the complete meaning of information in the text, but instead aim to capture limited relevant elements of the text. This process involves several

representational aspects: word sense, relevant information that modifies or changes the underlying meaning of the word senses, well-defined relations in the domain, and relevant information that modifies the relations.

Representation of word senses is usually achieved by means of the many controlled vocabularies or **ontologies** in the domain that associate words or terms with unique meanings, or concepts, and have corresponding codes. Therefore, semantic interpretation of a word or term entails mapping it to a code that represents its concept. As with parts of speech, many words have more than one semantic interpretation or sense; an NLP system must determine which of these is intended in the given context and map the sense to a well-defined concept. For example, *growth* can be either an abnormal physiologic process (e.g. for a tumor) or a normal one (e.g. for a child). The word *left* can indicate laterality (*pain in left leg*) or an action (*patient left hospital*).

Relations between words may be represented a number of different ways. One very general representational form is a frame-based representation in which the **frame** contains **slots** consisting of predefined types of information, which may be optional (Minsky 1975). In addition, relations between the slots are predetermined. Thus, a frame may be used to represent a simple concept along with its modifiers. For example, a frame representing a patient's condition, could have a slot for the condition, such as *cough*, and additional slots that modify *cough*, such as a slot for severity as in *severe cough*, a slot for temporal information, as in *cough for 4 days*, a slot for type of cough, as in *productive cough*, and a slot for negation, as in *denies cough* (Friedman et al. 2004). A frame may also contain more complex information associated with relations between entities. For example, an interaction frame could be defined to contain a slot for the interaction, a slot for the agent, a slot for the target, and slots that modify the relation, such as a negation slot to represent an interaction that is negated, or a degree slot to represent the strength of an interaction.

Another representation could be a predicate-argument form where the interpretation of the **predicate** and the roles of the **arguments** are specified. Representation of an interaction between biomolecular substances could be *Interaction(Agent,Target)*. For example, *Wnt blocks Pax-3* could be represented as *block(Wnt,Pax-3)* or the arguments could be codes uniquely defining those substances. Similarly, relations between medications and conditions can be represented as a predicate, such as *treat, prevent,* or *causes,* where the first argument could be the medication or a corresponding code, and the second argument could be the condition or its code.

8.5.4.2 Word Sense Interpretation
The problem of determining the correct sense of a term can involve matching a word to a concept in an ontology or controlled vocabulary in the given domain. For example, the UMLS identifies unique concepts, along with their variant and synonymous forms, and it would be straightforward to match the word *cough* in text to the concept cough (i.e. C0010200) in the UMLS. However, a word may have more than one sense, and the process of determining the correct sense is called **word sense disambiguation** (WSD). For example, *MS* could be mapped to C0026269, which corresponds to *mitral stenosis,* or to C0026769, which corresponds to *multiple sclerosis.* However, the underlying interpretation may not be in the UMLS, as in the sense *Ms* (the honorific title). WSD is much harder than syntactic disambiguation because there is no well-established notion of word sense, different lexicons or ontologies recognize different distinctions, and the space of word senses is substantially larger than that of syntactic categories. Words may be ambiguous within a particular domain, across domains, or in the natural language (e.g., English) in general. Abbreviations are notoriously ambiguous. The ambiguity problem is particularly troublesome in the biomolecular domain because biomolecular symbols in many model organism databases consist of three letters, and are ambiguous with other English words, and also with different gene symbols of different model organisms. For example, *nervous* and *to* are English words that are also the names of genes. When writing about a specific organism, authors use alias names that may correspond to different genes. For example,

in articles associated with the mouse, according to the Mouse Genome Database (MGD) (Blake et al. 2003), authors may use the term *fbp1* to denote different genes.

Semantic disambiguation of lexemes can be performed using similar rule-based or statistical methods described above for syntax. Rules can assign semantic types using contextual knowledge of other nearby words and their types. For example, *discharge from hospital* and *discharge from eye* can be disambiguated depending on whether the noun following *discharge* is an institution or a body location. However, statistical approaches are generally used to determine the most likely assignment of semantic types based on contextual information, such as surrounding words (Jurafsky and Martin 2009, pp 637–667). As with statistical methods for morphology and syntax, large amounts of training data are required to provide sufficient instances of the different senses for each ambiguous word. This is extremely labor intensive because it means that a large manually annotated corpus for each ambiguous word must be collected where optimally each sense occurs numerous times, although in certain cases automated annotation is possible.

8.5.4.3 Interpretation of Relations among Words
Similar to syntactic analysis of simple phrases, semantic analysis can also be achieved using regular expressions. An alternate, robust method for processing sentences with regular expressions, which is often employed in general, uses **cascading finite state automatas** (**FSAs**) (Hobbs et al. 1996). In this technique, a series of different FSAs are employed so that each performs a special tagging function. The tagged output of one FSA becomes the input to a subsequent FSA. For example, one FSA may perform tokenization and lexical lookup, another may perform partial parsing to identify syntactic phrases, such as noun phrases and verb phrases, the next may perform named entity recognition (NER), and the next may recognize semantic relations, determine the roles of the entities, and map the entities to a predicate-argument or frame-based structure. In some cases, the patterns for the semantic relations

will be based on a combination of syntactic phrases and their corresponding semantic classes, as shown below. The pattern for biomolecular interactions might then be represented using a combination of tags:

$$NP_{[GENE|PROT]} \cdot {}^* VP_{MFUN} \cdot {}^* NP_{[GENE|PROT]}$$

The advantage of cascading FSA systems is that they are relatively easy to adapt to different information extraction tasks because the FSAs that are domain independent (tokenizing and phrasal FSAs) remain the same while the domain-specific components (Semantic patterns) change with the domain and or the extraction task. These types of systems have been widely used in the 1990s to extract highly specific information, such as detection of terrorist attacks, identification of joint mergers, and changes in corporation management (Sundheim 1991, 1992, 1994, 1996, Grishman and Sundheim 1996). They are generally used to extract information from the literature, but they may not be accurate enough for clinical applications.

Complete parsing, similar to the methods used for syntactic parsing, can be used in systems that have a context-free semantic grammar. For example, the sentence *No increased tenderness* would be parsed correctly using the simple grammar shown in Fig. 8.4, where there is a finding that consists of a changephrase that has a negation (e.g. *no*) that modifies the change (e.g. *increased*), and the changephrase is followed by a symptom (e.g. *tenderness*). Therefore, *no* modifies the change and not the symptom. Note that ambiguity is possible in this grammar because a sentence such as *No/NEG increased/CHNG tenderness/SYMP* could be parsed by satisfying other rules. In an incorrect parse, the degreephrase (e.g. *no*) and the changephrase (e.g. *increased*) both modify *tenderness*; in this interpretation the symptom is negated and the change information is not.

8.5.5 Discourse

We focus in this section on one particular task as an example of discourse processing: automated resolution of referential expressions.

8.5.5.1 Automated Resolution of Referential Expressions

Coreference resolution can draw on both syntactic and semantic information in the text. Syntactic information for resolving referential expressions includes:

- Agreement of syntactic features between the referential phrase and potential referents
- Recency of potential referents (nearness to referential phrase)
- Syntactic position of potential referents (e.g. subject, direct object, object of preposition)
- The pattern of transitions of topics across the sentences

Syntactic features that aid the resolution include such distinctions as singular/plural, animate/inanimate, and subjective/objective/possessive. For example, pronouns in the text in Fig. 8.5 carry the following features: *he* (singular, animate, subjective), *his* (singular, animate, possessive) and *it* (singular, inanimate, subjective/objective). Animate pronouns (*he, she, her*) almost always refer humans. The inanimate pronoun *it* usually refers to things (e.g. *it had not invaded*), but sometimes does not refer to anything when it occurs in "cleft" constructions: *it was noted, it was decided to* and *it seemed likely that*.

Referential expressions are usually very close to their referents in the text. In *it had not invaded*, the pronoun refers to the immediately preceding noun phrase *area of tumor*. The pronoun in *it did partially occlude* has the same referent, but in this case there are two intervening nouns: *epithelium* or *trachea*. Thus, a rule that assigns pronouns to the most recent noun would work for the first case, but not for the second.

The syntactic position of a potential referent is an important factor. For example, a referent in subject position is a more likely candidate than the direct object, which in turn is more likely than an object of a preposition. In the fifth sentence of the text above, the pronoun *he* could refer to the patient or to the physician. The proper noun *Dr. Smith* is the more likely candidate, because it is the subject of the preceding sentence.

Centering theory accounts for reference by noting how the center (focus of attention) of each sentence changes across the discourse (Grosz et al. 1995). In our example text, the patient is the center of the first three sentences, the physician is the center of the fourth and fifth sentence, and the area of tumor is the center of the last sentence. In this approach, resolution rules attempt to minimize the number of changes in centers. Thus, in the above text it is preferable to resolve *he* in sentence five as the physician rather than the patient because it results in smoother transition of centers.

Semantic information for resolving referential expressions involves consideration of the semantic type of the expression, and how it relates to potential referents (Hahn et al. 1999):

- semantic type is the same as the potential referent
- semantic type is a subtype or a parent of the potential referent
- semantic type has a close semantic relationship with the potential referent

For example, in the example text, the definite noun phrase *the balloon* must be resolved. If the phrase *a balloon* occurred previously, this would be the most likely referent. Since there is no previous noun of similar type, it is necessary to establish a semantic relationship with a preceding noun. The word *dilation* is the best candidate because a balloon is a medical device used by that procedure.

8.5.6 Evaluation Metrics

Evaluating the performance of an NLP system is critical whether the NLP system is targeted for an end user directly or is part of a larger application. Evaluation generally involves obtaining a **reference standard** with which the system can be compared against. In the clinical domain, creating such reference standards can be a challenge, because of the need for anonymized patient information so the reference standard (also called gold standard) can be shared among researchers at different institutions. When a reference standard is created, it is important to further reliability and to reduce subjectivity and bias by relying on multiple experts, by measuring the inter-rater agreement, and by randomly selecting text instances (Friedman et al. 1998, Hripcsak and Wilcox 2002). There are basically two types of evaluation, **extrinsic** and **intrinsic**.

In an **extrinsic evaluation**, the NLP system is part of a bigger application that is intended to achieve a real-world task, and the aim of the evaluation is to measure performance of the overall task. Therefore, the output of the NLP system is not evaluated independently. A reference standard is generally created using domain experts, who manually perform the task by reading the text, or the reference standard may already exist from another study. For instance, an NLP system may be part of a clinical decision support system aimed at identifying patients with pneumonia based on textual radiology reports. A reference standard would be created consisting of radiology reports that would have been randomly selected and then reviewed manually as denoting or not denoting *pneumonia*. Domain experts are best to use to obtain a reference standard since they routinely read clinical reports and interpret the information in them. A substantial portion of the results of an extrinsic evaluation may be attributable to the decision support component, which generally will include reasoning based on the information extracted by the NLP system. For example, reasoning may be necessary in order to associate extracted findings, such as *infiltrate* and *consolidation*, with *pneumonia*. In such an evaluation, an error analysis would be needed to differentiate NLP errors from errors in the decision support component of the system.

In an **intrinsic evaluation**, the output of the NLP system is evaluated by comparing the output against a reference standard, which generally has been manually annotated so that it is deemed accurate. The extent of differences in results obtained by the NLP system and the reference standard are then computed. Evaluation may be performed for each component of the NLP system, or for the overall results. Depending on the evaluation design and NLP task, annotation generally requires linguistic expertise and may also require domain expertise. Therefore, an intrinsic evaluation that focuses on performance of the NLP system is helpful for advancing NLP development. However, generating the reference standard is generally time-consuming, and may not adequately reflect the information needed for a subsequent real-world application.

There are three basic quantitative measures used to assess performance in an extrinsic or intrinsic evaluation. They are all calculated from the number of **true positives** (TP), **true negatives** (TN), and **false negatives** (FN).

Recall is the percentage of results that should have been obtained according to the test set that actually were obtained by the system:

Recall = Number of correct results obtained by system (TP)/

Number of results specified in gold standard (TP + FN)

Precision is the percent of results that the system obtained that were actually correct according to the test set:

Precision = Number of correct results obtained by system (TP)/

Total number of results obtained by system (TP + FP)

There is usually a tradeoff between recall and precision, with higher precision usually being attainable at the expense of recall, and *vice versa*. The **F measure** is a combination of both measures and can be used to weigh the importance of one measure over the other by giving more weight to one. If both measures are equally important, the F measure is the **harmonic mean** of the two measures.

When reporting results, an **error analysis** provides much insight into ways to improve a system. This process involves determining reasons for errors in recall and in precision. In an extrinsic evaluation, some errors could be due to the NLP system and other errors could be due to the subsequent application component. Some NLP errors in recall (i.e. false negatives) could be due to failure of the NLP system to tokenize the text correctly, to recognize a word, to detect a relevant pattern, or to correctly interpret the meaning of a word or a structure correctly. Some errors in precision could be due to errors in interpreting the meaning of a word or structure or to loss of important information. Errors caused by the application component could be due to failure to access the extracted information properly or failure of the reasoning component.

8.6　Issues for NLP in Biomedicine and Health

Natural language processing is challenging for general language, but there are issues that are particularly germane to the domains of biomedicine and health. We list a few of them in this section.

8.6.1　Patient Privacy and Ethical Concerns

As an NLP system deals with patient information, its designers must remain cognizant of the privacy and ethical concerns entailed in handling protected health information. In the clinical domain for instance, the **Health Insurance Portability and Accountabiliy Act** (HIPAA; see Chap. 10) regulates the protection of patient-sensitive information (see Chap. 10 for a detailed description of privacy matters in the clinical domain). Online, patients provide much information about their own health in blogs and online communities. While there are no regulations in place concerning online patient-provided information, researchers have established guidelines for the ethical study and processing of patient-generated speech (Eysenbach and Till 2001).

8.6.2　Good System Performance

If the output of an NLP system is to be used to help manage and improve the quality of health care and to facilitate research, it must have high enough performance for the intended application. Evidently different applications require varying levels of performance; however, the performance must generally not be significantly worse than that of domain experts. This requirement means that before an NLP-based system can be used for a practical task, it must be evaluated carefully, both intrinsically and extrinsically, in the setting where the system will be used. For instance, if a system is designed for clinicians in the ICU, testing its use with primary care physicians might not be a reliable evaluation. This point is valid for the biological and health consumer domains as well (Caporaso et al. 2008).

8.6.3 System Interoperability

NLP-based systems are often part of larger applications. There must be seamless integration of the NLP component into its parent application. This point is valid for any domain, but becomes particularly relevant in the clinical domain, where NLP is typically part of the electronic record. In practice, the following might have to be ensured, depending on the particular task of the application:

- The system has to follow standards for interoperability among different health information technology systems, such as **Health Level 7** (**HL7**) and the **Clinical Document Architecture** (CDA; see Chap. 7). This is particularly important for information that pertains to a patient, but is not part of the notes per se. Similarly, the system has to be aware of the controlled terminologies in use in the institution (e.g. **SNOMED-CT** and **ICD-9-CM**; see Chap. 7), so that its input and output are understood by the clinical information system.
- The system has to be aware of the information storage strategies of the clinical information system. As of this date, there is no established structure across different institutions, and so care has to be given to understanding the structure of a particular institution in which the NLP system will be deployed. For instance, it is possible that different note types and reports are stored in different ways in the clinical information system, and the NLP system will have to acknowledge this in its workflow. Furthermore, within a given note, there might be institution-specific conventions concerning the overall format and use of abbreviations. Figure 8.8 shows portions of a cardiac catherization report. Some of the sections contain free text (i.e. procedures performed, comments, general conclusions), some consist of structured fields (i.e. height, weight) that are separated from each other by white space, and

Procedures performed: Right Heart Catheterization Pericardiocentesis

Complications: None
Medications given during procedure: None
Hemodynamic data
Height (cm): 180   Weight (kg): 74.0
Body surface area (sq. m): 1.93   Hemoglobin (gm/dL):
Heart rate: 102

Pressure (mmHg)

Sys	Dias	Mean	Sat	
RA	14	13	8	
RV	36	9	12	
PA	44	23	33	62%
PCW	25	30	21	

Conclusions: Post Operative Cardiac Transplant
Abnormal Hemodynamics
Pericardial Effusion
Successful Pericardiocentesis

General Comments:
  1600cc of serosanguinous fluid were drained from the pericardial sac with improvement in hemodynamics.

Fig. 8.8 A portion of a sample cardiac catherization report

some consist of tabular data (i.e. blood pressure). The NLP system has to be able to recognize and handle these different formats.

- The system has to generate output that can be stored in a **clinical data repository** (CDR) or **clinical data warehouse** (CDW). This is especially true for NLP systems that are deployed as part of an operational clinical application or research application. As for clinical information systems, there is no established database schema for the type of rich information found in clinical records. Depending on the type of NLP (i.e. information extraction vs. full syntactic parsing vs. semantic parsing), there might be some loss of information when storing the output of the NLP system in a database.

8.6.4 Misspellings and Typographical Errors

Clinicians, when typing free-text in the EHR, do so under time pressure and generally do not have the time to proofread their notes carefully.

In addition, they frequently use abbreviations (e.g. *HF* for *Hispanic female* or *heart failure*, *2/2* for *secondary to* or a date), many of which are non-standard and ambiguous. For patients and health consumers, when posting content online, misspellings, typographical errors, and non-standard abbreviations are pervasive like in the rest of the social Web. In a breast cancer online community, for instance, we found frequent spelling variations for the drug *tamoxifen* (e.g. *tamoxifin* and *tamaxifen*) as well as abbreviations. Ignoring these variations may cause an NLP system to lose or misinterpret information. At the same time, errors can be introduced when correcting the typos automatically. For instance, it is not trivial to correct *hyprtension* automatically without additional knowledge because it may refer to *hypertension* or *hypotension*. This type of error is troublesome not only for automated systems, but also for clinicians when reading a note, as this phenomenon is aggravated by the large amount of short, misspelled words in notes.

8.6.5   Expressiveness Vs. Ease of Access

Natural language is very expressive. There are often several ways to express a particular medical concept as well as numerous ways to express modifiers for that concept. For example, ways to express severity include *faint, mild, borderline, 1+, 3rd degree, severe, extensive, mild*, and *moderate*. This expressive power makes it challenging to build information extraction systems that capture all modifiers of a concept with high recall. Often, to complicate matters, modifiers can be composed or nested. For instance in the phrase "*no improvement in pneumonia,*" *improvement* is a change modifier that modifies the concept *pneumonia*, and *no* is a negation marker that modifies *improvement* (not *pneumonia*). In this situation, an information extraction system that detects changes concerned with pneumonia would have to look for primary findings associated with pneumonia, filter out cases not associated with a current episode, look for a change

modifier of the finding, and, if there is one, make sure there is no negation modifier on the change modifier. An alternative representation would facilitate retrieval by flattening the nesting. In this case, some information may be lost but ideally only information that is not critical. For example, *slightly improved* may not be clinically different from *improved* depending on the application. Since this type of information is fuzzy and imprecise, the loss of information may not be significant. However, the loss of a negation modifier would be significant, and those cases should be handled specially. Another such example concerns hedging, which frequently occurs in radiology reports as well as in scientific articles. This tradeoff between capturing the full expressive power of natural language and ease of access when extracting information influences design choices for an NLP system and depends on the overall task for which the system is built.

8.6.6   Reliance on Medical Knowledge and Reasoning

Whether in biomedical, clinical or health consumer texts, there is much implicit knowledge present in the text. In some systems, recovering the missing information can be important. For instance, the phrase "I have a temperature" as written by a patient online can mean I have a fever, but "I have a temperature of 98.6" means no fever. Inferring the presence of fever from the presence and/or value of a numerical modifier requires external medical knowledge. Similarly in the clinical domain, interpreting the findings extracted from a chest radiological report, or inferring that a patient is depressed based on the fact that an anti-depressant is prescribed (even though there is no explicit mention of depression in a note) requires extensive medical knowledge. Such knowledge can be quite complex. Ontologies contain some of this knowledge, encoded through entities and relations (e.g. parent–child, part of) between the entities. But the ontology may not be complete enough for particular tasks, both in the coverage of entities and relations, and such knowledge would have to be acquired. One way to do so is to leverage knowledge from experts and encode manual rules. For instance, a rule that detects a comorbidity of neoplastic disease based on information in a discharge summary, could consist of a Boolean combination of over 200 terms (Chuang et al. 2002). Another approach is to leverage machine-learning techniques and learn rules from examples of texts. In a supervised framework, for such rules to be learned, a large number of training and testing instances must be annotated. The cost (both from a financial and time standpoint) to annotate these instances depends on many factors, including the difficulty of the task and level of medical expertise needed to carry out accurate annotation, the degree of subjectivity entailed in the task, the number of instances needed to annotated and the easy access to annotators. Whether medical knowledge should be encoded directly or learned through examples is a question that is beyond the focus of this chapter. Thus far, the most promising approaches in NLP are hybrid ones that combine existing medical knowledge with knowledge mined from text.

8.6.7 Domains and Subdomains

As discussed earlier in this chapter, the fact that texts belong to a particular domain, be it clinical, biological or related to health consumers, allows us to capture domain-specific characteristics in the lexicon, the grammar, and the discourse structure. Thus, the more specific the domain of a text, the more knowledge can be encoded to help its processing, but the NLP system would then be very limited and specialized. For instance, in the domain of online patient discourse, patients discussing breast cancer among their peers online rely on a very different set of terms than caregivers of children on the autism spectrum. One could develop a lexicon for each subdomain, e.g. online breast cancer patients and online autism caregivers. But maintaining separate lexicons can be inefficient and error prone, since there can be a significant amount of overlap among terms across

subdomains. Conversely, if a single lexicon is developed for all subdomains, ambiguity can increase as terms can have different meanings in different subdomains. For example, in the emergency medicine domain *shock* will more likely refer to a procedure used for resuscitating a patient, or to a critical condition brought about by a drop in blood flow, whereas in psychiatry notes it will more likely denote an emotional response or electric shock therapy. Deciding on whether to model a domain as a whole or to focus on its subdomains independently of each other is a tradeoff. Careful determination of the use cases of a system can help determine the best choice for the system.

8.6.7.1 Dynamic Nature of Biomedical and Health Domains

Change is a natural phenomenon of human language. With time, new concepts enter the language and obsolete terms fall out of use. The biomedical and health domains are highly dynamic in the influx of new terms (e.g. new drug names, but also sometimes new disease names, like SARS and H1N1). The biomolecular domain is particularly dynamic. For example, for the week ending July 20, 2003, the Mouse Genome Informatics Website (Blake et al. 2003) reported 104 name changes related to the mouse alone. If the other organisms being actively sequenced were also considered, the number of name changes during that week would be much larger. Related to the language change is the sheer number of entities relevant to the biomolecular domain. Table 8.4 shows the approximate numbers for some different types of entities in the biomolecular domain. The number of entities is actually larger because not all types are shown in the table (i.e. small molecules, cell lines, genes and proteins of all organisms). Having such a large number of names means the NLP system must have a very large knowledge base of names or be capable of dynamically recognizing the type by considering the context. When entities are dynamically recognized without use of a knowledge source, identifying them within an established nomenclature system is not possible.

Table 8.4 The approximate number of some types of biomolecular entities

Type of entity	Number
Gene	3.5×10^4 (human only)
Protein	$>10^5$ (human only)
Cell type	10^6
Species	10^7

8.6.8 Polysemy

Biomedical and health terms are often ambiguous. This is particularly pervasive in the biomolecular domain because of the high number of acronyms and abbreviations. Short symbols consisting of two to three letters are frequently used that correspond to names of biomolecular entities. Since the number of different combinations consisting of only a few letters is relatively small, individual names often correspond to different meanings. For example, *to*, a very frequent English word, corresponds to two different Drosophila genes and to the mouse gene *tryptophan 2,3-dioxygenase*. *To further complicate matters*, the names of genes in different model organism groups are established independently of each other, leading to names that are the same but which represent different entities. The ambiguity problem is actually worse if the entire domain is considered. For example, *cad* represents over 11 different biomolecular entities in Drosophila and the mouse but it also represents the clinical concept *coronary artery disease*. Another contributing factor to the ambiguity problem is due to the different naming conventions for the organisms. These conventions were not developed for NLP purposes but for consistency within individual databases. For example, Flybase states that "Gene names must be concise. They should allude to the gene's function, mutant phenotype or other relevant characteristic. The name must be unique and not have been used previously for a Drosophila gene." This rule is fairly loose and leads to ambiguities.

8.6.9 Synonymy

Complementary to the phenomenon of polysemy, there are often terms that are different variations of the same concepts. For instance, the term *blood*

sugar is often used by health consumers to refer to a *glucose measurement*, but it is used rarely if ever in the clinical literature or in clinical notes. Synonymy occurs across domains, but is also present within a single domain. In the biomolecular domain, for instance, names are created within the model organism database communities, but they are not necessarily exactly the same as the names used by authors when writing journal articles. There are many ways authors vary names (particularly long names), which leads to difficulties in named entity recognition. This is also true in the medical domain but the problem is exacerbated in the biomolecular domain because of the frequent use of punctuations and other special types of symbols. Some of the more common types of variations are due to punctuations and use of blanks (*bmp-4*, *bmp 4*, *bmp4*), numerical variations (*syt4*, *syt IV*), variations containing Greek letters (*iga*, *ig alpha*), and word order differences (*phosphatidylinositol 3-kinase, catalytic, alpha polypeptide, catalytic alpha polypeptide phosphatidylinositol 3-kinase*). Low-level text processing can resolve some of these types of synonymy.

8.6.10 Complexity of Biological Language

The semantic interpretation of biological language is complex. In clinical text, the important source of information typically occurs in noun phrases that consist of descriptive information that corresponds to named entities and their modifiers. In biomolecular text, important information often involves interactions that are highly nested, corresponding to verb phrases, which are more complex structures than noun phrases and are often highly nested. Although syntactically the interaction may occur as a noun, it is generally a nominalized verb, and thus, has arguments that are important to capture along with their order (e.g. *Raf-1 activates Mek-1* has a different meaning than *Mek-1 activates Raf-1*). In addition, the argument may also be another interaction. Thus a typical sentence usually contains several nested interactions. For example, the sentence "*Bad phosphorylation induced by interleukin-3 (il-3) was inhibited by specific inhibitors of phosphoinositide 3-kinase*

Table 8.5 *Nested interactions extracted from the sentence* Bad phosphorylation induced by interleukin-3 (il-3) was inhibited by specific inhibitors of phosphoinositide 3-kinase (pi 3-kinase)

Interaction	Argument 1 (agent)	Argument 2 (target)	Interaction id
Phosphorylate	?	Bad	1
Induce	Interleukin-1	1	2
Inhibit	?	Phosphoinositide 3-kinase	3
Inhibit	3	1	

A '?' denotes that the argument was not present in the sentence

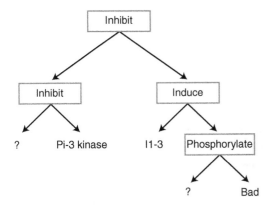

Fig. 8.9 A tree showing the nesting of biomolecular interactions that are in the sentence "*Bad phosphorylation induced by interleukin-3 (il-3) was inhibited by specific inhibitors of phosphoinositide 3-kinase (pi 3-kinase)*"

(*pi 3-kinase)*" consists of four interactions (and also two parenthesized expressions specifying abbreviated forms). The interaction and the arguments are illustrated in Table 8.5. The nested relations can be illustrated more clearly as a tree (see Fig. 8.9). Notice that the arguments of some interactions are also interactions (i.e. the second argument of *induce* is *phosphorylate*). Also note that an argument that is not specified in the sentence is represented by a "?" in the figure.

8.6.11 Interactions among Linguistic Levels

While the earlier sections of this chapter have introduced each linguistic level on its own, it should be clear through the many examples presented throughout the chapter that processing of language is not as simple as applying a pipeline of independent modules- one to determine tokens, one to assign part-of-speech tags to tokens and to parse the syntax, one to interpret the meaning of a sentence, one to resolve the discourse-level characteristics of the text, and so on. In reality, all linguis-

tic levels influence each other. Low-level decisions about how to tokenize a string impact named-entity recognition; determining which sense to attribute to a named entity depends on its place in the syntactic tree, the pragmatics of the text, and its place in the discourse structure. Determining how to model these interactions is one of the primary open research questions of natural language processing.

8.7   Resources for NLP in Biomedicine and Health

One of the ways for the field to make progress is for different teams of researchers to share their datasets, tools and resources. Shared datasets allow different research teams to test and compare their systems on the same data. Annotated shared datasets are critical, as they allow teams to train their systems as well. As such, they are very valuable to the community. In recent years, there has been a strong push in the biological and clinical NLP communities to create publicly available resources and tools, and to conduct community challenges. We present a few of them here but, because of the explosion of resources in the field, this list is bound to be obsolete. We therefore encourage the reader to check the literature and the Web for the latest.

8.7.1   Databases and Lexicons

- UMLS (Including the Metathesaurus, Semantic Network, the Specialist Lexicon) – Can be used as a knowledge base and resource for a lexicon. The Specialist lexicon provides detailed syntactic knowledge for words and phrases, and includes a comprehensive medical vocabulary. It also provides a set of tools to assist in NLP, such as a lexical variant generator, an index of words corresponding to UMLS terms, a file of derivational variants (e.g.

abdominal, abdomen), spelling variants (e.g. *fetal, foetal*), and a set of neoclassical forms (e.g. *heart, cardio*). The UMLS Metathesaurus provides the concept identifiers, while the Semantic Network specifies the semantic categories for the concepts. The UMLS also contains the terminology associated with various languages (e.g. French, German, Russian). The UMLS is the union of several vocabularies that are particularly useful for NLP, such as SNOMED-CT, LOINC, and MeSH.

- MedDRA and RxNorm are terminologies specific to adverse event terminology and medications. They are particularly helpful in the clinical domain, in pharmacovigilance and in pharmacogenomics.
- Biological databases. These include Model Organism Databases, such as Mouse Genome Informatics (Blake et al. 2003), the Flybase Database (FlyBase Consortium 2003), the WormBase Database (Harris et al. 2003), and the *Saccharomyces* Database (Issel-Tarver et al. 2001), as well as more general databases GenBank (Benson et al. 2003), Swiss-Prot (Boeckmann et al. 2003), LocusLink (Pruitt and Maglott 2001), and the Gene Ontology (GO 2003).

8.7.2 Corpora

- PubMed Central[2] provides full-text articles in biomedicine and health. PubMED provides abstracts and useful meta-information, such as MeSH indexes, and journal types.
- The MIMIC II database collects de-identified data about patients in the intensive care unit (Saeed et al. 2002). Along with ICU-specific structured data and times series, there are nursing notes, progress notes and reports available.
- The Pittsburgh Note Repository[3] provides de-identified clinical notes of many different types. Some of the notes have been annotated with specific semantic information as part of community challenges.

[2] http://www.ncbi.nlm.nih.gov/pmc (Accessed 4/26/13).
[3] http://www.dbmi.pitt.edu/nlpfront. (Accessed 4/26/13).

8.7.3 Community Challenges and Annotated Corpora

In biology, the GENIA corpus contains articles annotated with syntactic, semantic and discourse information (Kim et al. 2003). The BioCreAtIvE challenges have provided annotated articles with biologically relevant named-entities and entity-fact associations, such as protein-functional term association (Hirschman et al. 2005). The BioScope corpus provides texts annotated with hedging and negation information (Vincze et al. 2008). As part of yearly community challenges in the clinical domain, there are several corpora currently available with different types of annotations. The earliest is a collection of radiology reports with ICD-9-CM codes (Pestian et al. 2007). The i2b2 community challenges have provided clinical notes annotated with smoking status (Uzuner et al. 2008), obesity and co-morbidities (Uzuner 2009), medications mentions (Uzuner et al. 2010), assertions (Uzuner et al. 2011), and more recently co-references. There are several corpora specific to word sense disambiguation (WSD) for different semantic classes. The National Library of Medicine provides an annotated WSD dataset for 50 frequently occurring ambiguous terms based on the 1998 version of MEDLINE (Weeber et al. 2001).

8.7.3.1 Annotation Schema
In the same way terminologies like the UMLS provide an established organization for concepts in the language, community efforts have just started to create established representations for certain aspects of information, such as the different modifiers of concepts and the relations among concepts that can occur in texts. There had been early efforts by a large number of researchers called *The Canon group* to create such standard (Evans et al. 1994). That effort resulted in a common model for radiological reports of the chest (Friedman et al. 1995), but the model was not actually utilized by the different researchers.

8.7.3.2 Tools
Since the NLP field is currently a very active area of research, and new tools are continually

being developed; we point the reader to ORBIT (Online Registry of Biomedical Informatics Tools[4]). It provides a repository of tools, maintained by the community, and is a good place to get access to the most recent tools. In the general NLP domain, there are a few valuable suites of tools available, including NLTK,[5] LingPipe,[6] and OpenNLP.[7] Finally, UIMA[8] is a general framework for text analysis that is gaining popularity in NLP.

general domain, we refer the reader to the above three textbooks.

Kübler, S., McDonald, R., & Nivre, J. (2009). *Dependency parsing. Synthesis lecture on human language technology.* Morgan & Claypool. This book provides an in-depth review of dependency parsing in the general domain.

Palmer, M., Gilder, D., & Xue, N. (2010). *Semantic role labeling. Synthesis lectures in human language technology.* Morgan & Claypool. This book provides an in-depth discussion of semantic parsing.

Suggested Readings

Harris, Z., Gottfried, M., Ryckmann, T., Mattick, P., Jr., Daladier, A., Harris, T. N., & Harris, S. (1989). *The form of information in science: Analysis of an immunology sublanguage.* Reidel/Dordrecht: Boston Studies in the Philosophy of Science. This book offers an in-depth description of methods for analyzing the languages of biomedical science. It provides detailed descriptions of linguistic structures found in science writing and the mapping of the information to a compact formal representation. The book includes an extensive analysis of 14 full-length research articles from the field of immunology, in English and in French.

Sager, N., Friedman, C., & Lyman, M. S. (1987). *Medical language processing: Computer management of narrative data.* New York: Addison-Wesley. This book describes early techniques used by the Linguistic String Project, a pioneering language processing effort in the biomedical field, explaining how biomedical text can be automatically analyzed and the relevant content summarized.

Jurafsky, D., & Martin, J. H. (2009). *Speech and language processing. An introduction to natural language processing, computational linguistics and speech recognition.* Upper Saddle River: Prentice Hall.

Manning, C., Raghavan, P., & Schütze, H. (2008). *Introduction to information retrieval.* New York: Cambridge University Press.

Manning, C., & Schütze, H. (1999). *Foundations of statistical natural language processing.* Cambridge, MA: MIT Press. NLP is a very active field of research in the general domain. Many of the applications and techniques described in this chapter are investigated in other domains. For a review of NLP methods in the

Questions for Discussion

1. Develop a regular expression to regularize the tokens in lines four to nine of the cardiac catheterization report shown in Fig. 8.8 (*Complications* through *Heart Rate*).

2. Create a lexicon for the last seven lines of the cardiac catheterization report shown in Fig. 8.8 (*Conclusions* through the last sentence). For each word, determine all the parts of speech that apply, using the tags in Table 8.1. Which words have more than one part of speech? Choose eight clinically relevant words in that section of the report, and suggest appropriate semantic categories for them that would be consistent with the SNOMED-CT terminology and with the UMLS semantic network.

3. Using the grammar in Fig. 8.3, draw a parse tree for the last sentence of cardiac catheterization report shown in Fig. 8.8.

4. Using the grammar in Fig. 8.4, draw parse trees for the following sentences: *no increase in temperature; low grade fever; marked improvement in pain; not breathing.* (Hint: some lexemes have more than one word.)

5. Identify all the referential expressions in the text below and determine the correct referent for each. Assume that the compute attempts to identify referents by finding the most recent noun phrase. How well does this resolution rule work? Suggest a more effective rule.

The patient went to receive the AV fistula on December 4. However, he refuses transfusion. In the operating room it was determined upon initial incision that there was too much edema to successfully complete the operation and the incision was closed with staples. It was well tolerated by the patient.

6. In the two following scenarios, an out-of-the-shelf NLP system that identifies terms and normalizes them against UMLS concepts, is applied to a large corpus of texts. In the first scenario, the corpus consists of patient notes. Looking at the frequency of different concepts, you notice that there is a large number of patients with the concept C0019682 (HIV) present, much larger than the regular incidence of HIV in the population reported in the literature. In the second scenario, the corpus consists of full-text biology articles published in PubMED Central. Looking at the frequency of different concepts, you notice that the failed axon connection (fax) gene is one of the most frequently mentioned genes in your corpus. Describe how you would check the validity of these results. For both cases, discuss what could explain the high frequency counts.

Biomedical Imaging Informatics

9

Daniel L. Rubin, Hayit Greenspan,
and James F. Brinkley

After reading this chapter, you should know the answers to these questions:

- What makes images a challenging type of data to be processed by computers when compared to non-image clinical data?
- Why are there many different imaging modalities, and by what major two characteristics do they differ?
- How are visual and knowledge content in images represented computationally? How are these techniques similar to representation of non-image biomedical data?
- What sort of applications can be developed to make use of the semantic image content made accessible using the Annotation and Image Markup model?
- What are four different types of image processing methods? Why are such methods

assembled into a pipeline when creating imaging applications?
- What is an imaging modality with high spatial resolution? What is a modality that provides functional information? Why are most imaging modalities not capable of providing both?
- What is the goal in performing segmentation in image analysis? Why is there more than one segmentation method?
- What are two types of quantitative information in images? What are two types of semantic information in images? How might this information be used in medical applications?
- What is the difference between image registration and image fusion? What are examples of each?

9.1 Introduction

Imaging plays a central role in the health care process. The field is crucial not only to health care, but also to medical communication and education, as well as in research. In fact much of our recent progress, particularly in diagnosis, can be traced to the availability of increasingly sophisticated imaging techniques that not only show the structure of the body in incredible detail, but also show the function of the tissues within the body.

D.L. Rubin, MD, MS (✉)
Departments of Radiology and Medicine, Stanford University, 1201 Welch Road, P285,
Stanford 94305, CA, USA
e-mail: dlrubin@yahoo.com

H. Greenspan, PhD
Department of Biomedical Engineering, Faculty of Engineering, Tel-Aviv University,
Tel-Aviv 69978, Israel
e-mail: hayit@eng.tau.ac.il

J.F. Brinkley, MD, PhD
Departments of Biological Structure, Biomedical Education and Medical Education, Computer Science and Engineering, University of Washington, 357420,
Seattle 98195, WA, USA
e-mail: brinkley@u.washington.edu

This chapter is adapted from an earlier version in the third edition authored by James F. Brinkley and Robert A. Greenes.

E.H. Shortliffe, J.J. Cimino (eds.), *Biomedical Informatics*,
DOI 10.1007/978-1-4471-4474-8_9, © Springer-Verlag London 2014

Although there are many types (or modalities) of imaging equipment, the images the modalities produce are nearly always acquired in or converted to digital form. The evolution of imaging from analog, film-based acquisition to digital format has been driven by the necessities of cost reduction, efficient throughput, and workflow in managing and viewing an increasing proliferation in the number of images produced per imaging procedure (currently hundreds or even thousands of images). At the same time, having images in digital format makes them amenable to image processing methodologies for enhancement, analysis, display, storage, and even enhanced interpretation.

Because of the ubiquity of images in biomedicine, the increasing availability of images in digital form, the rise of high-powered computer hardware and networks, and the commonality of image processing solutions, digital images have become a core data type that must be considered in many biomedical informatics applications. Therefore, this chapter is devoted to a basic understanding of the unique aspects of images as a core data type and the unique aspects of imaging from an informatics perspective. Chapter 20, on the other hand, describes the use of images and image processing in various applications, particularly those in radiology since that field places the greatest demands on imaging methods.

The topics covered by this chapter and Chap. 20 comprise the growing discipline of biomedical imaging informatics (Kulikowski 1997), a subfield of biomedical informatics (see Chap. 1) that has arisen in recognition of the common issues that pertain to all image modalities and applications once the images are converted to digital form. Biomedical imaging informatics is a dynamic field, recently evolving from focusing purely on image processing to broader informatics topics such as representing and processing the semantic contents (Rubin and Napel 2010). At the same time, imaging informatics shares common methodologies and challenges with other domains in biomedical informatics. By trying to understand these common issues, we can develop general solutions that can be applied to all images, regardless of the source.

The major topics in biomedical imaging informatics include image acquisition, image content representation, management/storage of images, image processing, and image interpretation/computer reasoning (Fig. 9.1). **Image acquisition** is the process of generating images from the modality and converting them to digital form if they are not intrinsically digital. **Image content representation** makes the information in images accessible to machines for processing. **Image management/storage** includes methods for storing, transmitting, displaying, retrieving, and organizing images. **Image processing** comprises methods to enhance, segment, visualize, fuse, or analyze the images. **Image interpretation/computer reasoning** is the process by which the individual viewing the image renders an impression of the medical significance of the results of imaging study, potentially aided by computer methods. Chapter 20 is primarily concerned with information systems for image management and storage, whereas this chapter concentrates on these other core topics in biomedical imaging informatics.

An important concept when thinking about imaging from an informatics perspective is that images are an *unstructured data type*; as such, while machines can readily manage the raw image data in terms of storage/retrieval, they cannot easily access image contents (recognize the type of image, annotations made on the image, or anatomy or abnormalities within the image). In this regard, biomedical imaging informatics shares much in common with natural language processing (NLP; Chap. 8). In fact, as the methods of computationally representing and processing images is presented in this chapter, parallels to NLP should be considered, since there is synergy from an informatics perspective.

As in NLP, a major purpose of the methods of imaging informatics is to extract particular information; in biomedical informatics the goal is often to extract information about the structure of the body and to collect features that will be useful for characterizing abnormalities based on morphological alterations. In fact, imaging provides detailed and diverse information very useful for characterizing disease, providing an "imaging

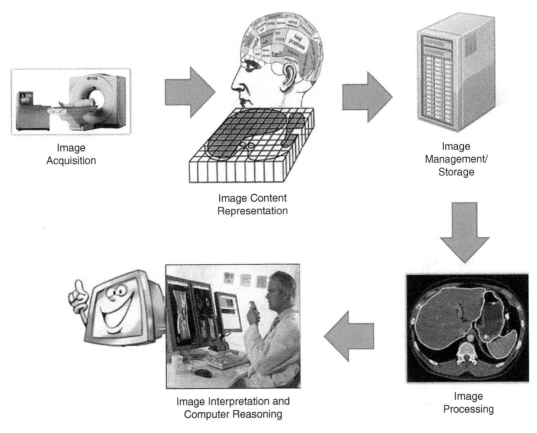

Image Acquisition

Image Content Representation

Image Management/ Storage

Image Interpretation and Computer Reasoning

Image Processing

Fig. 9.1 The major topics in biomedical imaging informatics follow a workflow of activities and tasks commencing with include image acquisition, followed by image content representation, management/storage of images, image processing, and image interpretation/computer reasoning

phenotype" useful for characterizing disease, since "a picture is worth a thousand words.[1]" However, to overcome the challenges posed by the unstructured image data type, recent work is applying semantic methods from biomedical informatics to images to make their content explicit for machine processing (Rubin and Napel 2010). Many of the topics in this chapter therefore involve how to represent, extract and characterize the information that is present in images, such as anatomy and abnormalities. Once that task is completed, useful applications that process the image contents can be developed, such as image search and decision support to assist with image interpretation.

While we seek generality in discussing biomedical imaging informatics, many examples in this chapter are taken from a few selected domains such as brain imaging, which is part of the growing field of **neuroinformatics** (Koslow and Huerta 1997). Though our examples are specific, we attempt to describe the topics in generic terms so that the reader can recognize parallels to other imaging domains and applications.

9.2   Image Acquisition

In general, there are two different strategies in imaging the body: (1) delineate *anatomic structure* (anatomic/structural imaging), and (2) determine *tissue composition or function* (functional imaging) (Fig. 9.2). In reality, one does not

---

[1] Frederick Barnard, "One look is worth a thousand words," Printers' Ink, December, 1921.

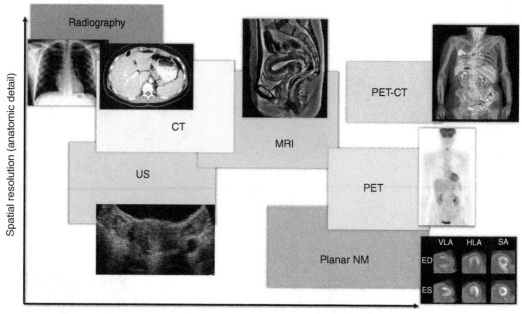

Fig. 9.2 The various radiology imaging methods differ according to two major axes of information of images, spatial resolution (anatomic detail) and functional infor- mation depicted (which represents the tissue composi- tion—e.g., normal or abnormal). A sample of the more common imaging modalities is shown

choose between anatomic and functional imag- ing; many modalities provide information about both morphology and function. However, in gen- eral, each imaging modality is characterized pri- marily as being able to render high-resolution images with good contrast resolution (anatomic imaging) or to render images that depict tissue function (functional imaging).

imaging, recognizing tissue function (e.g., tissue ischemia, neoplasm, inflammation, etc.) is not the goal, though this is crucial to functional imag- ing and to patient diagnosis. In most cases, imaging will be done using a combination of methods or modalities to derive both structural/ anatomic information as well as functional information.

9.2.1 Anatomic (Structural) Imaging

Imaging the structure of the body has been and continues to be the major application of medical imaging, although, as described in Sect. 9.2.2, functional imaging is a very active area of research. The goal of anatomic imaging is to accurately depict the structure of the body—the size and shape of organs—and to visualize abnor- malities clearly. Since the goal in anatomic imag- ing is to depict and understand the structure of anatomic entities accurately, high spatial resolu- tion is an important requirement of the imaging method (Fig. 9.2). On the other hand, in anatomic

9.2.2 Functional Imaging

Many imaging techniques not only show the structure of the body, but also the function, where for imaging purposes function can be inferred by observing changes of structure over time. In recent years this ability to image function has greatly accelerated. For example, ultrasound and angiography are widely used to show the func- tioning of the heart by depicting wall motion, and ultrasound Doppler can image both normal and disturbed blood flow (Mehta et al. 2000). Molecular imaging (Sect. 9.2.3) is increasingly able to depict the expression of particular genes superimposed on structural images, and thus can also be seen as a form of functional imaging.

A particularly important application of functional imaging is for understanding the cognitive activity in the brain. It is now routinely possible to put a normal subject in a scanner, to give the person a cognitive task, such as counting or object recognition, and to observe which parts of the brain light up. This unprecedented ability to observe the functioning of the living brain opens up entirely new avenues for exploring how the brain works.

Functional brain imaging modalities can be classified as *image-based* or *non-image based*. In both cases it is taken as axiomatic that the functional data must be mapped to the individual subject's anatomy, where the anatomy is extracted from structural images using techniques described in the previous sections. Once mapped to anatomy, the functional data can be integrated with other functional data from the same subject, and with functional data from other subjects whose anatomy has been related to a template or probabilistic atlas. Techniques for generating, mapping and integrating functional data are part of the field of Functional Brain Mapping, which has become very active in the past few years, with several conferences (Organization for Human Brain Mapping 2001) and journals (Fox 2001; Toga et al. 2001) devoted to the subject.

9.2.2.1 Image-Based Functional Brain Imaging

Image-based functional data generally come from scanners that generate relatively low-resolution volume arrays depicting spatially-localized activation. For example, **positron emission tomography** (PET) (Heiss and Phelps 1983; Aine 1995; Alberini et al. 2011) and **magnetic resonance spectroscopy** (MRS) (Ross and Bluml 2001) reveal the uptake of various metabolic products by the functioning brain; and **functional magnetic resonance imaging** (fMRI) reveals changes in blood oxygenation that occur following neural activity (Aine 1995). The raw intensity values generated by these techniques must be processed by sophisticated statistical algorithms to sort out how much of the observed

intensity is due to cognitive activity and how much is due to background noise.

As an example, one approach to fMRI imaging is language mapping (Corina et al. 2000). The subject is placed in the **magnetic resonance imaging** (MRI) scanner and told to silently name objects shown at 3-s intervals on a head-mounted display. The actual objects ("on" state) are alternated with nonsense objects ("off" state), and the fMRI signal is measured during both the on and the off states. Essentially the **voxel** values at the off (or control) state are subtracted from those at the on state. The difference values are tested for significant difference from non-activated areas, then expressed as t-values. The voxel array of t-values can be displayed as an image.

A large number of alternative methods have been and are being developed for acquiring and analyzing functional data (Frackowiak et al. 1997). The output of most of these techniques is a low-resolution 3-D image volume in which each voxel value is a measure of the amount of activation for a given task. The low-resolution volume is then mapped to anatomy guided by a high-resolution structural MR dataset, using one of the linear registration techniques described in Sect. 9.4.7.

Many of these and other techniques are implemented in the SPM program (Friston et al. 1995), the AFNI program (Cox 1996), the Lyngby toolkit (Hansen et al. 1999), and several commercial programs such as Medex (Sensor Systems Inc. 2001) and Brain Voyager (Brain Innovation B.V. 2001). The FisWidgets project at the University of Pittsburgh is developing an approach that allows customized creation of graphical user interfaces in an integrated desktop environment (Cohen 2001). A similar effort (VoxBox) is underway at the University of Pennsylvania (Kimborg and Aguirre 2002).

The ultimate goal of functional neuroimaging is to observe the actual electrical activity of the neurons as they perform various cognitive tasks. fMRI, MRS and PET do not directly record electrical activity. Rather, they record the results of electrical activity, such as (in the case of fMRI) the oxygenation of blood supplying the active neurons. Thus, there is a delay from the time of activity to the measured response. In other words these techniques have relatively poor temporal resolution (Sect. 9.2.4). **Electroencephalography** (EEG) or **magnetoencephalography** (MEG), on the other hand, are more direct measures of electrical activity since they measure the electromagnetic fields generated by the electrical activity of the neurons. Current EEG and MEG methods involve the use of large arrays of scalp sensors, the output of which are processed in a similar way to CT in order to localize the source of the electrical activity inside the brain. In general this "source localization problem" is under-constrained, so information about brain anatomy obtained from MRI is used to provide further constraints (George et al. 1995).

9.2.3 Imaging Modalities

There are many different approaches that have been developed to acquire images of the body. A proliferation in imaging modalities reflects the fact that there is no single perfect imaging modality; no single imaging technique satisfies all the desiderata for depicting the broad variety of types of pathology, some of which are better seen on some modalities than on others. The primary difference among the imaging modalities is the energy source used to generate the images. In radiology, nearly every type of energy in the electromagnetic spectrum has been used, in addition to other physical phenomena such as sound and heat. We describe the more common methods according to the type of energy used to create the image.

9.2.3.1 Light

The earliest medical images used visible light to create photographs, either of gross anatomic structures or, if a microscope was used, of histological specimens. Light is still an important source for creation of images, and in fact optical imaging has seen a resurgence of interest and application for areas such as molecular imaging (Weissleder and Mahmood 2001; Ray 2011) and imaging of brain activity on the exposed surface of the cerebral cortex (Pouratian et al. 2003).

Visible light is the basis for an emerging modality called "optical imaging" and has promising applications such as cancer imaging (Solomon, Liu et al. 2011). Visible light, however, does not allow us to see more than a short distance beneath the surface of the body; thus other modalities are used for imaging structures deep inside the body.

9.2.3.2 X-Rays

X-rays were first discovered in 1895 by Wilhelm Conrad Roentgen, who was awarded the 1901 Nobel Prize in Physics for this achievement. The discovery caused worldwide excitement, especially in the field of medicine; by 1900, there already were several medical radiological societies. Thus, the foundation was laid for a new branch of medicine devoted to imaging the structure and function of the body (Kevles 1997).

Radiography is the primary modality used in radiology departments today, both to record a static image (Fig. 9.3) as well as to produce a real-time view of the patient (fluoroscopy) or a movie (cine). Both film and fluoroscopic screens were used initially for recording X-ray images, but the fluoroscopic images were too faint to be used clinically. By the 1940s, however, television and image-intensifier technologies were developed to produce clear real-time fluorescent

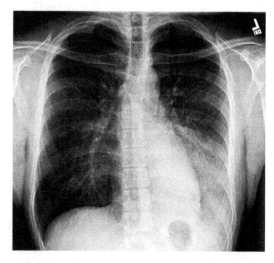

Fig. 9.3 A radiograph of the chest (Chest X-ray) taken in the frontal projection. The image is shown as if the patient is facing the viewer. This patient has abnormal density in the left lower lobe

images. Today, a standard procedure for many types of examinations is to combine real-time television monitoring of X-ray images with the creation of selected higher resolution film images. Until the early 1970s, film and fluoroscopy were the only X-ray modalities available. Recently, nearly all radiology departments have shifted away from acquiring radiographic images on film (analog images) to using digital radiography (Korner et al. 2007) to acquire digital images.

X-ray imaging is a projection technique; an X-ray beam—one form of ionizing radiation—is projected from an X-ray source through a patient's body (or other object) onto an X-ray array detector (a specially coated cassette that is scanned by a computer to capture the image in digital form), or film (to produce an non-digital image). Because an X-ray beam is differentially absorbed by the various body tissues based on the thickness and atomic number of the tissues, the X-rays produce varying degrees of brightness and darkness on the radiographic image. The differential amounts of brightness and darkness on the image are referred to as "image contrast;" differential contrast among structures on the image is the basis for recognizing anatomic structures. Since the image in radiography is a projection, radiographs show a superposition of all the structures traversed by the X-ray beam.

Computed radiography (CR) is an imaging technique that directly creates digital radiographs from the imaging procedure. Storage phosphor replaces film by substituting a reusable phosphor plate in a standard film cassette. The exposed plate is processed by a reader system that scans the image into digital form, erases the plate, and packages the cassette for reuse. An important advantage of CR systems is that the cassettes are of standard size, so they can be used in any equipment that holds film-based cassettes (Horii 1996). More recently, **Digital Radiography** (DR) uses charge-coupled device (CCD) arrays to capture the image directly.

Radiographic images have very high spatial resolution because a high photon flux is used to produce the images, and a high resolution detector (film or digital image array) that captures many line pairs per unit area is used. On the

other hand, since the contrast in images is due to differences in tissue density and atomic number, the amount of functional information that can be derived from radiographic images is limited (Fig. 9.2). Radiography is also limited by relatively poor contrast resolution (compared with other modalities such as **computed tomography** (CT) or MRI), their use of ionizing radiation, the challenge of spatial localization due to projection ambiguity, and their limited ability to depict physiological function. As described below, newer imaging modalities have been developed to increase contrast resolution, to eliminate the need for X-rays, and to improve spatial localization. A benefit of radiographic images is that they can be generated in real time (fluoroscopy) and can be produced using portable devices.

Computed Tomography (CT) is an important imaging method that uses X-ray imaging to produce cross sectional and volumetric images of the body (Lee 2006). Similar to radiography, X-rays are projected through the body onto an array of detectors; however, the beam and detectors rotate around the patient, making numerous views at different angles of rotation. Using computer reconstruction algorithms, an estimate of absolute density at each point (volume element or **voxel**) in the body is computed. Thus, the CT image is a computed image (Fig. 9.4); CT did not become practical for generating high quality images until the advent of powerful computers

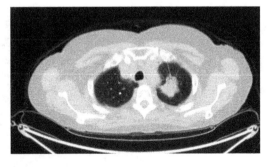

Fig. 9.4 A CT image of the upper chest. CT images are slices of a body plane; in this case, a cross sectional (axial) image of the chest. Axial images are viewed from below the patient, so that the patient's left is on viewer's right. This image shows a cancer mass in the left upper lobe of the lung

and development of computer-based reconstruction techniques, which represent one of the most spectacular applications of computers in all of medicine (Buxton 2009). The spatial resolution of images is not as high in CT as it is in radiography, however, due to the computed nature of the images, the contrast resolution and ability to derive functional information of tissues in the body is superior for CT than for radiography (Fig. 9.2).

9.2.3.3 Ultrasound

A common energy source used to produce images is **ultrasound**, which developed from research performed by the Navy during World War II in which sonar was used to locate objects of interest in the ocean. Ultrasonography uses pulses of high-frequency sound waves rather than ionizing radiation to image body structures (Kremkau 2006). The basis of image generation is due to a property of all objects called acoustical impedance. As sound waves encounter different types of tissues in a patient's body (particularly interfaces where there is a chance in acoustical impedance), a portion of the wave is reflected and a portion of the sound beam (which is now attenuated) continues to traverse into deeper tissues. The time required for the echo to return is proportional to the distance into the body at which it is reflected; the amplitude (intensity) of a returning echo depends on the acoustical properties of the tissues encoun-

tered and is represented in the image as brightness (more echoes returning to the source is shown as image brightness). The system constructs two-dimensional images (B-scans) by displaying the echoes from pulses of multiple adjacent one-dimensional paths (A-scans). Ultrasound images are acquired as digital images from the outset, and saved on computer disks. They may also be recorded as frames in rapid succession (cine loops) for real-time imaging. In addition, Doppler methods in ultrasound are used to measure and characterize the blood flow in blood vessels in the body (Fig. 9.5).

Since the image contrast in ultrasound is based on differences in the acoustic impedance of tissue, ultrasound provides functional information (e.g., tissue composition and blood flow). On the other hand, the flux of sound waves is not as dense as the photon flux used to produce images in radiography; thus ultrasound images are generally lower resolution images than other imaging modalities (Fig. 9.2).

Current ultrasound machines are essentially specialized computers with attached peripherals, with active development of three-dimensional imaging. The ultrasound transducer now often sweeps out a 3-D volume rather than a 2-D plane, and the data are written directly into a three-dimensional array memory, which is displayed using volume or surface-based rendering techniques (Ritchie et al. 1996).

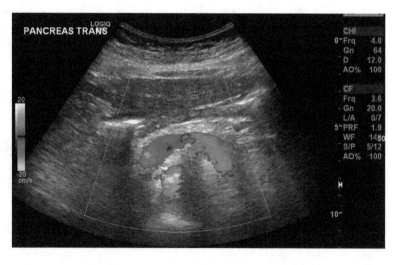

Fig. 9.5 An ultrasound image of abdomen. Like CT and MRI, ultrasound images are slices of a body, but because a user creates the images by holding a probe, any arbitrary plane can be imaged (so long as the probe can be oriented to produce that plane). This image shows an axial slice through the pancreas, and flow in nearby blood vessels (*in color*) is seen due to Doppler effects incorporated into the imaging method

9.2.3.4 Magnetic Resonance Imaging (MRI)

Creation of images from the resonance phenomena of unpaired spinning charges in a magnetic field grew out of **nuclear magnetic resonance** (NMR) **spectroscopy**, a technique that has long been used in chemistry to characterize chemical compounds. Many atomic nuclei within the body have a net magnetic moment, so they act like tiny magnets. When a small chemical sample is placed in an intense, uniform magnetic field, these nuclei line up in the direction of the field, spinning around the axis of the field with a frequency dependent on the type of nucleus, on the surrounding environment, and on the strength of the magnetic field.

If a radio pulse of a particular frequency is then applied at right angles to the stationary magnetic field, those nuclei with rotation frequency equal to that of the radiofrequency pulse resonate with the pulse and absorb energy. The higher energy state causes the nuclei to change their orientation with respect to the fixed magnetic field. When the radiofrequency pulse is removed, the nuclei return to their original aligned state (a process called "relaxation"), emitting a detectable radiofrequency signal as they do so. Characteristic parameters of this signal—such as intensity, duration, and frequency shift away from the original pulse—are dependent on the density and environment of the nuclei. In the case of traditional NMR spectroscopy, different molecular environments cause different frequency shifts (called chemical shifts), which we can use to identify the particular compounds in a sample. In the original NMR method, however, the signal is not localized to a specific region of the sample, so it is not possible to create an image.

Creation of medical images from NMR signals, known as Magnetic Resonance Imaging (MRI), had to await the development of computer-based reconstruction techniques, similar to CT. The basis of image formation in MRI is based on proton relaxation (referred to as T1 and T2 relaxation); differences in T1 and T2 are inherent properties of tissue and they vary among tissues. Thus, MRI provides detailed functional information about tissue and can be valuable in clinical

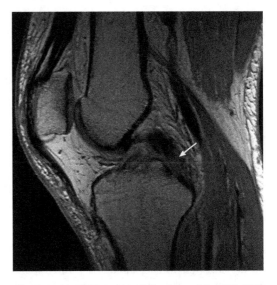

Fig. 9.6 An MRI image of the knee. Like CT, MRI images are slices of a body. This image is in the saggital plane through the mid knee, showing in a tear in the posterior cruciate ligament (*arrow*)

diagnosis (Fig. 9.6). At the same time, the flux of radiofrequency waves used to produce the images is high, and MRI thus has high spatial resolution (Fig. 9.2).

Many new modalities are being developed based on magnetic resonance. For example, magnetic resonance arteriography (MRA) and venography (MRV) are used to image blood flow (Lee 2003) and diffusion tensor imaging (DTI) is increasingly being used to image white matter fiber tracts in the brain (Le Bihan et al. 2001; Hasan et al. 2010; de Figueiredo et al. 2011; Gerstner and Sorensen 2011).

9.2.3.5 Nuclear Medicine Imaging

In **nuclear medicine imaging**, the imaging approach is a reverse of the radiographic imaging: instead of the imaging beam being outside the subject and projecting into the subject, the imaging source is inside the subject and projects out. Specifically, a radioactive isotope is chemically attached to a biologically active compound (such as an analogue of glucose) and then is injected into the patient's peripheral circulation. The compound collects in the specific body compartments or organs (such as metabolically-active tissues), where it is stored or processed by the body. The isotope emits radiation locally, and the radiation is measured using a special detector. The resultant nuclear-medicine image depicts the level of radioactivity that was measured at each spatial location of the patient. Because the counts are inherently quantized, digital images are produced. Multiple images also can be processed to obtain temporal dynamic information, such as the rate of arrival or of disappearance of isotope at particular body sites.

Nuclear medicine images, like radiographic images, are usually acquired as projections—a large planar detector is positioned outside the patient and it collects a projected image of all the radioactivity emitted from the patient. The images are similar in appearance to radiographic projection images. However, since the photon flux is extremely low (to minimize the radiation dose to the patient), the spatial resolution of nuclear medicine images is low. On the other hand, since the only places where radioisotope accumulates will be places in the body that are targeted by the injected agent, nearly all the information in nuclear medicine images is functional information; thus nuclear imaging methods have high functional information and low spatial resolution (Fig. 9.2). Nuclear medicine techniques have recently attracted much attention because of an explosion in novel imaging probes and targeting mechanisms to localize the imaging agent.

In addition to projection images, a computed tomography-like method called **single-photon emission computed tomography** (SPECT) (Alberini et al. 2011) has been developed. A camera rotates around the patient similar to CT, producing a computed volumetric image that may be viewed and navigated in multiple planes. A technique called Positron Emission Tomography (PET) uses a special type of radioactive isotope that emits positrons, which, upon encountering an electron, produces an annihilation event that sends out two gamma rays in opposite directions that are simultaneously detected on an annular detector array and used to compute a cross sectional slice through the patient, similar to CT and SPECT (Fig. 9.7). These volumetric nuclear medicine imaging methods, like the projection

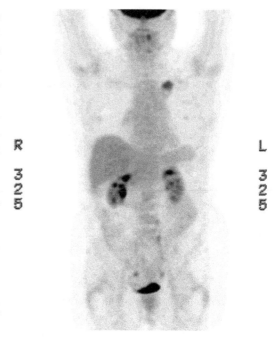

Fig. 9.7 A PET image of the body in a patient with cancer in the left lung (same patient as in Fig. 9.4). This is a projection image taken in the frontal plane after injection of a radioactive isotope that accumulates in cancers. A *small black spot* in the left upper lobe is abnormal and indicates the cancer mass in the upper lobe of the left lung

methods, have high functional information and low spatial resolution. However, recently a newer modality called PET/CT has been developed that integrates a PET scanner and CT with image fusion (discussed below) to get the best of both worlds—functional information about lesions in the PET image plus spatial localization of the abnormality on the CT image (Figs. 9.8 and 9.2).

A subdomain of nuclear imaging called **molecular imaging** has emerged that embodies this work on molecularly-targeted imaging (and therapeutic) agents (Weissleder and Mahmood 2001; Massoud and Gambhir 2003; Biswal et al. 2007; Hoffman and Gambhir 2007; Margolis et al. 2007; Ray and Gambhir 2007; Willmann et al. 2008; Pysz et al. 2010). Molecularly-tagged molecules are increasingly being introduced into the living organism, and imaged with optical, radioactive, or magnetic energy sources, often using reconstruction techniques and often in 3-D. It is becoming possible to combine gene sequence

Fig. 9.8 A PET/CT fused image. The axial slice from the PET study (Fig. 9.7) and the corresponding axial slice from the CT study (Fig. 9.4) are combined into a single image that has both good spatial resolution and functional information, showing that the lung mass has abnormal uptake of isotope, indicating it is metabolically active

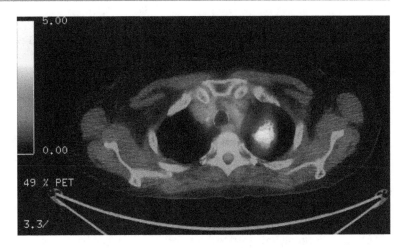

information, gene expression array data, and molecular imaging to determine not only which genes are expressed, but where they are expressed in the organism (Kang and Chung 2008; Min and Gambhir 2008; Singh et al. 2008; Lexe et al. 2009; Smith et al. 2009; Harney and Meade 2010). These capabilities will become increasingly important in the post-genomic era for determining exactly how genes generate both the structure and function of the organism.

9.2.4 Image Quality

9.2.4.1 Characteristics of Image Quality

The imaging modalities described above are complex devices with many parameters that need to be specified in generating the image, and most of the parameters can have substantial impact on the following key characteristics of the final image appearance: spatial resolution, contrast resolution, and temporal resolution, all of which have substantial impact on image quality and diagnostic value of the image. These characteristics provide an objective means for comparing images formed by digital imaging modalities.

- **Spatial resolution** is related to the sharpness of the image; it is a measure of how well the imaging modality can distinguish points on the object that are close together. For a digital image, spatial resolution is generally related to the number of pixels per image area.

- **Contrast resolution** is a measure of the ability to distinguish small differences in intensity in different regions of the image, which in turn are related to differences in measurable parameters, such as X-ray attenuation. For digital images, the number of bits per pixel is related to the contrast resolution of an image.

- **Temporal resolution** is a measure of the time needed to create an image. We consider an imaging procedure to be a real-time application if it can generate images concurrent with the physical process it is imaging. At a rate of at least 30 images per second, it is possible to produce unblurred images of the beating heart.

Other parameters that are specifically relevant to medical imaging are the degree of invasiveness, the dosage of ionizing radiation, the degree of patient discomfort, the size (portability) of the instrument, the ability to depict physiologic function as well as anatomic structure, and the availability and cost of the procedure at a specific location.

A perfect imaging modality would produce images with high spatial, contrast, and temporal resolution; it would be available, low in cost, portable, free of risk, painless, and noninvasive; it would use nonionizing radiation; and it would depict physiological function as well as anatomic structure. As seen above, the different modalities differ in these characteristics and none is uniformly strong across all the parameters (Fig. 9.2).

9.2.4.2 Contrast Agents

One of the major motivators for development of new imaging modalities is the desire to increase contrast resolution. A contrast agent is a substance introduced into the body to enhance the imaging contrast of structures or fluids in medical imaging. Contrast agents can be introduced in various ways, such as by injection, inspiration, ingestion, or enema. The chemical composition of contrast agents vary with modality so as to be optimally visible based on the physical basis of image formation. For example, iodinated contrast agents are used in radiography and CT because iodine has high atomic number, greatly attenuating X-rays, and thus greatly enhancing image contrast in any tissues that accumulate the contrast agent. Contrast agents for radiography are referred to as "radiopaque" since they absorb X-rays and obscure the beam. Contrast agents in radiography are used to highlight the anatomic structures of interest (e.g., stomach, colon, urinary tract). In an imaging technique called angiography, a contrast agent is injected into the blood vessels to opacify them on the images. In pathology, histological staining agents such as haematoxylin and eosin (H&E) have been used for years to enhance contrast in tissue sections, and magnetic contrast agents such as gadolinium have been introduced to enhance contrast in MR images.

Although these methods have been very successful, they generally are somewhat non-specific. In recent years, advances in molecular biology have led to the ability to design contrast agents that are highly specific for individual molecules. In addition to radioactively tagged molecules used in nuclear medicine, molecules are tagged for imaging by magnetic resonance and optical energy sources. Tagged molecules are imaged in 2-D or 3-D, often by application of reconstruction techniques developed for clinical imaging. Tagged molecules have been used for several years *in vitro* by such techniques as immunocytochemistry (binding of tagged antibodies to antigen) (Van Noorden 2002) and *in situ* hybridization (binding of tagged nucleotide sequences to DNA or RNA) (King et al. 2000). More recently, methods have been developed to image these molecules in the living organism, thereby opening up entirely new avenues for understanding the functioning of the body at the molecular level (Biswal et al. 2007; Hoffman and Gambhir 2007; Margolis et al. 2007; Ray and Gambhir 2007; Willmann et al. 2008; Pysz et al. 2010).

9.2.5 Imaging Methods in Other Medical Domains

Though radiology is a core domain and driver of many clinical problems and applications of medical imaging, several other medical domains are increasingly relying on imaging to provide key information for biomedical discovery and clinical insight. The methods of biomedical informatics presented in this chapter, while focusing on radiology in our examples, are generalizable and applicable to these other domains. We briefly highlight these other domains and the role of imaging in them.

9.2.5.1 Microscopic/Cellular Imaging

At the microscopic level, there is a rapid growth in **cellular imaging** (Larabell and Nugent 2010; Toomre and Bewersdorf 2010; Wessels et al. 2010), including use of computational methods to evaluate the features in cells (Carpenter et al. 2006). The confocal microscope uses electronic focusing to move a two-dimensional slice plane through a three-dimensional tissue slice placed in a microscope. The result is a three-dimensional voxel array of a microscopic, or even submicroscopic, specimen (Wilson 1990; Paddock 1994). At the electron microscopic level electron tomography generates 3-D images from thick electron-microscopic sections using techniques similar to those used in CT (Perkins et al. 1997).

9.2.5.2 Pathology/Tissue Imaging

The radiology department was revolutionized by the introduction of digital imaging and **Picture Archiving and Communication Systems** (PACS). Pathology has likewise begun to shift from an analog to a digital workflow (Leong and Leong 2003; Gombas et al. 2004). Pathology informatics is a rapidly emerging field (Becich 2000; Gabril and Yousef 2010), with goals and research problems similar to those in radiology, such as managing huge images, improving efficiency of workflow, learning new knowledge by mining historical cases, identifying novel imaging features through correlative quantitative imaging analysis, and decision support. A particularly promising area is deriving novel quantitative image features from pathology images to improve characterization and clinical decision making (Giger and MacMahon 1996; Nielsen et al. 2008; Armstrong 2010). Given that pathology and radiology produce images that characterize phenotype of disease, there is tremendous opportunity for information integration and linkage among pathology, radiology, and molecular data for discovery.

9.2.5.3 Ophthalmologic Imaging

Visualization of the retina is a core task of ophthalmology to diagnose disease and to monitor treatment response (Bennett and Barry 2009). Imaging modalities include retinal photography, autofluorescence, and fluorescein angiography. Recently, tomographic-based imaging has been introduced through a technique called **optical coherence tomography** (OCT; Fig. 9.9) (Figurska et al. 2010). This modality is showing great progress in evaluating a variety of retinal diseases (Freton and Finger 2012; Schimel et al. 2011; Sohrab et al. 2011). As with radiological

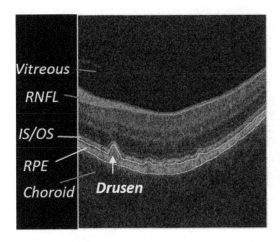

Fig. 9.9 An OCT image of the retina. Like ultrasound, OCT produces an image slice at any arbitrary angle (depending on how the light beam can be oriented), but it is limited to visualizing superficial structures due to poor penetration by light. In this image, the layered structure of the retina can be seen, as well as abnormalities (drusen)

imaging, a number of quantitative and automated segmentation methods are being created to evaluate disease objectively (Cabrera Fernandez et al. 2005; Baumann et al. 2010; Hu et al. 2010a, b). Likewise, image processing methods for image visualization and fusion are being developed, similar to those used in radiology.

9.2.5.4 Dermatologic Imaging

Imaging is becoming an important component of dermatology in the management of patients with skin lesions. Dermatologists frequently take photographs of patients with skin abnormalities, and while initially this was done for clinical documentation, increasingly this is done to leverage imaging informatics methods for training, to improve clinical care, for consultation, for monitoring progression or change in skin disease, and for image retrieval (Bittorf et al. 1997; Diepgen and Eysenbach 1998; Eysenbach et al. 1998; Lowe et al. 1998; Ribaric et al. 2001). Like radiology and pathology, recent work is being done to extract quantitative features from the images to enable decision support (Seidenari et al. 2003).

9.3   Image Content Representation

The image contents comprise two components of information, the *visual content* and the *knowledge content*. The visual content is the raw values of the image itself, the information that a computer can access in a digital image directly. The knowledge content arises as the observer, who has biomedical knowledge about the image content, views the visual information in the image. For example, a radiologist viewing a CT image of the upper abdomen immediately recognizes that the image contains the liver, spleen, and stomach (anatomic entities), as well as image abnormalities such as a mass in the liver with rim enhancement (imaging observation entities). Unlike the visual content, the knowledge content of images is not directly accessible to computers from the image itself. However, semantic methods are being developed to make this content machine-accessible (Sect. 9.3.2). In this section we describe imaging informatics methods for representing the visual and knowledge content of images.

9.3.1 Representing Visual Content in Digital Images

The visual content of digital images typically is represented in a computer by a two-dimensional array of numbers (a bit map). Each element of the array represents the intensity of a small square area of the picture, called a picture element (or pixel). Each **pixel** element corresponds to a volume element (or **voxel**) in the imaged subject that produced the pixel. If we consider the image of a volume, then a three-dimensional array of numbers is required. Another way of thinking of a volume is that it is a stack of two-dimensional images. However, it is also important to be aware of the voxel dimensions that correspond to the pixels when doing this. In many 2-D imaging applications, the in-plane resolution (the size of the voxels in the x, y plane) is higher than the resolution in the z-axis (i.e., the slice thickness). This creates a problem when re-sampling the volume data to create other projections, such as coronal or saggital from primary axial image data. If the dimensions

of the voxels (and pixels) are uniform in all dimensions, they are referred to as *isotropic*.

We can store any image in a computer as a matrix of integers (or real-valued numbers), either by converting it from an analog to a digital representation or by generating it directly in digital form. Once an image is in digital form, it can be handled just like all other data. It can be transmitted over communications networks, stored compactly in databases on magnetic or optical media, and displayed on graphics monitors. In addition, the use of computers has created an entirely new realm of capabilities for image generation and analysis: images can be computed rather than measured directly. Furthermore, digital images can be manipulated for display or analysis in ways not possible with film-based images.

In addition to the 2D (slice) and 3D (volume) representation for image data, there can be additional dimensions to representing the visual content of images. It is often the case that multi-modality data are required for the diagnosis; this can be a combination of varying modalities, (e.g., CT and PET, CT and MRI) and can be a combination of imaging sequences *within* a modality (e.g., T1, T2, or other sequences in MRI) (Fig. 9.10). Pixel (or voxel) content, from

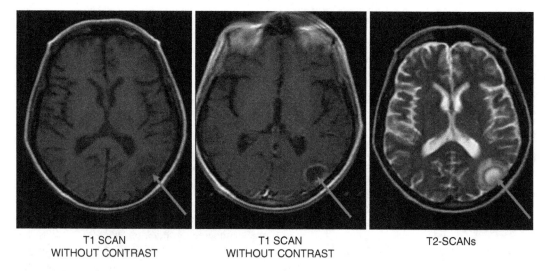

T1 SCAN
WITHOUT CONTRAST

T1 SCAN
WITHOUT CONTRAST

T2-SCANs

Fig. 9.10 Multi-modality imaging. Images of the brain from three modalities (T1 without contrast, T1 with contrast, and T2) are shown. The patient has a lesion in the left occipital lobe that has distinctive image features on each of these modalities, and the combination of these different features on different modalities establishes characteristic patterns useful in diagnosis

each of the respective acquisition modalities, are combined in what is known as a "feature-vector" in the multi-dimensional space. For example, a 3-dimensional intensity-based feature vector, based on three MRI pulse sequences, can be defined as a set of three values for each pixel in the image, where the intensity of each pixel in each of the three MRI images is extracted and recorded (e.g., [Intensity(Sequence 1), Intensity(Sequence 2), Intensity(Sequence 3)]. Any imaging performed over time (e.g., cardiac echo videos) can be represented by the set of values at each time point, thus the time is added as an additional dimension to the representation.

Finally, in addition to representing the visual content, medical images also need to represent certain information about that visual content (referred to as **image metadata**). Image metadata include such things as the name of the patient, date the image was acquired, the slice thickness, the modality that was used to acquire the image, etc. All image metadata are usually stored in the header of the image file. Given that there are many different types of equipment and software that produce and consume images, standards are crucial. For images, the Digital Imaging and Communications in Medicine (DICOM) standard is for distributing and viewing any kind of medical image regardless of the origin (Bidgood and Horii 1992). DICOM has become pervasive throughout radiology and is becoming a standard in other domains such as pathology, ophthalmology, and dermatology. In addition to specifying a standard file syntax and metadata structure, DICOM specifies a standard protocol for communicating images among imaging devices.

9.3.2 Representing Knowledge Content in Digital Images

As noted above, the knowledge content related to images is not directly encoded in the images, but it is recognized by the observer of the images. This knowledge includes recognition of the anatomic entities in the image, imaging observations and characteristics of the observations (sometimes called "findings"), and interpretations

(probable diseases). Representing this knowledge in the imaging domain is similar to knowledge representation in other domains of biomedical informatics (see Chap. 22). Specifically, for representing the entities in the domain of discourse, we adopt terminologies or ontologies. To make specific statements about individuals (images), we use information models that reference ontological entities as necessary.

9.3.2.1 Knowledge Representation of Anatomy

Given segmented anatomical structures, whether at the macroscopic or microscopic level, and whether represented as 3-D surface meshes or extracted 3-D regions, it is often desirable to attach labels (names) to the structures. If the names are drawn from a controlled terminology or ontology, they can be used as an index into a database of segmented structures, thereby providing a qualitative means for comparing structures from multiple subjects.

If the terms in the vocabulary are organized so as to assert relationships true of all individuals ("ontologies"), they can support systems that manipulate and retrieve image contents in "intelligent" ways. If anatomical ontologies are linked to other ontologies of physiology and pathology they can provide increasingly sophisticated knowledge about the *meaning* of the various images and other data that are increasingly becoming available in online databases. This kind of knowledge (by the computer, as opposed to the scientist) will be required in order to achieve the seamless integration of all forms of imaging and non-imaging data.

At the most fundamental level, *Nomina Anatomica* (International Anatomical Nomenclature Committee 1989) and its successor, *Terminologia Anatomica* (Federative Committee on Anatomical Terminology 1998) provide a classification of officially sanctioned terms that are associated with macroscopic and microscopic anatomical structures. This canonical term list, however, has been substantially expanded by synonyms that are current in various fields, and has also been augmented by a large number of new terms that designate structures omitted from

Terminologia Anatomica. Many of these additions are present in various controlled terminologies (e.g., MeSH (National Library of Medicine 1999), SNOMED (Spackman et al. 1997), Read Codes (Schultz et al. 1997), GALEN (Rector et al. 1993)). Unlike Terminologia these vocabularies are entirely computer-based, and therefore lend themselves for incorporation in computer-based applications.

The most complete primate *neuroanatomical* terminology is NeuroNames, developed by Bowden and Martin at the University of Washington (Bowden and Martin 1995). NeuroNames, which is included as a knowledge source in the National Library of Medicine's Unified Medical Language System (UMLS) (Lindberg et al. 1993), is primarily organized as a part-of hierarchy of nested structures, with links to a large set of ancillary terms that do not fit into the strict part-of hierarchy. Other neuroanatomical terminologies have also been developed (Paxinos and Watson 1986; Swanson 1992; Bloom and Young 1993; Franklin and Paxinos 1997; Bug et al. 2008). A challenge for biomedical informatics is either to come up with a single consensus terminology or to develop Internet tools that allow transparent integration of distributed but commonly agreed-on terminology, with local modifications.

Classification and ontology projects to date have focused primarily on arranging the terms of a particular domain in hierarchies. As noted with respect to the evaluation of Terminologia Anatomica (Rosse 2000), insufficient attention has been paid to the relationships among these terms. These relationships are named (e.g., "*is-a*" and "*part-of*") to indicate how the entities connected by them are related (e.g., Left Lobe of Liver *part-of* Liver). Linking entities with relations encodes knowledge and is used by computer reasoning applications in making inferences. Terminologia, as well as anatomy sections of the controlled medical terminologies, mix -*is a*- and -*part of*- relationships in the anatomy segments of their hierarchies. Although such heterogeneity does not interfere with using these term lists for keyword-based retrieval, these programs will fail to support higher level

knowledge (reasoning) required for knowledge-based applications. To meet this gap, the Foundational Model of Anatomy (FMA) was developed to define a comprehensive symbolic description of the structural organization of the body, including anatomical concepts, their preferred names and synonyms, definitions, attributes and relationships (Rosse et al. 1998a, b; Rosse and Mejino 2003) (Fig. 9.11).

In the FMA, anatomical entities are arranged in class-subclass hierarchies, with inheritance of defining attributes along the *is-a* link, and other relationships (e.g., parts, branches, spatial adjacencies) represented as additional descriptors associated with the concept. The FMA currently consists of over 75,000 concepts, represented by about 120,000 terms, and arranged in over 2.1 million links using 168 types of relationships. These concepts represent structures at all levels: macroscopic (to 1 mm resolution), cellular and macromolecular. Brain structures have been added by integrating NeuroNames with the FMA as a Foundational Model of Neuroanatomy (FMNA) (Martin et al. 2001).

The FMA can be useful for symbolically organizing and integrating biomedical information, particularly that obtained from images. But in order to answer non-trivial queries in neuroscience and other basic science areas, and to develop "smart tools" that rely on deep knowledge, additional ontologies must also be developed (e.g., for physiological functions mediated by neurotransmitters, and pathological processes and their clinical manifestations, as well for the radiological appearances with which they correlate). The relationships that exist among these concepts and anatomical parts of the body must also be explicitly modeled. Next-generation informatics efforts that link the FMA and other anatomical ontologies with separately developed functional ontologies will be needed in order to accomplish this type of integration.

9.3.2.2 Knowledge Representation of Radiology Imaging Features

While FMA provides a comprehensive knowledge representation for anatomy, it does not cover other portions of the radiology domain. As is

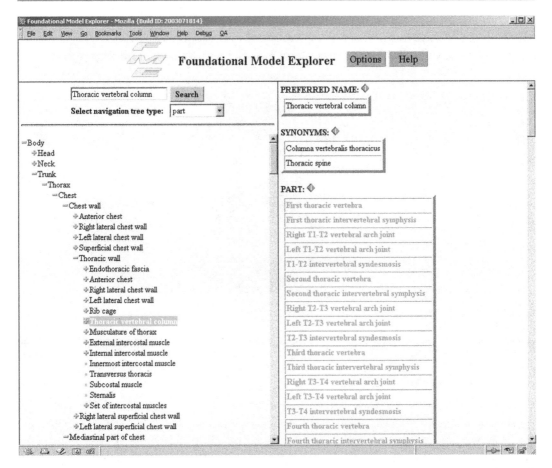

Fig. 9.11 The Foundational Model Explorer, a Web viewer for the frame-based University of Washington Foundational Model of Anatomy (FMA). The left panel shows a hierarchical view along the part of link. Hierarchies along other links, such as is-a, branch-of, tributary-of, can also be viewed in this panel. The right hand panel shows the detailed local and inherited attributes (slots) associated with a selected structure, in this case the thoracic vertebral column (Photograph courtesy of the Structural Informatics Group, University of Washington)

discussed in Chap. 7, there are controlled terminologies in other domains, such as MeSH, SNOMED, and related terminologies in the UMLS (Cimino 1996; Bodenreider 2008); however, these lack terminology specific to radiology for describing the features seen in imaging. The Radiological Society of North America (RSNA) recently developed RadLex, a controlled terminology for radiology (Langlotz 2006; Rubin 2008). The primary goal of RadLex is to provide a means for radiologists to communicate clear, concise, and orderly descriptions of imaging findings in understandable, unambiguous language. Another goal is to promote an orderly thought process and logical assessments and recommendations based on observed imaging features based on terminology-based description of radiology images and to enable decision support (Baker et al. 1995; Burnside et al. 2009). Another goal of RadLex is to enable radiology research; data mining is facilitated by the use of standard terms to code large collections of reports and images (Channin et al. 2009a, b).

RadLex includes thousands of descriptors of visual observations and characteristics for describing imaging abnormalities, as well as terms for naming anatomic structures, radiology imaging procedures, and diseases (Fig. 9.12).

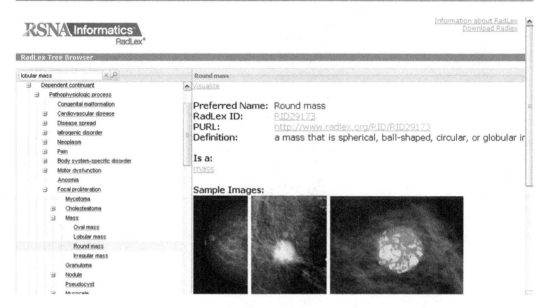

Fig. 9.12 RadLex contolled terminology (http://radlex. org). RadLex includes term hierarchies for describing anatomy ("anatomical entity"), imaging observations ("imaging observation") and characteristics ("imaging observation characteristic"), imaging procedures and procedure steps ("procedure step"), diseases ("pathophysio-logic process"), treatments ("treatment"), and components of radiology reports ("report"). Each term includes definitions, preferred name, image exemplars, and other term metadata and relationships such as subsumption (Figure reprinted with permission from Rubin 2011)

Each term in RadLex contains a unique identifier as well as a variety of attributes such as definition, synonyms, and foreign language equivalents. In addition to a lexicon of standard terms, the RadLex ontology includes term relationships—links between terms to relate them in various ways to encode radiological knowledge. For example, the *is-a* relationship records subsumption. Other relationships include part-of, connectivity, and blood supply. These relationships are enabling computer-reasoning applications to process image-related data annotated with RadLex.

RadLex has been used in several imaging informatics applications, such as to improve search for radiology information. RadLex-based indexing of radiology journal figure captions achieved very high precision and recall, and significantly improved image retrieval over keyword-based search (Kahn and Rubin 2009). RadLex has been used to index radiology reports (Marwede et al. 2008). Work is underway to introduce RadLex controlled terms into radiology reports to reduce radiologist variation in

use of terms for describing images (Kahn et al. 2009). Tools are beginning to appear enabling radiologists to annotate and query image databases using RadLex and other controlled terminologies (Rubin et al. 2008; Channin et al. 2009a, b).

In addition to RadLex, there are other important controlled terminologies for radiology. The Breast Imaging Reporting and Data System (BI-RADS) is a lexicon of descriptors and a reporting structure comprising assessment categories and management recommendations created by the American College of Radiology (D'Orsi and Newell 2007). Terminologies are also being created in other radiology imaging domains, including the Fleischner Society Glossary of terms for thoracic imaging (Hansell et al. 2008), the Nomenclature of Lumbar Disc Pathology (Appel 2001), terminologies for image guided tumor ablation (Goldberg et al. 2009) and transcatheter therapy for hepatic malignancy (Brown et al. 2009), and the CT Colonography Reporting and Data System (Zalis et al. 2005).

9.3.2.3 Semantic Representation of Image Contents

While ontologies and controlled terminologies are useful for representing knowledge related to images, they do not provide a means to directly encode assertions for recording the semantic content in images. For example, we may wish to record the fact that "there is a mass 4×5 cm in size in the right lobe of the liver." The representation of this semantic image content certainly will use ontologies and terminologies to record the entities to which such assertions refer; however, an **information model** is required to provide the required grammar and syntax for recording such assertions. There are two approaches to recording these assertions, no formal information model (narrative text) and a formal information model.

Narrative Text

In the current workflow, nearly all semantic image content is recorded in narrative text (radiology reports). The advantage of text reports is that they are simple, quick to produce (the radiologist speaks freely into a microphone), and they can be expressive, capturing the subtle nuances (and ambiguities) that the English language provides. There are several downsides, however. First, text reports are unstructured; there is no adherence to controlled terminology and not consistent structure that would permit reliable information extraction. Second, the reports may be incomplete, vague, or contradictory. Further, free text is challenging for computers (see Chap. 8), which makes it difficult to leverage free text in applications. Finally, radiology images and the corresponding radiologist report are currently disconnected; e.g., the report may describe a mass in an organ, and the image may contain a **region of interest** (ROI) measuring the lesion, but there is no information directly linking the description of the lesion in the report with the ROI in the image. Such linkage could enable applications such as content-based image retrieval, as described below.

Information Model

An information model provides an explicit specification of the types of data to be collected and the syntax by which it will be saved. So-called "semantic annotation" methods are being developed to adapt the semantic content about images that would have been put into narrative text so that it can instead be put in structured annotations compliant with the information model. The information model conveys the pertinent image information explicitly and in human-readable and machine accessible format. For example, a semantic annotation might record the coordinates of the tip of an arrow and indicate the organ (anatomic location) and imaging observations (e.g., mass) in that organ. These annotations can be recorded in a standard, searchable format, such as the Annotation and Image Markup (AIM) schema, recently developed by the National Cancer Institute's Cancer Biomedical Informatics Grid (caBIG) initiative (Channin et al. 2009a, b; Rubin et al. 2009b). AIM captures a variety of information about image annotations, e.g., ROIs, lesion identification, location, measurements, method of measurement, and other qualitative and quantitative features (Channin et al. 2009a, b).

The AIM information model includes use of controlled terms as semantic descriptors of lesions (e.g., RadLex). It also provides a syntax associating an ROI in an image with the aforementioned information, enabling raw image data to be linked with semantic information, and thus bridges the current disconnect between semantic terms and the lesions in images being described. In conjunction with RadLex, the AIM information model provides a standard syntax (in XML schema) to create a structured representation of the semantic contents of images (Fig. 9.13). Once the semantic contents are recorded in AIM (as XML instances of the AIM XML schema), applications can be developed for image query and analysis. Tools for creating semantic annotation of images as part of the routine clinical and research workflow is underway (Rubin et al. 2008). Automated semantic image annotation methods are also being pursued (Carneiro, Chan et al. 2007; Mechouche et al. 2008; Yu and Ip 2008) that will ultimately make the process of generating this structured information efficient.

In addition, tools to facilitate creating semantic annotations on images as part of the image viewing workflow are being developed. One such

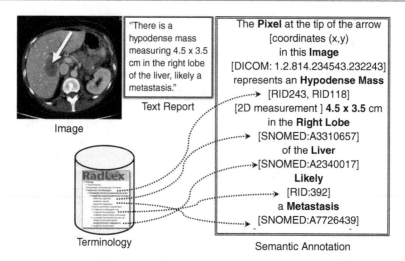

Fig. 9.13 Semantic annotation of images. The radiologist's image annotation (left) and interpretation (middle) associated with the annotation are not represented in a form such that the detailed content is directly accessible. The same information can be put into a structured representation as a semantic annotation (right), comprising terms from controlled terminologies (Systematized Nomenclature of Medicine (SNOMED) and RadLex) as well as numeric values (coordinates and measurements) (Figure reprinted with permission from (Rubin and Napel 2010)

tool, the electronic Imaging Physician Annotation Device (ePAD, formerly called iPAD; (Rubin et al. 2008)), a plug in to the Osirix image viewing program, is freely available. The ePAD tool permits the user to draw image annotations in a manner in which they are accustomed while viewing images, while simultaneously collecting semantic information about the image and the image region directly from the image itself as well as from the user using a structured reporting template (Fig. 9.14). The tool also features a panel to provide feedback so as to ensure complete and valid annotations. Image annotations are saved in the AIM XML format.

By making the semantic content of images explicit and machine-accessible, these structured annotations of images will help radiologists analyze data in large databases of images. For example, cancer patients often have many serial imaging studies in which a set of lesions is evaluated at each time point. Automated methods will be able to use semantic image annotations to identify the measurable lesions at each time point and produce a summary of, and automatically reason about, the total tumor burden over time, helping physicians to determine how well patients are responding to treatment (Levy and Rubin 2008).

9.3.2.4 Atlases

Spatial representations of anatomy, in the form of segmented regions on 2-D or 3-D images, or 3-D surfaces extracted from image volumes, are often combined with symbolic representations to form digital atlases. A digital atlas (which for this chapter refers to an atlas created from 3-D image data taken from real subjects, as opposed to artists' illustrations) is generally created from a single individual, which therefore serves as a "canonical" instance of the species. Traditionally, atlases have been primarily used for education, and most digital atlases are used the same way.

As an example in 2-D, the Digital Anatomist Interactive Atlases (Sundsten et al. 2000) were created by outlining ROIs on 2-D images (many of which are snapshots of 3-D scenes generated by reconstruction from serial sections) and labeling the regions with terminology from the FMA. The atlases, which are available on the web, permit interactive browsing, where the names of structures are given in response to mouse clicks; dynamic creation of "pin diagrams", in which selected labels are attached to regions on the images; and dynamically-generated quizzes, in which the user is asked to point to structures on the image (Brinkley et al. 1997).

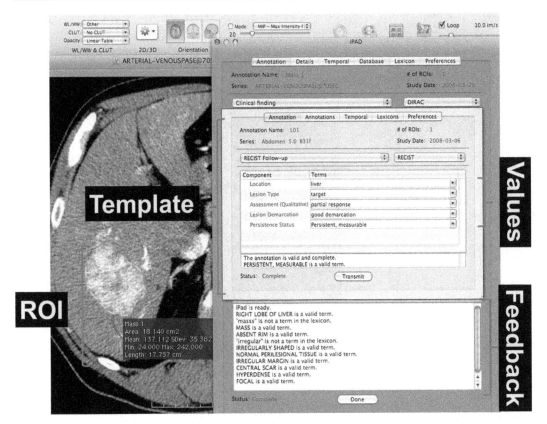

Fig. 9.14 The electronic Imaging Physician Annotation Device (ePAD). This tool creates structured semantic annotations on images using a graphical interface to minimize impact on image viewing workflow. The user views the image in and draws a region of interest (*left*). ePAD incorporates ontologies so that users can specify controlled terms as values in making their annotations (*pull down panel on right*). As they make their annotation, they receive feedback to ensure data entries are complete and that there are no violations of pre-specified annotation logic (*panel on lower right*). The ePAD tool saves image annotations in the AIM information model XML format

As an example 3-D, the Digital Anatomist Dynamic Scene Generator (DSG, Fig. 9.15) creates interactive 3-D atlases "on-the-fly" for viewing and manipulation over the web (Brinkley et al. 1999; Wong et al. 1999). In this case the 3-D scenes generated by reconstruction from serial sections are broken down into 3-D "primitive" meshes, each of which corresponds to an individual part in the FMA. In response to commands such as "Display the branches of the coronary arteries" the DSG looks up the branches in the FMA, retrieves the 3-D model primitives associated with those branches, determines the color for each primitive based on its type in the FMA is-a hierarchy, renders the assembled scene as a 2-D snapshot, then sends it to a web-browser, where the user may change the camera parameters, add new structures, or select and highlight structures.

An example of a 3-D brain atlas created from the Visible Human is Voxelman (Hohne et al. 1995), in which each voxel in the Visible Human head is labeled with the name of an anatomic structure in a "generalized voxel model" (Hohne et al. 1990), and highly-detailed 3-D scenes are dynamically generated. Several other brain atlases have also been developed, primarily for educational use (Johnson and Becker 2001; Stensaas and Millhouse 2001).

Atlases have also been developed for integrating functional data from multiple studies (Bloom and Young 1993; Toga et al. 1994, 1995; Swanson 1999; Fougerousse et al. 2000; Rosen et al. 2000; Martin and Bowden 2001). In their

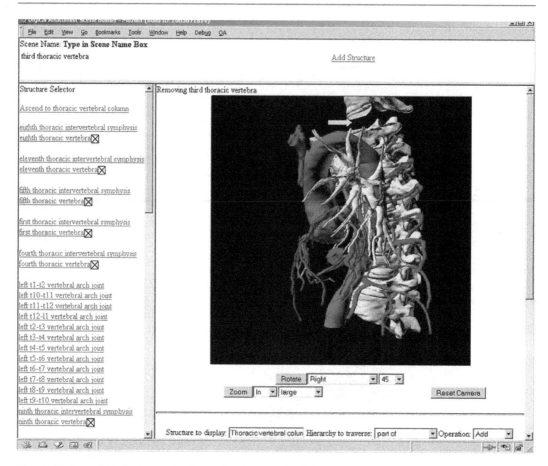

Fig. 9.15 The Digital Anatomist Dynamic Scene Generator. This-scene was created by requesting the following structures from the scene generator server: the parts of the aorta, the branches of the ascending aorta, the tributaries of the right atrium, the branches of the tracheobronchial tree, and the parts of the thoracic vertebral column. The server was then requested to rotate the camera 45°, and to provide the name of a structure selected with the mouse, in this case the third thoracic vertebra. The selected structure was then hidden (note the gap indicated by the *arrow*). The *left frame* shows a partial view of the FMA part of hierarchy for the thoracic vertebral column. Checked structures are associated with three-dimensional "primitive" meshes that were loaded into the scene (Photograph courtesy of the Structural Informatics Group, University of Washington)

original published form these atlases permit manual drawing of functional data, such as neurotransmitter distributions, onto hardcopy printouts of brain sections. Many of these atlases have been or are in the process of being converted to digital form. The Laboratory of Neuroimaging (LONI) at the University of California Los Angeles has been particularly active in the development and analysis of digital atlases (Toga 2001), and the California Institute of Technology Human Brain Project has released a web-accessible 3-D mouse atlas acquired with micro-MR imaging (Dhenain et al. 2001).

The most widely used human brain atlas is the Talairach atlas, based on post mortem sections from a 60-year-old woman (Talairach and Tournoux 1988). This atlas introduced a proportional coordinate system (often called "Talairach space") which consists of 12 rectangular regions of the target brain that are piecewise affine transformed to corresponding regions in the atlas. Using these transforms (or a simplified single affine transform based on the anterior and posterior commissures) a point in the target brain can be expressed in Talairach coordinates, and thereby related to similarly transformed points from other brains. Other human brain atlases have also been developed (Schaltenbrand and Warren 1977; Hohne et al. 1992; Caviness et al. 1996; Drury and Van Essen 1997; Van Essen and Drury 1997).

9.4   Image Processing

Image processing is a form of **signal processing** in which computational methods are applied to an input image to produce an output image or a set of characteristics or parameters related to the image. Most image processing techniques involve treating the image as a two-dimensional signal and analyzing it using signal-processing techniques or a variety of other transformations or computations. There are a broad variety of image processing methods, including transformations to enhance visualization, computations to extract features, and systems to automate detection or diagnose abnormalities in the images. The latter two methods, referred to as computer-assisted detection and diagnosis (CAD) is discussed in Sect. 9.5.2. In this section we discuss the former methods, which are more elemental and generic processing methods.

The rapidly increasing number and types of digital images has created many opportunities for image processing, since one of the great advantages of digital images is that they can be manipulated just like any other kind of data. This advantage was evident from the early days of computers, and success in processing satellite and spacecraft images generated considerable interest in biomedical image processing, including automated image analysis to improve radiological interpretation. Beginning in the 1960s, researchers devoted a large amount of work to this end, with the hope that eventually much of radiographic image analysis could be improved. One of the first areas to receive attention was automated interpretation of chest X-ray images, because, previously, most patients admitted to a hospital were subjected to routine chest X-ray examinations. (This practice is no longer considered cost effective except for selected subgroups of patients.) Subsequent research, however, confirmed the difficulty of completely automating radiographic image interpretation, and much of the initial enthusiasm stagnated long ago. Currently, there is less emphasis on completely automatic interpretation and more on systems that aid the user of images, except in specialized use cases.

Medical image processing utilizes tools similar to general image processing. But there are unique features to the medical imagery that present different, and often more difficult, challenges from those that exist in general image processing tasks. To begin with, the images analyzed all represent the 3D body; thus, the information extracted (be it in 2D or 3D) is based on a 3D volumetric object. The images themselves are often taken from multi-modalities (CT, MRI, PET), where each modality has its own unique physical characteristics, leading to unique noise, contrast and other issues that need to be addressed. The fusion of information across several modalities is a challenge that needs to be addressed as well.

When analyzing the data, it is often desirable to segment and characterize specific organs. The human body organs, or various tissue of interest within them, cannot be described with simple geometrical rules, as opposed to objects and scenes in non-medical images that usually can be described with such representations. This is mainly because the objects and free-form surfaces in the body cannot easily be decomposed into simple geometric primitives. There is thus very little use of geometric shape models that can be defined from *a-priori* knowledge. Moreover, when trying to model the shape of an organ or a region, one needs to keep in mind that there are large inter-person variations (e.g., in the shape and size of the heart, liver and so on), and, as we are frequently analyzing images of patients, there is a large spectrum of abnormal states that can greatly modify tissue properties or deform structures. Finally, especially in regions of interest that are close to the heart, complex motion patterns need to be accounted for as well. These issues make medical image processing a very challenging domain.

Although completely automated image-analysis systems are still in the future, the widespread availability of digital images, combined with image management systems such as PACS (Chap. 20) and powerful workstations, has led to many applications of image processing techniques. In general, routine techniques are available on the manufacturer's workstations (e.g., a vendor-provided console for an MR machine or an ultrasound machine), whereas more advanced image-processing algorithms are available as software packages that run on independent workstations.

The primary uses of image processing in the clinical environment are for image enhancement, screening, and quantitation. Software for such image processing is primarily developed for use on independent workstations. Several journals are devoted to medical image processing (e.g., *IEEE Transactions on Medical Imaging*, *Journal of Digital Imaging*, *Neuroimage*), and the number of journal articles is rapidly increasing as digital images become more widely available. Several books are devoted to the spectrum of digital imaging processing methods (Yoo 2004; Gonzalez et al. 2009), and the reader is referred to these for more detailed reading on these topics. We describe a few examples of image-processing techniques in the remainder of this section.

9.4.1 Types of Image-Processing Methods

Image processing methods are applied to representations of image content (Sect. 9.3). One may use the very low-level, pixel representation. The computational effort is minimal in the representation stage, with substantial effort (computational cost) in further analysis stages such as segmentation of the image, matching between images, registration of images, etc. A second option is to use a very high-level image content representation, in which each image is labeled according to its semantic content (medical image categories such as "abdomen vs chest", "healthy vs pathology"). In this scenario, a substantial computational effort is needed in the representation stage, including the use of automated image segmentation methods to recognize ROIs as well

as advanced learning techniques to classify the regions of image content. Further analysis can utilize knowledge resources such as ontologies, linked to the images using category labels. A mid-level representation exists, that balances the above two options, in which a transition is made from pixels to semantic features. Feature vectors are used to represent the spectrum of image content compactly and subsequent analysis is done on the feature vector representation.

Much of the current work uses the mid-level representation. In such work, a transition is made from pixel values to features, including: intensity, color, texture and in some cases also spatial coordinates or relative location features. Several main issues need to be addressed when selecting the feature set and the representation scheme: defining a global image representation (such as a histogram representation) or a more localized region-based representation, selecting a feature set that is robust or flexible to variability across the image archive, invariance issues such as the degree of sensitivity to rotation and scale. Some work has raised the issue of a hierarchical representation, such that images can be compared on the organ level in the categorization stage and on the pathology level in a higher-up stage of processing. In any scheme suggested, the representation needs to be general enough to accommodate multiple modalities and robust enough to handle the large variability of the data.

Image processing is the foundation for creating image-based applications, such as image enhancement to facilitate human viewing, to show views not present in the original images, to flag suspicious areas for closer examination by the clinician, to quantify the size and shape of an organ, and to prepare the images for integration with other information. To create such applications, several types of image processing are generally performed sequentially in an *image processing pipeline*, although some processing steps may feed back to earlier ones, and the specific methods used in a pipeline varies with the application. Most image processing pipelines and applications generalize from two-dimensional to three-dimensional images, though three-dimensional images pose unique image processing opportunities and challenges. Image processing pipelines are generally built using one or more of the following fundamental image processing methods: **global processing, image enhancement, image rendering/visualization, image quantitation**, image **segmentation**, image **registration**, and **image reasoning** (e.g., classification). In the remainder of this section we describe these methods, except for image reasoning which is discussed in Sect. 9.5.

9.4.2 Global Processing

Global processing involves computations on the entire image, without regard to specific regional content. The purpose is generally to enhance an image for human visualization or for further analysis by the computer ("pre-processing"). A simple but important example of global image processing is gray-scale windowing of CT images. The CT scanner generates pixel values (**Hounsfield numbers**, or CT numbers) in the range of −1,000 to +3,000. Humans, however, cannot distinguish more than about 100 shades of gray. To appreciate the full precision available with a CT image, the operator can adjust the mid-point and range of the displayed CT values. By changing the level and width (i.e., intercept and slope of the mapping between pixel value and displayed gray scale or, roughly, the brightness and contrast) of the display, radiologists enhance their ability to perceive small changes in contrast resolution within a subregion of interest.

Other types of global processing change the pixel values to produce an overall enhancement or desired effect on the image: *histogram equalization, convolution*, and *filtering*. In histogram equalization, the pixel values are changed, spreading out the most frequent intensity values to increase the global contrast of the image. It is most effective when the usable data of the image are represented by a narrow range of contrast values. Through this adjustment, the intensities can be better distributed on the histogram, improving image contrast by allowing for areas of lower local contrast to gain a higher contrast. In convolution and filtering, mathematical functions are applied to the entire image for a variety of purposes, such as de-noising, edge enhancement, and contrast enhancement.

9.4.3 Image Enhancement

Image enhancement uses global processing to improve the appearance of the image either for human use or for subsequent processing by computer. All manufacturers' consoles and independent image-processing workstations provide some form of image enhancement. We have already mentioned CT windowing. Another technique is unsharp masking, in which a blurred, or "unsharp," positive is created to be used as a "mask" that is combined with the original image, creating the illusion that the resulting image is sharper than the original. The technique increases local contrast and enhances the visibility of fine-detail (high-frequency) structures. Histogram equalization spreads the image gray levels throughout the visible range to maximize the visibility of those gray levels that are used frequently. Temporal subtraction subtracts a reference image from later images that are registered to the first. A common use of temporal subtraction is **digital-subtraction angiography** (DSA) in which a background image is subtracted from an image taken after the injection of contrast material.

9.4.4 Image Rendering/ Visualization

Image rendering and visualization refer to a variety of techniques for creating image displays, diagrams, or animations to display images more in a different perspective from the raw images. Image volumes are comprised of a stack of 2-D images. If the voxels in each image are isotropic, then a variety of arbitrary projections can be derived from the volume, such as a sagittal or coronal view, or even curved planes. A technique called maximum intensity projection (MIP) and minimum intensity projection (MinIP) can also be created in which imaginary rays are cast

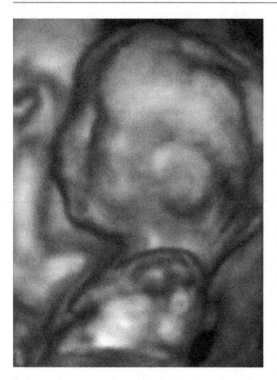

Fig. 9.16 Three-dimensional ultrasound image of a fetus, in utero. The ultrasound probe sweeps out a three-dimensional volume rather than the conventional two-dimensional plane. The volume can be rendered directly using volume-rendering techniques, or as in this case, fetal surfaces can be extracted and rendered using surface-rendering techniques (Source: http://en.wikipedia.org/wiki/File:3dultrasound_20_weeks.jpg)

ranging from cell images produced by confocal microscopy, to three-dimensional ultrasound images, to brain images created from MRI or PET.

Volume images can also be given as input to image-based techniques for warping the image volume of one structure to other. However, more commonly the image volume is processed in order to extract an explicit *spatial* (or quantitative) representation of anatomy (Sect. 9.4.5). Such an explicit representation permits improved visualization, quantitative analysis of structure, comparison of anatomy across a population, and mapping of functional data. It is thus a component of most research involving 3-D image processing.

9.4.5 Image Quantitation

Image quantitation is the process of extracting useful numerical parameters or deriving calculations from the image or from ROIs in the image. These values are also referred to as "quantitative imaging features." These parameters may themselves be informative—for example, the volume of the heart or the size of the fetus. They also may be used as input into an automated classification procedure, which determines the type of object found. For example, small round regions on chest X-ray images might be classified as tumors, depending on such features as intensity, perimeter, and area.

Mathematical models often are used in conjunction with image quantitation. In classic pattern-recognition applications, the mathematical model is a classifier that assigns a label to the image; e.g., to indicate if the image contains an abnormality, or indicates the diagnosis underlying an abnormality.

9.4.5.1 Quantitative Image Features
Quantitation uses global processing and segmentation to characterize regions of interest in the image with numerical values. For example, heart size, shape, and motion are subtle indicators of heart function and of the response of the heart to therapy (Clarysse et al. 1997). Similarly, fetal

through the volume, recording the maximum or minimum intensity encountered along the ray path, respectively, and displaying the result as a 2-D image.

In addition to these planar visualizations, the volume can be visualized directly in its entirety using **volume rendering** techniques (Foley et al. 1990; Lichtenbelt et al. 1998) (Fig. 9.16) which project a two-dimensional image directly from a three-dimensional voxel array by casting rays from the eye of the observer through the volume array to the image plane. Because each ray passes through many voxels, some form of segmentation (usually simple thresholding) often is used to remove obscuring structures. As workstation memory and processing power have advanced, volume rendering has become widely used to display all sorts of three-dimensional voxel data—

head size and femur length, as measured on ultrasound images, are valuable indicators of fetal well-being (Brinkley 1993b).

Image features/descriptors are derived from visual cues contained in an image. Two types of quantitative image features are *photometric* features, which exploit color and texture cues, derived directly from raw pixel intensities, and *geometric* features, which use shape-based cues. While color is one of the visual cues often used for content description (Hersh et al. 2009), most medical images are grayscale. Texture features encode spatial organization of pixel values of an image region. Shape features describe in quantitative terms the contour of a lesion and complement the information captured by color or texture. In addition, the histogram of pixel values within an ROI or transforms on those values is commonly performed to compute quantitative image features.

Quantitative image features are commonly represented by feature-vectors in a N-dimensional space, where each dimension of the feature vector describes an aspect of the individual pixel (e.g., color, texture, etc.) (Haralick and Shapiro 1992) Image analysis tasks that use the quantitative features, such as segmentation and classification are then approached in terms of distance measurements between points (samples) in the chosen N-dimensional feature space.

9.4.5.2 Image Patches

In the last several years, "patch-based" representations and "bag-of-features" classification techniques have been proposed and used as an approach to processing image contents (Jurie and Triggs 2005; Nowak et al. 2006; Avni 2009). An overview of the methodology is shown in Fig. 9.17. In these approaches, a shift is made from the pixel as being the atomic entity of computation to a "patch" – a small window centered on the pixel, thus region-based information is included. A very large set of patches is extracted from an image. Each small patch shows a localized "glimpse" at the image content; the collection of thousands and more such patches, randomly selected, have the capability to identify the entire image content (similar to a puzzle being formed from its pieces).

The patch size needs to be larger than a few pixels across, in order to capture higher-level semantics such as edges or corners. At the same time, the patch size should not be too large if it is to serve as a common building block of many images. Patch extraction approaches include using a regular sampling grid, a random selection of points, or the selection of points with high information content using salient point detectors, such as SIFT (Lowe 1999). Once patches are selected, the information content within a patch is extracted. It is possible to take the patch information as a collection of pixel values, or to shift the representation to a different set of features based on the pixels, such as SIFT features. Frequently, the dimensionality of the representation is reduced via dimensionality reduction techniques, such as principal-component analysis (PCA) (Duda et al. 2001). In addition to patch content information represented either by PCA coefficients or SIFT descriptors, it is possible to add the patch center coordinates to the feature vector. This addition introduces spatial information into the image representation, without the need to model explicitly the spatial dependency between patches. Special care needs to be taken when combining features of different units, such as coordinates and PCA coefficients. The relative feature weights are often tuned experimentally on a cross-validation set.

A final step in the process is to learn a dictionary of words over a large collection of patches, extracted from a large set of images. The vector represented patches are converted into "visual words" which form a representative "dictionary". A visual word can be considered as a representative of several similar patches. A frequently-used method is to perform K-means clustering (Bishop 1995) over the vectors of the initial collection, and then cluster them into K groups in the feature space. The resultant cluster centers serve as a vocabulary of K visual words, with K often in the hundreds and thousands).

Once a global dictionary is learned, each image is represented as a collection of words (also known as a "bag of words", or "bag of features"), using an indexed histogram over the defined words. Various image processing tasks

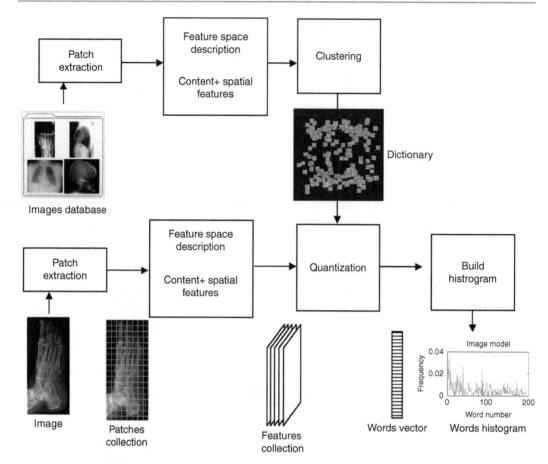

Fig. 9.17 A block diagram of the patch-based image representation. A radiographic image is shown with a set of patches indicated for processing the image data. Subsequent image processing is performed on each patch, and on the entire set of patches, rather than on individual pixels in the image. A dictionary of visual words is learned from a large set of images, and their respective patches. Further analysis of the image content can then be pursued based on a histogram across the dictionary words (Figure courtesy of Greenspan)

can then be undertaken, ranging from the categorization of the image content, giving the image a "high-level," more semantic label, the matching between images, or between an image and an image class, using patches for image segmentation and region-of-interest detection within an image. For these various tasks, images are compared using a distance measure between the representative histograms. In categorizing an image as belonging to a certain image class, well-known classifiers, such as the k- nearest neighbor and support-vector machines (SVM) (Vapnik 2000), are used.

In recent years, using patches or bags-of-visual-words (BoW) has successfully been applied to general scene and object recognition tasks (Fei-Fei and Perona 2005; Varma and Zisserman 2003; Sivic and Zisserman 2003; Nowak et al. 2006; Jiang et al. 2007). These approaches are now gradually emerging in medical tasks as well. For example, in (André et al. 2009) BoW is used as the representation of endomicroscopic images and achieves high accuracy in the tasks of classifying the images into neoplastic (pathological) and benign. In (Bosch et al. 2006) an application to texture representation for mammography tissue classification and segmentation is presented. The use of BoW techniques for large scale radiograph archive categorization can be found in the ImageCLEF competition, in a task to classify over 12,000 X-ray images to 196 different (organ-level) categories (Tommasi et al. 2010). This competition provides an important benchmarking tool to assess different feature sets as well as classification schemes on large archives of Radiographs. It is interesting to note that in the last few years, approaches based on local patch representation achieved the highest scores for categorization accuracy (Deselaers et al. 2006; Caputo et al. 2008; Greenspan et al. 2011). Current challenges entail extending from automatic classification of organs in X-ray data, to the identification and labeling of pathologies – achieving automatic healthy vs. pathology diagnostic-level categorization, as well as pathology level discrimination (e.g., work in Chest radiographs (Greenspan et al. 2011)).

9.4.6 Image Segmentation

Segmentation of images involves the extraction of ROIs from the image. The ROIs usually correspond to anatomically meaningful structures, such as organs or parts of organs, or they may be lesions or other types of regions in the image pertinent to the application. The structures may be delineated by their borders, in which case

edge-detection techniques (such as edge-following algorithms) are used, or by their composition in the image, in which case region-detection techniques (such as texture analysis) are used (Haralick and Shapiro 1992). Neither of these techniques has been completely successful as fully automated image segmentation methods; regions often have discontinuous borders or non-distinctive internal composition. Furthermore, contiguous regions often overlap. These and other complications make segmentation the most difficult subtask of the medical image processing problem. Because segmentation is difficult for a computer, it is usually performed either by hand or in a semi-automated manner with assistance by a human through operator-interactive approaches (Fig. 9.18). In both cases, segmentation is time intensive, and it therefore remains a major bottleneck that prevents more widespread application of image processing techniques.

A great deal of progress has been made in automated segmentation in the brain, partially because the anatomic structures tend to be reproducibly positioned across subjects and the contrast delineation among structures is often good. In addition, MRI images of brain tend to be high quality. Several software packages are currently available for automatic segmentation, particularly

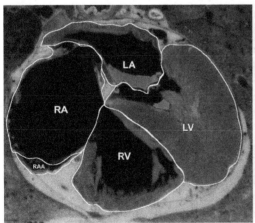
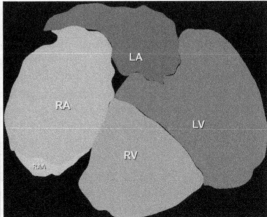
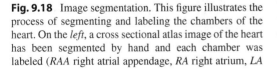

Fig. 9.18 Image segmentation. This figure illustrates the process of segmenting and labeling the chambers of the heart. On the *left*, a cross sectional atlas image of the heart has been segmented by hand and each chamber was labeled (*RAA* right atrial appendage, *RA* right atrium, *LA* left atrium, *RV* right ventricle, *LV* left ventricle). The boundary of each circumscribed anatomic region can be converted into a digital mask (*right*) which can be used in different applications where labeling anatomic structures in the image is needed

for normal macroscopic brain anatomy in cortical and sub-cortical regions (Collins et al. 1995; Friston et al. 1995; Subramaniam et al. 1997; Dale et al. 1999; MacDonald et al. 2000; Brain Innovation B.V. 2001; FMRIDB Image Analysis Group 2001; Van Essen et al. 2001; Hinshaw et al. 2002). The Human Brain Project's Internet Brain Segmentation Repository (Kennedy 2001) has been developing a repository of segmented brain images to use in comparing these different methods.

Popular segmentation techniques include reconstruction from serial sections, region-based methods, edge-based methods, model or knowledge-based methods, and combined methods.

9.4.6.1 Region-Based and Edge-Based Segmentation

In region-based segmentation, voxels are grouped into contiguous regions based on characteristics such as intensity ranges and similarity to neighboring voxels (Shapiro and Stockman 2001). A common initial approach to region-based segmentation is first to classify voxels into a small number of tissue classes. In brain MR images, a common class separation is into: gray matter, white matter, cerebrospinal fluid and background. One then uses these classifications as a basis for further segmentation (Choi et al. 1991; Zijdenbos et al. 1996). Another region-based approach is called region-growing, in which regions are grown from seed voxels manually or automatically placed within candidate regions (Davatzikos and Bryan 1996; Modayur et al. 1997). The regions found by any of these approaches are often further processed by mathematical morphology operators (Haralick 1988) to remove unwanted connections and holes (Sandor and Leahy 1997).

Edge-based segmentation is the complement to region-based segmentation: intensity gradients are used to search for and link organ boundaries. In the 2-D case, contour-following connects adjacent points on the boundary. In the 3-D case, isosurface-following or marching-cubes (Lorensen and Cline 1987) methods connect border voxels in a region into a 3-D surface mesh.

Both region-based and edge-based segmentation are essentially low-level techniques that only look at local regions in the image data.

9.4.6.2 Model- and Knowledge-Based Segmentation

A popular alternative method for medical image segmentation that is popular in brain imaging is the use of deformable models. Based on pioneering work called "Snakes" by Kass, Witkin and Terzopoulos (Kass et al. 1987), deformable models have been developed for both 2-D and 3-D. In the 2-D case the deformable model is a contour, often represented as a simple set of linear segments or a spline, which is initialized to approximate the contour on the image. The contour is then deformed according to a cost function that includes both intrinsic terms limiting how much the contour can distort, and extrinsic terms that reward closeness to image borders. In the 3-D case, a 3-D surface (often a triangular mesh) is deformed in a similar manner. There are several examples of using deformable models for brain segmentation (Davatzikos and Bryan 1996; Dale et al. 1999; MacDonald et al. 2000; Van Essen et al. 2001).

An advantage of deformable models is that the cost function can include knowledge of the expected anatomy of the brain. For example, the cost function employed in the method developed by MacDonald (MacDonald et al. 2000) includes a term for the expected thickness of the brain cortex. Thus, these methods can become somewhat knowledge-based, where knowledge of anatomy is encoded in the cost function.

An alternative knowledge-based approach explicitly records shape information in a geometric constraint network (GCN) (Brinkley 1992), which encodes local shape variation based on a training set. The shape constraints define search regions on the image in which to search for edges. Found edges are then combined with the shape constraints to deform the model and reduce the size of search regions for additional edges (Brinkley 1985, 1993a, b). The advantage of this sort of model over a pure deformable model is that knowledge is explicitly represented in the model, rather than implicitly represented in the cost function.

9.4.6.3 Combined Methods

Most brain segmentation packages use a combination of methods in a sequential pipeline. For example, a GCN model has been used to represent the overall cortical "envelope", excluding the detailed gyri and sulci (Hinshaw et al. 2002). The model is semi-automatically deformed to fit the cortex, then used as a mask to remove non-cortex such as the skull. Isosurface-following is then applied to the masked region to generate the detailed cortical surface. The model is also used on aligned MRA and MRV images to mask out non-cortical veins and arteries prior to isosurface-following. The extracted cortical, vein and artery surfaces are then rendered to produce a composite visualization of the brain as seen at neurosurgery (Fig. 9.9).

MacDonald et al. describe an automatic multi-resolution surface deformation technique called ASP (Anatomic Segmentation using Proximities), in which an inner and outer surface are progressively deformed to fit the image, where the cost function includes image terms, model-based terms, and proximity terms (MacDonald et al. 2000). Dale et al. describe an automated approach that is implemented in the FreeSurfer program (Dale et al. 1999; Fischl et al. 1999). This method initially finds the gray-white boundary, then fits smooth gray-white (inner) and white-CSF (outer) surfaces using deformable models. Van Essen et al. describe the SureFit program (Van Essen et al. 2001), which finds the cortical surface midway between the gray-white boundary and the gray-CSF boundary. This mid-level surface is created from probabilistic representations of both inner and outer boundaries that are determined using image intensity, intensity gradients, and knowledge of cortical topography. Other software packages also combine various methods for segmentation (Davatzikos and Bryan 1996; Brain Innovation B.V. 2001; FMRIDB Image Analysis Group 2001; Sensor Systems Inc. 2001; Wellcome Department of Cognitive Neurology 2001).

9.4.6.4 Parametric and Non-Parametric Clustering for Segmentation

The core operation in a segmentation task is the division of the image into a finite set of regions, which are smooth and homogeneous in their content and their representation. When posed in this way, segmentation can be regarded as a problem of finding clusters in a selected feature space.

The segmentation task can be seen as a combination of two main processes: (a) The generation of an image representation over a selected feature space. This can be termed the modeling stage. The model components are often viewed as groups, or *clusters* in the high-dimensional space. (b) The assignment of pixels to one of the model components or segments. In order to be directly relevant for a segmentation task, the clusters in the model should represent homogeneous regions of the image. In general, the better the image modeling, the better the segmentation produced. Since the number of clusters in the feature space is often unknown, segmentation can be regarded as an *unsupervised clustering* task in the high-dimensional feature space.

There is a large body of work on **clustering algorithms**. We can categorize them into three broad classes: (a) deterministic algorithms, (b) probabilistic model-based algorithms, and (c) graph-theoretic algorithms. The simplest of these are the deterministic algorithms such as k-means (Bishop 1995), mean-shift (Comaniciu and Meer 2002), and agglomerative methods (Duda et al. 2001). For certain data distributions, i.e., distributions of pixel feature vectors in a feature space, such algorithms perform well. For example, k-means provides good results when the data is convex or blob-like and the agglomerative approach succeeds when clusters are dense and there is no noise. These algorithms, however, have a difficult time handling more complex structures in the data. Further, they are sensitive to initialization (e.g., choice of initial cluster centroids). The probabilistic algorithms, on the other hand, model the distribution in the data using parametric models (McLachlan and Peel 2000). Such models include auto-regressive (AR) models, Gaussian mixture models (GMM), Markov random fields (MRF), conditional random fields, etc. Efficient ways of estimating these models are available using maximum likelihood algorithms such as the Expectation-maximization (EM) algorithm (Dempster et al. 1977). While probabilistic models offer a principled way to explain the structures present in the data, they could be restrictive when more complex structures are present. Another type of clustering algorithms is non-parametric in that this class imposes no prior shape or structure on the data. Examples of these are graph-theoretic algorithms based on spectral factorization (e.g., (Ng et al. 2001; Shi and Malik 2000)). Here, the image data are modeled as a graph. The entire image data along with a global cost function are used to partition the graph, with each partition now becoming an image segment. In this approach, global considerations determine localized decisions. Moreover, such optimization procedures are often compute-intensive.

Consider an example application in brain image segmentation using parametric modeling and clustering. The tissue and lesion segmentation problem in Brain MRI is a well-studied topic of research. In such images, there is interest in three main tissue types: white matter (WM), gray matter (GM) and cerebro-spinal fluid (CSF). The volumetric analysis of such tissue types in various part of the brain is useful in assessing the progress or remission of various diseases, such as Alzheimer's disease, epilepsy, sclerosis and schizophrenia. A segmentation example is shown in Fig. 9.19. In this example, images from three MRI imaging sequences are input to the system, and the output is a segmentation map, with different colors representing three different normal brain tissues, as well as a separate color to indicate regions of abnormality (multiple-sclerosis lesions).

Various approaches to the segmentation task are reviewed in (Pham et al. 2000). Among the approaches used are pixel-level intensity based clustering, such as K-means and Mixture of Gaussians modeling (e.g., (Kapur et al. 1996)). In this approach, the intensity feature is modeled by a mixture of Gaussians, where each Gaussian is assigned a semantic meaning, such as one of the tissue regions (or lesion). Using pattern recognition methods and learning, the Gaussians can be automatically extracted from the data, and once defined, the image can be segmented into the respective regions.

Algorithms for tissue segmentation using pixel-level intensity-based classification often exhibit high sensitivity to various noise artifacts, such as intra-tissue noise, inter-tissue intensity contrast reduction, partial-volume effects and others. Due to the artifacts present, classical voxel-wise intensity-based classification methods, including the K-means modeling and Mixture of Gaussians modeling, often give unrealistic results, with tissue class regions appearing granular, fragmented, or violating anatomical constraints. Specific works can be found addressing various aspects of these concerns (e.g., partial-volume effect quantification (Dugas-Phocion et al. 2004)).

One way to address the smoothness issue is to add spatial constraints. This is often done during a pre-processing phase by using a statistical atlas, or as a post-processing step via Markov Random Field models. A statistical atlas provides the prior probability for each pixel to originate from a particular

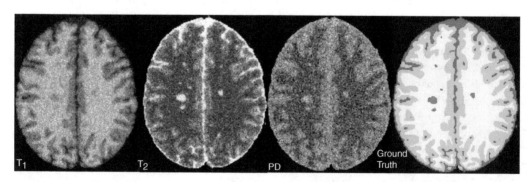

Fig. 9.19 Brain MRI segmentation example. Brain slice from multiple acquisition sequences (with 9 % noise) was taken from BrainWEB (http://www.bic.mni.mcgill.ca/brainweb/). From *left* to *right*: T1-, T2-, and proton den-sity (*PD*)-weighted image. Segmentation of the images is shown on the *right*: *Blue*: CSF, *Green*: Gray matter (GM), *Yellow*: white matter (WM), *Red*: Multiple-sclerosis lesions (MSL) (Friefeld et al. 2009)

tissue class (e.g., (Van Leemput et al. 1999; Marroquin et al. 2002; Prastawa et al. 2004)).

Algorithms exist that use the maximum-a-posteriori (MAP) criterion to augment intensity information with the atlas. However, registration between a given image and the atlas is required, which can be computationally prohibitive (Rohlfing and Maurer 2003). Further, the quality of the registration result is strongly dependent on the physiological variability of the subject and may converge to an erroneous result in the case of a diseased or severely damaged brain. Finally, the registration process is applicable only to complete volumes. A single slice cannot be registered to the atlas. Therefore it cannot be segmented using these state-of-the-art algorithms.

Segmentation can also be improved using a post-processing phase in which smoothness and immunity to noise can be achieved by modeling the interactions among neighboring voxels. Such interactions can be modeled using a Markov Random Field (MRF), and thus this technique has been used to improve segmentation (Held et al. 1997; Van Leemput et al. 1999; Zhang et al. 2001).

Finally, there are algorithms that use deformable models to incorporate tissue boundary information (McInerney and Terzopoulos 1997). They often imply inherent smoothness but require careful initialization and precisely calibrated model parameters in order to provide consistent results in the presence of a noisy environment.

In yet another approach, the image representation is augmented to include spatial information in the feature space, and GMM clustering is utilized to provide coherent clusters in feature space that correspond to coherent spatial localized regions in the image space. In this methodology, the atlas pre-processing step and the smoothing post-processing are not required components. For regions of complex shapes in the image plane, for which a single convex hull is not sufficient (will cover two or more different segments of the image), a plausible approach is to utilize very small spatial supports per Gaussian. This in turn implies the use of a large number of Gaussians, a modeling that was shown to be useful in the brain segmentation task (Greenspan et al. 2006) as well as extended to multiple-sclerosis lesion modeling task (Friefeld et al. 2009).

9.4.7 Image Registration

The growing availability of 3-D and higher dimensionality structural and functional images leads to exciting opportunities for realistically observing the structure and function of the body. Nowhere have these opportunities been more widely exploited than in brain imaging. Therefore, this section concentrates on 3-D brain imaging, with the recognition that many of the methods developed for the brain have been or will be applied to other areas as well.

The basic 2-D image processing operations of global processing, segmentation, feature detection, and classification generalize to higher dimensions, and are usually part of any image processing application. However, 3-D and higher dimensionality images give rise to additional informatics issues, which include image *registration* (which also occurs to a lesser extent in 2-D), *spatial* representation of anatomy, *symbolic* representation of anatomy, integration of spatial and symbolic anatomic representations in *atlases*, anatomical *variation*, and *characterization* of anatomy. All but the first of these issues deal primarily with anatomical structure, and therefore could be considered part of the field of structural informatics. They could also be thought of as being part of imaging informatics and **neuroinformatics**.

As noted previously, 3-D image volume data are represented in the computer by a 3-D volume array, in which each voxel represents the image intensity in a small volume of space. In order to depict anatomy accurately, the voxels must be accurately registered (or located) in the 3-D volume (*voxel registration*), and separately acquired image volumes from the same subject must be registered with each other (*volume registration*).

9.4.7.1 Voxel Registration
Imaging modalities such as CT, MRI, and confocal microscopy (Sects. 9.2.3 and 9.2.5) are inherently 3-D: the scanner generally outputs a series of image slices that can easily be reformatted as a 3-D volume array, often following alignment algorithms that compensate for any patient motion during the scanning procedure. For this

reason, almost all CT and MR manufacturers' consoles contain some form of three-dimensional reconstruction and visualization capabilities.

As noted in Sect. 9.4.4, two-dimensional images can be converted to 3-D volumes if they are closely spaced parallel sections through a tissue or whole specimen and contain isotropic voxels. In this case the problem is how to align the sections with each other. For whole sections (either frozen or fixed), the standard method is to embed a set of thin rods or strings in the tissue prior to sectioning, to manually indicate the location of these **fiducials** on each section, then to linearly transform each slice so that the corresponding fiducials line up in 3-D (Prothero and Prothero 1986). A popular current example of this technique is the Visible Human, in which a series of transverse slices were acquired, then reconstructed to give a full 3-D volume (Spitzer and Whitlock 1998) (Chap. 20).

It is difficult to embed fiducial markers at the microscopic level, so intrinsic tissue landmarks are often used as fiducials, but the basic principle is similar. However, in this case tissue distortion may be a problem, so non-linear transformations may be required. For example Fiala and Harris (Fiala and Harris 2001) have developed an interface that allows the user to indicate, on electron microscopy sections, corresponding centers of small organelles such as mitochondria. A non-linear transformation (warp) is then computed to bring the landmarks into registration.

An approach being pursued (among other approaches) by the National Center for Microscopy and Imaging Research[2] combines reconstruction from thick serial sections with electron tomography (Soto et al. 1994). In this case the tomographic technique is applied to each thick section to generate a 3-D digital slab, after which the slabs are aligned with each other to generate a 3-D volume. The advantages of this approach over the standard serial section method are that the sections do not need to be as thin, and fewer of them need be acquired.

An alternative approach to 3-D voxel registration from 2-D images is stereo-matching, a tech-nique developed in computer vision that acquires multiple 2-D images from known angles, finds corresponding points on the images, and uses the correspondences and known camera angles to compute 3-D coordinates of pixels in the matched images. The technique is being applied to the reconstruction of synapses from electron micrographs by a Human Brain Project collaboration between computer scientists and biologists at the University of Maryland (Agrawal et al. 2000).

9.4.7.2 Volume Registration

A related problem to that of aligning individual sections is the problem of aligning separate image volumes from the same subject, that is, *intra-subject* alignment. Because different image modalities provide complementary information, it is common to acquire more than one kind of image volume on the same individual. This approach has been particularly useful for brain imaging because each modality provides different information. For example, PET (Sect. 9.2.3) provides useful information about function, but does not provide good localization with respect to the anatomy. Similarly, MRV and MRA (Sect. 9.2.3) show blood flow but do not provide the detailed anatomy visible with standard MRI. By combining images from these modalities with MRI, it is possible to show functional images in terms of the underlying anatomy, thereby providing a common neuroanatomic framework.

The primary problem to solve in multimodality image fusion is volume registration—that is, the alignment of separately acquired image volumes. In the simplest case, separate image volumes are acquired during a single sitting. The patient's head may be immobilized, and the information in the image headers may be used to rotate and resample the image volumes until all the voxels correspond. However, if the patient moves, or if examinations are acquired at different times, other registration methods are needed. When intensity values are similar across modalities, registration can be performed automatically by intensity-based optimization methods (Woods et al. 1992; Collins et al. 1994). When intensity values are not similar (as is the case with MRA, MRV and MRI), images can be aligned to templates of the same modalities that are already

---

[2] http://ncmir.ucsd.edu/ (accessed 4/26/13).

aligned (Woods et al. 1993; Ashburner and Friston 1997). Alternatively, landmark-based methods can be used. The landmark-based methods are similar to those used to align serial sections (see earlier discussion of voxel registration in this section), but in this case the landmarks are 3-D points. The Montreal Register Program (MacDonald 1993) is an example of such a program.

9.5 Image Interpretation and Computer Reasoning

The preceding sections of this chapter as well as Chap. 20 describe informatics aspects of image generation, storage, manipulation, and display of images. Rendering an interpretation is a crucial final stage in the chain of activities related to imaging. *Image interpretation* is this final stage in which the physician has direct impact on the clinical care process, by rendering a professional opinion as to whether abnormalities are present in the image and the likely significance of those abnormalities. The process of image interpretation requires reasoning—to draw inferences from facts; the facts are the image abnormalities detected and the known clinical history, and the inferred information is the diagnosis and management decision (what to do next, such as another test or surgery, etc.). Such reasoning usually entails uncertainty, and optimally would be carried out using probabilistic approaches (Chap. 3), unless certain classic imaging patterns are recognized. In reality, radiology practice is usually carried out without formal probabilistic models that relate imaging observations to the likelihood of diseases. However, variation in practice is a known problem in image interpretation (Robinson 1997), and methods to improve this process are desirable.

Informatics methods can enhance radiological interpretation of images in two major ways: (1) image retrieval systems and (2) decision support systems. The concept of *image retrieval* is similar to that of information retrieval (see Chap. 21), in which the user retrieves a set of documents pertinent to a question or information need. The information being sought when doing image retrieval is images with specific content—typically to find images that are similar in some ways to a query image (e.g., to find images in the PACS containing similar-appearing abnormalities to that in an image being interpreted). Finding images containing similar content is referred to as **content based image retrieval** (CBIR). By retrieving similar images and then looking at the diagnosis of those patients, the radiologist can gain greater confidence in interpreting the images from patients whose diagnosis is not yet known.

As with the task of medical diagnosis (Chap. 22), radiological diagnosis can be enhanced using *decision support systems*, which assist the physician through a process called *computer reasoning*. In computer reasoning, the machine takes in the available data (the images and possibly other clinical information), performs a variety of image processing methods (Sect. 9.4), and uses one or more types of knowledge resources and/or mathematical models to render an output comprising either a decision or a ranked list of possible choices (e.g., diagnoses or locations on the image suspected of being abnormal).

There are two types of decision support in radiology, *computer-assisted detection* (CAD) and *computer-assisted diagnosis* (CADx). In the former, the computer locates ROIs in the image where abnormalities are suspected and the radiologist must evaluate their medical significance. In CADx, the computer is given an ROI corresponding to a suspected abnormality (possible with associated clinical information) and it outputs the likely diagnoses and possibly management recommendations (ideally with some sort of confidence rating as well as explanation facility).

In this section we describe informatics methods for image retrieval and decision support (computer reasoning with images).

9.5.1 Content-Based Image Retrieval

Since a key aspect of radiological interpretation is recognizing characteristic patterns in the imaging features which suggest the diagnosis, searching databases for similar images with known diagnoses could be an effective strategy to improving diagnostic accuracy. CBIR is the process of performing a match between images using their visual content. A query image can be presented as input to the system (or a combination of a query image and the patient's clinical record), and the system searches for similar cases in large archive settings (such as PACS) and returns a ranked list of such similar data (images). This task requires an informative representation for the image data, along with similarity measures across image data. CBIR methods are already useful in non-medical applications such as consumer imaging and on the Web (Wang et al. 1997; Smeulders et al. 2000; Datta et al. 2008).

There has also been ongoing work to develop CBIR methods in radiology. The approach generally is based on deriving quantitative characteristics from the images (e.g., pixel statistics, spatial frequency content, etc.; Sect. 9.4.5), followed by application of similarity metrics to search databases for similar images (Lehmann et al. 2004; Muller et al. 2004; Greenspan and Pinhas 2007; Datta et al. 2008; Deserno et al. 2009). The focus of the current work is on entire images, describing them with sets of numerical features, with the goal of retrieving similar images from medical collections (Hersh et al. 2009) that provide benchmarks for image retrieval. However, in many cases only a particular region of the image is of interest when seeking similar images (e.g., finding images containing similar-appearing lesions to those in the query image). More recently, "localized" CBIR methods are being developed in which a part of the image containing a region of interest is analyzed (Deselaers et al. 2007; Rahmani et al. 2008; Napel et al. 2010).

There are several unsolved challenges in CBIR. First, CBIR has been largely focused on query based on single 2-D images; methods need to be developed for 3D retrieval in which a volume is the query "image." A second challenge is the need to integrate images with non-image clinical data to permit retrieval based on entire patient cases and not single images (e.g., the CBIR method should take into consideration the clinical history in addition to the image appearance in retrieving a similar "case").

Another limitation of current CBIR is that image semantics is not routinely included. The information reported by the radiologist ("semantic features"), is complementary to the quantitative data contained in image pixels. One approach to capturing image semantics is analyzing and processing "visual words" in images, captured as image patches or codebooks (Sect. 9.4.5). These techniques have been shown to perform well in CBIR applications (Qiu 2002). Another approach to capture image semantics is to use the radiologist's imaging observations as image features. Several studies have found that combining the semantic information obtained from radiologists' imaging reports or annotations with the pixel-level features can enhance performance of CBIR systems (Ruiz 2006; Zhenyu et al. 2009; Napel et al. 2010). The knowledge representation methods described in Sects. 9.3.2 and 9.4.5 make it possible to combine these types of information.

9.5.2 Computer-Based Inference with Images and Knowledge

Though image retrieval described above (and information retrieval in general) can be helpful to a practitioner interpreting images, it does not directly answer a specific question at hand, such as, "what is the diagnosis in this patient" or "what imaging test should I order next?" Answering such questions requires reasoning, either by the physician with all the available data, or by a computer, using physician inputs and the images. As the use of imaging proliferates and the number of images being produced by imaging modalities explodes, it is becoming a major challenge for practicing radiologists to integrate the multitude of imaging data, clinical data, and soon molecular data, to formulate an accurate diagnosis and management plan for the patient. Computer-based inference systems (decision support systems) can help radiologists understand the biomedical import of this information and to provide guidance (Hudson and Cohen 2009).

There are two major approaches to computerized reasoning systems for imaging decision support, quantitative imaging-based methods (CAD/CADx) and knowledge-based computer reasoning systems.

9.5.2.1 Quantitative Imaging Computer Reasoning Systems (CAD/CADx)

The process of deriving quantitative image features was described in Sect. 9.4.5. Quantitative imaging applications such as CAD and CADx use these quantifiable features extracted from medical images for a variety of decision support applications, such as the assessment of an abnormality to suggest a diagnosis, or to evaluate the severity, degree of change, or status of a disease, injury, or chronic condition. In general, the quantitative imaging computer reasoning systems apply a mathematical model (e.g., a *classifier*) or other machine learning methods to obtain a decision output based on the imaging inputs.

CAD

In CAD applications, the goal is to scan the image and identify suspicious regions that may represent regions of disease in the patient. A common use for CAD is *screening*, the task of reviewing many images and identifying those that are suspicious and require closer scrutiny by a radiologist (e.g., mammography interpretation). Most CAD applications comprise an image processing pipeline (Sect. 9.4) that uses global processing, segmentation, image quantitation with feature extraction, and classification to determine whether an image should be flagged for careful review by a radiologist or pathologist. In CAD and in screening in general, the goal is to detect disease; thus, the tradeoff favors having false positive instead of missing false negatives. Thus CAD systems tend to flag a reasonable number of normal images (false positives) and they miss very few abnormal images (false negatives). If the number of flagged images is small compared with the total number of images, then automated screening procedures can be economically viable. On the other hand, too many false positives are time-consuming to review and lessens user confidence in the CAD system; thus for CAD to be viable, they must minimize the number of false positives as well as false negatives.

CAD techniques for screening have been applied successfully to many different types of images (Doi 2007), including mammography images for identifying mass lesions and clusters of microcalcifications, chest X-rays and CT of the chest to detect small cancerous nodules, and volumetric CT images of the colon ("virtual colonscopy") to detect polyps. In addition, CAD methods have been applied to Papanicolaou (Pap) smears for cancerous or precancerous cells (Giger and MacMahon 1996), as well as to many other types of non-radiologic images.

CADx

In CADx applications, a suspicious region in the image has already been identified (by the radiologist of a CAD application), and the goal is to evaluate it to render a diagnosis or differential diagnosis. CADx systems usually need to be provided an ROI, or they need to segment the image to locate specific organs and lesions in order to perform analysis of quantitative image features that are extracted from the ROI and use that to render a diagnosis. In general, a mathematical model is created to relate the quantitative (or semantic) features to the likely diagnoses. Probabilistic models have been particularly effective (Burnside et al. 2000, 2004a,b, 2006, 2007; Lee et al. 2009; Liu et al. 2009, 2011), because the image features are generated based on the underlying disease, so there is probabilistic dependence on the disease and the quantitative and perceived imaging features. In fact, it can be argued that radiological interpretation is fundamentally a Bayesian task (Lusted 1960; Ledley and Lusted 1991; Donovan and Manning 2007) (see Chaps. 3 and 22), and thus decision-support strategies based on Bayesian models may be quite effective.

CADx can be very effective in practice, reducing variation and improving positive predictive value of radiologists (Burnside et al. 2006). Deploying CADx systems, however, can be challenging. Since the inputs to CADx generally need to be structured (semantic features from the radiologist and/or quantitative features from the image), a means of capturing the structured image information as part of the routine clinical workflow is required. A promising approach is to combine structured reporting with CADx (Fig. 9.20); the radiologist records the imaging

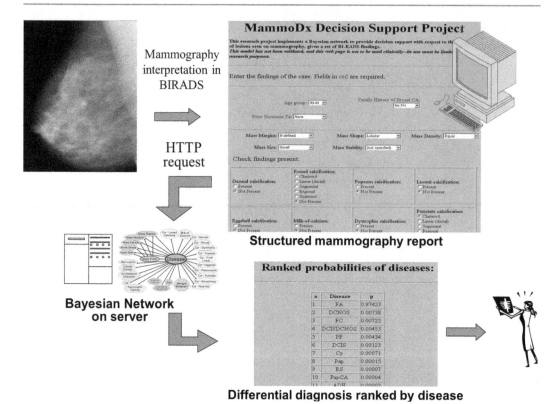

Mammography interpretation in BIRADS

HTTP request

Bayesian Network on server

Structured mammography report

Ranked probabilities of diseases:

Differential diagnosis ranked by disease

Fig. 9.20 Bayesian network-based system for decision support in mammography CADx. The radiologist interpreting the image enters the radiology observations and clinical information (patient history) in a structured reporting Web-based data capture form to render the report. This form is sent to a server which inputs the observations into the Bayesian network to calculate posterior probabilities of disease. A list of diseases, ranked by the probability of each disease, is return to the user who can make a decision based on a threshold of probability of malignancy, or based on shared decision making with the patient (Figure reprinted with permission from (Rubin 2011))

observations with a data capture form, which provides the structured image content required to the CADx system. Ideally the output would be presented immediately to the radiologist as the report is generated so that the output of decision support can be incorporated into the radiology report. Such implementations will be greatly facilitated by informatics methods to extract and record the image information in structured and standard formats and with controlled terminologies (Sect. 9.3.2).

9.5.2.2 Knowledge-Based Reasoning with Images

The CAD and CADx systems do not require processing radiological knowledge (e.g., anatomic knowledge) in order to carry out their tasks; they are based on quantitative modeling

of relationships of images features to diagnoses. However, not all image-based reasoning problems are amenable to this approach. In particular, knowledge-based tasks such as reasoning about anatomy, physiology, and pathology—tasks that entail symbolic manipulations of biomedical knowledge and application of logic—are best handled using different methods, such as ontologies and logical inference (see Chap. 22).

Knowledge-based computer reasoning applications use knowledge representations, generally ontologies, in conjunction with rules of logic to deduce information from asserted facts (e.g., from observations in the image). For example, an anatomy ontology may express the knowledge that "if a segment of a coronary artery is severed, then branches distal to the severed branch will not receive blood," and "the anterior and lateral portions of the right ventricle are supplied by branches of the right coronary artery, with little or no collateral supply from the left coronary artery." Using this knowledge, and recognition via image processing that the right coronary artery is severed in an injury, a computer reasoning application could deduce that the anterior and lateral portions of the right ventricle will become ischemic (among other regions; Fig. 9.21). In performing this reasoning task, the application uses the knowledge to draw correct conclusions by manipulating the anatomical concepts and relationships using the rules of logical inference during the reasoning process.

Computer reasoning with ontologies is performed by one of two methods: (1) *reasoning by ontology query* and (2) *reasoning by logical inference*. In reasoning by ontology query, the application traverse relationships that link particular entities in the ontology to directly answer particular questions about how those entities relate to each other. For example, by traversing the *part-of* relationship in an anatomy ontology, a reasoning application can infer that the left ventricle and right ventricle are part-of the chest (given that the ontology asserts they are each part of the heart, and that the heart is part of the chest), without our needing to specify this fact explicitly in the ontology.

In reasoning by logical inference, ontologies that encode sufficient information ("explicit semantics") to apply generic reasoning engines are used. The Web Ontology Language (OWL) (Bechhofer et al. 2004; Smith et al. 2004; Motik et al. 2008) is an ontology language recommended by the World Wide Web Consortium (W3C) as a standard language for the Semantic Web (World Wide Web Consortium W3C Recommendation 10 Feb 2004). OWL is similar to other ontology languages in that it can capture knowledge by representing the entities ("classes") and their attributes ("properties"). In addition, OWL provides the capability of defining "formal semantics" or meaning of the entities in the ontology. Entities are defined using logic statements that provide assertions about

entities ("class axioms") using **description logics** (DL) (Grau et al. 2008). DLs provide a formalism enabling developers to define precise semantics of knowledge in ontologies and to perform automated deductive reasoning (Baader et al. 2003). For example, an anatomy ontology in OWL could provide precise semantics for "hemopericardium," by defining it as a pericardial cavity that contains blood.

Highly optimized computer reasoning engines ("reasoners") have been developed for OWL, helping developers to incorporate reasoning efficiently and effectively in their applications (Tsarkov and Horrocks 2006; Motik et al. 2009). These reasoners work with OWL ontologies by evaluating the asserted logical statements about classes and their properties in the original ontology (the "asserted ontology"), and they create a new ontology structure that is deduced from the asserted knowledge (the "inferred ontology"). This reasoning process is referred to as "automatic classification." The inferences obtained from the reasoning process are obtained by querying the inferred ontology and looking for classes (or individuals) that have been assigned to classes of interest in the ontology. For example, an application was created to infer the consequences of cardiac injury in this manner (Fig. 9.21).

Several knowledge-based image reasoning systems have been developed that use ontologies as the knowledge source to process the image content and derive inferences from them. These include: (1) reasoning about the anatomic consequences of penetrating injury, (2) inferring and simulating the physiological changes that will occur given anatomic abnormalities seen in images, (3) automated disease grading/staging to infer the grade and/or stage of disease based on imaging features of disease in the body (4) surgical planning by deducing the functional significance of disruption of white matter tracts in the brain, (5) inferring the types of information users seek based on analyzing query logs of image searches, and (6) inferring the response of disease in patients to treatment based on analysis of serial imaging studies. We briefly describe these applications.

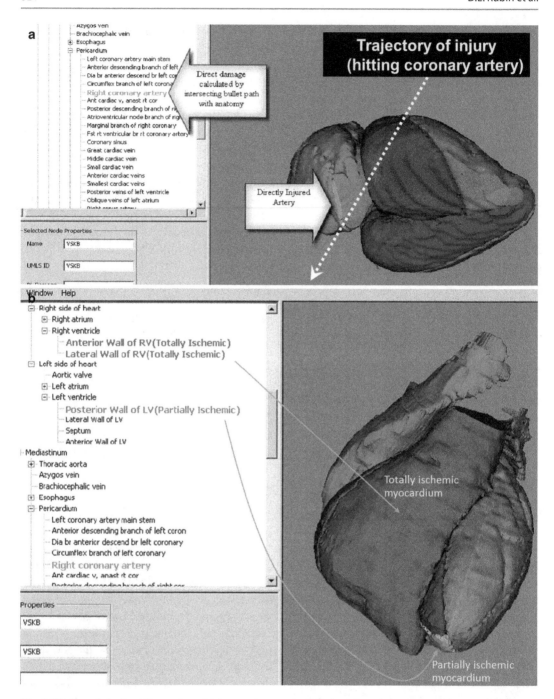

Fig. 9.21 Knowledge-based reasoning with images in a task to predict the portions of the heart that will become ischemic after a penetrating injury that injures particular anatomic structures. The application allows the user to draw a trajectory of penetrating injury on the image, a 3-D rendering of the heart obtained from segmented CT images. The reasoning application automatically carries out two tasks. (**a**) The application first deduces the anatomic structures that will be injured consequent to the trajectory (*arrow*, *right*) by interrogating semantic annotations on the image based on the trajectory of injury (injured anatomic structures shown in bold in the left panel). (**b**) The anatomic structures that are predicted to be initially injured are displayed in the volume rendering (*dark gray* = total ischemia; *light gray* = partial ischemia). In this example, the right coronary artery was injured, and the reasoning application correctly inferred there will be total ischemia of the anterior and lateral wall of the right ventricle and partial ischemia of the posterior wall of the left ventricle

Reasoning About Anatomic Consequences of Penetrating Injury

In this system, images were segmented and semantic annotations applied to identify cardiac structures. An ontology of cardiac anatomy in OWL was used to encode knowledge about anatomic structures and the portions of them that are supplied by different arterial branches. Using knowledge about part-of relationships and connectivity, the application uses the anatomy ontology to infer the anatomic consequences of injury that are recognized on the input images (Fig. 9.21) (Rubin et al. 2004, 2005, 2006b).

Inferring and Simulating the Physiological Changes

Morphological changes in anatomy have physiological consequences. For example, if a hole appears in the septum dividing the atria or ventricles of the heart (a septal defect), then blood will flow abnormally between the heart chambers and will produce abnormal physiological blood flow. The simulation community has created mathematical models to predict the physiological signals, such as time-varying pressure and flow, given particular parameters in the model such as capacitance, resistance, etc. The knowledge in these mathematical models can be represented ontologically, in which the entities correspond to nodes in the simulation model; the advantage is that a graphical representation of the ontology, corresponding to a graphical representation of the mathematical model, can be created. Morphological alterations seen in images can be directly translated into alterations in the ontological representation of the anatomic structures, and simultaneously can update the simulation model appropriately to simulate the physiological consequences of the morphological anatomic alteration (Rubin et al. 2006a). Such knowledge-based image reasoning methods could greatly enable functional evaluation of the static abnormalities seen in medical imaging.

Automated Disease Grading/Staging

A great deal of image-based knowledge is encoded in the literature and not readily available to clinicians needing to apply it. A good example of this is the criteria used to grade and stage disease based on imaging criteria. For example, there are detailed criteria specified for staging tumors and grading the severity of disease. This knowledge has been encoded in OWL ontologies and used to automate grading of brain gliomas (Marquet et al. 2007) and staging of cancer (Dameron et al. 2006) based on the imaging features detected by radiologists. This ontology-based paradigm could provide a good model for delivering current biomedical knowledge to practitioners "just-in-time" to help them grade and stage disease as they view images and record their observations.

Surgical Planning

Understanding complex anatomic relationships and their functional significance in the patient is crucial in surgical planning, particular for brain surgery, since there are many surgical approaches possible, and some will have less severe consequences to patients than others. It can be challenging to be aware of all these relationships and functional dependencies; thus, surgical planning is an opportune area to develop knowledge-based image reasoning systems. The anatomic and functional knowledge can be encoded in an ontology and used by an application to plan the optimal surgical approach. In recent work, such an ontological model was developed to assess the functional sequelae of disruptions of motor pathways in the brain, which could be used in the future to guide surgical interventions (Talos et al. 2008; Rubin et al. 2009a)

Inferring Types of Information Users Seek from Images

Knowledge-based reasoning approaches have been used to evaluate image search logs on Web sites that host image databases to ascertain the types of queries users submit. RadLex (Sect. 9.3.2) was used as the ontology, and by mapping the queries to leaf classes in RadLex and then traversing the subsumption relations, the types of queries could be deduced by interrogating the higher-level classes in RadLex (such as "visual observation" and "anatomic entity") (Rubin et al. 2011).

Inferring the Response of Disease Treatment

As mentioned above, the complex knowledge required to grade and stage disease can be represented using an ontology. Similarly, the criteria used to assess the response of patients to treatment is also complex, evolving, and dependent on numerous aspects of image information. The knowledge needed to apply criteria of disease response assessment have been encoded ontologically, specifically in OWL, and used to determine automatically the degree of cancer response to treatment in patients (Levy et al. 2009; Levy and Rubin 2011). The inputs to the computerized reasoning method are the quantitative information about lesions seen in the images, recorded as semantic annotations using the AIM information model (Sect. 9.3.2). This application demonstrates the potential for a streamlined workflow of radiology image interpretation and lesion measurement automatically feeding into decision support to guide patient care.

9.6   Conclusions

This chapter focuses on methods for computational representation and for processing images in biomedicine, with an emphasis on radiological imaging and the extraction and characterization of anatomical structure and abnormalities. It has been emphasized that the content of images is complex—comprising both quantitative and semantic information. Methods of making that content explicit and computationally-accessible have been described, and they are crucial to enable computer applications to access the "biomedical meaning" in images; presently, the vast archives of images are poorly utilized because the image content is not explicit and accessible. As the methods to extract quantitative and semantic image information become more widespread, image databases will be as useful to the discovery process as the biological databases (they will even likely become linked), and an era

of "data-driven" and "high-throughput imaging" will be enabled, analogous to modern "high-throughput" biology. In addition, the computational imaging methods will lead to applications that leverage the image content, such as CAD/CADx and knowledge-based image reasoning that use image content to improve physicians' capability to care for patients.

Though this chapter has focused on radiology, we stress that the biomedical imaging informatics methods presented are generalizable and either have been or will be applied to other domains in which visualization and imaging are becoming increasingly important, such as microscopy, pathology, ophthalmology, and dermatology. As new imaging modalities increasingly become available for imaging other and more detailed body regions, the techniques presented in this chapter will increasingly be applied in all areas of biomedicine. For example, the development of molecular imaging methods is analogous to functional brain imaging, since functional data, in this case from gene expression rather than cognitive activity, can be mapped to an anatomical substrate.

Thus, the general biomedical imaging informatics methods described here will increasingly be applied to diverse areas of biomedicine. As they are applied, and as imaging modalities continue to proliferate, a growing demand will be placed on leveraging the content in these images to characterize the clinical phenotype of disease and relate it to genotype and clinical data from patients to enhance research and clinical care.

Suggested Readings

Brinkley, J. F. (1991). Structural informatics and its applications in medicine and biology. *Academic Medicine, 66*(10), 589–591. Short introduction to the field.

Brinkley, J. F., & Rosse, C. (2002). Imaging and the human brain project: A review. *Methods of Information in Medicine, 41*, 245–260. Review of image processing work related to the brain. Much of the brain-related material for this chapter was adapted from this article.

Deserno, T. M. (2011). *Biomedical image processing.* Berlin: Springer. Edited book of current approaches to variety of biomedical image processing tasks.

Foley, D. D., Van Dam, A., Feiner, S. K., Hughes, J. F. (1990). *Computer Graphics: Principles and Practice. Reading,* MA: Addison-Wesley.

Gonzalez, R. C., Woods, R. E., et al. (2009). *Digital image processing using MATLAB.* Knoxville: S.I. Gatesmark Publishing. A comprehensive overview of image processing methods focusing on MATLAB examples.

Horii, S. C. (1996). *Image acquisition: Sites, technologies and approaches.* In Greenes, R. A. and Bauman, R. A. (eds.) Imaging and information management: computer systems for a changing health care environment. The Radiology Clinics of North America, 34(3):469–494.

Pham, D. L., Xu, C., & Prince, J. L. (2000). Current methods in medical image segmentation. *Annual Review of Biomedical Engineering, 2,* 315–337. Overview of medical image segmentation.

Potchen, E. J. (2000). Prospects for progress in diagnostic imaging. *Journal of Internal Medicine, 247*(4), 411–424. Nontechnical description of newer imaging methods such as cardiac MRI, diffusion tensor imaging, fMRI, and molecular imaging. Current and potential use of these methods for diagnosis.

Robb, R. A. (2000). *Biomedical imaging, visualization, and analysis.* New York: Wiley. Overview of biomedical imaging modalities and processing techniques.

Shapiro, L. G., & Stockman, G. C. (2001). *Computer vision.* Upper Saddle River: Prentice-Hall. Detailed description of many of the representations and methods used in image processing. Not specific to medicine, but most of the methods are applicable to medical imaging.

Sonka, M., & Fitzpatrick, J. M. (2000). *Handbook of medical imaging* (Medical image processing and analysis, Vol. 2). Bellingham: SPIE Press. Overview of biomedical imaging modalities and processing techniques.

Yoo, T. S. (2004). *Insight into images: Principles and practice for segmentation, registration, and image analysis.* Wellesley: A K Peters. Comprehensive overview of digital image processing methods with examples from the Insight Toolkit (ITK).

Questions for Discussion

1. How might you create an image processing pipeline to build an image-analysis program looking for abnormal cells in a PAP smear? How would you collect and incorporate semantic features into the program?

2. Why is segmentation so difficult to perform? Give two examples of ways by which current systems avoid the problem of automatic segmentation.

3. How might you build a decision-support system that is based on searching the hospital image archive for similar images and returning the diagnosis associated with the most similar images? How might you make use of the semantic information in images in images to improve the accuracy of retrieval?

4. Give an example of how knowledge about the problem to be solved (e.g., local anatomy in the image) could be used in future systems to aid in automatic segmentation.

5. Both images and free text share the characteristic that they are unstructured information; image processing methods to make the biomedical content in images explicit are very similar to related problems in natural language processing (NLP; Chap. 8). How are image processing methods and NLP similar in terms of (1) computer representation of the raw content? (2) representation of the semantic content? (3) processing of the content (e.g., what is the NLP equivalent of segmentation, or the image processing equivalent of named entity recognition)?

Ethics in Biomedical and Health Informatics: Users, Standards, and Outcomes

10

Kenneth W. Goodman, Reid Cushman, and Randolph A. Miller

After reading this chapter, you should know the answers to these questions:

- Why is ethics important to informatics?
- What are the leading ethical issues that arise in health care informatics?
- What are examples of appropriate and inappropriate uses and users for health-related software?
- Why does the establishment of standards touch on ethical issues?
- Why does system evaluation involve ethical issues?
- What challenges does informatics pose for patient and provider confidentiality?
- How can the tension between the obligation to protect confidentiality and that to share data be minimized?
- How might computational health care alter the traditional provider–patient relationship?

- What ethical issues arise at the intersection of informatics and managed care?
- What are the leading ethical and legal issues in the debate over governmental regulation of health care computing tools?

10.1 Ethical Issues in Biomedical and Health Informatics

More and more the tendency is towards the use of mechanical aids to diagnosis; nevertheless, the five senses of the doctor do still, and must always, play the preponderating part in the examination of the sick patient. Careful observation can never be replaced by the tests of the laboratory. The good physician now or in the future will never be a diagnostic robot. – Scottish surgeon Sir William Arbuthnot-Lane (Lane 1936)

Human values should govern research and practice in the health professions. Health care informatics, like other health professions, encompasses issues of appropriate and inappropriate behavior, of honorable and disreputable actions, and of right and wrong. Students and practitioners of the health sciences, including informatics, share an important obligation to explore the moral underpinnings and ethical challenges related to their research and practice.

Although ethical questions in medicine, nursing, human subjects research, psychology, social work, and affiliated fields continue to evolve and increase in number, the key issues are generally well known. Major questions in bioethics have been addressed in numerous professional,

K.W. Goodman, PhD (✉)
University of Miami Bioethics Program, 1400 NW 10th Ave., Suite 916 (M-825), Miami 33136, FL, USA
e-mail: kgoodman@med.miami.edu

R. Cushman, PhD
Department of Medicine, University of Miami, 1400 NW 10th Ave, NW, Suite 912, Miami 33136, FL, USA
e-mail: rcushman@med.miami.edu

R.A. Miller, MD
Department of Biomedical Informatics, Vanderbilt University Medical Center, 2209 Garland Avenue, B003C Eskind Biomedical Library, Nashville 37232-8340, TN, USA
e-mail: randolph.a.miller@vanderbilt.edu

E.H. Shortliffe, J.J. Cimino (eds.), *Biomedical Informatics*,
DOI 10.1007/978-1-4471-4474-8_10, © Springer-Verlag London 2014

scholarly, and educational contexts. Ethical matters in health informatics are, in general, less familiar, even though certain of them have received attention for decades (Szolovits and Pauker 1979; Miller et al. 1985; de Dombal 1987). Indeed, informatics now constitutes a source of some of the most important and interesting ethical debates in all the health professions.

People often assume that the confidentiality of electronically stored patient information is the most important ethical issue in informatics. Although confidentiality and privacy are indeed of vital interest and significant concern, the field is rich with other ethical issues, including the appropriate selection and use of informatics tools in clinical settings; the determination of who should use such tools; the role of system evaluation; the obligations of system developers, maintainers, and vendors; the appropriate standards for interacting with industry; and the use of computers to track clinical outcomes to guide future practice. In addition, informatics engenders many important legal and regulatory questions.

To consider ethical issues in health care informatics is to explore a significant intersection among several professions—health care informatics per se, health care delivery and administration, applied computing and systems engineering, and ethics—each of which constitutes a vast field of inquiry. Fortunately, growing interest in bioethics and computation-related ethics has produced a starting point for such exploration. An initial ensemble of guiding principles, or ethical criteria, has emerged to orient decision making in health care informatics. These criteria are of practical utility to health informatics, and often have broader implications for all of biomedical informatics.

10.2 Health-Informatics Applications: Appropriate Use, Users, and Contexts

Application of computer-based technologies in the health professions can build on previous experience in adopting other devices, tools, and methods. Before clinicians perform most health-related interventions (e.g., diagnostic testing, prescription of medication, surgical and other therapeutic procedures), they generally evaluate appropriate evidence, standards, available technologies, presuppositions, and values. Indeed, the very evolution of the health professions entails the evolution of evidence, of standards, of available technologies, of presuppositions, and of values.

To answer the clinical question, "What should be done in this case?" one must pay attention to a number of subsidiary questions, such as:

1. What is the problem?
2. What resources are available and what am I competent to do?
3. What will maintain or improve this patient's care?
4. What will otherwise produce the most desirable results (e.g., in public health)?
5. How strong are my beliefs in the accuracy of my answers to questions 1 through 4, above.

Similar considerations determine the appropriate use of informatics tools.

10.2.1 The Standard View of Appropriate Use

Excitement and enthusiasm often accompany initial use of new tools in clinical settings. Negative emotions are also common (Sittig et al. 2005). Based on the uncertainties that surround any new technology, scientific evidence counsels caution and prudence. As in other clinical areas, evidence and reason determine the appropriate level of caution. For instance, there is considerable evidence that electronic laboratory information systems improve access to clinical data when compared with manual, paper-based test-result distribution methods. To the extent that such systems improve care at an acceptable cost in time and money, there is an obligation to use computers to store and retrieve clinical laboratory results. There is a small but growing body of evidence that existing **clinical expert systems** can improve patient care in a small number of practice environments at an acceptable cost in time and money (Kuperman and Gibson 2003). Nevertheless, such systems cannot yet uniformly improve care in typical, more general practice settings, at least not without careful attention to the full range of managerial as well as technical issues affecting the particular care delivery setting in which they are used (Kaplan and Harris-Salamone 2009; Holroyd-Leduc et al. 2011; Shih et al. 2011).

Clinical expert systems (see Chap. 22) attempt to provide decision support for diagnosis, therapy, and/or prognosis in a more detailed and sophisticated manner than do simple reminder systems (Duda and Shortliffe 1983). A necessary adjunction of expert systems – creation and maintenance of their related knowledge bases – still involves leading-edge research and development. One must recognize that humans for the most part remain superior to electronic systems in understanding patients and their problems, in efficiently interacting with patients to ascertain pertinent past history and current symptoms across the spectrum of clinical practice, in the interpretation and representation of data, and in clinical synthesis. Humans might not always hold the upper hand in these tasks, and claims of their superiority must continually be tested empirically.

What has been called the "standard view" of computer-assisted clinical diagnosis (Miller 1990; cf. Friedman 2009) holds in part that human cognitive processes, being more suited to the complex task of diagnosis than machine intelligence, should not be overridden or trumped by computers. The standard view states that when adequate (and even exemplary) decision-support tools are developed, they should be viewed and used as supplementary and subservient to human clinical judgment. Quite literally: they *support* decisions; they do not make them. Progress should be measured in terms of whether clinicians using a CDS tool perform better on specific tasks than the same clinicians without the tool (Miller 1990; cf. Friedman 2009). These tools should assume subservient roles because the clinician caring for the patient knows and understands the patient's situation and can make compassionate judgments better than computer programs. Furthermore, clinicians, and not machine algorithms, are the entities whom the state licenses, and specialty boards accredit, to practice medicine, surgery, nursing, pharmacy, and other health-related activities.

Corollaries of the standard view are that (1) practitioners have an obligation to use any computer-based tool responsibly, through adequate user training and by developing an understanding of the system's abilities and limitations; and (2) practitioners must not abrogate their clinical judgment reflexively when using computer-based decision aids. Because the skills required for diagnosis are in many respects different from those required for the acquisition, storage, and retrieval of laboratory data, there is no contradiction in urging extensive use of electronic health records (as became U.S. policy under the HITECH act of 2009, discussed in Chap. 27), and, for the time being, cautious deployment of expert diagnostic decision-support tools (i.e., not permitting their use in settings in which knowledgeable clinicians cannot immediately override faulty advice).

The standard view addresses one aspect of the question, "How and when should computers be used in clinical practice?" by capturing important moral intuitions about error avoidance and evolving standards. Error avoidance and the benefits that follow from it shape the obligations of practitioners. In computer-software use, as in all other areas of clinical practice, good intentions alone are insufficient to insulate recklessness from culpability. Thus, the standard view may be seen as a tool for both error avoidance and ethically optimized action.

Ethical software use should be evaluated against a broad background of evidence for actions that produce favorable outcomes. Because informatics is a science in extraordinary ferment, system improvements and evidence of such improvements are constantly emerging. Clinicians have an obligation to be familiar with this evidence after attaining minimal acceptable levels of familiarity with informatics in general and with the clinical systems they use in particular (Fig. 10.1).

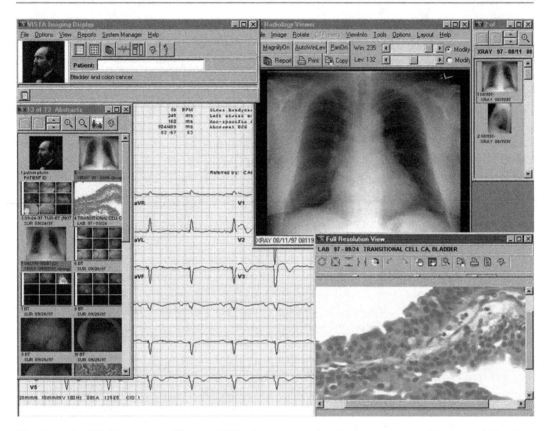

Fig. 10.1 The U.S. Department of Veterans Affairs has developed "Veterans Health Information Systems and Technology Architecture" (VistA), the largest electronic health record system in the United States. This fictitious screen shot demonstrates some of the system's functions and utilities (Credit: Courtesy of U.S. Department of Veterans Affairs, Veterans Health Administration Office of Informatics and Analytics)

10.2.2 Appropriate Users and Educational Standards

Efficient and effective use of health care informatics systems requires prior system evaluations demonstrating utility, then education and training of new users, monitoring of experience, and appropriate, timely updating. Indeed, such requirements resemble those for other tools used in health care and in other domains. Inadequate preparation in the use of tools is an invitation to catastrophe. When the stakes are high and the domain large and complex—as is the case in the health professions—education and training take on moral significance.

Who should use a health care-related computer application? Consider expert decision-support systems as an example. An early paper on ethical issues in informatics noted that potential users of such systems include physicians, nurses, physicians' assistants, paramedical personnel, students of the health sciences, patients, and insurance and government evaluators (Miller et al. 1985). Are members of all these groups appropriate users? One cannot answer the question until one precisely specifies the intended use for the system (i.e., the exact clinical questions the system will address). The appropriate level of training must be correlated with the question at hand. At one end of an appropriate-use spectrum, we can posit that medical and nursing students should employ decision-support systems for educational purposes; this assertion is relatively free of controversy once it has been verified that such tools convey accurately a sufficient quantity and quality of educational content. But it is less clear that patients, administrators, or managed-care gatekeepers, for example, should use expert decision-support systems for assistance in making diagnoses, in selecting therapies, or in evaluating the appropriateness of health professionals' actions. To the extent that some systems present general medical advice in generally understandable but sufficiently nuanced formats, such as was once the case with Dr. Benjamin Spock's 1950s era print-based child-care primer, one might condone system use by laypersons. There are additional legal concerns related to negligence and product liability, however, when health-related products are sold directly to patients rather than to licensed practitioners, and when such products give patient-specific counsel rather than general clinical advice (Miller et al. 1985).

Suitable use of a software program that helps a user to suggest diagnoses, to select therapies, or to render prognoses must be carray of goals and best practices for achieving those goals, including consideration of the characteristics and requirements of individual patients. For example, the multiple, interconnected inferential strategies required for arriving at an accurate diagnosis depend on knowledge of facts; experience with procedures; and familiarity with human behavior, motivation, and values. **Diagnosis** is a process rather than an event (Miller 1990), so even well-validated diagnostic systems must be used appropriately in the overall context of patient care.

To use a **diagnostic decision-support system** (Chap. 22), a clinician must be able to recognize when the computer program has erred, and, when it is accurate, what the output means and how it should be interpreted. This ability requires knowledge of both the diagnostic sciences and the software applications, and the strengths and limitations of each. After assigning a diagnostic label, the clinician must communicate the diagnosis, prognosis, and implications to a patient, and must do so in ways both appropriate to the patient's educational background and conducive to future treatment goals. It is not enough to be able to tell patients that they have cancer, human immunodeficiency virus (HIV), diabetes, or heart disease and then simply hand over a prescription.

The care provider must also offer context when available, comfort when needed, and hope as appropriate. The reason many jurisdictions have required pretest and posttest HIV counseling, for instance, is not to vex busy health professionals but rather to ensure that comprehensive, high-quality care—rather than mere diagnostic labeling—has been delivered.

This discussion points to the following set of ethical principles for appropriate use of decision-support systems:

1. A computer program should be used in clinical practice only after appropriate evaluation of its efficacy and the documentation that it performs its intended task at an acceptable cost in time and money.
2. Users of most clinical systems should be health professionals who are qualified to address the question at hand on the basis of their licensure, clinical training, and experience. Software systems should be used to augment or supplement, rather than to replace or supplant, such individuals' decision making.
3. All uses of informatics tools, especially in patient care, should be preceded by adequate training and instruction, which should include review of applicable product evaluations.

Such principles and claims should be viewed as analogous to other standards or rules in clinical medicine and nursing.

10.2.3 Obligations and Standards for System Developers and Maintainers

Users of clinical programs must rely on the work of other people who are often far removed from the context of use. As with all complex technologies, users depend on the developers and maintainers of a system and must trust evaluators who have validated a system for clinical use. Health care software applications are among the most complex tools in the technological armamentarium. Although this complexity imposes certain obligations on end users, it also commits a system's developers, designers, and maintainers to adhere to reasonable standards and, indeed, to acknowledge their moral responsibility for doing so.

10.2.3.1 Ethics, Standards, and Scientific Progress

The very idea of a **standard of care** embodies a number of complex assumptions linking ethics, evidence, outcomes, and professional training. To say that nurses or physicians must adhere to a standard is to say, in part, that they ought not stray from procedures previously shown or generally believed to work better than alternatives. The difficulty lies in how to determine if a procedure or device "works better" than another. Such determinations in the health sciences constitute progress, and provide evidence that we now know more. Criteria for weighing such evidence, albeit short of proof in most cases, are applied. For example, evidence from well-designed randomized controlled trials merits greater trust than evidence derived from uncontrolled retrospective studies (see Chap. 11). Typically, verification by independent investigators must occur before placing the most recent study results into common practice.

People who develop, maintain, and sell health care computing systems and their components have obligations that parallel those of system users. These obligations include holding patient care as the foremost value. The duty to limit or prevent harm to patients applies to system developers as well as to practitioners. Although this principle is easy to suggest and, generally, to defend, it invites subtle, and sometimes overt, resistance from people for whom profit or fame are primary motivators. (This is of course also true for other medical devices, processes and industries.) To be sure, quests for fame and fortune often produce good outcomes and improved care, at least eventually. Even so, some approaches fail to take into account the role of intention as a moral criterion.

In medicine, nursing, and psychology, a number of models of the **professional–patient relationship** place trust and advocacy at the apex of a hierarchy of values. Such a stance cannot be maintained if goals and intentions other than patient well-being are (generally) assigned

primacy. The same principles apply to those who produce and attend to health care information systems. Because these systems are health care systems—and are not devices for accounting, entertainment, real estate, and so on—and because system under performance can cause pain, disability, illness, and death, it is essential that the threads of trust run throughout the fabric of clinical system design and maintenance.

System purchasers, users, and patients must rely upon developers and maintainers to recognize the potentially grave consequences of errors or carelessness, trust them to care about the uses to which the systems will be put, and rely upon them to value the reduced suffering of other people at least as much as they value their own personal gain. This reliance emphatically does not entail that system designers and maintainers are blameworthy or unethical if they hope and strive to profit from their diligence, creativity, and effort. Rather, it implies that no amount of financial benefit for a designer can counterbalance bad outcomes or ill consequences that result from recklessness, avarice, or inattention to the needs of clinicians and their patients. Purchasers and users should require demonstrations that systems are worthy of such trust and reliance before placing patients at risk, and that safeguards (human and mechanical) are in place to detect, alert, and rectify situations in which systems underperform.

Quality standards should stimulate scientific progress and innovation while safeguarding against system error and abuse. These goals might seem incompatible, but they are not. Let us postulate a standard that requires timely updating and testing of knowledge bases that are used by decision-support systems. To the extent that database accuracy is needed to maximize the accuracy of inferential engines, it is trivially clear how such a standard will help to prevent or reduce decision-support mistakes. Furthermore, the standard should be seen to foster progress and innovation in the same way that any insistence on best possible accuracy helps to protect scientists and clinicians from pursuing false leads, or wasting time in testing poorly wrought hypotheses. It will not do for database maintainers to insist that they are busy doing the more productive or scientifically stimulating work of improving knowledge representation, say, or database design. Although such tasks are important, they do not supplant the tasks of updating and testing tools in their current configuration or structure. Put differently, scientific and technical standards are perfectly able to stimulate progress while taking a cautious or even conservative stance toward permissible risk in patient care.

This approach has been described as **progressive caution**. "Medical informatics is, happily, here to stay, but users and society have extensive responsibilities to ensure that we use our tools appropriately. This might cause us to move more deliberately or slowly than some would like." (Goodman 1998b).

A more recent concern, with both ethical and legal implications, is the responsibility of software developers to design and implement software programs that cannot easily be hacked by malicious code writers. This concern goes beyond privacy and confidentiality issues (discussed below), and includes the possibility that medical devices with embedded software might be nefariously "reprogrammed" in a manner that might cause harm to patients. (See, for example, Robertson 2011). A more detailed discussion of this topic appears under the Sect. 10.5 below.

10.2.3.2 System Evaluation as an Ethical Imperative

Any move toward "best practices" in biomedical informatics is shallow and feckless if it does not include a way to measure whether a system performs as intended. This and related measurements provide the ground for quality control and, as such, are the obligations of system developers, maintainers, users, administrators, and perhaps other players (see Chap. 11).

Medical computing is not merely about medicine or computing. It is about the introduction of new tools into environments with established social norms and practices. The effects of computing systems in health care are subject to analysis not only of accuracy and performance but of acceptance by users, of consequences for social and professional interaction, and of the context of use. We suggest that system evaluation can illuminate social and ethical issues in medical computing, and in so doing improve patient care. That being the case, there is an ethical imperative for such evaluation (Anderson and Aydin 1998).

To give a flavor of how a comprehensive evaluation program can ethically optimize implementation and use of an informatics system, consider these ten criteria for system scrutiny (Anderson and Aydin 1994):

1. Does the system work as designed?
2. Is it used as anticipated?
3. Does it produce the desired results?
4. Does it work better than the procedures it replaced?
5. Is it cost effective?
6. How well have individuals been trained to use it?
7. What are the anticipated long-term effects on how organizational units interact?
8. What are the long-term effects on the delivery of medical care?
9. Will the system have an impact on control in the organization?
10. To what extent do effects depend on practice setting?

Another way to make this important point is by emphasizing that *people* use computer systems. Even the finest system might be misused, misunderstood, or mistakenly allowed to alter or erode previously productive human relationships. Evaluation of health information systems in their contexts of use should be taken as a moral imperative. Such evaluations require consideration of a broader conceptualization of "what works best" and must look toward improving the overall health care delivery system rather than only that system's technologically based components. These higher goals entail the creation of a corresponding mechanism for ensuring institutional oversight and responsibility (Miller and Gardner 1997a, b).

10.3 Privacy, Confidentiality, and Data Sharing

Some of the greatest challenges of the Information Age arise from placing computer applications in health care settings while upholding traditional principles and values. One challenge involves balancing two competing values: (1) free access to information, and (2) protection of patients' privacy and confidentiality.

Only computers can efficiently manage the now-vast amount of information generated during clinical encounters and other health care transactions (see Chap. 2); at least in principle, such information should be easily available to health professionals and others involved in the administration of the care-delivery system, so that they can provide effective, efficient care for patients. Yet, making this information readily available creates greater opportunities for inappropriate access. Such access may be available to curious health care workers who do not need the information to fulfill job-related responsibilities, and, even more worrisome, to other people who might use the information to harm patients physically, emotionally, or financially. Clinical system administrators must balance the goals of protecting confidentiality by restricting use of computer systems and improving care by assuring the integrity and availability of data. These objectives are not incompatible, but there are trade-offs that cannot be avoided.

10.3.1 Foundations of Health Privacy and Confidentiality

Privacy and confidentiality are necessary for people to evolve and mature as individuals, to form relationships, and to serve as functioning members of society. Imagine what would happen if the local newspaper or gossip blog produced a daily report detailing everyone's actions, meetings, and conversations. It is not that most people have terrible secrets to hide but rather that the concepts of solitude, intimacy, and the desire to be left alone make no sense without the expectation that at least some of our actions and utterances will be kept private or held in confidence among a limited set of persons.

The "average" sentiment about the appropriate sphere of private vs. public may vary considerably from culture to culture, and even from generation to generation within any particular

culture; and it may differ widely among persons within a culture or generation, and evolve for any particular person over a lifetime. Even the "born digital" generation, for which Facebook and other social networking is a fact of everyday life, has its boundaries (Palfrey and Gasser 2010).

The terms privacy and confidentiality are not synonymous. As commonly used, "privacy" generally applies to people, including their desire not to suffer eavesdropping, whereas "confidentiality" is best applied to information. One way to think of the difference is as follows. If someone follows you and spies on you entering an AIDS (acquired immunodeficiency syndrome) clinic, your privacy is violated; if someone sneaks into the clinic without observing you in person and looks at your health care record, your record's confidentiality is breached. In discussions of the electronic health record, the term privacy may also refer to individuals' desire to restrict the disclosure of personal data (National Research Council 1997).

There are several important reasons to protect privacy and confidentiality. One is that privacy and confidentiality are widely regarded as rights of all people, and such protections help to accord them respect. On this account, people do not need to provide a justification for limiting access to their identifiable health data; privacy and confidentiality are entitlements that a person does not need to earn, to argue for, or to defend. Another reason is more practical: protecting privacy and confidentiality benefits both individuals and society. Patients who know that their identifiable health care data will not be shared inappropriately are more comfortable disclosing those data to clinicians. This trust is vital for the successful physician–patient, nurse–patient, or psychologist-patient relationship, and it helps practitioners to do their jobs.

Privacy and confidentiality protections also benefit public health. People who fear disclosure of personal information are less likely to seek out professional assistance, increasing the risks that contagion will be spread and maladies will go untreated. In addition, and sadly, people still suffer discrimination, bias, and stigma when certain health data do fall into the wrong hands. Financial harm may occur if insurers are given unlimited access to family members' records, or access to patient data, because some insurers might be tempted to increase the price of insurance for individuals at higher risk of illness or discriminate in other ways if such price differentiation were forbidden by law.

The ancient idea that physicians should hold health care information in confidence is therefore applicable whether the data are written on paper or embedded in silicon. The obligations to protect privacy and to keep confidences fall to system designers and maintainers, to administrators, and, ultimately, to the physicians, nurses, and others who elicit the information in the first place. The upshot for all of them is this: protection of privacy and confidentiality is not an option, a favor, or a helping hand offered to patients with embarrassing health problems; it is a duty, regardless of the malady or the medium in which information about it is stored.

Some sound clinical practice and public health traditions run counter to the idea of absolute confidentiality. When a patient is hospitalized, it is expected that all appropriate (and no inappropriate) employees or affiliates of the institution—primary physicians, consultants, nurses, therapists, and technicians—will have access to the patient's medical records, when it is in the interest of the patient's care to do so. In most communities of the United States, the contacts of patients who have active tuberculosis or certain sexually transmitted diseases are routinely identified and contacted by public health officials so that the contacts may receive proper medical attention. Such disclosures serve the public interest and are and should be legal because they decrease the likelihood that more widespread harm to other individuals might occur through transmission of an infection unknowingly.

A separate but important public health consideration (discussed in more detail below) involves the ability of health care researchers to anonymously pool data (i.e., pool by removing individual persons' identifying information) from patient cases that meet specified conditions to determine the natural history of the disease and the effects of various treatments. Examples of benefits from such pooled data analyses range from the ongoing results generated by regional collaborative chemotherapy trials to the discovery, nearly four decades ago, of the appropriateness of shorter lengths of stay for patients with myocardial infarction (McNeer et al. 1975). Most recently, the need for robust **syndromic surveillance** has been asserted as necessary for adequate bioterrorism preparedness, as well as for earlier detection of naturally occurring disease outbreaks (see Chap. 16).

10.3.2 Electronic Clinical and Research Data

Access to electronic patient records holds extraordinary promise for clinicians and for other people who need timely, accurate patient data (see Chap. 12). Institutions that do not deploy electronic health record systems are falling behind, a position that may soon become blameworthy. Failure to use such systems may also disqualify institutions for reimbursements from public and private insurance, making it effectively an organizational death sentence. Conversely, systems that make it easy for clinicians to access data also make it easier for people in general to access the data, and electronic systems generally magnify number of persons whose information becomes available when a system security breach occurs. Some would consider failure to prevent inappropriate access as at least as blameworthy as failure to provide adequate and appropriate access.

Nonetheless, there is no contradiction between the obligation to maintain a certain standard of care (in this case, regarding minimal levels of computer use) and ensuring that such a technical standard does not imperil the rights of patients. Threats to confidentiality and privacy are fairly well known. They include economic abuses, or discrimination by third-party payers, employers, and others who take advantage of the burgeoning market in health data; insider abuse, or record snooping by hospital or clinic workers who are not directly involved in a patient's care but examine a record out of curiosity, for blackmail, and so on; and malevolent hackers, or people who, via networks or other means, copy, delete, or alter confidential information (National Research Council 1997). Identity theft to commit insurance or other financial fraud could now be added to the list. Moreover, widespread dissemination of information throughout the health care system often occurs without explicit patient consent. Health care providers, third-party payers, managers of pharmaceutical benefits programs, equipment suppliers, and oversight organizations collect large amounts of patient-identifiable health information for use in managing care, conducting quality and utilization reviews, processing claims, combating fraud, and analyzing markets for health products and services (National Research Council 1997).

The proper approach to such challenges is one that will ensure both that appropriate clinicians and other people have rapid, easy access to patient records and that others do not have access. Is that a contradictory burden? No. Is it easy to achieve both? No. There are many ways to restrict inappropriate access to electronic records, but all come with a cost. Sometimes the cost is explicit, as when it comes in the form of additional computer software and hardware; sometimes it is implicit, as when procedures are required that increase the time commitment by system users.

One way to view the landscape of protective measures is to divide it into technological methods and institutional or policy approaches (Alpert 1998):

10.3.2.1 Technological Methods

Computers can provide the means for maximizing their own security, including authenticating system users with passwords, tokens or biometrics, to make sure that they are who they say they are; using access controls to prohibit people without a professional need from accessing particular health information within a system; and using audit trails, or logs, of people who do inspect confidential records so that automated security auditors, authorized facility administrators, as well as patients can review who accessed what. Encryption can protect data in transit and at rest (in storage). These technical means are complemented by protecting the elements of the electronic infrastructure with physical barriers when operations allow it. Auditing works best when appropriately severe punishments are widely known to be policy, and when policy breaches are uniformly punished in a semi-public manner.

10.3.2.2 Policy Approaches

In its landmark report, the National Research Council (1997) recommended that hospitals and other health care organizations create security and confidentiality committees and establish education and training programs. These recommendations parallel an approach that had worked well elsewhere in hospitals for matters ranging from infection control to bioethics. The Health Insurance Portability and Accountability Act (HIPAA) requires the appointment of privacy and security officials, special policies, and the training of health care workforce members who have access to health information systems.

Such measures are all the more important when health data are accessible through networks. The rapid growth of **integrated delivery networks** (**IDNs**) (see Chap. 14) and Health Information Exchanges, for example, illustrate the need not to view health data as a well into which one drops a bucket but rather as an irrigation system that makes its contents available over a broad—sometimes an extremely broad—area. It is not yet clear whether privacy and confidentiality protections that are appropriate in hospitals will be fully effective in a ubiquitously networked environment, but it is a start. System developers, users, and administrators are obliged to identify appropriate measures in light of the particular risks associated with a given implementation. There is no excuse for failing to make this a top priority throughout the data storage and sharing environment.

10.3.2.3 Electronic Data and Human Subjects Research

The use of patient information for **clinical research** and for quality assessment raises interesting ethical challenges. The presumption of a right to confidentiality seems to include the idea that patient records are inextricably linked to patient names or to other identifying data. In an optimal environment, then, patients can monitor who is looking at their records. But if all unique identifiers have been stripped from the records, is there any sense in talking about confidentiality?

The benefits to **public health** loom large in considering record-based research (Chap. 16). A valuable benefit of the electronic health record is the ability to access vast numbers of patient records to estimate the incidence and prevalence of various maladies, to track the efficacy of clinical interventions, and to plan efficient resource allocation (see Chap. 16). Such research and planning would, however, impose onerous or intractable burdens if informed, or valid consent had to be obtained from every patient whose record was represented in the sample. Using confidentiality to impede or forbid such research fails to benefit patients at the same time it sacrifices potentially beneficial scientific investigations.

A more practical course is to establish safeguards that better balance the ethical obligations to privacy and confidentiality against the social goals of public health and systemic efficiency. This balancing can be pursued via a number of paths. The first is to establish mechanisms to **anonymize** the information in individual records or to decouple the data contained in the records from any unique patient identifier. This task is not always straightforward; it can be remarkably difficult to anonymize data such that, when coupled with other data sets, the individuals are not at risk of re-identification. A relatively rare disease diagnosis coupled with demographic data such as age and gender, or geographic data such as a postal code, may act as a surrogate unique identifier; that is, detailed information can in combination serve as a data fingerprint that picks out an individual patient even though the patient's name, Social Security number, or other (official) unique identifiers have been removed from the record. Challenges and opportunities related to de-identifying and re-identifying data are among the most interesting, difficult and important in all health computing (Atreya et al. 2013; Benitez and Malin 2010; Malin and Sweeney 2004; Malin et al. 2011; Sweeney 1997; Tamersoy et al. 2012).

Such challenges point to a second means of balancing ethical goals in the context of database research: the use of institutional panels, such as **medical record committees** or **institutional review boards**. Submission of database research to appropriate institutional scrutiny is one way to make the best use of more or less anonymous electronic patient data. Competent panel members should be educated in the research potential of electronic health records, as well as in ethical issues in epidemiology and public health. Scrutiny by such committees can also give appropriate weight to competing ethical concerns in the context of internal research for quality control, outcomes monitoring, and so on (Goodman 1998b; Miller and Gardner 1997a, b).

10.3.2.4 Challenges in Bioinformatics

Safeguards are increasingly likely to be challenged as genetic information makes its way into the health care record (see Chaps. 24 and 25). The risks of bias, discrimination, and social stigma increase dramatically as **genetic data** become available to clinicians and investigators. Indeed, genetic information "goes beyond the ordinary varieties of medical information in its predictive value" (Macklin 1992). Genetic data also may be valuable to people predicting outcomes, allocating resources, and the like. In addition, genetic data are rarely associated with only a single person; they may provide information about relatives, including relatives who do not want to know about their genetic risk factors or potential maladies, as well as relatives who would love dearly to know more about their kin's genome. There is still much work to be done in sorting out and addressing the ethical issues related to electronic storage, sharing, and retrieval of genetic data (Goodman 1996).

Bioinformatics or **computational biology** provides an exciting ensemble of new tools to increase our knowledge of genetics, genetic diseases, and public health. Use of these tools is accompanied by responsibilities to attend to the ethical issues raised by new methods, applications, and consequences (Goodman and Cava 2008). Identifying and analyzing these issues are among the key tasks of those who work at the intersection of ethics and health information technology. The future of genetics and genomics is utterly computational, with data storage and analysis posing some of greatest financial and scientific challenges. For instance:

- How, to what extent, and by whom should genomic databases be used for clinical or public health decision support?
- Are special rules needed to govern the study of information in digital genetic repositories (or are current human subjects research protection rules adequate)?
- Does data mining software present new challenges when applied to human genetic information?
- What policies are required to guide and inform the communication of patient-specific and incidental findings?
- Are special protections and precautions needed to address and transmit findings about population subgroups?

It might be that the tools and uses of computational biology will eventually offer ethical challenges—and opportunities—as important, interesting and compelling as any technology in the history of the health sciences. Significantly, this underscores the importance of arguments to the effect that attention to ethics must accompany attention to science. Victories of health science research and development will be undermined by any failures to address corresponding ethical challenges. We must strive to identify, analyze, and resolve or mitigate important ethical issues.

10.4   Social Challenges and Ethical Obligations

The expansion of **evidence-based medicine** and, in the United States, of managed care (now sometimes called **accountable care** since the passage of health reform legislation in 2010; see Chap. 27) places a high premium on the tools of health informatics. The need for data on clinical outcomes is driven by a number of important social and scientific factors. Perhaps the most important among these factors is the increasing unwillingness

of governments and insurers to pay for interventions and therapies that do not work or that do not work well enough to justify their cost.

Health informatics helps clinicians, administrators, third-party payers, governments, researchers, and other parties to collect, store, retrieve, analyze, and scrutinize vast amounts of data—though the task of documenting this is itself a matter of research on what has come to be called "meaningful use." The functions of health informatics might be undertaken not for the sake of any individual patient but rather for cost analysis and review, quality assessment, scientific research, and so forth. These functions are critical, and if computers can improve their quality or accuracy, then so much the better.

Challenges arise when intelligent applications are mistaken for decision-making surrogates or when institutional or public policy recommends or favors computer output over human cognition. This may be seen as a question or issue arising under the rubric of "appropriate uses and users." That is, by whom, when, and under what constraints may we elicit and invoke computational analysis in shaping or applying public policy? The question whether an individual physician or multispecialty group, say, should be hired or retained or reimbursed or rewarded is information-intensive. The question that follows, however, is the key one: How should the decision-making skills of human and machine be used, and balanced (cf. Glaser 2010)?

10.4.1   Vendor Interactions

Motivated if not inspired by both technological necessity and financial opportunity, humble private practices and sprawling medical centers have—or should have—begun the transition from a paper patient record to an electronic one. The need to make such a transition is not in dispute: paper (and handwriting) are hard to store, find, read and analyze. **Electronic Health Records** (EHR) are not, or should not be. While there are important debates about the speed of the transition and regarding software quality, usability and ability to protect patient safety, it is widely agreed that the recording and storage of health information must be electronic.

Public policy has attempted to overcome some of the reluctance to make the change because of financial concerns. Notably, the U.S. Health Information Technology for Economic and Clinical Health (HITECH) Act, a part of the American Recovery and Reinvestment Act of 2009 (Blumenthal 2010), authorizes some $27 billion in incentives for EHR adoption. These incentives help address but do not eliminate financial concerns in that they offset only some of the cost of converting to an e-system. Still, while a number of companies had previously found opportunity in developing hospital and other clinical information systems, HITECH accelerated the pace (see Chap. 27).

The firms that make and sell EHRs are not regulated in the same way as those that manufacture pharmaceutical products or medical devices (see Sect. 10.5.3). In an increasingly competitive environment, this has led to controversy about the nature of vendor interactions with the institutions that buy their products. An EHR system for a mid-sized hospital can cost upwards of $100 million over time, including consulting services, hardware and training. It follows that it is reasonable to ask what values should guide such vendor interactions with clients, and whether they should be similar to or different from values that govern other free-market dealings.

While many or most contracts between vendors and hospitals are confidential, it has been reported that some HIT vendors require contract language that indemnifies system developers for personal injury claims or malpractice, even if the vendor is at fault; some vendors require system purchasers to agree not to disclose system errors except to the vendor (Koppel and Kreda 2009). Such provisions elicit concern to the extent they place or appear to place corporate interests ahead of patient safety and welfare. In this case, a working group chartered by AMIA, the society for informatics professionals (see Chap. 1), issued a report that provided guidance on a number of vendor interaction issues (Goodman et al. 2010). Importantly, the working group comprised industry representatives as well as scientists and other academics. The group's recommendations included these:

- Contracts should not contain language that prevents system users, including clinicians and others, from using their best judgment about what actions are necessary to protect patient safety. This includes freedom to disclose system errors or flaws, whether introduced or caused by the vendor, the client, or a third party. Disclosures made in good faith should not constitute violations of HIT contracts. This recommendation neither entails nor requires the disclosure of trade secrets or of intellectual property….

- Because vendors and their customers share responsibility for patient safety, contract provisions should not attempt to circumvent fault and should recognize that both vendors and purchasers share responsibility for successful implementation. For example, vendors should not be absolved from harm resulting from system defects, poor design or usability, or hard-to-detect errors. Similarly, purchasers should not be absolved from harm resulting from inadequate training and education, inadequate resourcing, customization, or inappropriate use.

While some of the debates that led to those conclusions were about political economy (regulation vs. free enterprise) as much as ethics (right vs. wrong), the opportunity for rapprochement in the service of a patient-centered approach may be seen as an affirmation of the utility of an applied ethics process in the evolution of health information technology.

10.4.2 Informatics and Managed Care

Consider the utility of **prognostic scoring systems** that use physiologic and mortality data to compare new critical-care patients with thousands of previous patients (Knaus et al. 1991). Such systems allow hospitals to track the performance of their critical-care units by, say, comparing the previous year's outcomes to this year's or by comparing one hospital to another. If, for instance,

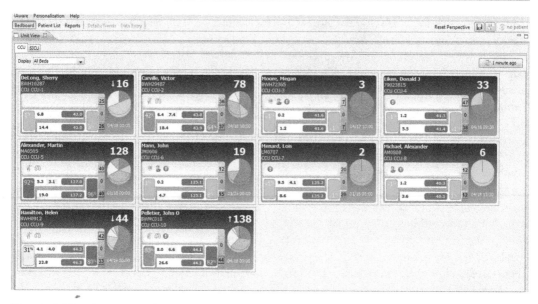

Fig. 10.2 "Severity adjusted daily data" in fictitious APACHE® Outcomes screen shot. Using prognostic scoring systems, clinicians in critical-care units can monitor events and interventions and administrators can manage staffing based on patient acuity. Clinicians can also use such systems to predict mortality, raising a number of ethical issues. This image shows 10 CCU patients. For the second one in the leftmost column, for instance, the "acute physiology score" is 128; the risk of hospital mortality is 96 % and the risk of ICU mortality is 92 % (Credit: Courtesy of Cerner Corporation, with permission)

patients with a particular profile tend to survive longer than their predecessors, then it might be inferred that **critical care** has improved. Such scoring systems can be useful for internal research and for quality management (Fig. 10.2).

Now suppose that most previous patients with a particular physiologic profile have died in critical-care units; this information might be used to identify ways to improve care of such patients—or it might be used in support of arguments to contain costs by denying care to subsequent patients fitting the profile (since they are likely to die anyway).

An argument in support of such an application might be that decisions to withdraw or withhold care are often and customarily made on the basis of subjective and fragmented evidence; so it is preferable to make such decisions on the basis of objective data of the sort that otherwise underlie sound clinical practice. Such **outcomes data** are precisely what fuels the engines of managed care, wherein health professionals and institutions compete on the basis of cost and outcomes. Why should society, or a managed-care organization,

or an insurance company pay for critical care when seemingly objective evidence exists that such care will not be efficacious? Contrarily, consider the effect on future scientific insights of denying care to such patients. Scientific progress is often made by noticing that certain patients do better under certain circumstances, and investigation of such phenomena leads to better treatments. If all patients meeting certain criteria were denied therapy on the basis of a predictive tool, it would become a self-fulfilling prophecy for a much longer time that all such patients would not do well (Miller 1997).

Now consider use of a decision-support system to evaluate, review, or challenge decisions by human clinicians; indeed, imagine an insurance company using a diagnostic expert system to determine whether a physician should be reimbursed for a particular procedure. If the expert system has a track record for accuracy and reliability, and if the system "disagrees" with the human's diagnosis or treatment plan, then the insurance company can contend that reimbursement for the procedure would be a mistake. Why pay for a procedure that is not indicated, at least according to a computational analysis?

In the two examples just offered (a prognostic scoring system is used to justify termination of treatment to conserve resources, and a diagnostic expert system is used to deny a physician reimbursement for procedures deemed inappropriate), there seems to be justification for adhering to the computer output. There are, however, three reasons why it is problematic to rely exclusively on clinical computer programs to guide policy or practice in these ways:

1. As we argued earlier with the standard view of computational diagnosis (and, by easy extension, prognosis), human cognition is, at least for a while longer, still superior to machine intelligence. Moreover, the act of rendering a diagnosis or prognosis is not merely a statistical or computational operation performed on un-interpreted data. Rather, identifying a malady and predicting its course requires understanding a complex ensemble of causal relations, interactions among a large number of variables, and having a store of salient background knowledge—considerations that have thus far failed to be grasped, assessed, and effectively blended into decisions made by computer programs.

2. Decisions about whether to treat a given patient are often value laden and must be made relative to treatment goals. In other words, it might be that a treatment will improve the quality of life but not extend life, or vice versa (Youngner 1988). Whether such treatment is appropriate cannot be determined scientifically or statistically (Brody 1989). The decisions ultimately depend on human preferences—those of the provider or, even more importantly, the patient.

3. Applying computational operations on aggregate data to individual patients runs the risk of including individuals in groups they resemble but to which they do not actually belong. Of course, human clinicians run this risk all the time—the challenge of inferring correctly that an individual is a member of a set, group, or class is one of the oldest problems in logic and in the philosophy of science. The point is that

computers have not solved this problem, yet, and allowing policy to be guided by simple or unanalyzed correlations constitutes a conceptual error.

The idea is not that diagnostic or prognostic computers are always wrong—we know that they are not—but rather there are numerous instances in which we do not know whether they are right. It is one thing to allow aggregate data to guide policy; doing so is just using scientific evidence to maximize good outcomes. But it is altogether different to require that a policy disallow individual **clinical judgment** and expertise.

Informatics can contribute in many ways to health care reform. Indeed, computer-based tools can help to illuminate ways to reduce costs, to optimize clinical outcomes, and to improve care. Scientific research, quality assessment, and the like are, for the most part, no longer possible without computers. But it does not follow that the insights from such research apply in all instances to the myriad variety of actual clinical cases at which competent human clinicians excel.

10.4.3   Effects of Informatics on Traditional Relationships

Ill patients are often scared and vulnerable. Treating illness, easing fear, and respecting vulnerability are among the core obligations of physicians, nurses, and other clinicians. Health informatics has the potential at some future time to complement these traditional duties and the relationships that they entail. We have pointed out that medical decisions are shaped by nonscientific considerations. This point is important when we assess the effects of informatics on human relationships. Thus:

> The practice of medicine or nursing is not exclusively and clearly scientific, statistical, or procedural, and hence is not, so far, computationally tractable. This is not to make a hoary appeal to the "art and science" of medicine; it is to say that the science is in many contexts inadequate or inapplicable: Many clinical decisions are not exclusively medical—they have social, personal, ethical, psychological, financial, familial, legal, and other components; even art might play a role. (Miller and Goodman 1998)

10.4.3.1 Professional–Patient Relationships

If computers, databases, and networks can improve physician–patient or nurse–patient relationships, perhaps by improving communication, then we shall have achieved a happy result. If reliance on computers impedes the abilities of health professionals to establish trust and to communicate compassionately, however, or further contributes to the dehumanization of patients (Shortliffe 1993, 1994), then we may have paid too dearly for our use of these machines.

Suppose that a physician uses a decision-support system to test a diagnostic hypothesis or to generate differential diagnoses, and suppose further that a decision to order a particular test or treatment is based on that system's output. A physician who is not able to articulate the proper role of computational support in his decision to treat or test will risk alienating those patients who, for one reason or another, will be disappointed, angered, or confused by the use of computers in their care. To be sure, the physician might just withhold this information from patients, but such deception carries its own threats to trust in the relationship.

Patients are not completely ignorant about the processes that constitute human decision making. What they do understand, however, may be subverted when their doctors and nurses use machines to assist delicate cognitive functions. We must ask whether patients should be told the accuracy rate of decision support automata—when they have yet to be given comparable data for humans. Would such knowledge improve the informed-consent process, or would it "constitute another befuddling ratio that inspires doubt more than it informs rationality?" (Miller and Goodman 1998).

To raise such questions is consistent with promoting the responsible use of computers in clinical practice. The question whether computer use will alienate patients is an empirical one; it is a question for which, despite many initial studies, we lack conclusive data to answer. (For example, we cannot yet state definitively whether all categories of patients will respond well to all specific types of e-mail messages from their doctors. Nevertheless, as a moral principle discussed above, one should not convey a new diagnosis of a malignancy via email.) To address the question now anticipates potential future problems. We must ensure that the exciting potential of health informatics is not subverted by our forgetting that the practice of medicine, nursing, and allied professions is deeply human and fundamentally intimate and personal.

10.4.3.2 Consumer Health Informatics

The growth of the World Wide Web and the commensurate evolution of clinical and health resources on the Internet also raise issues for professional–patient relationships. **Consumer health informatics**—technologies focused on patients as the primary users—makes vast amounts of information available to patients (see Chap. 17). There is also, however, misinformation—even outright falsehoods and quackery—posted on some sites. If physicians and nurses have not established relationships based on trust, the erosive potential of apparently authoritative Internet resources can be great. Physicians once accustomed to newspaper-inspired patient requests for drugs and treatments now face ever increasing demands that are informed by Web browsing. Consequently, the following issues will gain in ethical importance with each passing year:

- Peer review: How and by whom is the quality of a Web site to be evaluated? Who is responsible for the accuracy of information communicated to patients?

- Online consultations: There is no standard of care yet for online medical consultations. What risks do physicians and nurses run by giving advice to patients whom they have not met or examined in person? This question is especially important in the context of **telemedicine** or **remote-presence health care**, the use of video teleconferencing, image transmission, and other technologies that allow clinicians to evaluate and treat patients in other than face-to-face situations (see Chap. 18).

- Support groups: Internet support groups can provide succor and advice to the sick, but there is a chance that someone who might benefit from seeing a physician will not do so because of anecdotes and information otherwise attained. How should this problem be addressed?

That a resource is touted as worthwhile does not mean that it is. We lack evidence to illuminate the utility of consumer health informatics and its effects on professional–patient relationships. Such resources cannot be ignored given their ubiquity, and they often are useful for improving health. But we insist that here—as with decision support, appropriate use and users, evaluation, and privacy and confidentiality—there is an ethical imperative to proceed with caution. Informatics, like other health technologies, will thrive if our enthusiasm is open to greater evidence and is wed to deep reflection on human values.

10.4.3.3 Personal Health Records

At the same time as institutions have moved to computer-based health records systems, the tools available to individuals to keep their own health records have been making a similar transition. Electronic **personal health record** (PHR) systems, whether designed for use on a decoupled storage device or accessible over the Web, are now available from a rapidly expanding set of organizations (see Chap. 17) (Figs. 10.3 and 10.4).

PHRs provide a storage base for data once kept on paper (or in the patient's head) and repeatedly extracted with each institutional encounter for inclusion in that entity's records system, typically:

- Allergies, current medications
- Current health status and major health issues (if any)
- Major past health episodes and the condition of oneself and (sometimes) relatives
- Vaccinations, surgeries and other treatments

All these data can be kept on something simple (and un-networked) like a flash drive. It is becoming more common to store the data on a Web site, where PHR data can also be linked to other health information relevant to the person. The PHR data can also be linked to a health care provider institution's records, to allow updating in both directions, or be free of any such tie. A flash drive can be forgotten or lost, whereas a Web site can be centrally updated and uniformly available via any properly authenticated device on the Internet.

Traditional insurers and health care providers are duty-bound by privacy laws and regulations to protect the information under their control. PHRs have a somewhat shakier set of protections

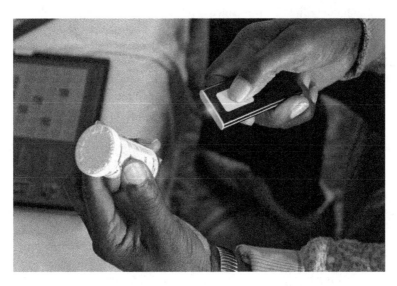

Fig. 10.3 Project HealthDesign is a program sponsored by the Robert Wood Johnson Foundation's Pioneer Portfolio and intended to foster development of personal health records. Here is a barcode scanner that recognizes medication labels. Designed by researchers at the University of Colorado at Denver, the "Colorado Care Tablet" allows elderly users to track prescriptions with such scanners and portable touch-screen tablets (Credit: Courtesy of Project HealthDesign (http://projecthealthdesign.org); Creative Commons Attribution 3.0 Unported License)

Fig. 10.4 A portable blood glucose communicator is part of the personal health record system developed by the T.R.U.E. Research Foundation of Washington, DC. The diabetes management application analyzes, summarizes, displays and makes individualized recommendations on nutritional data, physical activity data, prescribed medications, continuous blood glucose data, and self-reported emotional state (Credit: Courtesy of Project HealthDesign (http://projecthealthdesign.org); Creative Commons Attribution 3.0 Unported License)

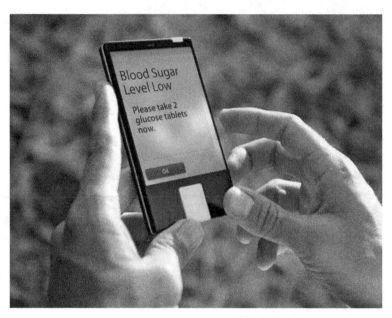

given their relatively short history. The legal obligations of institutions that provide PHRs, but do not fully manage the content of those records nor their use, as well as the obligations (if any) of the individuals who "manage" their own health records, remain to be sorted out (Cushman et al. 2010).

PHRs are now commonly linked to so-called "personal health applications" (PHAs) which provide ways of moving beyond simple static storage of one's medical history. Most provide some sort of primitive decision support, if only in linking to additional information about a particular disease or condition. Others include more ambitious decision-support functionality. All the concerns about the accuracy of Web-based information recur in this context, with concerns about the reliability of decision support added to that. Compounding concerns about accuracy are the inherent limitations of the "owner-operator": If it can be difficult for trained health care providers to evaluate the quality of advice rendered by a decision support system, the challenges for patients will be commensurately greater.

Traditional health care institutions may see the PHR as a device for patient empowerment because it adds a way for persons to keep track of their own data; but they can also be used as a way of preserving "loyalty" to a particular institution in the health care system. It has been proposed that PHRs be subject to standards allowing "interoperability"—in this case, easy movement from one type of PHR to another—to prevent leveraging it as an impediment to patients' movements when they wish to change providers or other preferences change. Whether such standards will evolve enough to make it easy to move from one PHR to another remains to be seen, given economic incentives to impede patient movement (provided the patient is economically desirable in terms of insurance status or personal wealth).

It is also unclear whether PHRs will reach the majority of patients. PHRs and their associated applications may be compelling for persons who must manage for themselves or a dependent a chronic health condition with complex treatment regimes. Persons who deal with less complex current conditions or histories may prefer to leave records management to their providers. There is also a concern that PHRs may replicate the "digital divide" in the context of health care, exacerbating rather than reducing health disparities. That is, PHRs are likely to be differentially beneficial to persons with the income and education to make full use of them.

10.5 Legal and Regulatory Matters

The use of clinical computing systems in health care raises a number of interesting and important legal and regulatory questions.

10.5.1 Difference Between Law and Ethics

Ethical and legal issues often overlap. Ethical considerations apply in attempts to determine what is good or meritorious and which behaviors are desirable or correct in accordance with higher principles. Legal principles are generally derived from ethical ones but deal with the practical regulation of morality or behaviors and activities. Many legal principles deal with the inadequacies and imperfections in human nature and the less-than-ideal behaviors of individuals or groups. Ethics offers conceptual tools to evaluate and guide moral decision making. Laws directly tell us how to behave (or not to behave) under various specific circumstances and prescribe remedies or punishments for individuals who do not comply with the law. Historical precedent, matters of definition, issues related to detectability and enforceability, and evolution of new circumstances affect legal practices more than they influence ethical requirements.

10.5.2 Legal Issues in Biomedical Informatics

Prominent legal issues related to the use of software applications in clinical practice and in biomedical research include liability under tort law; potential use of computer applications as expert witnesses in the courtroom; legislation governing privacy and confidentiality; and copyrights, patents, and intellectual property issues.

10.5.2.1 Liability Under Tort Law

In the United States and in many other nations, principles of tort law govern situations in which harm or injuries result from the manufacture and sale of goods and services (Miller et al. 1985). Because there are few, if any, U.S. legal precedents directly involving harm or injury to patients resulting from use of clinical software applications (as opposed to a small number of well-documented instances where software associated with medical devices has caused harm), the following discussion is hypothetical. The principles involved are, however, well established with voluminous legal precedents outside the realm of clinical software.

A key legal distinction is the difference between products and services. **Products** are physical objects, such as stethoscopes, that go through the processes of design, manufacture, distribution, sale, and subsequent use by purchasers. **Services** are intangible activities provided to consumers at a price by (presumably) qualified individuals.

The practice of clinical medicine has been deemed a service through well-established legal precedents. On the other hand, clinical software applications can be viewed as either goods ("products") (software programs designed, tested, debugged, placed on DVDs or other media, and distributed physically to purchasers) or services (applications that present data or provide advice to practitioners engaged in a service such as delivering health care). There are few legal precedents to determine unequivocally how software will be viewed by the courts, and it is possible that clinical software programs will be treated as goods under some circumstances and as services under others. It might be the case that software purchased and running in a private office to handle patient records or billing would be deemed a product, but the same software mounted on shared, centralized computers and accessed over the Internet (and billed on a monthly basis) would be offering a service.

Three ideas from tort law potentially apply to the clinical use of software systems:

(1) **Harm by intention**—when a person injures another using a product or service to cause the damage, (2) the **negligence theory**, and (3) **strict product liability** (Miller et al. 1985). Providers of goods and services are expected to uphold the standards of the

community in producing goods and delivering services. When individuals suffer harm due to substandard goods or services, they may sue the service providers or goods manufacturers to recover damages. **Malpractice** litigation in health care is based on negligence theory.

Because the law views delivery of health care as a service (provided by clinicians), it is clear that negligence theory will provide the minimum legal standard for clinicians who use software during the delivery of care. Patients who are harmed by clinical practices based on imperfect software applications may sue the health care providers for negligence or malpractice, just as patients may sue attending physicians who rely on the imperfect advice of a human consultant (Miller et al. 1985). Similarly, a patient might sue a practitioner who has not used a decision-support system when it can be shown that use of the decision-support system is part of the current standard of care, and that use of the program might have prevented the clinical error that occurred (Miller 1989). It is not clear whether the patients in such circumstances could also successfully sue the software manufacturers, as it is the responsibility of the licensed practitioner, and not of the software vendor, to uphold the standard of care in the community through exercising sound clinical judgment. Based on a successful malpractice suit against a clinician who used a clinical software system, it might be possible for the practitioner to sue the manufacturer or vendor for negligence in manufacturing a defective clinical software product, but cases of this sort have not yet been filed. If there were such suits, it might be difficult for a court to discriminate between instances of improper use of a blameless system and proper use of a less-than-perfect system.

In contrast to negligence, strict product liability applies only to harm caused by defective products and is not applicable to services. The primary purpose of strict product liability is to compensate the injured parties rather than to deter or punish negligent individuals (Miller et al. 1985). For strict product liability to apply, three conditions must be met:

1. The product must be purchased and used by an individual.
2. The purchaser must suffer physical harm as a result of a design or manufacturing defect in the product.
3. The product must be shown in court to be "unreasonably dangerous" in a manner that is the demonstrable cause of the purchaser's injury.

Note that negligence theory allows for adverse outcomes. Even when care is delivered in a competent, caring, and compassionate manner, some patients with some illnesses will not do well. Negligence theory protects providers from being held responsible for all individuals who suffer bad outcomes. As long as the quality of care has met the prevailing standards, a practitioner should not be found liable in a malpractice case (Miller et al. 1985). Strict product liability, on the other hand, is not as forgiving or understanding.

No matter how good or exemplary a manufacturer's designs and manufacturing processes might be, if even one in ten million products is defective, and that one product defect is the cause of a purchaser's injury, then the purchaser may collect damages (Miller et al. 1985). The plaintiff needs to show only that the product was unreasonably dangerous and that its defect led to harm. In that sense, the standard of care for strict product liability is 100-percent perfection. To some extent, appropriate product labeling (e.g., "Do not use this metal ladder near electrical wiring") may protect manufacturers in certain strict product liability suits in that clear, visible labeling may educate the purchaser to avoid "unreasonably dangerous" circumstances. Appropriate labeling standards may similarly benefit users and manufacturers of clinical expert systems (Geissbuhler and Miller 1997).

Health care software programs sold to clinicians who use them as decision-support tools in their practices are likely to be treated under negligence theory as services. When advice-giving clinical programs are sold directly to patients, however, and there is less opportunity for intervention by a licensed practitioner, it is more likely that the courts will treat them as products, using strict product liability, because the purchaser of the program is more likely to be the individual who is injured if the product is defective. (As personal health records become more common, this legal theory may well be tested.)

A growing number of software "bugs" in medical devices have been reported to cause injury to patients (Majchrowski 2010). The U.S. Food and Drug Administration (FDA) views software embedded within medical devices, such as cardiac pacemakers and implantable insulin pumps, as part of the physical device, and so regulates such software as part of the device (FDA 2011). The courts are likely to view such software using principles of strict product liability (Miller and Miller 2007)

Corresponding to potential strict product liability for faulty software embedded in medical devices is potential negligence liability if such software can easily be "hacked" (Robertson 2011). Malicious code writers might mimic external software-based "radio" controllers for pacemakers and insulin pumps and reprogram them to cause harm to patients. While such "hackers" should face criminal prosecution if they cause harm by intention, the device manufacturers have a responsibility to make it difficult to change the software code embedded in devices without proper authorization.

10.5.2.2 Privacy and Confidentiality

The ethical basis for privacy and confidentiality in health care is discussed in Sect. 10.3.1. For a long time, the legal state of affairs for privacy and confidentiality of electronic health records was chaotic (as it remains for written records, to some extent). This state of affairs in the U.S. had not significantly changed in the three decades since it was described in a classic New England Journal of Medicine article (Curran et al. 1969).

However, a key U.S. law, the Health Insurance Portability and Accountability Act (HIPAA), has prompted significant change. HIPAA's privacy standards became effective in 2003 for most health care entities, and its security standards followed 2 years later. A major impetus for the law was that the process of "administrative simplification" via electronic recordkeeping, prized for its potential to increase efficiency and reduce costs, would also pose threats to patient privacy and confidentiality. Coming against a backdrop of a variety of noteworthy cases in which patient data were improperly—and often embarrassingly—disclosed, the law was also seen as a badly needed tool to restore confidence in the ability of health professionals to protect confidentiality. While the law has been accompanied by debate both on the adequacy of its measures and the question whether compliance was unnecessarily burdensome, it nevertheless established the first nationwide health privacy protections. At its core, HIPAA embodies the idea that individuals should have access to their own health data, and more control over uses and disclosures of that health data by others. Among its provisions, the law requires that patients be informed about their privacy rights, including a right of access; that uses and disclosures of "protected health information" generally be limited to exchanges of the "minimum necessary"; that uses and disclosures for other than treatment, payment and health care operations be subject to patient authorization; and that all employees in "covered entities" (institutions that HIPAA legally affects) be educated about privacy and information security.

As noted above, the HITECH Act provided substantial encouragement for Electronic Health Record (EHR) development, particularly the encouragement of billions of dollars in federal subsidies for "meaningful use" of EHRs. However HITECH also contained many changes to HIPAA privacy and security requirements, strengthening the regulations that affect the collection, use and disclosure of health information not only by covered entities, but also the "business associates" (contractors) of those covered entities, and other types of organizations engaged in health information exchange.

The Office of Civil Rights in the U.S. Department of Health and Human Services remains the entity primarily charged with HIPAA enforcement, but there is now a role for states' attorneys general as well as other agencies such as the Federal Trade Commission. HITECH increases penalty levels under HIPAA and includes a mandate for investigations and periodic audits, shifting the enforcement balance away from voluntary compliance and remediation plans.

HITECH's changes to HIPAA, those from other federal laws such as the Genetic Information Nondiscrimination Act of 2008 (GINA) and the Patient Safety and Quality Improvement Act of 2005, and the new attention to information privacy and security in most states' laws, comprise significant changes to the legal-regulatory landscape for health information.

10.5.2.3 Copyright, Patents, and Intellectual Property

Intellectual property protection afforded to developers of software programs, biomedical knowledge bases, and World Wide Web pages remains an underdeveloped area of law. Although there are long traditions of copyright and patent protections for non-electronic media, their applicability to computer-based resources is not clear. **Copyright law** protects intellectual property from being copied verbatim, and **patents** protect specific methods of implementing or instantiating ideas. The number of lawsuits in which one company claimed that another copied the functionality of its copyrighted program (i.e., its "look and feel") has grown, however, and it is clear that copyright law does not protect the "look and feel" of a program beyond certain limits. Consider, for example, the unsuccessful suit in the 1980s by Apple Computer, Inc., against Microsoft, Inc., over the "look and feel" of Microsoft Windows as compared with the Apple Macintosh interface (which itself resembled the earlier Xerox Alto interface).

It is not straightforward to obtain copyright protection for a list that is a compilation of existing names, data, facts, or objects (e.g., the telephone directory of a city), unless you can argue that the result of compiling the compendium creates a unique object (e.g., a new organizational scheme for the information) (Tysyer 1997). Even when the compilation is unique and copyrightable, the individual components, such as facts in a database, might not be copyrightable. That they are not copyrightable has implications for the ability of creators of biomedical databases to protect database content as intellectual property. How many individual, unprotected facts can someone copy from a copyright-protected database before legal protections prevent additional copying?

A related concern is the intellectual-property rights of the developers of materials made available through the World Wide Web. Usually, information made accessible to the public that does not contain copyright annotations is considered to be in the public domain. It is tempting to build from the work of other people in placing material on the Web, but copyright protections must be respected. Similarly, if you develop potentially copyrightable material, the act of placing it on the Web, in the public domain, would allow other people to treat your material as not protected by copyright. Resolution of this and related questions may await workable commercial models for electronic publication on the World Wide Web, whereby authors could be compensated fairly when other people use or access their materials. Electronic commerce might eventually provide copyright protection (and perhaps revenue) similar to age-old models that now apply to paper-based print media; for instance, to use printed books and journals, you must generally borrow them from a library, purchase them or access them under Creative Commons or similar open-access platforms.

10.5.3 Regulation and Monitoring of Computer Applications in Health Care

In the mid-1990s, the U.S. Food and Drug Administration (FDA) held public meetings to discuss new methods and approaches to regulating clinical software systems as medical devices. In response, a consortium of professional organizations related to health care information (AMIA, the Center for Health Care Information Management, the Computer-Based Patient Record Institute, the American Health Information Management Association, the Medical Library Association, the Association of Academic Health Science Libraries, and the American Nurses Association) drafted a position paper published in both summary format and as a longer discussion with detailed background and explanation (Miller and Gardner 1997a, b). The position paper was subsequently endorsed by the boards of directors of all the organizations (except the Center for Health Care Information Management) and by the American College of Physicians Board of Regents.

The recommendations from the consortium include these:

- Recognition of four categories of clinical system risks and four classes of monitoring and regulatory actions that can be applied based on the level of risk in a given setting.
- Local oversight of clinical software systems, whenever possible, through the creation of autonomous **software oversight committees**, in a manner partially analogous to the institutional review boards that are federally mandated to oversee protection of human subjects in biomedical research. Experience with prototypical software-oversight committees at pilot sites should be gained before any national dissemination.
- Adoption by health care-information system developers of a code of good business practices.
- Recognition that budgetary, logistic, and other constraints limit the type and number of systems that the FDA can regulate effectively.
- Concentration of FDA regulation on those systems posing highest clinical risk, with limited opportunities for competent human intervention, and FDA exemption of most other clinical software systems.

The recommendations for combined local and FDA monitoring are summarized in Table 10.1. Even as the question of regulation continues to challenge the health information technology community, there has been a noteworthy move to attempt to certify and accredit software. Whether such certification efforts will have a meaningful impact on health care outcomes mediated by clinical systems has yet to be determined. Similarly, we do not yet know whether improved outcomes would occur if vendors were to give qualified (i.e., informatics-capable) institutional purchasers greater local control over system functionality.

10.5.4   Software Certification and Accreditation

If, as above, (1) there is an ethical obligation to evaluate health information systems in the contexts in which they are being used, and if, as we just saw, (2) there are good reasons to consider the adoption of software oversight committees or something similar, then it is worthwhile to consider the ethical utility of efforts to review and endorse medical software and systems.

Established in 2004, the Certification Commission for Health Information Technology, in collaboration with the Office of the National Coordinator for health information technology, assesses electronic health records according to an array of criteria, in part to determine their success in contributing to "meaningful use." These criteria address matters ranging from electronic provider order entry and electronic problem lists to decision support and access control (cf. Classen et al. 2007; Wright et al. 2009). The criteria, tests and test methods are developed in concert with the National Institute of Standards and Technology. Practices and institutions that want to receive government incentive payments must adopt certified electronic health record technologies.

Conceived under the American Recovery and Reinvestment Act, these processes aim to improve outcomes, safety and privacy. Whether they can accomplish this—as opposed to celebrate technology for its own sake—is an excellent source of debate (Hartzband and Groopman 2008). What should be uncontroversial is that any system of regulation, review or certification must be based on and, as a matter of process emphasize, certain values. These might include, among others, patient-centeredness, ethically optimized data management practices, and what we have here commended as the "standard view," that is, human beings and not machines practice medicine, nursing and psychology.

The move to certification has unfortunately engendered precious little in the way of ethical analysis, however. To make any system of regulation, review or certification ethically credible, government and industry leaders must eventually make explicit that attention to ethics is a core component of their efforts.

Table 10.1 Consortium recommendations for monitoring and regulating clinical software systems[a]

Variable	Regulatory class			
	A	B	C	D
Supervision by FDA	Exempt from regulation	Excluded from regulation	Simple registration and postmarket surveillance required	Premarket approval and postmarket surveillance required
Local software oversight committee	Optional	Mandatory	Mandatory	Mandatory
Role of software oversight committee	Monitor locally	Monitor locally instead of monitoring by FDA	Monitor locally and report problems to FDA as appropriate	Assure adequate local monitoring without replicating FDA activity
Software risk category				
0: Informational or generic systems[b]	All software in category	—	—	—
1: Patient-specific systems that provide low-risk assistance with clinical problems[c]	—	All software in category	—	—
2: Patient-specific systems that provide intermediate-risk support on clinical problems[d]	—	Locally developed or locally modified systems	Commercially developed systems that are not modified locally	—
3: High-risk, patient-specific systems[e]	—	Locally developed, non commercial systems	—	Commercial systems

Source: Miller and Gardner (1997a)

[a]FDA5Food and Drug Administration

[b]Includes systems that provide factual content or simple, generic advice (such as "give flu vaccine to eligible patients in mid-autumn") and generic programs, such as spreadsheets and databases

[c]Systems that give simple advice (such as suggesting alternative diagnoses or therapies without stating preferences) and give ample opportunity for users to ignore or override suggestions

[d]Systems that have higher clinical risk (such as those that generate diagnoses or therapies ranked by score) but allow users to ignore or override suggestions easily; net risk is therefore intermediate

[e]Systems that have great clinical risk and give users little or no opportunity to intervene (such as a closed-loop system that automatically regulates ventilator settings)

10.6 Summary and Conclusions

Ethical issues are important in biomedical informatics, and especially so in the clinical arena. An initial ensemble of guiding principles, or ethical criteria, has emerged to orient decision making:

1. Specially trained human beings remain, so far, best able to provide health care for other human beings. Hence, computer software should not be allowed to overrule a human decision.

2. Practitioners who use informatics tools should be clinically qualified and adequately trained in using the software products.

3. The tools themselves should be carefully evaluated and validated.

4. Health informatics tools and applications should be evaluated not only in terms of performance, including efficacy, but also in terms of their influences on institutions, institutional cultures, and workplace social forces.

5. Ethical obligations should extend to system developers, maintainers, and supervisors as well as to clinician users.

6. Education programs and security measures should be considered essential for protecting confidentiality and privacy while improving appropriate access to personal patient information.

7. Adequate oversight should be maintained to optimize ethical use of electronic patient information for scientific and institutional research.

New sciences and technologies always raise interesting and important ethical issues. Much the same is true for legal issues, although in the absence of precedent or legislation any legal analysis will remain vague. Similarly important challenges confront people who are trying to determine the appropriate role for government in regulating health care software. The lack of clear public policy for such software underscores the importance of ethical insight and education as the exciting new tools of biomedical and health informatics become more common.

Suggested Readings

Cushman, R., Froomkin, M. A., Cava, A., Abril, P., & Goodman, K. W. (2010). Ethical, legal and social issues for personal health records and applications. *Journal of Biomedical Informatics, 43*, S51–S55. This article provides an overview of ethical issues related to the use of personal health records. Topics include privacy and confidentiality, decision support and the clinician-patient relationship.

Goodman, K. W. (Ed.). (1998). *Ethics, computing, and medicine: Informatics and the transformation of health care*. Cambridge: Cambridge University Press. (2nd edn in press.) This volume, the first devoted to the intersection of ethics and informatics, contains chapters on informatics and human values, responsibility for computer-based decisions, evaluation of medical information systems, confidentiality and privacy, decision support, outcomes research and prognostic scoring systems, and meta-analysis.

Goodman, K. W., Berner, E. S., Dente, M. A., Kaplan, B., Koppel, R., Rucker, D., Sands, D. Z., & Winkelstein, P. (2011). Challenges in ethics, safety, best practices, and oversight regarding HIT vendors, their customers, and patients: a report of an AMIA special task force. *Journal of the American Medical Informatics Association, 18*(1), 77–81. This document is one of the first to examine issues related to the manufacturers and vendors of electronic health records, including their relationships with hospitals.

Miller, R. A. (1990). Why the standard view is standard: People, not machines, understand patients' problems. *Journal of Medicine and Philosophy, 15*, 581–591. This contribution lays out the standard view of health informatics. This view holds, in part, that because only humans have the diverse skills necessary to practice medicine or nursing, machine intelligence should never override human clinicians.

Miller, R. A., Schaffner, K. F., & Meisel, A. (1985). Ethical and legal issues related to the use of computer programs in clinical medicine. *Annals of Internal Medicine, 102*, 529–536. This article constitutes a major early effort to identify and address ethical issues in informatics. By emphasizing the questions of appropriate use, confidentiality, and validation, among others, it sets the stage for all subsequent work.

National Research Council. (1997). *For the record: Protecting electronic health information*. Washington, DC: National Academy Press. A major policy report, this document outlines leading challenges for privacy and confidentiality in medical information systems and makes several important recommendations for institutions and policymakers.

Questions for Discussion

1. What is meant by the "standard view" of appropriate use of medical information systems? Identify three key criteria for determining whether a particular use or user is appropriate.

2. Can quality standards for system developers and maintainers simultaneously safeguard against error and abuse and stimulate scientific progress? Explain your answers. Why is there an ethical obligation to adhere to a standard of care?

3. Identify (a) two major threats to patient data confidentiality, and (b) policies or strategies that you propose for protecting confidentiality against these threats.

4. Many prognoses by human beings are subjective and are based on faulty memory or incomplete knowledge of previous cases. What are the two drawbacks to using objective prognostic scoring systems to determine whether to allocate care to individual patients?

5. People who are educated about their illnesses tend to understand and to follow instructions, to ask insightful questions, and so on. How can the World Wide Web improve patient education? How, on the other hand, might Web access hurt traditional physician–patient and nurse–patient relationships?

Evaluation of Biomedical and Health Information Resources

Charles P. Friedman and Jeremy C. Wyatt

After reading this chapter, you should know the answers to these questions:

- Why are empirical studies based on the methods of evaluation and technology assessment important to the successful implementation of information resources to improve health?
- What challenges make studies in informatics difficult to carry out? How are these challenges addressed in practice?
- Why can all evaluations be classified as empirical studies?
- What features do all evaluations have in common?
- What are the key factors to take into account as part of a process of deciding what are the most important questions to use to frame a study?
- What are the major assumptions underlying objectivist and subjectivist approaches to evaluation? What are the strengths and weaknesses of each approach?

- How does one distinguish measurement and demonstration aspects of objectivist studies, and why are both aspects necessary? In the demonstration aspect of objectivist studies, how are control strategies used to draw inferences?
- What steps are followed in a subjectivist study? What techniques are employed by subjectivist investigators to ensure rigor and credibility of their findings?
- Why is communication between investigators and clients central to the success of any evaluation?

11.1 Introduction

Most people understand the term evaluation to mean an assessment of an organized, purposeful activity. Evaluations are usually conducted to answer questions or in anticipation of the need to make decisions (Wyatt and Spiegelhalter 1990). Evaluations may be informal or formal, depending on the characteristics of the decision to be made and, particularly, how much is at stake. But all activities labeled as evaluation involve the empirical process of collecting information that is relevant to the decision at hand. For example, when choosing a holiday destination, members of a family may informally ask friends which

C.P. Friedman, PhD, FACMI (✉)
Schools of Information and Public Health,
University of Michigan, 105 S State St,
Ann Arbor, MI 48109, USA
e-mail: cpfried@umich.edu

J.C. Wyatt, MB BS, FRCP, FACMI
Leeds Institute of Health Sciences,
University of Leeds, Charles Thackrah Building,
101 Clarendon Road, Leeds LS2 9LJ, UK
e-mail: j.c.wyatt@leeds.ac.uk

This chapter is adapted from an earlier version in the third edition authored by Charles P. Friedman, Jeremy C. Wyatt, and Douglas K. Owens.

E.H. Shortliffe, J.J. Cimino (eds.), *Biomedical Informatics*,
DOI 10.1007/978-1-4471-4474-8_11, © Springer-Verlag London 2014

Hawaiian island they prefer and browse various websites including those that provide ratings of specific destinations. After factoring in costs and convenience, the family reaches a decision. More formally, when a health care organization faces the choice of a new electronic health record system, the leadership will develop a plan to collect comparable data about competing systems, analyze the data according to the plan, and ultimately, again through a predetermined process, make a decision.

The field of biomedical and health informatics focuses on the collection, processing, and communication of health related information and the implementation of **information resources**—usually consisting of digital technology designed to interact with people—to facilitate these activities. These information resources can collect, store, and process data related to the health of individual persons (institutional or personal electronic health records), manage and reason about biomedical knowledge (knowledge acquisition tools, knowledge bases, decision-support systems, and intelligent tutoring systems), and support activities related to public health (disease registries and vital statistics, disease outbreak detection and tracking). Thus, there is a vast range of biomedical and health information resources that can be foci of evaluation.

Information resources have many different aspects that can be studied (Friedman and Wyatt 2005, Chap. 3). Where safety is an issue, as it often is, (Fox 1993), we might focus on inherent characteristics of the resource, asking such questions as, "Are the code and architecture compliant with current software engineering standards and practices?" or "Is the data structure the optimal choice for this type of application?" Clinicians, however, might ask more pragmatic questions such as, "Is the knowledge in this system completely up-to-date?" or "Can I retrieve all the information about a patient or just the information generated in my own clinic?" Executives and public officials might wish to understand the effects of these resources on individuals and populations, asking questions such as, "Has this resource improved the quality of care?" or "What effects will a patient portal have

on working relationships between practitioners and patients?" Thus, evaluation methods in biomedical informatics must address a wide range of issues, from technical characteristics of specific systems to systems' effects on people and organizations. The outcomes or effects attributable to the use of health information resources will almost always be a function of how individuals choose to use them, and the social, cultural, organizational, and economic context in which these uses take place (Lundsgaarde 1987).

For these reasons, there is no formula for designing and executing evaluations; every evaluation, to some significant degree, must be custom-designed. In the end, decisions about what evaluation questions to pursue and how to collect and analyze data to pursue them, are exquisitely sensitive to each study's special circumstances and constrained by the resources that are available for it. Evaluation is very much the art of the possible. But neither is evaluation an exercise in alchemy, pure intuition, or black magic. There exist many methods for evaluation that have stood the test of time and proved useful in practice. There is a literature on what works and where, and there are numerous published examples of successful evaluation studies. In this chapter, we will introduce many of these methods, and present frameworks that guide the application of methods to specific decision problems and study settings.

11.2 Why Are Formal Evaluation Studies Needed?

11.2.1 Computing Artifacts Have Special Characteristics

Why are empirical studies of information resources needed at all? Why is it not possible, for example, to model (and thus predict) the performance of information resources, and thus save a lot of time and effort? The answer lies, to a great extent, in the complexity of computational artifacts and their use. For some disciplines, specification of the structure of an artifact allows one to predict how it will function, and engineers can even design new objects with known performance characteristics directly from functional requirements. Examples of such artifacts are elevators and conventional road bridges: The principles governing the behavior of materials and structures made of these materials are sufficiently well understood that a new elevator or bridge can be designed to a set of performance characteristics with the expectation that it will perform exactly as predicted. Laboratory testing of models of these devices is rarely needed. Field testing of the artifact, once built, is conducted to reveal relatively minor anomalies, which can be rapidly remedied, or to tune or optimize performance. However, when the object concerned is a computer-based resource, not a bridge, the story is different (Littlejohns et al. 2003). Software designers and engineers have theories linking the structure to the function of only the most trivial computer-based resources (Somerville 2002). Because of the complexity of computer-based systems themselves, their position as part of a complex socio-technical system including the users and the organization in which they work, and the lack of a comprehensive theory connecting structure and function, there is no way to know exactly how an information resource will perform until it is built and tested (Murray 2004); and similarly there is no way to know that any revisions will bring about the desired effect until the next version of the resource is tested.

In sum, the only practical way to determine if a reasonably complex body of computer code does what it is intended to do is to test it. This testing can take many shapes and forms. The informal design, test, and revise activity that characterizes the development of all computer software is one such form of testing and results in software that usually functions as expected *by the developers*. More formal and exhaustive approaches to software design, verification and testing using synthetic test cases (e.g., Scott et al. 2011) and other approaches help to guarantee that the software will do what it was designed to do. Even these approaches, however, do not guarantee the success of the software when put into the hands of the intended end-users. This requires more formal studies of the types that will be described in this chapter, which can be undertaken before, during, and after the initial development of an information resource. Such evaluation studies can guide further development; indicate if the resource is likely to be safe for use in real health care, public health, research, or educational settings; or elucidate if it has the potential to improve the professional performance of the users and disease outcomes in their clients.

Many other writings elaborate on the points offered here. Some of the earliest include Spiegelhalter (1983) and Gaschnig et al. (1983) who discussed these phases of evaluation by drawing analogies from the evaluation of new drugs or the conventional software life cycle, respectively. Wasson et al. (1985) discussed the evaluation of clinical prediction rules together with some useful methodological standards that apply equally to information resources. Many other authors since then have described, with differing emphases, the evaluation of health care information resources, often focusing on decision-support tools, which pose some of the most extreme challenges. One relevant book (Friedman et al. 2005) discusses the challenges posed by evaluation in biomedical informatics and offers a wide range of methods described in considerable detail to help investigators explore and resolve these challenges. Other books have explored more technical, health technology assessment or organizational approaches to evaluation methods (Szczepura and Kankaanpaa 1996; van Gennip and Talmon 1995; Anderson et al. 1994; Brender 2005).

11.2.2 The Special Issue of Safety

Before disseminating any biomedical information resource that stores and communicates health data or knowledge and is designed to influence real-world practice or personal health decisions, it is important to verify that the resource is safe when used as intended. In the case of new drugs, European and US regulators have imposed a statutory duty on developers to perform extensive in vitro testing, and in vivo testing in animals, before any human receives a dose of the drug.

Analogous testing is currently not required of information resources. However, since 2000, the safety of biomedical information resources has come increasingly into the spotlight (Rigby et al. 2001; Koppel et al. 2005). For biomedical information resources, safety tests analogous to those required for drugs would include assessment of the accuracy of the data stored and retrieved, determining whether and how easily end-users can employ the resource for its intended purposes, and estimating how often the resource furnishes misleading or incorrect information (Eminovic et al. 2004). It may be necessary to repeat these assessments following any substantial modifications to the information resource, as the correction of safety-related problems may itself generate new problems or uncover previously unrecognized ones.

Determining if an information resource is safe and effective goes fundamentally to the process of evaluation we address in this chapter. All of the methodological issues we raise apply to safety assessments. Casual assessments that fail to address these issues will not resolve the safety question, and will not reveal safety defects that can be remedied. Many of these issues are issues of sampling that we introduce in Sect. 11.4.2. For example, the advice or other "output" generated by most information resources depends critically on the quality and quantity of data available to it and on the manner in which the resource is used by patients or practitioners. People or practitioners who are untrained, in a hurry, or exhausted at 3 A.M., are more likely to fail to enter key data that might lead to the resource generating misleading advice, or to fail to heed an alarm that is not adequately emphasized by the user interface. Thus, to generate valid results, functional tests must put the resources in actual users' hands under the most realistic conditions possible, or in the hands of people with similar knowledge, skills and experience if real users are not available.

Other safety issues are, from a methodological perspective, issues of measurement that we address in Sect. 11.4.2. For example, should "usability" of an information resource be determined by documenting that the resource development process followed best practices to inculcate usability,

asking end-users if they believed the resource was usable, or by documenting and studying their "click streams" to determine if end-users actually navigated the resource as the designers intended? There is no single clear answer to this question (see Jacob Nielsen's invaluable resource on user testing[1]), but we will see that all measurement processes have features that make their results more or less dependable and useful. We will also see that the measurement processes built into evaluation studies can themselves be designed to make the results of the studies more helpful to all stakeholders, including those focused on safety.

11.3 Two Universals of Evaluation

11.3.1 The Full Range of What Can Be Formally Studied

Deciding what to study is fundamentally a process of winnowing down from a universe of potential questions to a parsimonious set of questions that can be realistically addressed given the priorities, time, and resources available. This winnowing process can begin with the full range of what can potentially be studied. To both ensure that the most important questions do get "on the table" and to help eliminate the less important ones, it can be useful to start with such a comprehensive list. While experienced evaluators do not typically begin study planning from this broadest perspective, it is always helpful to have the full range of options in mind.

There are five major aspects of an information resource, or an identified class of resources, that can be studied:

1. Need for the resource: Investigators study the status quo *absent* the resource, including the nature of problems the resource is intended to address and how frequently these problems arise. (When an information resource is already deployed, the "status quo" might be the currently deployed resource, and the resource under study is a proposed replacement for it or enhancement to it.)

---

[1] www.useit.com (Accessed 4/19/13).

2. Design and development process: Investigators study the skills of the development team, and the development methodologies employed by the team, to understand if the resulting resource is likely to function as intended.

3. Resource static structure: Here the focus of the evaluation includes specifications, flow charts, program code, and other representations of the resource that can be inspected without actually running it.

4. Resource usability and dynamic functions: The focus is on the usability of the resource and how it performs when it is used in pilots prior to full deployment.

5. Resource use, effect and impact: Finally, after deployment, the focus switches from the resource itself to the extent of its use and its effects on professional, patient or public users, and health care organizations.

In a theoretically "complete" evaluation, sequential studies of a particular resource might address all of these aspects, over the life cycle of the resource. In the real world, however, it is difficult, and rarely necessary, to be so comprehensive. Over the course of its development and deployment, a resource may be studied many times, with the studies in their totality touching on many or most of these aspects. Some aspects of an information resource will be studied informally using anecdotal data collected via casual methods. Other aspects will be studied more formally in ways that are purposefully designed to inform specific decisions and that involve systematic collection and analysis of data. Distinguishing those aspects that will be studied formally from those left for informal exploration is a task facing all evaluators.

11.3.2 The Structure of All Evaluation Studies, Beginning with a Negotiation Phase

If the list offered in the previous section can be seen as the universe of what can be studied, Fig. 11.1 can be used as a framework for planning all evaluation studies. The first stage in any study is negotiation between the individuals who will be carrying out the study (the "evaluators") and the "stakeholders" who have interests in or otherwise will be concerned about the study results. Before a study can proceed, the key stakeholders who are supporting the study financially and providing other essential resources for it—such as the institution where the information resource is deployed—must be satisfied with the general plan. The negotiation phase identifies the broad aim and objectives of the study, what kinds of reports and other deliverables will result and by when, where the study personnel will be based, the resources available to conduct the study, and any constraints on what can be studied.

The results of the negotiation phase are expressed in a document, generally known as a contract between the evaluators and the key stakeholders. The contact guides the planning and execution of the study and, in a very significant way, protects all parties from misunderstandings about intent and execution. Like any contract, an **evaluation contract** can be changed later with consent of all parties.

Following the negotiation process and its reflection in a contract, the planning of the evaluation proceeds in a sequence of logical steps, starting with the formulation of specific questions to be addressed, then the selection of the

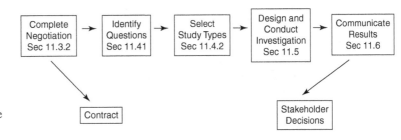

Fig. 11.1 Generic structure of all evaluation studies

type(s) of study that will be used, the investigation that entails the collection and analysis of data, and ultimately the communication of the findings back to the stakeholders, which typically inform a range of decisions. Although Fig. 11.1 portrays a one-way progression through this sequence of stages, in the real world of evaluation there are often detours and backtracks.

11.4 Deciding What to Study and What Type of Study to Do: Questions and Study Types

11.4.1 The Importance of Identifying Questions

Once the study's scope and other applicable "ground rules" have been established, the real work of study planning can begin. The next step, as suggested by Fig. 11.1, is to convert the perspectives of the concerned parties, and what these individuals or groups want to know, into a finite, specific set of questions. It is important to recognize that, for any evaluation setting that is interesting enough to merit formal evaluation, the number of potential questions is infinite. This essential step of identifying a tractable number of questions has a number of benefits:

- It helps to crystallize thinking of both investigators and key members of the audience who are the stakeholders in the evaluation.
- It guides the investigators and clients through the critical process of assigning priority to certain issues and thus productively narrowing the focus of a study.
- It converts broad statements of aim (e.g., *"to evaluate a new order communications system"*) into specific questions that can potentially be answered (e.g., *"What is the impact of the order communications system on how clinical staff spend their time, the rate and severity of adverse drug events and the length of patient stay?"*).
- It allows different stakeholders in the evaluation process—patients, professional groups,

managers – to see the extent to which their own concerns are being addressed, and to ensure that these feed into the evaluation process.

- Most important, perhaps, it is hard if not impossible to develop investigative methods without first identifying questions, or at least focused issues, for exploration. The choice of methods follows from the evaluation questions: not from the novel technology powering the information resource or the type of resource being studied. Unfortunately, some investigators choose to apply the same set of the methods to any study, irrespective of the questions to be addressed, or even to limit the evaluation questions addressed to those compatible with the methods they prefer. We do not endorse this approach.

Consider the distinction made earlier between informal evaluations that people undertake continuously as they make choices as part of their everyday personal or professional lives, and more formal evaluations that are planned and then executed according to that plan. In short, formal evaluations are those that conform to the architecture of Fig. 11.1. In these formal evaluations, the questions that actually get addressed survive a narrowing process that begins with a broad set of candidate questions. When starting a formal evaluation, therefore, a major decision is whom to consult to establish the questions that will get "on the table", how to log and analyze their views, and what weight to place on each of these views. There is always a wide range of potential players in any evaluation (see Box 11.1) and there is no formula that defines whom to consult or in what order. Through this process, the investigators apply their common sense and, with experience, learn to follow their instincts; it is often useful to establish a steering group to advise the evaluators to ensure that their efforts remain true to the interests and preferences of the stakeholders. The only universal mistake is to fail to consult one or more of the key stakeholders, especially those paying for the study or those ultimately making the key decisions to be informed by the evaluation.

more focused issues. For example, when evaluating an electronic lab notebook system for researchers, it is important to distinguish operational, low level issues, such as the time taken to enter data for equipment orders, from strategic issues such as the impact of the resource on research productivity. While this distinction may seem trivial in the abstract, in practice these issues often get muddled as different stakeholders argue for their particular needs and interests to be represented.

It is critical that the specific questions serving as the beacon guiding the study be determined and endorsed by all key stakeholders, before any significant decisions about the detailed design of the study are made. We will see later that evaluation questions can, in many circumstances, change over the course of a study; but that fact does not obviate the need to specify a set of questions at the outset.

Consider as an example a new information resource that sends SMS text messages to patients with chronic illnesses, reminding them of upcoming appointments, to take their medication (e.g. Lester et al. 2010) or about other key events (for example, recurring blood draws) that are important to their care. An example set of initial negotiated questions for this study is shown below, along with the stakeholder groups that will have direct or primary interest in each question.

Through discussions with various stakeholder groups, the hard decisions regarding the questions to be addressed in the study are made. A significant challenge for investigators is the risk of getting swamped by detail resulting from the multiplicity of questions that can be asked in any study. To manage through the process, reflect on the major issues identified after each round of discussions with stakeholders, and then identify the questions that map to these issues. Where possible keep questions at the same level of granularity. It is important to keep a sense of perspective, distinguishing the issues as they arise and organizing them into some kind of hierarchy, for example low or operational level issues, tactical or medium level and high level strategic issues. Interdependencies should be noted and care should be taken to avoid intermingling global issues with

11.4.2 Selecting a Study Type

After developing evaluation questions, the next step is to understand which study type(s) the evaluation questions naturally invoke. These study types are specific to the study of information resources, and are particularly informative to the design of evaluation studies in biomedical informatics. The study types are described below and also summarized in Table 11.1. The second column of Table 11.1 links the study types to the aspect of the resource that is studied, as introduced in Sect. 11.3.1. Each study type is likely to appeal to certain stakeholders in the evaluation process, as suggested in the rightmost column of the table. A wide range of data collection and analysis methods, as discussed in Sect. 11.5, can

Table 11.1 Classification of generic study types by broad study question and the stakeholders most concerned

Study type	Aspect studied	Broad study question	Audience/stakeholders primarily interested in results
1. Needs assessment	Need for the resource	What is the problem?	Resource developers, funders of the resource
2. Design validation	Design and development process	Is the development method in accord with accepted practices?	Funders of the resource; professional and governmental certification agencies e.g., Food and Drug Administration, Office of the National Coordinator for HIT
3. Structure validation	Resource static structure	Is the resource appropriately designed to function as intended?	Professional indemnity insurers, resource developers; professional and governmental certification agencies
4. Usability test	Resource dynamic usability and function	Can intended users navigate the resource so it carries out intended functions?	Resource developers, users, funders
5. Laboratory function study	Resource dynamic usability and function	Does the resource have the potential to be beneficial?	Resource developers, funders, users, academic community
6. Field function study	Resource dynamic usability and function	Does the resource have the potential to be beneficial in the real world?	Resource developers, funders, users
7. Lab user effect study	Resource effect and impact	Is the resource likely to change user behavior?	Resource developers and funders, users
8. Field user effect study	Resource effect and impact	Does the resource change actual user behavior in ways that are positive?	Resource users and their clients, resource purchasers and funders
9. Problem impact study	Resource effect and impact	Does the resource have a positive impact on the original problem?	The universe of stakeholders

be used to answer the questions embraced by all nine study types. *Choice of a study type typically does not constrain the methods that can be used to collect and analyze data.*

1. **Needs assessment** studies seek to clarify the information problem the resource is intended to solve. These studies take place before the resource is designed–usually in the setting where the resource is to be deployed, although simulated settings may sometimes be used. Ideally, these potential users will be studied while they work with real problems or cases, to understand better how information is used and managed, and to identify the causes and consequences of inadequate information flows. The investigator seeks to understand users' skills, knowledge and attitudes, as well as how they make decisions or take actions. An example is a study on 300 primary care physicians to understand their trade-offs

among the reliability of an electronic patient record, where they could access the resource, and who could have access to it (Wyatt et al. 2010). To ensure that developers have a clear model of how a proposed information resource will fit with working practices and structures, they may also need to study health care or research processes, team functioning, or relevant aspects of the larger organization in which work is done.

2. **Design validation** studies focus on the quality of the processes of information resource design and development, for example by asking experts to review these processes. The experts may review documents, interview the development team, compare the suitability of the software engineering methodology and programming tools used with others that are available, and generally apply their expertise to identify potential flaws in the approach

used to develop the software, as well as constructively to suggest how these might be corrected.

3. **Structure validation** studies address the static form of the software, usually after a first prototype has been developed. This type of study is most usefully performed by an expert or a team of experts with experience in developing software for the problem domain and concerned users. For these purposes, the investigators need access to both summary and detailed documentation about the system architecture, the structure and function of each module, and the interfaces among them. The expert might focus on the appropriateness of the algorithms that have been employed and check that they have been correctly implemented. Experts might also examine the data structures (e.g., whether they are appropriately normalized) and knowledge bases (e.g., whether they are evidence-based, up to date, and modelled in a format that will support the intended analyses or reasoning). Most of this will be done by inspection and discussion with the development team. Sometimes specialized software may be used to test the structure of the resource (Somerville 2002).

   Note that the study types listed up to this point do not require a functioning information resource. However, beginning with usability testing below, the study types require the existence of at least a functioning prototype.

4. **Usability testing** studies focus on system function and addresses whether intended users can actually operate or navigate the software, to determine whether the resource has the potential to be helpful to them (see also Chap. 4). In this type of study, use of a prototype by typical users informs further development and should improve its usability. Although usability testing is often performed by obtaining opinions of usability experts, usability can also be tested by deploying the resource in a laboratory or classroom setting, introducing users to it, and then allowing them either to navigate at will and provide unstructured comments or to attempt to complete some scripted tasks (see Nielsen, www.useit.com).

Data can be collected by the computer itself, from the user, by a live observer, via audio or video capture of users' actions and statements, or by specialized instrumentation such as eye-tracking tools. Many software developers have usability testing labs equipped with sophisticated measurement systems, staffed by experts in human computer interaction to carry out these studies—an indication of the importance increasingly attached to this type of study.

5. **Laboratory function studies** go beyond usability to explore more specific aspects of the information resource, such as the quality of data captured, the speed of communication, the validity of the calculations carried out, or the appropriateness of advice given. These functions relate less to the basic usability of the resource and more to how the resource performs in relation to what it is trying to achieve for the user or the organization. When carrying out any kind of function testing, the results will depend crucially on what problems the users are asked to solve, so the "tasks" employed in these studies should correspond as closely as possible to those to which the resource will be applied in real working life.

6. **Field function studies** are a variant of laboratory function testing in which the resource is "pseudo-deployed" in a real work place and employed by real users, up to a point. However, in field function tests, although the resource is used by real users with real tasks, there is no immediate access by the users to the output or results of interaction with the resource that might influence their decisions or actions, so no effects on these can occur. The output is recorded for later review by the investigators, and perhaps by the users themselves.

   Studies of the effect or impact of information resources on users and problems are in many ways the most demanding. As the focus of its study moves from its functions to its possible effects on health decisions or care processes, the conduct of research, or educational practice, there is often the need to establish cause and effect.

7. In **laboratory user effect studies**, simulated user actions are studied. Practitioners employ the resource and are asked what they "would do" with the results or advice the resource generates, but no action is taken. Laboratory user effect studies are conducted with prototype or released versions of the resource, outside the practice environment. Although such studies involve individuals who are representative of the "end-user" population, the primary results of the study derive from simulated actions, so the care of patients or conduct of research is not affected by a study of this type. An example is a study in which junior doctors viewed realistic prescribing scenarios and interacted with a simulated prescribing tool while they were exposed to simulated prescribing alerts of various kinds (Scott 2011).

8. In a **field user effect study**, the actual actions or decisions of the users of the resource are studied after the resource is formally deployed. This type of study provides an opportunity to test whether the resource is actually used by the intended users, whether they obtain accurate and useful information from it, and whether this use affects their decisions and actions in significant ways. In field user effect studies, the emphasis is on the behaviors and actions of users, and not the consequences of these behaviors. For example, one study examined the impact of SMS reminders on anti-retroviral medication adherence in Africans with HIV and showed a dramatic improvement (Lester et al. 2010).

9. **Problem impact studies** are similar to field user effect studies in many respects, but differ profoundly in the questions that are the focus of exploration. Problem impact studies examine the extent to which the original problem that motivated creation or deployment of the information resource has been addressed. Often this requires investigation that looks beyond the actions of care providers, researchers, or patients to examine the consequences of these actions. For example, an information resource designed to reduce medical errors may affect the behavior of some clinicians who employ the resource, but for a variety of reasons, the

error rate remains unchanged. The causes of errors may be system-level factors and the changes inculcated by the information resource may address only some of these factors. Patients may be motivated to exercise through interaction with an information resource, but fail to meet weight loss objectives because they cannot afford concomitant changes in their diets. In other domains, an information resource may be widely used by researchers to access biomedical information, as determined by a user effect study, but a subsequent problem impact study may or may not reveal effects on scientific productivity. New educational technology may change the ways students learn, but may or may not increase their performance on standardized examinations. In the Lester study of SMS alerts (Lester et al. 2010), increased adherence to antiretroviral therapy (a user action) was also accompanied by improved viral load suppression. Fully comprehensive problem impact studies will also be sensitive to unintended consequences. Sometimes, the solution to the target problem creates other, unintended and unanticipated problems that can affect perceptions of success. As electronic mail became an almost universal mode of communication, almost no one anticipated the problems of "spam" or "phishing".

11.4.3 Factors Distinguishing the Nine Study Types

Table 11.2 further distinguishes the nine study types, as described above, using a set of key differentiating factors discussed in detail in the paragraphs that follow.

The setting in which the study takes place: Studies of the design process, the resource structure, and many resource functions are typically conducted outside the active practice or decision environment, in a "laboratory" setting. Studies to elucidate the need for a resource and studies of its impact on users would usually take place in ongoing practice settings—known generically as the "field"—where health care practitioners, researchers, students, or administrators are doing

Table 11.2 Factors distinguishing the nine generic study types

Study type	Study setting	Version of the resource	Sampled users	Sampled tasks	What is observed
1. Needs assessment	Field	None, or pre-existing resource to be replaced	Anticipated resource users	Actual tasks	User skills, knowledge, decisions or actions; care processes, costs, team function or organization; patient outcomes
2. Design validation	Development lab	None	None	None	Quality of design method or team
3. Structure validation	Lab	Prototype or released version	None	None	Quality of resource structure, components, architecture
4. Usability test	Lab	Prototype or released version	Proxy, real users	Simulated, abstracted	Speed of use, user comments, completion of sample tasks
5. Laboratory function study	Lab	Prototype or released version	Proxy, real users	Simulated, abstracted	Speed and quality of data collected or displayed; accuracy of advice given…
6. Field function study	Field	Prototype or released version	Proxy, real users	Real	Speed and quality of data collected or displayed; accuracy of advice given…
7. Lab user effect study	Lab	Prototype or released version	Real users	Abstracted, real	Impact on user knowledge, simulated/pretend decisions or actions
8. Field user effect study	Field	Released version	Real users	Real	Extent and nature of resource use. Impact on user knowledge, real decisions, real actions
9. Problem impact study	Field	Released version	Real users	Real	Care processes, costs, team function, cost effectiveness

real work in the real world. The same is true for studies of the impact of a resource on persons and organizations. These studies can take place only in a setting where the resource is available for use at the time and where professional activities occur and/or important decisions are made. To an investigator planning studies, an important consideration that determines the kind of study possible is the degree of access to users in the field setting. If, as a practical matter, access to the field setting is very limited, then several study types listed in Tables 11.1 and 11.2 are not possible, and the range of evaluation questions that can be addressed is limited accordingly.

The version of the resource used: For some kinds of studies, a simulated or prototype version of the resource may be sufficient (Scott et al. 2011), whereas for studies in which the resource is employed by intended users to support real decisions and actions, a fully robust and reliable version is needed (e.g., Lester et al. 2010).

The sampled resource users: Most biomedical information resources are not autonomous agents that operate independently of users. More typically, information resources function through interaction with one or more such "users" who often bring to the interaction their own domain knowledge and knowledge of how to operate the resource. In some types of evaluation studies, the users of the resource are not the end users for whom the resource is ultimately designed, but are members of the development or evaluation teams, or other individuals we can call "proxy users" who are chosen because they are conveniently available or because they are affordable. In other types of studies, the users are sampled from the end-users for whom the resource is ultimately designed. The type of users employed gives shape to a study and can affect its results profoundly. The usability of a resource is easily overestimated if the "users" in a usability study are those who designed the system. Volunteer users of a consumer-oriented website may be more literate than the general population the resource is designed to benefit.

The sampled tasks: For function and effect studies, the resource is actually "run." The users included in the study actually interact with the resource. This requires tasks, typically clinical or scientific case or problems, for the users to undertake. These tasks can be invented or simulated; they can be abstracted versions of real cases or problems, shortened to suit the specific purposes of the study; or they can be live cases or research problems as they present to resource users in the real world. Clearly, the kinds of tasks employed in a study have serious implications for the study results and the conclusions that can be drawn from them.

The observations that are made: All evaluation studies entail observations that generate data that are subsequently analyzed to make decisions. As seen in Table 11.2, many different kinds of observations[2] can be made.

In the paragraphs above we have introduced the term "sampling" for both tasks and users. It is important to establish that in real evaluation studies, tasks and users are always sampled from some real or hypothetical populations. Sampling of users and tasks are major challenges in evaluation study design since it is never possible, practical, or desirable to try to study everyone doing everything possible with an information resource. Sampling issues are addressed later in this chapter.

11.5 Conducting Investigations: Collecting and Drawing Conclusions from Data

11.5.1 Two Grand Approaches to Study Design, Data Collection, and Analysis

Several authors have developed classifications, or **typologies**, of evaluation methods or approaches. Among the best is that developed in 1980 by

Ernest House (1980). A major advantage of House's typology is that each approach is linked elegantly to an underlying philosophical model, as detailed in his book. This classification divides current practice into eight discrete approaches, four of which may be viewed as **objectivist** and four of which may be viewed as **subjectivist**. While the distinctions between the eight approaches House describes are beyond the scope of this chapter, the grand distinction between objectivist and subjectivist approaches is very important. Note that these approaches are not entitled "objective" and "subjective", because those labels carry strong and fundamentally misleading connotations of scientific precision in the former case and of idiosyncratic imprecision in the latter. We will see in this section how both objectivist (often called quantitative) and subjectivist (often called qualitative) approaches find rigorous application across the range of study types described earlier.

To appreciate the fundamental difference between the approaches, it is necessary to address their very different philosophical roots. The objectivist approaches derive from a **logical–positivist** philosophical orientation—the same orientation that underlies the classic experimental sciences. The major premises underlying the objectivist approaches are as follows:

- In general, attributes of interest are properties of the resource under study. More specifically, this position suggests that the merit and worth of an information resource—the attributes of most interest in evaluation—can in principle be measured with all observations yielding the same result. It also assumes that an investigator can measure these attributes without affecting how the resource under study functions or is used.
- Rational persons can and should agree on what attributes of a resource are important to measure and what results of these measurements would be identified as a most desirable, correct, or positive outcome. In medical informatics, making this assertion is tantamount to stating that a gold standard of resource performance can always be identified and that all rational individuals can be brought to consensus on what this gold standard is.

[2] We use "observations" here very generically to span a range of activities that includes watching someone work with an information resource as well as highly-instrumented tracking or measurement.

- Because numerical measurement allows precise statistical analysis of performance over time or performance in comparison with some alternative, numerical measurement is prima facie superior to a verbal description. Verbal, descriptive data (generally known as qualitative data) are useful in only preliminary studies to identify hypotheses for subsequent, precise analysis using quantitative methods.
- Through these kinds of comparisons, it is possible to demonstrate to a reasonable degree that a resource is or is not superior to what it replaced or to a competing resource.

Contrast these assumptions with a set of assumptions that derives from an **intuitionist–pluralist** or de-constructivist philosophical position that spawns a set of subjectivist approaches to evaluation:

- What is observed about a resource depends in fundamental ways on the observer. Different observers of the same phenomenon might legitimately come to different conclusions. Both can be objective in their appraisals even if they do not agree; it is not necessary that one is right and the other wrong.
- Merit and worth must be explored in context. The value of a resource emerges through study of the resource as it functions in a particular patient care or educational environment.
- Individuals and groups can legitimately hold different perspectives on what constitutes the most desirable outcome of introducing a resource into an environment. There is no reason to expect them to agree, and it may be counterproductive to try to lead them to consensus. An important aspect of an evaluation would be to document the ways in which they disagree.
- Verbal description can be highly illuminating. Qualitative data are valuable, in and of themselves, and can lead to conclusions as convincing as those drawn from quantitative data. The value of qualitative data, therefore, goes far beyond that of identifying issues for later "precise" exploration using quantitative methods.
- Evaluation should be viewed as an exercise in argument or rhetoric, rather than as a demonstration, because any study can appear equivocal when subjected to serious scrutiny.

The approaches to evaluation that derive from this subjectivist philosophical perspective may seem strange, imprecise, and unscientific when considered for the first time. This perception stems in large part from the widespread acceptance of the objectivist worldview in biomedicine. Over the last two decades, however, thanks to some early high quality studies (e.g., Forsythe et al. 1992; Ash et al. 2003) the importance and utility of these subjectivist approaches in evaluation has been established within biomedical informatics. As stated earlier, the evaluation mindset includes methodological eclecticism. It is important for people trained in classic experimental methods at least to understand, and possibly even to embrace, the subjectivist worldview if they are to conduct fully informative evaluation studies.

Some of these issues are further considered in Appendix B, which describes some more recent perspectives on evaluation.

11.5.2 Conduct of Objectivist Studies

Figure 11.2 expands the generic process for conducting evaluation studies to illustrate the steps involved in conducting an objectivist study. Figure 11.2 illustrates the linear sequence in which the investigation portion of an evaluation study is typically carried out. We will focus in this chapter on issues of study design that are the biggest challenge to the validity of objectivist studies and we will further focus on that subset of objectivist study designs which are comparative in nature. More details on the other aspects of objectivist studies are available in a textbook on the subject (Friedman et al. 2005) and in standard references on experimental design (Campbell & Stanley 1963).

11.5.2.1 Structure and Terminology of Comparative Studies

Most objectivist evaluations performed in the world make a comparison of some type. For informatics, aspects of performance of individuals, groups, or organizations *with* the

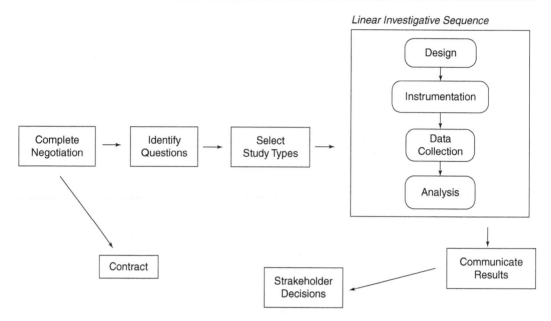

Fig. 11.2 Generic structure depicting an objectivist investigation

information resource are compared to those same aspects *without* the resource or with some alternative resource. After identifying a sample of participants for the study, the researcher assigns each participant, often randomly, to one or a set of conditions. Some outcomes of interest are measured for each participant. The averaged values of these outcomes are then compared across the conditions. If all other factors are controlled, then any measured difference in the averaged outcomes can be attributed to the resource.

This relatively simple description of a comparative study belies the many issues that affect their design, execution, and ultimate usefulness. To understand these issues, we must first develop a precise terminology.

The **participants** in a study are the entities about which data are collected. It is key to emphasize that participants are often people—for example, care providers or recipients—but also may be information resources, groups of people, or organizations. Because many of the activities in informatics are conducted in hierarchical settings with naturally occurring groups (a "doctor's patients"; the "researchers in a laboratory"), investigators

must, for a particular study, define the participants carefully and consistently.

Variables are specific characteristics of the participants that either are measured purposefully by the investigator or are self-evident properties of the participants that do not require measurement. Some variables take on a continuous range of values. Others have a discrete set of levels corresponding to each of the possible measured values. For example, in a hospital setting, physician members of a ward team can be classified as residents, fellows, or attending physicians. In this case, the variable "physician's level of qualification" is said to have three "levels".

The **dependent variables** are those variables in the study that captures the outcomes of interest to the investigator. (For this reason, dependent variables are also called **outcome variables**.) A study may have one or more dependent variables. In a typical study, the dependent variables will be computed, for each participant, as an average over a number of tasks. For example, clinicians' diagnostic performance may be measured over a set of cases, or "tasks", that provide a range of diagnostic challenges.

The **independent variables** are included in a study to try and explain the measured values of the dependent variables. For example, whether an information resource is available, or not, to support certain clinical tasks could be the major independent variable in a study designed to evaluate the effects of that resource.

Measurement challenges almost always arise in the assessment of the outcome or dependent variable for a study (Friedman 2003). Often, for example, the dependent variable is some type of performance measure that invokes concerns about reliability (precision) and validity (accuracy) of measurement. The independent variables may also raise measurement challenges. When the independent variable is patient gender, for example, the measurement problems are relatively straightforward—though in some studies classifying trans-gender individuals may need some thought. If the independent variable is an attitude or other "state of mind", profound measurement challenges can arise.

11.5.2.2 Issues of Measurement

Measurement is the process of assigning a value corresponding to the presence, absence, or degree of a specific attribute in a specific object, as illustrated in Fig. 11.3. When we speak specifically of measurement, it is customary to use the term "object" to refer to the entity on which measurements are made. Measurement usually results in either (1) the assignment of a numerical score representing the extent to which the attribute of interest is present in the object, or (2) the assignment of an object to a specific category. Taking the temperature (attribute) of a patient (object) is an example of the process of measurement.

From the premises underlying objectivist studies (see Sect. 11.5.1), it follows that proper execution of such studies requires careful and specific attention to methods of measurement. It can never be assumed, particularly in informatics, that attributes of interest are measured without error. Accurate and precise measurement must not be an afterthought. Measurement is of particular importance in biomedical informatics because, as a relatively young field, informatics does not have a well-established tradition of "variables worth measuring" or proven instruments for measuring them (Friedman 2003). By and large, people planning studies in informatics are faced first with the task of deciding what to measure and then with that of developing their own measurement methods. For most researchers, these tasks prove to be harder and more time-consuming than initially anticipated.

We can underscore the importance of measurement by establishing a formal distinction between studies undertaken to develop methods

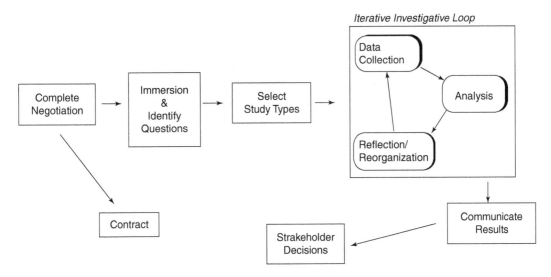

Fig. 11.3 Generic structure depicting a subjectivist investigation

for making measurements, which we call measurement studies, and the subsequent use of these methods to address questions of direct importance in informatics, which we call demonstration studies. **Measurement studies** seek to determine how accurately and precisely an attribute of interest can be measured in a population of objects. In an ideal objectivist measurement, all observers will agree on the result of the measurement. Any disagreement is therefore due to error, which should be minimized. The more agreement among observers or across observations, the better the measurement. Measurement procedures developed and validated through measurement studies provide researchers with what they need to conduct **demonstration studies** that directly address questions of substantive and practical concern to the stakeholders for an evaluation study. Once we know how accurately we can measure an attribute using a particular procedure, we can employ the measured values of this attribute as a variable in a demonstration study to draw inferences about the performance, perceptions, or effects of an information resource. For example, once measurement studies have determined how accurately and precisely the usability of a class of information resources can be measured, a subsequent demonstration study could explore which of two resources that are members of this class has greater usability.

A detailed discussion of measurement issues is beyond the scope of this chapter. The bottom line is that investigators should know that their measurement methods will be adequate before they collect data for their studies. It is necessary to perform a measurement study, involving data collection on a small scale, to establish the adequacy of all measurement procedures if the measures to be used do not have an established track record (e.g., Ramnarayan et al. 2003; Demiris et al. 2000). Even if the measurement procedures of interest do have a track record in a particular health care environment and with a specific mix of cases and care providers, they may not perform equally well in a different environment, so measurement studies may still be necessary. Researchers should always ask themselves, "How good are my measures in this particular

setting?" whenever they are planning a study, before they proceed to the demonstration phase. The importance of measurement studies for informatics was explained in 1990 by Michaelis and co-workers (Michaelis et al. 1990). Another study (Friedman et al. 2003) has demonstrated that studies of clinical information systems have not systematically addressed the adequacy of the methods used to measure the specific outcomes reported in these studies.

Whenever possible, investigators planning studies should employ established measurement methods with a "track record", rather than developing their own. While there exist relatively few compendia and measurement instruments specifically for health informatics, a web-based resource listing over 50 instruments associated with the development, usability, and impact of management information systems is available on the Internet.[3]

11.5.2.3 Sampling Strategies
Selection of Participants

The participants selected for objectivist studies must resemble those to which the evaluator and others responsible for the study wish to apply the results. For example, when attempting to quantify the likely impact of a clinical information resource on clinicians at large, there is no point in studying its effects on the clinicians who helped develop it, especially if they built it, as they are likely to be more familiar with the resource than average practitioners. Characteristics of clinical participants that typically need to be taken into account include age, experience, role, attitude toward digital information resources, and extent of their involvement in the development of the resource. Analogous factors would apply to patients or health care consumers as participants.

Volunteer Effect

A common bias in the selection of participants is the use of volunteers. It has been established in many areas that people who volunteer as participants, whether to complete questionnaires, partici-

---

[3] http://www.misq.org/skin/frontend/default/misq/surveys98/surveys.html#toc (Accessed January 27, 2013).

pate in psychology experiments, or test-drive new cars or other technologies, are atypical of the population at large (e.g., Pinsky et al. 2007). Although volunteers may make willing participants for pilot studies, they should be avoided in definitive demonstration studies, as they considerably reduce the generality of findings. One strategy is to include all participants meeting the selection criteria in the study. However, if this would result in too many participants, rather than asking for volunteers, it is better randomly or otherwise systematically to select a representative sample of all eligible clinicians, following up invitation letters with telephone calls to achieve as near 100 % recruitment of the selected sample as possible.

Number of Participants Needed

The financial investment required for an evaluation study depends critically on the number of participants needed. The required number in turn depends on the precision of the answer required from the study and the risk investigators are willing to take of failing to detect a significant effect. (All other things being equal, the larger the sample size, the greater the likelihood of detecting an effect against a predetermined criterion for statistical significance.) Statisticians can advise on this point and carry out sample-size calculations to estimate the number of participants required. Sometimes, in order to recruit the required number of participants, an element of volunteer effect must be tolerated; often there is a trade-off between obtaining a sufficiently large sample and ensuring that the sample is representative. Also, the impact of sample size on effect detection is non-linear. The value of adding, say, 10 more representative participants to a sample of 100 is far less than that of adding 10 more participants to a sample of 30.

Selection of Tasks

In the same way that participants must be carefully selected to resemble the people likely to use the information resource, any tasks the participants complete must also resemble those that will generally be encountered in the field setting where the information resource is deployed. Thus when evaluating a clinical order-entry system

intended for general use, it would be unwise to use only complex cases from, for example, a pediatric intensive care setting. Although the order-entry system might well be of considerable benefit in intensive care cases, it is inappropriate to generalize results from such a limited sample to the full range of cases seen in ambulatory pediatrics. An instructive example is provided by the study of Van Way et al. (1982) who developed a scoring system for diagnosing appendicitis and studied the resource's accuracy using exclusively patients who had undergone surgery for suspected appendicitis. Studying this group of patients had the benefit of allowing the true cause of the abdominal pain to be obtained with near certainty as a by-product of the surgery itself. However, in these patients who had all undergone surgery for suspected appendicitis the symptoms were more severe and the incidence of appendicitis was five to ten times higher than for the typical patient for whom such a scoring system would be used. Thus the accuracy obtained with postsurgical patients would be a poor estimate of the system's accuracy in routine clinical use.

If the performance of an information resource is measured on a small number of hand-picked cases, the functions it performs may appear spuriously complete and its usability overestimated. This is especially likely if these cases are similar to, or even identical with, the training set of cases used to develop or tune the information resource before the evaluation is carried out. When a statistical model that powers an information resource is carefully adjusted to achieve maximal performance on training data, this adjustment may worsen its accuracy on a fresh set of data due to a phenomenon called over fitting (Wasson 1985). Thus it is important to obtain a new set of cases and evaluate performance on this new test set. Sometimes developers omit cases from a sample if they do not fall within the scope of the information resource, for example if the final diagnosis for a case is not represented in a diagnostic system's knowledge base. This practice violates the principle that a test set should be representative of all cases in which the information resource will be used, and will overestimates its effectiveness with unseen data.

11.5.2.4 Control Strategies in Comparative Studies

One of the most challenging questions in comparative study design is how to obtain control (Liu et al. 2011). We need a way to account for all the other changes taking place that are not attributable to the information resource. In the following sections we review a series of control strategies. We employ, as a running example of an information resource under study, a reminder system that prompts doctors to order prophylactic antibiotics for orthopedic patients to prevent postoperative infections. In this example, the intervention is the installation and commissioning of the reminder system; the participants are the physicians; and the tasks are the patients cared for by the physicians. The dependent variables derive from the outcome measurements made and would include physicians' ordering of antibiotics and the rate of postoperative infections averaged across the patients cared for by each physician.

Descriptive (Uncontrolled) Studies

In the simplest possible design, an uncontrolled or **descriptive study**, we install the reminder system, allow a suitable period for training, and then make our measurements. There is no independent variable. Suppose that we discover that the overall postoperative infection rate is 5% and that physicians order prophylactic antibiotics in 60 % of orthopedic cases. Although we have two measured dependent variables, it is hard to draw meaningful conclusions from these figures. It is possible that there has been no change due to the system.

Historically Controlled Experiments

As a first improvement to a descriptive study, let us consider a **historically controlled experiment**, sometimes called a **before–after study**. The investigator makes baseline measurements of antibiotic ordering and postoperative infection rates before the information resource is installed, and then makes the same measurements after the information resource is in routine use. The independent variable is time and has two levels: before and after resource installation. Let us say

Table 11.3 Results from a hypothetical before-after study of the impact of reminders on post operative infection rates

	Reminder group
Baseline infection rate	10 %
Post-intervention infection rate	5 %

that, at baseline, the postoperative infection rates were 10 % and doctors ordered prophylactic antibiotics in only 40 % of cases; the post-intervention figures are the same as before (see Table 11.3).

The investigators may claim that the halving of the infection rate can be safely ascribed to the information resource, especially because it was accompanied by a 20 % improvement in doctors' antibiotic prescribing. Many other factors might, however, have changed in the interim to cause these results, especially if there was a long interval between the baseline and postintervention measurements. New staff could have taken over, the case mix of patients could have changed, new prophylactic antibiotics may have been introduced, or clinical audit meetings may have highlighted the infection problem and thus caused greater clinical awareness. Simply assuming that the reminder system alone caused the reduction in infection rates is naive. Other factors, known or unknown, could have changed meanwhile, making untenable the simple assumption that our intervention is responsible for all of the observed effects (Liu et al. 2011). An improvement on this design is to add either internal or external controls—preferably both. The internal control should be a measure likely to be affected by any nonspecific changes happening in the local environment, but unaffected by the intervention. The external control can be exactly the same measure as in the target environment, but in a similar external setting, e.g., another hospital. If the measure of interest changes while there is no change in either internal or external controls, a skeptic needs to be quite resourceful to claim that the system is not responsible (Wyatt and Wyatt 2003).

Simultaneous Nonrandomized Controls

To address some of the problems with historical controls, we might use **simultaneous controls**, which requires us to make our outcome measure-

Table 11.4 Results of a hypothetical non-randomized parallel group study of reminders and post op infection rates

	Reminder group (%)	Control group (%)
Baseline rate	10	10
Post-intervention rate	5	11

ments in doctors and patients who are not influenced by the prophylactic antibiotic reminder system but who are subject to the other changes taking place in the environment. Taking measurements both before and during the intervention strengthens the design, because it gives an estimate of the changes due to the nonspecific factors taking place during the study period.

This study design would be a parallel group comparative study with simultaneous controls. Table 11.4 gives hypothetical results of such a study, focusing on postoperative infection rates as a single outcome measure or dependent variable. The independent variables are time and group, both of which have two levels of intervention and control.

There is the same improvement in the group where reminders were available, but no improvement—indeed a slight deterioration—where no reminders were available. This design provides suggestive evidence of an improvement that is most likely to be due to the reminder system. This inference is stronger if the same doctors worked in the same wards during the period the system was introduced, and if similar kinds of patients, subject to the same nonspecific influences, were being operated on during the whole time period.

Even though the controls in this example are simultaneous, skeptics may still refute our argument by claiming that there is some systematic, unknown difference between the clinicians or patients in the two groups. For example, if the two groups comprised the patients and clinicians in two adjacent wards, the difference in the infection rates could be attributable to systematic or chance differences between the wards. Perhaps hospital-staffing levels improved in some wards but not in others, or there was cross infection by a multiple-resistant organism only among the

patients in the control ward. To overcome such criticisms, we could expand the study to include all wards in the hospital—or even other hospitals—but that would clearly take considerable resources. We could try to measure everything that happens to every patient in both wards and to build complete psychological profiles of all staff to rule out systematic differences. We would still, however, be vulnerable to the accusation that some variable that we did not measure—did not even know about—explains the difference between the two wards. A much simpler strategy is to ensure that the controls really are comparable by randomizing them.

Simultaneous Randomized Controls

The crucial problem in the previous example is that, although the controls were simultaneous, there may have been systematic, unmeasured differences between them and the participants receiving the intervention (Liu and Wyatt 2011). A simple and effective way of removing systematic differences, whether due to known or unknown factors, is to randomize the assignment of participants to control or intervention groups. Thus, we could randomly allocate one-half of the doctors on both wards to receive the antibiotic reminders and the remaining doctors to work as they did before. We would then measure and compare postoperative infection rates in patients managed by doctors in the reminder and control groups. Provided that the doctors never look after one another's patients, any difference that is statistically "significant" (conventionally, a result that is statistically determined to have a probability of 0.05 or less of occurring by chance) can be attributed reliably to the reminders.

Table 11.5 shows the hypothetical results of such a study. The baseline infection rates in the patients managed by the two groups of doctors are similar, as we would expect, because the patients were allocated to the groups by chance. There is a greater reduction in infection rates in patients of reminder physicians compared with those of control physicians. Because random assignment means that there was no systematic difference in patient characteristics between groups, the only systematic difference between

Table 11.5 Results of a hypothetical randomized controlled trial of the impact of reminders on post op infection rates

	Reminder physicians (%)	Control physicians (%)
Baseline infection rate	11	10
Post intervention infection rate	6	8
Difference in infection rate	−5	−2

the two groups of patients is receipt of reminders by their doctors.

Provided that the sample size is large enough for these results to be statistically significant, we might begin to conclude with some confidence that providing doctors with reminders caused the reduction in infection rates. One lingering question is why there was also a small reduction, from baseline to installation, in infection rates in control cases, even though the control group should have received no reminders.

11.5.3 Conduct of Subjectivist Studies

The objectivist approaches to evaluation, described in the previous section, are useful for addressing some, but not all, of the interesting and important questions that challenge investigators in medical informatics. The subjectivist approaches described here address the problem of evaluation from a different set of premises. They use different but equally rigorous methods. Figure 11.3 expands the generic process for conducting evaluation studies to illustrate the stages involved in conducting a subjectivist study, and emphasizes the "iterative loop" of data collection, analysis and reflection as the major distinguishing characteristic of a subjectivist investigation. Another distinctive feature of subjectivist studies is an immersion in the environment where the resources is being or will be deployed. Because subjectivist approaches may be less familiar to readers of this chapter, we describe subjectivist studies in more detail than we did their objectivist counterparts.

11.5.3.1 The Rationale for Subjectivist Studies

Subjectivist methods enable us to address the deeper questions that arise in informatics: the detailed "whys" and "according to whoms" in addition to the aggregate "whethers" and "whats." Subjectivist approaches seek to represent the viewpoints of people who are users of the resource or are otherwise significant participants in the environment where the resource operates. The goal is illumination rather than judgment. The investigators seek to build an argument that promotes deeper understanding of the information resource or environment of which it is a part. The methods used derive largely from **ethnography** (Forsythe 1992). The investigators immerse themselves physically in the environment where the information resource is or will be operational, and they collect data primarily through observations, interviews, and reviews of documents. The designs—the data-collection plans—of these studies are not rigidly predetermined and do not unfold in a fixed sequence. They develop dynamically and nonlinearly as the investigators' experience accumulates.

11.5.3.2 A Rigorous, but Different, Methodology

The subjectivist approaches to evaluation, like their objectivist counterparts, are empirical methods. Although it is easy to focus only on their differences, these two broad classes of evaluation approaches share many features. In all empirical studies, for example, evidence is collected with great care; the investigators are always aware of what they are doing and why. The evidence is then compiled, interpreted, and ultimately reported. Investigators keep records of their procedures, and these records are open to audit by the investigators themselves or by individuals outside the study team. The principal investigator or evaluation-team leader is under an almost sacred scientific obligation to report their methods. Failure to do so will invalidate a study. Both classes of approaches also share a dependence on theories that guide investigators to explanations of the observed phenomena, as well as to a dependence on the pertinent empirical literature such as published studies that address similar phenomena or similar settings. In both approaches, there are rules of good practice that are generally accepted; it is therefore possible to distinguish a good study from a bad one.

There are, however, fundamental differences between objectivist and subjectivist approaches. First, subjectivist studies are **emergent** in design. Objectivist studies typically begin with a set of hypotheses or specific questions, and with a plan for addressing each member of this set. The investigator assumes that, barring major unforeseen developments, the plan will be followed exactly. Deviation, in fact, might introduce bias. The investigator who sees negative results emerging from the exploration of a particular question or use of a particular measurement instrument might change strategies in hope of obtaining more positive findings. In contrast, subjectivist studies typically begin with general **orienting issues** that stimulate the early stages of investigation. Through these initial investigations, the important questions for further study emerge. The subjectivist investigator is willing, at virtually any point, to adjust future aspects of the study in light of the most recent information obtained. Subjectivist investigators tend to be **incrementalists**; they change their plans from day-to-day and have a high tolerance for ambiguity and uncertainty. In this respect, they are much like good software developers. Also like software developers, subjectivist investigators must develop the ability to recognize when a project is finished, when further benefit can be obtained only at too great a cost in time, money, or work.

A second feature of subjectivist studies is a **naturalistic** orientation, a reluctance to manipulate the setting of the study, which in most cases is the environment in to which the information resource is introduced. They do not alter the environment to study it. Control groups, placebos, purposeful altering of information resources to create contrasting interventions, and other techniques that are central to the construction of objectivist studies typically are not used. Subjectivist studies will, however, employ quantitative data for descriptive purposes and may offer quantitative comparisons when the research

setting offers a "natural experiment" where such comparisons can be made without deliberate intervention. For example, when physicians and nurses both use a clinical system to enter orders, their differing experiences with the system offer a natural basis for comparison (Ash 2003). Subjectivist researchers are opportunists where pertinent information is concerned; they will use what they see as the best information available to illuminate a question under investigation.

A third important distinguishing feature of subjectivist studies is that their end product is a report written in narrative prose. These reports may be lengthy and may require significant time investment from the reader; no technical understanding of quantitative research methodology or statistics is required to comprehend them. Results of subjectivist studies are therefore accessible— and may even be entertaining—to a broad community in a way that results of objectivist studies are not. Objectivist study reports often can be results of inferential statistical analyses that most readers will not find easy to read and will typically not understand. Reports of subjectivist studies seek to engage their audience.

11.5.3.3 Natural History of a Subjectivist Study

Figure 11.3 illustrates the stages that characterize a subjectivist study (see also Chap. 9 in Friedman et al. 2005). These stages constitute a general sequence, but, as we mentioned, subjectivist investigators must always be prepared to revise their thinking and possibly to return to earlier stages in light of new evidence. Backtracking is a legitimate step in this model.

1. *Negotiation of the ground rules of the study*: In any empirical research, and particularly in evaluation studies, it is important to negotiate an understanding between the study team and the people commissioning the study. This understanding should embrace the general aims of the study; the kinds of methods to be used; the access to various sources of information, including health care providers, patients, and various documents; and the format for interim and final reports. The aims of the study may be formulated in a set of initial

orienting questions. Ideally, this understanding will be expressed in a **memorandum of understanding**, analogous to a contract.

2. *Immersion into the environment*: At this stage, the investigators begin spending time in the work environment. Their activities range from formal introductions to informal conversations, or to silent presence at meetings and other events. Investigators use the generic term **field** to refer to the setting, which may be multiple physical locations, where the work under study is carried out. Trust and openness between the investigators and the people in the field are essential elements of subjectivist studies to ensure full and candid exchange of information.

   Even as immersion is taking place, the investigator is already collecting data to sharpen the initial questions or issues guiding the study. Early discussions with people in the field, and other activities primarily targeted toward immersion, inevitably begin to shape the investigators' views. Almost from the outset, the investigator is typically addressing several aspects of the study simultaneously.

3. *Iterative loop*: At this point, the procedural structure of the study becomes akin to an iterative loop, as the investigator engages in cycles of data collection, analysis and reflection, member checking, and reorganization. Data collection involves interview, observation, document analysis, and other methods. Data are collected on planned occasions, as well as serendipitously or spontaneously. The data are recorded carefully and are interpreted in the context of what is already known. Analysis and reflection entail the contemplation of the new findings during each cycle of the loop. **Member checking** is the sharing of the investigator's emerging thoughts and beliefs with the participants themselves. Reorganization results in a revised agenda for data collection in the next cycle of the loop.

   Although each cycle within the iterative loop is depicted as linear, this representation is misleading. Net progress through the loop is clockwise, as shown in Fig. 11.3, but backward steps are natural and inevitable. They are

not reflective of mistakes or errors. An investigator may, after conducting a series of interviews and studying what participants have said, decide to speak again with one or two participants to clarify their positions on a particular issue.

4. *Communicate results*: Subjectivist students tend to have a multi-staged reporting and communication process. The first draft of the study report should itself be viewed as a research instrument. By sharing this report with a variety of individuals, the investigator obtains a major check on the validity of the findings. Typically, reactions to the preliminary report will generate useful clarifications and a general sharpening of the study findings. Because the report usually includes a prose narrative, it is vitally important that it be well written in language understandable by all intended audiences. Circulation of the report in draft can ensure that the final document communicates as intended. Use of anonymous quotations from interviews and documents makes a report highly vivid and meaningful to readers.

   The final report, once completed, should be distributed as negotiated in the original memorandum of understanding. Distribution is often accompanied by "meet the investigator" sessions that allow interested persons to ask the author of the report to expand or explain what has been written.

11.5.3.4 Subjectivist Data-Collection and Data-Analysis Methods

What data-collection strategies are in the subjectivist researcher's black bag? There are several, and they are typically used in combination. We shall discuss each one, assuming a typical setting for a subjectivist study in medical informatics, the introduction of an information resource into patient care activities in a hospital.

Observation

The investigators typically immerse themselves into the setting under study in one of two ways. The investigator may act purely as a detached observer, becoming a trusted and unobtrusive feature of the environment but not a participant in the day-to-day work and thus reliant on multiple "informants" as sources of information. True to the naturalistic feature of this kind of study, great care is taken to diminish the possibility that the presence of the observer will skew the work activities that occur or that the observer will be rejected outright by the team. An alternative approach is participant observation, where the investigator becomes a member of the work team. Participant observation is more difficult to engineer; it may require the investigator to have specialized training in the study domain. It is time consuming but can give the investigator a more vivid impression of life in the work environment. During both kinds of observation, data accrue continuously. These data are qualitative and may be of several varieties: statements by health care providers and patients, gestures and other nonverbal expressions of these same individuals, and characteristics of the physical setting that seem to affect the delivery of health care.

Interviews

Subjectivist studies rely heavily on interviews. Formal interviews are occasions where both the investigator and interviewee are aware that the answers to questions are being recorded (on paper or tape) for direct contribution to the evaluation study. Formal interviews vary in their degree of structure. At one extreme is the **unstructured interview**, where there are no predetermined questions. Between the extremes is the **semi structured interview**, where the investigator specifies in advance a set of topics that he would like to address but is flexible as to the order in which these topics are addressed, and is open to discussion of topics not on the prespecified list. At the other extreme is the **structured interview**, with a schedule of questions that are always presented in the same words and in the same order. In general, the unstructured and semi structured interviews are preferred in subjectivist research. Informal interviews—spontaneous discussions between the investigators and members of a team that occur during routine observation—are also part of the data collection process. Informal interviews are invariably considered a source of important data. Group interviews, akin to focus groups, may also be employed (e.g., Haddow et al. 2011). Group interviews are very efficient ways to reach large numbers of participants, but investigators should not assume that individual participants will express in a group setting the same sentiments they will express if interviewed one-on-one.

Sampling also enters into the interview process. There are usually more participants to interview than resources. Unlike in objectivist studies, where random sampling is a form of gold standard to inform statistical inference, subjectivist studies employ more purposeful strategies. Investigators might actively seek interviewees they suspect to have unique or particularly insightful opinions. They might remain in more frequent contact with key informants who, for various reasons, have the most insight into what is happening.

Document and Artifact Analysis

Every project produces a trail of papers and other artifacts. These include patient charts, the various versions of a computer program and its documentation, memoranda prepared by the project team, perhaps a cartoon hung on the office door by a ward clerk. Unlike the day-to-day events of patient care, these artifacts do not change once created or introduced. They can be examined retrospectively and referred to repeatedly, as necessary, over the course of a study. Also included under this heading are **unobtrusive measures**, which are the records accrued as part of the routine use of the information resource. They include, for example, user trace files of an information resource. Data from these measures are often quantifiable.

Anything Else That Seems Useful

Subjectivist investigators are supreme opportunists. As questions of importance to a study emerge, the investigators will collect any information that they perceive as bearing on these questions. This data collection could include clinical chart reviews, questionnaires, tests, simulated patients, and other methods more commonly associated with the objectivist approaches.

When to end data collection is another challenge in otherwise open-ended subjectivist studies. "Saturation" is important principle to help investigators know when to stop. Stated simply, a data collection process is saturated when it becomes evident that, as more data are collected, no new findings or insights are emerging.

Analysis of Subjectivist Data

There are many alternative procedures for analysis of qualitative data. The important point is that the analysis is conducted systematically. In general terms, the investigator looks for insights, themes or trends emerging from several different sources. She collates individual statements and observations by theme, as well as by source. Some investigators transfer these observations to file cards so they can be sorted and resorted in a variety of ways. Others use software especially designed to facilitate analysis of qualitative data (Fielding and Lee 1991). Because they allow electronic recording of the data while the investigator is "in the field", tablets, smartphone Apps and other hand-held devices are changing the way subjectivist research is carried out.

The subjectivist analysis process is fluid, with analytic goals shifting as the study matures. At an early stage, the goal is primarily to focus the questions that themselves will be the targets of further data elicitation. At the later stages of study, the primary goal is to collate data that address these questions. Conclusions derive credibility from a process of "triangulation", which is the degree to which information from different independent sources generate the same theme or point to the same conclusion. Subjectivist analysis also employs a strategy known as "member checking" whereby investigators take preliminary conclusions back to the persons in the setting under study, asking if these conclusions make sense, and if not, why not. In subjectivist investigation, unlike objectivist studies, the agenda is never completely closed. The investigator is constantly on the alert for new information that can require a significant reorganization of the findings and conclusions that have been drawn to date.

11.6 Communicating Evaluation Results

Once a study is complete, the results need to be communicated to the stakeholders and others who might be interested. In many ways, communication of evaluation results, a term we prefer over "reporting", is the most challenging aspect of evaluation. Elementary theory tells us that, in general, successful communication requires a sender, one or more recipients, and a channel linking them, along with a message that travels along this channel (Ong and Coiera 2011).

Seen from this perspective, successful communication of evaluation results is challenging in several respects. It requires that the recipient of the message actually receive it. That is, for evaluations, the recipient must read the written report or attend the meeting intended to convey evaluation results, and the investigator is challenged to create a report the stakeholders will want to read or to choreograph a meeting they will be motivated to attend. Successful communication also requires that the recipient understand the message, which challenges investigators to draft written documents at the right reading level, with audience-appropriate technical detail. Sometimes there must be several different forms of the written report to match several different audiences. Overall, we encourage investigators to recognize that their obligation to communicate does not end with the submission of a written document comprising their technical evaluation report. The report is one means or channel for communication, not an end in itself.

Depending on the nature, number, and location of the recipients, there are a large number of options for communicating the results of a study, including:
- Written reports
  - Document(s) prepared for specific audience(s)
  - Internal newsletter article
  - Published journal article, with appropriate permissions
  - Monograph, picture album, or book

- One-to-one or small group meetings
  - With stakeholders or specific stakeholder groups
  - With general public, if appropriate
- Formal oral presentations
  - To groups of project stakeholders
  - Conference presentation with poster or published paper in proceedings
  - To external meetings or seminars
- Internet
  - Project Web site or blog
  - Web "chat", forum or Twitter feed to socialize results
  - Online preprint
  - Internet based journal
- Other
  - Video or podcast describing study and information resource
  - Interview with journalist on newspaper, TV, radio

A written, textual report is not the sole medium for communicating evaluation results. Verbal, graphical, or multimedia approaches can be helpful as ways to enhance communication with specific audiences. Another useful strategy is to hold a "town meeting" to discuss a traditional written report after it has been released. Photographs or videos can portray the work setting for a study, the people in the setting, and the people using the resource. If appropriate permissions are obtained, these images—whether included as part of a written report, shown at a town meeting, or placed on a Web site—can be worth many thousands of words. The same may be true for recorded statements of resource users. If made available, with permission, as part of a multimedia report, the voices of the participants can convey a feeling behind the words that can enhance the credibility of the investigator's conclusions (Fig. 11.4).

In addition to the varying formats for communication described above, investigators have other decisions to make after the data collection and analysis phases of a study are complete. One key decision is what personal role they will adopt after the formal investigative aspects of the work are complete. They may elect only to communicate the results, but they may also choose to persuade stakeholders to take specific actions in

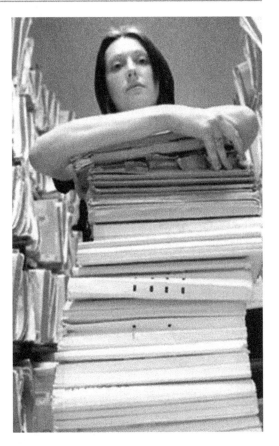

Fig. 11.4 A picture is worth 1000 words: in the report of a study to establish the need for an electronic patient record, a casual photograph like this may prove much more persuasive than a table of data or paragraphs of prose

response to the study results, and perhaps even assist in the implementation of these actions. This raises a key question: Is the role of an evaluator simply to record and communicate study findings and then to move on to the next study, or is it to engage with the study stakeholders and help them change how they work as a result of the study?

To answer this question about the role of an evaluator, we need to understand that an evaluation study, particularly a successful one, has the potential to trigger a series of events, starting with the analysis of study results through communication to interpretation, recommendation, and even implementation. Some evaluators— perhaps enthused by the clarity of their results and an opportunity to use them to improve health care, biomedical research, or education—prefer to go beyond reporting the results and conclusions to making recommendations, and then helping the stakeholders to implement them. The dilemma often faced by evaluators is whether to retain their scientific detachment and merely report the study results, or to stay engaged somewhat longer. Evaluators who choose to remain may become engaged in helping the stakeholders interpret what the results mean, guiding them in reaching decisions and perhaps even in implementing the actions decided upon. The longer they stay, the greater the extent to which evaluators must leave behind their scientific detachment and take on a role more commonly associated with change agents. Some confounding of these roles is inevitable when the evaluation is performed by individuals within the organization that developed the information resource under study. There is no hard-and-fast rule for deciding on the most appropriate role for the evaluator; the most important realization for investigators is that the different options exist and that a decision among them must inevitably be made.

11.7 Conclusion: Evaluation as an Ethical and Scientific Imperative

Evaluation takes place, either formally or informally, throughout the resource development cycle: from defining the need to monitoring the continuing impact of a resource once it is deployed (Stead et al. 1994). We have seen in this chapter that different issues are explored, at different degrees of intensity, at each stage of resource development. For meaningful evaluation to occur, adequate resources must be allocated for studies when time and money are budgeted for a development effort. Evaluation cannot be left to the end of a project. While formal evaluations, as we have described them here, are still seen as optional for resources of the types that are the foci of biomedical and health informatics, the increasing complexity and prevalence of these resources have raised concerns about

their safety and effectiveness when used in the real world (e.g., Koppel et al. 2005). For the moment, we would argue that formal evaluations, using the range of methods described in this chapter, are mandated by the professional ethics of biomedical informatics as an applied scientific discipline (see Chap. 10).

Formal evaluations of biomedical information resources may someday be a statutory or regulatory requirement in many or all parts of the world, as they are already for new drugs or medical devices. If and when that day comes, the wide variety of questions to be addressed and the diversity of legitimate methods available to address those questions, as described in this chapter, will make it difficult to describe with exactitude how these studies should be done. There have been some published academic checklists or guidelines describing things to study and report in such studies (Talmon et al. 2009), but this is a bridge to be crossed in the future. We express the hope that writers of such guidelines and regulations will not overprescribe the methods to be used, while insisting on rigor in drawing conclusions from data collected using study designs thoughtfully matched to carefully identified questions. We hope the reader has learned from this chapter that rigor in evaluation is achievable in many ways, that information resources differ from drugs in many ways, and that overly rigid prescription of evaluation methods for informatics, however well intentioned, could defeat the well-intentioned purpose. However, it is also clear that the intensity of the evaluation effort should be closely matched to the resource's maturity (Stead et al. 1994). For example, one would not wish to conduct an expensive field trial of an information resource that is barely complete, is still in prototype form, may evolve considerably before taking its final shape, or is so early in its development that it may fail because simple programming bugs have not been eliminated. Seen from this perspective, biomedical information resources are merely a subset of complex intervention, and their development and evaluation needs to follow a logical pathway, such as the MRC Framework for Complex Interventions (Campbell et al. 2000).

Suggested Readings

Anderson, J. G., & Aydin, C. E. (Eds.). (2005). *Evaluating the organizational impact of health care Information systems*. New York: Springer. This is an excellent edited volume that covers a wide range of methodological and substantive approaches to evaluation in informatics.

Brender, J. (2006). *Handbook for evaluation for health informatics*. Burlington: Elsevier Academic Press. Along with the Friedman and Wyatt text cited below, one of few textbooks available that focuses on evaluation in health informatics.

Cohen, P. R. (1995). *Empirical methods for artificial intelligence*. Cambridge, MA: MIT Press. This is a nicely written, detailed book that is focused on evaluation of artificial intelligence applications, not necessarily those operating in medical domains. It emphasizes objectivist methods and could serve as a basic statistics course for computer science students.

Fink, A. (2004). *Evaluation fundamentals: Insights into the outcomes, effectiveness, and quality of health programs* (2nd ed.). Thousand Oaks: Sage Publications. A popular text that discusses evaluation in the general domain of health.

Friedman, C. P., & Wyatt, J. C. (2006). *Evaluation methods in biomedical informatics*. New York: Springer. This is the book on which the current chapter is based. It offers expanded discussion of almost all issues and concepts raised in the current chapter.

Jain, R. (1991). *The art of computer systems performance analysis: Techniques for experimental design, measurement, simulation, and modelling*. New York: Wiley. This work offers a technical discussion of a range of objectivist methods used to study computer systems. The scope is broader than Cohen's book (1995) described earlier. It contains many case studies and examples and assumes knowledge of basic statistics.

Lincoln, Y. S., & Guba, E. G. (1985). *Naturalistic inquiry*. Thousand Oaks: Sage Publications. This is a classic book on subjectivist methods. The work is very rigorous but also very easy to read. Because it does not focus on medical domains or information systems, readers must make their own extrapolations.

Rossi, P. H., Lipsey, M. W., & Freeman, H. E. (2004). *Evaluation: A systematic approach* (7th ed.). Thousand Oaks: Sage Publications. This is a valuable textbook on evaluation, emphasizing objectivist methods, and is very well written. It is generic in scope, and the reader must relate the content to biomedical informatics. There are several excellent chapters addressing pragmatic issues of evaluation. These nicely complement the chapters on statistics and formal study designs.

Questions for Discussion

1. Associate each of the following hypothetical evaluation scenarios with one or more of the nine types of studies listed in Table 11.1. Note that some scenarios may include more than one type of study.

   (a) An order communication system is implemented in a small hospital. Changes in laboratory workload are assessed.

   (b) The developers of the order communication system recruit five potential users to help them assess how readily each of the main functions can be accessed from the opening screen and how long it takes users to complete them.

   (c) A study team performs a thorough analysis of the information required by psychiatrists to whom patients are referred by a community social worker.

   (d) A biomedical informatics expert is asked for her opinion about a PhD project on a new bioinformatics algorithm. She requests copies of the student's code and documentation for review.

   (e) A new intensive care unit system is implemented alongside manual paper charting for a month. At the end of this time, the quality of the computer-derived data and data recorded on the paper charts is compared. A panel of intensive care experts is asked to identify, independently, episodes of hypotension from each data set.

   (f) A biomedical informatics professor is invited to join the steering group for a series of apps to support people living with diabetes. The only documentation available to critique at the first meeting is a statement of the project goal, description of the planned development method, and the advertisements and job descriptions for team members.

(g) Developers invite educationalists to test a prototype of a computer-aided learning system as part of a user-centered design workshop

(h) A program is devised that generates a predicted 24-h blood glucose profile using seven clinical parameters. Another program uses this profile and other patient data to advise on insulin dosages. Diabetologists are asked to prescribe insulin for a series of "paper patients" given the 24-h profile alone, and then again after seeing the computer-generated advice. They are also asked their opinion of the advice.

(i) A program to generate alerts to prevent drug interactions is installed in a geriatric clinic that already has a computer-based medical record system. Rates of clinically significant drug interactions are compared before and after installation of the alerting program.

2. Choose any alternative area of biomedicine (e.g., drug trials) as a point of comparison, and list at least four factors that make studies in medical informatics more difficult to conduct successfully than in that area. Given these difficulties, discuss whether it is worthwhile to conduct empirical studies in medical informatics or whether we should use intuition or the marketplace as the primary indicators of the value of an information resource.

3. Assume that you run a philanthropic organization that supports biomedical informatics. In investing the scarce resources of your organization, you have to choose between funding a new system or resource development, or funding empirical studies of resources already developed. What would you choose? How would you justify your decision?

5. To what extent is it possible to be certain how effective a medical informatics resource really is? What are the most important criteria of effectiveness?

4. Do you believe that independent, unbiased observers of the same behavior or outcome should agree on the quality of that outcome?

5. Many of the evaluation approaches assert that a single unbiased observer is a legitimate source of information in an evaluation, even if that observer's data or judgments are unsubstantiated by other people. Give examples drawn from our society where we vest important decisions in a single experienced and presumed impartial individual.

6. Do you agree with the statement that all evaluations appear equivocal when subjected to serious scrutiny? Explain your answer.

Appendices

Appendix A: Two Evaluation Scenarios

Here we introduce two scenarios that collectively capture many of the dilemmas facing those planning and conducting evaluations in biomedical informatics:

1. A prototype information resource has been developed, but its usability and potential for benefit need to be assessed prior to deployment;

2. A commercial resource has been deployed across a large enterprise, and there is need to understand its impact on users as well as on the organization.

These scenarios do not address the full scope of evaluations in biomedical informatics, but they cover a lot of what people do. For each, we introduce sets of evaluation questions that frequently arise and examine the dilemmas that investigators face in the design and execution of evaluation studies.

Scenario 1: A Prototype Information Resource has Been Developed, but its Usability and Potential for Benefit Need to Be Assessed Prior to Deployment

The primary evaluation issue here is the upcoming decision to continue with the development of the prototype information resource. Validation of the design and structure of the resource will have been conducted, either formally or informally, but not yet a usability study. If this looks promising, a laboratory evaluation of key functions is also advised before making the substantial investment required to turn a promising prototype into a system that is stable and likely to bring more benefits than problems to users in the field. Here, typical questions will include:

- Who are the target users, and what are their background skills and knowledge?
- Does the resource make sense to target users?
- Following a brief introduction, can target users navigate themselves around important parts of the resource?
- Can target users carry out a selection of relevant tasks using the resource, in reasonable time and with reasonable accuracy?
- What user characteristics correlate with the ability to use the resource and achieve fast, accurate performance with it?
- What other kinds of people can use it safely?
- How to improve the layout, design, wording, menus etc.
- Is there a long learning curve? What user training needs are there?
- How much on-going help will users require once they are initially trained?
- What concerns do users have about the system – e.g., accuracy, privacy, effect on their jobs, other side effects
- Based on the performance of prototypes in users' hands, does the resource have the potential to meet user needs?

These questions fall within the scope of the usability and laboratory function testing approaches listed in Table 11.1. A wide range of techniques–borrowed from the human-computer interaction field and employing both objectivist and subjectivist approaches–can be used, including:

- Seeking the views of potential users after both a demonstration of the resource and a hands-on exploration. Methods such as focus groups may be very useful to identify not only immediate problems with the software and how it might be improved, but also potential broader concerns and unexpected issues that may include user privacy and long term issues around user training and working relationships.
- Studying users while they carry out a list of pre-designed tasks using the information resource. Methods for studying users includes watching over their shoulder, video observation (sometimes with several video cameras per user); think aloud protocols (asking the user to verbalize their impressions as they navigate and use the system); and automatic logging of keystrokes, navigation paths, and time to complete tasks.
- Use of validated questionnaires to capture user impressions, often before and after an experience with the system, one example being the Telemedicine Preparedness questionnaire (Demiris et al. 2000).
- Specific techniques to explore how users might improve the layout or design of the software. For example, to help understand what users think of as a "logical" menu structure for an information resource, investigators can use a card sorting technique. This entails listing each function available on all the menus on a separate card and then asking users to sort these cards into several piles according to which function seems to go with which [www.useit.com].

Depending on the aim of a usability study, it may suffice to employ a small number of potential users. Nielsen has shown that, if the aim is to identify only major software faults, the proportion identified rises quickly up to about 5 or 6 users then much more slowly to plateau at about 15–20 users (Nielsen 1994). Five users will often identify 80 % of software problems. However, investigators conducting such small studies, useful though they may be for software development, cannot then expect to publish them in a scientific journal. The achievement in this case is having found answers to a very specific question about a specific software prototype. This kind of local reality test is unlikely to appeal to the editors or readers of a journal. By contrast, the results of formal laboratory function studies, that typically employ more users, are more amenable to journal publication.

Scenario 2: A Commercial Resource Has Been Deployed Across a Large Enterprise, and There Is Need to Understand its Impact on Users as Well as on the Organization

The type of evaluation questions that arise here include:

- In what fraction of occasions when the resource could have been used, was it actually used?
- Who uses it, why, are these the intended users, and are they satisfied with it?
- Does using the resource improve influence information/communication flows?
- Does using the resource influence their knowledge or skills?
- Does using the resource improve their work?
- For clinical information resources, does using the resource change outcomes for patients?
- How does the resource influence the whole organization and relevant sub units?
- Do the overall benefits and costs or risks differ for specific groups of users, departments, the whole organization?
- How much does the resource really cost the organization?
- Should the organization keep the resource as it is, improve it or replace it?
- How can the resource be improved, at what cost, and what benefits would result?

To each of the above questions, one can add: "Why, or why not ?", to get a broader understanding of what is happening as a result of use of the resource.

This evaluation scenario, suggesting a problem impact study, is often what people think of first when the concept of evaluation is introduced. However, we have seen in this chapter that it is one of many evaluation scenarios, arising relatively late in the life cycle of an information resource. When these impact-oriented evaluations are undertaken, they usually result from a realization by stakeholders, who have invested significantly in an information resource, that the benefits of the resource are uncertain and there is need to justify recurring costs. These stakeholders usually vary in the kind of evaluation methods that will convince them about the impacts that the resource is or is not having. Many such stakeholders will wish to see quantified indices of benefits or harms from the resource, for example the number of users and daily uses, the amount the resource improves productivity or reduces costs, or perhaps other benefits such as reduced waiting times to perform key tasks or procedures, lengths of hospital stay or occurrence of adverse events. Such data are collected through objectivist studies as discussed earlier. Other stakeholders may prefer to see evidence of perceived benefit and positive views of staff, in which case staff surveys, focus groups and unstructured interviews may prove the best evaluation methods. Often, a combination of many methods is necessary to extend the investigation from understanding what impact the resource has to why this impact occurs – or fails to occur.

If the investigator is pursuing objectivist methods, deciding which of the possible effect variables to include in an impact study and developing ways to measure them can be the most challenging aspect of an evaluation study design. (These and related issues receive the attention of five full chapters of a textbook by the authors of this chapter (Friedman and Wyatt 2005).) Investigators usually wish to limit the number of effect measures employed in a study for many reasons: limited evaluation resources, to minimize manipulation of the practice environment, and to avoid statistical analytical problems that result from a large number of measures.

Effect or impact studies can also use subjectivist approaches to allow the most relevant "effect" issues to emerge over time and with increasingly deep immersion into the study environment. This emergent feature of subjectivist work obviates the need to decide in advance which effect variables to explore, and is considered by proponents of subjectivist approaches to be among their major advantages.

In health care particularly, every intervention carries some risk, which must be judged in comparison to the risks of doing nothing or of providing an alternative intervention. It is difficult to decide whether an information resource is an improvement unless the performance of the current decision-takers is also measured in a comparison-based evaluation. For example, if physicians' decisions are to become more accurate following introduction of a decision-support tool, the resource needs to be "right" when the user would usually be "wrong" This could mean that the tool's error rate is lower than that of the physician, or its errors are in different cases, or they should be of a different kind or less serious than those of the clinician, so as not to introduce new errors caused by the clinician following resource advice even when that advice is incorrect – "automation bias" (Goddard et al. 2012).

For effect studies, it is often important to know something about how the practitioners carry out their work prior to the introduction of the information resource. Suitable measures include the accuracy, timing, and confidence level of their decisions and the amount of information they require before making a decision. Although data for such a study can sometimes be collected by using abstracts of cases or problems in a laboratory setting (Fig. 11.2), these studies inevitably raise questions of generalization to the real world. We observe here one of many trade-offs that occur in the design of evaluation studies. Although control over the mix of cases possible in a laboratory study can lead to a more precise estimate of practitioner decision making, ultimately it may prove better to conduct a baseline study while the individuals are doing real work in a real practice setting. Often this audit of current decisions and actions provides useful input to the design of the information resource, and a reference against which resource performance may later be compared.

When conducting problem impact studies in health care settings, investigators can sometimes save themselves much time and effort without sacrificing validity by measuring effect in terms of certain health care processes, rather than patient outcomes (Mant and Hicks 1995). For example, measuring the mortality or complication rate in patients with heart attacks requires data collection from hundreds of patients, as complications and death are (fortunately) rare events. However, as long as large, rigorous trials or meta-analyses have determined that a certain procedure (e.g., giving heart attack patients streptokinase within 24 h) correlates closely with the desired patient outcome, it is perfectly valid to measure the rate of performing this procedure as a valid "surrogate" for the desired outcome. Mant and Hicks demonstrated that measuring the quality of care by quantifying a key process in this way may require one tenth as many patients as measuring outcomes (Mant and Hicks 1995).

Appendix B: Other Views of Evaluation that Bear on Informatics

The field of evaluation continues to evolve. We describe briefly below two perspectives on evaluation that reflect the goals of making evaluation relevant and useful. Biomedical informatics has inherited from the culture of biomedical research a default vision of evaluation that reflects the fully randomized clinical trial as the gold-standard for determining the truth expressed as cause and effect relationships, and which, in the parlance of this chapter, puts objectivist comparison-based studies on a pedestal. In the limited space of this chapter, while devoting the most space to objectivist studies, we have introduced the complementary subjectivist approaches. Overall, objectivist comparison-based studies are limited by the time and expense of conducting them. This can be particularly problematic in a field like informatics where the information resources themselves change very rapidly and yet, paradoxically, have to be "frozen" for the full duration of an objectivist study if the study is going to be internally valid. Readers interested in addressing this challenge are encouraged to read further about the two methods described below, and other emerging alternatives – if only to consider for themselves whether and how these approaches might apply their work, and perhaps dismiss them.

Realist Evaluation

"Realist" or "Realistic" evaluation is based on Pawson and Tilley's work (Pawson and Tilley 1997) and has started to influence the design and interpretation of a handful of studies in biomedical informatics. This approach is based on a subset of the philosophical school of realism called scientific realism, which asserts that both material and social worlds are 'real', in the sense that they can have real effects. The aims of realist evaluation are thus to work towards a better understanding of material and social elements which can cause change, to acknowledge that change can occur in both material and social dimensions, and that both are important. Some of the insights made by Pawson and Tilley which underlie the realist approach to evaluation include:

- Many interventions are an attempt to address a social problem – that is, to create some level of social change.
- Many interventions, such as information resources, work by enabling participants to make different choices, although these choices are usually constrained by participants' previous experiences, beliefs and attitudes, opportunities and access to resources.
- Making and sustaining different choices requires a change in participant's reasoning (for example, values, beliefs, attitudes, or the logic they apply to a particular situation) and/or the resources (e.g. information, skills, material resources, support) they have available to them. This combination of "reasoning and resources" is what causes the impact of the intervention and is known in realist evaluation as the intervention "mechanism".

- Interventions work in different ways for different people, i.e. Interventions can trigger different change mechanisms in different participants.
- The contexts in which interventions are delivered often makes a difference to the outcomes they achieve. Relevant contexts may include social, economic and political structures, organizational context, participants, staffing, geographical and historical context, and so on.
- Some factors in the context may enable particular mechanisms to be triggered, while other factors may prevent this. There is always an interaction between context and mechanism, and that interaction is what creates the intervention's impacts or outcomes: Context + Mechanism = Outcome.
- Because interventions work differently in different contexts and through different change mechanisms, they cannot simply be replicated from one context to another and automatically achieve the same outcomes. Good understanding about "what works for whom, in what contexts, and how" is, however, portable.
- Therefore, one of the tasks of evaluation is to learn more about "what works for whom", "in which contexts particular interventions do and don't work", and "what mechanisms are triggered by what interventions in what contexts".

It is important to note that Realist Evaluation is derived from – and is largely applied to – social and educational programs, where the context (rather than the intervention) is likely to be a much more important determinant of the outcome. We believe that this rarely applies in the study of biomedical informatics and information resources. In addition, the message of realist evaluation – that each study's results can only be applied in the context in which they were derived – will seem rather pessimistic, even deconstructivist, to most scientists. This is because the aim of science is to progressively develop better grounded theories that we can confidently use to predict the impact of interventions in a wide range of – though not necessarily all – contexts. Arguably, if Pawson and Tilley's realist approach applied throughout biomedical informatics, we could not confidently generalize about the impact of any intervention from the results of any evaluation studies. This in turn would make biomedical informatics a discipline in which progress based on the work and findings of others was difficult, if not impossible. This is manifestly untrue – as this book amply demonstrates. However, there may be some biomedical informatics settings in which the context is more important – and more variable – than the intervention, so Realist evaluation methods would then be more appropriate.

Utilization Focused Evaluation

Based on pragmatism rather than theory, Utilization-Focused Evaluation begins with the assumption that evaluations should be judged by their utility and the actual use and impact of the results (Patton 1999). The implication is that evaluators should facilitate the evaluation process and design any evaluation with careful consideration of how everything that is done, *from beginning to end*, will affect the use of the results. Use concerns how real people in the real world apply evaluation findings and experience the evaluation process. Therefore, the *focus* in utilization-focused evaluation is on intended use by intended users.

Since no evaluation study is entirely value-free, utilization-focused evaluation addresses the question, "*Whose values should frame the evaluation ?*" by working with clearly identified, primary intended users, who in turn have the responsibility to apply the evaluation findings and implement the recommendations. Any study based on the principles of utilization-focused evaluation is thus highly personal and situational. The evaluation facilitator develops a working relationship with intended users of the results to help them determine what kind of evaluation they need. This requires negotiation with the evaluator offering a menu of possibilities within the framework of established evaluation methods, approaches and principles.

As a result, utilization-focused evaluation does not advocate any particular evaluation content, model, method, theory, or even use. Instead, it is a process for helping primary intended users select the most appropriate model, methods, theory, and uses for their particular situation. The need to respond to the situation guides the interaction between the evaluator and primary intended users. A utilization-focused evaluation can therefore include any evaluative purpose (e.g. formative, summative, developmental), any kind of data (e.g. quantitative, qualitative, mixed), any kind of design (e.g., naturalistic, experimental), and any kind of focus (e.g. processes, outcomes, impacts, costs, and cost-benefit). Utilization-focused evaluation is a process for helping evaluators to make decisions about these issues in collaboration with an identified group of primary users of the study results, focusing on the intended uses of the evaluation. Collaborative evaluation is a further development of this approach (Rodriguez-Campos 2012).

Part II

Biomedical Informatics Applications

Electronic Health Record Systems

12

Clement J. McDonald, Paul C. Tang, and George Hripcsak

After reading this chapter, you should know the answers to these questions:

- What is the definition of an electronic health record (EHR)?
- How does an EHR differ from the paper record?
- What are the functional components of an EHR?
- What are the benefits of an EHR?
- What are the impediments to development and use of an EHR?

12.1 What Is an Electronic Health Record?

The preceding chapters introduced the conceptual basis for the field of biomedical informatics, including the use of patient data in clinical practice and research. We now focus attention on the

C.J. McDonald, MD (✉)
Office of the Director, Lister Hill National Center for Biomedical Communications, National Library of Medicine, National Institutes of Health,
8600 Rockville Pike 38a 7n707,
Bethesda 20894, MD, USA
e-mail: clemmcdonald@mail.nih.gov

P.C. Tang, MD, MS
Internal Medicine, Palo Alto Medical Foundation,
2350 W. El Camino Real, Mountain View 94040,
CA, USA
e-mail: paultang@stanford.edu

G. Hripcsak, MD, MS
Department of Biomedical Informatics, Columbia University Medical Center, 622 W 168th St, VC5,
New York 10032, NY, USA
e-mail: hripcsak@columbia.edu

patient record, commonly referred to as the patient's chart, medical record, or health record. In this chapter, we examine the definition and use of electronic health record (EHR) systems, discuss their potential benefits and costs, and describe the remaining challenges to address in their dissemination.

12.1.1 Purpose of a Patient Record

Stanley Reiser (1991) wrote that the purpose of a patient record is "to recall observations, to inform others, to instruct students, to gain knowledge, to monitor performance, and to justify interventions." The many uses described in this statement, although diverse, have a single goal—to further the application of health sciences in ways that improve the well-being of patients, including the conduct of research and public health activities that address population health. A modern electronic health record (EHR) is designed to facilitate these uses, providing much more than a static view of events.

An **electronic health record** (**EHR**) is a repository of electronically maintained information about an individual's health status and health care, stored such that it can serve the multiple legitimate uses and users of the record. Traditionally, the patient record was a record of care provided when a patient was ill. Health care is evolving to encourage health care providers to focus on the continuum of health and health care from wellness to illness and recovery.

E.H. Shortliffe, J.J. Cimino (eds.), *Biomedical Informatics*,
DOI 10.1007/978-1-4471-4474-8_12, © Springer-Verlag London 2014

Consequently, we anticipate that eventually it will carry all of a person's health related information from all sources over their lifetime. The Department of Veterans Affairs (VA) has already committed to keeping existing patient electronic data for 75 years. In addition, the data should be stored such that different views of those data can be presented to serve the many different uses described in Chap. 2.

The term **electronic health record system** (also referred to as a computer-based patient-record system) includes the active tools that are used to manage the information, but in common use, the term EHR can refer to the entire system. EHRs include information management tools to provide clinical reminders and alerts, linkages with knowledge sources for health care decision support, and analysis of aggregate data both for care management and for research. The EHR helps the reader to organize, interpret, and react to data. Examples of tools provided in current EHRs are discussed in Sect. 12.3.

12.1.2   Ways in Which an Electronic Health Record Differs from a Paper-Based Record

Compared to the historical paper medical record, whose functionality is constrained by its recording media, and the fact that only one physical copy of it exists—the EHR is flexible and adaptable (see also Sect. 2.3 in Chap. 2). Data may be entered in one format to simplify the input process and then displayed in many different formats according to the user's needs. The entry and display of dates is illustrative. Most EHRs can accept many date formats, i.e. May 1, 1992, 1 May 92, or 1/5/92, as input; store that information in one internal format, such as 1992-05-01; and display it in different formats according to local customs. The EHR can incorporate multimedia information, such as radiology images and echocardiographic video loops, which were never part of the traditional medical record. It can also analyze a patient's record, call attention to trends and dangerous conditions and suggest corrective actions much like an airplane flight control computer. EHRs can organize data about one patient to facil-

itate his or her care or about a population of patients to assist management decisions or answer epidemiologic questions. When considering the functions of an EHR, one must think beyond the constraints of paper records. An EHR system can capture, organize, analyze, and display patient data in many ways.

Inaccessibility is a problem with paper records. They can only be in one place and with at most one user at one point in time. In large organizations, medical record departments often would sequester the paper medical record for days after the patient's hospital discharge while the clinician completed the discharge summary and signed every form. Individual physicians may borrow records for their own administrative or research purposes, during which times the record will also be unavailable. In contrast, many users, including patients, can read the same electronic record at once. So it is never unavailable. With today's secure networks, clinicians and patients can access a patient's EHR from geographically distributed sites, such as the emergency room, their office, or their home. Such availability can also support health care continuity during disasters. Brown et al. (2007) found a "stark contrast" between the care VA versus non-VA patients obtained after Hurricane Katrina, because "VA efforts to maintain appropriate and uninterrupted care were supported by nationwide access to comprehensive electronic health record systems." While EHR systems make data more accessible to authorized users, they also provide greater control over access and enforce applicable privacy policies as required by the Health Insurance Portability and Accountability Act (HIPAA) (see Chaps. 10 and 27).

The EHR's content is more legible and better organized than the paper alternative and the computer can increase the quality of data by applying validity checks as data is being entered. The computer can reduce typographical errors through restricted input menus and spell checking. It can require data entry in specified fields, conditional on the value of other fields. For example, if the user answers yes to current smoker, the computer, guided by rules, could then ask how many packs per day smoked or how soon after awakening does the patient take their first smoke? So the

EHR not only stores data but can also conditionally enforce the capture of certain data elements. This enforcement power should be used sparingly, however. As part of the ordering process, the computer can *require* the entry of data that may not be available (e.g., the height of a patient with leg contractures), and thus prevent the clinician from completing an important order (Strom et al. 2010); and overzealous administrators can ask clinicians to answer questions that are peripheral to clinical care and slow the care process.

The degree to which a particular EHR achieves benefits depends on several factors:

Comprehensiveness of information. Does the EHR contain information about health as well as illness? Does it include information from all organizations and clinicians who participated in a patient's care? Does it cover all settings in which care was delivered (e.g., office practice, hospital)? Does it include the full spectrum of clinical data, including clinicians' notes, laboratory test results, medication details, and so on?

Duration of use and retention of data. EHRs gain value over time because they accumulate a greater proportion of the patients' medical history. A record that has accumulated patient data over 5 years will be more valuable than one that contains only the last month's records.

Degree of structure of data. Narrative notes stored in electronic health records have the advantage over their paper counterparts in that they can be searched by word, although the success of such searches is subject to the wide variations in the author's choice of medical words and abbreviations. Computer-supported decision making, clinical research, and management analysis of EHR data require structured data. One way to obtain such data is to ask the clinical user to enter information through structured forms whose fields provide dropdown menus or restrict data entry to a controlled vocabulary (see Chap. 7).

Ubiquity of access. A system that is accessible from a few sites will be less valuable than one accessible by an authorized user from anywhere (see Chap. 5).

An EHR system has some disadvantages. It requires a larger initial investment than its paper counterpart due to hardware, software, training, and support costs. Physicians and other key personnel have to take time from their work to learn how to use the system and to redesign their workflow to use the system. Although it takes time to learn how to use the system and to change workflows, clinicians increasingly recognize that EHR systems are important tools to assist in the clinical, regulatory, and business of practicing medicine.

Computer-based systems have the potential for catastrophic failures that could cause extended unavailability of patients' computer records. However, these risks can be mitigated by using fully redundant components, mirrored servers, and battery backup. Even better is to have a parallel site located remotely with **hot fail over**, which means that a failure at the primary site would not be noticed because the remote site could support users with, at most, a momentary pause. Yet, nothing provides complete protection; contingency plans must be developed for handling brief or longer computer outages. Moreover, paper records are also subject to irretrievable loss, caused by, for example, human error (e.g. misfiling), floods, or fires.

12.2 Historical Perspective

The development of automated systems was initially stimulated by regulatory and reimbursement requirements. Early health care systems focused on inpatient charge capture to meet billing requirements in a fee-for-service environment.

The Flexner report on medical education was the first formal statement made about the function and contents of the medical record (Flexner 1910). In advocating a scientific approach to medical education, the Flexner report also encouraged physicians to keep a patient-oriented medical record. Three years earlier, Dr. Henry Plummer initiated the "unit record" for the Mayo Clinic (including its St. Mary's Hospital), placing all the patient's visits and types of information in a single folder. This innovation represented the first longitudinal medical record (Melton 1996). The Presbyterian Hospital (New York) adopted the unit record for its inpatient and outpatient care in 1916, studying the effect of the unit record on length of stay and quality of care (Openchowski

1925) and writing a series of letters and books about the unit record that disseminated the approach around the nation (Lamb 1955).

The first record we could find of a computer-based medical record was a short newspaper article describing a new "electronic brain" – to replace punched and file index cards and to track hospital and medical records (Brain 1956). Early development of hospital information systems (HIS)—that used terminals rather than punched cards for data entry—emerged around 1970 at varying degrees of maturity (Lindberg 1967; Davis et al. 1968; Warner 1972; Barnett et al. 1979). Weed's problem-oriented medical record (POMR) (1968) shaped medical thinking about both manual and automated medical records. His computer-based version of the POMR employed touch screen terminals, a new programming language and networking—all radical ideas for the time (Schultz et al. 1971). In 1971, Lockheed's hospital information system (HIS) became operational at El Camino Hospital in Mountain View, CA. Technicon, Inc. then propagated it to more than 200 hospitals (see also Chap. 14) (Coffey 1979).

Hospital-based systems provided feedback (decision support) to physicians, which affected clinical decisions and ultimately patient outcomes. The HELP system (Pryor 1988) at LDS Hospital, the Columbia University system (Johnson et al. 1991), the CCC system at Beth Israel Deaconess Medical Center (Slack and Bleich 1999), the Regenstrief System (Tierney et al. 1993; McDonald et al. 1999) at Wishard Memorial Hospital, and others (Giuse and Mickish 1996; Halamka and Safran 1998; Hripcsak et al. 1999; Teich et al. 1999; Cheung et al. 2001; Duncan et al. 2001; Brown et al. 2003) are long-standing systems that add clinical functionality to support clinical care, and set the stage for future systems.

The ambulatory care medical record systems emerged around the same time as inpatient systems but were slower to attract commercial interest than hospital information systems. COSTAR (Barnett et al. 1978; Barnett 1984), the Regenstrief Medical Record System (RMRS) (McDonald et al. 1975), STOR (Whiting-O'Keefe et al. 1985), and TMR (Stead and Hammond 1988) are

among the examples. Costar and RMRS are still in use today. The status of ambulatory care records was reviewed in a 1982 report (Kuhn et al. 1984). There are now hundreds of vendors who offer ambulatory care EHRs, and a number of communities have begun to adopt EHRs on a broad scale for ambulatory care (Goroll et al. 2009; Menachemi et al. 2011). Morris Collen, who also pioneered the multiphasic screening system (1969), wrote a readable 500-page history of medical informatics (1995) that provides rich details about these early medical records systems, as does a three decade summary of computer-based medical record research projects from the U.S. Agency for Health Care Policy and Research (AHCPR, now called the Agency for Health Care Research and Quality (AHRQ)) (Fitzmaurice et al. 2002).

12.3 Functional Components of an Electronic Health Record System

As we explained in Sect. 12.1.2, an EHR is not simply an electronic version of the paper record. A medical record that is part of a comprehensive EHR system has linkages and tools to facilitate communication and decision making. In Sects. 12.3.1, 12.3.2, 12.3.3, 12.3.4, and 12.3.5, we summarize the components of a comprehensive EHR system and illustrate functionality with examples from systems currently in use. The five functional components are:

1. Integrated view of patient data
2. Clinician order entry
3. Clinical decision support
4. Access to knowledge resources
5. Integrated communication and reporting support

12.3.1 Integrated View of Patient Data

Providing an integrated view of all relevant patient data is an overarching goal of an EHR. However, capturing *everything* of interest is not

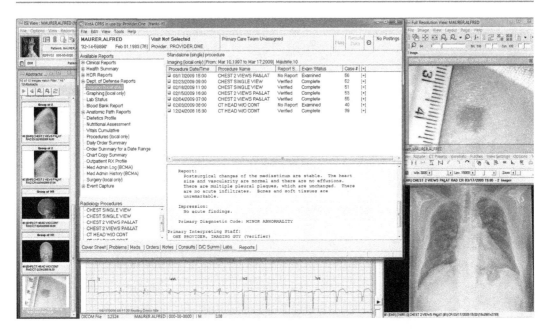

Fig. 12.1 A screenshot of the combined WorldVistA Computer Based Patient Record System (CPRS) and ISI Imaging system. These systems are derived from the Department of Veterans Affairs VistA and VistA Imaging systems (http://www.va.gov/vista_monograph/). The image illustrates the opportunity to present clinical images as well as laboratory test results, medications, notes and other relevant clinical information in a single longitudinal medical record (Source: Courtesy of WorldVistA (world-vista.org) and ISI Group (www.isigp.com), 2012)

yet possible because: (1) Some patient data do not exist in electronic form anywhere, for example, the hand-written data in old charts. (2) Much of the clinical data that do exist in electronic form are sequestered in isolated external computer systems, for example, office practices, free-standing radiology centers, home-health agencies, and nursing homes that do not yet have operational links to a given EHR or each other. (3) Even when electronic and organizational links exist, a fully integrated view of the data may be thwarted by the difference in conceptualization of data among systems from different vendors, and among different installations of one vendor's system in different institutions.

An integrated EHR must accommodate a broad spectrum of data types ranging from text to numbers and from tracings to images and video. More complex data types such as radiology images are usually delivered for human viewing—standards like DICOM[1] exist for displaying most of these complex data types, and JPEG[2] display of images is universally available for any kind of image (see also Chaps. 7 and 9). Figure 12.1 shows the VistA CPRS electronic health record system, which integrates a variety of text data and images into a patient report data screen including: demographics, a detailed list of the patient's procedures, a DICOM chest x-ray image, and JPG photo of a skin lesion. Other tabs in the system provide links to: problems, medications, orders, notes, consults, discharge summary, and labs. An important challenge to the construction of an integrated view is the lack of a national patient identifier in the United States. Because each organization assigns its own medical record number, a receiving organization cannot directly file a patient's data that is only identified by a medical record number from an external care organization. Linking schemes based on name, birth date and other patient characteristics must be implemented and monitored (Zhu et al. 2009).

---

[1] Digital Imaging and Communications in Medicine, http://dicom.nema.org/ (Accessed 1/2/2013).

[2] JPEG from Wikipedia, the free encyclopedia, http://en.wikipedia.org/wiki/JPEG (Accessed 1/2/2013).

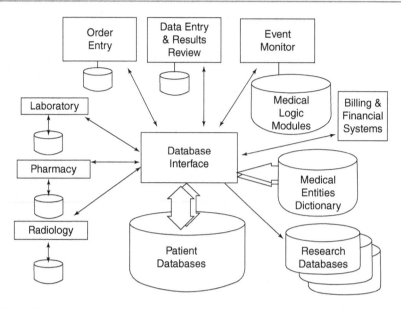

Fig. 12.2 A block diagram of multiple-source-data systems that contribute patient data, which ultimately reside in a computerized patient record (CPR). The database interface, commonly called an interface engine, may perform a number of functions. It may simply be a router of information to the central database. Alternatively, it may provide more intelligent filtering, translating, and alerting functions, as it does at Columbia University Medical Center (Source: Courtesy of Columbia University Medical Center, New York)

The idiosyncratic, local terminologies used to identify clinical variables and their values in many source systems present major barriers to integration of health record data within EHRs. However, those barriers will shrink as institutions adopt code standards (Chap. 7) such as LOINC[3] for observations, questions, variables, and assessments (McDonald et al. 2003; Vreeman et al. 2010); SNOMED CT[4] (Wang et al. 2002) for diagnoses, symptoms, findings, organisms and answers; UCUM[5] for computable units of measure; and RxNorm[6] and RxTerms[7] for clinical drug names, ingredients, and orderable drug names. Federal regulations from CMS and ONC for **Meaningful Use** 2 (MU2) encourage or require the use of LOINC, RxNorm and SNOMED CT for various purposes. (Final Rule: CMS 2012; Final Rule: ONC 2012) (see also Chaps. 7 and 27). Now most laboratory instrument vendors specify what LOINC codes to use for each test result generated by their instruments.

Today, most clinical data sources and EHRs can send and receive clinical content as version 2.x **Health Level 7** (**HL7**)[8] messages. Larger organizations use interface engines to send, receive, and, when necessary, translate the format of, and the codes within, such messages (see Chap. 7); Fig. 12.2 shows an example of architecture to integrate data from multiple source systems. The Columbia University Medical Center computerized patient record (CPR) interface depicted in this diagram not only provides message-handling capability but can also automatically translate codes from the external source to the preferred codes of the receiving EHR. And although many vendors now offer single systems that serve "all" needs, they never escape the need

---

[3] Logical Observation Identifiers Names and Codes (LOINC®). http://loinc.org/ (Accessed 1/2/2013).

[4] SNOMED Clinical Terms® (SNOMED CT®). http://www.ihtsdo.org/snomed-ct/ (Accessed 1/2/2013).

[5] The Unified Code for Units of Measure. http://unitsofmeasure.org/ (Accessed 1/2/2013).

[6] RxNorm Overview. http://www.nlm.nih.gov/research/umls/rxnorm/overview.html (Accessed 1/2/2013).

[7] RxTerms. https://wwwcf.nlm.nih.gov/umslicense/rxtermApp/rxTerm.cfm (Accessed 1/2/2013).

[8] Health Level Seven International, http://www.hl7.org/ (Accessed 1/2/2013).

for HL7 interfaces to capture data from some systems, e.g., EKG carts, cardiology systems, radiology imaging systems, anesthesia systems, off-site laboratories, community pharmacies and external collaborating health systems. At least one high-capability open-source interface engine, Mirth Connect,[9] is now available. One of us, (CM), used it happily, for example, in a project that links a local hospital's emergency room to Surescripts' medication history database.[10]

12.3.2 Clinician Order Entry

One of the most important components of an EHR is order entry, the point at which clinicians make decisions and take actions, and the computer can provide assistance. Electronic order entry can improve health care at several levels. An electronic order entry system can potentially reduce errors and costs compared to a paper system, in which orders are transcribed manually from one paper form (e.g., the paper chart) to another (e.g., the nurse's work list or a laboratory request form). Orders collected directly from the decision maker can be passed in a legible form to the intended recipient without the risk of transcription errors or the need for additional personnel. Order entry systems also provide opportunities to deliver decision support at the point where clinical decisions are being made. Most order entry systems pop up alerts about any interactions or allergies associated with a new drug order. But implementers should be selective about which alerts they present and which ones are interruptive, to avoid wasting provider time on trivial or low-likelihood outcomes (Phansalkar et al. 2012a, b). This capability is discussed in greater detail in the next section. Order entry systems can facilitate the entry of simple orders like "vital signs three times a day," or very complicated orders such as total parenteral nutrition (TPN) which requires specification of many additives, and

many calculations and checks to avoid physically impossible or dangerous mixtures and to assure that the prescribed goals for the number of calories and the amount of each additive are met. Figure 12.3 shows an example of a TPN order entry screen from Vanderbilt (Miller 2005b). Once a clinician order-entry system is adopted by the practice, simply changing the default drug or dosing based on the latest scientific evidence can shift the physician's ordering behavior toward the optimum standard of care, with benefits to quality and costs. Because of the many potential advantages for care quality and efficiency, care organizations are adopting computerized physician order entry (CPOE) (Khajouei and Jaspers 2010).

12.3.3 Clinical Decision Support

Clinical trials have shown that reminders from decision support improve the care process (Haynes 2011; Damiani et al. 2010; Schedlbauer et al. 2009). The EHR can deliver decision support in batch mode at intervals across a whole practice population in order to identify patients who are not reaching treatment targets, are past due for immunizations or cancer screening, or have missed their recent appointments, to cite a few examples. In this mode, the practice uses the batch list of patients generated by decision support to contact the patient and encourage him or her to reach a goal or to schedule an appointment for the delivery of suggested care. This is the only mode that can reach patients who repeatedly miss appointments.

Decision support—especially related to prevention—is most efficiently delivered when the patient comes to the care site for other reasons (e.g., a regularly scheduled visit). In addition, many kinds of computer suggestions are best delivered during the physician order entry process. For example, order entry is the only point in the workflow at which to discourage or countermand an order that might be dangerous or wasteful. It is also a convenient point to offer reminders about needed tests or treatments, because they will usually require an order for their initiation.

---

[9] Mirth Corporation Community Overview. http://www.mirthcorp.com/community/overview. (Accessed 1/2/2013).

[10] Surescripts: The Nation's e-Prescription Network http://www.surescripts.com/ (Accessed 1/2/2013).

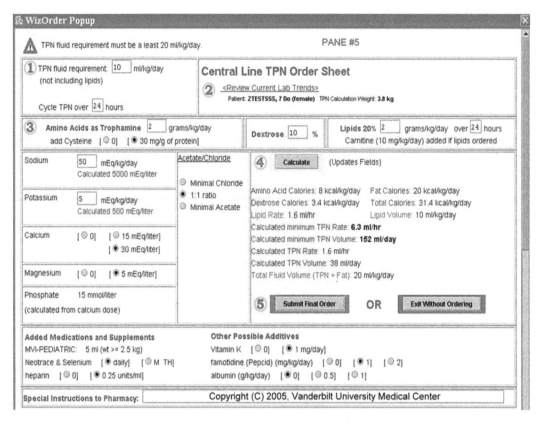

Fig. 12.3 Neonatal Intensive Care Unit (NICU) Total Parenteral Nutrition (TPN) Advisor provides complex interactive advice and performs various calculations in response to the provider's prescribed goal for amount of fluid, calories, nutrition, and special additives (Source: Miller et al. (2005b). Elsevier Reprint License No. 2800411402464)

The best way for the computer to suggest actions that require an order is to present a pre-constructed order to the provider who can confirm or reject it with a single key stroke or mouse click. It is best to annotate such suggestions with their rationale, e.g., "the patient is due for his pneumonia vaccine because he has emphysema and is over 65," so the provider understands the suggestion.

Figure 12.4a, b show the suggestions of a sophisticated inpatient decision support system from Intermountain Health Care that uses a wide range of clinical information to recommend antibiotic choice, dose, and duration of treatment. Decision support from the system improved clinical outcomes and reduced costs of infections among patients managed with the assistance of this system (Evans et al. 1998; Pestotnik 2005). Vanderbilt's inpatient "WizOrder" order entry (CPOE) system also addresses antibiotic orders,

as shown in Fig. 12.5; it suggests the use of Cefepine rather than ceftazidine, and provides choices of dosing by indication.

Clinical alerts attached to a laboratory test result can include suggestions for appropriate follow up or treatments for some abnormalities (Ozdas et al. 2008; Rosenbloom et al. 2005). Physician order-entry systems can warn the physician about allergies (Fig. 12.6a) and drug interactions (Fig. 12.6b) before they complete a medication order, as exemplified by screenshots from Partner's outpatient medical record orders.

Reminders and alerts are employed widely in outpatient care. Indeed, the outpatient setting is where the first clinical reminder study was performed (McDonald 1976) and is still the setting for the majority of such studies (Garg et al. 2005). Reminders to physicians in outpatient settings quadrupled the use of certain vaccines in eligible patients compared with those who did not receive

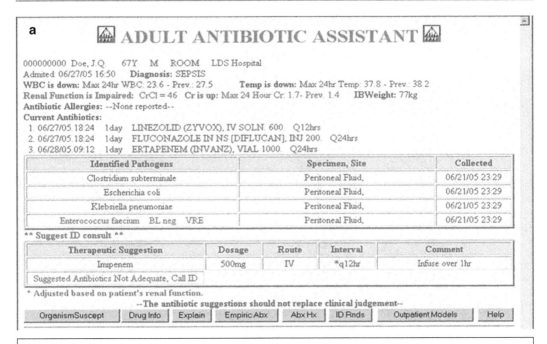

Fig. 12.4 Example of the main screen (a) from the Intermountain Health Care Antibiotic Assistant program. The program displays evidence of an infection-relevant patient data (e.g., kidney function, temperature), recommendations for antibiotics based on the culture results, and (b) disclaimers (Source: Courtesy of R. Scott Evans, Robert A. Larsen, Stanley L. Pestotnik, David C. Classen, Reed M. Gardner, and John P. Burke, LDS Hospital, Salt Lake City, UT (Larsen et al. 1989))

reminders (McDonald et al. 1984b; McPhee et al. 1991; Hunt et al. 1998; Teich et al. 2000). Reminder systems can also suggest needed tests and treatments for eligible patients. Figure 12.7 shows an Epic system screen with reminders to consider ordering a cardiac echocardiogram and starting an ACE inhibitor—in an outpatient patient with a diagnosis of heart failure but no record of a cardiac echocardiogram or treatment with one of the most beneficial drugs for heart failure.

Though the outpatient setting is the primary setting for preventive care reminders, preventive reminders also can be influential in the hospital (Dexter et al. 2001). And reminders directed to inpatient nurses can improve preventive care as much or more than reminders directed to physicians (Dexter et al. 2004).

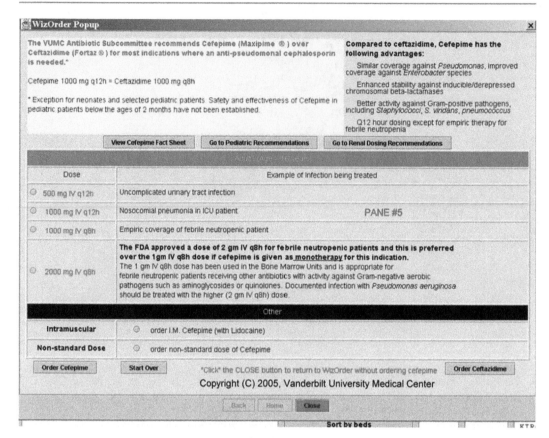

Fig. 12.5 User ordered an antibiotic for which the Vanderbilt's inpatient "WizOrder" order entry (CPOE) system, based on their Pharmaceuticals and Therapeutics (PandT) Committee input, recommended a substitution. This educational advisor guides clinician through ordering an alternative antibiotic. Links to "package inserts" (via buttons) detail how to prescribe recommended drug under various circumstances (Source: Miller, et al. (2005b). Elsevier Reprint License No. 2800411402464)

12.3.4 Access to Knowledge Resources

Most clinical questions, whether addressed to a colleague or answered by searching through text books and published papers, are asked in the context of a specific patient (Covell et al. 1985). Thus, an appropriate time to offer knowledge resources to clinicians is while they are writing notes or orders for a specific patient. Clinicians have access to a rich selection of knowledge sources today, including those that are publically available, e.g. the National Library of Medicine's (NLM) PubMed and MedlinePlus, the Centers for Disease Control and Prevention's (CDC) vaccines and international travel information, the Agency for Healthcare Research and Quality's (AHRQ) National Guideline Clearinghouse, and those produced by commercial vendors such as UpToDate, Micromedex, and electronic textbooks, all of which can be accessed from any web browser at any point in time. Some EHR systems are proactive and present short informational nuggets as a paragraph adjacent to the order item that the clinician has chosen. EHRs can also pull literature, textbook or other sources of information relevant to a particular clinical situation through an **Infobutton** and present that information to the clinician on the fly (Del Fiol et al. 2012), an approach being encouraged by the CMS MU2 regulations (see Fig. 12.8) (Final Rule: CMS 2012).

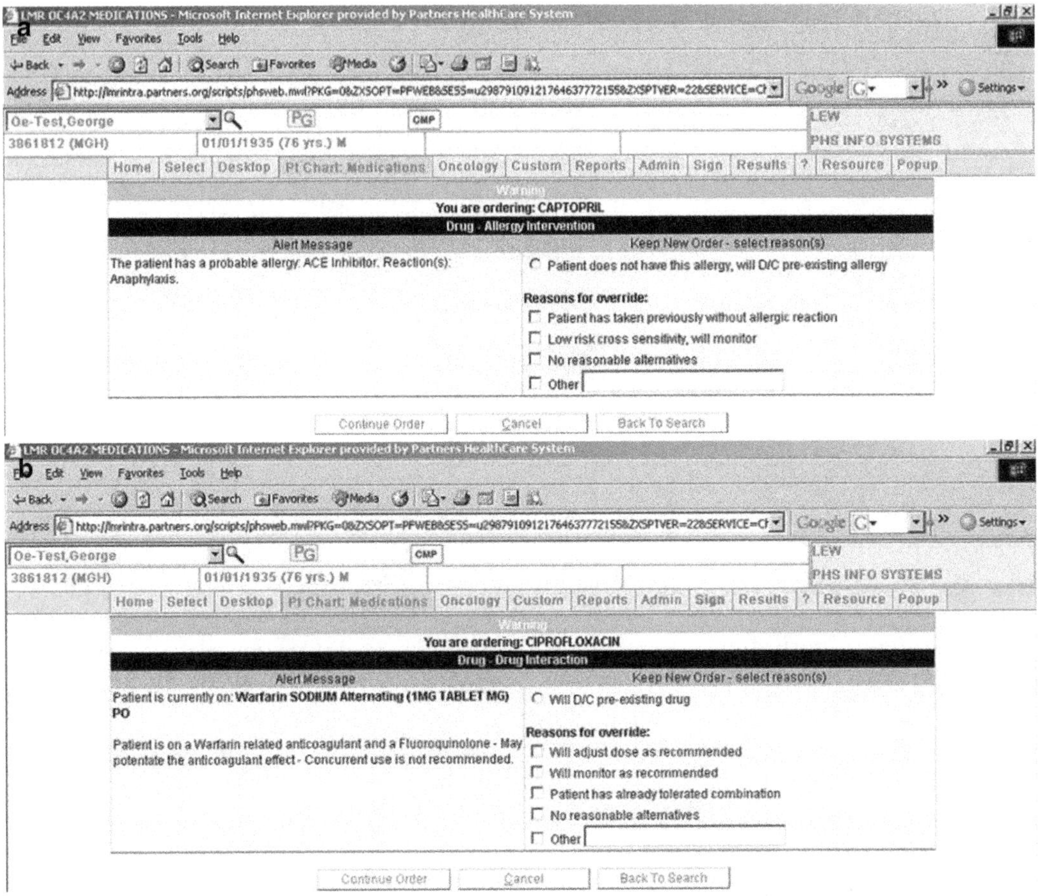

Fig. 12.6 Drug-alert display screens from Partners outpatient medical record application (Longitudinal Medical Record, LMR). The screens show (**a**) a drug-allergy alert for captopril, and (**b**) a drug-drug interaction between ciprofloxacin and warfarin (Source: Courtesy of Partners Health Care System, Chestnut Hill, MA)

12.3.5   Integrated Communication and Reporting Support

Increasingly, the delivery of patient care requires multiple health care professionals and may cross many organizations; thus, the effectiveness, efficiency, and timeliness of communication among such team members and organizations are increasingly important. Such communications usually focus on a single patient and may require a care provider to read content from his or her local EHR or from an external clinical system or to send information from his system to an external system. Therefore, communication tools should be an integrated part of the EHR system.

Ideally providers' offices, the hospital, and the emergency room should all be linked together—not a technical challenge with today's Internet, but still an administrative challenge due to organizational barriers. Connectivity to the patient's home will be increasingly important to patient-provider communication: for delivery of reminders directly to patients (Sherifali et al. 2011), and for home health monitoring, such as home blood pressure (Earle 2011; Green et al. 2008), and glucose monitoring. The patient's personal health record (PHR) will also become an important destination for clinical messages and test results (see Chap. 17). Relevant information can be "pushed" to the user via e-mail or pager services (Major et al. 2002; Poon et al. 2002) or "pulled" by users on demand during their routine interactions with the computer.

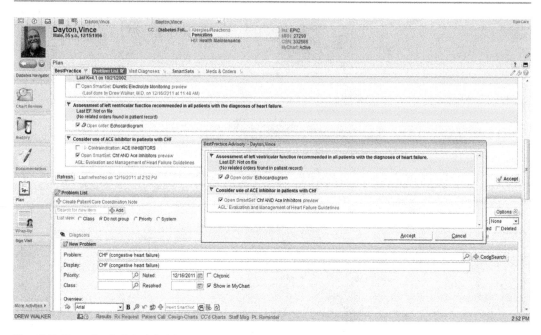

Fig. 12.7 Example of clinical decision support alerts to order an echocardiogram and to start an ACE inhibitor in a patient with diagnosed congestive heart failure (Source: Courtesy of Epic Systems, Madison, WI)

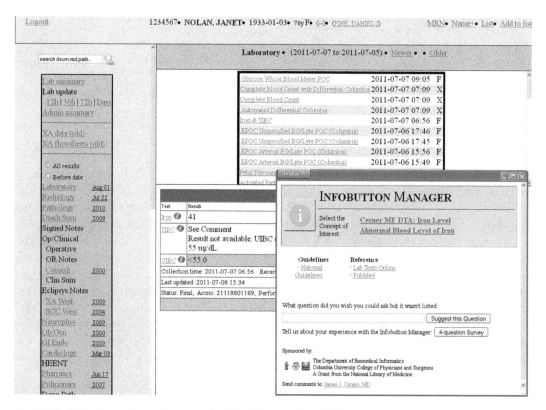

Fig. 12.8 This figure shows the use of Columbia University Medical Center's info-buttons during results review. Clicking on the info-button adjacent to the Iron result generates a window (image) with a menu of questions. When the user clicks on one of the questions, the info button delivers the answers (Source: Courtesy of Columbia University Medical Center, New York)

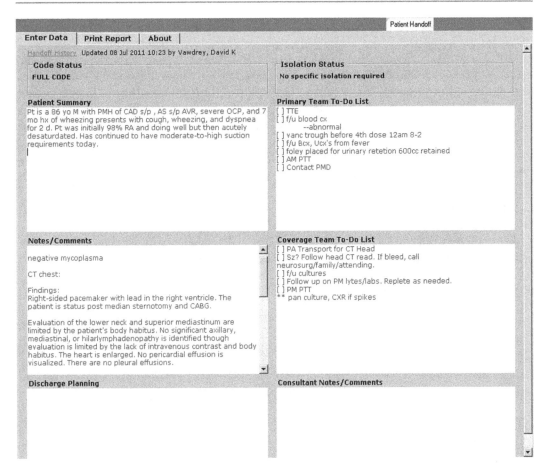

Fig. 12.9 Patient handoff report—a user-customizable hard copy report with automatic inclusion of patient allergies, active medications, 24-h vital signs, recent common laboratory test results, isolation requirements, code status, and other EHR data. This system was developed by a customer within a vendor EHR product (Sunrise Clinical Manager, Allscripts, Chicago, IL) and was disseminated among other customers around the nation (Source: Courtesy of Columbia University Medical Center, New York)

EHR systems can also help with patient hand-offs, during which the responsibility for care is transferred from one clinician to another. Typically the transferring clinician delivers a brief verbal or written turn-over note to help the receiving clinician understand the patient's problems and treatments. Figure 12.9 shows an example of a screen that presents a "turn-over report" with instructions from the primary physician, as well as relevant system-provided information (e.g., recent laboratory test results) and a "to-do" list, that ensures that critical tasks are not dropped (Stein et al. 2010). Such applications support communication among team members and improve coordination.

Although a patient encounter is usually defined by a face-to-face visit (e.g., outpatient visit, inpatient bedside visit, home health visit), provider decision making also occurs during patient telephone calls, prescription renewal requests, and the arrival of new test results; so the clinician and key office personnel should be able to respond to these events with electronic renewal authorizations, patients' reports about normal test results, and back-to-work forms as appropriate. In addition, when the provider schedules a diagnostic test such as a mammogram, an EHR system can keep track of the time since the order was written and can notify the physician that a test result has not appeared in a specified time so that the provider can investigate and correct the obstacle to fulfillment.

EHRs are usually bounded by the institution in which they reside. The National Health Information Infrastructure (NHII) (NCVHS, 2001) proposed a future in which a provider caring for a patient could reach beyond his or her local institution to automatically obtain patient information from any place that carried data about the patient (see Chap. 13). Today, examples of such community-based "EHRs," often referred to as **Health Information Exchanges (HIE)**, serve routine and emergency care, public health and/or other functions. A few examples of long-existing HIEs are those in: Indiana (McDonald et al. 2005), Ontario, Canada (electronic Child Health Network),[11] Kentucky (Kentucky Health Information Exchange),[12] and Memphis (Frisse et al. 2008).[13] A study from this last system showed that the extra patient information provided by this HIE reduced resource use and costs (Frisse et al. 2011). The New England Health care Exchange Network (NEHEN)[14] has created a community-wide collaborative system for managing eligibility, preauthorization, and claim status information (Fleurant et al. 2011).

The **Office of the National Coordinator (ONC)** has developed two communication tools to support the **Nationwide Health Information Network (NwHIN)**[15] and health data exchange (see Chaps. 13 and 27). NwHIN Connect[16] is an HHS project designed for pulling information from any site within a national network of health care systems. It offers a sophisticated consenting system by which patients can control who can use

and see their information, but has only been used in a few pairs of communicating institutions. **NwHIN Direct**[17] is a much simpler approach that uses standard Web Email, **domain name system (DNS)** and **public-private keys** to push patient reports as encrypted email messages from their source (e.g. laboratory system) to clinicians and hospitals. It could also be used to link individual care organizations to an HIE. Microsoft, among others, has implemented NwHIN Direct.

Communication tools that support timely and efficient communication between patients and the health care team can enhance coordination of care and disease management, and eHealth applications can provide patients with secure online access to their EHR and integrated communication tools to ask medical questions or conveniently perform other clinical (e.g., renew a prescription) or administrative tasks (e.g., schedule an appointment) (Tang 2003).

12.4 Fundamental Issues for Electronic Health Record Systems

All health record systems must serve the same functions, whether they are automated or manual. From a user's perspective, the major difference is the way data are entered into, and delivered from, the record system. In this section, we explore the issues and alternatives related to data entry and then describe the options for displaying and retrieving information from an EHR.

12.4.1 Data Capture

EHRs use two general methods for **data capture**: (1) electronic interfaces from systems, such as laboratory systems that are already fully automated, and (2) direct manual data entry, when no such electronic source exists or it cannot be accessed.

[11] eCHN electronic Child Health Network. http://www.echn.ca/ (Accessed 1/2/2013).

[12] Kentucky Health Information Exchange Frequently Asked Questions. http://khie.ky.gov/Pages/faq.aspx?fc=010 (Accessed 1/2/2013).

[13] MidSoutheHealth Alliance. http://www.midsoutheha.org (Accessed 1/2/2013).

[14] New England Health care Exchange Network (NEHEN). www.nehen.net (Accessed 1/2/2013).

[15] http://www.healthit.gov/policy-researchers-implementers/nationwide-health-information-network-nwhin (Accessed 1/3/2013).

[16] http://www.healthit.gov/policy-researchers-implementers/connect-gateway-nationwide-health-information-network (Accessed 1/3/2013).

[17] Office of the National Coordinator for Health Information Technology. Direct Project http://directproject.org/ (Accessed 1/2/2013).

12.4.1.1 Electronic Interfaces

The preferred method of capturing EHR data is to implement an electronic interface between the EHR and the existing electronic data sources such as laboratory systems, pharmacy systems, electronic instruments, home monitoring devices, registration systems, scheduling systems, etc.

The creation of interfaces requires effort to implement as described under Sect. 12.3.1, but, once implemented they provide near-instant availability of the clinical data without the labor costs and error potential of manual transcription. Interfacing is usually easier when the organization that owns the EHR system also owns, or is tightly affiliated with, the source system. Efforts to interface with systems outside the organizational boundary can be more difficult. However, interfaces between office practice systems and major referral laboratories for exchanging laboratory test orders and results, and between hospitals and office practices to pharmacies for e-prescribing, are now relatively easy and quite common.

The above discussion about interfacing concerns data produced, or ordered, by a home organization. However, much of the information about a patient will be produced or ordered by an outside organization and will not be available to a given organization via any of the conventional interfaces described above. For example, a hospital-based health care system will not automatically learn about pediatric immunizations done in private pediatric offices, or public health clinics, around town. So, special procedures and extra work are required to collect all relevant patient data. The promotion of health information exchange stimulated by passage of the Health Information Technology for Economic and Clinical Health (HITECH) Act of 2009 (see Chap. 27) and other information exchange mechanisms (e.g. NwHIN Direct) described in Sect. 12.3.5 will facilitate the capture of such information from any source (see Chaps. 7 and 13).

12.4.1.2 Manual Data Entry

Data may be entered as narrative free-text, as codes, or as a combination of codes and free text annotation. Trade-offs exist between the use of codes and narrative text. The major advantage of coding is that it makes the data "understandable" to the computer and thus enables selective retrieval, clinical research, quality improvement, and clinical operations management. The coding of diagnoses, allergies, problems, orders, and medications is of special importance to these purposes; using a process called auto complete, clinicians can code such items by typing in a few letters of an item name, then choosing the item they need from the modest list of items that match the string they have entered. This process can be fast and efficient when the computer includes a full range of synonyms for the items of interest, and has frequency statistics for each item, so that it can present a short list of the most frequently occurring items that match the letters the user has typed so far.

Natural-language processing (NLP) (see Chap. 8) offers hope for automatic encoding of narrative text (Nadkarni et al. 2011). There are many types of NLP systems, but in general, such systems first regularize the input to recognize sections, sentences, and tokens like words or numbers. Through a formal grammar or a statistical technique, the tokens are then mapped to an internal representation of concepts (e.g., specific findings), their modifiers (e.g., whether a finding was asserted as being present or denied, and the timing of the finding), and their relations to other concepts. The internal representation is then mapped to a standard terminology and data model for use in a data warehouse or for automated decision support.

12.4.1.3 Physician-Entered Data

Physician-gathered patient information requires special comment because it presents the most difficult challenge to EHR system developers and operators. Physicians spend about 20 % of their time documenting the clinical encounter (Gottschalk and Flocke 2005; Hollingsworth et al. 1998). And the documentation burden has risen over time, because patient's problems are more acute, care teams are larger, physicians order more tests and treatments, and billing regulatory bodies demand more documentation.

Many believe that clinicians themselves should enter all of this data directly into the EMR under the assumption that the person who collects the data should enter it. This tactic makes the most sense for prescriptions, orders, and perhaps diagnoses and procedure codes, whose immediate entry during the course of care will speed service to the patient and provide crucial grist for decision support. Direct entry by clinicians may not be as important for visit notes because the time cost of physician input is high and the information is not a pre-requisite to the check-out process.

Physicians' notes can be entered into the EHR via one of three general mechanisms: (1) transcription of dictated or written notes, (2) clinic staff transfer or coding of some or all of the data by clinicians on a paper encounter form, and (3) direct data entry by physicians into the EHR (which may be facilitated by electronic templates or macros). Dictation with **transcription** is a common approach for entering narrative information into EHRs. If physicians dictate their reports using standard formats (e.g., present illness, past history, physical examinations, and treatment plan), the transcriptionist can maintain a degree of structure in the transcribed document via section headers, and the structure can also be delivered as an HL7 CDA document (Ferranti et al. 2006).

Some practices have employed scribes (a variant on the stenographers of old) to some of the physicians' data entry work (Koshy et al. 2010), and CMS's MU2 regulation (Final Rule: CMS 2012) allows credentialed medical assistants to take on this same work. **Speech recognition** software offers an approach to "dictating" without the cost or delay of transcription. The computer translates the clinician's speech to text automatically. However, even with accuracy rates of 98 %, users may have to invest important amounts time to find and correct these errors.

Some dictation services use speech recognition to generate a draft transcription, which the transcriptionist corrects while listening to the audio dictation, thus saving transcriptionist time; others are exploring the use of natural language processing (NLP) to auto-encode transcribed text, and employ the transcriptionist to correct any NLP coding errors (see Chap. 8).

The second data-entry method is to have physicians record information on a **structured encounter form**, from which their notes are transcribed or possibly scanned (Downs et al. 2006; Hagen et al. 1998). One system (Carroll et al. 2011) uses paper turn-around documents to capture visit note data in one or more steps. First, the computer generates a child-specific data-capture form completed by the mother and the nursing staff. The computer scans the completed form (Fig. 12.10a), reads the hand-entered numeric data (top of form), check boxes (middle of form) and the bar codes (bottom of form), and stores them in the EHR. Next, the computer generates a physician encounter form that is also child-specific. The physician completes this form (Fig. 12.10b) and the computer processes it the same way it processed the nursing form.

The third alternative is the **direct entry** of data into the computer by care providers. This alternative has the advantage that the computer can immediately check the entry for consistency with previously stored information and can ask for additional detail or dimensions conditional on the information just entered. Some of this data will be entered into fields which require selection from pre-specified menus. For ease of entry, such menus should not be very long, require scrolling, or impose a rigid hierarchy (Kuhn et al. 1984). A major issue associated with direct physician entry is the physician time cost. Studies document that structured data entry consumes more clinician time than the traditional record keeping (Chaudhry et al. 2006), as much as 20s per SNOMED CT coded diagnoses (Fung et al. 2011)—which may be a function of the interface terminology used (or not used), and a small study suggests that the EHR functions taken together may consume up to 60 min of the physician's free time per clinic day (McDonald and McDonald 2012). So, planners must be sensitive to these time costs. In one study, the computer system was a primary cause of clinician dissatisfaction (Edgar 2009) and their reason for leaving military medicine.

The use of templates and menus can speed note entry, but they can also generate excessive boilerplate and discourage specificity, i.e., it is easier to pick an available menu option than to a 1618149875 **CHICA Pre-Screening**

MRN: #9999999-7
Name: Patient, Jenny D
Age: 2 yo DOB: Nov 18 2009
Date: Nov 29 2011

Height: 84.5 cm. Uncooperative / Unable to Screen: ☐ Vision ☐ Hearing ☐ BP

Weight: 14.2 kg. Vision Left: 20/

HC: . cm. Vision Right: 20/ Pulse Ox: %

BP: / Left Ear @ 25db: P ☐ F ☐ Right Ear @ 25db: P ☐ F ☐

Temp: . deg. F

Pulse: /min RR:

☐ Sick Visit
☐ Two IDs checked
☐ Patient refused to complete form
☐ Patient left without treatment

Box For Nursing Use Only - Box For Nursing Use Only - Box For Nursing Use Only - Box For Nursing Use Only

Parents: Thank you for answering these questions about your child. The answers will help your doctor provide better quality of care. If your child is age 11 or older, he/she should answer the questions privately. Answers are confidential, but if you prefer not to answer that is allowed. You may want to talk about these questions with your doctor.

Please fill in the circles completely with a pencil or pen.

Y	N	
	X	Is Jenny having pain today?
	X	Does Jenny take prescription or over-the-counter medicine, herbal medicine or vitamins, or use an inhaler or medicated creams or lotions?
X		Does Jenny say six or more words other than 'Mama', 'Dada' and names of family members or pets?
X		Has your partner kicked, hit, or slapped you?
X		Does Jenny always wear a helmet when riding her bike or tricycle?
X		Does Jenny usually watch TV or computer more than 2 hours a day?
X		Do you know what to do if Jenny is choking?
	X	Has your partner or another adult threatened or hurt your children?
	X	Has Jenny seen a dentist this year?
	X	Are any firearms or guns kept in Jenny's home?

Y	N	
X		Please fill out the attached form about Jenny's development.
X		Can Jenny take off any of her clothes, such as pajamas (tops or bottoms) or pants? Do not count diapers, hats, socks, or shoes.
X		Do you feel safe in your home?
	X	Jenny has sickle cell disease (HbSS). Is she taking antibiotics twice a day, every day?
X		Does Jenny have a TV in her room?
X		Does anyone in Jenny's home smoke?
	X	Has Jenny ever been around water when an adult has not been within an arm's length?
	X	Does Jenny ever use a bottle?
X		Is Jenny on the WIC program?
X		Has Jenny spent more than a week in Asia, Africa, Latin America or Eastern Europe?

Preguntas en español al otro lado.

Fig. 12.10 (**a**) Nurse/mother completes the first form with questions tailored to patient's age. An OCR system reads the hand written numbers at top, the check boxes in center and bar code identifiers at the bottom and passes the content to the EHR. (**b**) The computer generates a physician encounter form based on the contents of the first form and adds reminders. The OCR system interprets the completed form, encodes the answers given in the check boxes, and stores the hand writing as image as part of the visit note (Source: Courtesy of Regenstrief Institute, Indianapolis, IN)

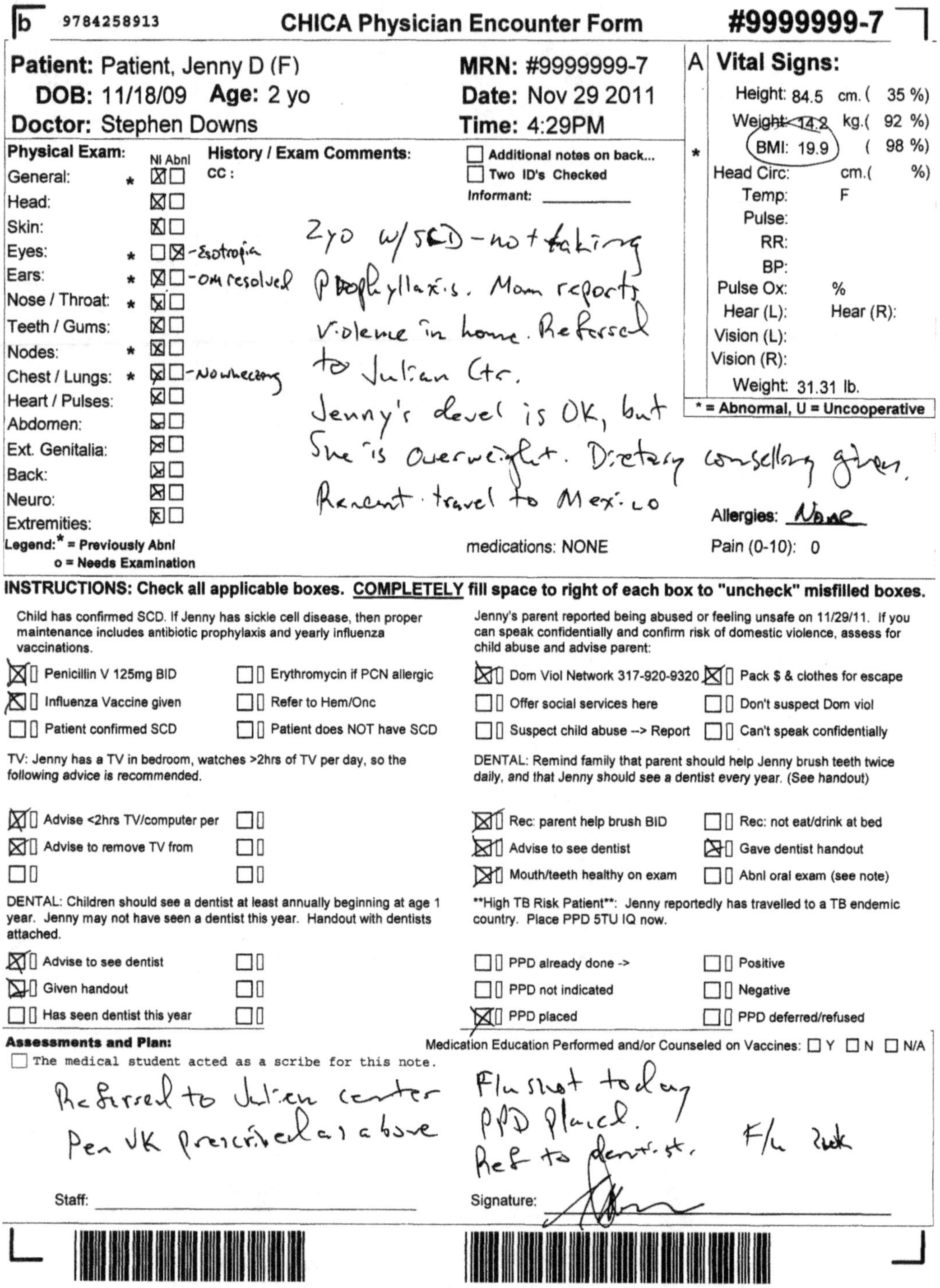

b 9784258913 **CHICA Physician Encounter Form** **#9999999-7**

Patient: Patient, Jenny D (F)
DOB: 11/18/09 **Age:** 2 yo
Doctor: Stephen Downs

MRN: #9999999-7
Date: Nov 29 2011
Time: 4:29PM

A **Vital Signs:**
Height: 84.5 cm. (35 %)
Weight: ~~14.2~~ kg.(92 %)
* BMI: 19.9 (98 %)
Head Circ: cm.(%)
Temp: F
Pulse:
RR:
BP:
Pulse Ox: %
Hear (L): Hear (R):
Vision (L):
Vision (R):
Weight: 31.31 lb.
* = Abnormal, U = Uncooperative

Physical Exam:		Nl	Abnl	
General:	*	☒	☐	
Head:		☒	☐	
Skin:		☒	☐	
Eyes:	*	☐	☒	-Esotropia
Ears:	*	☒	☐	-OM resolved
Nose / Throat:	*	☒	☐	
Teeth / Gums:		☒	☐	
Nodes:	*	☒	☐	
Chest / Lungs:	*	☒	☐	-No wheezing
Heart / Pulses:		☒	☐	
Abdomen:		☒	☐	
Ext. Genitalia:		☒	☐	
Back:		☒	☐	
Neuro:		☒	☐	
Extremities:		☒	☐	

Legend: * = Previously Abnl
o = Needs Examination

History / Exam Comments:
CC :
☐ Additional notes on back...
☐ Two ID's Checked
Informant: ________

2yo w/SCD - not taking prophylaxis. Mom reports violence in home. Referral to Julian Ctr.
Jenny's level is OK, but she is overweight. Dietary counseling given.
Recent travel to Mexico

medications: NONE

Allergies: None
Pain (0-10): 0

INSTRUCTIONS: Check all applicable boxes. COMPLETELY fill space to right of each box to "uncheck" misfilled boxes.

Child has confirmed SCD. If Jenny has sickle cell disease, then proper maintenance includes antibiotic prophylaxis and yearly influenza vaccinations.

☒ Penicillin V 125mg BID ☐ Erythromycin if PCN allergic
☒ Influenza Vaccine given ☐ Refer to Hem/Onc
☐ Patient confirmed SCD ☐ Patient does NOT have SCD

Jenny's parent reported being abused or feeling unsafe on 11/29/11. If you can speak confidentially and confirm risk of domestic violence, assess for child abuse and advise parent:

☒ Dom Viol Network 317-920-9320 ☒ Pack $ & clothes for escape
☐ Offer social services here ☐ Don't suspect Dom viol
☐ Suspect child abuse --> Report ☐ Can't speak confidentially

TV: Jenny has a TV in bedroom, watches >2hrs of TV per day, so the following advice is recommended.

☒ Advise <2hrs TV/computer per ☐
☒ Advise to remove TV from ☐
☐ ☐

DENTAL: Remind family that parent should help Jenny brush teeth twice daily, and that Jenny should see a dentist every year. (See handout)

☒ Rec: parent help brush BID ☐ Rec: not eat/drink at bed
☒ Advise to see dentist ☒ Gave dentist handout
☒ Mouth/teeth healthy on exam ☐ Abnl oral exam (see note)

DENTAL: Children should see a dentist at least annually beginning at age 1 year. Jenny may not have seen a dentist this year. Handout with dentists attached.

☒ Advise to see dentist ☐
☒ Given handout ☐
☐ Has seen dentist this year ☐

High TB Risk Patient: Jenny reportedly has travelled to a TB endemic country. Place PPD 5TU IQ now.

☐ PPD already done -> ☐ Positive
☐ PPD not indicated ☐ Negative
☒ PPD placed ☐ PPD deferred/refused

Assessments and Plan:
☐ The medical student acted as a scribe for this note.

Medication Education Performed and/or Counseled on Vaccines: ☐ Y ☐ N ☐ N/A

Referred to Julian center
Pen VK prescribed as above

Flu shot today
PPD placed.
Ref to dentist. F/u 2wk

Staff: ________
Signature: ________

Fig. 12.10 (continued)

describe a finding or event in detail. Further, with templates, the user may also accept default values too quickly so notes written via templates may not convey as clear a picture of the patient's state as a note that is composed free-form by the physician and may contain inaccurate information.

Free-form narrative entry—by typing, dictation, or speech recognition—allows the clinician to express whatever they deem to be important. When clinicians communicate, they naturally prioritize findings and leave much information implicit. For example, an experienced clinician often leaves out "pertinent negatives" (i.e., findings that the patient does not have but that nevertheless inform the decision making process) knowing that the clinician who reads the record will interpret them properly to be absent. The result is usually a more concise history with a high signal-to-noise ratio that not only shortens the data capture time but also lessens the cognitive burden on the reading clinician. Weir and colleagues present compelling evidence about these advantages, especially when narrative is focused and vivid, and emphasize that too much information interferes with inter-provider communication (Weir et al. 2011).

Most EHRs let physicians cut and paste notes from previous visits and other sources. For example, a physician can cut and paste parts of a visit note into a letter to a referring physician and into an admission note, a most appropriate use of this capability. However, this cutting and pasting capability can be over-used and cause 'note bloat.' In addition, without proper attention to detail, some information may be copied that is no longer pertinent or true. In one study, 58 % of the text in the most recent visit notes duplicated the content of a previous note (Wrenn et al. 2010), although of course some repetition from note to note can be appropriate.

Tablets and smart phones provide new opportunities for data capture by clinical personnel including physicians. The University of Washington (Hartung et al. 2010) has developed a sophisticated suite of open source tools called the Open Data Interface (ODI) that includes form design and deployment to smart phones as well as delivery of captured data to a central resource. Data capture can be fast, and physicians and health care assistants in some third-world countries are using these tools eagerly. Figure 12.11 shows four screen shots from a medical record application of ODI. The first (Fig. 12.11a) is the patient selection screen. After choosing a patient, the user can view a summary of the patient's medical record. Scrolling is usually required to view the whole summary. Figure 12.11b, c show screen shots of two portions of the summary. Users can

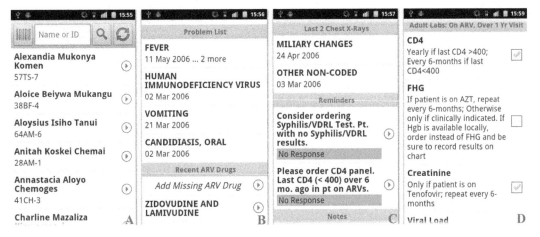

Fig. 12.11 ODK Clinic is a mobile clinical decision support system that helps providers make faster and better decisions about care. Providers equipped with ODK Clinic on a mobile phone or tablet can (**a**) access a list of patients (**b**) and (**c**) download patient summaries that include data from one patient record about diagnoses, diseases, reminders, and (**d**) specific lab data from an OpenMRS electronic medical record system. Summaries can be customized for specific diseases (i.e., for a provider treating a adult HIV patient). Users can also print lab orders on nearby printer and enter clinical data into some applications. The application is the result of a collaboration between USAID-AMPATH, the University of Washington, and the Open Data Kit project (Used with permission of Univ. of Washington. Find out more at: http://opendatakit.org)

choose to see the details of many kinds of information. Figure 12.11d shows the details of a laboratory test result. ODI ties into the OpenMRS project (Were et al. 2011), which has also been adopted widely in developing countries.

The long-term solution to data capture of information generated by clinicians is still evolving. The current ideal is the semi-structured data entry, which combines the use of narrative text fields and formally structured fields that are amenable to natural language processing combined with structured data entry fields where needed. With time and better input devices, direct computer entry will become faster and easier. In addition, direct entry of some data by patients will reduce the clinician's data entry (Janamanchi et al. 2009).

12.4.1.4 What to Do About Data Recorded on Paper Before the Installation of the EHR

Care organizations have used a number of approaches to load new EHR systems with pre-existing patient data. One approach is to interface the EHR to available electronic sources—such as a dictation service, pharmacy systems, and laboratory information systems—and load data from these sources for 6–12 months before going live with the EHR. A second approach is to abstract selected data, e.g., key laboratory results, the problem lists, and active medications from the paper record and hand enter those data into the EHR prior to each patient's visit when the EHR is first installed. The third approach is to scan and store 1–2 years of the old paper records. This approach does solve the availability problems of the paper chart, and can be applied to any kind of document, including handwritten records, produced prior to the EHR installation. Remember that these old records will have to be labeled with the patient ID, date information, and, preferably, the type of content (e.g., laboratory test, radiology report, provider dictation, and discharge summary, or, even better, a precise name, such as chest x-ray or operative note) and this step requires human effort. **Optical Character Recognition (OCR)** capability is built into most document scanners today, and converts typed text

within scanned documents to computer understandable text with 98–99 % character accuracy.

12.4.1.5 Data Validation

Because of the chance of transcription errors with the hand entry of data, EHR systems must apply **validity checks** scrupulously. A number of different kinds of checks apply to clinical data (Schwartz et al. 1985). **Range checks** can detect or prevent entry of values that are out of range (e.g., a serum potassium level of 50.0 mmol/L—the normal range for healthy individuals is 3.5–5.0 mol/L). The computer can ask the users to verify results beyond the absolute range. **Pattern checks** can verify that the entered data have a required pattern (e.g., the three digits, hyphen, and four digits of a local telephone number). **Computed checks** can verify that values have the correct mathematical relationship (e.g., white blood cell differential counts, reported as percentages, must sum to 100). **Consistency checks** can detect errors by comparing entered data (e.g., the recording of cancer of the prostate as the diagnosis for a female patient). **Delta checks** warn of large and unlikely differences between the values of a new result and of the previous observations (e.g., a recorded weight that changes by 100 lb in 2 weeks). **Spelling checks** verify the spelling of individual words.

12.4.2 Data Display

Once stored in the computer, data can be presented in numerous formats for different purposes without further entry work. In addition, computer-stored records can be produced in novel formats that are unavailable in manual systems.

Increasingly, EHRs are implemented on web browser technology because of the ease of deployment to any PC or smart device (including smart phone and tablets; see Chap. 14) so health care workers (e.g., physicians on call) can view patient data off-site. Advanced web security features such as **Transport Layer Security (TLS)** (NIST 2005)—a revised designation for **Secure**

Sockets Layer (SSL)—can ensure the confidentiality of any such data transmitted over the Internet.

Here, we discuss a few helpful formats. Clinicians need more than just integrated access to patient data; they also need various views of these data: in chronologic order as flowsheets or graphs to highlight changes over time, and as snapshots that show a computer view of the patients' current status and their most important observations.

12.4.2.1 Timeline Graphs

A graphical presentation can help the physician to assimilate the information quickly and draw conclusions (Fafchamps et al. 1991; Tang and Patel 1994; Starren and Johnson 2000). An anesthesia system vendor provides an especially good example of the use of numbers and graphics in a timeline to convey the patient's state in form that can be digested at a glance (Vigoda and Lubarsky 2006). Sparklines—"small, high resolution graphics embedded in a context of words, numbers, images" (Tufte 2006), which today's browsers and spreadsheets can easily generate—provide a way to embed graphic timelines into any report. One study found that with sparklines, "physicians were able to assess laboratory data faster … enable more information to be presented in a single view (and more compactly) and thus reduce the need to scroll or flip between screens" (Bauer et al. 2010). The second column of the flowsheet in Fig. 12.12a displays sparklines that include all of the data points for a given variable. The yellow band associated with those sparklines highlights the reference range. Clicking on one or more sparklines produces a pop-up that displays a standard graph for all of the selected variables. The user can expand the timeline of this graph to spread out points that are packed too closely together as shown in Fig. 12.12b.

12.4.2.2 Timeline Flowsheets

Figure 12.13a shows an integrated view of a flowsheet of the radiology impressions with the rows representing different kinds of radiology examinations and the columns representing study dates. Clicking on the radiology image icon brings up the radiology images, e.g., the quarter resolution chest X-ray views in Fig. 12.13b. An analogous process applies to electrocardiogram (ECG) measurements where clicking on the ECG icon for a particular result brings up the full ECG tracing in Portable Document Format (PDF) form. Figure 12.14 shows the popular pocket rounds report that provides laboratory and nursing measurements as a very compact flowsheet that fits in a white coat pocket (Simonaitis et al. 2006).

Flowsheets can be specialized to carry information required to manage a particular problem. A flowsheet used to monitor patients who have hypertension (high blood pressure) for example might contain values for weight, blood pressure, heart rate, and doses of medications that control hypertension as well as results of laboratory tests that monitor complications of hypertension, or the medications used to treat it. Systems often permit users to adjust the time granularity of flowsheets on the fly. An ICU user might view results at minute-by-minute intervals, and an out-patient physician might view them with a month-by-month granularity.

12.4.2.3 Summaries and Snapshots

EHRs can highlight important components (e.g., active allergies, active problems, active treatments, and recent observations) in clinical summaries or snapshots (Tang et al. 1999b). Figure 12.15 from Epic's product shows an example that presents the active patient problems, active medications, medication allergies, health maintenance reminders, and other relevant summary information. These views are updated automatically with any new data entry so they are always current. In the future, we can expect more sophisticated summarizing strategies, such as automated detection of adverse events (Bates et al. 2003b) or automated time-series events (e.g., cancer chemotherapy cycles). We may also see reports that distinguish abnormal changes that have been explained or treated from those that have not, and displays that dynamically organize the supporting evidence for existing problems (Tang and Patel 1994; Tang et al. 1994a).

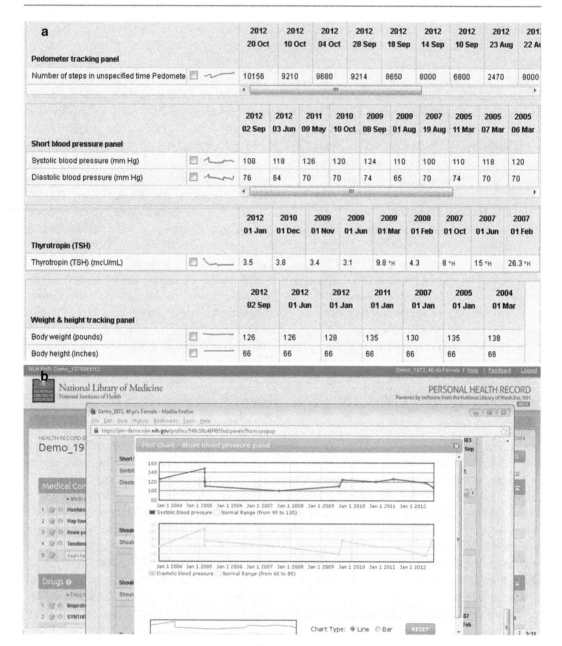

Fig. 12.12 The National Library of Medicine Personal Health Record (PHR) flow sheet (**a**) allows the consumer to track test, treatments and symptoms over time. Clicking on a sparklines graph in the flow sheet table opens a larger plot chart view (**b**) consumers can click on multiple sparklines to obtain full-sized graphs of the selected variables on one page. They can also mouse over a specific data point on the chart to expand the timeline, as shown shaded in *pink* (Source: Courtesy of Clement J. McDonald, Lister Hill National Center for Biomedical Communications, National Library of Medicine, Bethesda, MD)

Ultimately, computers should be able to produce concise and flowing summary reports that are like an experienced physician's hospital discharge summary.

12.4.2.4 Dynamic Search

Anyone who has reviewed a patient's chart knows how hard it can be to find a particular piece of information. From 10 % (Fries 1974) to

81 % (Tang et al. 1994b) of the time, physicians do not find patient information that has been previously recorded in a paper medical record. Furthermore, the questions clinicians routinely ask are often the ones that are difficult to answer from perusal of a paper-based record. Common questions include whether a specific test has ever been performed, what kinds of medications have been tried, and how the patient has responded to particular treatments (e.g., a class of medications) in the past. Physicians constantly ask these questions as they flip back and forth in the chart searching for the facts to support or refute one in a series of evolving hypotheses. Search tools (see Sect. 12.4.3) help the physician to locate relevant data. The EHR can

then display these data as specialized presentation formats (e.g., flowsheets or graphics) to make it easier for them to draw conclusions from the data. A graphical presentation can help the physician to assimilate the information quickly and to draw conclusions (Fafchamps et al. 1991; Tang et al. 1994a; Starren and Johnson 2000).

12.4.3 Query and Surveillance Systems

The **query** and **surveillance** capabilities of computer-stored records have no counterpart in manual systems. Medical personnel, quality

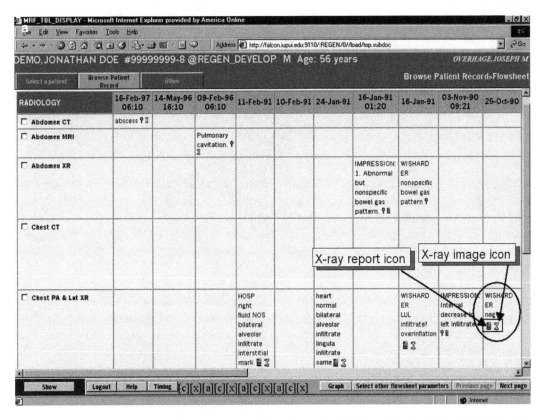

Fig. 12.13 Web resources. (**a**) Web-browser flow sheet of radiology reports. The rows all report one kind of study, and the columns report one date. Each cell shows the impression part of the radiology report as a quick summary of the content of that report. The cells include two icons. Clicking on the report icon provides the full radiology report. Clicking on the radiology image icon provides the images. (**b**) The chest X-ray images on radiology images

obtained by clicking on the "bone" icon. What shows by default is a quarter-sized view of both the PA and lateral chest view X-ray. By clicking on various options, users can obtain up to the full (2,000×2,300) resolution, and window and level the images over the 12 bits of a radiographic image, using a control provided by Medical Informatics Engineering (MIE), Fort Wayne Indiana (Source: Courtesy of Regenstrief Institute, Indianapolis, IN)

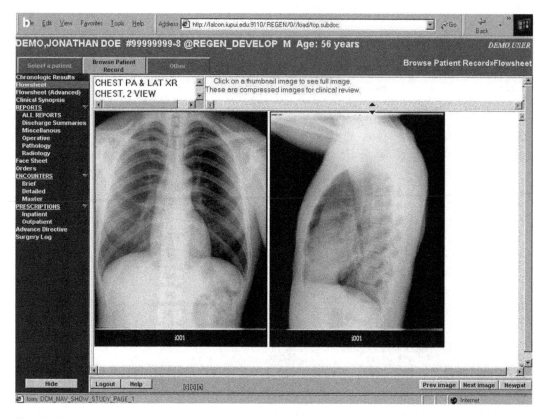

Fig. 12.13 (continued)

and patient safety professionals, and administrators can use these capabilities to analyze patient outcomes and practice patterns. Public health professionals can use the reporting functions of computer-stored records for surveillance, looking for emergence of new diseases or other health threats that warrant medical attention.

Although these functions of decision support on the one hand, and query surveillance systems, on the other, are different, their internal logic is similar. In both, the central procedure is to find records of patients that satisfy pre-specified criteria and export selected data when the patient meets those criteria. Surveillance queries generally address a large subset, or all, of a patient population; the output is often a tabular report of selected raw data on all the patient records retrieved or a statistical summary of the values contained in the records. Decision support generally addresses only those patients

under active care; its output is an **alert** or **reminder message** (McDonald 1976). Query and surveillance systems can be used for clinical care, clinical research, retrospective studies, and administration.

12.4.3.1 Clinical Care

A query can also identify patients who are due for periodic screening examinations such as immunizations, mammograms, and cervical Pap tests and can be used to generate letters to patients or call lists for office staff to encourage the preventive care. Query systems are particularly useful for conducting ad hoc searches such as those required to identify and notify patients who have been receiving a recalled drug. Such systems can also facilitate quality management and patient safety activities. They can identify candidate patients for concurrent review and can gather many of the data required to complete such audits.

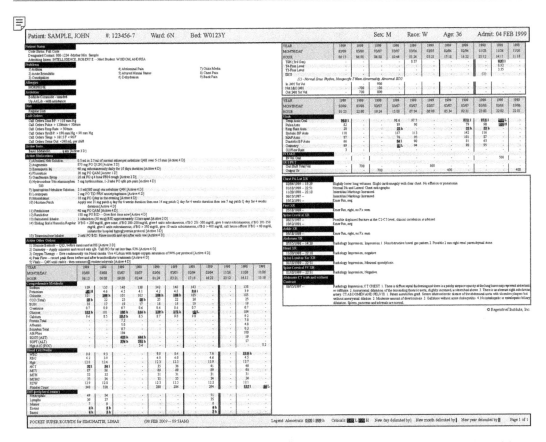

Fig. 12.14 The Pocket rounds report—so called because when folded from top to bottom, it fits in the clinician's white coat pocket as a booklet. It is a dense report (12 lines per inch, 36 characters per inch), printed in landscape mode on one 8 1/2 × 11 in. page), and includes the all active orders (including medications), recent laboratory results, vital signs and the summary impressions of radiology, endoscopy, and cardiology reports (Source: Courtesy of L. Simonaitis, Regenstrief Institute, Indianapolis, IN)

12.4.3.2 Clinical Research

Query systems can be used to identify patients who meet eligibility requirements for prospective clinical trials. For example, an investigator could identify all patients seen in a medical clinic who have a specific diagnosis and meet eligibility requirements while not having any exclusionary conditions. These approaches can also be applied in real time. At one institution, the physician's work station was programmed to ask permission to invite the patient into a study, when that physician entered a problem that suggested the patient might be a candidate for a local clinical trial. If the physician gave permission, the computer would send an electronic page to the nurse recruiter who would then invite the patient to participate in the study. It was first applied to a study of back pain (Damush et al. 2002).

12.4.3.3 Quality Reporting

Query systems can also play an important role in producing quality reports that are used for both internal quality improvement activities and for external public reporting. And, although it would be difficult for paper-based records to incorporate patient-generated input, and would require careful tagging of data source, an EHR could include data contributed by patients (e.g., functional status, pain scores, symptom reports). These patient-reported data may be incorporated in future quality measures. With the changing reimbursement payment models focusing more on outcomes measures instead of volume of transactions, generating efficient and timely reports of clinical quality measures will play an increasingly important role in management and payment.

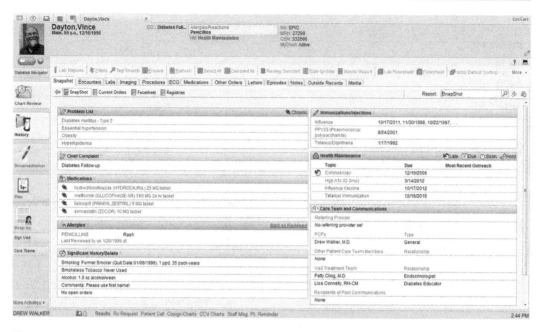

Fig. 12.15 Summary record. The patient's active medical problems, current medications, and drug allergies are among the core data that physicians must keep in mind when making any decision on patient care. This one-page screen provides an instant display of core clinical data elements as well as reminders about required preventive care. (Source: Courtesy of Epic Systems, Madison, WI)

12.4.3.4 Retrospective Studies

Randomized **prospective studies** are the gold standard for clinical investigations, but **retrospective studies** of existing data have contributed much to medical progress (See Chap. 11). Retrospective studies can obtain answers at a small fraction of the time and cost of comparable prospective studies.

EHR systems can provide many of the data required for a retrospective study. They can, for example, identify study cases and comparable control cases, and provide data needed for statistical analysis of the comparison cases (Brownstein et al. 2007). Combined with access to discarded specimens, they also offer powerful approaches to retrospective genome association studies that can be accomplished much faster and at cost magnitudes lower than comparable prospective studies (Kohane 2011; Roden et al. 2008).

Computer-stored records do not eliminate all the work required to complete an epidemiologic study; chart reviews and patient interviews may still be necessary. Computer-stored records are likely to be most complete and accurate with respect to drugs administered, laboratory test results, and visit diagnoses, especially if the first two types of data are entered directly from automated laboratory and pharmacy systems. Consequently, computer-stored records are most likely to contribute to research on a physician's practice patterns, on the efficacy of tests and treatments, and on the toxicity of drugs. However, NLP techniques make the content of narrative text more accessible to automatic searches (see Chap. 8).

12.4.3.5 Administration

In the past, administrators had to rely on data from billing systems to understand practice patterns and resource utilization. However, claims data can be unreliable for understanding clinical practice because the source data are coarse and often entered by non-clinical personnel not directly involved with the care decisions. Furthermore, relying on claims data as proxies for clinical diagnoses can produce inaccurate information and lead to inappropriate policymaking (Tang et al. 2007). Medical query systems in conjunction with administrative systems can provide information about the relationships among diagnoses, indices of severity of illness, and resource consumption. Thus, query systems are important tools for administrators who wish to make informed decisions in the increasingly cost-sensitive world of health care. On the other hand, the use of EHR data for billing and administration can produce incentives for clinicians to steer their documentation to optimize payment and resource allocation, potentially making that documentation less clinically accurate. It may therefore be best to base financial decisions on variables that are not open to interpretation.

12.5   Challenges Ahead

Although many commercial products are labeled as EHR systems, they do not all satisfy the criteria that we defined at the beginning of this chapter. Even beyond matters of definition, however, it is important to recognize that the concept of an EHR is neither unified nor static. As the capability of technology evolves, the function of the EHR will expand. Greater involvement of patients in their own care, for example, means that **personal health records** (**PHRs**) should incorporate data captured at home and also support two-way communication between patients and their health care team (see also Chap. 17). The potential for patient-entered data includes history, symptoms, and outcomes entered by patients as well as data uploaded automatically by home monitoring devices such as scales, blood pressure monitors, glucose meters, and pulmonary function devices. By integrating these patient-generated data into the EHR, either by uploading the data into the EHR or by linking the EHR and the PHR, a number of long-term objectives can be achieved: patient-generated data may in some circumstances be more accurate or complete, the time spent entering data during an office visit by both the provider and the patient may be reduced, and the information may allow the production of outcomes measures that are better attuned to patients' goals. One caveat in this vision is the perception that this may lead to a deluge of data that the

provider will never have time to sort through yet will be legally responsible for. A review of current products would be obsolete by the time that it was published. We have included examples from various systems in this chapter, both developed by their users and commercially available, to illustrate a portion of the functionality of EHR systems currently in use.

The future of EHR systems depends on both technical and nontechnical considerations. Hardware technology will continue to advance, with processing power doubling every 2 years according to Moore's law (see Chap. 1). Software will improve with more powerful applications, better user interfaces, and more integrated decision support. New kinds of software that support collaboration will continue to improve; social media are growing rapidly both inside and outside of health care. For example, as both providers and patients engage increasingly in social media, new ways to capture data, share data, collaborate, and share expertise may emerge. Perhaps the greater need for leadership and action will be in the social and organizational foundations that must be laid if EHRs are to serve as the information infrastructure for health care. We touch briefly on these challenges in this final section.

12.5.1   Users' Information Needs

We discussed the importance of clinicians directly using the EHR system to achieve maximum benefit from computer-supported decision making. On the one hand, organizations that require providers to enter all of their order, notes, and data directly into the EHR will gain substantial operational efficiency. On the other hand, physicians will bear the time costs of entering this information and may lose efficiency. Some balance between the organization's and providers' interests must be found. This balance is easiest to reach when physicians have a strong say in the decision.

Developers of EHR systems must thoroughly understand clinicians' information needs and workflows in the various settings where health care is delivered. The most successful systems have been developed either by clinicians or through close collaborations with practicing clinicians.

Studies of clinicians' information needs reveal that common questions that physicians ask concerning patient information (e.g., Is there evidence to support a specific patient diagnosis? Has a patient ever had a specific test? Has there been any follow up because of a particular laboratory test result?) are difficult to answer from the perusal of the paper-based chart (Tang et al. 1994b)). Regrettably, most clinical systems in use now cannot easily answer many of the common questions that clinicians ask. Developers of EHR systems must have a thorough grasp of users' needs and workflows if they are to produce systems that help health care providers to use these tools efficiently to deliver care effectively.

12.5.2 Usability

An intuitive and efficient user interface is an important part of the system. Designers must understand the cognitive aspects of the human and computer interaction and the professional workflow if they are to build interfaces that are easy-to-learn and easy-to-use (see Chap. 4). Improving human–computer interfaces will require changes not only in how the system behaves but also in how humans interact with the system. User interface requirements of clinicians entering patient data are different from the user interfaces developed for clerks entering patient charges. Usability for clinicians means fast computer response times, and the fewest possible data input fields. *A system that is slow or requires too much input is not usable by clinicians.* The menus and vocabularies that constrain user input must include synonyms for all the ways health professionals name the items in the vocabularies and menus, and the system must have keyboard options for all inputs and actions because switching from mouse to keyboard steals user time. To facilitate use by busy health care professionals, health care applications developers must focus

on clinicians' unique information needs. What information the provider needs and what tasks the provider performs should influence what and how information is presented. Development of human-interface technology that matches the data-processing power of computers with the cognitive capability of human beings to formulate insightful questions and to interpret data is still a rate-limiting step (Tang and Patel 1994). For example, one can imagine an interface in which speech input, typed narrative, and mouse-based structured data entry are accepted and seamlessly stored into a single data structure within the EHR, with a hybrid user display that shows both a narrative version of the information and a structured version of the same information that highlights missing fields or inconsistent values.

12.5.3 Standards

We alluded to the importance of standards earlier in this chapter, when we discussed the architectural requirements of integrating data from multiple sources. Standards are the focus of Chap. 7. Here, we stress the critical importance of national standards in the development, implementation, and use of EHR systems (Miller and Gardner 1997b). Health information should follow patients as they interact with different providers in different care settings. Uniform standards are essential for systems to interoperate and exchange data in meaningful ways. Having standards reduces development costs, increases integration, and facilitates the collection of meaningful aggregate data for quality improvement and health policy development. The HIPAA legislation has mandated standards for administrative messages, privacy, security, and clinical data. Regulations based on this legislation have already been promulgated for the first three of these categories.[18] Incentives provided by the HITECH Act (see Chaps. 7 and 27) stimulated a number of efforts including a report by the ONC

---

[18] http://www.hhs.gov/ocr/privacy/hipaa/administrative/index.html (Accessed 1/2/2012).

HIT Standards Committee (Health IT Standards Committee 2011) and Meaningful Use 2 (MU2) federal regulations (Final Rules: CMS 2012; Final Rule: ONC 2012) defining message and vocabulary standards for clinical data and encouraging EHR vendors and users to adopt them (see Sect. 12.3.1).[19] The US Department of Health and Human Services (HHS) maintains the current status of its HITECH programs on their Web site.[20]

12.5.4 Privacy and Security

Privacy and security policies and technology that protect individually identifiable health data are important foundational considerations for all applications that store and transmit and display health data. HIPAA established key regulations, and HITECH enhanced them, to protect the confidentiality of individually identifiable health information. With appropriate laws and policies computer-stored data can be more secure and confidential than those data maintained in paper-based records (Barrows and Clayton 1996).

12.5.5 Costs and Benefits

The Institute of Medicine (IOM) declared the EHR an essential infrastructure for the delivery of health care, and the protection of patient safety (IOM Committee on Improving the Patient Record 2001). Like any infrastructure project, the benefits specifically attributable to infrastructure are difficult to establish; an infrastructure plays an enabling role in all projects that take advantage of it. Early randomized controlled clinical studies showed that computer-based decision-support systems reduce costs and improve quality compared with usual care sup-

ported with a paper medical record (Tierney et al. 1993; Bates et al. 1997, 2003b; Classen et al. 1997), and recent meta-analyses of health information technology have demonstrated quality benefits (Buntin et al. 2011; Lau et al. 2010); however, Romano and Stafford (2011) did not find any "consistent association between EHRs and CDS and better quality."

Because of the significant resources needed and the significant broad-based potential benefits, the decision to implement an EHR system is a strategic one. Hence, the evaluation of the costs and benefits must consider the effects on the organization's strategic goals, as well as the objectives for individual health care (Samantaray et al. 2011). Recently, the federal government and professional organizations have both expressed interest in **Open Source** options for EHR software (Valdes 2008).

12.5.6 Leadership

Leaders from all segments of the health care industry must work together to articulate the needs, to define the standards, to fund the development, to implement the social change, and to write the laws to accelerate the development and routine use of EHR systems in health care. Because of the prominent role of the federal government in health care—as a payer, provider, policymaker, and regulator—federal leadership to create incentives for developing and adopting standards and for promoting the implementation and use of EHRs is crucial. Recently, Congress and the administration have acted to accelerate the adoption and meaningful use of health information technology based on some of the foundational research done in the informatics community (see Chap. 27). Technological change will continue to occur at a rapid pace, driven by consumer demand for entertainment, games, and business tools. Nurturing the use of information technology in health care requires leaders who promote the use of EHR systems and work to overcome the obstacles that impede widespread use of computers for the benefit of health care.

---

[19] http://www.healthit.gov/sites/default/files/standards-certification/HITSC_CQMWG_VTF_Transmit_090911.pdf (Accessed 1/3/2012).

[20] http://www.healthit.gov/policy-researchers-implementers/health-it-rules-regulations (Accessed 1/3/2012).

Suggested Readings

Barnett, G. O. (1984). The application of computer-based medical-record systems in ambulatory practice. *New England Journal of Medicine, 310*(25), 1643–1650. This seminal article compares the characteristics of manual and automated ambulatory patient record systems, discusses implementation issues, and predicts future developments in technology.

Bates, D. W., Kuperman, G. J., Wang, S., et al. (2003). Ten commandments for effective clinical decision support: Making the practice of evidence-based medicine a reality. *Journal of the American Medical Informatics Association, 10*(6), 523–530. The authors present ten very practical tips to designers and installers of clinical decision support systems.

Berner, E. S. (Ed.). (2010). *Clinical decision support systems, theory and practice: Health informatics series* (3rd ed.). New York: Springer. This text focuses on the design, evaluation, and application of Clinical Decision Support systems, and examines the impact of computer-based diagnostic tools both from the practitioner's and the patient's perspectives. It is designed for informatics specialists, teachers or students in health informatics, and clinicians.

Collen, M. F. (1995). *A history of medical informatics in the United States, 1950–1990*. Indianapolis: American Medical Informatics Association, Hartman Publishing. This rich history of medical informatics from the late 1960s to the late 1980s includes an extremely detailed set of references.

Gauld, R., & Goldfinch, S. (2006). *Dangerous enthusiasms: E-government, computer failure and information system development*. Dunedin: Otago University Press. Gauld and Goldfinch describe a number of large-scale **information and communications technology (ICT)** projects with an emphasis on health information systems, emphasizes the high failure rates of mega projects that assume they can create a design denovo, build from the design and deploy successfully. It also highlights the advantages of starting with more modest scopes and growing incrementally based on experience with the initial scope.

Institute of Medicine (IOM) Roundtable on Value and Science-Driven Health Care. (2011). *Digital infrastructure for the learning health system: The foundation for continuous improvement in health and health care – workshop series summary*. Washington, DC: National Academy Press. This report summarizes three workshops that presented new approaches to the construction of advanced medical record system that would gather the crucial data needed to improve the health care system.

Kuperman, G. J., Gardner, R. M., & Pryor, T. A. (1991). *The HELP system*. Berlin/Heidelberg: Springer-Verlag GmbH and Co. K. The HELP (Health Evaluation through Logical Processing) system was a computerized hospital information system developed by the authors at the LDS Hospital at the University of Utah, USA. It provided clinical, hospital administration and financial services through the use of a modular, integrated design. This book thoroughly documents the HELP system. Chapters discuss the use of the HELP system in intensive care units, the use of APACHE and APACHE II on the HELP system, various clinical applications and inactive or experimental HELP system modules. Although the HELP system has now been retired from routine use, it remains an important example of several key issues in EHR implementation and use that continue in the commercial systems of today.

Osheroff, J., Teich, J., Levick, D., et al. (2012). *Improving outcomes with clinical decision support: An implementers guide* (2nd ed.). Scottsdale: Scottsdale Institute, AMIA, AMDIS and SHM. This text provides guidance on using clinical decision support interventions to improve care delivery and outcomes in a hospital, health system or physician practice. The book also presents considerations for health IT software suppliers to effectively support their CDS implementer clients.

Walker, J. M., Bieber, E. J., & Richards, F. (2006). *Implementing an electronic health record system*. London: Springer. This book provides rich details, including the process plans, for implementing an EHR in a large provider setting. It is a great resource for anyone trying to learn about EHR deployments, covering topics related to preparation, support, and implementation.

Weed, L. L. (1969). *Medical records, medical evaluation and patient care: The problem-oriented record as a basic tool*. Chicago: Year Book Medical Publishers. In this classic book, Weed presents his plan for collecting and structuring patient data to produce a problem-oriented medical record.

Questions for Discussion

1. What is the definition of an EHR? What, then, is an EHR system? What are five advantages of an EHR over a paper-based record? Name three limitations of an EHR.

2. What are the five functional components of an EHR? Think of the information systems used in health care institutions in which you work or that you have seen. Which of the components that you named do those systems have? Which are missing? How do the missing elements limit the value to the clinicians or patients?

3. Discuss three ways in which a computer system can facilitate information transfer between hospitals and ambulatory care facilities, thus enhancing continuity of care for previously hospitalized patients who have been discharged and are now being followed up by their primary physicians.

4. Much of medical care today is practiced in teams, and coordinating the care delivered by teams is a major challenge. Thinking in terms of the EHR functional components, describe four ways that EHRs can facilitate care coordination. Describe two ways in which EHRs are likely to create additional challenges in care coordination.

5. How does the health care financing environment affect the use, costs, and benefits of an EHR system? How has the financing environment affected the functionality of information systems? How has it affected the user population?

6. Would a computer scan of a paper-based record be an EHR? What are two advantages and two limitations of this approach?

7. Among the key issues for designing an EHR system are what information should be captured and how it should be entered into the system. Physicians may enter data directly or may record data on a paper worksheet (encounter form) for later transcription by a data-entry worker. What are two advantages and two disadvantages of each method? Discuss the relative advantages and disadvantages of entry of free text instead of entry of fully coded information. Describe an intermediate or compromise method.

8. EHR data may be used in clinical research, quality improvement, and monitoring the health of populations. Describe three ways that the design of the EHR system may affect how the data may be used for other purposes.

9. Identify four locations where clinicians need access to the information contained in an EHR. What are the major costs or risks of providing access from each of these locations?

10. What are three important reasons to have physicians enter orders directly into an EHR system? What are three challenges in implementing such a system?

11. Consider the task of creating a summary report for clinical data collected over time and stored in an EHR system. Clinical laboratories traditionally provide summary test results in flowsheet format, thus highlighting clinically important changes over time. A medical record system that contains information for patients who have chronic diseases must present serial clinical observations, history information, and medications, as well as laboratory test results. Suggest a suitable format for presenting the information collected during a series of ambulatory-care patient visits.

12. The public demands that the confidentiality of patient data must be maintained in any patient record system. Describe three protections and auditing methods that can be applied to paper-based systems. Describe three technical and three nontechnical measures you would like to see applied to ensure the confidentiality of patient data in an EHR. How do the risks of privacy breaches differ for the two systems?

Health Information Infrastructure 13

William A. Yasnoff

After reading this chapter you should know the answers to these questions:

- What is the vision and purpose of Health Information Infrastructure (HII)?
- What kinds of impacts will HII have, and in what time periods?
- Why is architecture so crucial to HII success?
- What are the political and technical barriers to HII implementation?
- What are the desirable characteristics of HII evaluation measures?

13.1 Introduction

This chapter addresses **health information infrastructure** (**HII**), community level informatics systems designed to make comprehensive electronic patient records available when and where needed for the entire population. There are numerous difficult and highly interdependent challenges that HII systems must overcome, including privacy, stakeholder cooperation, assuring all-digital information, and providing financial sustainability. As a result, while HII has been pursued for years with myriad approaches in many countries, progress has been slow and no proven formula for success has yet been identified.

W.A. Yasnoff, MD, PhD
NHII Advisors, 1854 Clarendon Blvd.,
Arlington 22201, VA, USA
e-mail: william.yasnoff@nhiiadvisors.com

While the discussion here is focused on the development of the HII in the United States, many other countries are involved in similar activities and in fact have progressed further along this road. Canada, Australia, and a number of European nations have devoted considerable time and resources to their own national HIIs. The United Kingdom, for example, has spent several billion pounds over the last few years to upgrade substantially its health information system capabilities. It should be noted, however, that all of these nations have centralized, government-controlled health care systems. This organizational difference from the multifaceted, mainly private health care system in the U.S. results in a somewhat different set of issues and problems. One can hope that the lessons learned from HII development activities across the globe can be effectively shared to ease the difficulties of everyone who is working toward these important goals.

13.2 Vision and Benefits of HII

The vision of HII is comprehensive electronic patient information when and where needed, allowing providers to have complete and current information upon which to base clinical decisions. In addition, clinical decision support (see Chap. 22) would be integrated with information delivery. In this way, both clinicians and patients could receive reminders of the most recent **clinical guidelines** and research results. This would

Fig. 13.1 Estimated value vs.
completeness of health
information. Medical
information of any given type
for a patient typically needs to
be over 85 % complete before
it starts being truly valuable to
clinicians

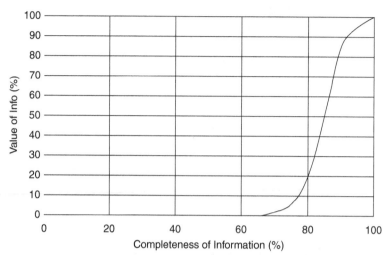

avoid the need for clinicians to have superhuman memory capabilities to assure the effective practice of medicine, and enable patients more easily to adhere to complex treatment protocols and to be better informed. Patients could also review and add information to their record and thereby become more active participants in their care. In addition, the availability of comprehensive records for each patient would enable value-added services, such as immediate electronic notifications to patients' family members about emergency care, as well as authorized queries in support of medical research, public health, and public policy decisions.

In considering HII, it is extremely important to appreciate that medical information for a given patient must, in general, be relatively complete before it is truly valuable for clinical use (see Fig. 13.1). For example, if a physician has access to an electronic information system that can retrieve half of each patient's list of medications, it is unlikely such a system will be actively used. Knowing that the information is incomplete, the physician will still need to rely on other traditional sources of information to fill in the missing data (including questioning the patient). So there is little added benefit for investing the time to obtain the partial information from the new system. Similarly, applying clinical decision support to incomplete patient data may produce erroneous, misleading, or even potentially dangerous results. Therefore, HII systems must reliably

provide reasonably complete information to be valuable to clinicians for patient care, and to make their use worthwhile.

The potential benefits of HII are both numerous and substantial. Perhaps most important are error reduction and improved quality of care. Many studies have shown that the complexity of present-day medical care results in very frequent errors of both omission and commission (Institute of Medicine 1999). The source of this problem was clearly articulated by Masys, who observed that current medical practice depends upon the "clinical decision-making capacity and reliability of autonomous practitioners for classes of problems that routinely exceed the bounds of unaided human cognition." (Masys 2002). Electronic health information systems can contribute significantly to alleviating this problem by reminding practitioners about recommended actions at the point of care. This can include both notifications of actions that may have been missed and warnings about planned treatments or procedures that may be harmful or unnecessary. Literally dozens of research studies have shown that such reminders improve safety and reduce costs (Bates 2000; Kass 2001). In one such study, medication errors were reduced by 55 % (Bates et al. 1998). Another study by the RAND Corporation showed that only 55 % of U.S. adults were receiving recommended care (McGlynn et al. 2003). The same techniques used to reduce medical errors with electronic health information systems also contribute substantially to ensuring that recommended care is provided. This is becoming increasingly important as the population ages and the prevalence of chronic disease increases.

Guidelines and reminders also can improve the effectiveness of dissemination of new research results. At present, widespread application of a new research in the clinical setting takes an average of 17 years (Balas and Boren 2000). Patient-specific reminders delivered at the point of care, highlighting important new research results, could substantially accelerate this adoption rate.

Another important contribution of HII to the research domain is improving the efficiency of clinical trials. At present, most clinical trials require the creation of a unique information infrastructure to insure protocol compliance and to collect essential research data. With an effective HII, every practitioner would have access to a fully functional **electronic health record (EHR)**, so clinical trials could routinely be implemented through the dissemination of guidelines that specify the research protocol. Data collection would occur automatically in the course of administering the protocol, reducing time and costs. In addition, there would be substantial value in analyzing **de-identified aggregate data** from routine patient care to assess the outcomes of various treatments, and monitor the health of the population.

Another critical function for HII is early detection of patterns of disease, particularly early detection of outbreaks from newly-virulent microorganisms or possible bioterrorism. Our current system of disease **surveillance**, which depends on alert clinicians diagnosing and reporting unusual conditions, is both slow and potentially unreliable. These problems are illustrated by delayed detection of the anthrax attacks in the Fall of 2001, when seven cases of cutaneous anthrax in the New York City area 2 weeks before the so-called "index" case in Florida went unreported (Lipton and Johnson 2001). Since all the patients were seen by different clinicians, the pattern could not have been evident to any of them even if the correct diagnosis had immediately been made in every case. Wagner et al. described nine categories of requirements for surveillance systems for potential bioterrorism outbreaks—several categories must have immediate electronic reporting to ensure early detection (Wagner et al. 2003).

HII would allow immediate electronic reporting of both relevant clinical events and laboratory results to public health (see Chap. 16). Not only would this be an invaluable aid in early detection of bioterrorism, it would also serve to improve the detection of the much more common naturally occurring disease outbreaks. In fact, early results from a number of electronic reporting demonstration projects show that disease outbreaks can routinely be detected sooner than was ever possible using the current system (Overhage et al. 2001). While early detection has been shown to be a key factor in reducing morbidity and mortality from bioterrorism (Kaufmann et al. 1997), it will also be extremely helpful in reducing the negative consequences from other disease outbreaks.

Finally, HII can substantially reduce health care costs. The inefficiencies and duplication in our present paper-based health care system are enormous. One study showed that the anticipated nationwide savings from implementing advanced **computerized physician order entry** (CPOE) systems in the outpatient environment would be $44 billion/year (Johnston et al. 2003), while a related study (Walker et al. 2004) estimated $78 billion more in savings from **health information exchange** (HIE) (for a total of $122 billion/ year). Substantial additional savings are possible in the inpatient setting—numerous hospitals have reported large net savings from implementation of EHRs. Another example, electronic prescribing, would not only reduce medication errors from transcription, but also drastically decrease the administrative costs of transferring prescription information from provider offices to pharmacies. Another analysis concluded that the total efficiency and patient safety savings from HII would be in range of $142–371 billion each year (Hillestad et al. 2005), and a survey of the recent literature found predominantly positive benefits from HII (Buntin et al. 2011). It is important to note that much of the savings depends not just on the widespread implementation of EHRs, but the effective interchange of this information to insure that the complete medical record for every patient is immediately available in every care setting.

Inasmuch as the current cost trend of health care is unsustainable, particularly in the face of our aging population, this issue is both important and urgent. Without comprehensive electronic information, any health care reform is largely guesswork in our current "black box" health care environment where the results of interventions often take years to understand. We do not currently have mechanisms for timely monitoring of health care outcomes to inform needed course corrections in any proposed reform. In essence, health care must be "informed" before it can be "reformed."

13.3   History

In the U.S., the first major report to address HII was issued by the Institute of Medicine of the National Academy of Sciences in 1991 (IOM 1991). This report, "The Computer-Based Patient Record," was the first in a series of national expert panel reports recommending transformation of the health care system from reliance on paper to electronic information management (see Chap. 12). In response to the IOM report, the Computer-based Patient Record Institute (CPRI), a private not-for-profit corporation, was formed for the purpose of facilitating the transition to computer-based records. A number of **community health information networks** (CHINs) were established around the country in an effort to coalesce the multiple community stakeholders in common efforts towards electronic information exchange. The Institute of Medicine updated its original report in 1997 (IOM 1997), again emphasizing the urgency to apply information technology to the information intensive field of health care.

However, most of the CHINs were not successful. Perhaps the primary reason for this was that the standards and technology were not yet ready for cost-effective community-based electronic HIE. Another problem was the focus on

availability of aggregated health information for secondary uses (e.g., policy development), rather than individual information for the direct provision of patient care. Also, there was neither a sense of extreme urgency nor were there substantial funds available to pursue these endeavors. However, at least one community (Indianapolis, Indiana) continued to move forward throughout this period and has now emerged as an a national example of the application of information technology to health care both in individual health care settings and throughout the community (McDonald et al. 2005).

Widespread attention was focused on this issue with the IOM report "To Err is Human" (IOM 1999). This landmark study documented the accumulated evidence of the high error rate in the medical care system, including an estimated 44,000–98,000 preventable deaths each year in hospitals alone. It has proven to be a milestone in terms of public awareness of the negative consequences of paper-based information management in health care. Along with the follow-up report, "Crossing the Quality Chasm" (IOM 2001), the systematic inability of the health care system to operate at a high degree of reliability has been thoroughly elucidated. These reports clearly place the blame on the system, not on the dedicated health care professionals who work in an environment without effective tools to promote quality and to minimize errors.

Several additional national expert panel reports have emphasized the IOM findings. In 2001, the President's Information Technology Advisory Committee (PITAC) issued a report entitled "Transforming Health Care Through Information Technology" (PITAC 2001). That same year, the Computer Science and Telecommunications Board of the National Research Council (NRC) released "Networking Health: Prescriptions for the Internet" (NRC 2001), which emphasized the potential for using the Internet to improve electronic exchange of health care information. Finally, the National Committee on Vital and Health Statistics (NCVHS) outlined a vision for building a National HII in its report, "Information for Health" (NCVHS 2001). NCVHS, a statutory advisory body to the U.S.

Department of Health and Human Services (DHHS), indicated that Federal government leadership was needed to facilitate further development of HII. In response, DHHS began an HII initiative, organizing a large national conference in 2003 to develop a consensus agenda to guide progress (DHHS 2003; Yasnoff et al. 2004).

In April, 2004, a Presidential Executive Order created the Office of the National Coordinator for Health Information Technology (ONC) in DHHS (see also Chap. 27). The initial efforts of ONC focused on promoting standards and certification to support adoption of EHRs by physicians and hospitals. It also promoted implementation of an "institution centric" model for HIE by **Regional Health Information Organizations** (**RHIOs**), wherein electronic records for a given patient stored at sites of past care episodes are located, assembled, and delivered in real time when needed for patient care. Four demonstration projects implementing this model were funded, but did not lead to sustainable systems.

In 2008, ONC was codified in law by the Health Information Technology for Economic and Clinical Health (HITECH) portion of the ARRA statute (Chap. 27). In addition, $20+ billion was appropriated including $2 billion for ONC and the remainder for payment of EHR incentives through Medicare and Medicaid to providers who achieve "Meaningful Use" of these systems. The ONC used its resources to establish **regional extension centers** (**RECs**) to subsidize assistance to providers adopting and using EHRs ($677 million), fund states to establish HIEs ($564 million), and initiate several research programs.

In December, 2010, the President's Council of Advisors on Science and Technology (PCAST) issued a report expressing concern about ONC strategy, specifically indicating that its HIE efforts through the states "*will not solve the fundamental need for data to be universally accessed, integrated, and understood while also being protected*" (PCAST 2010). Findings of a recent survey of HIEs "*call into question whether RHIOs in their current form can be self-sustaining and effective*"(Adler-Milstein et al. 2011). It is clear that more than two decades after the 1991

IOM report urging universal adoption of EHRs, the U.S. still lacks a clear and feasible roadmap leading to the widespread availability of comprehensive electronic patient information when and where needed. Despite much progress, no one in the U.S. as yet receives their medical care with the assured, immediate availability of all their records across multiple providers and provider organizations.

13.4 Requirements for HII

As with any informatics system development project, it is critical at the outset to understand the desired end result. In the case of a large, extremely complex system such as HII, this is especially important because there are many stakeholders with conflicting incentives and agendas, as well as challenging policy and operational issues. The ultimate goal is the "availability of comprehensive electronic patient records when and where needed." In transforming this goal into a design specification, it is critical to understand the issues and constraints that must be addressed. Then any proposed system design must demonstrate (on paper) how the objectives will be achieved within those limitations.

13.4.1 Privacy and Trust

The most important and overriding requirement of HII is privacy. Clearly, health records are very sensitive – perhaps the most sensitive personal information that exists. In addition to our natural desire to keep our medical information private, improper disclosure can lead to employment discrimination. Furthermore, failure to assure the privacy of records will naturally result in patient unwillingness to disclose important personal details to their providers – or even to avoid seeking care at all. In addition to the contents of the records, the very existence of certain records (e.g., a visit to psychiatric hospital) is sensitive even if no details are available. Therefore, extraordinary care must be taken to ensure that information is protected from unauthorized disclosure and use.

In general, U.S. Federal law (the HIPAA Privacy Rule as introduced in Chap. 10) requires patient consent for disclosure and use of medical records. However, consent is not required for record release for treatment, payment, and health care operations. These "TPO" exceptions have, as a practical matter, allowed health care organizations to utilize medical records extensively while bypassing patient consent. The organization that holds medical information has sole discretion to make the decision whether a proposed disclosure is or is not a TPO exception. Until recently, TPO disclosures did not even need to be recorded, effectively preventing discovery of improper disclosures. Even under the recent HITECH legislation that requires records of TPO disclosures, such records are not automatically available to the subjects of the disclosures. The net effect is that individuals not only lack control over the dissemination of their medical records, but are not even informed when they are disclosed beyond where they were created.

It seems appropriate to question whether this disclosure regime is adequate for electronic health records. The general public understands that making electronic patient records available for good and laudable purposes simultaneously makes them more available for evil and nefarious purposes, thereby necessitating higher levels of protection to avoid abuses. Assigning decision-making for disclosure of personal medical records to anyone other than the patient or the patient's representative inherently erodes trust. In essence, the patient is being told, "we are going to decide for you where your medical records should go because we know what's in your interest better than you do." Patients may wonder why, if a given disclosure is in their interest, their consent would not be sought. Furthermore, failing to seek such consent inevitably leads to suspicion that the disclosure is in fact not in the patient's interest, but rather in the interest of the organization deciding that the records should be released.

The concern about privacy of medical records is not at all theoretical or insignificant. In two recent consumer surveys, 13–17 % of consumers indicated that they already employ "information hiding" behaviors with respect to their medical records (CHCF 2005; Harris Interactive 2007). This includes activities such as obtaining laboratory tests under an assumed name or seeking out-of-state treatment to conceal an illness from their primary care provider. Even assuming that everyone engaged in such behaviors was willing to admit to them in such a survey, this represents a substantial proportion of consumers who would, at a minimum, refuse to participate in an electronic medical information system that did not provide them with control over their own records. Of even greater concern, such a large percentage of consumers would likely organize and use their political power to halt the deployment and operation of such a system. Indeed, it was a much smaller percentage of concerned citizens that, citing the threat to privacy, convinced Congress to repeal the provisions in the original HIPAA legislation calling for a unique medical identifier for all U.S. residents (see Chap. 10).

In view of this, there are those who argue that all decisions about release of patient records need to be entrusted to the patient (with rare exceptions, such as mental incompetence). They also suggest that attention to these concerns may be especially important for enabling HII, because patients must trust that their records are not being misused in such a system. Some argue that patients are not sufficiently informed to make such decisions and may make mistakes that are harmful to them, whereas others believe that the negative consequences of delegating this decision-making to others than the patient could be much greater. Advocates of patient control of medical information argue, by analogy, that society has accepted that individuals retain the right to make decisions about how their own money is spent, even though this can lead to adverse consequences when those decisions prove to be unwise. In considering these issues, it should be noted that prior to the 2002 HIPAA Privacy Rule that established the TPO exceptions, both law and practice had always required patient consent for all access to medical records. While acknowledging the need for consumer education about decisions relating to release of medical records, patient-control advocates believe that the same freedom and personal responsibility that applies to an individual's financial decisions may need to be applied to the medical records domain. These medical information privacy policy issues may be even more urgent in the context of the enhanced trust necessary when seeking to implement an effective and accepted HII.

13.4.2 Stakeholder Cooperation

To ensure the availability of comprehensive patient records, all health care stakeholders that generate such records must consistently make them available. While it would be ideal if such cooperation were voluntary, assuring long-term collaboration of competing health care stakeholders is problematic. Indeed, only a handful of communities have succeeded in developing and maintaining an organization that includes the active participation of the majority of health care providers. Even in these communities, the system could be disrupted at any time by the arbitrary withdrawal of one or more participants. The unfortunate reality is that health care stakeholders are often quite reluctant to share patient records, fearing loss of competitive advantage.

Therefore, some would argue that mandating health care stakeholder participation in a system for sharing electronic patient records is highly desirable, since it would result in consistently more comprehensive individual records. Since imposing a new requirement on health care stakeholders would be a daunting political challenge, such an approach would be most feasible as part of an existing mandate. Proponents of this approach have noted that one such mandate that could be utilized is the HIPAA Privacy Rule itself, which requires all providers to respond to patient requests for their own records (U.S. 45 CFR 164.524(a)). Furthermore, if patients request their records in electronic form, and they are available in electronic form, this regulation also requires that they be delivered in electronic form. Although not well known, this latter provision is included in the original HIPAA Privacy Rule (U.S. 45 CFR 164.524(c)(2)), and has been reinforced by HITECH. It is also being promoted by

the more recent "blue button" initiative that seeks to allow patients to retrieve their own records electronically (Chopra et al. 2010).

Advocates argue that patient control, in addition to being an effective approach to privacy, could also serve to ensure ongoing, consistent health care stakeholder participation. Of course, in order for this approach to be practical, the rights of patients to electronic copies of their records under HIPAA would need to be enforced. Such enforcement has to date been inconsistent, and, until recently, exclusively dependent on the Office of Civil Rights at DHHS (since patients do not have a private right of action). Under HITECH, state attorneys general may also bring legal action, which may be helpful in improving compliance.

13.4.3 Ensuring Information in Electronic Form

It is self-evident that the electronic exchange of health information cannot occur if the information itself is not in electronic form. While medication information and laboratory results are already predominantly electronic, patient records, particularly for office-based physicians, are not. While estimates vary, it is clear that the majority of office-based physicians still do not utilize EHR systems, even though there is a major effort to incentivize the adoption of such records (see Chaps. 12 and 27). Furthermore most of those who do have electronic records utilize systems with limited capabilities (DesRoches et al. 2008).

The major obstacle for physician adoption of EHRs is not merely cost, as is often cited, but the very unfavorable ongoing cost/benefit ratio. Most of the benefits of EHRs in physician offices accrue not to the physician, but to other stakeholders. In one study, 89 % of the economic benefit was attributed to other stakeholders (Hersh 2004). It is unreasonable to expect physicians to shoulder 100 % of the cost of systems while accruing only 11 % of the benefits.

While the substantial physician subsidies in HITECH ($44,000–$63,750) are helpful (Chap. 27), they do not cover the majority of costs for physician EHR systems. This is particularly evident when including the substantial conversion costs related to reduced revenue from lost productivity during the transition from paper to electronic records. In addition, the HITECH subsidies are one time only, while the costs of EHRs continue indefinitely for physicians. To assure EHR adoption by the vast majority of practices, many observers believe it will be necessary to provide permanent reimbursement and/or other offsetting benefits to allow physicians to recoup their costs. At the very least, any proposed approach to building a sustainable HII will be more effective if it includes mechanisms that result in a favorable cost/benefit ratio for physician EHRs.

As for hospitals, they also have not uniformly adopted EHRs. However, hospitals have a more substantial economic incentive to do so, since reducing their costs improves financial performance under the **diagnosis-related groups (DRG)** reimbursement system that pays a fixed amount for a specific condition. While it remains to be seen if the HITECH incentives for hospitals are sufficient to induce widespread adoption, it appears that their effectiveness will be substantially greater than for office-based physicians. In addition, once patients are admitted to the hospital, coordinating their records is largely an internal problem that cannot be greatly aided by external HII. Furthermore, the large majority of health care encounters do not involve hospitals, and therefore HII should focus primarily on the outpatient environment.

It is important to note that EHRs alone, even if adopted by all health care providers, are a necessary but not sufficient condition for achieving HII. Indeed, each EHR simply converts an existing paper "silo" of information to electronic form. These provider-based systems manage the *provider* information on the patient in question, but do not have *all* the information for each patient. To achieve the goal of availability of comprehensive patient information, there must also be an efficient and cost-effective mechanism to aggregate the scattered records of each patient from all their various providers. Major gains in quality and efficiency of care will be attainable

only through HII that ensures the availability of every patient's comprehensive record when and where needed.

13.4.4 Financial Sustainability

There are three fundamental approaches that can be used individually or in combination to provide long-term financial sustainability for HII: (1) public subsidy; (2) leveraging anticipated future health care cost savings; or (3) leveraging new value created. The first approach has been advocated by those who assert, with some justification, that HII represents a public good that benefits everyone. They compare HII to other publicly available infrastructure, such as roads, and suggest that taxation is an appropriate funding mechanism. Of course, new taxes are consistently unpopular and politically undesirable, and other key infrastructures such as public utilities and the Internet, although regulated, are funded through user fees rather than taxation. Note, however, that at least two states (Maryland and Vermont) are using this mechanism to help fund their HII.

The most common approach suggested for long-term HII sustainability is leveraging anticipated health care cost savings. This is based on the substantial and growing body of evidence that the availability of more comprehensive electronic patient records to providers results in higher quality and lower cost care (AHRQ 2006; Buntin et al. 2011). Some of the best examples include large, mostly closed health care systems such as Kaiser, Group Health and the Veterans Administration, where the conversion of records into electronic form over time has been consistently associated with both cost savings and better care. While the case for HII reducing health care costs is compelling, the distribution and timing of those savings is difficult to predict. In addition, cost savings to the health care system means revenue losses to one or more stakeholders – clearly an undesirable result from their perspective. Finally, the allocation of savings for a given population of patients is unknown, with the result that organizations are reluctant to make specific financial commitments that could be larger than their own expected benefits.

The final but least frequently mentioned path to financial sustainability of HII is utilizing the new value created by the availability of comprehensive electronic information. While it is widely recognized that this information will be extremely valuable for a wide variety of purposes, this option has remained largely unexplored. One example of such new value is the potential reduction in cost for delivering laboratory results to ordering physicians. The expenses borne by individual laboratories for their own infrastructure providing this essential service can be greatly reduced by a single uniform community infrastructure providing electronic delivery to physicians through one mechanism. Another example is availability of medical information for research – both to find eligible subjects for clinical trials and to utilize the data itself for research queries. While this latter application has the potential to defray a substantial portion of the costs of HII, it requires efficient mechanisms for both searching data and recording and maintaining patient consent that have not generally been incorporated into HII systems.

Perhaps the most lucrative HII revenue source lies in the development of innovative applications that rely on the underlying information to deliver compelling value to consumers and other health care stakeholders. For example, HII allows the delivery of timely and accurate reminders and alerts to patients for recommended preventive services, needed medication refills, and other medically related events of immediate interest to patients and their families. It also would allow deployment of applications that assist consumers automatically with management of their chronic diseases. Microsoft recognized and identified such an "application ecosystem" as the ultimate business model that could support HII when it introduced its HealthVault™ personal health record system (Microsoft 2012). Utilizing new value to finance HII avoids the prediction and allocation problems inherent in attempts to leverage expected health care cost savings, with the added incentive that any such savings would fully accrue to whoever achieves them.

13.4.5 Community Focus

Most observers believe that successful HII must be focused on the community. An essential element in HII is trust, which is inherently local. Furthermore, health care itself is predominantly local, since the vast majority of medical care for residents of a given community is provided in that community. Indeed, people traveling away from home who are injured or become ill inevitably will return home at their earliest opportunity if their condition permits (and does not resolve quickly). Since medical care is predominantly local, creating a system that delivers comprehensive electronic patient information in a community solves the overwhelming majority of information needs in that community. While movement of health information over long distances has some value and ultimately must be addressed to assure completeness of records, its contribution to a total solution is marginal.

The lack of any examples of working HII in communities larger than about ten million people provides additional evidence of the need for local focus. Keeping the scope of such projects relatively small also increases their likelihood of success by reducing complexity, thereby avoiding the huge increases in failure rates of extremely large-scale IT projects. For example, the need for local focus was a key part in planning for HII in the U.K., which was divided into five regions of approximately 12 million people in an attempt to facilitate addressing HII development through multiple systems, each working at a feasible scale (Granger 2004).

In thinking about HII, analogies are often made to the international financial system that efficiently transfers and makes funds available to individuals anywhere in the world. However, it is often forgotten that these financial institutions, that also are heavily dependent on trust, began as "building and loan funds" in small communities designed to share financial resources among close neighbors. It took many decades of building trust before large-scale national and international financial institutions emerged.

13.4.6 Governance and Organizational Issues

Trust is arguably the most important element in considering the appropriate governance for HII. Even in a system where patients exert full control over their own records, the organization that operates the HII must earn the full faith and confidence of consumers for the security, integrity, and protection of the records, as well as ensuring that records are appropriately available for purposes that consumers specify. Furthermore, the organization ideally must be devoid of any biases or hidden agendas that would favor one category of health care stakeholders over another, or favor specific stakeholders within a given category.

None of the existing health care stakeholders seem well suited to meet the trust requirement. Many argue that government cannot operate an HII because it is inherently not trusted with sensitive personal records, and furthermore needs to assume the role of providing regulatory oversight for whatever organization does take the HII responsibility. Similarly, it seems problematic for employers to be responsible for the HII since one of the primary concerns of consumers is to avoid disclosing sensitive medical information to their employers. Health plans and insurers are typically not trusted by consumers because their incentives are not aligned–they have a financial incentive to deny care, which is a natural concern to consumers. Hospitals are in competition with each other and therefore are not in a good position to cooperate in a long-term HII effort. Physicians are the most trusted health care stakeholders, from a consumer perspective, but are not organized in a way to facilitate the creation of HII. Furthermore, they are also in competition with each other and, most importantly, do not generally have the informatics capabilities necessary for such a complex endeavor.

Therefore, many believe that an independent (perhaps entirely new) organization is needed to operate HII in communities. This organization would have no direct connections to existing health care stakeholders and therefore would be unbiased. Its sole function would be to protect

and make available comprehensive electronic patient records on behalf of consumers. Such an independent organization would also ideally facilitate cooperation among all existing stakeholders, who would know that the HII activity was completely neutral and designed primarily to serve consumers.

13.5 Architecture for HII

13.5.1 Institution-Centric Architecture

With rare exceptions, most existing HII systems have chosen an institution-centric approach to data storage, leaving patient records wherever they are created (Fig. 13.2). Although records are not stored centrally, there is a need to maintain at least a central index of where information can be found for a particular patient; without such an index, finding information about each patient would require queries to every possible source of medical information worldwide – clearly an impractical approach. When a given patient's record is requested, the index is used to generate queries to the locations where information is stored. The responses to those queries are then aggregated (in real time) to produce the patient's complete record. After the patient encounter, the new data is entered into the clinician's EHR system and another pointer (to that system) is added to the index so it will be queried (in addition to all the other prior locations) next time that patient's record is requested.

While this architecture is appealing to health care stakeholders because they continue to "control" the records they generate, one can argue that it fails to meet several key requirements, does not scale effectively, and is complex and expensive to operate. The most critical requirement that is not addressed by this architecture is searching the data, e.g., to find all patients with a cholesterol level above 300. To do such a search, the records of every patient must be assembled from their various locations and examined one at a time. This is known as a sequential search, and has a very long completion time that increases linearly

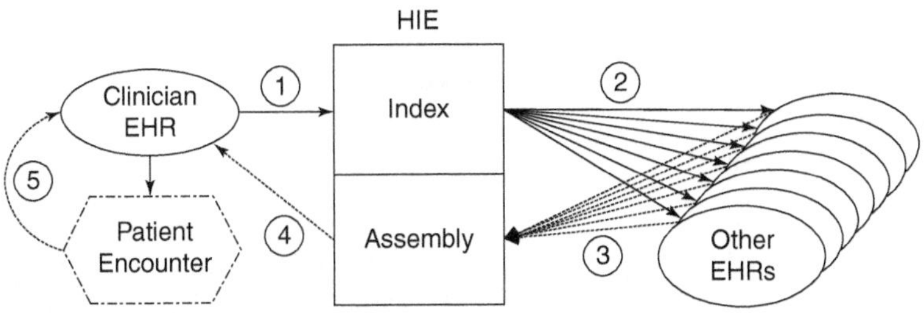

Fig. 13.2 Institution-centric HII architecture. *1.* The clinician EHR requests prior patient records from the HIE; this clinician's EHR is added to the index for future queries for this patient (if not already present). *2.* Queries are sent to EHRs at all sites of prior care recorded in the HIE index. *3.* EHRs at each prior site of care return records for that patient to the HIE; the HIE must wait for all responses. *4.* The returned records are assembled and sent to the clinician EHR; any inconsistencies or incompatibilities between records must be resolved in real time. *5.* After the care episode, the new information is stored in the clinician EHR only (© Health Record Banking Alliance, 2013. Used with permission)

with the size of the population. For example, in a modest-sized HIE with 500,000 patients, assuming retrieval and processing of each patient's records requires just 2 s (a very low estimate), each such search would take at least 12 days (1 million seconds). Furthermore, every such search would require that each provider record system connected to the HIE retrieve and transmit all its information – a very substantial computing and communications burden (that also increases the risk of interception of information). In standard database systems, impractical sequential search times are reduced by pre-indexing the contents of the records. However, such pre-indexing would in essence create a central repository of indices that could be used to reconstruct most of the original data, and therefore is inconsistent with this architectural approach.

It may be argued that the searches could themselves be distributed to the provider systems, and then the results aggregated into a coherent result. However, this approach also fails for this architecture because individual patient records are incomplete in each system. Therefore, searches that require multiple items of patient data (e.g., patients with chest pain who have taken a certain medication in the past year), will produce anomalous results unless all the instances of the relevant data for a given patient are in a single provider system (i.e., if one system finds a patient with chest pain, but without any indication of the medication of interest [which is in another provider's system], that patient will not be reported

as satisfying the conditions). It is possible to limit searches to a single criterion and then combine the results from each such search to generate a correct result. However, this would mean that such searches would require multiples of the completion time for a single criterion (e.g., 12 days ×2=24 days for the two criteria example), making the retrieval times and processing burdens even more untenable.

In addition to the scaling issues for this architecture related to searching, there is also a problem with response time for assembling a patient record. When a given patient record is requested, the locations where the patient has available records are found using the central index. Then, a **query-response cycle** is required for each location where patient records are available. Following completion of the query-response cycles, all the information obtained must be integrated into a comprehensive record and made available to the requestor. While the query-response cycles can all be done in parallel, the final integration of results must wait for the slowest response. As the number of connected systems increases, so does the probability of a slow (or absent) response from one of them when queried for patient records. In addition, more systems mean more processing time to integrate multiple sources of information into one coherent record. Thus, the response time will become slower as the number of connected systems increases.

The institution-centric architecture also introduces high levels of operational complexity.

Fig. 13.3 Example of a
Network Operations Center
(NOC) (Reproduced with
permission from Evans
Consoles Corporation)

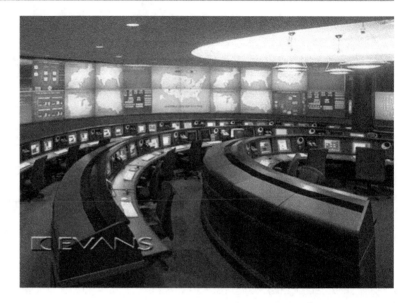

Since the completeness of retrieval of a given patient's records is dependent on the availability of all the systems that contain information about that patient, ongoing real-time monitoring of all connected information sources is essential. This translates into a requirement for a 24×7 **network operations center** (**NOC**), that constantly monitors the operational status of every medical information system and is staffed with senior IT personnel who can immediately troubleshoot and correct any problems detected (Fig. 13.3). Even with modest system failure rates (e.g., 1/1000), a community with thousands of EHRs will typically have a handful of systems that are unresponsive to queries for patient records and require immediate expert attention to restore to full operation. The cost of this around-the-clock monitoring is very substantial, since a staff of at least five full-time network engineers is required to assure that at least one person is always available for every shift 7 days a week.

In addition to the cost of the NOC, every EHR system in an institution-centric model must always be able to respond to queries in real-time. In addition to the cost of assuring 24×7 operation of all these systems, which will be extremely problematic for physician offices, every system will need additional hardware, software, and telecommunications capabilities to simultaneously support such queries while also serving its local

users. Clearly, the transaction volumes generated will be substantial, since each patient's records will be queried whenever they receive care at any location. Contrast this to a central repository model where the information from a care episode is transmitted once to the repository and no further queries to the source system are ever needed. This analysis has recently been confirmed by a simulation study of the institution-centric architecture demonstrating that both the transaction volume and probability of incomplete records (from missing data due to a malfunctioning network node) increase exponentially with the average number of sites where each patient's data is located (Lapsia et al. 2012).

13.5.2 Patient-Centric Architecture (Health Record Banking)

Health record banking is a patient-centric approach to developing community HII that both addresses the key requirements and can overcome the challenges that have stymied current efforts (Yasnoff 2006). A **health record bank** (**HRB**) is defined as "an independent organization that provides a secure electronic repository for storing and maintaining an individual's lifetime health and medical records from multiple sources and assures that the individual always

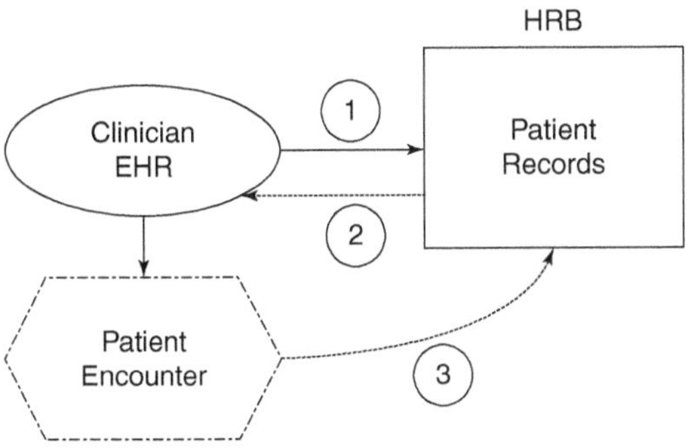

HRB

Fig. 13.4 Patient-centric HII architecture. *1*. The clinician EHR requests prior patient records from the HRB. *2*. The prior patient records are immediately sent to the clinician EHR. *3*. After the care episode, the new information is stored in the clinician EHR and sent to the HRB; any inconsistencies or incompatibilities with prior records in the HRB need to be resolved before that patient's records are requested again (but not in real time). (Note: this process is repeated whenever care is provided, resulting in the accumulation of each patients's records from all sources in the HRB) (© Health Record Banking Alliance, 2013. Used with permission)

has complete control over who accesses their information" (HRBA 2008).

Using a community HRB to provide patient information for medical care is straightforward (Fig. 13.4). Prior to seeking care (or at the time of care in an emergency), the patient gives permission for the caregiver to access his/her HRB account records (either all or part) through a secure Internet portal. The provider then accesses (and optionally, downloads) the records through a similar secure web site. When the care episode is completed, the caregiver then transmits any new information generated to the HRB to be added to the account-holder's lifetime health record. The updated record is then immediately available for subsequent care.

The health record banking concept has been evolving for nearly two decades since it was initially proposed (Szolovits et al. 1994). The term "health information bank" was introduced in 1997 in the U.K. (Dodd 1997), and was subsequently described as the "bank of health"(Ramsaroop and Ball 2000). A legal analysis of the implications of a "health record trust" was published in 2002 (Kostyack 2002), an Italian system known as the "health current account" was described in 2004

(Saccavini and Greco 2004), and the "health record bank" concept was described by Dyson in 2005 (Dyson 2005). In 2006, a Heritage Foundation policy paper endorsed health record banking (Haislmaier 2006), additional papers described HRBs in more detail (Ball and Gold 2006; Shabo 2006), the non-profit Health Record Banking Alliance was formed (HRBA 2006), the State of Washington endorsed the concept after a 16-month study (State of Washington 2006), and the non-profit Dossia consortium was formed by several large employers to implement and operate an HRB for their employees (Dossia 2006). In 2007, the Information Technology and Innovation Foundation recommended that the health record banking approach be used to build the U.S. HII (Castro 2007), while Gold and Ball described the "health record banking imperative" (Gold and Ball 2007). That same year, both Microsoft and Google introduced patient-controlled medical record repositories. In 2009, three pilot HRBs were funded by the State of Washington, another one was started in Rotterdam, Netherlands,[1]and the role of HRBs in protecting privacy was described (Kendall 2009). The HRB concept, although not always named as such, is now appearing with greater frequency in articles discussing the need for comprehensive EHRs (Steinbrook 2008; Mandl and Kohane 2008; Kidd 2008; Miller et al. 2009; Krist and Woolf 2011).

13.5.2.1 Patient Control Ensures Privacy and Stakeholder Cooperation

In an HRB, everything is done with *consumer consent*, with account-holders controlling their copy of all their records and deciding who gets to see any or all of it. This protects privacy (since each consumer sets their own customized privacy policy), promotes trust, and ensures stakeholder cooperation since all holders of medical information must provide it when requested by the patient (Kendall 2009). Of course, the operations of an HRB must be open and transparent with

---

[1]http://webwereld.nl/nieuws/54340/rotterdam-start-eigen-versie-elektronisch-pati--ntendossier.html. Posted January 14, 2009. (accessed 21 Apr 2013).

independent auditing of privacy practices. World-class state-of-the-art computer security is needed to protect the HRB, which will be a natural target for hackers. However, this is no different from any other system design for HII, even if the information is not stored centrally, since by definition any such system must be capable of immediately assembling a complete patient record on request.

Natural concerns arise from the ability of the patient to suppress any or all of their HRB account information, which could lead to misdiagnosis and dangerous treatment. This capability could be abused by patients who, for example, may seek multiple prescriptions for controlled substances for the purpose of diversion for illegal sale. With respect to the possibility of medical errors resulting from incomplete information, the patient would be clearly and unmistakably warned about this when choosing not to disclose any specific information (e.g., "Failure to disclose any of your medical information may lead to serious medical problems, including your death"). The expectation is that few people will choose to do this, particularly after such a warning. However, as noted earlier, 13–17 % of patients already engage in this practice, leading many observers to conclude that the general public may not be comfortable with a system that provides easy access to their records unless they are in control of such access. This issue ultimately becomes one of public policy and may also be a subject of discussion between the doctor and the patient (i.e., the doctor will want to be assured by the patient that all information is being provided). Clearly, physicians should not be liable for the consequences of the patient's choice to withhold information.

With respect to patients who use their power to withhold information as a way to facilitate improper or illegal activity, there is clearly an overriding public policy concern. For example, in the case of controlled substances, it may be necessary to report to the physician (or, if legislatively mandated, to regulatory authorities) whenever a patient suppresses any information about controlled substance prescriptions. The information itself would still be under the patient's control, but the physician would be alerted with a notice such as "some controlled substance prescription information has been withheld at the patient's request." There may be other situations where such warnings are needed.

13.5.2.2 Assuring the Information Is in Electronic Form and Complies with Standards

HRBs can provide ongoing incentives for EHR adoption by clinicians. To ensure electronic information, all providers must have EHRs. As indicated earlier, since most of the economic benefits of office-based EHRs do not accrue to providers, high levels of outpatient EHR adoption will most likely require some kind of ongoing compensation or value for their costs. For physicians who already have EHR systems, a per-encounter or per-month payment system can be used. Those physicians who do not currently have EHRs could receive no-cost Internet-accessible EHR systems (at HRB expense) with the understanding that information from patient encounters will be automatically transferred to the HRB. "Meaningful Use" of those EHRs is assured and can be easily audited on an ongoing basis since the information from each patient encounter must be deposited in the HRB. It is even possible to link reimbursement for medical services to HRB deposits – i.e., providers would not be paid unless the medical record information generated from those services is transmitted to an HRB. This makes sense economically, as the value of medical services is greatly limited if the information about patients is not readily available for their ongoing care.

HRBs also serve to ensure compliance with data standards, both initially and on an ongoing basis. Clearly, any EHR provided through the HRB can, by definition, transmit information back to the HRB in a standard format (since the HRB only provides systems that can do so). For physicians who already have EHRs, HRB reimbursements for those systems naturally require standard transactions to be used to send encounter data to the HRB. Over time, higher levels of encoding of medical information can be promoted through the gradual introduction of more stringent standards requirements (with plenty of lead time to allow for system upgrades).

Compliance with such changes in standards can also be assured through the direct relationship to reimbursement.

13.5.2.3 Business Model

Health record banking has advantages on both the cost and revenue sides of the business model; the cost is lower and the revenue opportunities greater. Because of the lower operating costs and additional functionality for searching records, one can envision a variety of business models for HRBs that do not depend on public subsidies or attempt to capture any health care savings, but are solely funded through new value created for consumers and other stakeholders (HRBA 2012).

Due to the simplicity of HRB operations, the cost is substantially less than an equivalent institution-centric architecture. For an HRB, providing access at the point of care only involves a single retrieval from the bank's repository of records. In an institution-centric model, the records for a given patient are located at an arbitrary number of dispersed sites, and must be assembled in real-time and integrated into a comprehensive record before they can be used for patient care. Not only is this process of assembly complex, time-consuming, and prone to error, it necessitates, as noted above, the creation of a fully staffed 24×7 NOC to monitor the availability of all information sources as well as troubleshoot and correct those that are malfunctioning.

The estimated cost for the NOC in an institution-centric model is substantial. For example, given a population of 1,000,000, at least 1,000 systems would need monitoring (1 for every 1,000 patients). Assuming a reasonable failure rate for fully functional query connectivity to each system of once/year (representing a **mean time between failures [MTBF]** of over 8,700 h), there would be an average of 2.73 failures/day or 0.91 failures per 8-h shift that would need troubleshooting attention. A minimum staff for the NOC would be 1 person 24×7; given 21 shifts/week plus leeway for vacations and sick leave, this would require at least 5 full-time equivalent staff costing about $200,000 each including equipment, overhead and fringe benefits. Assuming an additional $500,000/year for hardware and software to operate the institution-centric system (over and above the data repository needed for an HRB) yields an annual cost of $1.5 million or $1.50/person/year. This would add nearly 20 % for the institution-centric model to the estimated $8/person/year needed to operate an HRB (Kaelber et al. 2008).

Beyond this, the additional costs imposed in the institution-centric model for each connected EHR for additional hardware, software, telecommunications capability, and additional operational expenses to maintain 24×7 system availability must also be included. Even if such costs were only a very modest $1,000/year/system (less than $100/month), this would result in an additional $1,000,000 or $1/person/year. Adding this to the $1.50/person/year for the NOC gives a total estimated cost of $2.50/person/year, resulting in over 30 % higher costs for the institution-centric model than a basic HRB. Added to this would be the costs and complexity of establishing and maintaining data sharing agreements among all the entities, which would be substantial.

On the revenue side, the inability of the institution-centric model to efficiently search the data impedes generation of potentially significant revenue from consumer applications and research. For example, generating medication refill reminders to consumers alone could potentially yield $20/year of revenue per consumer, paid by pharmaceutical firms as a completely ethical and appropriate mechanism to improve both compliance and their own bottom line. Even if only 20 % of consumers used this service, potential average revenue from this application alone would be $4/person/year, half the estimated HRB cost.

Another key source of revenue could be targeted advertising to consumers (based on the information in their accounts), which could generate an estimated $6/person/year or more. Consumers would also be allowed to opt-out of such advertising by paying the $6/year. To protect privacy, advertisers would not be allowed to identify anyone viewing their ads unless the consumer voluntarily provided contact information.

Revenue from searching the data (with consumer permission) could also be substantial. Finding eligible subjects for clinical trials is quite

Table 13.1 Comparison of the institution-centric and patient-centric approaches to Health Information Infrastructure

Issue	Institution-centric	Patient-centric (HRB)
Cooperation needed	Extensive; community-wide	Unifying; HIPAA mandates records on patient request
Organizational complexity	High; ongoing collaboration of multiple competing stakeholders necessary	Low; HRB is neutral and independent of all stakeholders
Privacy	Patient consent difficult to implement; many complex data sharing agreements needed	Simple; patients in control of all access to their own records; consent easy to implement
Startup funding	Substantial (due to high complexity)	Minimal
Business model	Complex; no clear approach has emerged	Flexible; many options possible funded by patients/payers/purchasers
Clinician EHR incentives	Not included	Easy to include
Clinician EHR processing burden	Extensive; incoming query each time current patients seen anywhere	Minimal; information deposited once in HRB; no incoming queries
Interoperability (data standards)	Compliance voluntary	Compliance can be assured with financial incentives
IT system design	Complex; requires queries to multiple entities, real-time reconciliation of inconsistencies, and NOC	Simple; no secondary queries or real-time reconciliation needed; NOC unnecessary
Completeness of patient records	Requires data source queries each time a patient's records are requested; all must respond for completeness	Comprehensive data available at all times for each patient

expensive, and could be greatly facilitated by sending electronic invitations directly to qualified patients identified through an HRB (to protect privacy, the identities of the recipients of the invitations could be hidden from the researchers). Also, anonymized reports from searches of HRB data would be very valuable to medical researchers, public health officials, and policymakers. Reasonable fees for such reports would therefore be another important revenue source. While it is difficult to estimate the magnitude of this revenue, it seems likely that it would be at least a few dollars per patient each year.

Finally, the low cost of HRBs allows them to subsidize outpatient EHRs. To cover fully the expense of office-based EHRs costs about $10/person/year. This is based on a cost of $5,000/year/physician for an internet-accessible EHR (a high estimate) allocated to 500 people (300 million U.S. population divided by 600,000 physicians needing EHRs). Given the strong revenue potential for HRBs, this additional $10/person/year expense could be included in operating costs over and above the expected $8/person/year anticipated as baseline expenditures. There are several key advantages if the HRB assumes these costs: (1) it promotes much higher levels of EHR adoption, thereby ensuring that more patient information is electronic; (2) it allows the HRB to ensure that EHRs submit data using standards (by subsidizing only compliant EHRs); (3) it provides a mechanism for ensuring updates to standards as they are needed; and (4) it creates a mutually beneficial relationship with clinicians that facilitates their cooperation as a marketing channel for HRB (by offering no-cost accounts to their patients). While the additional $10/person/year for EHRs is a substantial cost burden, revenue opportunities from value-added applications, consumer advertising, and research could more than cover the resultant total operating costs of $18/person/year without the need to quantify or capture any potential health care savings.

Table 13.1 summarizes the characteristics of the institution-centric approach to HII compared to the patient-centric (health record bank) model. The patient-centric model is simpler and more straightforward, and deals directly with the issue of privacy by putting patients in control of their own information. Interoperability is much more easily accomplished in the patient-centric model since standards compliance can be reinforced with financial incentives, and reconciliation of inconsistencies between records need not be real-time. The patient centric approach is financially sustainable with a variety of business models, and can provide powerful incentives to clinicians to acquire EHRs. Finally, the patient-centric model avoids the substantial processing burden on clinician EHRs from queries each time any patient whose record is stored is seen anywhere.

13.6 HII Evaluation

The last element in the strategy for promoting a complex and lengthy project such as the HII is evaluation to both gauge progress and define a complete system. Evaluation measures should have several key features. First, they should be sufficiently sensitive so that their values change at a reasonable rate (a measure that only changes value after 5 years will not be particularly helpful). Second, the measures must be comprehensive enough to reflect activities that affect most of the stakeholders and activities needing change. This ensures that efforts in every area will be reflected in improved measures. Third, the measures must be meaningful to policymakers. Fourth, periodic determinations of the current values of the measures should be easy so that the measurement process does not detract from the actual work. Finally, the totality of the measures must reflect the desired end state so that when the goals for all the measures are attained, the project is complete.

A number of different types or dimensions of measures for HII progress are possible. Aggregate measures assess HII progress over the entire nation. Examples include the percentage of the population covered by an HII and the percentage of health care personnel who utilize EHRs. Another type of measure is based on the setting of

care. Progress in implementation of EHR systems in the inpatient, outpatient, long-term care, home, and community environments could clearly be part of an HII measurement program. Yet another dimension is health care functions performed using information systems support, including, for example, registration systems, decision support, and CPOE. Finally, it is also important to assess progress with respect to the semantic encoding of EHRs. Clearly, there is a progression from the electronic exchange of images of documents, where the content is only readable by the end user viewing the image, to fully encoded EHRs where all the information is indexed and accessible in machine-readable form using standards.

Sadly, the evidence is now overwhelming that U.S. HIEs in their current form are, with rare exceptions, not succeeding. Labkoff and Yasnoff described four criteria for the quantitative evaluation of HII progress in communities: (1) completeness of information, (2) degree of usage, (3) types of usage, and (4) financial sustainability (Labkoff and Yasnoff 2007). Using these criteria, four of the most advanced community HII projects in the U.S. achieved scores of 60–78 % (on a 0–100 scale), indicating substantial additional work was required before the HII could be viewed as complete.

The 2010 PCAST report stated, *"HIEs have drawbacks that make them ill-suited as the basis for a national health information architecture"* (PCAST 2010). Among those drawbacks, PCAST cited administrative burdens (data sharing agreements to ensure stakeholder cooperation), financial sustainability, interoperability, and an architecture that cannot be scaled effectively. The most recent (Adler-Milstein et al. 2011) of a series of surveys of HIEs (Adler-Milstein et al. 2008, 2009) found only 13 HIEs in the U.S. (covering 3 % of hospitals and 0.9 % of physician practices) capable of meeting Stage 1 Meaningful Use criteria, and even those metrics by no means ensure the availability of comprehensive electronic patient information when and where needed. Of those, only six were reported to be financially viable. More importantly, *none* of the HIEs surveyed had the capabilities of a comprehensive system as specified by an expert panel.

Overall, the current approaches to building HII consistently fail to meet one or more of the requirements described above: privacy, stakeholder cooperation, ensuring fully electronic information, financial sustainability, and independent governance. While these problems are highly interdependent, it is useful to consider them in the context of the decisions that communities have made about HII architecture, privacy, and business model that, while appearing attractive to stakeholders in the short term, have so far been largely unsuccessful. Exploration and large-scale testing of alternative approaches that directly address the requirements, such as health record banking, seem both necessary and increasingly urgent.

13.7 Conclusion

While progress has been made and efforts are continuing, successful development and operation of comprehensive HII systems remains a largely unsolved problem. The extensive focus on building HII systems has greatly improved our understanding of the requirements, barriers, and challenges, as well as potential solutions. Despite the daunting obstacles, the benefits of HII are sufficiently urgent and compelling to ensure major ongoing work in this domain. Through these activities, the HII path to comprehensive electronic patient records when and where needed is becoming clearer, and substantial advances are likely in the next few years.

Suggested Readings

Aanestad, M., & Jensen, T.B. (2011). Building nationwide information infrastructures in healthcare through modular implementation strategies. *Journal of Strategic Information Systems, 20*(2), 161–176. An interesting study comparing two large-scale HII implementations, one of which failed, suggesting that both a gradual transition of the installed base and a modular approach are needed for success.

Adler-Milstein, J., Bates, D.W., & Jha, A.K. (2011). A survey of health information exchange organizations in the United States: Implications for meaningful use. *Annals of Internal Medicine, 154*, 666–671. The recent comprehensive survey of 179 HIEs that found that none of them had comprehensive capabilities and concluded that the current development path was unlikely to succeed.

Castro D. (2007) *Improving health care: Why a dose of IT may be just what the doctor ordered*. Information Technology and Innovation Foundation. Available at http://www.itif.org/publications/improving-health-care-why-dose-it-may-be-just-what-doctor-ordered. Accessed 17 Dec 2012. This is the first independent report that endorsed patient-centric architecture (HRBs) as an effective approach to HII. It describes clearly the problems and challenges of HIEs.

Krist, A.H., & Woolf, S.H. (2011). A vision for patient-centered health information systems. *JAMA: The Journal of the American Medical Association, 305*(3), 300–301. A vision of how fully functional patient-centric electronic medical record systems could be the basis for an effective HII.

Miller, R.H., & Miller, B.S. (2007). The Santa Barbara County Care Data Exchange: What happened? *Health Affairs, 26*(5), 568w–580w. This paper describes the history of one of the earliest HIEs, including details about the factors leading to its failure.

National Committee on Vital and Health Statistics. (2001). *Information for health: A strategy for building the National Health Information Infrastructure. Report and recommendations from the National Committee on Vital and Health Statistics*. Available at http://www.ncvhs.hhs.gov/nhiilayo.pdf. Accessed 17 Dec 2012. This seminal work was the first to call for a national HII, coining the term. It comprehensively describes the need for HII, the problems it would solve, and the necessity for government investment to incentivize its development.

Steinbrook, R. (2008). Personally controlled online health data—The next big thing in medical care? *The New England Journal of Medicine, 358*(16), 1653–1656. A physician's perspective on the need for patients to control their own electronic health data.

Yasnoff, W.A., Humphreys, B.L., Overhage, J.M., Detmer, D.E., Brennan, P.F., Morris, R.W., Middleton, B., Bates, D.W., & Fanning, J.P. (2004). A consensus action agenda for achieving the national health information infrastructure. *Journal of the American Medical Informatics Association, 11*(4), 332–338. This paper describes the results of the first national consensus conference on HII held in Washington, DC, in 2003. This was the meeting that led to the creation of ONC in 2004.

Questions for Discussion

1. Make the case for and against investing $billions in the HII. How successful have the HITECH Meaningful Use incentives been in promoting HII development? What could be done to make them more effective?

2. What organizational options would you consider if you were beginning the development of HII? What are the pros and cons of each? How would you proceed with making a decision about which one to use?

3. Estimate the required bandwidth and transaction rate for central (HRB) vs. institution-centric HII architecture.

4. Consider the policy implications of universal availability of comprehensive electronic patient records. What are the risks and how could they be mitigated?

5. Given the architectural and other advantages of HRBs, why have most communities adopted institution-centric architectures up to now? What are some steps that might be helpful in encouraging communities to evaluate alternative architectures such as HRBs?

6. Show specifically the potential locations where patient consent functionality could be added to the institution-centric and patient-centric HII architectures in Figs. 13.2 and 13.4 and describe the granularity of consent that would be possible at each proposed location. After eliminating any redundant functionality, compare and contrast the consent implementation issues for the two alternative architectures, describing the advantages and disadvantages of each. Which architecture more efficiently addresses the issue of patient consent? Why?

Management of Information in Health Care Organizations

14

Lynn Harold Vogel

After reading this chapter, you should know the answers to these questions:

- What are the primary information requirements of health care organizations (HCOs)?
- What are the clinical, financial, and administrative functions provided by health care information systems (HCISs), and what are the potential benefits of implementing such systems?
- How have changes in health care delivery models changed the scope and requirements of HCISs over time?
- How do differences among business strategies and organizational structures influence information systems choices?
- What are the major challenges to implementing and managing HCISs?
- How are ongoing health care reforms, technological advances, and changing social norms likely to affect HCIS requirements in the future?

14.1 Overview

Health care organizations (HCOs), like many other business entities, are information-intensive enterprises. Health care personnel require sufficient data and information management tools to make appropriate decisions. At the same time, they need to care for patients and manage and run the enterprise; they also need to document and communicate plans and activities, and to meet the requirements of numerous regulatory and accrediting organizations. Clinicians assess patient status, plan patient care, administer appropriate treatments, and educate patients and families regarding clinical management of various conditions. They are also concerned about evaluating the clinical outcomes, quality, and increasingly, the cost of health services provided. Administrators determine appropriate staffing levels, manage inventories of drugs and supplies, and negotiate payment contracts for services. Governing boards make decisions about whether to invest in new business lines, how to partner with other organizations, and how to eliminate underutilized services. Collectively, health care professionals comprise a heterogeneous group with diverse objectives and information requirements.

The purpose of **health care information systems** (HCISs) is to support the access and management of the information that health professionals need in order to perform their jobs effectively and efficiently. HCISs facilitate communication, integrate information, and coordinate action among multiple health care professionals.

L.H. Vogel, PhD
LH Vogel Consulting, LLC,
371 Beveridge Road, Ridgewood, NJ 07450, USA
e-mail: lynn@lhvogelconsulting.com

This chapter is adapted from an earlier version in the third edition authored by Lynn Harold Vogel and Leslie E. Perreault.

E.H. Shortliffe, J.J. Cimino (eds.), *Biomedical Informatics*,
DOI 10.1007/978-1-4471-4474-8_14, © Springer-Verlag London 2014

In addition, they assist in the organization and storage of data, and they support certain record-keeping and reporting functions. Many of the clinical information functions of an HCIS were detailed in our discussion of the computer-based patient record (CPR) in Chap. 12; systems to support nurses and other care providers are discussed in Chap. 15. Furthermore, HCISs are key elements that interface with the health information infrastructure (HII), as discussed in Chap. 13. An HCIS also supports the financial and administrative functions of a health organization and associated operating units, including the operations of ancillary and other clinical-support departments. The evolving complexities of HCOs place great demands on an HCIS. Many HCOs are broadening their scope of activities to cover the care continuum, partially in response to **Accountable Care Organization** (ACO) initiatives from the federal government. HCISs must organize, manage, and integrate large amounts of clinical and financial data collected by diverse users in a variety of organizational settings (from physicians' offices to hospitals to health care systems) and must provide health care workers (and, increasingly, patients) with timely access to complete, accurate, and up-to-date information presented in a useful format.

14.1.1 Evolution from Automation of Specific Functions to Health care System Information Systems

Over time, changes in the health care economic and regulatory environments have radically transformed the structure, strategic goals, and operational processes of health care organizations through a gradual shifting of financial risk from third party payers (e.g., traditional insurance companies such as Blue Cross and Blue Shield, Medicare and Medicaid programs that emerged in the 1960s and 1970s, and subsequently managed care companies that became quite prominent in the 1980s) to the providers themselves. This shifting of risk initially brought about a consolidation of health care providers

into **integrated delivery networks** (IDNs) in the 1990s. Subsequently, there was a retreat from the most restrictive models of managed care toward greater consumer choice, a slowing of mergers and acquisitions activities, several high profile IDN failures (Shortell et al. 2000, Weil 2001, Kastor 2001), and major new regulatory requirements aimed at improved efficiency and greater patient privacy and safety. Most recently, the pendulum has swung back as IDNs acquire both physician practices and hospitals while shifting their focus to becoming identified as an **ACO**. All these changes have tremendous implications for HCISs.

The evolution of HCISs has paralleled—and in many ways responded to—the organizational evolution of the health care industry itself. The earliest HCISs were largely focused on the automation of specific functions within hospitals including, initially, patient registration and billing. The justification for these systems was relatively straightforward since large mainframe computers were easily capable of performing the clerical tasks associated with tracking patients and sending out bills. In the 1960s and 1970s, seeing the benefits coming from more highly automated financial systems, hospital departments began to focus on installing computer systems to support ancillary activities such as those found in radiology, the pharmacy, and the laboratories. Hardware vendors such as the Digital Equipment Corporation (DEC) responded with smaller computing platforms known as **minicomputers**, which enabled individual departments to remain quite separate not only in function but in terms of computer hardware, operating systems, and even programming languages—even though collectively they were now known as **hospital information systems** (HISs). The lack of connectivity among these various systems created significant obstacles to keeping track of where patients were located in a hospital, and more importantly, what kind of care was being provided and the clinical results of that care. It was not uncommon for caregivers to have to log on to several different computer systems just to learn the status of specific clinical results from different laboratories or departments. By the late 1980s, **clinical information system** (CIS) components of HISs offered clinically oriented capabilities, such as order writing and results communications. During the same period, **ambulatory medical record systems** (AMRSs) and **practice management systems** (PMSs) were being developed to support large outpatient clinics and physician offices, respectively. These systems performed functions analogous to those of hospital systems, but were generally less complex, reflecting the lower volume and complexity of patient care delivered in outpatient settings. Increasingly, these various systems were implemented within organizational boundaries, but with little or no integration between hospital and ambulatory settings.

The development of so many different, functionally specific information systems is one of the unique attributes of HCOs and one of the drivers of the complexity of HCOs. These systems were often developed in isolation from one another as vendors focused on developing as much highly specialized functionality as possible—in effect, striving for a "**best of breed**" designation in the marketplace for their particular type of system. The isolation of these systems, even within a single organizational structure, was overcome in part by the development of interfaces between the various systems. Initially these interfaces focused on delivering patient demographic information from registration systems to the ancillary systems and data on specific clinical events (e.g., laboratory tests, radiology exams, medications ordered) from the ancillary systems to the billing system. However, as more information systems were added to the HCIS environment, the challenge of moving data from one system to another became overwhelming. In response, two unique developments occurred: (1) the **interface engine**; and (2) **Health Level Seven** (HL7), a standard for the content of the data messages that were being sent from one information system to another as discussed in Chap. 7.

The challenge of sharing data among many different information systems that emerged in the 1980s and 1990s was daunting. As we noted earlier, the various components of the HCISs were

in most cases developed by different vendors, using different hardware (e.g., DEC, IBM), operating systems (e.g., PICK, Altos, DOS, VMS, MUMPS on minicomputers, and IBM's 360 OS on mainframes) and programming languages (e.g., BASIC, PL1, COBOL, MUMPS and even assembler). Sharing data among two different systems typically required a two-way interface—one to send data from System A to System B, the other to send data or acknowledge receipt from B back to A. Adding a third system didn't require simply one additional interface because the new system would in many cases have to be interfaced to both of the original systems, resulting in the possibility of six interfaces. Introducing a fourth system into the HCIS environment increased the complexity further, since it often meant the need for two-way interfaces to *each* of the original three systems, for a total of twelve (Fig. 14.1). With the prospect of interfaces increasing exponentially as new systems were added (represented by the formula, $I = n\,(n-1)$ where I represents the number of interfaces

Systems   # Interfaces

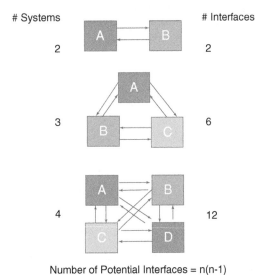

2   2

3   6

4   12

Number of Potential Interfaces = n(n-1)

Fig. 14.1 The challenge of moving data from one system to another becomes complicated with the addition of each new system. Considering that even small size hospitals may have several hundred applications, interfacing is a major challenge. While in reality not all systems need to have two-way interfaces to every other system, this figure illustrates the challenges that even small numbers of systems bring

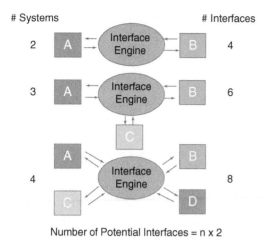

Systems   # Interfaces

2   A ← Interface Engine ← B   4

3   A ← Interface Engine → B   6

   C

4   A, B, C, Interface Engine, D   8

Number of Potential Interfaces = n x 2

Fig. 14.2 The introduction of the Interface Engine (*IE*) made system interfaces much more manageable, particularly so with the implementation of HL7 data messaging standards. With an IE, each additional system only added two additional interfaces to the mix, one to send data and one to acknowledge receipt of the data

needed and *n* represents the number of systems), it was clear that a new solution was needed to address the complexity and cost of interfacing. In response, an industry niche was born in the late 1980s which focused on creating a software application designed specifically to manage the interfacing challenges among disparate systems in the HCIS environment. Instead of each system having to interface to every other system independently, the interface engine served as the central connecting point for all interfaces (Fig. 14.2). Each system had only to connect to the interface engine; the engine would then manage the sending of data to and from any other system that needed it. The interface engine concept, which originated in health care, has given rise to a whole series of strategies for managing multiple systems. Many of the vendors who got their start in health care interfacing subsequently found new markets in financial services as well as other industries.

The creation of HL7 (see Chap. 7) was yet another response to the challenge of moving data among disparate health care systems. HL7 is a health care-based initiative, also started in the late 1980s, to develop standards for the sharing of data among the many individual systems that

comprise an HCIS. The basic idea was to use messaging standards so that data could be sent back and forth using standard formats within the HCIS environment. Most of the departmental systems that were introduced at this time were the products of companies focused on specific niche markets, including laboratories, pharmacies and radiology departments. Consequently there was strong support for both the interface engine and the HL7 efforts as mechanisms to permit smaller vendors to compete successfully in the marketplace. In recent years, many of these pioneering vendors have been purchased and their products included as components of larger product families.

The decade of the 1990s was marked by a large number of mergers and affiliations among previously independent and often competing HCOs designed to drive excess capacity from the system (e.g., an oversupply of hospital beds) and to secure market share. Hospitals and medical centers began to build satellite ambulatory-care clinics and to reach out to community physician practices in an attempt to secure patient referrals to their specialty services and to fill their increasingly vacant inpatient beds. Later, facing competition with **vertically integrated** for-profit health care chains and with other integrating organizations, hospitals started at first affiliating and then more tightly integrating into regional aggregates of health care service providers—the Integrated Delivery Networks (IDNs) mentioned earlier (See Fig. 14.3).

By 2000, IDNs were prominent in almost every health care market in the United States and in several cases, spanned large geographic regions and multiple states. Each IDN typically consisted of multiple acute-care facilities, satellite ambulatory health centers, and owned or managed physicians' practice groups. In addition, larger IDNs might have skilled nursing homes, hospices, home-care agencies, and for-profit sub-corporations to deliver support services back to the health care providers, including regional laboratories, separate organizations for purchasing and distributing drugs and medical supplies, and remote billing services. A major goal of such IDNs was cost reduction (both internally and from suppliers), as well as to retain or

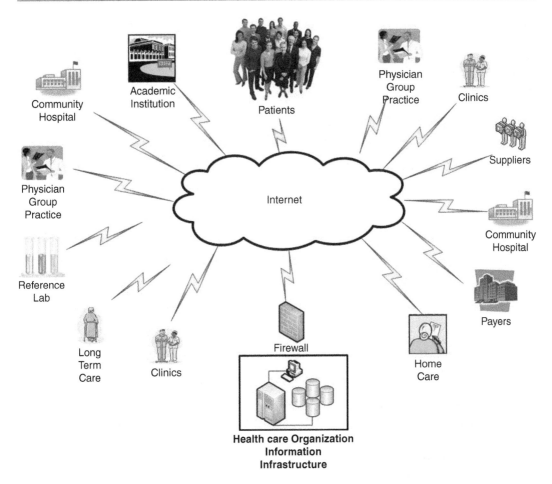

Fig. 14.3 Major organizational components of an integrated delivery network (IDN). A typical IDN might include several components of the same type (e.g., clinics, community hospitals. Physician group practices, etc.). Components within the same geographic area may have direct data connections, but increasingly the Internet is the preferred way to connect organizational components

increase revenues by improving their negotiating strength with third party payers. Because they controlled a significant regional market share and were positioned to provide and manage comprehensive health services, IDNs expected to negotiate favorable purchasing contracts with suppliers and competitive service contracts with payers or directly with large employers. Some IDNs went further and affiliated with a regional **health maintenance organization** (**HMO**) or developed their own health-plan organizations to act as their own insurance carriers. The largest IDNs had annual revenues approaching several billions of dollars, were contracting with thousands of physicians and nurses, and managed contracts to provide comprehensive care for more than one million patients.

One of the major expectations was that IDNs could reduce costs by leveraging economies of scale; for example, by consolidating administrative and financial functions and combining clinical services. Such IDNs were challenged to coordinate patient care and manage business operations throughout an extensive network of community and regional resources. As a result, HCISs were developed to share information and coordinate activities not only within, but among multiple hospitals, ambulatory care sites, physicians' practice groups, and other affiliated organizations.

Although IDNs are still a prominent feature in many health care markets, there had been a decrease in the rate of market consolidation and some highly visible IDN failures. While the most successful of IDNs have achieved a measure of structural and operational integration, gains from the integration of clinical activities and from the consolidation of information systems have been much more difficult. Many IDNs scaled back their original goals for integrating clinical activities and actually began to shed home care services, physician practices, health plans and managed care entities, although as noted earlier in this chapter, we are now seeing a return to consolidation, mergers and acquisitions as reimbursement constraints and federal ACO initiatives strive to improve both the efficiency and effectiveness of HCOs. It appears that the expertise gained from managing an inpatient-driven organization producing a relatively large amount of revenue from a relatively small set of events (e.g., a hospital) did not translate easily to the successful management of other organizational activities that in many cases required many more events to produce a similar level of revenue (e.g., from outpatient clinics). In some cases, it was even a challenge to translate management processes from inpatient operations to outpatient clinics, or one hospital to another. Attempts to apply hospital management principles to ambulatory clinics have been challenged because hospitals generate a relatively small number of patient bills with high dollar amounts whereas ambulatory clinics do just the opposite—generate a relatively large number of patient bills, each with a relatively small dollar amount. To date, it is fair to say that few IDNs have gained the degree of cost savings and efficiencies they had originally projected. The immense up-front costs of implementing (or integrating) the required HCISs in particular have contributed to this limited success. Regardless of organizational structure, all health care organizations are striving toward greater information access and integration, including improved information linkages with physicians and patients. The "typical" IDN is a melding of diverse organizations, and the associated information systems infrastructure is still far from integrated; rather, it remains in many cases an amalgam of heterogeneous systems, processes, and data stores.

14.1.2　Information Requirements

The most important function of any HCIS is to present data to decision makers so that they can improve the quality and timeliness of the decisions they need to make. From a clinical perspective, the most important function of an HCIS is to present patient-specific data to care givers so that they can easily interpret the data for diagnostic and treatment planning purposes, and support the necessary communication among the many health care workers who cooperate in providing health services to patients. From an administrative perspective, the most pressing information needs are those related to the daily operation and management of the organization—bills must be generated accurately and rapidly, employees and vendors must be paid, supplies must be ordered, and so on. In addition, administrators need information to make short-term and long-term planning decisions.

Since clinical system information requirements are discussed in Chaps. 12, 13, 15, and 22, we focus here on operational information needs, and specifically on four broad categories: daily operations, planning, communication, and documentation and reporting.

- *Operational requirements.* Health care workers—both care givers and administrators—require detailed and up-to-date factual information to perform the daily tasks that keep a hospital, clinic, or physician practice running—the bread-and-butter tasks of the institution. Here are examples of queries for operational information: Where is patient John Smith? What drugs is he receiving? What tests are scheduled for Mr. Smith after his discharge? Who will pay his bill? Is the staffing skill mix sufficient to handle the current volume and special needs of patients in Care Center 3 West? What are the names and telephone numbers of patients who have appointments for tomorrow and need to be called for a reminder? What authorization is needed to perform an ultrasound procedure on Jane Blue under the terms of her health insurance coverage? HCISs can support these operational requirements for information by organizing data for prompt and easy access. Because the HCO may have developed product-line specialization within a particular facility (e.g., a diagnostic imaging center or women's health center), however, answering even a simple request may require accessing information stored in different systems at several different facilities.

• *Planning requirements.* Health professionals also require information to make short-term and long-term decisions about patient care and organizational management. The importance of appropriate clinical decision-making is obvious—we devote all of Chaps. 3 and 22 to explaining methods to help clinicians select diagnostic tests, interpret test results, and choose treatments for their patients. The decisions made by administrators and managers are no less important in their choices concerning the acquisition and use of health care resources. In fact, clinicians and administrators alike must choose wisely in their use of resources to provide high-quality care and excellent service at a competitive price. HCISs should help health care personnel to answer queries such as these: What are the organization's clinical guidelines for managing the care of patients with this condition? Have similar patients experienced better clinical outcomes with medical treatment or with surgical intervention? What are the financial and medical implications of closing the maternity service? If we added six care managers to the outpatient-clinic staff, can we improve patient outcomes and reduce emergency admissions? Will the proposed contract to provide health services to Medicaid patients be profitable given the current cost structure and current utilization patterns? Often, the data necessary for planning are generated by many sources. HCISs can help planners by aggregating, analyzing, and summarizing the information relevant to decision-making.

• *Communication requirements.* Communication and coordination of patient care and operations across multiple personnel, multiple business units, and far-flung geography is not possible without investment in an underlying technology infrastructure. For example, the routing of paper medical records, a cumbersome process even within a single hospital, is an impossibility for a regional network of providers trying to act in coordination. Similarly, it is neither timely nor cost effective to copy and distribute hard copy documents to all participants in a regionally distributed organization. An HCO's technology infrastructure can enable information exchange via web-based access to shared databases and documents, electronic mail, standard document-management systems, and on-line calendaring systems, as well as providing and controlling access for authorized users at the place and time that information is required.

• *Documentation and reporting requirements.* The need to maintain records for future reference or analysis and reporting makes up the fourth category of informational requirements. Some requirements are internally imposed. For example, a complete record of each patient's health status and treatment history is necessary to ensure continuity of care across multiple providers and over time. External requirements create a large demand for data collection and record keeping in HCOs (as with mandated reporting of vaccination records to public health agencies). As discussed in Chap. 12, the medical record is a legal document. If necessary, the courts can refer to the record to determine whether a patient received proper care. Insurance companies require itemized billing statements, and medical records substantiate the clinical justification of services provided and the charges submitted to them. The **Joint Commission (JC)**, which certifies the qualifications and performance of many health care organizations, has specific requirements concerning the content and quality of medical records, as well as requirements for organization-wide information-management processes. Furthermore, to qualify for participation in the

Medicare and Medicaid programs, the JC requires that hospitals follow standardized procedures for auditing the medical staff and monitoring the quality of patient care, and they must be able to show that they meet the safety requirements for infectious disease management, buildings, and equipment. Employer and consumer groups are also joining the list of external monitors.

14.1.3 Integration Requirements

If an HCO is to manage patient care effectively, project a focused market identity, and control its operating costs, it must perform in a unified and consistent manner. For these reasons, information technologies to support data and process integration are recognized as critical to an HCO's operations. From an organizational perspective, information should be available when and where it is needed; users must have an integrated view, regardless of system or geographic boundaries; data must have a consistent interpretation; and adequate security must be in place to ensure access only by authorized personnel and only for appropriate uses. Unfortunately, these criteria are much easier to describe than to meet.

14.1.3.1 Data Integration

In hospitals, clinical and administrative personnel have traditionally had distinct areas of responsibility and performed many of their functions separately. Thus, it is not surprising that administrative and clinical data have often been managed separately—administrative data in business offices and clinical data in medical-records departments. When computers were first introduced, the hospital's information processing was often performed on separate computers with separate databases, thus minimizing conflicts about priorities in services and investment. As we have seen earlier in this chapter, information systems to support hospital functions and ambulatory care historically have, due to organizational boundaries, developed independently. Many hospitals, for example, have rich databases for inpatient data but maintain less information for outpatients—often including only billing data such as diagnosis and procedure codes and charges for services provided. Even today, relatively few clinical data are available in electronic format for most ambulatory-care clinics and physician offices in the United States, although this disparity is beginning to diminish as hospitals and physician practices continue a long term trend toward greater integration and increasing investments in HCISs. As **fee-for-service** reimbursement models continue to be challenged for their focus on activity-driven care, alternatives such as Accountable Care Organizations (ACOs), **bundled payments** for services, and **pay for performance** proposals will stimulate efforts toward greater data integration.

The historical lack of integration of data from diverse sources creates a host of problems. If clinical and administrative data are stored on separate systems, then data needed by both must either be entered separately into each system, be copied from one system to another, or data from both sources transferred to yet another location in order to be analyzed. In addition to the expense of redundant data entry and data maintenance incurred by these approaches (see also the related discussion for the health information infrastructure in Chap. 13), the consistency of information tends to be poor because data may be updated in one place and not in the other, or information may be copied incorrectly from one place to another. In the extreme example, the same data may be represented differently in different settings. As we noted earlier within the hospital setting, many of these issues have been addressed through the development of automated interfaces to transfer demographic data, orders, results, and charges between clinical systems and billing systems. Even with an interface engine managing data among disparate systems, however, an organization still must solve the thorny issues of synchronization of data and comparability of similar data types.

With the development of IDNs and other complex HCOs, the sharing of data elements among operating units becomes more critical and more problematic. Data integration issues are further compounded in IDNs by the acquisition of previously independent organizations that have clinical and administrative information systems incompatible with those of the rest of the IDN. It is still not unusual to encounter minimal automated information exchange among organizations even within an IDN. Patients register and reregister at the physician's office, diagnostic imaging center, ambulatory surgery facility, and acute-care hospital—and sometimes face multiple registrations even within a single facility. Each facility may continue to keep its own clinical records, and shadow files may be established at multiple locations with copies of critical information such as operative reports and hospital discharge summaries. Inconsistencies in these multiple electronic and manual databases can result in inappropriate patient management and inappropriate resource allocation. For example, medications that are first given to a patient while she is a hospital inpatient may inadvertently be discontinued when she is transported to a rehabilitation hospital or nursing home. Also, information about a patient's known allergies and medication history may be unavailable to physicians treating an unconscious patient in an emergency department.

The objectives of coordinated, high-quality, and cost-effective health care cannot be completely satisfied if an organization's multiple computer systems operate in isolation. Unfortunately, free-standing systems within HCOs are still common, although HCOs and IDNs are increasingly investing in the implementation of new more consistent systems across all of their facilities or in integrating existing systems to allow data sharing. The capital investment required to pursue a strategy of system-wide data integration can be significant, and with ongoing challenges to reimbursement rates for both hospitals and physicians, the funding to pursue this strategy is often limited either due to competing investment requirements (e.g., acquiring or maintaining buildings and equipment) or the continued downward trend in reimbursement for services. In Sect. 14.4, we discuss architectural components and strategies for data integration.

14.1.3.2 Process Integration

To be truly effective, information systems must mesh smoothly with the people who use them and with the specific operational workflows of the organization. But **process integration** poses a significant challenge for HCOs and for the HCIS's as well. Today's health care-delivery models represent a radical departure from historical models of care delivery. Changes in reimbursement and documentation requirements may lead, for example, to changes in the responsibilities and work patterns of physicians, nurses, and other care providers; the development of entirely new job categories (such as care managers who coordinate a patient's care across facilities or between encounters); and the more active participation of patients in their own personal health management (Table 14.1). Process integration is further complicated in that component entities typically have evolved different operational policies and procedures, which can reflect different historical and leadership experiences from one office to another, or in the extreme example, from one floor to another within a single hospital. The most progressive HCOs are developing new enterprise-wide processes for providing easy and uniform access to health services, for deploying consistent clinical guidelines, and for coordinating and managing patient care across multiple care settings throughout the organization. Integrated information technologies are essential to supporting such enterprise-wide processes. Mechanisms for information management aimed at integrating operations across entities must address not only the migration from legacy systems but also the migration from legacy work processes to new, more consistent and more standardized policies and processes within and across entities.

The introduction of new information systems almost always changes the workplace. In fact research has shown that in most cases the real value from an investment in information systems comes only when underlying work processes are changed to take advantage of the new information technology (Vogel 2003; see Figs. 14.4 and 14.5). At times, these changes can be substantial. The implementation of a new system offers an

Table 14.1 The changing health care environment and its implications for an IDN's core competencies

Characteristics	Old care model	New care model
Goal of care	Manage sickness	Manage wellness
Center of delivery system	Hospital	Primary-care providers/ambulatory settings
Focus of care	Episodic acute and chronic care	Population health, primary and preventive care
Driver of care decisions	Specialists	Primary-care providers/patients
Metric of system success	Number of admissions	Number of enrollees
Performance optimization	Optimize individual provider performance	Optimize system-wide performance
Utilization controls	Externally controlled	Internally controlled
Quality measures	Defined as inputs to system	Defined as patient outcomes and satisfaction
Physician role	Autonomous and independent	Member of care team; user of system-wide guidelines of care
Patient role	Passive receiver of care	Active partner in care

Source: Copyright CSC. Reprinted with permission

Order Entry Management Tasks Before Automation

Physician Tasks	Nursing Tasks	Clerk Tasks
Locate patient chart		Locate patient chart
Review clinical results (lab, radiology, etc.)		Transcribe orders-to clerk kardex, to nurse kardex
	Locate patient chart	
Jot notes from clinical results	Verify orders transcribed correctly	If clarification is needed,contact nurse
Examine patient (s)	"Note"new med orders correct on medication records	Complete requisitions-lab, radiology,etc.
Locate patient chart		
Review record again	Sign off on each set of orders	Send requisitions to depts or put in a pick up area
Open "orders" tab	Close chart	
Write orders	"Unflag"chart indicating orders complete	Send via fax or call depts for new orders- diet, respiratory,etc
If writing discharge order-write discharge prescriptions	Put chart back in chart rack	Locate medication records
Sign orders	Carry out orders or assign to staff to complete	Enter new medication orders
"Flag" chart that new orders are present	Educate patient on new orders as needed	Note status/completion of each item on order
Replace chart in rack		Close chart
If wrote STAT orders, notify clerk and nurse		"Flag" chart that orders have been transcribed
		Put chart back in rack
13 steps	**9 steps**	**12 steps**

Fig. 14.4 The process of managing the manual creation of orders requesting services on behalf of patients in a hospital involves numerous tasks performed not only by the ordering physician, but by nursing and clerical staff

opportunity to rethink and redefine existing work processes to take advantage of the new information-management capabilities, thereby reducing costs, increasing productivity, or improving service levels. For example, providing electronic access to information that was previously accessible only on paper can shorten the overall time required to complete a multistep activity by enabling conversion of serial processes (completed by multiple workers using the

Benefits from reduced tasks for Provider
require additional "complementary"
management changes

Physician Tasks

| Logon to system |
| Select a patient |
| Review Clinical Results |
| Enter new order(s) |
| Sign orders electronically |
| Logoff |

**Reduce 13 steps
To 6**

Change role of Provider

Change job description of Clerk

Change job description of Nurse

Change order intake workflow
for all ancillaries

Change order notification
procedures for Nursing

Change order notification
procedures for Clerks

Consider new role: Medical
Assistant

Change clinical results
notification process

Develop new reports on orders
processing, completion
timeliness, etc.

Change to role-based
authentication process for all
providers

**Changes for Staff Roles
and Tasks**

Develop and periodically test
downtime procedures

Ensure sufficient ordering
hardware: desktops, laptops,
tablets, etc.

Ensure sufficient network
bandwidth

Develop 7x24 HELP desk
availability

Ensure 7x24 Desktop Support

Ensure 7x24 Network Support

Ensure 7x24 Application Support

**Changes for
IS Department**

Fig. 14.5 The implementation of an electronic physician order entry system reduces the number of tasks that a physician needs to perform in order to enter an order, but such a system will only be successful if a number of other "complementary" changes are made to both the workflow of staff and the responsibilities of the IS Department

same record sequentially) to concurrent processes (completed by the workers accessing an electronic record simultaneously). More fundamental business transformation is also possible with new technologies; for example, direct entry of medication orders by physicians, linked with a decision-support system, allows immediate checking for proper dosing and potential drug interactions, and the ability to recommend less expensive drug substitutes.

Few health care organizations today have the time or resources to develop entirely new information systems and redesigned processes on their own; therefore, most opt to purchase commercial software products and to use consultants to assist them in the implementation of industry "best practices". Although these commercial systems allow some degree of custom tailoring, they also reflect an underlying model of work processes that may have evolved through development in other health care organizations with different underlying operational policies and procedures. In order to be successful, HCO's typically must adapt their own work processes to those embodied in the systems they are installing (For example, some commercial systems require care providers to discontinue and then reenter all orders when a patient is admitted to the hospital after being monitored in the emergency department). Furthermore, once the systems are installed and workflow has been adapted to them, they become part of the organization's culture—and any subsequent change to the new system may be arduous because of these workflow considerations. Decision-makers should take great care when selecting and configuring a new system to support and enhance desired work processes. Such organizational workflow adaptation represents a significant challenge to the HCO and its systems planners. Too often organizations are unable to realize the full potential return on their information-technology investments when they attempt to change the system to accommodate historical work flows, even before the new system is installed. Such management practices can significantly reduce much of the potential gains from the HCO's IT investment.

To meet the continually evolving financial and quality documentation requirements of today's health care environment, HCOs must continually evolve as well—and the analogy between changing an HCO and turning an aircraft carrier seems apt. Although an HCO's business plans and information-systems strategies may be reasonable and necessary, changing ingrained organizational behavior can be much more complex than changing the underlying information systems. Technology capabilities often exceed an HCO's ability to use them effectively and efficiently. Successful process integration requires not only successful deployment of the technology but also sustained commitment of resources to use that technology well; dedicated leadership with the willingness to make difficult, sometimes unpopular decisions; education; and possibly new performance incentives to overcome cultural inertia and politics. Government incentives to stimulate HCOs toward the **meaningful use** of information technology, which emerged from the 2010 Health care Reform legislation (Chap. 27), are a recent example of attempts to bring process integration and data integration together.

14.1.4 Security and Confidentiality Requirements

The protection of health information from unwanted or inappropriate use is governed not only by the trust of patients in their health providers but also by law. In accordance with the **Health Insurance Portability and Accountability Act (HIPAA) of 1996** (Chap. 10), the Secretary of Health and Human Services recommended that "Congress enact national standards that provide fundamental privacy rights for patients and define responsibilities for those who serve them." This law and subsequent federal regulations now mandate standardized data transactions for sending data to payer organizations, the development and adherence to formal policies for securing and maintaining access to patient data, and under privacy provisions, prohibit disclosure of patient-identifiable information by most providers and health plans, except as authorized by the patient or explicitly permitted by legislation. Recent changes to the HIPAA regulations have strengthened considerably the requirements for security and privacy protections and have also given patients the right to pursue actions against both organizations and individuals when they feel that their personal information has been compromised. HIPAA also provides consumers with significant rights to be informed about how and by whom their health information will be used, and to inspect and sometimes amend their health information. Stiff criminal penalties including fines and possible imprisonment are associated with noncompliance or the knowing misuse of patient-identifiable information.

Computer systems can be designed to provide security, but only people can promote the trust necessary to protect the confidentiality of patients' clinical information. In fact, most breeches and inappropriate disclosures stem from human actions rather than from computer system failures. To achieve the goal of delivering coordinated and cost-effective care, clinicians need to access information on specific patients from many different locations. Unfortunately, it is difficult to predict in advance which clinicians will need access to which patient data and from which locations. Therefore, an HCIS must strike a balance between restricting information access and ensuring the accountability of the users of patient information. To build trust with its patients and meet HIPAA requirements, an HCO should adopt a three-pronged approach to securing information. First, the HCO needs to designate a security officer (and typically a privacy officer as well) and develop uniform security and confidentiality policies, including specification of sanctions, and to enforce these policies rigorously. Second, the HCO needs to train employees so they understand the appropriate uses of patient-identifiable information and the consequences of violations. Third, the HCO must use electronic tools such as intrusion detection, access controls and audit trails not only to discourage misuse of information, but also to inform employees and patients that people who access confidential information without proper authorization or a "need to know", can be tracked and will be held accountable.

14.1.5 The Benefits of Health care Information Systems

On average, health care workers in administrative departments spend about three-fourths of their time handling information; workers in nursing units spent about one-fourth of their time on these tasks. The fact is that information management in health care organizations, even with significant computerization, is a costly activity. The collection, storage, retrieval, analysis, and dissemination of the clinical and administrative information necessary to support the organization's daily operations, to meet external and internal requirements for documentation and reporting, and to support short-term and strategic planning remain important and time-consuming aspects of the jobs of health-care workers.

Today, the justifications for implementing HCISs include cost reduction, productivity enhancement, and quality and service improvement, as well as strategic considerations related to competitive advantage and regulatory compliance (Vogel 2003):

- *Cost reduction*. Much of the historical impetus for implementing HCISs was their potential to reduce the costs of information management in hospitals and other facilities. HCOs continue to make tactical investments in information systems to streamline administrative processes and departmental workflow. Primary benefits that may offset some information-systems costs include reductions in labor requirements, reduced waste (e.g., dated surgical supplies that are ordered but unused or food trays that are delivered to the wrong destination and therefore are wasted), and more efficient management of supplies and other inventories. Large savings can be gained through efficient scheduling of expensive resources such as operating suites and imaging equipment. In addition, HCISs can help to eliminate inadvertent ordering of duplicate tests and procedures. Once significant patient data are available online, information systems can reduce the costs of storing, retrieving, and transporting charts in the medical-records department.

- *Productivity Enhancements*. A second area of benefit from an HCIS comes in the form of improved productivity of clinicians and other staff. With continuing (and at times increasing) constraints on reimbursements, HCOs are continually faced with the challenge of doing more with less. Providing information systems support to staff can in many cases enable them to manage a larger variety of tasks and data than would otherwise be possible using strictly manual processes. Interestingly, in some cases hospital investments in an HCIS support the productivity improvement of staff that are not employed by the hospital, namely the physicians, and can even extend to payers by lowering their costs. One of the major challenges with introducing a new HCIS is that the productivity of users may actually decrease in the initial months of the implementation. With complex clinical applications in particular, learning new ways of working can lead to high levels of user dissatisfaction in addition to lowered productivity.

- *Quality and service improvement*. As HCISs have broadened in scope to encompass support for clinical processes, the ability to improve the quality of care has become an additional benefit. Qualitative benefits of HCISs include improved accuracy and completeness of documentation, reductions in the time clinicians spend documenting (and associated increases in time spent with patients), fewer drug errors and quicker response to adverse events, and improved provider-to-provider communication. Through telemedicine and remote linkages (see Chap. 18), HCOs are able to expand their geographical reach and improve delivery of specialist care to rural and outlying areas. Once patient data are converted from a purely transaction format to a format better suited for analytic work, the use of **clinical decision-support systems** in conjunction with a clinically focused HCIS can produce impressive benefits, namely improving the quality of care while reducing costs (Chap. 22) (Bates and Gawande 2003; James and Savitz 2011; Goldzweig, et al. 2009; Himmelstein and Woolhandler 2010; McCullough et al. 2010).

- *Competitive advantage*. Information technologies must be deployed appropriately and effectively; however, with respect to HCISs, the question is no longer whether to invest, but rather how much and what to buy. Although some organizations still attempt to cost justify all information-systems investments, many HCOs have recognized that HCISs are "**enabling technologies**" which means that the value comes not from the system itself but from what it "enables" the organization to do differently and better. If workflow and processes are not changed to take advantage of the technology, the value of the investment will largely go unrealized. And it is not just the ratio of financial benefits to costs that is important; access to clinical information is necessary not only to carry out patient management, but also to attract and retain the loyalty of physicians who care for (and thus control much of the HCO's access to) the patients. The long-term benefits of clinical systems include the ability to influence clinical practices by reducing large unnecessary variations in medical practices, to improve patient outcomes, and to reduce costs—although these costs might be more broadly economic and societal than related to specific reductions for the hospital itself (Leatherman et al. 2003, James and Savitz 2011). Physicians ultimately control the great majority of the resource-utilization decisions in health care through their choices in prescribing drugs, ordering diagnostic tests, and referring patients for specialty care. Thus, providing physicians with access to information on "best practices" based on the latest available clinical evidence, as well as giving them other clinical and financial data to make appropriate decisions, is an essential HCIS capability.

- *Regulatory compliance*. Health care is among the most heavily regulated industries in our economy. State and federal regulatory agencies perform a variety of oversight activities, and these require increasingly sophisticated and responsive HCISs to provide the necessary reports. For example, the Food and Drug Administration now mandates the use of barcodes on all drugs. Similarly, HIPAA rules specify the required content and format for certain electronic data transactions for those HCOs that exchange data electronically. OSHA, the Department of Labor, the Environmental Protection Agency, the Nuclear Regulatory Commission, and a host of other agencies all have an interest in seeing that the health care provided by HCOs is consistent with standards of safety and fairness.

14.1.6 Managing Information Systems in a Changing Health Care Environment

Despite the importance of integrated information systems, implementation of HCISs has proved to be a daunting task, often requiring a multiyear capital investment of tens (and at times, hundreds) of millions of dollars and forcing fundamental changes in the types and ways that health care professionals perform their jobs. To achieve the potential benefits, health organizations must plan carefully and invest wisely. The grand challenge for an HCO is to implement an HCIS that is sufficiently flexible and adaptable to meet the changing needs of the organization. Given the rapidly changing environment and the multiyear effort involved, people must be careful to avoid implementing a system that is obsolete functionally or technologically before it becomes operational. Success in implementing an HCIS entails consistent and courageous handling of numerous technical, organizational, and political challenges.

14.1.6.1 Changing Technologies

As we discussed in Chaps. 5 and 6, past decades have seen dramatic changes in computing and networking technologies. These advances are important in that they allow quicker and easier information access, less expensive computational power and data storage, greater flexibility, and other performance advantages. A major challenge for many HCOs is how to decide whether to support a best of breed strategy, with its requirement either to upgrade individual systems and interfaces to newer products or to migrate from their patchwork of legacy systems to a more integrated systems environment. Such migration requires integration and selective replacement of diverse systems that are often implemented with closed or nonstandard technologies and medical vocabularies. Unfortunately the trade-off between migrating from best of breed to more integrated systems is that vendors offering more integrated approaches seldom match the functionality of the best of breed environment. However, this strategy is becoming less of an option since commercial vendors are broadening and deepening the scope of their application suites in order to minimize the challenges of building and managing interfaces and to protect their market share. In a sense, it is the information content of the systems and the ability to implement them that is much more important than the underlying technology—as long as the data are accessible, the choice of specific technology is less critical.

14.1.6.2 Changing Culture

In the current health care environment, physicians are confronted with significant obstacles to the practice of medicine as they have historically performed it. With a long history of entrepreneurial practice, physicians face significant adjustments as they are confronted by pressures to practice in accordance with institutional standards aimed at reducing variation in care, and to focus on the costs of care even when those costs are borne either by hospitals or by third party payers. They are expected to assume responsibility not simply for healing the sick, but for the wellness of people who come to them not as patients but as members of health plans and health maintenance organizations. In addition, they must often work as members of collaborative patient-care teams. The average patient

length of stay in a hospital is decreasing; at the same time, the complexity of the care provided both during and after discharge is increasing. The time allotted for an individual patient visit in an ambulatory setting is decreasing as individual clinicians face economic incentives to increase the number of patients for whom they care each day. Some HCOs, aided by federal funding incentives, are now instituting **pay-for performance** incentives to reward desired work practices. At the same time, it is well known that the amount of knowledge about disease diagnosis and treatment increases significantly each year, with whole new areas of medicine being added from major breakthroughs in areas such as genomic and imaging research. To cope with the increasing workload, greater complexity of care, extraordinary amounts of new medical knowledge, new skills requirements, and the wider availability of medical knowledge to consumers through the Internet, both clinicians and health executives must become more effective information managers, and the supporting information systems must meet their workflow and information requirements. As the health care culture and the roles of clinicians and health executives continue to change, HCOs must constantly reevaluate the role of information technology to ensure that the implemented systems continue to match user requirements and expectations.

14.1.6.3 Changing Processes

Developing a new vision of how health care will be delivered and managed, designing processes and implementing supporting information systems are all critical to the success of evolving HCOs. Changes in process affect the jobs that people do, the skills required to do those jobs, and the fundamental ways in which they relate to one another. For example, models of care management that cross organizational or specialty boundaries encourage interdisciplinary care teams to work in harmony to promote health as well as treat illness. Although information systems are not the foremost consideration for people who are redesigning processes, a poor information-systems implementation can institutionalize bad processes.

HCOs periodically undertake various process redesign initiatives (following models such as **Six Sigma** or **LEAN**), and these initiatives can lead to fundamental transformations of the enterprise. Indeed, work process redesign is essential if information systems are to become truly valuable "enablers" in HCOs. Too often, however, the lack of a clear understanding of existing organizational dynamics leads to a misalignment of incentives—a significant barrier to change—or to the assumption that simply installing a new computer system will be sufficient to generate value. Moreover, HCOs, like many organizations, are collections of individuals who often have natural fears about and resistance to change. Even under the best of circumstances, there are limits to the amount of change that any organization can absorb. The magnitude of work required to plan

and manage organizational change is often underestimated or ignored. The handling of people and process issues has emerged as one of the most critical success factors for HCOs as they implement new work methods and new and upgraded information systems.

14.1.6.4 Management and Governance

Figure 14.6 illustrates the information-technology environment of an HCO composed of two hospitals, an owned physician practice, affiliated nursing homes and hospice, and several for-profit service organizations. Even this relatively simple environment presents significant challenges for the management and governance of information systems. For example, to what extent will the information management function be controlled centrally versus decentralized to the individual operating units

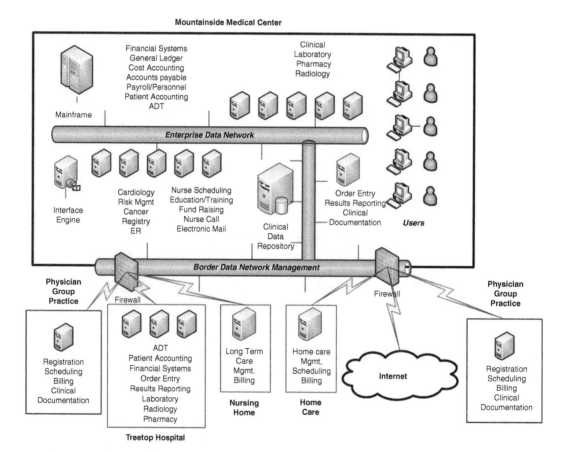

Fig. 14.6 An example of an information systems environment for a small integrated delivery network (IDN). Even this relatively simply IDN has a complex mix of

information systems that pose integration and information management challenges for the organization and departments? How should limited resources be allocated between new investment in strategic projects (such as office-based data access for physicians) and the often critical operational needs of individual entities (e.g., replacement of an obsolete laboratory information system)? Academic medical centers with distinct research and educational needs raise additional issues for managing information across operationally independent and politically powerful constituencies.

Trade-offs between functional and integration requirements, and associated contention between users and information-systems departments, will tend to diminish over time with the development and widespread adoption of technology standards and common clinical-data models and vocabulary. On the other hand, an organization's information-systems "wants" and "needs" will always outstrip its ability to deliver these services. Political battles will persist, as HCOs and their component operating units wrestle with the age-old issues of how to distribute scarce resources among competing, similarly worthy projects.

A formal HCIS governance structure with representation from all major constituents provides a critical forum for direction setting, prioritization, and resource allocation across an HCO. Leadership by respected clinical peers has proved a critical success factor for clinical systems planning, implementation, and acceptance. In addition, the creation of an Information Systems Advisory or Steering Committee composed of the leaders of the various constituencies within the HCO, can be a valuable exercise if the process engages the organization's clinical, financial, and administrative leadership and users and results in their gaining not only a clear understanding of the highest-priority information technology investment requirements but also provides a sense of accountability and ownership over the HCISs and their various functions (Vogel 2006). This supports one of the principles of information technology governance: *how* an institution makes IT investment decisions is often more important than *what* specific decisions are made (Weill and Ross 2004). Because of the dynamic nature of both health care business strategies and the supporting technologies, many HCOs have seen the timeframes of their strategic

information-management thinking shrink from 5 years to three, and then be changed yet again through annual updates.

14.2 Functions and Components of a Health Care Information System

Carefully designed computer-based information systems can increase the effectiveness and productivity of health professionals, improve the quality and reduce the costs of health services, and improve levels of service and of patient satisfaction. As described in Sect. 14.1, the HCISs support a variety of functions, ranging from the delivery and management of patient care to the administration of the health organization. From a functional perspective, HCISs typically consist of components that support five distinct purposes: (1) patient management and billing, (2) ancillary services, (3) care delivery and clinical documentation, (4) clinical decision support, (5) institutional financial and resource management.

14.2.1 Patient Management and Billing

Systems that support patient management functions perform the basic HCO operations related to patients, such as registration, scheduling, admission, discharge, transfer among locations, and billing. Historically within HCOs, maintenance of the hospital census and a patient billing system were the first tasks to be automated—largely because a patient's location determined not only the daily room/bed charges (since an ICU bed was more expensive than a regular medical/surgical bed) but where medications were to be delivered, and where clinical results were to be posted. Today, virtually all hospitals and ambulatory centers and many physician offices use a computer-based **master patient index** (**MPI**) to store patient-identification information that is acquired during the patient-registration process, and link to simple encounter-level information such as dates and locations where services were provided. The MPI can also be integrated within the registration module of an ambulatory care or physician-practice system or even elevated to an **enterprise master patient index** (**EMPI**) across several facilities. Within the hospital setting, the census is maintained by the **admission–discharge–transfer** (**ADT**) module, which is updated whenever a patient is admitted to the hospital, discharged from the hospital, or transferred from one bed to another.

Registration and patient census data serve as a reference base for the financial programs that perform billing functions. When an HCIS is extended to other patient-care settings—e.g., to the laboratory, pharmacy, and other ancillary departments—patient-management systems provide a common reference base for the basic patient demographic data needed by these systems. Without access to the centralized database of patient financial, demographic, registration and location data, these subsystems would have to maintain duplicate patient records. In addition, the transmission of registration data can trigger other activities, such notification of hospital housekeeping when a bed becomes available after a patient is discharged. The billing function in these systems serves as a collection point for all of the chargeable patient activity that occurs in a facility, including room/bed charges, ancillary service charges, and supplies used during a patient's stay.

Scheduling in a health care organization is complicated because patient load and resource utilization can vary by day, week, or season or even through the course of a single day simply due to chance, emergencies that arise, or to patterns of patient and physician behavior. Effective resource management requires that the appropriate resources be on hand to meet such fluctuations in demand. At the same time, resources should not remain unnecessarily idle since that would result in their inefficient use. The most sophisticated scheduling systems have been developed for the operating rooms and radiology departments, where scheduling challenges include matching the patient not only with the providers but also with special equipment and support staff such as technicians. **Patient-tracking applications** monitor patient movement in multistep

processes; for example, they can monitor and manage patient wait times in the emergency department.

Within a multi-facility HCO, the basic tasks of patient management are compounded by the need to manage patient care across multiple settings, some of which may be supported by independent information systems. Is the Patricia C. Brown who was admitted last month to Mountainside Hospital the same Patsy Brown who is registering for her appointment at the Seaview Clinic? Integrated delivery networks ensure unique patient identification either through conversion to common registration systems or, more frequently, through implementation of an enterprise EMPI (see Sect. 14.4) that links patient identifiers and data from multiple registration systems.

14.2.2 Ancillary Services

Ancillary departmental systems support the information needs of individual clinical departments within an HCO. From a systems perspective, those areas most commonly automated are the laboratory, pharmacy, radiology, blood-bank, operating rooms, and medical-records departments, but can also include specialized systems to support cardiology (for EKGs), respiratory therapy and social work. Such systems serve a dual purpose within an HCO. First, ancillary systems perform many dedicated tasks required for specific departmental operations. Such tasks include generating specimen-collection lists and capturing results from automated laboratory instruments in the clinical laboratory, printing medication labels and managing inventory in the pharmacy, and scheduling examinations and supporting the transcription of image interpretations in the radiology department. In addition, information technology coupled with robotics can have a dramatic impact on the operation of an HCO's ancillary departments, particularly in pharmacies (to sort and fill medication carts) and in clinical laboratories (where in some cases the only remaining manual task is the collection of the specimen and its transport to the laboratory's robotic system). Second, the ancillary systems contribute major data components to online patient records, including laboratory-test results and pathology reports, medication profiles, digital images (see Chap. 20), records of blood orders and usage, and various transcribed reports including history and physical examinations, operating room and radiology reports. HCOs that consolidate ancillary functions outside hospitals to gain economies of scale—for example, creating outpatient diagnostic imaging centers and reference laboratories—increase the complexity of integrated patient management, financial, and billing processes.

14.2.3 Care Delivery and Clinical Documentation

Electronic health record (EHR) systems that support care delivery and clinical documentation are discussed at length in Chap. 12. Although comprehensive EHRs are the ultimate goal of most HCOs, many organizations today are still building more basic clinical-management capabilities. Automated **order entry** and **results reporting** are two important functions provided by the clinical components of an HCIS. Health professionals can use the HCIS to communicate with ancillary departments electronically, eliminating the easily misplaced paper slips or the transcription errors often associated with translating hand-written notes into typed requisitions, thus minimizing delays in conveying orders. The information then is available online, where it is easily accessible by any authorized health professional that needs to review a patient's medication profile or previous laboratory-test results. Ancillary departmental data represent an important subset of a patient's clinical record. A comprehensive clinical record, however, also includes various data that clinicians have collected by questioning and observing the patient, including the history and physical report, progress notes and problem lists. In the hospital, an HCIS can help health personnel perform an initial assessment when a patient is admitted to a unit, maintain patient-specific care plans, chart vital signs, maintain medication-administration records, record diagnostic and therapeutic information, document patient and family teaching,

and plan for discharge (also see Chap. 15). Many organizations have developed diagnosis-specific **clinical pathways** that identify clinical goals, interventions, and expected outcomes by time period. Using clinical pathways, case managers or care providers can document actual versus expected outcomes and are alerted to intervene when a significant unexpected event occurs. More hospitals are now implementing systems to support what are called **closed loop medication management systems** in which every task from the initial order for medication to its administration to the patient is recorded in an HCIS—one outcome of increased attention to patient safety issues.

With the shift toward delivering more care in outpatient settings, clinical systems have become more common in ambulatory clinics and physician practices. Numerous vendors have introduced **smart phones**, **tablets**, and other mobile devices with software designed specifically for physicians in ambulatory settings, so that they can access appropriate information even as they move from one exam room to another. Such systems allow clinicians to record problems and diagnoses, symptoms and physical examinations, medical and social history, review of systems, functional status, active and past prescriptions, provide access to therapeutic and medication guidelines, etc. The most successful systems are integrated with a practice management system, providing additional support for physician workflow and typical clinic functions, for example, by documenting telephone follow-up calls or printing prescriptions. In addition, specialized clinical information systems have been developed to meet the specific requirements of intensive-care units (see Chap. 19), long-term care facilities, home-health organizations, and specialized departments such as cardiology and oncology.

14.2.4 Clinical Decision Support

Clinical decision-support systems (Chap. 22) directly assist clinical personnel in data interpretation and decision-making. Once the basic clinical components of an HCIS are well developed, clinical decision-support systems can use the information stored there to monitor patients and issue alerts, to make diagnostic suggestions, to provide limited therapeutic guidance, and to provide information on medication costs. These capabilities are particularly useful when they are integrated with other information-management functions. For example, a useful adjunct to **computer-based physician order-entry (CPOE)** is a decision-support program that alerts physicians to patient food or drug allergies; helps physicians to calculate patient-specific drug-dosing regimens; performs advanced order logic, such as recommending an order for prophylactic antibiotics before certain surgical procedures; automatically discontinues drugs when appropriate or prompts the physician to reorder them; suggests more cost-effective drugs with the same therapeutic effect; or activates and displays applicable clinical-practice guidelines (see Chap. 22). **Clinical-event monitors** integrated with results-reporting applications can alert clinicians to abnormal results and drug interactions by electronic mail, text message or page. In the outpatient setting, these event monitors may produce reminders to provide preventive services such as screening mammograms and routine immunizations. The same event monitors might trigger access to the HCO's approved formulary, displaying information that includes costs, indications, contraindications, approved clinical guidelines, and relevant online medical literature (Perreault and Metzger 1999; Teich et al. 1997; Kaushal et. al. 2003).

14.2.5 Financial and Resource Management

Financial and administrative systems assist with the traditional business functions of an HCO, including management of the payroll, human resources, general ledger, accounts payable, and materials purchasing and inventory. Most of these data-processing tasks are well structured, and have been historically labor intensive and repetitious—ideal opportunities for substitution with computers. Furthermore, with the exception of patient-billing functions, the basic financial tasks of an HCO do not differ substantially from those of organizations in other industries. Not surprisingly, financial and administrative applications have typically been among the first systems to be standardized and centralized in IDNs.

Conceptually, the tasks of creating a patient bill and tracking payments are straightforward, and financial transactions such as claims submission and electronic funds transfer have been standardized to allow **electronic data interchange (EDI)** among providers and payers. In operation, however, patient accounting requirements are complicated by the myriad and oft-changing reimbursement requirements of government and third-party payers. These requirements vary substantially by payer, by insurance plan, by type of facility where service was provided, and often by state. As the burden of financial risk for care has shifted from third party payers to providers (through **per diem** or **diagnosis-based reimbursements**), these systems have become even more critical to the operation of a successful HCO. As another example, managed care contracts add even more complexity, necessitating processes and information systems to check a patient's health-plan enrollment and eligibility for services, to manage referrals and preauthorization for care, to price claims based on negotiated contracts, and to create documentation required to substantiate the services provided.

As HCOs increasingly go "at risk" for delivery of health services by negotiating **per diem**, **diagnosis-based**, **bundled** and **capitated payments**, their incentives need to focus not only on reducing the cost per unit service but also on maintaining the health of members while using health resources effectively and efficiently. Similarly, the HCO's scope of accountability broadens from a relatively small population of sick patients to a much larger population of plan members (such as might be found in ACOs), most of whom are still well.

Provider-profiling systems support utilization management by tracking each provider's resource utilization (costs of drugs prescribed, diagnostic tests and procedures ordered, and so on) compared with severity-adjusted outcomes of that provider's patients such as their rate of hospital readmission and mortality by diagnosis.

Such systems are also being used by government bodies and consumer advocate organizations as they publicize their findings, often through the Internet. **Contract-management systems** have capabilities for estimating the costs and payments associated with potential managed care contracts and comparing actual with expected payments based on the terms of the contracts. More advanced managed-care information systems handle **patient triage** and medical management functions, helping the HCOs to direct patients to appropriate health services and to proactively manage the care of chronically ill and high-risk patients. Health plans, and IDNs that incorporate a health plan, also must support payer and insurance functions such as claims administration, premium billing, marketing, and member services.

14.3 Historical Evolution of the Technology of Health care Information Systems (HCISs)

Technological advances and changes in the information and organizational requirements of HCOs have driven many of the changes in system architecture, hardware, software, and functionality of HCISs over time. The tradeoff between functionality and ease of integration is another important factor that accounts for choices that vendors have made in systems design (see Fig. 14.7).

14.3.1 Central and Mainframe-based Systems

The earliest HCISs (typically found in hospitals) were designed according to the philosophy that a single comprehensive or **central computer system** could best meet an HCO's information processing requirements. Advocates of the centralized approach emphasized the importance of first identifying all the hospital's information needs and then designing a single, unified framework to meet these needs. As we have seen, patient management and billing functions were the initial focus of such efforts. One result of this design goal was the development of systems in which a single, large computer performed all information processing and managed all the data files using application-independent file-management programs—although focusing almost exclusively on financial and billing data. Users accessed these systems via general-purpose **video-display terminals (VDTs)** affectionately known as "green screens" because the displayed numbers and text were often green on a dark background.

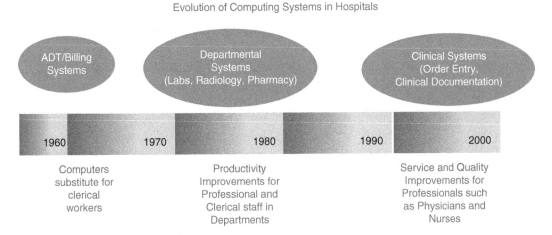

Fig. 14.7 The evolution of computing systems in hospitals has followed a path that parallels the evolution of computing systems in general. From mainframes to minicomputers to desktops, and more recently mobile devices, the purpose and function of systems in hospitals has followed a path from financial systems to departmental systems to systems designed specifically to enhance the productivity and raise the quality of health care services

One of the first clinically-oriented HCISs was the Technicon Medical Information System. System development began in 1965 as a collaborative project between the Lockheed Corporation and El Camino Hospital, a community hospital in Mountain View, California. By 1987, the system had been installed in more than 85 institutions by Technicon Data Systems (TDS), which had purchased the system from Lockheed in 1971. TDS was one of the earliest examples of a large, centrally operated, and clinically focused HCIS. Depending on the size of the central machine, the TDS center could support from several hundred to a few thousand hospital beds. Because of this high capacity, one computer installation could serve multiple hospitals in an area. The hospitals were connected via high-speed dedicated telephone lines linked to the central computer. Within a hospital, a switching station connected the telephone lines to an onsite network connecting to stations on every patient-care unit. Each unit had at least one VDT and one printer which enabled users to display, and print patient information. Initially, TDS sold proprietary terminals, printers, light pens and even implemented their own data transmission protocols, but as more general purpose PCs became prominent and data networking protocols more standardized, the proprietary nature of the system diminished to where the focus was entirely on the software. Because the TDS system was designed for use by both nurses and physicians it was one of the first systems to support both nursing clinical documentation and physician order entry.

The Center for Clinical Computing (CCC) system, developed by Howard Bleich and Warner Slack as a centralized clinical computing system, was first deployed in 1978 at the Beth Israel Medical Center in Boston (now part of the Beth Israel Deaconess Medical Center and the CareGroup IDN). Still in operation, this system is designed around a single common registry of patients, with tight integration of all its departmental systems. It was remarkable in the breadth of its functionality to support physicians and the intensity of its use by clinicians. It was the first system to offer hospital-wide electronic mail, as well as end-user access to Medline via PaperChase. In addition, CCC was among the first to employ audit trails on who was looking at patient data, a feature now common in clinical systems (and a HIPAA requirement). In ambulatory clinics, an electronic patient record including support for problem lists, clinic notes, prescription writing, and other functions supported over 1,000 clinicians in more than 30 primary-care and specialty areas (Safran et al. 1991). On the other hand, the system provided only limited support for order entry, alerts, and reminders. The CCC also featured a MUMPS database functioning as a clinical-data repository and an online data warehouse, called ClinQuery (Safran et al. 1989) with complete data on all test results and medications, as well as **ICD-9-CM** and **SNOMED** diagnosis codes. The CCC was transferred to the Brigham and Women's Hospital in 1983 and was subsequently developed separately as the Brigham Integrated Computer System (BICS), a distributed client–server system. In 2012, Partners Health care, of which Brigham and Women's Hospital is a member organization, made the decision to replace BICS and other in-house developed systems with a commercial vendor product.

Central systems integrated and communicated information well because they provided users with a centralized data store and a single, standardized method to access information simply and rapidly. On the other hand, the biggest limitation of central systems was their inability to accommodate the diverse needs of individual departments. There is a tradeoff between the uniformity (and relative simplicity) of a generalizable system and the nonuniformity and greater responsiveness of custom-designed systems that solve specific problems. Generality—a characteristic that enhances communication and data integration in a homogeneous environment—can be a drawback in an HCO because of the complexity and heterogeneity of the information-management tasks. In general, central systems have proved too unwieldy and inflexible to support current HCO requirements, except in smaller facilities. The development of smaller but powerful computing platforms subsequently led to software development that focused more on specific departmental requirements.

14.3.2 Departmental Systems

By the 1970s, departmental systems began to emerge. Decreases in the price of hardware and improvements in software made it feasible for individual departments within a hospital to acquire and operate their own computers. In a **departmental system**, one or a few computers can be dedicated to processing specific functional tasks within the department. Distinct software application modules carry out specific tasks, and a common framework, which is specified initially, defines the interfaces that will allow data to be shared among the modules. Radiology (Chap. 20) and Laboratory systems are examples of this type of system.

The most ambitious project based on the departmental approach was the Distributed Hospital Computer Program (DHCP) for the Veterans Administration (VA) hospitals which was initially announced in 1982, although based on work begun at the VA in the 1970s. The system had a common database (Fileman), which was written to be both hardware- and operating-system-independent. A small number of support centers in the VA developed the software modules in cooperation with user groups. The CORE—the first set of applications to be developed and installed—consisted of modules for patient registration, ADT, outpatient scheduling, laboratory, outpatient pharmacy, and inpatient pharmacy. Modules to support other clinical departments (such as radiology, dietetics, surgery, nursing, and mental health) and administrative functions (such as financial and procurement applications) were developed subsequently. By 1985, the VA had installed DHCP in more than one-half of its approximately 300 hospitals and clinics. The software was in the public domain and was also used in private hospitals and other government facilities (Kolodner and Douglas 1997). Interestingly, one of the reasons for the success of the VA system was its ability to focus on the clinical environment. Given the nature of government reimbursement for the care of veterans at the time, there was no need to develop or integrate a billing function into the DHCP system.

The departmental approach responded to many of the challenges of central systems. Although individual departmental systems are constrained to function with predefined interfaces, they do not have to conform to the general standards of an overall system, so they can be designed to accommodate the special needs of specific areas. For example, the processing capabilities and file structures suitable for managing the data acquired from a patient-monitoring system in the intensive-care unit (analog and digital signals acquired in real time) differ from the features that are appropriate for a system that reports radiology results (text storage and text processing). Furthermore, modification of departmental systems, although laborious with any approach, is simpler because of the smaller scope of the system. The price for this greater flexibility is increased difficulty in integrating data and communicating among modules of the HCISs. In reality, installing a subsystem is never as easy as simply plugging in the connections.

Also in the early 1980s, researchers at the University of California, San Francisco (UCSF) Hospital successfully implemented one of the first **Local Area Networks** (**LANs**) to support communication among several of the hospital's standalone systems in the early 1980s. Using technology developed at the Johns Hopkins University, they connected minicomputers that supported patient registration, medical records, radiology, the clinical laboratory, and the outpatient pharmacy. Interestingly, each of the four computer systems was different from the other three: the computers were made by different manufacturers and ran different operating systems (McDonald, Wiederhold et al. 1984a) but were able to communicate with each other through standardized communications protocols.

By the late1980s, HCISs based on evolving network-communications standards were being developed and implemented in HCOs. As **distributed computer systems**, connected through electronic networks, these HCISs consisted of a federation of independent systems that had been tailored for specific application areas. The computers operated autonomously and shared data (and sometimes programs and other resources, such as printers) by exchanging information over a local area network (LAN; see Chap. 5) using standard protocols such as **TCP/IP** and Health Level 7(HL7) for communication and in many cases utilizing the interface engine strategy we discussed earlier in Sect. 14.1.1.

The University of Michigan Hospital in Ann Arbor later adopted a hybrid strategy to meet its information needs. The hospital supported a central model of architecture and operated a mainframe computer to perform core HCIS functions. In 1986, however, it installed a local area network (LAN) to allow communication among all its internal clinical laboratories and to allow physicians to obtain laboratory-test results directly from the laboratory information system. At the time of installation, more than 95 % of all the peripheral devices in the laboratories were connected to the network rather than hardwired directly to the laboratory computer. A second clinical host computer, which supported the radiology information system, was later added to the LAN, allowing physicians to access radiology reports as well. Although the mainframe HCIS initially was not connected to the LAN, the hospital later adopted the strategy of installing universal workstations that could access both the mainframe computer and the clinical hosts via the LAN (Friedman and Dieterle 1987).

One advantage of LAN-connected distributed systems was that individual departments could have greater flexibility in choosing hardware and software that optimally suited their specific needs. Even smaller ancillary departments such as Respiratory Therapy, which previously could not justify a major computer acquisition, could now purchase microcomputers and participate in the HCIS environment. Health care providers in nursing units or at the bedside, physicians in their offices or homes, and managers in the administrative offices could eventually access and analyze data locally using what were initially termed microcomputers (later known as desktop personal computers or PCs). On the downside, the distribution of information processing capabilities and responsibility for data among diverse systems made the tasks of data integration, communication, and security more difficult—a fact

that continues to the present day. Development of industry-wide standard network and interface protocols such as TCP/IP and HL7 has eased the technical problems of electronic communication considerably. Still, there are problems to overcome in managing and controlling access to a patient database that is fragmented over multiple computers, each with its own file structure and method of file management. Furthermore, when no global architecture or vocabulary standards are imposed on the HCISs, individual departments and entities may encode data values in ways that are incompatible with the definitions chosen by other areas of the organization. The promise of sharing among independent departments, entities, and even independent institutions has increased the importance of defining clinical data standards (see Chap. 7). As noted earlier, some HCOs pursue a best of breed strategy in which they choose the best system, regardless of vendor and technology, then work to integrate that system into their overall HCIS environment. Some HCOs modify this strategy by choosing suites of related applications (e.g., selecting all ancillary systems from a single vendor, also known as **best of cluster**), thereby reducing the overall number of vendors they work with and, in theory, reducing the costs and difficulty of integration. Commercial software vendors have supported this strategy by broadening their offerings of application suites and managing the integration at the suite level rather than at the level of individual applications. Cerner and Epic are examples of clinical systems vendors who have pursued this strategy, and Oracle's PeopleSoft and Lawson are examples on the financial/administrative side.

The complexity and variety of information processing requirements across today's HCOs and IDNs, means that some level of distributed architecture is often required. Simply put, no single vendor has been able to develop and implement applications that support the entire range of an HCO's information processing requirements. So in general, all large commercial systems support some type of distributed model. PC-based universal workstations are the norm as well. In fact, some HCOs and IDN's now support thousands of PCs in enterprise-wide networked environments. The requirement for direct access to independent ancillary systems has been largely eliminated not only by enterprise data networks, but by interfaces that join such systems to a core clinical system or a centralized clinical data repository that receives clinical data from each ancillary system. For example, whereas staff working in the laboratory may access the laboratory system directly, clinicians may view all clinical results (laboratory, radiology, and so on) stored in a centralized **clinical data repository**. The ability to access patient databases (by clinicians), human resources documents (by employees), financial information (by administrators) and basic information about facilities, departments, and staff (by the public) is enabled through a single enterprise-wide data network (See Fig. 14.3).

14.3.3   Integrated Systems from Single Vendors

Many smaller HCOs have opted for implementation of turnkey systems, in which commercial vendors have bundled a number of functional capabilities into a single application suite (MEDITECH is a good example of this type of offering).

These systems offer a way to achieve reasonable function and integration, although they typically permit minimal customization to meet institution-specific workflows and requirements. In addition, they may not have the depth of specialized functions compared to systems designed for specific departmental functions. Numerous debates have been held at national conferences regarding the desirability of an integrated system versus best of breed approaches in which the various systems have to be interfaced in order to function. In the late 1990s, several large IDNs developed their IT strategies based on the use of integrated systems from vendors historically focused on smaller hospitals. This provided greater credibility to these vendors and at the same time challenged the long held assumption that the greater functionality of best of breed strategies, with their inherently greater cost and interface requirements, is the only viable strategy for large IDNs.

14.4   Architecture for a Changing Environment

As the complexity of the health care business continues to increase, HCOs and IDNs present new challenges to information systems developers. As we described in Sect. 14.1, most IDNs have developed through the merger or acquisition of independent organizations. Thus, the information systems environment of a new or evolving IDN can be a jumble of disparate legacy systems, technologies, and architectures. In such an environment, the challenge is for the IDN's information systems team to configure systems and processes to support new business strategies (such as a diabetes management program or a central call center) and provide integrated information access throughout the IDN, while maintaining uninterrupted operational support for the IDN's existing business units, and do so within the financial constraints of reimbursement levels that seem to decline almost annually.

Sometimes, an IDN will selectively replace specific systems to fit its new organizational structure and strategies (e.g., consolidation of the finance and human resources departments and migration to common corporate general ledger, accounts payable, payroll, and human resources systems for all business entities). As always, resources (both money and staff) are limited; and often it is simply not feasible for an IDN to replace all legacy systems with new common systems, so specific HCISs may remain relatively isolated for long periods of time.

Legacy systems environments and business strategies in both large HCOs and IDNs present unique information challenges. Nonetheless, a few lessons can be learned from past efforts. First, a strategy for data preservation must be developed by providing access to data and implementing an approach for standardizing the meaning of those data. Second, to the extent possible, IDNs and HCOs should separate three conceptual layers—data management, applications and business logic, and user interface—to allow greater flexibility (See Fig. 14.8).

The first layer of architecture is the **data layer**. Data—the results of transactions that the

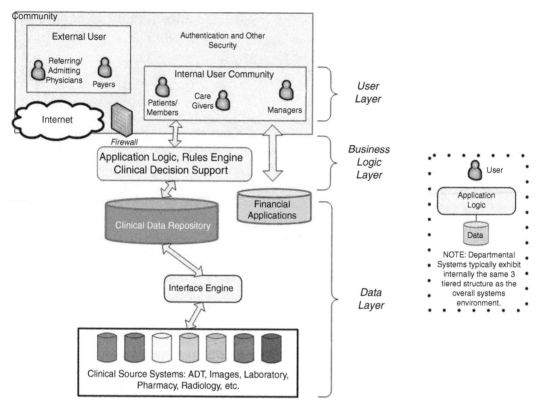

Fig. 14.8 Three conceptual layers of an information systems architecture illustrate the separation that occurs among the data, business logic and presentation layers. Over time, changes in the presentation and business logic layers may be made while retaining the data layer. As noted in the figure, the three layers can typically be found even within a single application (e.g., a laboratory or radiology system)

HCO generates—are of central importance. One fundamental mistake that a health care organization can make is to fail to provide access to its data. Organizations that choose information systems based on the functionality available to meet short-term needs may find that these needs are no longer as important as the HCO or IDN continues to evolve. For this reason, a long-term data strategy needs to be a separate component of the information-management plan. This plan must include access to data for applications and a method to ensure that demographic, clinical, and financial data collected across business units are consistent and comparable. Security and confidentiality safeguards (see Sect. 14.1.4) should also be part of the data strategy.

With respect to clinical data, HCOs and IDNs need data for both real-time operations and retrospective data analysis. These needs generate different requirements for data management. In the first case, detailed data need to be stored and optimized for retrieval for the individual patient. In the second case, the data need to be optimized for aggregation across a population of patients. Although the terms are sometimes used interchangeably, the distinction should be made between a **clinical data repository** (**CDR**), which typically stores "transaction" data and serves the needs of patient care and day-to-day operations, and an **enterprise information warehouse** (**EIW**) which serves as the foundation for analytic tasks for both retrospective and longer term business and clinical planning such as contract management and outcomes evaluation. Both the CDR and data warehouse should be purchased or developed for their ability to model, store, and retrieve efficiently the organization's data. Quite often, vendors of a CDR or warehouse include programs to view and manipulate these data. Conceptually, this packaging makes sense.

The second component of a clinical data strategy is an ability to keep patient information comparable. At the simplest level one needs to uniquely identify each patient. When a health organization consisted of only one hospital and one major information system, the authority over patient identification was relatively simple and usually resided in the HCIS's admitting or registration module (see Sect. 14.2.1). As HCOs evolve into IDNs, there is no one authority that can identify the patient or resolve a conflicting identification. Thus, as we noted earlier, a new architectural component, the enterprise master patient index (EMPI), has arisen as the **name authority**. In its simplest form, the EMPI is an index of patient names and identification numbers used by all information systems in the IDN that store a patient registry. Using this type of EMPI requires considerable manual intervention to ensure data synchrony, but it does enable an IDN to uniquely identify its patients and link their data. Alternatively, an EMPI can be configured as the name authority for all systems that hold patient information even within a single HCO. Then each system must interact with the EMPI in order to get a patient-identification number assigned. This type of EMPI requires that all other systems disable their ability to assign identification numbers and use the external—and unique—EMPI-generated identification numbers.

Uniquely identifying patients within the HCO and the IDN is just a necessary first step in ensuring data comparability and consistency. Health care providers also may want to know which of their patients are allergic to penicillin, which patients should be targeted for new cardiac-disease prevention services, or which patients are likely to need home services when they are discharged from the hospital or emergency room. To store and evaluate the data that could be used to make such determinations, a consistent approach must be developed for naming data elements and defining their values (see Chaps. 7 and 8). Some institutions, such as Columbia University

Medical Center (CUMC) in New York City, have developed their own internal vocabulary standards, or **terminology authority**. CPMC separates the storage and retrieval of data from the meaning of the terms in the database using a **medical entities dictionary** that defines valid database terms and synonyms for use by its clinical applications. An alternative approach is to develop a set of **terminology services**. These services fall into three categories: (1) linking or normalizing the data contained within the HCO's or IDN's legacy databases before these data are copied to a CDR; (2) reregistering all terms used by new applications and linking them to external authoritative vocabulary terms, such as those contained within the Unified Medical Language System's **Metathesaurus** (see Chap. 8); and (3) providing real-time help in selecting the appropriate term to describe a clinical situation.

The second layer of architecture is the **business logic layer**. As we discussed in Sect. 14.1.6, once a system has been installed, its users will usually resist change. The reason for this inertia is not just that there is a steep learning curve for a new system but also that historical systems embody institutional workflow. Separating the workflow or business logic from the database will enable more natural migrations of systems as the HCO or IDN evolves. Organizations should not, however, assume that old workflow is correct or should necessarily be embodied in new information systems. The point here is that a modern architecture that separates the workflow from the data allows prior data to be carried forward as the systems migrate. This also enables organizations to change workflow as new features and functions become available in newer products or product releases.

The third layer, the **user-interface layer**, is how users "see" the data, and most often the layer most subject to frequent change. The cost of desktop devices and support represents a significant portion of HCO and IDN information systems budgets—often as much as one-third of the total budget. For example, an IDN that supports 10,000 workstations will incur ongoing costs for hardware and software alone of close to $10 million per year, assuming a $3,000 unit cost and a

3-year life span per workstation. **Thin clients,** and **web-based technologies,** which minimize processing at the workstation level, can substantially reduce this cost by allowing simpler maintenance and support as well as decreased cost per device.

Future network and computer systems architectures such as **Services Oriented Architecture (SOA)** will likely increasingly rely on the tools and technological developments driven by the ubiquity of the Internet. Smart phones, tablets, **pagers** and other mobile devices continue to shrink in size while increasing in functionality. However, often due to size limitations (and specifically the **form factor** limits of keyboards and display screens available on smaller devices), these systems are currently better suited for one-way retrieval and presentation of information and do not adequately support clinicians' requirements for data input where free text entry continues to be used. But even with shrinking size, these devices are still suitable for accessing electronic schedule and contact lists and have (modified) handwriting recognition capabilities, and support other productivity tools which have become popular. Voice-entry devices have found some utility where noncontinuous speech is supported by good screen design (see Chap. 5). The introduction of computer tablets with handwriting recognition show promise for use in specialized clinical applications. Most likely, clinicians will require a variety of devices—some that are application specific and some that vary with personal preference. The important design consideration is that, if possible, the design of the display and the nature of the input devices should not be so tied to the application that change and modification are difficult.

14.5   Forces That Will Shape the Future of Health Care Information Systems

As we have discussed throughout this chapter, the changing landscape of the health-care industry and the strategic and operational requirements of HCOs and IDNs have accelerated the acquisition and implementation of HCISs. The acquisition and implementation of **Electronic Medical Records (EMRs)** have been a particular focus, especially with the availability of federal stimulus funding through the provisions of the **Health Information Technology for Economic and Clinical Health (HITECH)** Act under the **American Recovery and Reinvestment Act of 2009 (ARRA)**. Although there are many obstacles to implementation and acceptance of smoothly functioning, fully integrated HCISs, few people today would debate the critical role that information technology plays in an HCO's success or in an IDN's efforts at clinical and operational management.

We have emphasized the dynamic nature of today's health care environment and the associated implications for HCISs. A host of new requirements loom that will challenge today's available solutions. We anticipate additional expectations and requirements associated with the changing organizational landscape, technological advances, and broader societal changes.

14.5.1   Changing Organizational Landscape

Although the concepts underlying HCOs and IDNs are no longer new, the underlying organizational forms and business strategies of these complex organizations continue to evolve. The success of individual HCOs varies widely. Some, serving target patient populations such as those with heart disease or cancer or age-defined groups such as children, have been relatively more successful financially that those attempting to serve patients across a wide range of illnesses or those attempting to combine diverse missions of clinical care, teaching and research. IDNs, on the other hand, have by and large failed to achieve the operational improvements and cost reductions they were designed to deliver. It is possible that entirely new forms of HCOs and IDNs will emerge in the coming years. Key to understanding the magnitude of the information systems challenge for IDNs in particular is recognizing the extraordinary pace of change—IDNs reorganize, merge, uncouple, acquire, sell off, and strategically align services and organizational units in a matter of weeks. While information technology is itself changing with accelerating frequency, today's state-of-the-art systems (computer systems and people processes) typically require months or years to build and refine.

All too frequently, business deals are cut with insufficient regard to the cost and time required to create the supporting information infrastructure. For IDNs even in the best of circumstances, the cultural and organizational challenges of linking diverse users and care-delivery settings will tax their ability to change their information systems environments quickly enough. These issues will increase in acuity as operational budgets continue to shrink—today's HCOs and IDNs are spending significant portions of their capital budgets on information-systems investments. In turn, these new investments translate into increased annual operating costs (costs of regular system upgrades, maintenance, user support, and staffing). Still most health care organizations devote at most 3–4 % of their total revenues to their information systems operating budgets; in other information-intensive industries (e.g., financial services, air transportation), the percentage of operating budgets devoted to information technology investment can be three to four times higher.

14.5.2 Technological Changes Affecting Health Care Organizations

Future changes in technology are hard to predict. For example, although we have heard for over two decades that voice-to-text systems are 5 years away from practical use, with the introduction of controlled vocabularies in areas such as radiology and pathology, we are beginning to see commercial products that can "understand" dictated speech and represent it as text that can then be structured for further analysis. First, the emergence of increasingly powerful processor and memory chips, and the decreasing cost of storage media will continue to be a factor in future health-systems design—although the tsunami of data coming from genomic medicine sequencing and analysis may be a significant challenge (see Chaps. 2, 25, and 26). Second, the ever expanding availability of Internet access, the increasing integration of voice, video, and data, and the availability of ever smaller platforms like tablets and smart phones, will challenge HCOs and IDNs to have communications capacity not only within their traditional domain but also to an extended enterprise that may include patients' homes, schools, and workplaces. Third, the design of modern software based on the replicability of code, code standards such as **XML**, and frameworks such as Services Oriented Architecture (SOA) should eventually yield more flexible information technology systems.

One of the most significant technological challenges facing HCOs and IDNs today occurs because, while much of the health care delivered today is within the four walls of a physician's office or a hospital, as the population ages, patients may seek care from both primary and specialty practices, may have multiple hospital visits (and even visits to multiple hospitals) and may increasingly be monitored in their homes. Health care information technologies (and clinical systems in particular) have focused historically on what happens within a physician's office or within a hospital, and not across physicians' office nor between the physicians' office and the hospital nor in the home of the patient.

In general, EHR products on the market today started with a single purpose: to automate the workflow of clinicians within a particular organizational setting. Among other features, EHRs focus on making data from previous encounters or activities easier to access, and assuring that orders for tests and x-rays have the correct information, or that the next shift knows what went on previously. In spite of visible successes and failures for all manner of products, EHRs in general can facilitate the automation of a complex workflow—of automating intra-organizational clinical processes.

Architectures that focus on what happens *within* organizational boundaries do not easily facilitate access to data *across* organizational boundaries. This is the challenge of **interoperability**. Recognizing that patients often receive care in a variety of organizational settings—hospitals, physicians offices, rehabilitation facilities, pharmacies, etc.—the challenge is to extend the internal workflow beyond the boundaries of individual organizations so that data is available across a continuum of care. Interoperability then is not so much about what happens *within* an organization (although there can be challenges here as well), but what happens *across* organizational boundaries.

The architectural requirements for automating *intra*-organizational clinical workflows are very different from the architectural requirements for facilitating *inter*-organizational interoperability. An *intra*-organizational architecture focuses on facilitating real time communications among providers, on optimizing the process of collecting data at the point of care, and on ensuring that clinical tasks are carried out in an appropriate sequence. An *inter*-organizational architecture needs to be designed to minimize the duplicate collection of data in different care settings, to facilitate quick searches of relevant data from a variety of (often external) sources, and to rank data in terms of relevance to a particular clinical question. Transitioning from *intra*- to *inter-organizational* data sharing is a significant technological challenge. While Health Information Exchanges (HIEs) and Health Record Banks (HRBs) are at the forefront of this transition (see Chap. 13), over time we can expect that the architectures of clinical systems that currently focus on what happens *within* an organization will need to transition to facilitate what happens *across* organizations.

Security and confidentiality concerns will likely increase as the emergence of a networked society profoundly changes our thinking about the nature of health care delivery. Health services are still primarily delivered locally—we seldom leave our local communities to receive health care except under the most dire circumstances. In the future, providers and even patients will have access to health care experts that are dispersed over state, national, and even international boundaries. Distributed health care capabilities will need to support the implementation of collaborative models that could include virtual house calls and routine **remote monitoring** via telemedicine linkages (see Chap. 18).

14.5.3 Societal Change

At the beginning of the twenty-first century, clinicians find themselves spending less time with each patient and more time with administrative and regulatory concerns. This decrease in clinician–patient contact has contributed to declining patient and provider satisfaction with care-delivery systems. At the same time, empowered health consumers interested in self-help and unconventional approaches have access to more health information than ever before. These factors are changing the interplay among physicians, care teams, patients, and external (regulatory and financial) forces. The changing model of care, coupled with changing economic incentives to deliver high quality care at lower cost, places a greater focus on wellness and preventative and lifelong care. Although we might agree that aligning economic incentives with wellness is a good thing, this alignment also implies a shift in responsibility from care givers to patients.

Like the health care environment, the technological context of our lives is also changing. The Internet has already dramatically changed our approaches to information access and system design. Concurrent with the development of new standards of information display and exchange is a push led by the entertainment industry (and others) to deliver broadband multimedia into our homes. Such connectivity has the potential to change care models more than any other factor we can imagine by bringing fast, interactive, and multimedia capabilities to the household level. Finally, vast amounts of information can now be stored efficiently on movable media such as **memory sticks**, which brings more flexibility as well as more risk, as such devices are both more convenient and more susceptible to being lost or misplaced. With the increase in the availability of consumer-oriented health information, including, for example, video segments that show the appearance and sounds of normal and abnormal conditions or demonstrate common procedures for home care and health maintenance, we can expect even more changes in the traditional doctor/patient relationship.

With societal factors pushing our HCOs and IDNs to change, cost constraints looming larger, and the likely availability of extensive computing and communication capacity in the home, in the work place, and in the schools, HCOs and health providers are increasingly challenged to rethink the basic operating assumptions about how to deliver care. The traditional approach has been facility and physician centric—patients usually come to the hospital or to the physician's office at a time convenient for the hospital or the physician. The HCO and IDN of the twenty-first century may have to be truly "patient centric", operating within a health care delivery system without walls, where routine health management is conducted in nontraditional settings, such as homes and workplaces, using the power of telemedicine and consumer informatics.

Suggested Readings

Christensen, C., Grossman, J., & Hwang, J. (2009). *The innovator's prescription*. New York: McGraw-Hill. This book builds on the author's previous work on disruptive innovation with specific applications to the health care industry. Christensen uses terms such as "precision medicine" to describe the advent of more personalized approaches to medical diagnosis and treatment, and builds on his analysis of disruptive business models in other industries to analyze both the underlying problems and challenges of our health care delivery system.

Lee, T., & Mongan, J. (2009). *Chaos and organization in health care*. Cambridge, MA: The MIT Press. The authors describe the current health care situation as one simply of "chaos". Among the solutions they propose are increasing the use of electronic medical records and information technology in general for sharing knowledge.

Ong, K. (2011). *Medical informatics: an executive primer* (2nd ed.). Chicago: Health care and Management Information Systems Society. An excellent overview of the challenges facing information technology applications in hospitals, physicians' offices, and in the homes of patients. Also includes a discussion of recent federal legislation intended to stimulate the use of electronic medical records and the challenges of measuring how to determine whether such investments are in fact "meaningfully used".

Porter, M., & Teisberg, E. (2006). *Redefining health care: creating value-based competition on results*. Cambridge, MA: Harvard Business School Press. The authors begin with a very straightforward assumption, which is that "the way to transform health care is to realign competition with *value for patients*" (p. 4), and proceed with an exhaustive discussion of the historical failures at reforming the health care system, the challenges inherent in physician-provider organization relationships, and how the only likely solution set to the current high cost of health care is to focus our efforts on what brings value to the patients.

Questions for Discussion

1. Briefly explain the differences among an HCO's operational, planning, communications, and documentary requirements for information. Give two examples in each category. Choose one of these categories, and discuss similarities and differences in the environments of an integrated delivery network, a community-based ambulatory-care clinic, and a specialty-care physician's office. Describe the implied differences in these units' information requirements.

2. Describe three situations in which the separation of clinical and administrative information could lead to inadequate patient care, loss of revenue, or inappropriate administrative decisions. Identify and discuss the challenges and limitations of two methods for improving data integration.

3. Describe three situations in which lack of integration of information systems with clinicians' workflow can lead to inadequate patient care, reduced physician productivity, or poor patient satisfaction with an HCO's services. Identify and discuss the challenges and limitations of two methods for improving process integration.

4. Describe the trade-off between functionality and integration. Discuss three

strategies currently used by HCOs to minimize this tradeoff.

5. Assume that you are the chief information officer of multi-facility HCO. You have just been charged with planning a new clinical HCIS to support a large tertiary care medical center, two smaller community hospitals, a nursing home, and a 40-physician group practice. Each organization currently operates its own set of integrated and standalone technologies and applications. What technical and organizational factors must you consider? What are the three largest challenges you will face over the next 24 months?

6. How do you think the implementation of clinical HCISs will affect the quality of relationships between patients and providers? Discuss at least three potential positive and three potential negative effects. What steps would you take to maximize the positive value of these systems?

Patient-Centered Care Systems

15

Judy Ozbolt, Suzanne Bakken, and Patricia C. Dykes

After reading this chapter, you should know the answers to these questions:

- What is patient-centered care? How does it differ from traditional, clinician-centric care?
- What are the information management challenges in patient-centered care?
- What are the roles of electronic health records and other informatics applications in supporting patient-centered care?
- What forces and developments have led to the emergence of patient-centered care systems?
- What collaborative processes are required to design patient-centered care systems and the electronic health records to support such care?
- How is current informatics research advancing progress toward collaborative, interdisciplinary, patient-centered care?

J. Ozbolt, PhD, RN, FAAN, FACMI, FAIMBE (✉)
Department of Organizational Systems and Adult Health, University of Maryland School of Nursing, 655 West Lombard Street,
Baltimore 21201, MD, USA
e-mail: judy.ozbolt@gmail.com

S. Bakken, RN, PhD, FAAN, FACMI
Department of Biomedical Informatics,
School of Nursing, Columbia University,
630 W. 168th Street, New York 10032, NY, USA
e-mail: sbh22@columbia.edu

P.C. Dykes, PhD, MA
Center for Patient Safety Research & Practice,
Brigham and Women's Hospital, 1 Brigham Circle,
Boston 02124, MA, USA
e-mail: pdykes@partners.org

15.1 Information Management in Patient-Centered Care

Patient care is the focus of many clinical disciplines—medicine, nursing, pharmacy, nutrition, therapies such as respiratory, physical, and occupational, and others. Although the work of the various disciplines sometimes overlaps, each has its own primary focus, emphasis, and methods of care delivery. Each discipline's work is complex in itself, and collaboration among disciplines, an essential component of patient-centered care, adds another level of complexity. In all disciplines, the quality of clinical decisions depends in part on the quality of information available to the decision-maker. The systems that manage information for patient-centered care are therefore a critical tool. Their fitness for the job varies, and the systems enhance or detract from patient-centered care accordingly. This chapter describes information management issues in patient-centered care, the emergence of patient-centered care systems in relation to these issues, the interdisciplinary collaboration required to develop patient-centered care systems, and current research. In so doing, it will demonstrate the necessity of a patient-centered perspective in the design of electronic health records.

As described later in this chapter, reports of the National Academy of Sciences, Federal Government mandates, and a variety of social forces have called for transformation in the organization, delivery, financing, and quality of health care. The demand is for evidence-based,

E.H. Shortliffe, J.J. Cimino (eds.), *Biomedical Informatics*,
DOI 10.1007/978-1-4471-4474-8_15, © Springer-Verlag London 2014

cost-effective, **patient-centered care**. Informatics is seen as essential to the provision, monitoring, and improvement of such care.

15.1.1 From Patient Care to Patient-Centered Care

Patient-centered care is a collaborative, interdisciplinary process focused on the care recipient in the context of the family, significant others, and community. A distinguishing feature of patient-centered care is the patient's active collaboration in shared decision-making, as contrasted to traditional clinician-centered care where the clinician holds the preponderance of power and authority. Patient-centered care empowers patients to actively participate in care by presenting treatment options that are consistent with patient values and preferences and in a format or context that is understandable and actionable (Krist and Woolf 2011; Payton et al. 2011). Typically, patient care includes the services of physicians, nurses, and members of other health disciplines according to patient needs: physical, occupational, and respiratory therapists; nutritionists; psychologists; social workers; and many others. Each of these disciplines brings specialized perspectives and expertise. Specific cognitive processes and therapeutic techniques vary by discipline, but all disciplines share certain commonalities in the provision of care.

In its simplest terms, the process of patient-centered care begins with collecting data and assessing the patient's current status and expressed concerns in comparison to criteria or expectations of normality. Through cognitive processes specific to the discipline, diagnostic labels are applied, therapeutic goals are identified with timelines for evaluation, and therapeutic interventions are selected and implemented. The patient participates, as he or she is able, in determining therapeutic goals and selecting personally acceptable interventions from the options and their potential consequences as described by the clinician. At specified intervals, the patient is reassessed, the effectiveness of care is evaluated, and therapeutic goals and interventions are continued or adjusted as needed. If the reassessment shows that the patient no longer needs care, services are terminated. This process was illustrated for nursing in 1975 (Goodwin and Edwards 1975) and was updated and made more general in 1984 (Ozbolt et al. 1984). The flowchart reproduced in Fig. 15.1 could apply equally well to other patient-care disciplines.

Although this linear flowchart helps to explain some aspects of the process of care, it is, like the solar-system model of the atom, a gross simplification. Frequently, for example, in the process of collecting data for an initial patient assessment, the nurse may recognize (diagnose) that the patient is anxious about her health condition. Simultaneously with continuing the data collection, the nurse sets a therapeutic goal that the patient's anxiety will be reduced to a level that increases the patient's comfort and ability to participate in care. The nurse selects and implements therapeutic actions of modulating the tone of voice, limiting environmental stimuli, maintaining eye contact, using gentle touch, asking about the patient's concerns, and providing information. All the while, the nurse observes the effects on the patient's anxiety and adjusts his behavior accordingly. Thus, the complete care process can occur in a microcosm while one step of the care process—data collection—is underway. This simultaneous, nonlinear quality of patient care poses challenges to informatics in the support of patient care and the capture of clinical data.

Each caregiver's simultaneous attention to multiple aspects of the patient is not the only complicating factor. Just as atoms become molecules by sharing electrons, the care provided by each discipline becomes part of a complex molecule of interdisciplinary, patient-centered care. Caregivers and developers of informatics applications to support care must recognize that true patient-centered care is as different from the separate contributions of the various disciplines as an organic molecule is from the elements that go into it. The contributions of the various disciplines are not merely additive; as a therapeutic force acting upon and with the patient, the work of each discipline is transformed by its interaction with the patient and the other disciplines in the larger unity of patient-centered care.

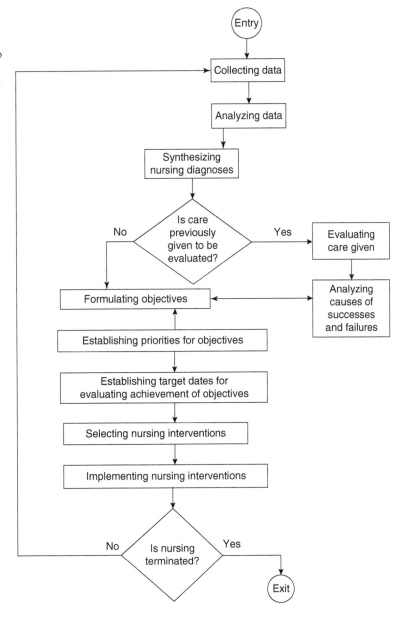

Fig. 15.1 The provision of nursing care is an iterative process that consists of steps to collect and analyze data, to plan and implement interventions, and to evaluate the results of interventions (Source: Adapted with permission from Ozbolt, J.G. et al. (1985). A proposed expert system for nursing practice. *Journal of Medical Systems*, 9:57–68)

15.1.2 Patient-Centered Care in Action

A 75-year-old woman with osteoarthritis, high blood pressure, and urinary incontinence is receiving care from a physician, a home-care nurse, a nutritionist, a physical therapist, and an occupational therapist. From a clinician-centered, additive perspective, each discipline could be said to perform the following functions:

1. Physician: diagnose diseases, prescribe appropriate medications, authorize other care services

2. Nurse: assess patient's understanding of her condition and treatment and her self-care abilities and practices; assess patient's concerns, values, and preferences regarding the management of her health; teach and counsel as needed; help patient to perform exercises at home; report findings to physician and other caregivers

3. Nutritionist: assess patient's nutritional status and eating patterns; prescribe and teach appropriate diet to control blood pressure and build physical strength
4. Physical therapist: prescribe and teach appropriate exercises to improve strength and flexibility and to enhance cardiovascular health, within limitations of arthritis
5. Occupational therapist: assess abilities and limitations for performing activities of daily living; prescribe exercises to improve strength and flexibility of hands and arms; teach adaptive techniques and provide assistive devices as needed

In a collaborative, interdisciplinary, patient-centered practice, the nurse discovers that the patient is not taking walks each day as prescribed because her urinary incontinence is exacerbated by the diuretic prescribed to treat hypertension, and the patient is embarrassed to go out. The nurse reports this to the physician and the other clinicians so that they can understand why the patient is not carrying out the prescribed regime. The physician then changes the strategy for treating hypertension while initiating treatment for urinary incontinence. The nurse helps the patient to understand the interaction of the various treatment regimes, provides practical advice and assistance in dealing with incontinence, and helps the patient to find personally acceptable ways to follow the prescribed treatments. The nutritionist works with the patient on the timing of meals and fluid intake so that the patient can exercise and sleep with less risk of urinary incontinence. The physical and occupational therapists adjust their recommendations to accommodate the patient's personal needs and preferences while moving toward the therapeutic goals. Finally, the patient, rather than being assailed with the sometimes conflicting demands of multiple clinicians, is supported by an ensemble of services that meet shared therapeutic goals in ways consistent with her preferences and values.

This kind of patient-centered collaboration requires exquisite communication and feedback. The potential for information systems to support or sabotage patient-centered care is obvious.

15.1.3 Coordination of Patient-Centered Care

When patients receive services from multiple clinicians, patient-centeredness requires coordinating those services. Coordination includes seeing that patients receive all the services they need in logical sequence without scheduling conflicts and ensuring that each clinician communicates as needed with the others. Sometimes, a **caseman-ager** or **care coordinator** is designated to do this coordination. In other situations, a physician or a nurse assumes the role by default. Sometimes, coordination is left to chance, and both the processes and the outcomes of care are put at risk. In recognition of this, the Institute of Medicine designated coordination of care as 1 of 14 priorities for national action to transform health care quality (Adams and Corrigan 2003). The Health Information Technology for Economic and Clinical Health Act (HITECH Programs 2009[1]) calls for patients to have a **medical home**, a primary care practice that will maintain a comprehensive problem list to make fully informed decisions in coordinating their care. Well-designed information systems with patient facing-technologies (e.g., personal health records and patient portals) enable care coordination as they ensure that patients and providers have immediate access to accurate health information at home and across care settings (Ahern et al. 2011).

15.1.4 Patient-Centered Care Across Multiple Patients

Delivering and managing interdisciplinary patient-centered care for an individual is challenging enough, but patient care has yet another level of complexity. Each clinician is responsible for the care of multiple patients. In planning and executing the work of patient-centered care, each professional must consider the competing demands of all the patients for whom she is responsible, as well as the exigencies of all the

---

[1] http://healthit.hhs.gov/portal/server.pt/community/heal-thit_hhs_gov__hitech_programs/1487 (Accessed: 4/26/13).

other professionals involved in each patient's care. Thus, the nurse on a post-operative unit must plan for scheduled treatments for each of her patients to occur near the optimal time for that patient. She must take into account that several patients may require treatments at nearly the same time and that some of them may be receiving other services, such as imaging or physician's visits, at the time when it might be most convenient for the nurse to administer the treatment. When unexpected needs arise, as they often do—an emergency, an unscheduled patient, observations that could signal an incipient complication—the nurse must set priorities, organize, and delegate to be sure that at least the critical needs are met. Similarly, the physician must balance the needs of various patients who may be widely dispersed throughout an institution. Decision-support systems have the potential to provide important assistance for both the care of individual patients and the organization of the clinician's workload.

15.1.5 Integrating Indirect-Care Activities

Finally, clinicians not only deliver services to patients, with all the planning, documenting, collaborating, referring, and consulting attendant on direct care; they are also responsible for **indirect-care** activities, such as teaching and supervising students, attending staff meetings, participating in continuing education, and serving on committees. Each clinician's plan of work must allow for both the direct-care and the indirect-care activities. Because the clinicians work in concert, these plans must be coordinated.

In summary, patient care is an extremely complex undertaking with multiple levels. To achieve patient-centered care, each clinician's contributions to the care of every patient must take into account not only that patient's values, preferences, and concerns, but also the ensemble of contributions of all clinicians involved in the patient's care and the interactions among them, and this entire suite of care must be coordinated to optimize effectiveness and efficiency. These

very complex considerations are multiplied by the number of patients for whom each clinician is responsible. Patient care is further complicated by the indirect-care activities that caregivers must intersperse among the direct-care responsibilities and coordinate with other caregivers. The resulting cognitive workload frequently overwhelms human capacity. Systems that effectively assist clinicians to manage, process, and communicate the data, information, and knowledge essential to patient-centered care are critical to the quality and safety of that care.

15.1.6 Information to Support Patient-Centered Care

As complex as patient care is, the essential information for direct, patient-centered care is defined in the answers to the following questions:

- What are the patient's needs, concerns, preferences, and values?
- Who is involved in the care of the patient?
- What information does each clinician require to make decisions in his or her professional domain?
- From where, when, and in what form does the information come?
- What information does each clinician generate? Where, when, and in what form is it needed?

The framework described by Zielstorff, Hudgings, and Grobe (1993) provides a useful heuristic for understanding the varied types of information required to answer each of these questions. As listed in Table 15.1, this framework delineates three information categories: (1) patient-specific data about a particular patient acquired from a variety of data sources; (2) agency-specific data relevant to the specific organization under whose auspices the health care is provided; and (3) domain information and knowledge specific to the health care disciplines.

The framework further identifies four types of information processes that information systems may apply to each of the three information categories. *Data acquisition* entails the methods

Table 15.1 Framework for design characteristics of a patient-care information system with examples of patient-specific data, agency-specific data, and domain information and knowledge for patient care

Types of data	System processes			
	Acquiring	Storing	Transforming	Presenting
Domain-specific	Downloading relevant scientific or clinical literature or practice guidelines	Maintaining information in electronic journals or files, searchable by key words	Linking related literature or published findings; updating guidelines based on research	Displaying relevant literature or guidelines in response to queries
Agency-specific	Scanning, downloading, or keying in agency policies and procedures; keying in personnel, financial, and administrative records	Maintaining information in electronic directories, files, and databases	Editing and updating information; linking related information in response to queries; analyzing information	Displaying on request continuously current policies and procedures; sharing relevant policies and procedures in response to queries; generating management reports
Patient-specific	Point-of-care entry of data about patient assessment, diagnoses, treatments planned and delivered, therapeutic goals, and patient outcomes	Moving patient data into a current electronic record or an aggregate data repository	Combining relevant data on a single patient into a cue for action in a decision-support system; performing statistical analyses on data from many patients	Displaying reminders, alerts, probable diagnoses, or suggested treatments; displaying vital signs graphically; displaying statistical results

Source: Framework adapted with permission from *Next Generation Nursing Information Systems*, 1993, American Nurses Association, Washington, DC

by which data become available to the information system. It may include data entry by the care provider or acquisition from a medical device or from another computer-based system. *Data storage* includes the methods, programs, and structures used to organize data for subsequent use. Standardized coding and classification systems useful in representing patient-centered care concepts are discussed in greater detail in Chaps. 2, 7, and 12. *Data transformation* (or *data processing*) comprises the methods by which stored data or information are acted on according to the needs of the end-user—for example, calculation of a pressure ulcer risk-assessment score at admission or calculation of critically ill patients' acute physiology and chronic health evaluation (APACHE) scores. Figure 15.2 illustrates the transformation (abstraction, summarization, aggregation) of patient-specific data for multiple uses. *Presentation* encompasses the forms in which information is delivered to the end-user after processing.

Transformed patient-specific data can be presented in a variety of ways. Numeric data may be best presented in chart or graph form to allow the user to examine trends, whereas the compilation of potential diagnoses generated from patient-assessment data is better presented in an alphanumeric-list. Different types of agency-specific data lend themselves to a variety of presentation formats. Common among all, however, is the need for presentation at the point of patient care. For example, the integration of upto-the-minute patient-specific data with agency-specific guidelines or parameters can produce alerts, reminders, or other types of notifications for immediate action. See Chap. 19, on patient-monitoring systems, for an overview of this topic. Presentation of domain information and knowledge related to patient care is most frequently accomplished through interaction with databases and knowledge bases, such as Medline or Micromedex (see Chap. 21). Commercial applications such as UpToDate™ are popular among

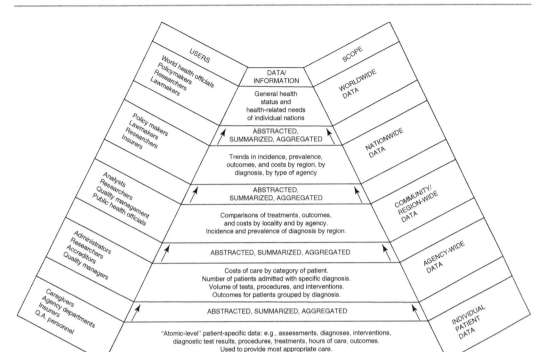

Fig. 15.2 Examples of uses for atomic-level patient data collected once but used many times (Source: Reprinted with permission from Zielstorff, R. D., Hudgings, C. I., Grobe S. J. & The National Commission on Nursing Implementation Project Task Force on Nursing Information Systems. Next-Generation Nursing Information Systems, © 1993 American Nurses Publishing, American Nurses Foundation/American Nurses Association, Washington, DC. Reproduced with permission of the publisher)

clinicians because they provide easy access to knowledge resources at the point of care. The Infobutton, developed at New York-Presbyterian Hospital, is in the public domain. Incorporated into electronic health records, Infobuttons can integrate data about the patient and the clinical context to provide immediate, point-of-care access to relevant knowledge resources (Cimino et al. 2002a).

To support patient-centered care, information systems must be geared to the needs of all the clinicians involved in care. The systems should acquire, store, process, and present each type of information (patient-, agency-, and domain-specific) where, when, and how the information is needed by each clinician in the context of his or her professional domain. Systems designed for patient-centered care have the potential to go beyond supporting the collaborative, interdisciplinary care of individual patients. Through appropriate use of patient-specific information

(care requirements), agency-specific information (clinicians and their responsibilities and agency policies and procedures), and domain information (guidelines), such systems can greatly aid the coordination of interdisciplinary services for individual patients and the planning and scheduling of each caregiver's work activities. Patient acuity is taken into account in scheduling nursing personnel, but historically has most often been entered into a separate system rather than derived directly from care requirements as recorded in the electronic health record. Fully integrated, patient-centered systems—still an ideal today—would enhance our understanding of each patient's situation, needs, and values, improve decision-making, facilitate communications, aid coordination, and use clinical data to provide feedback for improving clinical processes.

Clearly, when electronic health records and other information systems designed to support patient-centered care fulfill their potential, they will not merely replace oral and paper-based methods of recording and communicating. They will be an integral and essential part of the transformation of health care to apply evidence-based interventions in accordance with patient needs and values. How far have we come toward the ideal? What must we do to continue our progress?

15.2　The Emergence of Patient-Centered Care Systems

Events in the first decade of the Twenty-first Century planted the seeds of transformative change in patient care and clinical informatics. Over 10 years, the shared ideal of health care began to move from the Twentieth Century "doctor knows best" model toward a new vision of health care based on interdisciplinary teams drawing on a variety of knowledge and information resources to collaborate with one another and with patients and families to resolve or alleviate health problems and to achieve health goals. Recursive and iterative developments grew from reports of the National Research Council and the Institute of Medicine (components of the National Academy of Sciences); from government policies and initiatives; from changes in organizational and financial structures for health care delivery; and from advances in the informatics methods and technologies that have become integral to the provision, management, reimbursement, and improvement of health care. During the second decade, much remains to be done to nurture continuing development, but with care and patience, before this decade ends we can begin to harvest the benefits of better health care and better health for individuals and populations.

15.2.1　Publications of the National Academy of Sciences

With its seminal publication, *To Err is Human: Building a Safer Health System* (Kohn et al. 2000), the Institute of Medicine startled the world by estimating that clinical errors were killing up to 98,000 hospitalized Americans each year. The report called for a national focus to advance knowledge about safety, reporting efforts to identify and learn from errors, higher standards and expectations for safety, and implementation of safe practices and systems within health care organizations.

The follow-on report, *Crossing the Quality Chasm: A New Health System for the 21st Century* (Committee on Quality of Health Care in America 2001), addressed the need for fundamental change in the health care delivery system. The report noted that the provision of health care had not kept pace with advances in science and technology and did not make the best use of resources. Moreover, health systems had not been restructured to raise quality, control costs, and employ information technologies to improve clinical and administrative processes. Nor had clinical infrastructures been developed to provide the full range of services needed by persons with chronic conditions, the leading causes of illness. Significantly, the report placed the blame for these shortcomings not on individual health care professionals, but on inadequate and broken systems of care.

Crossing the Quality Chasm outlined a call for action by government, payers, providers, and the public to embrace a statement of purpose for the health care system as a whole—to reduce illness and improve health and functioning—and to adopt a shared agenda to achieve health care that would be safe, effective, patient-centered, timely, efficient, and equitable. The report recommended Federal Government funding and initiatives to track progress toward these aims. It also advised the redesign of care processes to achieve continuity in care relationships; customization in accordance with patient needs and values; the sharing of knowledge, information, and decision-making with patients; evidence-based decision-making; safety as a system property; transparency of information to facilitate informed decision-making by patients and families; anticipation of patient needs; continuous decrease in waste; and cooperation among clinicians. Since achievement of these aims could be predicted to improve health and thereby reduce fee-for-service revenues, the report urged government and private payers to devise approaches to health care financing that would support quality.

The report gave considerable attention to informatics as an essential methodology to achieve these aims and called for a renewed national commitment to a national health information infrastructure, with the elimination of most hand-written clinical information by 2010. Finally, the report noted that the changes in practice it recommended would require new approaches to the education of clinicians.

The following year, the Institute of Medicine produced a set of *Priority Areas for National Action* (Adams and Corrigan 2003) to transform the quality of health care. In addition to identifying a number of diseases and health conditions as foci, the report recommended efforts to advance three cross-cutting strategies: care coordination, self-management/health literacy, and medication management. It saw these strategies as essential to ensuring that care be evidence-based, adequate, appropriate, and patient-centered.

In *Patient Safety: Achieving a New Standard for Care* (Committee on Data Standards for Patient Safety 2004), the Committee highlighted the fact that a national health information infrastructure – a foundation of systems, technology, applications, standards, and policies - is required for error prevention and capture of data that facilitate local and global learning from adverse events, near misses, and hazards. The need for data interchange standards as an essential building block was emphasized.

The National Academy of Sciences followed these four reports with a number of others that explored in greater depth aspects of the problems and recommendations described within them and made further recommendations for public and private actions to improve health care and its costs and outcomes. In 2009, The National Research Council published *Computational Technology for Effective Health Care: Immediate Steps and Strategic Directions* (Stead & Lin, Eds.). This report noted that many health information technologies in the current marketplace lacked the functionality to achieve the goals of improving health care. It addressed the challenges of implementing the best of today's health information technologies to achieve short-term gains and of identifying advances in those technologies

needed to reach the ultimate aims of health care as described in the other reports cited. The central finding was that computer scientists, experts in health and biomedical informatics, and clinicians would need to collaborate to create technologies that would provide cognitive support to clinicians, patients, and family members as they sought to understand, resolve, or alleviate health challenges. The report recommended that Federal and state governments and clinicians join forces to require vendors to provide systems that offer such "meaningful" support.

15.2.2 Federal Government Initiatives

The Health Information Technology for Economic and Clinical Health (HITECH) Act provided an unprecedented federal investment in HIT through a series of initiatives aimed at ensuring that all Americans benefit from EHR-supported patient-centered care. Administered by the Office of the National Coordinator for Health Information Technology, the activities are designed:

- To support the health care workforce through Regional Extension Centers for technical assistance for implementation of EHRs and training initiatives to ensure meaningful use of EHRs
- To enable coordination and alignment within and among states (State Health Information Exchange Cooperative Agreement Program)
- To establish connectivity to the public health community in case of emergencies (Beacon Community Program)
- To achieve breakthrough advances, overcoming factors that have hindered EHR adoption (Strategic Health IT Research Projects (SHARP) Program[2]; "HITECH Programs").

In addition, two federal rules support meaningful use of EHRs. The Incentive Programs for Electronic Health Records rule from the Centers

---

[2] http://healthit.hhs.gov/portal/server.pt/community/strategic_health_it_advanced_research_projects/1436/home/16979. (Accessed: 4/26/13).

for Medicare & Medicaid Services (CMS) defines minimum requirements that hospitals and eligible professionals must meet through their use of certified technology to qualify for incentive payments. Criteria related to providing patients with an electronic copy of their own health information and ability to electronically exchange key clinical information are particularly important to patient-centered care. The complementary Standards and Certification Criteria for Electronic Health Records rule defines the criteria for certification of the technology. Also relevant to patient-centered care are NHIN Direct and NHIN CONNECT, which support health information exchange to enable patient-centered care. These are described in more detail in Chap. 13.

The Agency for Health care Research and Quality (AHRQ) has also invested in advancing patient-centered care through investments in health information technology. A particular focus is the re-use of EHR data for comparative effectiveness research with an emphasis on underserved populations. This in reflected in the AHRQ PROSPECT (Prospective Outcome Systems using Patient-specific Electronic Data to Compare Tests and Therapies) grant portfolio. For example, the Washington Heights/Inwood Informatics Infrastructure for Comparative Effectiveness Research (WICER) integrates EHR data with data from home health care, long-term care, and a community household survey to examine research questions related to hypertension management.

Given these major investments in promoting EHR adoption and use for patient-centered care and research, the vision of every American reaping the benefits of EHRs is moving closer to reality. However, this will be heavily influenced by associated changes in health care financial and organizational structures.

15.2.3 Financial and Organizational Structures in Health Care

The historical evolution of information systems that support patient care, and eventually patient-centered care, is not solely a reflection of the available technologies (e.g. Web 2.0, cloud computing). Societal forces—including delivery-system structure, practice model, payer model, and quality focus—have influenced the design and implementation of patient-care systems (Table 15.2).

15.2.3.1 Delivery-System Structure

Authors have noted the significant influence of the organization and its people on the success or failure of informatics innovations (Massaro 1993; Campbell et al. 2006; Ash et al. 2007). Others have documented unintended consequences of implementation of health information technology and called for applications of models of processes, such as Iterative Sociotechnical Analysis, that take into account, health care organizations' workflow, social interactions, culture, etc. to further elucidate the relationship between organizations and technology (Harrison et al. 2007; Koppel et al. 2005). As delivery systems shifted from the predominant single-institution structure of the 1970s to the **integrated delivery networks** of the 1990s to the complex linkages of the twenty-first century, the information needs changed, and the challenges of meeting those information needs increased in complexity. The **patient centered medical home** (PCMH)[3] (also known as primary care medical home, advanced primary care, and health care home) is a model of primary care that delivers care that is patient-centered, comprehensive, coordinated, accessible, and continuously improved through a systems-based approach to quality and safety ("Patient Centered Medical Home Resource Center" 2011).[4] AHRQ and others (Bates and Bitton 2010) have noted the seminal role of health information technology (e.g., health information exchange, disease registries, alerts and reminders) to support tasks related to NCQA PCMH standards for enhancing access and continuity, identifying and managing patient populations, planning and managing care, providing self-care and community support, tracking and coordinating care, and measuring and improving performance ("Patient Centered Medical

---

[3] http://www.ncqa.org/ (Accessed: 4/26/13).

[4] http://www.pcmh.ahrq.gov/portal/server.pt/community/pcmh__home/1483 (Accessed 4.26.13).

Table 15.2 Societal forces that have influenced the design and implementation of patient-centered systems

	1970s	1980s	1990s	2000s	2010s
Delivery-system structure	Single institution	Single organization	Integrated delivery systems		Patient-centered medical home
Professional-practice model	Team nursing	Primary nursing	Patient-focused care, multi-disciplinary care, case management	Patient-centered care	Expansion of nurse and advanced practice nurse roles to legal scope of practice
	Single or small group physician practice	Group models for physicians	Variety of constellations of physician group practice models		
Payer model	Fee for service	Fee for service	Capitation	CMS P4P hospital initiative	Affordable Care Act of 2010
		Prospective payment	Managed care		Accountable Care Organizations
		Diagnosis-related groups			
Quality focus	Professional Standards Review Organizations (PSROs)	Continuous quality improvement	Risk-adjusted outcomes	Patient safety	Value-driven health care
	Retrospective chart audit	Joint Commission on Accreditation of Health Care Organization (JCAHO) 's Agenda for Change	Benchmarking	Learning organizations	Patient-centered outcomes
			Practice guidelines	Consumer-driven	
			Critical paths/care maps		
			Health Employer Data and Information Set ((HEDIS)		
General technology trends			World Wide Web (Web 1.0)	Web 2.0	Cloud computing
				Social media	
				"Smart" mobile devices	

Home 2011"). See Chaps. 14, 15, and 16 for discussions of managing clinical information in integrated delivery systems, in consumer-provider partnerships in care, and in the public health information infrastructure.

15.2.3.2 Professional Practice Models

Professional practice models have also evolved for nurses and physicians. In the 1970s, team nursing was the typical practice model for the hospital, and the nursing care plan—a document for communicating the plan of care among nursing team members—was most frequently the initial computer-based application designed for use by nurses. The 1990s were characterized by a shift to interdisciplinary-care approaches necessitating computer-based applications such as critical paths to support case management of aggregates of patients, usually with a common medical diagnosis, across the **continuum of care**. The twenty-first century sees advanced practice nurses increasingly taking on functions previously provided by physicians while maintaining a nursing perspective on collaborative, interdisciplinary care. This trend is likely to accelerate given the recommendations for facilitating full scope of practice for nurses and advanced practice nurses (e.g., certified nurse midwives, nurse practitioners) in the 2010 Institute of Medicine report on *The Future of Nursing*: *Leading Change, Advancing Health* (Committee on the Robert Wood Johnson Foundation Initiative on the Future of Nursing at the Institute of Medicine 2010). These changes broaden and diversify the demands for decision support, feedback about clinical effectiveness, and quality improvement as a team effort.

Physician practice models have shifted from single physician or small group offices to complex constellations of provider organizations. The structure of the model (e.g., staff model health-maintenance organization, captive-group model health-maintenance organization, or independent-practice association; see Chap. 14) determines the types of relationships among the physicians and the organizations. These include issues— such as location of medical records, control of practice patterns of the physicians, and data-reporting

requirements—that have significant implications for the design and implementation of patient-care systems. In addition, the interdisciplinary and distributed care approaches of the 1990s and the 2000s have given impetus to system-design strategies, such as the creation of a single patient problem list, around which the patient-care record is organized, in place of a separate list for each provider group (e.g., nurses, physicians, respiratory therapists). Electronic whiteboards, wikis, and other communication tools have been advocated to address concerns that clinicians may not all be on the same page in regards to a patients' care goals and to promote common ground among the members of the interdisciplinary care team (Collins et al. 2011b).

15.2.3.3 Payer Models

Changes in payer models have been a significant driving force for information-system implementation in many organizations. With the shift from fee for service to prospective payment in the 1980s, and then toward capitation in the 1990s, information about costs and quality of care has become an essential commodity for rational decision-making in the increasingly competitive health care marketplace. Because private, third-party payers often adopt federal standards for reporting and regulation, health care providers and institutions have struggled in the early 2000s to keep up with the movement toward data and information system standards accelerated by the Health Insurance Portability and Accountability Act (HIPAA)[5] and the initiatives to develop a National Health Information Network. With the advent of pay for performance (P4P), CMS has eliminated reimbursement for preventable conditions (e.g., catheter-associated urinary tract infections) that occur during hospitalizations ("CMS P4P,"). In this decade, there is no doubt that the implementation of the highly controversial Affordable Care Act of 2010 and evolving Accountable Care Organizations will profoundly impact patient-centered care and the information systems needed to support it. See Chap. 14 for a thorough discussion of the effects of health care financing on health-care information systems.

---

[5] http://hhs.gov/ocr/privacy/ (Accessed: 4/26/13).

15.2.3.4 Quality Focus

Demands for information about quality of care have also influenced the design and implementation of patient-care systems. The quality-assurance techniques of the 1970s were primarily based on retrospective chart audit. In the 1980s, continuous quality improvement techniques became the modus operandi of most health care organizations. The quality-management techniques of the 1990s were much more focused on concurrently influencing the care delivered than on retrospectively evaluating its quality. In the Twenty-first Century, patient-centered systems-based approaches—such as practice guidelines, alerts, and reminders tailored on patient clinical data and, in some instances, genomic data (i.e., personalized medicine) —are an essential component of **quality management**. In addition, institutions must have the capacity to capture data for benchmarking purposes and to report process and outcomes data to regulatory and accreditation bodies, as well as to any voluntary reporting programs to which they belong. Increasingly, concurrent feedback about the effectiveness of care guides clinical decisions in real time and "dashboards" are used to display indicators related to different dimensions of quality.

15.2.4 Advances in Patient-Centered Care Systems

The design and implementation of patient-care systems, for the most part, occurred separately for hospital and ambulatory-care settings. Early patient-care systems in the hospital settings included the University of Missouri-Columbia System (Lindberg 1965), the Problem-Oriented Medical Information System (PROMIS) (Weed 1975), the TriService Medical Information System (TRIMIS) (Bickel 1979), the Health Evaluation Logical Processing (HELP) System (Kuperman et al. 1991), and the Decentralized Hospital Computer Program (DHCP) (Ivers et al. 1983). The Computer-Stored Ambulatory Record (COSTAR), the Regenstrief Medical Record System (McDonald 1976), and The Medical Record (TMR) were among the earliest ambulatory care systems. For a comprehensive review, see Collen (1995).

According to Collen (1995), the most commonly used patient-care systems in hospitals of the 1980s were those that supported nursing care planning and documentation. Systems to support capture of physicians' orders, communications with the pharmacy, and reporting of laboratory results were also widely used. Some systems merged physician orders with the nursing care plan to provide a more comprehensive view of care to be given. This merging, such as allowing physicians and nurses to view information in the part of the record designated for each other's discipline, was a step toward integration of information. It was still, however, a long way from support for truly collaborative interdisciplinary practice.

Early ambulatory-care systems most often included paper-based patient encounter forms that were either computer-scannable mark-sense format or were subsequently entered into the computer by clerical personnel. Current desktop, laptop, or handheld systems use keyboard, mouse, touchpad, or pen-based entry of structured information, with free text kept to a minimum. These systems also provide for retrieval of reports and past records. Some systems provide decision support or alerts to remind clinicians about needed care, such as immunizations or screening examinations, and to avoid contraindicated orders for medications or unnecessary laboratory analyses. The best provide good support for traditional medical care. Support for comprehensive, collaborative care that gives as much attention to health promotion as to treatment of disease presents a challenge not only to the developers of information systems but also to practitioners and health care administrators who must explicate the nature of this practice and the conditions under which agencies will provide it.

Patient-care information systems in use today represent a broad range in the evolution of the field. Versions of some of the earliest systems are still in use. These systems were generally designed to speed documentation and to increase legibility and availability of the records of patients currently receiving care. Most lack the capacity to aggregate data across patients, to query the data about subsets of patients, or to use data collected for clinical purposes to meet informational needs of administrators or researchers. These shortcomings seem glaring today, but they were not apparent when the very idea of using computers to store and communicate patient information required a leap of the imagination.

More recently developed systems attempt with varying success to respond to the edict "collect once, use many times." Selected items of data from patient records are abstracted manually or electronically to aggregate databases where they can be analyzed for administrative reports, for quality improvement, for clinical or health-services research, and for required patient safety and public health reporting. Such functionality is a key aspect of meaningful use. See Chap. 16 for a full discussion of public health informatics.

Some recently developed systems offer some degree of coordination of the information and services of the various clinical disciplines into integrated records and plans. Data collected by one caregiver can appear, possibly in a modified representation, in the "view" of the patient record designed for another discipline. When care-planning information has been entered by multiple caregivers, it can be viewed as the care plan to be executed by a discipline, by an individual, or by the interdisciplinary team. Some patient-care systems offer the option to organize care temporally into clinical pathways and to have variances from the anticipated activities, sequence, or timing reported automatically. Others offer a patient "view" so that individuals can view and contribute to their own records. For example, patients hospitalized for cardiac conditions can review selected aspects of their records and enter data such as pain ratings into CUPID (Computerized Unified Patient Interaction Device), an iPad-based application (Vawdrey et al. 2011).

Electronic documentation of clinician progress notes has lagged behind other functions in electronic health records (Doolan et al. 2003). The process of entering notes may occur through dictation, selecting words and phrases from structured lists, use of templates, and typing free text. Amid concerns that salience may be lost in electronic notes (Siegler 2010), Johnson et al. (2008) advocated for a hybrid approach that combines semi-structured data entry and natural language processing within a standards-based and computer-processible document structure. Thus, ability for data re-use is preserved while maintaining clinician efficiency and expressivity.

The publication of the Institute of Medicine's reports *To Err is Human* (2000) and *Crossing the Quality Chasm* (2001) resulted in increasing demands from health care providers for information systems that reduce errors in patient care. Information system vendors are responding by developing such systems themselves and by purchasing the rights to patient care systems developed in academic medical centers that have demonstrated reductions in errors and gains in quality of care and cost control. **Closed loop** medication systems use technologies such as bar codes and decision support to guard against errors throughout the process of prescribing, dispensing, administering, and recording and have been identified as a key intervention to improve medication safety. In a before-and-after evaluation of the closed loop electronic medication administration system at Brigham and Women's Hospital (BWH), investigators found a significant reduction in the rates of transcription errors, medication errors, and potential adverse events (Poon et al. 2010). In other contexts, decision support systems offer "best practice" guidelines, protocols, and order sets as a starting point for planning individualized patient care; provide alerts and reminders; use knowledge bases and patient data bases to assess orders for potential contraindications; and offer point-and-click access to knowledge summaries and full-text publications. See Chap. 21 for more information about these systems.

Many health care agencies have substantial investment in legacy systems and cannot simply switch to more modern technology. Finding ways to phase the transition from older systems to newer and more functional ones is a major challenge to health informatics. To make the transition from a patchwork of systems with self-contained functions to truly integrated systems with the capacity to meet emerging information needs is even more challenging (see Chap. 14). Approaches to making this transition are described in the Proceedings of the 1996 IAIMS Symposium (Stead et al. 1996) and in the Journal of the American Medical Informatics Association (Stead et al. 1996). More recently, some institutions have applied Web 2.0 approaches to create configurable user interfaces to legacy systems. For example, MedWISE integrates a set of features that supports custom displays, plotting of selected clinical data, visualization of temporal trends, and self-updating templates as mechanisms for facilitating cognition during the clinical decision making and documentation process (Senathirajah and Bakken 2009).

If patient-centered care systems are to be effective in supporting better care, health care professionals must possess the informatics competencies to use the systems. Consequently, many are integrating informatics competencies into health science education (See Chap. 23). For example, the Quality and Safety Education for Nurses (QSEN) initiative has produced competencies and associated curriculum to support patient-centered care competencies including those related to quality, safety, team work, and collaboration (Cronenwett et al. 2009).

To what degree do patient-care disciplines need to prepare their practitioners for roles as informatics specialists? To the degree that members of the discipline use information in ways unique to the discipline, the field needs members prepared to translate the needs of clinicians to those who develop, implement, and make decisions about information systems. If the information needs are different from those of other disciplines, some practitioners should be prepared as system developers.

The mere existence of information systems does not improve the quality of patient care. The adoption and use of advanced features (such as clinical decision support) that are sensitive to both workflow and human factors are needed to improve the quality of care (Stead and Lin 2009; Zhou et al. 2009). Recent safety reports, public policy, and reimbursement incentives raise awareness of the need for patient-centered care systems. Because traditional requirements for electronic health records (EHR) were provider-centric, existing information systems rarely provide the comprehensive suite of advanced features needed to support patient-centered care. However, the ability of systems to support patient-centered care is essential for achieving the vision of health care reform. What are the requirements for patient-centric information systems? How do these requirements drive the design of systems that will support patient-centered care?

15.3 Designing Systems for Patient-Centered Care

In the second decade of the twenty-first century, the vision for systems that support patient-centered care practices such as inter-professional care planning, care coordination, quality reporting, and patient engagement is becoming more widely shared. This evolution is fueled in part by meaningful use requirements that aim to engage patients and families in their health care and to improve care coordination and the overall quality of care provided. Traditional EHR functionality must be expanded to support new features, functions and care practices including seamless communication, inter-professional collaboration, and patient access to information. To achieve sound human factors and integration of systems and workflow, these features must be built into information systems as core requirements, rather than as an afterthought.

The *Principles to Guide Successful Use of Health Care Information Technology* described by the National Research Council (Stead and Lin 2009) provide a comprehensive framework for defining a set of core requirements that will support the design of systems for patient-centered care. This framework defines nine principles related to both evolutionary (i.e., iterative, long-term improvements) and radical (i.e., revolutionary, new-age improvements) changes occurring in the United States' health care system. The principles and associated system design prerequisites are included in Table 15.3.

Table 15.3 Principles to guide successful use of health care information technology

	Principle	System design prerequisites
Evolutionary change	1. Focus on improvements in care—technology is secondary	Gaps in patient-centered care are clearly defined and operationalized. Health care IT is employed to enable the process changes needed to close gaps in patient-centered care.
	2. Seek incremental gain from incremental effort	An organization's portfolio of health care IT projects has varying degrees of investment. Each project is linked to measurable process changes to provide ongoing visible success with closing gaps in patient-centered care.
	3. Record available data so they can be used for care, process improvement, and research	Health care IT systems support auto capture of data about people, processes, and outcomes at the point of care. Data are used in the short term to support incremental improvements in patient-centered care processes. An expandable data collection infrastructure is employed that is responsive to future needs that cannot be anticipated today.
	4. Design for human and organizational factors	Clear consideration is given to sociological, psychological, emotional, cultural, legal, economic and organizational factors that serve as barriers and incentives to providing patient-centered care. Health care IT should eliminate the barriers and enable the incentives, making it easy to provide patient-centered care.
	5. Support the cognitive functions of all caregivers, including health professionals, patients, and their families	Health care IT systems include advanced clinical decision support for high-level decision-making that is sensitive to both workflow and human factors.
Radical change	6. Architect information and workflow systems to accommodate disruptive change	Health care IT systems are designed using standard interconnection protocols that support the patient-centered care processes and roles of today while accommodating rapidly changing requirements dictated by new knowledge, care venues, policy, and increasing patient engagement.
	7. Archive data for subsequent re-interpretation	Health care IT systems support archival of raw data to enable ongoing review and analysis in the context of advances in biomedical science and patient-centered care practices.
	8. Seek and develop technologies that identify and eliminate ineffective work processes	Health care IT system design is preceded by a thorough investigation of current and future state work processes of all stakeholders (including patients and their families). Health care IT systems support efficient workflows that leverage ubiquitous access to information and communication and are not constrained by existing care venues or provider-centric practice patterns.
	9. Seek and develop technologies that clarify the context of data	Health care IT systems facilitate patient-centered care by presenting information in context with patient values and preferences and in a format that is understandable and actionable.

15.4 Current Research Toward Patient-Centered Care Systems

Friedman (1995) proposed a typology of the science in medical informatics. His four categories build from fundamental conceptualization to evaluation as follows:

- Formulating models for acquisition, representation, processing, display, or transmission of biomedical information or knowledge
- Developing innovative computer-based systems, using these models, that deliver information or knowledge to health care providers

- Installing such systems and then making them work reliably in functioning health care environments
- Studying the effects of these systems on the reasoning and behavior of health-care providers, as well as on the organization and delivery of health care

While the Friedman typology continues to be useful more than 15 years after its inception, we propose extending the second and third categories in Sects. 15.4.2 and 15.4.3 to expand the focus from clinical informatics as a provider-centric discipline to a discipline that enables and supports patient-centric care. Following are examples of recent research with implications for patient-centered care.

15.4.1 Formulation of Models

For several decades, standards development organizations (SDOs) and professional groups alike have focused on the formulation of models that describe the patient care process and the formal structures that support management and documentation of patient care. The efforts of SDOs are summarized in Chap. 7. Early SDO efforts focused primarily on representing health care concepts such as professional diagnoses (e.g., medical diagnoses, nursing diagnoses) and actions (e.g., procedures, education, referrals). These efforts were complemented by professional efforts such as those of the Nursing Terminology Summit (Ozbolt 2000). As a result of multi-national efforts, SNOMED CT became an international standard that provides a formal model for concepts that describe clinical conditions and the actions of the multidisciplinary health care team (International Health Terminology Standards Development Organization 2011). Toward the goal of patient-centered care, attention has also been paid to approaches for formal representation of terms that patients use to describe their problems and actions (Doing-Harris and Zeng-Treitler 2011).

In more recent years, the focus has turned to the development of information models and formal document structures that support sharing of data across heterogeneous information systems.

In regards to the latter, the Continuity of Care Document (CCD) standard is of particular importance to patient-centered care because it provides a formal structure for representing a core set of data elements across the life span. Dolin and colleagues demonstrated its relevance to a key patient safety issue, medication reconciliation (Dolin et al. 2007). Moreover, the CCD standard serves as the foundation for some personal health records and as an output format for data accessed through regional health information organizations. For example, a CCD designed specifically for socioeconomically disadvantaged persons living with HIV/AIDS (PLWH) was implemented for viewing by PLWH members of an HIV special needs plan, their clinicians, and case managers to promote coordination and quality of care (Schnall et al. 2011a, b).

Supporting interdisciplinary, collaborative, patient-centered care requires information systems that adequately represent the concepts of practice of all the professions involved in patient care. In addition, in the home care setting it is essential to include relevant concepts for domestic help, social services, and family caregivers. In Sweden, a shared care plan was developed to include all these elements (Hagglund et al. 2011). The concepts and relationships in the shared care plan were then compared with those represented in two standards, the European continuity of care model (CONTsys) and *open* EHR, to determine the semantic interoperability of the shared care plan. The investigators found that additional archetypes were needed in both standards to represent some of the concepts and relationships in the shared care plan. It is to be expected that much additional work will be needed around the world to model and represent concepts and relationships in the transition from clinician-centered care to patient-centered care.

Through the Strategic Health IT Advanced Research Projects (SHARP) Program, the Mayo Clinic is leading ONC-initiated efforts to create and advance models that promote integration and re-use of electronic health data ("Strategic Health IT Advanced Research Projects (SHARP) Program,"). Such efforts are essential to enable patient-centered care systems.

15.4.2 Development of Innovative Systems

For the purposes of developing innovative *patient-centered* computer-based systems, the second category of the Friedman Typology described in 15.4 is expanded to address the use of models that deliver information or knowledge to both health care providers *and* patients. Consumers regularly use information and communication technology to support decision making in all aspects of their lives. However, access to tools to support health care decision making is suboptimal (Krist and Woolf 2011). Krist, Woolf, & Rothemich (2010) proposed five levels of functionality for patient-centered health information systems.

- Level 1: Collects patient information related to health status, behaviors, medications, symptoms, and diagnoses (e.g., electronic version of traditional paper records maintained by patients)
- Level 2: Integrates patient information with clinical information (e.g., personal health record tethered to an EHR)
- Level 3: Interprets information to provide context in an appropriate level of health literacy
- Level 4: Provides tailored recommendations based on patient information, clinical information and evidence-based guidelines
- Level 5: Facilitates patient decision-making, ownership and action

The levels of functionality needed to support patient-centered health information systems relate directly to several of the *Principles to Guide Successful Use of Health Care Information Technology* described by the National Research Council (Stead and Lin 2009) and outlined in Sect. 15.3; specifically principles 5, 8 and 9 (see Table 15.3).

Partners Health Care System (PHS) in Boston, MA, developed Patient Gateway, a secure patient portal serving over 65,000 patient users from primary and specialty care practices affiliated with the Dana Farber Cancer Institute, Brigham and Women's Hospital (BWH), and Massachusetts General Hospital (MGH). Patient Gateway is a

tethered personal health record (see Chap. 17) that provides functionality in line with the five levels described by Krist and Woolf. For example, tools for management of chronic illness are used by patients and providers to promote adherence with evidence-based health maintenance guidelines and to improve collaboration on diabetes self-management plans (Grant et al. 2006; Wald et al. 2009). Research on patient response and satisfaction with Patient Gateway suggests that patients appreciate the ability to communicate electronically with providers, they welcome greater access to their health information including test results and they believe that Patient Gateway enables them to better prepare for visits (Grant et al. 2006; Schnipper et al. 2008b; Wald et al. 2009). Evaluations of patient satisfaction with personal health records with similar levels of functionality at other sites including Geisinger Health System (Hassol et al. 2004), Group Health Cooperative (Ralston et al. 2007), and Virginia Commonwealth University (Krist et al. 2010) are consistent with the results reported at PHS.

The involvement of end-users has been identified as fundamental to well designed systems that are usable and useful in the context of busy patient care workflows (Rahimi et al. 2009). Some examples of development activities where end-user involvement is needed are content standardization, workflow modeling, and usability testing.

- *Content standardization*: Content standardization includes identifying EHR content needed to support documentation of care provided and identification of data needed for reuse (e.g., decision support, quality reporting, and research). Content that is shared across disciplines and patients is identified. Content is modeled using standards to ensure data reuse and interoperability (Principle 3, Table 15.3) (Chen et al. 2008; Dykes et al. 2010; Kim et al. 2011).
- *Workflow modeling*: Sound modeling of the clinical workflow that underlies an electronic system is essential to designing systems that are usable by care team members (Peute et al. 2009). Workflow models are based on

observations of current state clinical workflows including interactions with patients, staff, equipment, and supplies. Understanding of workflow interactions, including current state inefficiencies, is leveraged to inform effective and efficient future state workflows, use-case development, and system prototypes (Rausch and Jackson 2007). Workflow modeling of patient-centered systems includes clear evaluation of ways to use technology to identify and eliminate ineffective work processes (Principle 8, Table 15.3). Design of new systems is an opportunity to provide ubiquitous access to information and communication by all care team members including patients. Therefore, future state workflows are not constrained by existing care venues or provider-centric practice patterns.

- *Usability testing*: A key lesson learned from CPOE implementations is electronic systems with poor usability interfere with clinical workflow. The unintended consequences of poorly designed systems are well known and some widely disseminated papers (Ash et al. 2004, 2009; Koppel et al. 2005) have called into question the safety of using such systems with patients. Examples of common usability problems include overly cluttered screen design, poor use of available screen space, and inconsistencies in design. Involving end-users in design and enforcing usability design standards when building clinical systems prevents implementing systems that are difficult to use and interfere with, rather than support, patient-centered care (Principles 4, 5 and 8, Table 15.3).

Innovative systems to support patient care often take advantage of information entered in one context for use in other contexts. For example, the Brigham Integrated Computing System (BICS), a PC-based client–server HIS developed at BWH in Boston, used information from the order entry, scheduling, and other systems to prepare drafts of the physician's discharge orders and the nurse's discharge abstract, thus minimizing the information to be entered manually. The professionals reviewed the drafts and edited as needed (O'Connell et al. 1996). The BICS system's success in this and other functions led to its acquisition for commercial deployment.

The principle of entering information once for multiple uses also drove development of the low-cost bedside workstations for intensive-care units at the University Hospital of Giessen, Germany (Michel et al. 1996). The client–server architecture combined local data-processing capabilities with a central relational patient database, permitting, for example, clinical nursing data to be used in calculating workload. These workstations also combined data from many sources, including medical devices, to support the integrated care of physicians, nurses, and other caregivers.

Even as systems such as these begin to fulfill some of the promises of informatics to support patient-centered care, research and development continue to address the demands that the complexities of patient care place on information systems. Hoy and Hyslop (1995) reported a series of projects directed toward the development of a person-based health record. They found problems with traditional approaches to automating paper-based care-planning systems that resulted in loss of data detail, inability to use data for multiple purposes, and limitations in the capacity to aggregate and query patient data. Hoy and Hyslop (1995) recommended:

- Making the structure of the clinical record (including the care plan) more flexible and extensible to allow summarized higher-level data, with lower-level details where appropriate
- Simplifying the elements of that structure to make data entry and retrieval easier and more effective

Hoy and Hyslop (1995) built a prototype system to demonstrate their recommendations. Like other investigators, they concluded that "the issues of language and structures must be dealt with before the integration of person-based systems can be realized." As noted in Chap. 7, significant headway has been made in this regard during the last 5 years.

At Vanderbilt University Medical Center, patient-care systems have evolved since the mid-1990s to support patient safety and quality of care in a variety of ways. Clinical teams, assisted by specially trained clinical librarians, develop evidence-based order sets as templates for interdisciplinary care. These order sets are instantiated in Vanderbilt's order-entry system, where they serve as the starting point for planning and documenting each patient's care. When a patient is admitted to the hospital, a decision-support tool helps the physician to identify the appropriate evidence-based order set and then to edit the template to produce an individualized plan of care. In this way, the most current clinical knowledge provides the basis for each patient's care. Özdas et al. (2006) demonstrated that use of the evidence-based order set increased physician compliance with quality indicators for treating acute myocardial infarction. Other research opportunities are to explore the impact (positive or negative) of deviations from the template order sets in the context of different patient characteristics and comorbidities, thereby refining the evidence base and adding to clinical knowledge. Patient care systems like this make it possible to learn from data collected in the course of patient care about the effectiveness and safety of specific care practices and to integrate that emerging knowledge in continual quality improvement (Ozbolt et al. 2001; Ozbolt 2003).

At Partners Health Care, system developers are working with clinical teams to identify system requirements, to iteratively develop, and to test patient-centric systems that integrate decision support into the clinical workflow. For example, Dykes et al. (2010) developed a fall prevention toolkit that reuses fall risk assessment data entered into the clinical documentation system by nurses and automatically generates a tailored set of tools that provide decision support to all care team members, including patients and their family members at the bedside (Dykes et al. 2009). The fall prevention toolkit logic was developed from focus groups of professional and paraprofessional caregivers (Dykes et al. 2009), and of patients and family members (Carroll et al. 2010). As nurses complete and file the routine fall risk assessment scale, the documentation system automatically generates a tailored bed poster that alerts all team members about each patient's fall risk status and patient-appropriate

interventions to mitigate risk. In addition, a patient education handout is generated that identifies why each individual patient is at risk for falls and what the patient and family members can do while in the hospital to prevent a fall. In a randomized control trial of over 10,000 patients, the toolkit was associated with significantly fewer falls than usual fall prevention practices (Dykes et al. 2010). This work is currently being expanded to reuse data from provider order entry and the clinical documentation systems to display icon-based alerts on an electronic white board at each patient's bedside to communicate the core set of information needed by care team members to safely care for individual patients.

15.4.3 Implementation of Systems

Much has been written about health information technology failures and associated costs and consequences (Bloxham 2008; Booth 2000; McManus and Wood-Harper 2007; Ornstein 2003; Rosencrance 2006). Higgins and associates (see Rotman et al. 1996) described the lessons learned from a failed implementation of a computer-based physician workstation that had been designed to facilitate and improve ordering of medications. Those lessons are not identical to, but are consistent with, the recommendations of Leiner and Haux (1996) in their protocol for systematic planning and execution of projects to develop and implement patient-care systems.

As these experiences demonstrate, the implementation of patient-care systems is far more complex than the replacement of one technology with another. Such systems transform work and organizational relationships. If the implementation is to succeed, attention must be given to these transformations and to the disruptions that they entail. Southon and colleagues (1997) provided an excellent case study of the role of organizational factors in the failed implementation of a patient-care system that had been successful in another site.

To realize the promise of informatics for health and clinical management, people who develop and promote the use of applications must anticipate, evaluate, and accommodate the full range of consequences. In early 2003, these issues came to the attention of the public when a large academic medical center decided to temporarily halt implementation of its CPOE system due to mixed acceptance by the physician staff (Chin 2003; Ornstein 2003). A case series study by Doolan, Bates, and James (2003) identified five key factors associated with successful implementation: (1) having organizational leadership, commitment, and vision; (2) improving clinical processes and patient care; (3) involving clinicians in the design and modification of the system; (4) maintaining or improving clinical productivity; and (5) building momentum and support amongst clinicians. A collaboration of ten **American Medical Informatics Association** (AMIA) working groups and the **International Medical Informatics Association** (IMIA) Working Group on Organizational and Social Issues cosponsored a workshop to review factors that lead to implementation failure. These include poor communication, complex workflows, and failure to engage end-users in clearly defining system requirements. Recognizing that the problems encountered in failed implementations tend to be more administrative than technical, they recommended the following set of managerial strategies to overcome implementation barriers; (1) provide incentives for adoption, remove disincentives; (2) identify and mitigate social, IT, and leadership risks; (3) allow adequate resources and time for training before and after implementation (i.e., ongoing); (4) learn from the past and from others about implementation successes and failures and about how failing situations were turned around (Kaplan and Harris-Salamone 2009).

For the purposes of promoting successful implementation of patient-centered systems, the third category of the Friedman typology is expanded to provide access to information to all team members including patients and their families or caregivers outside of traditional health care settings as follows: *Installing such systems and then making them work reliably in functioning health care environments and other settings where information is needed to promote health and well being*. The majority of self-care occurs outside of traditional health care settings. As noted in Table 15.3, a prerequisite for patient-centered systems is that they support efficient workflows that leverage ubiquitous access to information and communication and are not constrained by existing care venues or provider-centric practice patterns (Principle #8). Strategies to involve end-users in system design or selection and customization will support successful implementation of systems that meet user expectations (Burley et al. 2009; Rahimi et al. 2009; Saleem et al. 2009b). End-user involvement in defining future state workflows contributes to a shared understanding about the impact of information systems on clinical tasks and workflows (Leu et al. 2008).

Careful attention to the *Principles to Guide Successful Use of Health Care Information Technology* during system design will support successful implementation. For example, the principles related to evolutionary health care changes keep the focus on designing and implementing usable systems that enable patient-centered care practices. Principles related to radical change focus on development of flexible, adaptable systems that are architected to accommodate disruptive change and iterative development based on end-user feedback.

15.4.4 Effects of Clinical Information Systems on the Potential for Patient-Centered Care

Electronic health records (EHRs) and computer-based provider order-entry (CPOE) systems are intended to support safe, evidence-based, patient-centered care by examining patient-specific information, agency-specific information, and domain-specific information in the clinical context and proposing appropriate courses of action or alerting clinicians to potential dangers. Many current systems, however, fail to follow design principles that take into account the real contingency-driven, non-linear, highly interrupted, collaborative, cognitive, and operational workflow of clinical practice (Ash et al. 2004). These flaws can lead to errors in entering and retrieving information, cognitive overload, fragmentation of the clinical overview of the patient's situation, lack of essential operational flexibility, and breakdown of communication. Physicians, in particular, have found themselves chagrined by changes in the power structure as they have devoted more time to entering information and orders while other members of the health team have gained greater access to information and the concomitant capacity to make certain decisions without consulting the physician. Clinicians across the range of professions have expressed concern about the decrease in face-to-face communication with its verbal and non-verbal richness, negotiation, and redundant safety checks as more and more clinical information is exchanged via the computer (Campbell et al. 2006; Ash et al. 2007). These and other unintended consequences of EHRs and CPOE systems are the subject of ongoing research. Detecting and finding ways to prevent or mitigate the adverse, unintended consequences of these systems will be critical for supporting patient-centered care.

A number of unintended consequences stem from the incompatibility of system design with the clinician's cognitive workflow. For example, systems that make it difficult to find and retrieve information can interfere with patient-centered care. In a hospital preparing to implement a commercial CPOE system, investigators compared the efficiency, usability, and safety of information retrieval using the vendor's system, the current paper form, and a prototype CPOE developed on principles of User Centered Design. They found the prototype system to be similar to the paper form and both to be significantly superior to the vendor's system in efficiency, usability, and safety (Chan et al. 2011).

Other unintended consequences arise from over-reliance on the information system because of limited understanding of its design and capacities. To date, many clinical decision support systems are somewhat limited in their ability to incorporate patient-specific data into their decision algorithms. A synthesis of 17 systematic reviews conducted with sound methodology found that clinical decision support systems often improved providers' performance, especially in medication orders and preventive care. The reviewers noted, "These outcomes may be explained by the fact that these types of CDSS require a minimum of patient data that are largely available before the advice is (to be) generated: at the time clinicians make the decisions" (Jaspers et al. 2011, p. 327).

On the other hand, many systems offer functionalities that support patient-centered care. An important component of patient-centered care is the application of evidence in a plan of care tailored to the patient's needs. To increase the use of evidence-based order sets, investigators at Sinai-Grace Hospital in Detroit, Michigan, embedded order sets for the most common primary and secondary diagnoses for patients admitted to their medical service into the general admission order set. The result was a fivefold increase in the use of evidence-based order sets in the 16-month period following implementation (Munasinghe et al. 2011).

As in the examples above, most systems to support the cognitive workload have been directed toward physicians. Patient-centered care requires a broader perspective. A study of the information needs of case managers for persons living with HIV found that the most frequent needs were for patient education resources (33 %), patient data (23 %), and referral resources (22 %) (Schnall et al. 2011b). The investigators recommended that targeted resources to meet these information needs be provided in EHRs and continuity of care records through mechanisms such as the Infobutton Manager.

Key to patient-centered care is communication among all the health care professionals on the patient's team. A study at one academic medical center (Hripcsak et al. 2011) reviewed electronic medical records of hospitalized patients, along with usage logs, to make inferences about time spent writing and viewing clinical notes and patterns of communication among team members. In this setting, the core team for each patient consisted of one or more attending physicians, residents, and nurses, with social workers, dieticians, and various therapists joining the team later. Results showed that clinical notes were more likely to be reviewed within the same professional group, with attending physicians and residents viewing notes from nurses or social workers less than a third of the time. The investigators proposed that it might be useful to develop ways for EHRs "to summarize information and make it readily available, perhaps with the ability of the author to highlight information that may be critical and that has a high priority for communication" (p. 116). They also noted that their study was limited to communications within the EHR and did not take into account face-to-face or telephone communications that might have occurred, especially in urgent situations. They suggested further research involving direct observation of clinicians, time-motion analyses, and think-aloud methods to develop deeper knowledge of how clinicians communicate about patient care, especially across the professions.

The quality of documentation tools can have a profound effect on whether information, even if communicated face-to-face, is acted upon in clinical care (Collins et al. 2011b). In a neurovascular intensive care unit, therapeutic goals for patients were stated during daily interdisciplinary rounds. In this setting, the interdisciplinary team treated the attending physician's note as a common patient-focused source of information. Although the attending physician's note contained 81 % of the stated ventilator weaning goals, it included only 49 % of the stated sedation weaning goals. Overall, nearly a quarter of stated goals were not documented in the note. If a goal was not documented, it was 60 % less likely to have a related action documented. Nurses' documentation rarely mentioned the goals, even if actions recorded were consistent with the goals as stated during rounds. Notably, the nurses' structured documentation system did not support sedation-related goals, even though sedation weaning was a nursing responsibility in this setting. The authors noted that the frequent omission of sedation goals from the attending physician's note might be because this nursing function was not a billable goal or act. They also expressed concern that the omission from the EHR of evidence of important clinical judgments nurses make could impair patient safety, quality improvement, and development of nursing knowledge. Thus, in this example, although the interdisciplinary team was collaborating in setting and reaching therapeutic goals, deficiencies in their processes and in the nurses' documentation system limited their achievement of patient-centered care.

A study at Vanderbilt University Medical Center also demonstrated both strengths and shortcomings in the ability of a clinical information system to support patient-centered care. Attending physicians in the Trauma and Surgical ICUs established protocols for Intensive Insulin Therapy (IIT) that were built into a CDSS to advise nurses on insulin doses based on a patient's blood glucose and insulin resistance trends. In 94.4 % of studied instances, nurses administered the recommended dose. When nurses over-rode the recommended dose, they overwhelmingly administered less insulin than the recommended dose, leading to a higher incidence of hyperglycemia than when the recommended dose was administered. Nurses appeared more concerned about hypoglycemia than hyperglycemia and to consider the patient's blood glucose but not the insulin resistance trend. They also noted that their workflow was impeded by the need to record information about the blood glucose, insulin dose, and primary dextrose source in two places—the CPOE that included the CDSS and the separate nurse charting system. The investigators' recommendations included displaying information about insulin resistance trends on screen (provided that this did not produce clutter and confusion) and developing clinical information systems that do not require double documentation. Strengths of this example for supporting patient-centered care include the collaboration of physicians and nurses in maintaining blood glucose in the desired range based on patient data. Shortcomings include the failure to present nurses with information about the patient's insulin resistance trend to aid their decision-making and the requirement that they record the same data in two places, thereby reducing time for direct patient care (Campion et al. 2011).

Patient-centered care systems not only support the cognitive work and communications of clinicians; they also take into account the resources patients and families use to manage their health concerns. Increasingly, patients and family members engaged in promoting their own health turn to social networking sites on the Internet. An examination of ten sites focused on diabetes mellitus, however, found significant gaps in quality and safety (Weitzman et al. 2011b). On only half the sites was content aligned with current medical science. Of nine sites that carried advertising, only four made a clear distinction between advertising and editorial content; two sites contained advertisements about a "cure" for diabetes. Six sites, including four moderated sites, contained member-posted misinformation about a "cure" for diabetes. Privacy practices were generally poor. The authors offered straightforward, readily implementable recommendations for improving the quality and safety of health-related social networking sites, but they noted that there is no authority or agency empowered to enforce them.

To provide patients with high quality information resources, many health care organizations are offering their own Web sites and portals. Atkinson et al. (2011) demonstrated the importance of involving users in evaluating the design of such resources, including giving them more than one version to evaluate and varying the order of presentation. Notably, they found that users liked the opportunity to explore the site and assess its credibility and authoritativeness before registering and entering personal information. A survey of individuals using health-related social networking sites provided by three major medical centers found that the most important factor determining the degree of empathy that people perceived they received from the site was the effectiveness of seeking information, as compared with social support or personal similarity of participants (Nambisan 2011). The investigator recommended that health care organizations providing such sites take pains to make it easy for participants to find the information they need.

Although such sites can be helpful to patients, they are not readily accessible to everyone. An examination of the usage of Kaiser Permanente's patient portal by adults in northern California

with a diagnosis of diabetes found that African Americans and Latinos had a higher probability of never logging on compared to Caucasians. Similarly, those with a college degree were much more likely to log on to the site than those without a college degree (Sarkar et al. 2011b). The investigators expressed concern that already disadvantaged populations might be further deprived of needed health information and education as providers turn increasingly to the Internet for patient communication and education.

When patients are willing and able to use electronic communications with providers, clinicians have special responsibilities to assure safe, ethical, patient-centered care. Mittal et al. (2010) measured 18 indicators of response quality to a fictional patient email. The respondents were 50 first- or second-year rheumatology residents from six different fellowship programs over a period of 4 years (2005–2008). Responses tended to be concise (74 %) and courteous (68 %). However, the residents did less well on two other dimensions: understanding the role of email as a complement to a visit and not for urgent matters, and understanding the administrative and legal aspects of email, such as the need for proper documentation and encryption. Thus, even though 92 % of the residents acknowledged that the patient's condition (as described in the fictional email) required immediate medical attention, few (30 %) took steps to contact the patient other than by email response. None of the residents encrypted their messages. The investigators acknowledged that the residents might have responded differently to an email from a real patient but concluded that there is a need for more formal training in the proper use of email in the provider-patient relationship.

In patient-centered care, **personal health records** (PHRs; see Chap. 17) are often viewed as a means of communication between patients and providers and as a method of engaging patients in understanding and acting in the interests of their own health. The Military Health System (MHS), charged with providing patients with access to their health information through an interoperable system, initiated a pilot project in 2008 to allow patients a choice of platforms, Google Health (now-defunct) or Microsoft HealthVault, as the repository for their health data (Nahn et al. 2011). A portal called MiCare was created as the gateway to the repository of choice and to other PHR functionalities. MiCare also provided the platform for transferring data, at the patient's request, from various Department of Defense sources to the PHR repository of choice. Users were generally satisfied with MiCare as a portal to their information, but they wanted more functionalities, such as secure messaging and appointment scheduling. The investigators cited four important lessons learned. First, although most patients requested automatic transfer of all their data to the repository, this slowed response time to an unacceptable level. The designers then changed the model to transfer data only upon specific patient request. Second, although the patient representatives to the project requested instant access to all their data, providers insisted on a 7-day publication delay for routine information, to give them time to contact the patient and explain the results. For sensitive information such as pregnancy, positive cancer findings, and sexually transmitted diseases, the providers required direct contact with the patient, with publication happening only with patient request and provider concurrence. Third, providers found that accessing the PHR impeded their workflow and that lack of complete information from the MHS might pose a danger of ill-informed clinical decisions. A dashboard that integrated patient requests with full MHS data on the patient might have helped. Fourth, giving patients the power to determine what medical information to share with the provider could similarly lead to clinical decisions made in the absence of vital information, with resulting harm to patients. The investigators concluded that while there is broad agreement on desired functionalities for PHRs, challenging tensions remain between patients' desire for access to and control of health information and providers' needs for full information about the patient and for appropriate opportunities for ethical disclosure of information to patients.

Electronic health records and other computer-based information resources can influence the provision of patient-centered care even when the patient and the provider are in the same room. A study of computer use during acute pediatric outpatient visits found that female physicians were more likely than males to be communicating with patients and families while using the computer (Fiks et al. 2011). An observational study involving 20 primary care physicians and 141 of their adult patients showed how the inclusion of the computer in the clinical consultation can help patients shift the balance of power and authority toward shared decision-making and patient-centered care (Pearce et al. 2011). This Australian study found that about one-third of the patients actively included the computer as a party to the consultation, drawing the physician's attention to it as a source of information or authority. They concluded, "In the future, computers will have greater agency, not less, and patients will involve themselves in the three-way consultation in more creative ways—for example, through online communication, or through the plugging into computers of their own electronic records, creating a situation where they co-own the information in the computer …. By democratizing and commoditizing information flows and authority in the consultation, we may in fact create truly patient-centered medicine, with the patient directing the action" (p. 142).

As these examples illustrate, the complexity of collaborative, interdisciplinary, patient-centered care poses serious challenges to the design of clinical information systems. Many systems fall short in supporting cognitive work, even from a clinician-centric perspective. Supporting communications among clinicians, between clinicians and patients, and among patient and family support groups presents myriad technical and ethical problems. Still, researchers and clinicians increasingly share a vision of patient-centered care that drives them to push the frontiers and develop support for this emerging model of care.

15.5 Outlook for the Future

Social and political forces have begun to transform health care in the United States, and health information technology is advancing to support the changes. The transformation is rapid, disruptive, and not always smooth, but mandates and incentives are aligning with social and economic imperatives to maintain progress.

To meet demands for patient-centered care, changes must occur in clinician practice patterns and processes, in the organization and management of health services, and in the education of health care professionals and the public. To support patient-centered care, clinicians, informatics professionals, and computer scientists must develop health information and communication technologies that support collaboration; cognitive processes and operational workflow; communication and shared decision making between and among clinicians, patients, and family members; and trustworthy tools for the management of personal and family health.

Transformational change is daunting, and resistance is inevitable. Still, the chances for success have never been better. The vision of health care articulated by the National Academy of Sciences is guiding policy, research, and practical action by government agencies, health care providers, and the public.

Suggested Readings

Adams, K., & Corrigan, J.M. (Eds.). (2003). *Priority areas for national action*: *Transforming health care quality*. A report of the Institute of Medicine. Washington, DC: National Academy Press. This book outlines a plan for transforming health care, identifying specific chronic diseases and conditions as targets for initial work and describing cross-cutting changes, including the widespread use of health information technologies, to achieve a better health care system.

Ahern, D. K., Woods, S. S., Lightowler, M. C., Finley, S. W., & Houston, T. K. (2011). Promise of and potential for patient-facing technologies to enable meaningful use. *American Journal of Preventive Medicine, 40*(5 Suppl 2), S162–S172. This article describes specific technologies that patients can use in the interests of their health and that support patient-centered care.

Committee on Quality of Health Care in America. (2001). *Crossing the quality chasm*: *A new health system for the 21st century*. A report of the Institute of Medicine. Washington, DC: National Academy Press. This book articulates a vision of better health care and emphasizes the importance of health information technology in creating and maintaining better systems of care.

Dykes, P. C., Carroll, D. L., Hurley, A., Lipsitz, S., Benoit, A., Chang, F., et al. (2010). Fall prevention in acute care hospitals: a randomized trial. *Journal of the American Medical Association, 304*(17), 1912–1918. This article describes development and testing of an electronic fall prevention toolkit integrating decision support into clinical workflow at the bedside and intended for use by all team members including patients and family.

Kohn, L.T., Corrigan, J.M., & Donaldson, M.S. (Eds.). (2000). *To err is human*: *Building a safer health system*. A report of the Institute of Medicine. Washington, DC: National Academy Press. This book describes flaws in the American health care system that result in unnecessary death and suffering.

Stead, W.W., & Lin, H.S. (Eds.). (2009). *Computational technology for effective health care*: *Immediate steps and strategic directions*. A report of the National Research Council. Washington, DC: National Academy Press. This book proposes principles and methods to achieve the best functionality from existing health information technologies and proposes collaboration to advance technologies to the level needed for a transformed health care system.

Questions for Discussion

1. What is the utility of a linear model of patient care as the basis for a decision-support system? What are two primary limitations? Discuss two challenges that a nonlinear model poses for representing and supporting the care process in an information system.

2. Compare and contrast additive, clinician-centered versus coordinated, patient-centered models of interdisciplinary patient care. What are the advantages and disadvantages of each model as a mode of care delivery? What are the broad implications for design of information systems to support clinician-centered versus patient-centered models of care?

3. Imagine a patient-care information system that assists in planning the care of each patient independently of all the other patients in a service center or patient-care unit. What are three advantages to the developer in choosing such an information architecture? What would

be the likely result in the real world of practice? Does it make a difference whether the practice setting is hospital, ambulatory care, or home care? What would be the simplest information architecture that would be sufficiently complex to handle real-world demands? Explain.

4. Zielstorff et al. (1993) proposed that data routinely recorded during the process of patient care could be abstracted, aggregated, and analyzed for management reports, policy decisions, and knowledge development. What are three advantages of using patient care data in this way? What are three significant limitations?

5. A number of patient-care information systems designed in the 1970s are still in use. How do the practice models, payer models, and quality focus of today differ from those of the past? What differences do these changes require in information systems? What are two advantages and two disadvantages of "retrofitting" these changes on older systems versus designing new systems "from scratch"?

6. What challenges exist in modeling information for patient-centered care? What considerations are important in designing patient-facing health information and communication technologies?

Public Health Informatics

16

Martin LaVenture, David A. Ross,
and William A. Yasnoff

After reading this chapter you should know the answers to these questions:

- What are the three core functions of public health, and how do they help to shape the different foci of public health and medicine?
- What are the current and potential effects on public health informatics from a) the use of electronic health records and b) global disease outbreaks?
- What are the potential value and benefits for patients and clinicians to exchange data with public health agencies?
- What factors influence the use of immunization information systems (IIS) and how can this model apply to other areas of the health system?

M. LaVenture, MPH, PhD (✉)
Minnesota Department of Health,
Office of HIT and e-Health,
Center for Health Informatics, 85 East 7th Place,
Suite 220, P.O. Box 64882, St. Paul, MN, USA
e-mail: martin.laventure@state.mn.us

D.A. Ross, DSc
Public Health Informatics Institute/The Task Force
for Global Health, 325 Swanton Way,
Decatur 30092, GA, USA
e-mail: dross@phii.org

W.A. Yasnoff, MD, PhD
NHII Advisors, 1854 Clarendon Blvd, Arlington
22201, VA, USA
e-mail: william.yasnoff@nhiiadvisors.com

16.1 Introduction

Biomedical informatics includes health interventions at the population level. This chapter focuses on the public health system and specifically the role of governmental public health to improve the health of the entire population such as city, county, state or national level and how it relies upon an informatics infrastructure. Chapter 13 describes **health information infrastructure** (**HII**), including its role in supporting public health.

Population-level informatics has its own special challenges and considerations. Creating information systems that inform health policy or support an understanding of the health of sub-populations usually requires a large number of cases and multiple data elements. Population health involves understanding the social determinants of health related to the environment, behavior, and socio-economic status.

Rapid increases in the number of data sources available to assess and understand aspects of health and determinants of disease in the population, improved analytical and visualization software like GIS, and the ability to integrate health data with other information makes public health

The authors gratefully acknowledge the co-authors of the third edition version of this chapter, Patrick W. O'Carroll, and Andrew Friede. In addition, we very much appreciate the substantial contribution of Bill Brand through his thoughtful edits, comments and suggestions and to Pat Kuruchitthan for his careful review and assistance with the materials.

informatics a foundational science for public health. Public health informatics can support primary prevention and disease interventions and public health research, while also informing public policy. However, much work remains to fully achieve the potential of systems that support healthier communities and populations.

16.1.1 Chapter Overview

This chapter primarily deals with the aspect of public health informatics that relates to the medical care of populations. The chapter will not discuss areas of public health like detecting threats to health from the food supply, water systems, unsafe roads or how informatics assists in human-caused or natural disaster management. Monitoring the environment for health risks due to biological, chemical, and radiation exposures (natural and human-made) has been of increased concern for protecting the public's health. Although they do not directly relate to medical care, such technologies are designed to protect human health and should properly be considered within the domain of public health informatics.

16.2   What Is Public Health?

Public health is a complex and varied discipline, encompassing a wide variety of specialty areas. The broad scope and diversity of activities make it difficult readily and concisely to define and explain public health. A common theme of all the activities is a primary focus on prevention.

One useful conceptualization defines public health in terms of its three core functions of assessment, policy development, and assurance (Institute of Medicine (IOM) 1988).

Assessment involves monitoring and tracking the health status of populations including identifying and controlling disease outbreaks and epidemics. By relating health status to a variety of demographic, geographic, environmental, and other factors, it is possible to develop and test hypotheses about the etiology, transmission, risk factors and control options that contribute to health problems in a population.

Policy development is the second core function of public health. It utilizes the results of assessment activities and etiologic research in concert with local values and culture (as reflected via citizen input) to recommend interventions and public policies that improve health status. For example, the relationship between fatalities in automobile accidents and ejection of passengers from vehicles led to recommendations, and eventually laws mandating seat belt use. It is in the area of policy development that information technology may have its greatest impact.

Because public health is primarily a governmental activity, it depends upon and is informed by the consent of those governed. Policy development in public health is (or should be) based on science, but it is also derived from the values, beliefs, and opinions of the society it serves. Today, e-mail, Web sites, on-line discussion groups, and social media sites are the most heavily used Internet applications. Public health officials who wish to promote certain health behaviors, or to promulgate regulations concerning, say, fluoridated water or bicycle helmets, would do well to tap into the online marketplace of ideas—both to understand the opinions and beliefs of their citizenry, and (hopefully) to inform and influence them.

The third core function of public health is assurance, which refers to the duty of public health agencies to assure their constituents that services necessary to achieve agreed upon goals are available. Note that the services in question (including medical care) might be provided directly by the public health agency or by encouraging or requiring (through regulation) other public or private entities to deliver the services. For example, in some communities, local public health agencies provide a great deal of direct clinical care to underserved or at risk populations. The health department in Multnomah County, Oregon, for example, currently offers health care services in 7 primary care clinics, 3 county jails, 13 schools, 4 community sites and in people's homes. In other communities (e.g., Pierce County, Washington), local public health

Table 16.1 Ten essential services of public health (DHHS 1994)

1. Monitor the health status of individuals in the community to identify community health problems
2. Diagnose and investigate community health problems and community health hazards
3. Inform, educate, and empower the community with respect to health issues
4. Mobilize community partnerships in identifying and solving community health problems
5. Develop policies and plans that support individual and community efforts to improve health
6. Enforce laws and rules that protect the public health and ensure safety in accordance with those laws and rules
7. Link individuals who have a need for community and personal health services to appropriate community and private providers
8. Ensure a competent workforce for the provision of essential public health services
9. Research new insights and innovate solutions to community health problems
10. Evaluate the effectiveness, accessibility, and quality of personal and population-based health services in a community

agencies have sought to minimize or eliminate direct clinical care services, instead working with and relying on community partners to provide such care. Though there is great variation across jurisdictions, the fundamental function is unchanged: to assure that all members of the community have adequate access to needed services, especially prevention services.

The assurance function is frequently associated with clinical care, but also refers to assurance of the conditions that allow people to be healthy and free from avoidable threats to health—which include access to clean water, a safe food supply, well-lighted streets, responsive and effective public safety entities, and so forth.

This "core functions" framework has proven to be useful in clarifying the fundamental, overarching responsibilities of public health. The three core functions contain a set of ten essential public health services (Table 16.1) (Department of Health and Human Services (DHHS) 1994). Although there is great variation in capacity to implement the ten services, they represent types of activities that public health uses to achieve its

mission to assure the conditions in which people can be healthy.

Whether one views public health through the lens of the core functions or the ten essential services, managing and using information is at the core of public health effectiveness. Assessment, and several of the essential public health services rely heavily on public health **surveillance**, the ongoing collection, analysis, interpretation, and dissemination of data on health conditions (e.g., breast cancer) and threats to health (e.g., smoking prevalence). Surveillance data represent one of the fundamental means by which priorities for public health action are set. Surveillance data serve short term (e.g., in surveillance for acute infectious diseases) and also longer term, (e.g., in determining leading causes of premature death, injury, or disability) purposes. In either case, surveillance data are collected for the purposes of action, either to guide a public health response as in the case of an outbreak investigation, or to help direct public health policy. A recent example of the latter is the surveillance data showing the dramatic rise in obesity in the United States. A tremendous amount of energy and public focus has been brought to bear on this problem, including a major DHHS program, the Childhood Overweight and Obesity Prevention Initiative (DHHS 2011) driven largely by compelling surveillance data.

16.3 Public Health Informatics

Public health informatics has been defined as the systematic application of information science, computer science, and technology to public health practice, research, and learning (Friede et al. 1995; Yasnoff et al. 2000). Public health informatics is distinguished by its focus on populations (versus the individual), its orientation to prevention (rather than diagnosis and treatment), and its governmental context, because public health nearly always involves government agencies. It is a large and complex area that is the focus of another entire textbook in this series (O'Carroll et al. 2003).

The differences between public health informatics and other informatics specialty areas relate to the contrast between public health and medical care itself (Friede and O'Carroll 1998; Yasnoff et al. 2000). Public health focuses on the health of the community as opposed to that of the individual patient. In the medical care system, individuals with specific diseases or conditions are the primary concern. In public health, issues related to the community as the patient may require "treatment" such as disclosure of the disease status of an individual to prevent further spread of illness or even quarantining some individuals to protect others. Environmental factors, especially ones that affect the health of populations over the long term (e.g., air quality), are also a special focus of the public health domain. Public health places a large emphasis on the prevention of disease and injury versus intervention after the problem has already occurred. To the extent that traditional medical care involves prevention, its focus is primarily on delivery of preventive services to individual patients.

Public health actions are not limited to the clinical encounter—in fact, actions can take place at one or more points in the entire causal chain. In public health, the nature of a given intervention is not predetermined by professional discipline, but rather by the cost, expediency, and social acceptability of intervening at any potentially effective point in the series of events leading to disease, injury, or disability. Public health interventions have included (for example) wastewater treatment and solid waste disposal systems, housing and building codes, fluoridation of municipal water supplies, removal of lead from gasoline, food sanitation and smoke alarms. Contrast this with the modern health care system, which generally accomplishes its mission through medical and surgical encounters.

Public health also generally operates directly or indirectly through government agencies that must be responsive to legislative, regulatory, and policy directives, carefully balance competing priorities, and openly disclose their activities. In addition, certain public health actions involve authority for specific (sometimes coercive) measures to protect the community. Examples include closing a contaminated swimming beach, or a restaurant that fails inspection.

16.4 Information Systems in Public Health

The fundamental science of public health is **epidemiology**, which is the study of the prevalence and determinants of injury, disability and disease in populations. Hence, most public health information systems focus on information about aggregate populations. Disease or risk factor surveillance is the key tool that epidemiologists use to study populations and hence many public health information systems are designed for disease surveillance.

Almost all medical information systems focus almost exclusively on supporting the processes of care for individuals. For example, almost any clinical laboratory system can quickly find a patient's culture results whereas public health practitioners would want to know the time trend of antibiotic resistance for the population served by the clinic.

Most health care professionals are surprised to learn that there is no uniform national routine reporting–never mind information system–for most diseases, injuries, disabilities, risk factors, or prevention activities in the United States. In contrast, France, Great Britain, Denmark, Norway and Sweden have comprehensive systems in selected areas, such as occupational injuries, infectious diseases, and cancer; no country, however, has complete reporting for every problem. In fact, it is only births, deaths, and–to a lesser extent–fetal deaths that are uniformly and relatively completely reported in the U.S. by the National Vital Statistics System, operated by the states and the Centers for Disease Control and Prevention (CDC). If you have an angioplasty (an intravascular procedure to relieve a narrowing in one of the arteries feeding the heart muscle) and survive, nobody at the state or federal level necessarily knows.

The Federal, State or Local (city or county) government settings are responsible for implementing public health information systems in the United States. The information requirements for each setting vary by the degree of information granularity and type of system functionality needed.

Table 16.2 Example types of information systems at a state health department that exchange individual level data with clinics, hospitals and others in the community when required for public health – (Minnesota 2010)

1. Women, Infants and Children (WIC)
2. Children with Special Health Needs
3. Newborn Hearing Screening/Early Hearing Detection and Intervention
4. Birth Defects Information System
5. Blood Lead Information System
6. Infectious Disease Surveillance System
7. Immunization Information System
8. Tuberculosis Control System
9. Refugee/Immigrant Health Information System
10. Sexually Transmitted Infections (STD/SDI) Surveillance System
11. AIDS/HIV Surveillance system
12. Vital Statistics System (e.g. birth and death records)
13. Cancer Surveillance System
14. Breast/Cervical Cancer Screening system
15. Traumatic Brain and Spinal Cord Injury System
16. Public Health Laboratory Information System
17. Newborn Metabolic Screening System

The Federal systems often are large scale such as the National Notifiable Disease Surveillance System (NNDSS) that collects counts of diseases from each state and in this case advanced analysis, reporting and mapping functions are essential.

State health department information systems are often dedicated to a particular disease or condition such as infections disease, cancer or injury registries, immunization information systems and the like. In Minnesota, for example, there are at least 17 such information systems that maintain individual level information and exchange information with hospitals, clinics and other health settings in the community (Table 16.2). These database systems have both analytical capability and case-based management functions. Use of this information is essential to characterize the health of the state population.

The County/City public health departments often interact closely with individuals and families and thus must maintain information systems that support detailed data on public health activities, such as client medication observed therapy

follow-up for a TB case or exposed person or coordination of an asthma action plan.

Public health information systems are designed with special features for population-level analysis and context. These systems involve indexing multiple variables in a database coupled with sophisticated statistical and **Geographic Information System** (**GIS**) support capabilities often found in a data warehouse. For example, they are optimized for retrieval from very large (multi-million) record databases, and to quickly cross-tabulate, study seasonal and secular trends, and look for patterns by person, place, and time (see example in Fig. 16.1).

Public health agencies retain personal identifiers only as needed by the use of the data and as the law allows. Thus, data submitted to federal agencies often omit personal identifiers. Examples of systems designed to support population-level analysis include CDC's HIV/AIDS reporting system and the NNDSS.

At the national level, the use of personal identifiers in these systems is very limited, and their use is generally restricted to linking data from different sources (e.g., data from a state laboratory and a disease surveillance form). A few examples of these kinds of population-focused systems include CDC systems such as the HIV/AIDS reporting system, which collects millions of observations concerning people infected with the Human Immunodeficiency Virus (HIV) and those diagnosed with Acquired Immunodeficiency Syndrome (AIDS) and is used to conduct dozens of studies (and which does not collect personal identifiers; individuals are tracked by **pseudo-identifier**); the NNDSS operated by CDC in collaboration with the Council of State and Territorial Epidemiologists (CSTE) in which state epidemiologists report some 77 conditions (for 2011; the exact number is set each year and varies as conditions wax and wane) every week to the CDC (and which makes up the center tables in the Morbidity and Mortality Weekly Report [MMWR]).

Assessment of the magnitude of non-reportable health conditions and surveillance for these conditions, usually managed by state health departments and federal health agencies (largely

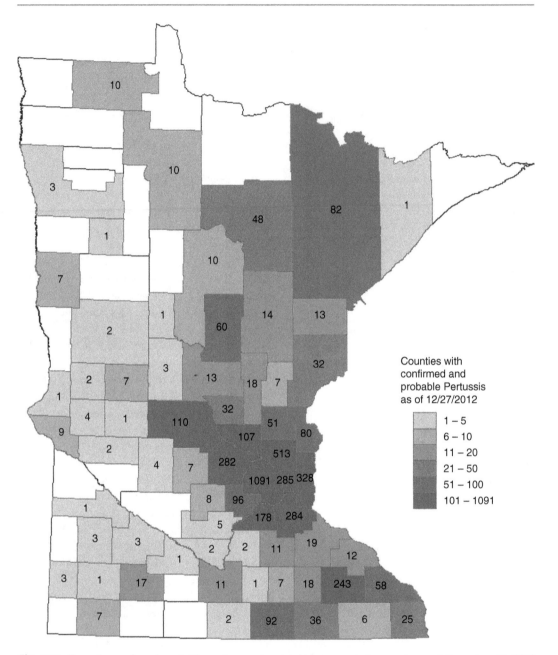

Fig. 16.1 Example: confirmed, probable, and suspect pertussis case counts by county as of December 13, 2012 (Source: Minnesota Department of Health; Immunization Program, 2012)

the CDC), provide periodic estimates of risk factors, incidence and prevalence of diseases. Because these data derive largely from population samples, it is often impossible to obtain estimates at a level of geographic detail finer than a region or state. Moreover, many of the behavioral indices are patient self-reported (although extensive validation studies have shown that they are good for trends and sometimes are more reliable than data obtained from clinical systems). In the case of special surveys, such as CDC's National Health and Nutrition Examination Survey (NHANES), there is primary data entry into a CDC system. The data are complete, but the survey costs many millions of dollars, is done only every few years, and requires years for the data to be made available.

Disease registries track, often completely, the incidence of certain conditions, especially cancers, birth defects, injuries, and conditions associated with environmental contamination. They tend to focus on one topic or to cover certain diseases for specific time periods. Most of these surveillance systems rely on health care providers to submit the data, thereby leading to incomplete reporting (Overhage et al. 2008), even as it becomes increasingly automated from laboratory information and EHR systems.

While separate disease-specific information systems served their purposes well for many years, issues of duplicate data entry and increasing pressures to exchange data electronically with clinical and other systems led to the creation of the Public Health Information Network (PHIN). The PHIN addresses this issue by promoting the use of data and information system standards to advance the development of efficient, integrated, and interoperable surveillance systems at federal, state and local levels (CDC 2011). This activity is designed to facilitate standards-based electronic transfer of information between systems (see Chap. 7), reduce provider burden in submitting the information, and enhance both the timeliness and quality of information provided. Standards for immunization transactions, reportable electronic laboratory results and transactions for syndromic surveillance, are being integrated into the requirements for achieving the various stages of **meaningful use**. Submission of data such as immunizations and disease reports from EHRs to public health is part of the meaningful use incentive program (see Chaps. 12, 14, and 22) with the ultimate goal of bi-directional communications between public health departments and clinicians.

Now that historical and epidemiological forces are making the world smaller and causing lines between medicine and public health to blur, systems will need to be multifunctional, and clinical and public health systems will, of necessity, coalesce. Public health systems need to inform the state of the health ecology. To fill that need, pub-

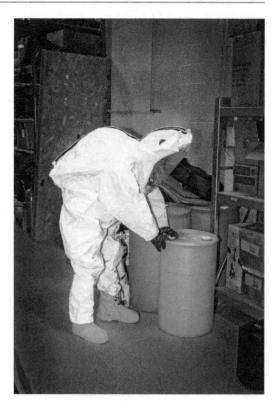

Fig. 16.2 Example: public health officials respond to potential bio-terrorism event or exposure bio-threat as a result of a natural disaster (Source: LaVenture M, Minneapolis, Minnesota 2013)

lic health and clinical informaticians will need to work closely together to build the tools to study and control new and emerging infectious diseases, bioterrorism threats, and support efforts to respond to and manage natural disasters and other environmental effects on health (see photo in Fig. 16.2). For example, in the late 1990's, Columbia Presbyterian Medical Center and the New York City Department of Health collaborated on the development of a tuberculosis registry for northern Manhattan, and the Emory University System of Health Care and the Georgia Department of Public Health built a similar system for tuberculosis monitoring and treatment in Atlanta. It is not by chance that these two cities each developed tuberculosis systems; rather, tuberculosis is a perfect example of what was once a public health problem (that affected primarily the poor and underserved) coming into the mainstream population as a result of an emerging infectious disease (AIDS), immigration, increased international travel, multidrug resistance, and our growing prison population. Hence, the changing ecology of disease, coupled with revolutionary changes in how health care is managed and paid for, will necessitate information systems that serve both individual medical and public health needs.

16.5 Immunization Information Systems: A Public Health Informatics Example

Immunization Information Systems (IIS) are confidential, computerized, population-based systems that collect and consolidate vaccination data from vaccine providers and offer tools for designing and sustaining effective immunization strategies at the provider and program levels (MMWR 2011).[1]

IIS represent a good example for illustrating the principles of public health informatics. In addition to their orientation to prevention, they can function properly only through continuing interaction with the health care system; in fact, they were designed for use primarily in the clinical setting. Although IIS are among the largest and most complex public health information systems, the many successful implementations show conclusively that it is possible to overcome the challenging informatics problems they present. The maturity and value of IIS is reflected in the inclusion of provider and hospital reporting to IIS as a "Meaningful Use" objective.

The major functions of IIS include the ability to accept immunization records either through manual entry or electronically using a variety of file formats and messaging standards (see below), providing on-line secure access to patient immunization records 24/7, providing vaccine forecasting/decision support based on patient age and immunization history, supporting vaccine inventory management and vaccine ordering, producing official immunization records for school and other enrollment, generating immunization coverage reports for an individual provider, clinical

practice or jurisdiction, and supporting Vaccine Adverse Event Reporting.

16.5.1 History and Background of IIS

Childhood immunizations have been among the most successful public health interventions, resulting in the near elimination of nine vaccine preventable diseases that historically extracted a major toll in terms of both morbidity and mortality (IOM, 2000). The need for IIS stems from the challenge of assuring complete immunization protection for the approximately 10,800 children born each day in the United States in the context of three complicating factors: the scattering of immunization records among multiple providers; an immunization schedule that has become increasingly complex as the number of vaccines has grown; and the conundrum that the very success of mass immunization has reduced the incidence of disease, lulling parents and providers into a sense of complacency.

IIS must be able to exchange a high volume of immunization information accurately and consistently, so they were the first public health information systems to develop HL7 messaging guides (see Chap. 7), beginning in 1995.

In addition to messaging standards, the CDC and IIS community also developed functional standards (Table 16.3), codifying years of experience in refining system requirements. CDC and state IIS have established a detailed measurement system containing about 100 measures for tracking progress that annually assesses adherence to the 12 functions and other functional and use metrics (see example in Fig. 16.3). Further formalizing the public policy commitment to the development of IIS, the national Healthy People 2020 objective is to increase to 95 % the percentage of children aged <6 years whose immunization records are housed in a fully operational IIS (DHHS 2010). In 2011, 20 states and 3 of 6 major cities measured had met this objective (Fig. 16.4)

Numerous best practice guidelines have been developed by the IIS community's American Immunization Registry Association (AIRA) to help ensure ongoing quality improvement, efficiency and increased standardization.

---

[1] http://www.cdc.gov/mmwr/ (accessed 4/26/13).

Table 16.3 Twelve functional standards for immunization registries (CDC, 2002)

1. Electronically store data regarding all National Vaccine Advisory Committee-approved core data elements
2. Establish an IIS record within 6 weeks of birth for each child born in the catchment area
3. Enable access to vaccine information from the IIS at the time of the encounter
4. Receive and process vaccine information within 1 month of vaccine administration
5. Protect the confidentiality of medical information
6. Protect the security of medical information
7. Exchange vaccination records by using Health Level 7 standards
8. Automatically determine the immunization(s) needed when a person is seen by the health care provider for a scheduled vaccination
9. Automatically identify persons due or late for vaccinations to enable the production of reminder and recall notices
10. Automatically produce vaccine coverage reports by providers, age groups, and geographic areas
11. Produce authorized immunization records
12. Promote accuracy and completeness of IIS data

16.5.2 Key Informatics Issues in Immunization Information Systems

The implementation, upgrading and management of IIS present challenging informatics issues in at least four areas: (1) interdisciplinary communications; (2) organizational and collaborative issues; (3) funding and sustainability; and (4) system design and interoperability. While the specific manifestations of these issues are unique to IIS, these four areas represent the typical domains that must be addressed and overcome in most public health informatics projects.

16.5.2.1 Interdisciplinary Communications

Interdisciplinary communications is a key challenge in any biomedical informatics project—it is certainly not specific to public health informatics. To be useful, a public health information system must accurately represent and enable the complex concepts and processes that underlie the specific business functions required. Information systems represent a highly abstract and complex

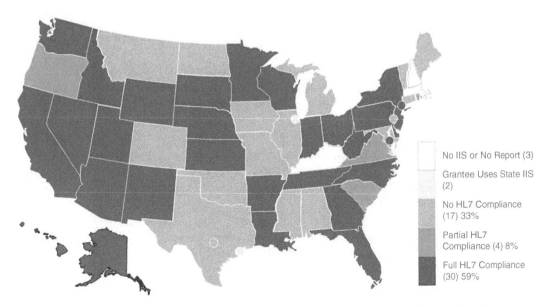

No IIS or No Report (3)

Grantee Uses State IIS (2)

No HL7 Compliance (17) 33%

Partial HL7 Compliance (4) 8%

Full HL7 Compliance (30) 59%

Fig, 16.3 Example: compliance with HL7 Messaging Standards in a Grantee Immunization Information System – United States and six cities, 2011 (Source: Urquhart, GA, Centers for Disease Control and Prevention, Chief, Immunization systems Support Branch; presentation to the Association of Immunization Managers, 2010 program managers meeting)

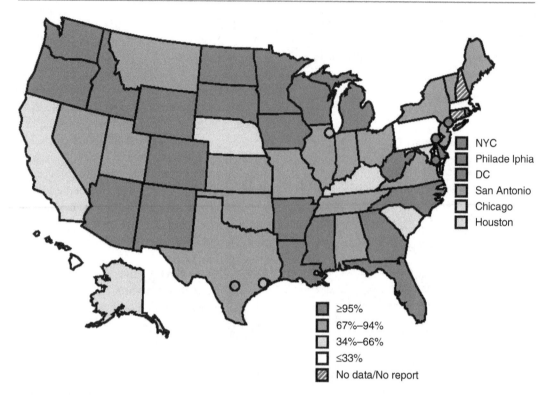

Fig. 16.4 Example: percentage of children aged <6 years participating in an Immunization Information System — United States, five cities,† and the District of Columbia, 2011 (Source: CDC. Progress in immunization information systems—United States 2011. *MMWR* 2013;62(03):48–51)

set of data, processes, and interactions. This complexity needs to be discussed, specified, and understood in detail by a variety of personnel with little or no expertise in the terminology and concepts of information technology. Therefore, successful IIS implementation and enhancements require clear communication among public health specialists, immunization specialists, providers, IT specialists, and related disciplines, an effort complicated by gaps in a shared vocabulary and differences in the usage of common terms from the various domains.

To deal with the communications challenges, particularly between IT and public health specialists, it is essential to identify an interlocutor who has familiarity with both information technology and public health. The interlocutor should spend sufficient time in the user environment to develop a deep understanding of the information processing context of both the current and proposed systems. It is also important for individuals from all the disciplines related to the project to have representation in the decision-making processes.

16.5.2.2 Organizational and Collaborative Issues

The organizational and collaborative issues involved in operating and upgrading an IIS are challenging because of the large number and wide variety of users, most of whom are outside the IIS organization. Each of the user groups has distinct needs, including clinicians (to ensure age-appropriate vaccination and for vaccine management and ordering), schools (to ensure student adherence to state school immunization laws), health plans (to measure immunization coverage among beneficiaries and perhaps by provider), local health departments (to assess immunization coverage in their jurisdiction and identify children who have fallen behind and require outreach), and CDC (for accountability of federally-funded vaccines and IIS funding).

Ensuring these diverse needs are understood, balanced and effectively met can be daunting on the typically slim governmental budgets on which IIS must operate.

Governance

Governance issues are also critical to success of implementation or enhancements to IIS. All the key stakeholders need to be represented in the ongoing, open and transparent decision-making processes, guided by a mutually acceptable governance mechanism. IIS require established rules for identifying needed enhancements, prioritizing them across the often disparate needs of diverse users, and effectively managing and communicating the changes as they are developed and implemented. Governance can also be used for establishing metrics for progress, such as provider sites enrolled and trained, setting other priorities, and for review of confidentiality policies.

Legislative and Policy Issues

Legislative and policy issues are important aspects of the informatics challenges of IIS. State laws typically govern who has access to IIS data for what purposes, so system design must accommodate multiple levels of role-based authorized access to functionality. A major issue is whether patient/parent consent is required before submission of immunization data to IIS, and, if so, how that consent is communicated and managed in the system. IIS must also be able to record that the patient has declined to receive vaccines for religious or other reasons as defined in state law, and use that indicator to suppress vaccine forecasting/decision support messages and reminder-recall notices. Some jurisdictions have enacted regulations requiring providers to submit immunization data to IIS. Such a regulatory approach to ensuring information completeness is less burdensome as automated electronic file submissions have largely replaced manual data entry. Negotiating policy for interstate access and data exchange is another key issue.

16.5.2.3 Funding and Sustainability

Funding and sustainability are continuing challenges for all IIS. Naturally, an important tool for securing funding is development of a business case that shows the anticipated costs and benefits of IIS. A substantial body of evidence now shows benefits, effectiveness and costs of IIS (Guide to Community Preventive Services 2010). However, many of the currently operational IIS had to develop their business cases prior to the availability of good quantitative data.

Specific benefits associated with IIS include preventing duplicative immunizations, eliminating the necessity to review the vaccination records for school and day care entry, and efficiencies in provider offices from the immediate availability of complete immunization history information and patient-specific vaccine schedule recommendations. The careful review of the evidence on effectiveness, costs and benefits of specific immunization IIS functions may also be helpful in prioritizing system enhancement requirements.

16.5.2.4 System Design and Interoperability

System design and interoperability are important factors in the success of IIS. Difficult design issues include data acquisition, database organization, identification and matching of individuals, generating immunization recommendations, access to data, protocols for electronic exchange and interoperability, and reports related to clinic practice and community rates of immunization. Acquiring immunization data is a challenging system design issue and an area of considerable IIS change as electronic health record use becomes more common, new adolescent and adult immunizations are added to IIS, and a broader scope of settings like pharmacies submit information. Within the context of busy pediatric and primary care practices (where the majority of immunizations are given) the data acquisition strategy must of necessity be extremely efficient and should result in no additional work for participating providers. Use of certified EHR systems can support this strategy; however, only a minority of physician practices is currently using EHRs and few EHR vendors have integrated IIS query and exchange into their software.

Database design must support the desired IIS functions and allow efficient implementation of these capabilities. The design must consider operational needs for data access for an individual record and calculating individual forecasts of needed immunizations, and the requirements for population-based immunization assessment, management of vaccine inventory, and generating recall and reminder notices. One example of a particularly important database design decision for IIS is whether to represent immunization information by vaccine or by antigen. Vaccine-based representations map each available preparation, including those with multiple antigens, into its own specific data element. Antigen-based representations translate multi-component vaccines into their individual antigens prior to storage. In some cases, it may be desirable to represent the immunization information both ways. Specific consideration of required response times for specific queries must also be factored into key design decisions.

Identification and matching of individuals within IIS is another critical issue. Because it is relatively common for an individual to receive immunizations from multiple providers, any system must be able to match information from multiple sources to assemble a complete record of immunizations. In the absence of a national unique patient identifier, most IIS assign an arbitrary number to each individual and use a matching algorithm, which utilizes multiple items of demographic information to assess the probability that two records are really from the same person and can detect duplicate reports of an immunization. Development of such algorithms and optimization of their parameters has been the subject of active investigation in the context of IIS, particularly with respect to **deduplication** (Miller et al. 2001).

Another critical design issue is generating vaccine recommendations from an individual's prior immunization history, based on guidance from the CDC's Advisory Committee on Immunization Practices (ACIP). As more vaccines have become available, both individually and in various combinations, the immunization schedule has become increasingly complex, especially if any delays occur in receiving doses, an individual has a contraindication, or local issues require special consideration. The language used in the written guidelines can be ambiguous with respect to definitions, e.g., for ages and intervals, making implementation of decision support systems problematic. Considering that the recommendations are updated relatively frequently, maintaining software that produces accurate immunization recommendations is a continuing challenge. Accordingly, the implementation, testing, and maintenance of decision support systems to produce vaccine recommendations has been the subject of extensive study (Yasnoff and Miller 2003).

Finally, easy access to the information in IIS is essential. While independent web based interfaces are common, the ideal is to provide a seamless query launched within the context of the provider's EHR workflow and having IIS information and forecast returned and incorporated into the EHR. Similarly the design should support efficient access to summary reports on immunization rates for a clinic or community, reports on children who are behind schedule and support delivery of electronic reminder or recall notices to support prevention. Consumer direct access to their own immunization record is desirable; however, there are design considerations regarding security, allowable data views and editing rights.

16.6 Conclusions and Future Challenges

Public health informatics may be viewed as the application of biomedical informatics to populations. In a sense, it is the ultimate evolution of biomedical informatics, which has traditionally focused on applications related to individual patients. Public health informatics highlights the potential of the health informatics disciplines as a group to integrate information from the molecular to the population level. Effective public health information systems can help to assure prevention actions, timely monitoring of disease patterns, and rapid responses to outbreaks, thereby saving lives and money.

Public health informatics and the development of **health information infrastructure** (see Chap. 13) are closely related. Public health informatics supports the population assessment, assurance and policy development roles of public health. In contrast, health information infrastructures focus on medical care to individuals but connect providers and patients within a population. Ideally these two areas work together supporting both community health assessment and individual care. In the past, public health and health care have not traditionally interacted as closely as they should. In a larger sense, both really focus on the health of communities—public health does this directly, while the medical care system does it one patient at a time. However, it is now clear that medical care must also focus on the community to integrate the effective delivery of services across all care settings for all individuals (Institute of Medicine 2011a). Public health informatics confronts many challenges including the varied ways governments organize public health practice, the legal issues involved in inter-institutional information systems and defining user information and system needs in a multi-stakeholder discipline that is public health.

Public health systems frequently involve non-health organizations such as law enforcement and parks and recreation departments. Thus public health informaticians must adopt methodologies that bridge professional and organizational divides. The Public Health Informatics Institute's Collaborative Requirements Methodology is one such example (PHII 2011)

Despite the focus of many current public health informatics activities on population-based extensions of the medical care system (leading to the orientation of this chapter), applications beyond this scope are both possible and desirable. Indeed, the phenomenal contributions to health made by the hygienic movement of the nineteenth and early twentieth centuries suggest the power of large-scale environmental, legislative, and social changes to promote human health (Rosen 1993). Public health informatics must explore these dimensions as energetically as those associated with prevention and clinical care at the individual level.

The effective application of informatics to populations through public health is a key challenge of the twenty-first century. It is a challenge we must accept, understand, and overcome if we want to create an efficient and effective health care system as well as truly healthy communities for all.

Suggested Readings

American Immunization Registry Association (AIRA). Best practice guidelines for IIS; available at http://www.immregistries.org/resources/aira-mirow (Accessed 15 Dec 2012). A practical set of consensus-based practices for implementation and operation of IIS.

CDC (Centers for Disease Control and Prevention). (2002). Immunization Registry Progress — United States. Morbidity and Mortality Weekly Report. 51(34): 760–762.

Friede, A., Blum, H. L., & McDonald, M. (1995). Public health informatics: how information-age technology can strengthen public health. *Annual Review of Public Health, 16,* 239–252. The seminal article on public health informatics.

Guide to Community Preventive Services (2010). *Universally recommended vaccinations: immunization information systems.* Atlanta: Guide to Community Preventive Services. Available at http://www.thecommunityguide.org/vaccines/universally/imminfosystems.html. (Accessed 29 Nov 2012). A practical guide to the benefit and value of Immunizations and other preventive services.

Hallestad, R., Bigelow, J., Bower, A., Girosi, F., Meili, R., Scoville, R., & Taylor, R. (2005). Can electronic medical record systems transform health care? Potential health benefits, savings, and costs. *Health Affairs, 24,* 1103–1117. A summary of the real and potential value of electronic health records.

Hinman, A. R., & Ross, D. A. (2010). Immunization registries can be building blocks for national health information systems. *Health Affairs, 29*(4), 676–682. Describes the components of IIS and how they are also key elements in the national health infrastructure.

IOM (Institute of Medicine). 2011. Engineering a learning healthcare system: A look at the future: Workshop summary. Washington, DC: The National Academies Press. A report on the future opportunities and a vision for the health system.

IOM Institute of Medicine (2000). Calling the Shots — Immunization Finance Policies and Practices. Washington, DC: National Academy Press.

Koo, D., O'Carroll, P. W., & LaVenture, M. (2001). Public health 101 for informaticians. *Journal of the American Medical Informatics Association, 8*(6), 585–597. An accessible document that introduces public health thinking.

Miller P.L., Frawley SJ, Sayward FG (2001). Exploring the utility of demographic data and vaccination history data in the deduplication of immunization registry patient records. J Biomed Inform, 34(1):37–50.

O'Carroll, P. W., Yasnoff, W. A., Ward, M. E., Ripp, L. H., & Martin, E. L. (Eds.). (2003). *Public health informatics and information systems.* New York: Springer. A comprehensive textbook.

Overhage, M., Grannis, S., & McDonald, C. J. (2008). A comparison of the completeness and timeliness of automated electronic laboratory reporting and spontaneous reporting of notifiable conditions. *American*

Journal of Public Health, 98(2), 344–350. This study documents the improved quality and timeliness of electronic lab reporting of diseases to public health.

US Department of Health and Human Services. (2010). *Healthy people 2020.* Washington, DC: US Department of Health and Human Services. Available at http://healthypeople.gov/2020/topicsobjectives2020/objectiveslist.aspx?topicid=23. (Accessed 29 Nov 2012). The essential guide to the national public health goals.

Yasnoff, W. A., O'Carroll, P. W., Koo, D., Linkins, R. W., & Kilbourne, E. M. (2000). Public health informatics: Improving and transforming public health in the information age. *Journal of Public Health Management and Practice, 6*(6), 67–75. A concise yet comprehensive introduction to the field.

Questions for Discussion

1. How might the trend of widespread adoption of electronic health records and increasing consumer interest in health information affect public health informatics?

2. How can the successful model of immunization registries be used in other domains of public health (be specific about those domains)? How might it fail in others? Why?

3. A significant and increasing percentage of the US GDP is spent on medical care. How could public health informatics help to use those monies more efficiently? Or lower the figure absolutely?

4. Compare and contrast the database desiderata for clinical versus public health information systems. Explain it from non-technical and technical perspectives.

5. If public health informatics (PHI) involves the application of information technology in any manner that improves or promotes human health, does this necessarily involve a human "user" that interacts with the PHI application? For example, could the information technology underlying anti-lock braking systems be considered a public health informatics application? Provide other examples.

6. What is the relationship between public health informatics and the developing health information infrastructure (HII) (see Chap. 13)? How might public health inform the developing HII?

7. How will cloud computing (shared configurable computing resources including networks, servers, storage, applications, and services), and mobile technology transform public health informatics?

Consumer Health Informatics and Personal Health Records

17

Kevin Johnson, Holly Brugge Jimison, and Kenneth D. Mandl

After reading this chapter, you should know the answers to these questions:

- What is the central tenet of consumer health informatics?
- What are the issues that biomedical informatics research can address relating to consumer communication, decision-making, and information access needs?
- Although technology is a major focus of the discussion around consumer health informatics, we realize that any technology of interest today will be obsolete in the next 10 years. However, the issues this technology is trying to address will continue to be prevalent. With that in mind, what are the larger biomedical informatics topics this technology is being used to address?

- Define patient portals, personal health records, patient-controlled health records, and personal health applications.

17.1 Introduction

Complexity and collaboration characterize health care in the early twenty-first century. Complexity arises from a deeper or more sophisticated understanding of health and diseases, wherein etiological models must take into account both molecular processes and physical environments. Collaboration reflects not only inter-professional collaboration, but also a realization that successful attainment of optimal well being and effective management of disease processes necessitate active engagement of clinicians, lay persons, concerned family members, and society as a whole. This chapter introduces technologies forming the foundation of **consumer health informatics**, including **personal health records** (PHR), **patient portals**, **personal health applications**, and **social networking**. We will illustrate how each of these tools embraces the complexity of health care and makes possible the collaborations necessary to engage consumers in health promotion, disease management, and preventive

K. Johnson, MD, MS (✉)
Department of Biomedical Informatics,
Vanderbilt University School of Medicine,
2209 Garland Ave, Nashville 37232, TN, USA
e-mail: kevin.johnson@vanderbilt.edu

H.B. Jimison, PhD, FACMI
Consortium on Technology for Proactive Care,
Colleges of Computer & Information Sciences
and Health Sciences, Northeastern University,
360 Huntington Ave, WVH 476,
Boston 02115, MA, USA
e-mail: h.jimison@neu.edu

K.D. Mandl, MD, MPH
Children's Hospital Informatics Program,
Harvard Medical School, Boston Children's Hospital,
300 Longwood Avenue, Boston 02446, MA, USA
e-mail: kenneth_mandlh@arvard.edu

The authors acknowledge and thank the co-authors of the previous chapter edition, Patricia Flatley Brennan and Justin Starren.

E.H. Shortliffe, J.J. Cimino (eds.), *Biomedical Informatics*,
DOI 10.1007/978-1-4471-4474-8_17, © Springer-Verlag London 2014

care. In the first part of this chapter, we introduce four common health care challenges that consumer health informatics addresses: consumer engagement, information sharing, communication and decision facilitation. We then describe the history of consumer health informatics and the tools commonly available to address the above challenges. We conclude the chapter by describing many of the emerging trends in the discipline and some of the continuing opportunities.

17.1.1 The Challenge of Improving Consumer Engagement

Contemporary consumers are under greater pressure to participate in their own care than have patients at any time since the emergence of modern health care. Patient participation takes many forms, including shared decision-making, self-care, and collaborative practices (Mead and Bower 2000). The role of the consumer as a full partner in health promotion and disease management has never been more necessary than now. In the distributed managed-care models of health care, consumers serve as their own case managers, brokering care from generalists, specialists, and ancillary groups. Rarely do consumers receive all of their clinical services from a single provider. Although health information technology, such as the electronic health record, provides an integrated data repository and communication service, the view of the patient from a single electronic health record often will not include a record of services provided through the continuum of care. Moreover, for some patients, the inability to access this record may represent a barrier to optimal care delivery (Detmer 2003). Consumer health informatics as a subdiscipline is founded on this need for access. A central tenet of consumer health informatics is that although not all patients will participate, patients participating in their health care leads to higher quality care than that which is achievable without patient participation.

Patient engagement is not purely driven by the patient. Seminal work by sociologists such as Goffman (1959) and psychologists such as Skinner (1938) and Deci and Ryan (1985) observed that consumers may become engaged because of an innate desire to be rewarded by participation or through external rewards. These observers of human behavior have reinforced the notion that in many individuals, innate desire motivates engagement without the apparent presence of an extrinsic reward or punishment as a consequence of engaging in the activity. These observers also note, importantly, that not every person will have an innate desire to engage, or may lack the desire as the perception of the cost of engaging increases. For these individuals, extrinsic motivators (money, material goods, and praise) may catalyze behavior change. It is also the case for many of these individuals that peers, family members, and even others in their social network may provide a surrogate for the patient's lack of engagement by actively participating in information gathering and health care decision making. All of these observations may be addressed by consumer health informatics researchers.

17.1.2 The Challenge of Improving the Information Available to Consumers

It has long been recognized that information sharing can lead to improved decision making and health care system vigilance. Pamplets, newpaper articles, and phone communication about disease outbreaks were once the only methods to accomplish information dissemination. These methods were suboptimal in their ability to address challenges with health literacy, numeracy, widespread access, appropriately timed access, or proper formatting/tailoring (for example, so that they could benefit adolescents as well as adults, or men as well as women.) The advent of the Internet, **interactive television** and a host of widely available home technologies provide a rich source of tools to address this challenge.

17.1.3 The Challenge of Improving the Communication Among Consumers and Providers

Consumer health informatics also strives to improve consumer-provider interactions by both helping to prepare patients for meaningful discussions with their clinicians and by facilitating shared decision making. A full discussion of the efforts in this area may be found in the chapter on Telemedicine (Chap. 18).

Consumer-to-consumer communication has been an important source of relevant information for patients with diseases of all sorts. Before the Internet became available, this type of communication was difficult, though many health care institutes, churches, and communities developed support groups for common diseases or interests (Lieberman 1988).

17.1.4 The Challenge of Improving Consumer Decision-Making

One of the most important aspects of consumer health informatics has to do with moving beyond providing background health information toward helping consumers make quality health decisions and appropriate actions. Before the increased availability of home computing and the Internet, patients facing difficult decisions used information available in public libraries or sent to them (via stamped, self-addressed envelopes!) They relied on conversations and advice from family, close friends, church members, other patients, or doctors. Importantly, they made decisions often with no attention given to the evidence supporting each treatment alternative, without an objective assessment of risks and benefits, and without recognizing their own personal characteristics that might impact the outcome of the chosen approach.

Each of these challenges to consumer engagement has rationalized work in the field of consumer health informatics since its inception. We will now briefly review the history of this sub discipline.

17.2 Historical Perspective of Consumer Health Informatics

17.2.1 The Rise of Consumer-Oriented Health Communications

In essence, what we think of as consumer engagement reflects a shift from the patient as the silent recipient of ministrations from a wise, beneficent clinician to an active collaborator whose values, preferences, and lifestyle not only alter predisposition to certain illnesses but also shape the characteristics of desirable treatments.

Patients, family members and the general public have long-played an active role in health care and have actively sought information from health professionals and government agencies. During the early twentieth century, the US Federal Children's Bureau served as a major source of health information for the public. Mothers could write to this federal agency, asking questions about normal child development, nutrition, and disease management. Written materials, such as letters and pamphlets served as the primary mechanism for delivering information that supported lay people in their handling of health challenges. Patient education companies such as Krames[1] would partner with organizations like the American Heart Association to provide general printed material on heart disease or with the American Cancer Society to provide information on cancer. As television became commonplace, broadcast and reproduction media including television, videotapes and audiotapes, were quickly harnessed by health professionals as a means for presenting complex information and health care instructions to people in their homes. Consumer health broadcasts, and eventually dedicated channels covering topics such as nutrition, fitness, and women's health issues, became common and were broadcast on local daytime television and radio networks. This mechanism continues today, and often uses consumer panels, live phoned in

---

[1] www.krames.com (accessed 4/23/13).

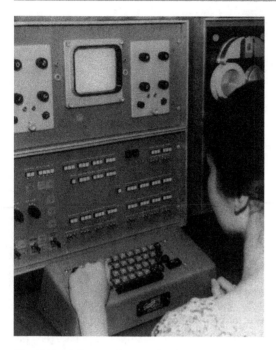

Fig. 17.1 Early use of computing in consumer health informatics, here taking a medical history directly from a patient (Slack, WV, et al. (1966). *NEJM* with permission)

questions, expert guests, audience participation, and other ways to provide general advice for consumers.

Computers and telecommunications have been used since the early 1940's for patient assessment, patient education, and clinical information sharing. In the 1950's Collen and colleagues at Kaiser Permanente created a health appraisal system that prompted for patient data and returned a systematic risk appraisal (Collen et al. 1964). Then in the 1960's Warner Slack and colleagues at the University of Wisconsin used a mainframe computer system as a health assessment tool. Patients sat at a cathode ray tube (CRT) terminal and responded to text questions, receiving a printed summary of their health appraisal at the end of the session (Slack et al. 1967). Figure 17.1 shows an early example of the mainframe-based tool developed by Slack. At Massachusetts General Hospital in the late 1950's, computer-driven telephone systems were used to conduct home-based follow-up with post-surgery cardiac patients, calling them daily to obtain pulse readings. From the very beginning,

these advocates for integrating technology into the examination room were intrigued by the aspect of computer use both by patients for their needs, as well as by patients to assist with health care professional needs.

17.2.2 Early Advances in Consumer Information Sharing and Decision Making

The legacy of the self-help movement of the 1970s and the consumerism of the 1980s was growth in the importance of the patient as a full participant in health care. At the time, the failure of bioscience research to produce definitive evidence-based guidelines for most common diseases required that medical science be combined with patient preferences (e.g., between surgical and radiation therapies). Patients participated by self-monitoring, by evaluating and choosing therapeutic strategies from a set of acceptable alternatives, by implementing the therapies, and by evaluating their effects. In addition, social and clinical changes in the manner in which care was provided shifted activities that were once the purview of licensed professionals to patients and their family caregivers. Furthermore, there was growing belief that behavioral interventions and alternative therapies held great promise as adjuncts, or even replacements, for traditional medical therapies.

In the 1980s clinicians and health educators capitalized on the increasingly common personal computers as vehicles for health education. Initially, computers were used primarily for computer-assisted learning programs, providing general coaching regarding topics such as nutrition and home care of the elderly. As shown in Fig. 17.2, The Body Awareness Resource Network (BARN), developed in the 1980s by Gustafson and colleagues at the University of Wisconsin, engaged adolescents in game-like interactions to help them learn about growth and development, develop healthy attitudes towards avoidance of risky behaviors, and rehearse strategies for negotiating the complex interpersonal world of adolescence (Bosworth et al. 1983). Later developments in the 1980s and 1990s moved beyond computer

Fig. 17.2 BARN topic index and use by teens. Bosworth (1983). This picture shows teens interacting with a game on the an early graphical computer. The figure on the left is the topic index as displayed on the screen (With permission from Gustafson, D, personal communication)

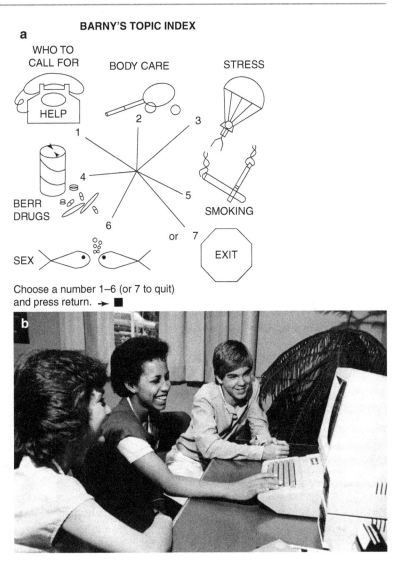

BARNY'S TOPIC INDEX

a

WHO TO CALL FOR

BODY CARE

STRESS

HELP

1

2

3

4

5

BERR DRUGS

6

SMOKING

SEX

or 7

EXIT

Choose a number 1–6 (or 7 to quit) and press return. ➤ ■

b

aided learning to values clarification and risk appraisal exercises, thus capitalizing on the computational power as well as the visual display capabilities of the computer. As the Internet became more available in homes, Internet support groups gathered momentum. One such example, Hopkins Teen Central developed by Ravert and colleagues (2001), allowed otherwise isolated children with cystic fibrosis to meet virtually and to discuss health and developmental issues that impacted healthy decision making. This additional computational power eventually found its way into computer games (Kato and Beale 2006). Although these games were both time-consuming

and expensive to build, they were relatively easy to disseminate, and were associated with measurable changes in knowledge (Lieberman 2001) and, in some cases, symptom management—such as with nausea in pediatric cancer (Redd et al. 1987) and anxiety management (Patel et al. 2006).

17.2.3 Early Advances in Consumer-Consumer Communication

Early electronic newsgroups, bulletin boards, and a precursor to the World Wide Web known as Gopher connected patients to information about various rare and chronic diseases (Grunfeld and Ho 1997; Grunfeld et al. 1996; National Research Council (U.S.). Committee on Enhancing the Internet for Health and Biomedical Applications: Technical Requirements and Implementation Strategies. 2000) One of the earliest such examples was patient handouts made available through the National Heart, Lung, and Blood Institute (Grunfeld and Ho 1997). This medium of distribution was attractive to many health care institutions because of the nature of the Internet, which allowed patients to retrieve information that was of interest without requiring the author to actively disseminate this information to a previously-identified group of people. Ferguson was heavily influential in the 1980's and 90's in creating and analyzing online social support groups for patients (Ferguson 1996). Later, Gustafson and colleagues in Wisconsin demonstrated that online social support could reduce anxiety and hopelessness, with suggestive evidence for improving coping skills and life expectancy (Ferguson 1997). Soon, the idea of the Internet support group became an active area of development, continuing through today (Eysenbach et al. 2004).

At the same time, this increasing use of the Internet raised concerns about the quality of the material available to consumers (Kershaw 2003). This concern, in turn, fueled an industry of groups consisting of content editors, clinicians, and technologists charged with creating legible and responsive consumer information that could be subscribed to on the Web, as well as others focused on rating the quality of this information. One notable group that promotes the deployment of useful online health information is the **Health on the Net Foundation** (HON),[2] pioneered by an international panel of experts and supported by the numerous European groups. Although many of these pioneering companies have long since vanished, the access to consumer health information has remained a core function of the Internet—with 56 % of American adults seeking information about a personal health concern annually (Tu and Cohen 2008).

17.2.4 Early Advances in Consumer Decision-Facilitation

Given that most health care activities actually take place in the home, away from clinics and hospitals (Ferguson 1996), it has always been important that individuals be active and informed participants in their own care. A variety of approaches have been used to provide "just-in-time" information and decision assistance to consumers. As noted above, pamphlets and videos were created to explain treatment options and medical procedures to patients, as background for decision-making. This was followed by an era of interactive video systems to help patients understand the risks and benefits associated with treatment options, but also to help define their values for possible future health outcomes. The prime examples of this type of system originated with the Foundation for Informed Medical Decision Making.[3] As early as 1973, Wennberg and others discovered that the rates of many expensive surgeries and other treatments would vary from location to location throughout the U.S. (Wennberg and Gittelsohn 1973). This variation seemed to occur for medical conditions where there were multiple viable treatment options and choices depended more on physician and resource availability than need or patient characteristics. Wennberg and Mulley focused on developing interactive video consumer decision aids that focused on these conditions (e.g., prostate cancer, breast cancer, back pain, etc.), discovering that patient preferences and priorities for possible health outcomes could vary dramatically from person to person, and could be critical to defining an optimal decision.

17.3 Current Trends

17.3.1 Consumer-Facing Software

There is an enormous amount of momentum in consumer activation. In part, this momentum is fueled by lessons discovered by pioneers in the

---

[2] www.hon.ch (accessed 4/23/13).

[3] www.informedmedicaldecisions.org (accessed 4/23/13).

Table 17.1 Various modes of consumer engagement with health care technology

Mode of engagement	Definition	Examples
Communication	Support for patient-to-patient, computer-to-patient and patient-to-provider knowledge or information dissemination	Patient portals Patient-physician secure email Online support groups Social networking sites
Data storage	A patient-centered and managed repository for patient-entered data or "liquid" health-related information	Personal health records Data portals for devices, health systems and, pharmaceutical companies
Behavior management	Tools to support personal health goals, often by combining data storage, care protocols, information dissemination, and communication	Weight management tools Physical activity tools Medication reminder systems
Decision aids	Prepare people to participate in 'close call' decisions that involve weighing benefits, harms, and scientific uncertainty	Interactive tools for Breast Ca, Prostate Ca, Back Pain, End of Life, Heart Disease

field. In addition, this momentum is the consequence of a contemporary health care environment that is more diffuse and involves more people than ever before. The home and the community are fast becoming the most common sites where health care is provided. Information technologies necessary to support patients and their family caregivers must not only migrate from the inpatient institution to the community but also be populated with information resources that help to guide patients in complex health care decision-making, to communicate with health professionals and to access the clinical records and health science knowledge necessary to help them comprehend their health states and participate in appropriate treatments.

With the ready availability of home computers and cellular phone platforms that support Web browsing and extensible software via "apps," there is a wealth of what is called "consumer-facing" software now available to consumers. Although the types of consumer-facing health technology will come and go over the years, these technologies can be categorized into four modes in which consumers engage with health care through the use of technology. Table 17.1 summarizes these modes. Each mode of engagement will be discussed below, along with some examples illustrating the potential for this mode of engagement.

17.3.2 Communication

17.3.2.1 Patient-Centered Communication

For decades, as the health care system has had to wrestle with chronic illness and as an increasing knowledge base required practicing technically sophisticated and high quality care, the process of disease management has become more and more specialized. It is not uncommon for a patient to see up to seven different providers to manage the average chronic illness. Patients frequently express frustration about the inability for electronic health records to support record-sharing. This frustration has led to recommendations by the **Institute of Medicine** (IOM) that recognize the central role of patients as a repository of their own medical information in their "To Err is Human" book series (Aspden and Institute of Medicine (U.S.). Committee on Data Standards for Patient Safety. 2004; Institute of Medicine Committee on Improving the Patient Record (2001); Kohn et al. 2000), culminating the explicit notion that quality health care should be "patient-centered" among other attributes, and noting that six out of ten rules to improve health care quality depend on patient involvement in their care (Institute of Medicine (U.S.). Committee on Quality of Health Care in America. 2001). The role of patients in communicating also was a central component of early visions for the **National Health Information**

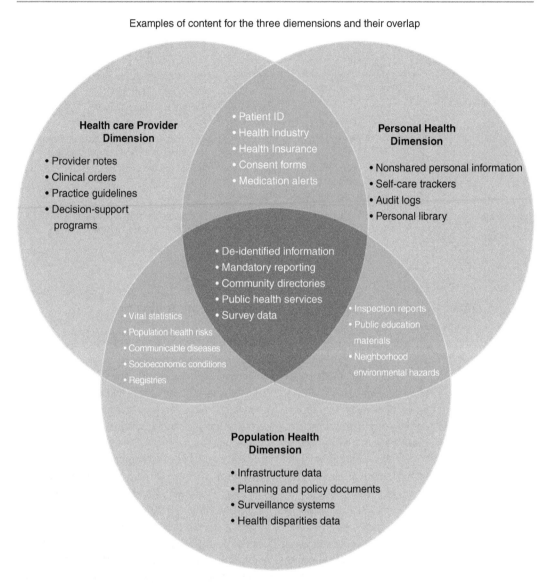

Examples of content for the three diemensions and their overlap

Health care Provider Dimension
- Provider notes
- Clinical orders
- Practice guidelines
- Decision-support programs

- Patient ID
- Health Industry
- Health Insurance
- Consent forms
- Medication alerts

Personal Health Dimension
- Nonshared personal information
- Self-care trackers
- Audit logs
- Personal library

- De-identified information
- Mandatory reporting
- Community directories
- Public health services
- Survey data

- Vital statistics
- Population health risks
- Communicable diseases
- Socioeconomic conditions
- Registries

- Inspection reports
- Public education materials
- Neighborhood environmental hazards

Population Health Dimension
- Infrastructure data
- Planning and policy documents
- Surveillance systems
- Health disparities data

Fig. 17.3 Information dimensions. *Information for health: a strategy for building the National Health Information Infrastructure* (2001) (Source: http://aspe. hhs.gov/sp/nhii/documents/NHIIReport2001/ default.htm)

Infrastructure. Figure 17.3 depicts the information dimensions outlined in this work, which included a personal health dimension that emphasized data required for patients to communicate among or on behalf of their providers.

In addition to this lack of what has been termed "data liquidity" (Courtney 2011) – representing the ideal state of fast, free-flowing, and interoperable data - there are data important to health that may not be in the typical electronic

health record. For example, patient over-the-counter medications, home therapy for allergies or trauma, many health screening forms, and data derived in physiologic monitoring in the home may provide valuable information to caregivers.

Part of the STEEEP ("Safe, Timely, Effective, Efficient, Equitable, Patient-Centered") care framework by the IOM (Institute of Medicine (U.S.). Committee on Quality of Health Care in America. 2001), patient-centeredness implies that liquidity is facilitated by patients being able to access and direct other's access to their information according to clearer laws and protocols that provide consistency and transparency. This ensures that clinicians will have the right information to make informed decisions at the point of care.

17.3.2.2 Electronic Support Groups

As mentioned above, concomitant with the era of home computers and later, the Internet, there was an immediate recognition that technology had removed geographic and physiologic obstacles to communication. Patients who had rare diseases, or people in need of support to help make tough decisions or to face lifestyle altering conditions suddenly had a way to communicate with one another. One of the earliest electronic support groups was developed by Johnson and Ravert, who recognized the ease with which adolescents adopted technology. Hopkins Teen Central was an internet support group developed initially using a device known as WebTV™, which provided Internet access via phone lines and household televisions (Johnson et al. 2001). This project proved extremely successful. It demonstrated, for example, the power of patient-to-patient email, as well as the role of moderated health discussions in answering questions common to patients with a shared medical need.

Electronic support groups, also known as **Internet Support Groups** (ISGs), have since become an almost ubiquitous way for patients comfortable with the Internet to communicate with each other. One study has suggested that over 28 % of Internet users have visited at least one ISG (Horrigan et al. 2001). ISGs use four modes of communication alone or in combination: e-mail lists, instant messaging, bulletin boards, and chat rooms. While the sustained availability of these sites suggests their value to patients, a recent meta-analysis of ISGs for depression noted the poor quality of the evidence. Chat room use appeared to be associated with lower levels of depression. Patients with breast cancer appeared to get the most value from ISGs, although the results all came from one site. These equivocal results will benefit from more sophisticated multicenter trials; however, the lack of

negative findings, coupled with the widespread acceptance of ISGs among consumer organizations suggests that this mode of communication should be considered as a part of armamentarium for biomedical informatics research and health information technology tools. Further research in this area includes the use of group videoconferencing and socialization interventions to more closely simulate the face-to-face support groups that have been shown to be effective.

17.3.2.3 Social Networks

The phenomenon of **social networking** has grown rapidly and is a new form of patient-patient communication. Such sites, epitomized by Facebook (www.facebook.com), are online virtual communities where participants describe themselves with member-entered attributes, establish or break connections to other members, communicate, and share information. This simple strategy results in an exponential number of community members sharing one or more attributes, allowing users to connect with people with similar conditions. The for-profit online health-related social networking community Patients Like Me has demonstrated that individuals with a severe chronic disease—amyotrophic lateral sclerosis—are highly willing, even without compensation, to contribute data and observations to a patient community (Frost and Massagli 2008) to accelerate learning about their disease. The site has no ties to the conventional health care system and short-circuits the traditional research enterprise, rewarding participants, not just researchers, with knowledge. The patient outcomes of diverse therapies are collected using crowd sourcing, where patients contribute their information to a common database that can be queried to obtain summaries of an aggregated experience of their peers.

Social networking Web sites share most or all of the features of electronic support groups, and even some data commonly provided through a portal (through creating an affiliation with a group who externalizes public or private information). Social networking platforms combined with personal health records provide a means for social network members to share and aggregate data obtained from the traditional health system,

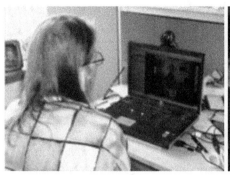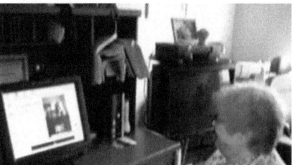

Fig. 17.4 These computer users are part of a cognitive health coaching study where they use their home computers to communicate with their coach, receive feedback from home monitoring data on cognitive exercise, sleep, physical exercise, and socialization. These photos show two study participants communicating with each other from their homes using Skype as part of the socialization protocol (Jimison et al. (2007) with permission)

and to do so in a private manner (Eysenbach 2008; Weitzman et al. 2011a).

One of the features of health-related online social networks is the rapid dissemination of information across a network; however, there is great variability in the quality of discourse on health-related social networking sites. As shown in Fig. 17.4, conversations may be moderated (in this case by a health coach). Conversations also may be unmoderated and commercial influences may enter the discourse without transparency. There are also concerns around privacy. Compared with the restrictive institutional consents and compacts with patients that limit use of data and specimens under federal regulations applicable to much federally sponsored research, online social networks are generally governed by no more than a terms of use statement, often subject to change without notice in 30 days. These privacy policies may be difficult to find and not written in language accessible by a population with a broad range of health literacy (Weitzman et al. 2011b). Industry standards governing safety and privacy of online health-related social networking are yet to emerge.

17.3.3 Patient Access to Health Information

Szolovits' **Guardian Angel Proposal** represents one of the first, if not the first, example of recognizing the role of the patient as a curator of his or her lifetime of health data (Riva et al. 2001). The Guardian Angel "Manifesto" was posted when the Web was only 2 years old at the then readily available 2-letter domain name www.ga.org. The Manifesto presented a comprehensive vision of a Web-based process that would be spawned at a person's birth and care for them through management of health records, decision support, insurance benefits, education and communication. Over the past two decades, this vision has been realized through advances in personal health records.

17.3.3.1 Portals

As the electronic health record gains acceptance, its relevance to individual patients also grows. Many hospitals and clinics have begun providing direct patient access to the clinical record. These **portals** are defined as consumer-facing systems tethered to electronic health records, allowing patient views of clinical or claims data in a single institutional electronic health record system or payer system (Conn and Lubell 2006). Portals provide motivated individuals with a way to electronically access sections of their records to recall salient instructions or obtain results of tests (Markle Foundation 2004). Some of the first such personal health records (PHRs) were Columbia's PatCIS system (Cimino et al. 1998) and Beth Israel Deaconess's PatientSite, developed in 1999 (Weingart et al. 2006). Some of the most widely deployed are Epic's MyChart (which is used

Fig. 17.5 Example screen snapshot from PatCIS, a portal developed at Columbia University. Cimino (1998) (Source: Cimino, J, personal communication, 2011)

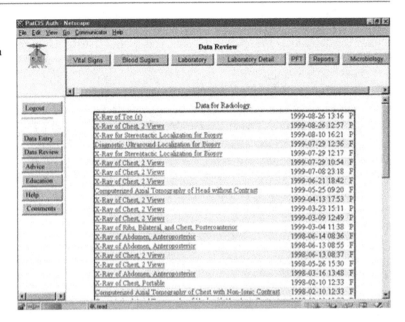

across large HMO's with Epic electronic health record deployments, including Kaiser and Group Health Cooperative) and My HealtheVet (used by over half a million US Veterans (Nazi et al. 2008)). Many of these portals also include functions besides viewing EHR information, such as secure physician-patient messaging, appointment scheduling, and viewing and managing medical bills. Users of the Group Health Cooperative patient portal most frequently viewed test results, requested medication refills, participated in secure messaging with their provider(s), and viewed after-visit summaries (Ralston et al. 2007). The range of functions available in patient portal systems varies widely.

Figure 17.5 shows the PatCIS system developed at Columbia University (Cimino et al. 2002) Critical aspects of security, privacy and accurate identification of patients must be addressed, as well as compliance with government regulations (see Chap. 5). Additionally, designers must take special care to insure that the language used in presenting personal health data enhances the patient's understanding of his or her health concerns. Many of these portals also provide secure messaging systems, allowing patients to communicate concerns about their clinical record to their health care providers. One article comparing four patient portals (Halamka et al. 2008) demonstrated

the challenges and opportunities associated with deploying this technology, noting important issues such as authentication, policies around minors desiring patient portal access to a PHR, decisions about how much of the EHR should be available, and a host of other issues. This article, as well as two by Osborn et al. (2010, 2011) articulates the pervasive way that even simple shifts from a provider-centric to patient-centric view precipitate ripples in the processes and culture of health care.

17.3.3.2 Personal Health Records

The PHR has become the foundation for developing tools to store data and to facilitate its reuse in ways patients find engaging. According to the Markle Foundation, a PHR is "An electronic application through which individuals can access, manage and share their health information, and that of others for whom they are authorized, in a private, secure, and confidential environment"(Markle Foundation 2004).

The idea of a personal repository for medical information is far from new. Families with infants have used an immunization record book for decades. The immunization blue book is a quintessential, efficient system with portable information that supports entry by multiple providers and storage by the patient. Clayton Christensen, who invented the concept of "disruptive innovation," summarizes the widely held promise of this technology in his book, the *Innovator's Prescription: A Disruptive Solution for Health Care* (Christensen et al. 2009). "We cannot overstate how important PHRs are to the efficient functioning of a low-cost, high quality health care system…. We think that the Indivo system [described below], or something like it is a good place to start." PHRs are an inversion of the current approach to medical records in that they are created by, and reside with patients who grant permissions to institutions, clinicians, researchers, public health agencies, and other users of medical information. By contrast, electronic health records store data in thousands of individual silos which later need to be united through some form of health information exchange. PHRs are designed to enable users to acquire copies of their data from every site of care, a capability that will become commonly leveraged under the HHS's **Meaningful Use** certification requiring EHRs to provide an export to patients. In some ways, this model advances information flow far more than models requiring inter-institutional data sharing agreements. Hence, data from two competing health care networks may reside in the same PHR without cumbersome agreements between those two networks. The patient asserts her claim to the data for each network independently. This consumer-driven model of data aggregation may promote data liquidity far more than competing approaches, such as health information exchanges (Adler-Milstein et al. 2008), which require centralized management of data sharing agreements between networks and institutions.

17.3.3.3 Personally-Controlled Health Records

Closely replicating the patient-centered functionality and convenience of the immunization blue book is the **personally controlled health record** (PCHR), a special instance of personal health records (Halamka, et al. 2008; Pagliari et al. 2007). The first instance, called the **Personal Internetworked Notary and Guardian** or PING (Riva, et al. 2001) and was developed in 1998, with funding from the National Library of Medicine (National Institutes of Health) under the **Next Generation Internet Initiative** (National Library of Medicine) and the Advanced Networks programs (National Library of Medicine). PING was later renamed to Indivo (Mandl et al. 2007) in 2006. Figure 17.6 provides an overview of a PCHR architecture.

After diffusion of the PCHR model at two Harvard Medical School invitational conferences,[4] Indivo became the reference model for subsequent PCHRs, including Microsoft's HealthVault, which used Indivo software code, GoogleHealth (now defunct), which implemented the model on its own servers with its own code, and the Dossia consortium of large employers, which contracted with the Indivo creators to create a version for deployment to populations of employees of the consortium founders, including Wal-Mart, AT&T and Intel.

Despite the initial enthusiasm for the PCHR model, uptake of this technology has been gradual, primarily because PCHRs work best when they can readily obtain a copy of data from the EHR. Although many EHRs and other sources of patient data are willing to provide this access to patients, there are numerous barriers to the vision of the PCHR that have, to date, negated this willingness to share data. First and foremost, EHR vendors have been slow to allow data liquidity. Important data may reside in unstructured clinical notes, text blobs, or even scanned images—all formats that compromise liquidity. Data may be structured but may not be sufficiently demarcated to separate the entry into usable pieces. The evolution from a less to more structure prescribing standard in recent years is a good example of this barrier. Data within an EHR may not conform to published standards for interoperability. For example, although the system may share laboratory data, it may not code the data in a standard such as **LOINC**. Therefore, a receiving system may not be able to merge these data with other laboratory data. Finally, data may conform to a content standard, but may use a proprietary form of a messaging standard, making transit difficult.

---

[4] www.pchri2006.org and www.pchri2007.org (accessed 4/23/13).

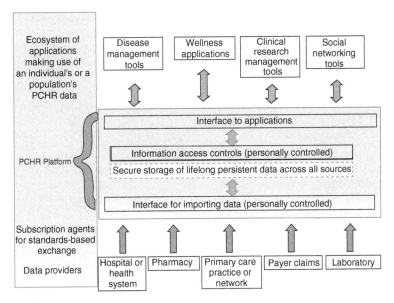

Fig. 17.6 An architecture for a personally controlled health record system. The personally controlled health record (PCHR) has a secure repository of data with subsequent accesses controlled by the patient or her proxy. PCHRs facilitate consumer-driven data aggregation in a manner analogous to a health care version of the financial Quicken product, thus advancing information flow far more than models requiring inter-institutional data-sharing agreements. PCHR users acquire copies of their data across sites of care. Importantly, patients can not only share data with family members and physicisins, but also with ecosystem of apps – modular, self-contained, software applications – that can interact with users and contribute to, analyze, and monitor their personal health data stores

The belief in the importance of an interoperable platform promoting data liquidity has been validated through Project HealthDesign (www.projecthealthdesign.org). The PCHR, similar to how Quicken and MINT.com function for financial data, is a tool enabling a patient to collect copies of her data across sites of care and over time. This functionality is similar to that provided by PHRs. Where PCHRs diverge is the notion of "control" of the data. First, PCHR data can be given attributes based on the semantics of the information content or based on the patient preferences. The patient may, for example, hide specific encounter data, or may allow only a subset of authorized users to see all data in the PCHR. For example, the PCHR model enables the patient to authorize access to individuals including clinical providers, family members, health care proxies, and researchers information (views or even copies of the record) or to intelligent software agents ("apps"). Thus, beyond its properties as a "data sponge", the PCHR is envisioned as a consumer gateway to a rich ecosystem built around data stored in individual health records. Analogous to the iPhone™ and Android™ platforms, PCHRs expose those data, under patient control, to third party apps across an open application programming interface (Mandl and Kohane 2008, 2009). Hence, PCHRs are designed to spawn apps that provide additional functionality without stifling innovation. A platform promoting market competition among apps is intended to address shortcomings of current HIT in terms of user interface and utility (Kim and Johnson 2004). The major PCHR platform providers offer a programming interface that third parties can use to provide "value-added" software-based applications and services such as interpretation of laboratory tests, referrals, and customized medical advice. Employers, governmental and nongovernmental organizations and health centers can create substitutable applications that connect to PCHRs, upon patient approval, through the interface. Healthvault lists scores of such Web apps on its site. The SMART (Substitutable Medical Applications, Reusable

Technologies) Platforms project (www.smart-platforms.org), a part of the Strategic Health IT Advanced Research Projects (SHARP) Program, extends the Indivo PCHR model and seeks to develop a common application programming interface across EHRs and PCHRS that supports the ready creation and use of substitutable applications across the health care system.

17.3.4 Behavior Management

Tools to assist in the achievement of personal health goals have had a long history of development in the consumer sector. Many patients have believed in the concept of health prevention through wellness activities (active lifestyle development, stress reduction, weight control) long before health care professionals endorsed this mode of self-care. However, with the advent of preventive medicine and data supporting the role that wellness activities can play in maintaining health, many of these tenets have become a part of the armamentarium for disease management and are an area of discovery supported by the Agency for Health care Research and Quality (AHRQ) and other Federal institutes.

A complete discussion of foundational models of behavior change is beyond the scope of this chapter, but key works are listed in Table 17.2. Researchers and educators capitalize on these theories in helping to reduce risky behaviors (e.g., cigarette smoking, unprotected sexual intercourse, and unhealthy eating) and to promote desirable health behaviors (i.e., referred to as behavior change.)

Many of the early games targeted at behavior change (described above) attempted to remove the stigma (attitude) associated with engaging in healthy behaviors (such as taking medications to combat a chronic illness.)

Beginning in 2007, the Robert Wood Johnson Foundation, in the Project HealthDesign Initiative (Brennan et al. 2007) catalyzed the development of personal health applications, with the belief that a properly developed common platform would be essential to the spread of intelligent,

Table 17.2 Models of health behavior change

Name and source	Summary
Self-efficacy (Bandura 1977)	An individual's impression of one's own knowledge and skill to perform any task, based on prior success, physical ability, and outside sources of persuasion. Predicts the amount of effort a person will expend to change behavior. It is a key component of other theories, such as the Theory of Planned Behavior.
Social cognitive theory (Bandura 1989)	Behavior change is determined by personal, environmental and behavioral elements, which are interdependent.
Theory of planned behavior (Ajzen 1985)	A link between attitudes and behavior. It asserts that behaviors viewed positively and supported by others (subjective norm) are more likely to have higher levels of motivation and more likely to be performed.
Transtheoretical/ stages of change model (Prochaska 2005)	This model asserts that behavioral change is a 5-step process, between which a person may oscillate before achieving complete change.

interoperable and theoretically-based behavior change tools. This initiative demonstrated many tools that could help consumers with behavior change, as will be discussed later. These demonstrations leveraged the widespread adoption of "smart" phone technology across geographic and socio-economic divides. This widespread adoption, coupled with easy to use software development environments, enables the development of personal health applications that operate as stand-alone or integrated tools available to most consumers.

17.3.5 Consumer Decision-Making

Social trends, coupled with the introduction of managed care and the rapid growth of computer tools, networks, and multimedia, led to both an explosion of need for health care information by the lay public and a dramatic rise in the use of information technology to meet that need. Lay persons need information about health promotion, illness prevention, and disease management. At present, special computer programs, health-focused CD-ROMs, and health-related Internet-based Web sites all provide information likely to be useful to the lay public in participating in health care management and treatment decisions. These applications of medical informatics technologies focus on the patient as the primary user.

We have seen decision tools develop for helping parents know when to take their child to the doctor or start treatment at home, decision tools for helping someone decide to have a screening test, and tools for deciding between surgery or drug therapy. Simpler decision aids are offered in paper form. These consumer health decision aids sometimes take the form of decision trees, where answers to questions lead patients to a recommendation. Many of the newer tools provide dynamic assistance for health behavior change interventions through mobile devices. Other systems, typically offered on the Web, are based on complex decision models that support tailored risk information and utility assessment tools aimed at measuring individual patient preferences for multiple possible health outcomes. O'Connor and colleagues reviewed a variety of patient decision aids (O'Connor et al. 2009), defining these as tools that "prepare people to participate in 'close call' decisions that involve weighing benefits, harms, and scientific uncertainty." In their review of the literature they found that consumer decision aids improve knowledge, reduce decisional conflict (both in relation to feeling uninformed and in regard to personal values), reduce passivity, and reduce indecision. Tools such as Weight Watchers Online[5] represent more reference-based decision aids, while numerous tools, such as Vandemheen's decision aid to help patients with cystic fibrosis consider lung transplantation as an option, use more sophisticated approaches (Vandemheen et al. 2010).

These researchers noted that while the physicians and evidence from the literature provide expertise about the diagnosis and prognosis for a patient with a given condition and with treatment alternatives, it is the patient who must provide values and preferences associated with these possible outcomes. These interactive decision aids provide descriptions and testimonials about future outcomes from the patient perspective (usually video or quotes of patients describing their experiences). Evidence from the literature has shown that these types of decision aids increase consumers' knowledge (O'Connor et al. 2009) and satisfaction with their treatment decision (Whelan et al. 2004); in addition, when patients and physicians use these types of decision tools, the patients are more likely to choose the less invasive treatment.

Currently, consumer health decision aids are offered for the full spectrum from assistance for routine health decisions in the home to intricate sophisticated systems for serious conditions with complex treatment options. Many new health decision aids are still provided in paper-based form, but most are interactive and easily delivered in a Web format. Challenges still remain in integrating these systems into clinical work flow, easily explaining and assessing patient preferences, and in tailoring the risk and probability information and recommended protocols to individual patients.

17.3.6 Consumer Information Access

Patients need quick, private access to accurate information that can calm fears and ensure direct access to currently accepted treatment for their illness. Unfortunately, most existing health care delivery systems are not designed to satisfy these "just-in-time" information requests. Instead of providing this information just in time, it is provided "just in case", typically by a busy clinician as a part of a standardized monolog that covers frequently asked questions. Computer technology can supplement clinicians' teaching with more detailed information that can be referenced repeatedly by a patient in the privacy of his home, and at the time it is most relevant.

---

[5] www.weightwatchers.com (accessed 4/23/13).

17.3.6.1 Passive Information Access

Consumer health informatics resources provide substantive and procedural knowledge about health problems and promising interventions. These information resources may be derived from carefully conducted, theoretically grounded, resource-intensive processes, or they may be extracted from information published for other purposes to save time or money. For this reason, information resources vary in content and sophistication. Some of these resources are little more than digitized brochures, presenting in an electronic form exactly what can be found in available printed materials. Others include interactive or multimedia presentations of information about specific conditions and appropriate actions to prevent, cure, or ameliorate the problem. Multimedia presentations capitalize on the features of computer systems to enrich the presentation of health-related materials with pictures, short movies, and drawings.

Consumer health informatics resources provide patients with condition-specific and disease-specific information about the problems they face. Some resources explain the etiology and natural history of disease in terms comprehensible to lay people. Other resources provide procedural information, explain diagnostic procedures or services, detail expected treatment activities, and provide any relevant warnings and precautions. The presentation of CHI is heavily influenced by the perspective of the system developer. Medically oriented clinical resources demonstrate an emphasis on locally accepted medical practice. Community health-oriented resources are more likely to include information relevant to living in the community with a specific disease or condition.

Consumer health informatics resources originate from two major perspectives: professional and self-help. Professional-developed consumer resources are those developed by health care clinicians and their organizations. Health care organizations—such as HMOs, managed-care companies, and group practices—develop information resources as a service to the patient populations that they treat. These resources tend to complement and extend the clinical services offered by the professional group and may be based on a desire to ensure adherence with accepted therapies or to triage and manage access to care for common health problems. Examples include Kaiser Permanente Health Facts, a program designed to help Kaiser members answer questions about common health problems, and the Mayo Health Advisor, a commercially available CDROM that any interested person can purchase and use to help manage his health at home. Examples of other commercially available programs that have a professional orientation include Health Wise and Health Desk. Figure 17.7 shows an example of professional-developed CHI resources accessible via the Internet.

Consumer health informatics resources developed from a self-help perspective complement and augment those provided by the formal health care delivery system. A self-help perspective is generally more inclusive than a professional perspective. The information may address daily living concerns and lifestyle issues along with, or in place of, content deemed credible by established medical authorities.

Many CHI resources represent a combination of professional and self-help perspectives. Web-based resources, such as those provided by the Fred Hutchinson Cancer Research Center, provide pointers to other Web sites that represent professional or self-help perspectives. Commercial vendors, such as HealthGate Data Corporation, provide access via a Web site to professional-developed and self-help–oriented CHI resources for a subscription or transaction-based fee.

17.3.6.2 Active Information Access

In addition to the passive models that require patients to search for information, there is an increasing number of personal health applications that actively provide information based on specific patient needs. The Project HealthDesign teams developed many demonstrations of active

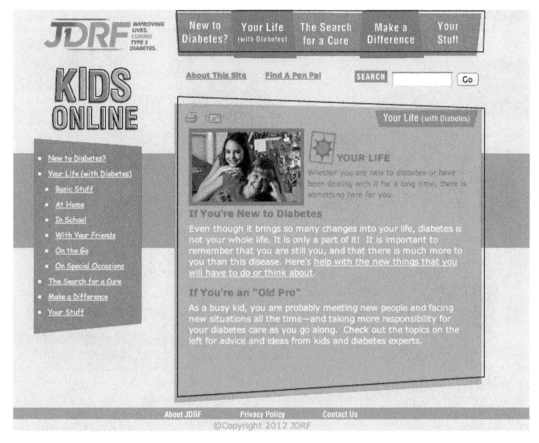

Fig. 17.7 Professionally developed consumer health information. Note the informal language style and easy navigation (*Photo provided courtesy of JDRF* (http://kids.jdrf.org/index.cfm))

access (Brennan, et al. 2007). For example, a team at the University of Rochester developed a "conversational assistant" to provide patients with a daily checkup and information to mitigate exacerbations of their heart disease (Ferguson et al. 2010). Another project, developed by Siek and Ross at the University of Colorado, allowed older adults to manage complex medication regimens at home, using active information access to denote possible side effects, duplicate therapies and special instructions related to dosing (Siek et al. 2011). Jimison and researchers at the Oregon Center for Aging & Technology additionally use monitoring data from sensors in the home to produce automated feedback and intelligent alerts for coaching interventions in the areas of cognitive exercise, physical exercise, sleep management,

socialization, and intelligent medication reminding. Figure 17.8 depicts the variety of sensors available for home care (Pavel et al. 2010; Jimison et al. 2007). With tailored interfaces to a common database, these new approaches enable coaches and informal caregivers to help manage large panels of patients remotely and enable patients and family members to participate as active and informed members of the care team.

Researchers also have begun leveraging text messaging as a medium to provide information actively to patients. For example, in the project MyMediHealth, Johnson and colleagues provide medication reminders to patients in real time using text messaging to their phones. When a dose is missed, MyMediHealth is able to escalate its medication reminder to a parent or other adult

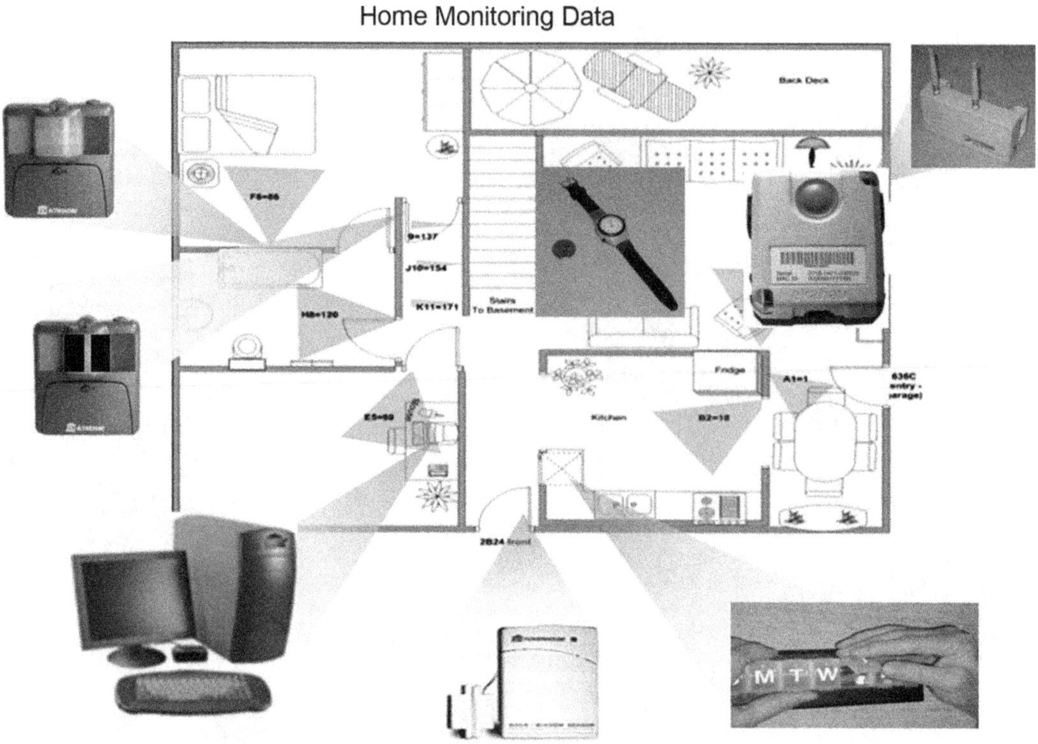

Home Monitoring Data

Fig. 17.8 A variety of sensors in the home can provide feedback for health behavior change coaching systems (motion sensors, pressure mats, contact switches, wireless medication dispensers, etc.). This figure shows a sample apartment layout with sensors for monitoring older adults in the home (Jimison et al. (2007) with permission)

(Slagle et al. 2010). Studies also have demonstrated the utility of appointment or preventive care reminders in reducing clinic no-show rates (Brannan et al. 2011; Leong et al. 2006)

17.4 Opportunities and Challenges

17.4.1 Health Information Technology for Economic and Clinical Health Act of 2009

The **Health Information Technology for Economic and Clinical Health Act of 2009** (HITECH) ("Health Information Technology for Economic and Clinical Health (HITECH) Act, Title XIII of Division A and Title IV of Division B of the American Recovery and Reinvestment Act of 2009 (ARRA).", 2009) may help increase the momentum behind this model. The HITECH Act provides that, for covered entities using or maintaining an EHR, "the individual shall have a right to obtain from such covered entity a copy of such information in an electronic format." By 2013, this feature of EHRs will be required under the final rule for meaningful use of certified electronic health record technology. In preparation for this, early stage efforts have arisen to promote data liquidity through the very well-marketed **Blue Button** initiative from the Department Veterans Affairs (Chopra et al. 2010), and the Direct Project, a federally initiated, health specific implementation of the **SMTP protocol** to enable point-to-point communication of health information in a secure, standards-based (www.directproject.org). Unfortunately these approaches to data liquidity came too late for the Google Health project, which was closed down after not gaining a foothold in the health space. While patients and institutions may have had issues viewing Google as a trusted intermediary to store and manage health data, an at least equally major issue for the service was that even the early adopters, the technophiles who wanted to make this work, experienced challenges populating their PHRs with data.

Hence we can expect that even before 2013 a "tectonic shift in the health information economy" (Mandl and Kohane 2008) will begin, mediated by a change in the locus of control of health information from institutions to individuals. While this shift will be largely driven by a need to improve clinical care processes, it will also have a deep impact on population health research. The ability to reach out to populations directly, thereby disintermediating traditional institutions, will produce very large cohorts of individuals who can share EHR data and provide detailed self-reported information about their care and health states. And patients are willing to share data for aggregate knowledge, research, and public health (Weitzman et al. 2010). A major area of focus for research and policy needs to be development of a properly aligned compact with patients to share data for research and public health by engaging them on their own terms; the PCHR is a technology designed to do just that.

As CHI and telehealth evolve from being research novelties, to being the way health care is delivered, many challenges must be overcome. Some of these challenges arise because the one patient, one doctor model no longer applies. Basic questions of identity and trust become paramount. At the same time, the shifting focus from treating illness to managing health and wellness requires that clinicians know not only the history of the individuals they treat but also information about the social and environmental context within which those individuals reside.

17.4.2 Information Credentialing

The amount of information available to consumers is growing rapidly. This volume of information can be overwhelming. Therefore, consumers may need help in sifting through the mass of available

resources. Furthermore, the quality of such information varies widely not only in terms of the extent to which it is accepted by the formal medical community but also in its basic clinical or scientific accuracy. Therefore, a key issue in CHI lies in determining the quality and relevance of health information found on Web sites. Credentialing or certification by recognized bodies, such as respected health care providers or clinical professional associations, represents one approach to ensuring the quality of health information available to consumers. This approach differs from the HON approach (see Sect. 17.2.3) in that it bases its quality ratings on reviews and evaluations conducted by established knowledgeable sources. It has the advantage of delivering an imprimatur to a Web site, which informs the user that the information presented meets a standard of quality. Credentialing is most useful when the credential itself is accompanied by a statement indicating the perspectives and biases of those granting it. Information presented by alternative therapies and other non-clinical groups is no less susceptible to bias than is information presented by professional sources.

Inherent in the credentialing approach are three disadvantages. First, the challenge to ensure that every information element—every link in a decision program or pathway in a Web site—is tested exceeds the resources available to do so. In many cases, the credentialing approach rests on certification of the group or individuals providing the information rather than approval of the content itself. Second, the credentialing approach leaves control of the authority for health care information in the hands of traditional care providers, reflecting both the expertise and the biases of established medical sources. Third, credentialing alone is inherently contradictory to healthcare consumerism, which empowers the consumer to make choices consistent with her own worldview. A source's credential is just an additional piece of information that may be considered in making personal health decisions.

An approach to evaluating the quality and relevance of CHI resources that is consistent with a philosophy of patient participation is based on teaching patients and lay people how to evaluate CHI resources. Consumers with sufficient literacy and evaluation skills can locate CHI resources and determine these resources' relevance to their individual health concerns.

17.4.3 Privacy and Security

Because of the public, shared nature of the Internet, its resources are widely accessible by citizens and health care organizations. This public nature also presents challenges to the security of data transmitted along the Internet. The openness of the Internet leaves the transmitted data vulnerable to interception and inappropriate access. In spite of significant improvements in the security of Web browsing several areas, including protection against viruses, authentication of individuals and the security of email, remain problematic.

One of the most important challenges and responsibilities associated with the new developments in interactive health systems for patients is ensuring the privacy and security of health information in a way that protects the security of the data and truly incorporates patient preferences for data sharing. Consumer health Web sites often offer users the capability of entering personal data in order to obtain tailored feedback. This ranges from calculators of body mass index to ongoing weight management or smoking cessation programs. These Web sites typically display their privacy practices. Consumers also can look for certificates of accreditation from organizations such as URAC,[6] TRUSTe[7] and HON.[8] These accreditation groups each have a set of policies to protect consumers' privacy and certify that processes that encourage high quality accurate information is presented. Given that the privacy policies for consumer health Web sites are often quite long and complicated; this approach allows consumers to feel confident that the site follows best practices. Privacy policies are also posted for search engines – the most common tool that consumers use for finding health information. Companies associated with the search engines have the capability to infer a good deal about the health status of the user or the user's family from the search terms used and from the sites visited. However, users very rarely investigate the privacy policies and also rarely understand the implications of how data about them might be used.

More complicated privacy situations arise with the new technologies for home monitoring. Data is collected in the home and then typically encrypted and transferred to a secure server in another location. A wide variety of data may be collected (blood pressures, blood glucose, activity, location, sleep quality, etc.) and then potentially shared with a variety of care team members (care manager, clinical, specialist, family caregiver, etc.). Not all care team members should necessarily have the same access to data. Role-based access representations are beginning to be used to make it easier and more meaningful for patients to indicate their preferences on who (if anyone) should see what data about them.

There has recently been a dramatic upsurge in the use of mobile applications for consumer health monitoring and data sharing. However, the privacy and security techniques for this area are still lagging behind the development and use of the systems. In 2010 there was a 250 % jump in mobile phone viruses and spyware, and 61 % of the reported smartphone infections were spyware that could monitor communication from the device (Bela and Hamel 2010). Health care systems are working rapidly to address the privacy and security issues as technology and consumers' way of using it change.

17.4.4 Technology Digital Divide

Ensuring every citizen access to the Internet represents a second important challenge to the ability to use it for public health and consumer health purposes. Access to the Internet presently requires computer equipment that may be out of reach for persons with marginal income levels.

---

[6] www.urac.org (accessed 4/23/13).

[7] www.truste.com (accessed 4/23/13).

[8] www.hon.ch (accessed 4/23/13).

The digital divide with respect to access to computer-based health care information occurs for many reasons, including economic disparity, unequal broadband access in various geographical locations, and cultural issues. Majority-language literacy and the physical capability to type and read present additional requirements for effective use of the Internet. Preventing unequal access to health care resources delivered via the Internet will require that health care agencies work with other social service and educational groups to make available the technology necessary to capitalize on this electronic environment for health care.

17.4.5 Workflow Integration

Systems that are designed to facilitate shared decision making with a physician are difficult to integrate into routine clinical workflow. This integration requires overcoming two main challenges. First, many care providers are reluctant to review patient-generated information until it is a reimbursable activity. Therefore, the preferred workflow is to have these data brought in by the patient for review at the time of a patient encounter. This approach may be helpful for many medical conditions, but is potentially less efficient for the patient who may be able to improve health outcomes sooner by more timely professional review of data.

The second challenge relates to the health information technology used by clinicians. Ideally, data that are created by patients should be easily imported into the physician's repository and provided as a view alongside clinician-generated data. However this model has yet to be standardized. This model would be a requirement to achieve clinician buy-in with timely data review, and is very important even for the visit-based data review if decisions are made based on these data.

Additionally, it has been difficult to reliably and meaningfully explain outcomes and probabilities to patients in a way that helps them weigh risks and benefits of complex scenarios. Finally, much more work needs to be done to improve the process of assessing patient preferences (utilities on outcomes) and communicating this to the clinician. These issues are all critical for improving health care decision-making.

17.5 Future Directions

The advances in consumer health informatics over the past 20 years have been made under assumptions about the availability of home computing power, the general willingness of patients to communicate, and the ways in which data informs knowledge. The future of the field is most likely to be shaped by disruptions in each of these assumptions.

17.5.1 Home Computing Power

In 1988, inspired by discussions with social scientists, philosophers, anthropologists, and computer scientists, Mark Weiser, then at Xerox PARC asserted that a "third wave" of computing would transform society. The first wave, mainframe computers, allowed many people to access one computer. This wave was complemented by the personal computer wave that supported one person on one computer. The third wave, "ubiquitous computing" further complemented the first and second waves by allowing one person to have many computers. This era will usher in "calm technology," where technology becomes embedded into all aspects of our life and allows us to focus on the task, not the tool. Examples of this technology have been incorporated into the plots of science fiction movies for years.

The average person now uses dozens of computer-enabled devices, ranging from smartphones and cars to coffee-makers, digital thermometers, HDTVs, and thermostats. The availability of computers, coupled with the power of the technology, will be leveraged by consumer health informatics researchers. Already, programs such as Robert Wood Johnson's Project HealthDesign[9] have demonstrated how home

---

[9] www.projecthealthdesign.org (accessed 4/23/13).

biosensors, mobile computing platforms, and other innovations can transform personal health applications.

As computer power increases and the integration of computer technology into everyday life becomes more commonplace, we anticipate that health information will follow suit. Why doesn't a pill container send data directly to a personal health record when opened? Why doesn't that pill container use wifi, speech recognition, and publically available and appropriately tagged data to answer consumer questions about side effects or special instructions? Why can't a need to refill that medication be transmitted to a schedule automatically, or included as a reminder when a car starts? It is likely that Federal groups such as the US Army's Telemedicine and Advanced Technology Resource Center (TATRC) or the National Science Foundation will lead the way toward this level of interoperability and seamless information dissemination to consumers. As data liquidity is increased, influential consumer health technologies will flourish. In the mean time, efforts such as Google Health™ stumble waiting for data from the health system to enter the hands of consumers. In fact, it is clear that Google Health and personal data repositories may follow the path of other notable technologies, such as personal digital assistants or the Apple Newton MessagePad™, which emerged before supporting technologies or market awareness was there to sustain them. In the case of personal health data repositories, the key driver may be these personal health applications integrated into daily life.

17.5.2 Patient Communication

It is estimated that 83 % of U.S. adults have a cell phone of some kind, and that 42 % of them own a smartphone (Smith 2011). In addition to cellular technology, social networking adoption has exploded in the past decade. The widespread use of these technologies affirms the belief that patients are more willing than ever to communicate about their health issues. In study after study about the tradeoff between communication and privacy, it has become clear that we value communication and hope that there is privacy through anonymity.

One example of patient willingness to communicate about health is the success of tools like researchmatch.org[10] developed by Harris and colleagues. This tool allows patients to voluntarily create a profile that is then used to alert them to studies in which they might be able to participate. Patients using this system trust that the security in place is sufficient and that any risk of a security breach is offset by the potential personal or societal gains associated with patient research.

We can expect various tools to leverage patient's willingness to communicate. For example, social networks might be used to connect a person with a home health need to a person who is willing to help. Online forums or classified advertisements that already connect patients to patients for physician referrals or durable equipment sales could do more to help patients find information or other commodities.

17.5.3 Data Informing Knowledge

One of the most exciting, though potentially alarming consequences of our extensive use of the Web for shopping, communicating, and learning is that each of us leaves behind a profile of who we are, what we like or dislike, what we know or don't know, and what we want or already have. When combined with data mining and natural language processing techniques, it is possible to create highly targeted and predictive personal knowledge. It is this ability that search engines exploit to create a profile of each searcher and to improve the relevance of retrieved results. This technology also is likely to improve the ways in which consumers and consumer-facing technologies operate. We can expect the use of these massive data sets (also called "big data") to impact how medical care is personalized. Data created by consumers, coupled with ubiquitous computing, might provide just–in–time nutritional consults, over the counter medication

---

[10] www.researchmatch.org (accessed 4/23/13).

advice, or advice that might prevent illnesses, such as convenient locations to receive a flu vaccine or when to begin medications for seasonal allergies.

While the direction that consumer health informatics will take in the future is at best, educated speculation, it is clear that as long as patient-provider partnerships are endorsed, technology will be a third partner in ensuring that activated consumers manage their health and disease effectively.

Suggested Readings

The 1994 Guardian Angel Manifesto. www.ga.org. This site describes a collaborative project begun in 1994 to "put power and responsibility for health care more into the hands of patients." It also provides a comprehensive set of references to many other personal health record projects.

Susanna Fox's blogs and reports. http://www.pewinternet.org/Experts/Susannah-Fox.aspx. This site provides a collection of presentations from form Pew Internet and American Life Project, which studies the technology-related cultural shifts in health care.

Mandl, K. D., & Kohane, I. S. (2008). The architecture of Personally Controlled Health Records. Tectonic shifts in the health information economy. *New England Journal of Medicine, 358*(16), 1732–1737. This is a recent review of the transformation taking place in health care as a result of widespread introduction of personally controlled health records.

Questions for Discussion

1. What is the role of the health system in monitoring the quality of discourse on online social networks?
2. What is the optimal model for personal health records? Should personal health records display advertisements?
3. Which populations of consumers would be most likely to use personal health records?
4. Which consumer technologies do you think will be most influential in consumer-focused health informatics?
5. What is the right balance between privacy of personal health information and ready access to it? For example for an unconscious patient in the emergency department?

Telehealth

18

Justin B. Starren, Thomas S. Nesbitt,
and Michael F. Chiang

After reading this chapter you should know the answers to these questions:

- What are the key informatics requirements for successful implementation of telehealth systems?
- What are some key benefits from and barriers to implementation of telehealth systems?
- What are the most promising application domains for telehealth?

18.1 Introduction

Complexity and collaboration characterize health care in the early twenty-first century. Complexity arises from increasing sophistication in the understanding of health and disease, wherein etiological models must take into account both molecular processes and physical environments. Collaboration reflects not only inter-professional collaboration, but also a realization that successful attainment of optimal well-being and effective management of disease processes necessitate active engagement of clinicians, lay persons, concerned family members, and society as a whole. This chapter introduces the concepts of **telemedicine** and **telehealth**, and illustrates how maturing computer networks like the Internet make possible the collaborations necessary to achieve the full benefits of our growing understanding of health promotion, disease management and disability prevention. Consider the following situation:

Samuel is a 76 year-old man with coronary artery disease, poorly-controlled Type II diabetes, and high blood pressure. In the past, he has been unable to keep medical appointments consistently because of difficulty arranging transportation. He had a recent acute hyperglycemic episode that required hospitalization. After 4 days he is medically stable and ready for discharge. He is able to measure his blood glucose and can safely administer the appropriate dose of insulin. The nurse notes that Samuel sometimes has trouble calibrating his insulin dose to the blood glucose reading.

J.B. Starren, MD, PhD (✉)
Division of Health and Biomedical Informatics,
Department of Preventive Medicine and Medical
Social Sciences, Northwestern University Feinberg
School of Medicine, 750 N. Lake Shore Dr.,
Chicago, IL 60611, USA
e-mail: justin.starren@northwestern.edu

T.S. Nesbitt, MD, MPH
Department of Family and Community Medicine,
School of Medicine, UC Davis Health System, 4610
X Street, Suite 3101m, Sacramento, CA 95817, USA
e-mail: thomasnesbitt@ucdmc.ucdavis.edu

M.F. Chiang, MD, MA
Department of Ophthalmology & Medical
Informatics and Clinical Epidemiology, Oregon
Health & Science University, 3375 SW Terwilliger
Boulevard, Portland, OR 97239, USA
e-mail: chiangm@ohsu.edu

This chapter is adapted from an earlier version in the third edition authored by Patricia Flatley Brennan and Justin B. Starren.

E.H. Shortliffe, J.J. Cimino (eds.), *Biomedical Informatics*,
DOI 10.1007/978-1-4471-4474-8_18, © Springer-Verlag London 2014

18.1.1 Telemedicine and Telehealth to Reduce the Distance Between the Consumer and the Health care System

Historically, health care has usually involved travel. Either the health care provider traveled to visit the patient, or more recently, the patient traveled to visit the provider. Patients with diabetes, like Samuel, typically meet with their physician every 2–6 months to review data and plan therapy changes. Travel has costs, both directly, in terms of gasoline or transportation tickets, and indirectly, in terms of travel time, delayed treatment, and lost productivity. In fact, travel has accounted for a significant proportion of the total cost of health care (Starr 1982). Because of this, both patients and providers have been quick to recognize that rapid electronic communications have the potential to improve care by reducing the costs and delays associated with travel. This has involved both access to information resources, as well as direct communication among various participants, including patients, family members, primary care providers and specialists.

As is the case with informatics, the formal definitions of telemedicine and telehealth tend to be very broad. **Telemedicine** involves the use of modern information technology, especially two-way interactive audio/video communications, computers and telemetry to deliver health services to remote patients and to facilitate information exchange between primary care physicians and specialists at some distance from each other (Bashshur 1997). **Telehealth** is a somewhat newer and broader term referring to remote health care that includes clinical services provided using telemedicine, as well as interactions with automated systems or information resources. Because of its broader scope, we are using the term telehealth in this chapter.

As is the case with Biomedical informatics, there are many different sub-domains within telehealth. For nearly every clinical domain, there is a "tele-X" or "X telehealth", where X is the clinical domain. Examples include: **Teleradiology** (see Sect. 18.3.4.1); **Teleophthalmology** (see Sect. 18.3.4.2); **Telepsychiatry** (see Sect. 18.3.5.1);

and, **telehealth** (see Sect. 18.3.5.3). Some sub-domains do not fit neatly into this naming paradigm. **Correctional Telehealth** (see Sect. 18.3.5.2) refers to the location of the patient in a correctional institution. It is discussed separately because of the different business model, and the fact that it represents an early and sustained success. **Remote Intensive Care** (see Sect. 18.3.5.5) is the term used to describe the use of telehealth technologies in an ICU setting. **Teleconsultation** is a general term describing the use of telehealth technologies to support discussions between clinicians, or between a clinician and a patient. The archetypal teleconsultation occurs when the patient and the generalist clinician are in a rural or remote location and a specialist is at a distant tertiary referral facility. **Telepresence** (see Sect. 18.3.6) refers to high-speed, multi-modality telehealth interactions, such as **Telesurgery**, that gives the feeling of "being there".

It is clear from the definition above that there is considerable overlap between telehealth and Biomedical informatics. In fact, one will frequently find papers on telehealth systems presented at Biomedical Informatics conferences and presentations on informatics at telehealth and telemedicine meetings. Some groups, especially in Europe, have adopted the rubric **health information and communication technology** (HICT). The major distinction is one of emphasis. Telehealth and telemedicine emphasize the distance, especially the provision of care to remote or isolated patients and communities. In contrast, Biomedical Informatics emphasizes methods for handling the information, irrespective of the distance between patient and provider.

Consumer health informatics (CHI) is a related domain that bridges the distance between patients and health care resources, and that typically emphasizes interactions with computer-based information such as websites or information resources. Collectively, CHI and telehealth deliver health care knowledge and expertise to where they are needed, and are ways to involve the patient as an active partner in care. Despite their similarities, CHI and telehealth come from very different historical foundations. Telehealth derived from traditional patient care, while CHI derived from the self-help movements of the 1970's. Largely owing to this historical separation, practitioners and researchers in the two fields tend to come from different backgrounds. For these reasons, we are presenting CHI and telehealth as two distinct, but closely related domains (see Chap. 17 for more on CHI).

18.2 Historical Perspectives

The use of communication technology to convey health-related information at a distance is nothing new. The earliest known example may be the use of so-called "leper bells" carried by individuals during Roman times. Sailing ships would fly a yellow flag to indicate a ship was under quarantine and awaiting clearance by a doctor, or a yellow and black "plague flag" to indicate that infected individuals were on board. By some accounts, when Alexander Graham Bell said "Mr. Watson. Come here. I need you" in 1876, it was because he had spilled acid on his hand and needed medical assistance. In 1879, only 3 years later, the first description of telephone use for clinical diagnosis appeared in a medical journal (Practice by Telephone 1879).

18.2.1 Early Experiences

One of the earliest and most long-lived telehealth projects is the Australian Royal Flying Doctor Service (RFDS), founded in 1928. In addition to providing air ambulance services, the RFDS provides telehealth consultations. These consultations first used Morse Code, and later voice, radio communications to the remote sheep stations in the Australian outback. Lay people played a significant role here, clearly communicating their concerns and clinical findings to the RFDS and carefully carrying out instructions while awaiting, if necessary, the arrival of the physician. The RFDS is most famous for its standardized medical chest, introduced in 1942. The chest contains diagnostic charts and medications, identified only by number. This allowed the consulting clinician to localize symptoms by number and then prescribe care, such as "take one number five and two number fours."

Modern telehealth can be traced to 1948 when the first transmission of a radiograph over a phone line was reported. Video-based telehealth can be traced to 1955 when the Nebraska Psychiatric Institute began experimenting with a closed-curcuit video network on its campus. In 1964 this was extended to a remote state mental health facility to support education and **teleconsultation**. In 1967, Massachusetts General Hospital (MGH) was linked to Logan International Airport via a microwave audio-video link (Bird 1972; Murphy et al. 1973). In 1971 the National Library of Medicine began the Alaska Satellite Biomedical Demonstration project linking 26 remote Alaskan villages utilizing NASA satellites (Hudson and Parker 1973)

The period from the mid 1970's to the late 1980's was a time of much experimentation, but few fundamental changes in telehealth. A variety of pilot projects demonstrated the feasibility and utility of video-based telehealth. The military funded a number of research projects aimed at developing tools for providing telehealth care on the battlefield. The early 1990's saw several important advances. Military applications developed during the previous decades began to be deployed. Military **teleradiology** was first deployed in 1991 during Operation Desert Storm. Telehealth in military field hospitals was first deployed in 1993 in Bosnia. Several states, including Georgia, Kansas, North Carolina and Iowa implemented statewide telehealth networks. Some of these were pure video networks, based on broadcast television technology. Others were built using evolving Internet technology. During this same period, correctional telehealth (see Sect. 18.3.5.2) became much more common. For example, in 1992 East Carolina University contracted with the largest maximum-security prison in North Carolina to provide telehealth consultation.

Telehealth projects in the early 1990s continued to be plagued by two problems that had hampered telehealth since its inception: high cost and poor image quality. Both hardware and **high-bandwidth** connections were prohibitively expensive. A single telehealth station typically cost over $50,000 and connectivity could cost thousands of dollars per month. Most programs were dependent on external grant funding for survival. Even with this, image resolution was frequently poor and **motion artifacts** were severe.

The Internet revolution that began in the late 1990s drove fundamental change in telehealth. Advances in computing power both improved image quality and reduced hardware costs to the point that, by 2000, comparable systems cost less than a tenth of what they had a decade earlier. Improvements in **image compression** made it possible to transmit low-resolution, full-motion video over standard telephone lines, enabling the growth of telehome care. With the increasing popularity of the World Wide Web, high-bandwidth connections became both more available and less expensive. Many telehealth applications that had relied on expensive, dedicated, point-to-point connections were converted to utilize commodity Internet connections. The availability of affordable hardware and connectivity also made access to health-related electronic resources from the home, school or work place possible and fueled the growth of consumer health information (see Chap. 17).

18.2.2 Recent Advances in Medical-Grade Broadband Technology

As telemedicine applications are being increasingly used in critical medical situations such as emergency care and remote surgery applications, quality of service (QOS) becomes extremely important. It is important to note that optimally provisioning a network for medical-grade QOS does not simply imply that the network will provide "quality" in the sense of reliability, consistency and bandwidth performance, although these characteristic are certainly important requirements. Any network, no matter the bandwidth available, can become congested – overwhelmed with the volume of traffic to the extent that sessions are interrupted and data lost. Bandwidth availability limitations are particularly prevalent in rural locations where high-capacity circuits may be unavailable or prohibitively expensive.

Newer network routing technologies such as **multiprotocol label switching** (MPLS) can, in addition to providing superior network throughput performance, permit explicit prioritization of clinical traffic while simultaneously providing access to lower priority administrative and other nonclinical traffic. The individual data packets of high priority traffic (e.g., telehealth or patient monitoring sessions) are "tagged" with a numerical priority flag. As the QOS-tagged packets traverse the network, each routing/switching device recognizes the priority tag and preferentially processes and forwards the packets. This explicit QOS combined with advanced security and privacy features within a broadband network has been characterized as "Medical Grade" broadband.

18.3 Bridging Distance with Informatics: Real-world Systems

There are many ways to categorize telehealth resources, including classifications based on participants, bandwidth, information transmitted, medical specialty, immediacy, health care condition, and financial reimbursement. The categorization in Table 18.1 is based loosely on bandwidth and overall complexity. This categorization was chosen because each category presents different challenges for informatics researchers and practitioners.

A second categorization of telehealth systems that overlaps the previous one is the separation into synchronous (or real-time) and asynchronous (or **store-and-forward** systems). Video conferencing is the archetypal synchronous telehealth application. Synchronous telehealth encounters are analogous to conventional office visits. Telephony, chat-groups, and **telepresence** (see Sect. 18.3.6) are also examples of synchronous telehealth. A major challenge in all synchronous telehealth is scheduling. All participants must be at the necessary equipment at the same time.

Store-and-forward, as the name implies, involves the preparation of a dataset at one site that is sent asynchronously to a remote recipient. Remote interpretation, especially teleradiology, is

Table 18.1 Categories of telehealth and consumer health informatics

Telehealth category	Bandwidth	Applications
Information resources	Low to moderate	Web-based information resources, patient access to electronic medical records
Messaging	Low	E-mail, chat groups, consumer health networks, personal clinical electronic communications (PCEC)
Telephone	Low	Scheduling, triage
Remote monitoring	Low to moderate	Remote monitoring of pacemakers, diabetes, asthma, hypertension, Congestive Health Failure (CHF).
Remote interpretation	Moderate	PACS, remote interpretation of radiographic studies and other images, such as dermatologic and retinal photographs.
Videoconferencing	Low to high	Wide range of applications, from low-bandwidth telehome care over telephone lines, to high-bandwidth telementoring and telepsychiatry
Telepresence	High	Remote surgery, telerobotics

the archetypal example of store-and-forward telehealth. Images are obtained at one site and then sent, sometimes over very low bandwidth connections, to another site where the domain expert interprets them. Other examples of store-and-forward include access to Web sites, e-mail and text messaging. Some store-and-forward systems support the creation of multimedia "cases" that contain multiple clinical data types, including text, scanned images, wave forms and videos.

18.3.1 The Forgotten Telephone

Until recently, the telephone was a forgotten component in teleheath. The field of telemedicine and telehealth focused on video and largely ignored the audio-only telehealth. Few studies were done and few articles written. This is paradoxical given that up to 25 % of all primary care encounters occur via the telephone. These include triage, case management, results review, consultation, medication adjustment and logistical issues, like scheduling. In part, this can be traced to the fact that telephone consultations are not reimbursed by most insurance carriers.

More recently, increased interest in cost control through case management has driven renewed interest in use of audio-only communication between patients and providers. Multiple articles have appeared on the value of telephone follow-up for chronic conditions. Several managed care companies have set up large telephone triage centers. The National Health Service in the UK is

investing £123 million per year in NHS Direct, a nation wide telephone information and triage system that handles 27,000 calls per day. With some insurance providers reimbursing for e-mails and text messaging, providers are asking why not reimburse for telephone calls also.

18.3.2 Electronic Messaging

Electronic text-based messaging has emerged as a popular mode of communication between patients and providers. It began with patients sending conventional e-mails to physicians. The popularity of this grew so rapidly that national guidelines were developed (Kane and Sands 1998). However, e-mail has a number of disadvantages for health related messaging: delivery is not guaranteed; security is problematic; e-mail is transient (there was no automatic logging or audit trail); and the messages are completely unstructured.

To address these limitations, a variety of Web-based messaging solutions, called **personal clinical electronic communications**, have been developed (Sarkar and Starren 2002). Because the messages never leave the Web site, many of the problems associated with conventional e-mail are avoided. Web-based messaging is a standard feature of **patient portals** see Chap. 17) associated with many EHRs. The inclusion of messaging as a Meaningful Use requirement for Certified EHRs is expected to significantly increase the use of web-based messaging to provide telehealth (Fig. 18.1).

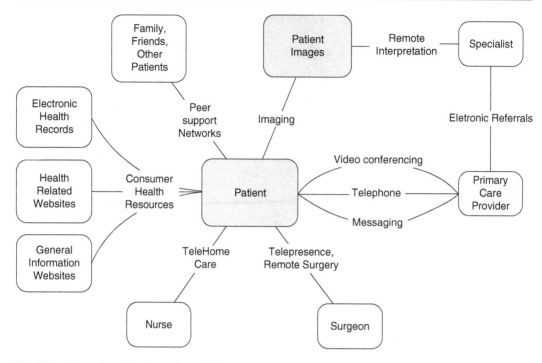

Fig. 18.1 Connections. The figure shows different ways that electronic communications can be used to link patients with various health resources. Only connections directly involving the patient are shown (e.g., use of the EHR by the clinician is not shown). Some of the resources, such as Web sites or telehome care, can be accessed from the patient's home. Other resources, such as remote surgery or imaging, would require the patient to go to a telehealth-equipped clinical facility

18.3.3   Remote Monitoring

Remote monitoring is a subset of telehealth focusing on the capture of clinically relevant data in the patients' homes or other locations outside of conventional hospitals, clinics or health care provider offices, and the subsequent transmission of the data to central locations for review. The conceptual model underlying nearly all remote monitoring is that clinically significant changes in patient condition occur between regularly scheduled visits and that these changes can be detected by measuring physiologic parameters.

The care model presumes that, if these changes are detected and treated sooner, the overall condition of the patient will be improved. An important distinction between remote monitoring and many conventional forms of telemedicine is that remote monitoring focuses on management, rather than on diagnosis. Typically, remote monitoring involves patients who have already been diagnosed with a chronic disease or condition.

Remote monitoring is used to track parameters that guide management. Any measurable parameter is a candidate for remote monitoring. The collected data may include continuous data streams or, more commonly, discrete measurements.

Another important feature of most remote monitoring is that the measurement of the parameter and the transmission of the data are typically separate events. The measurement devices have a memory that can store multiple measurements. The patient will send the data to the caregiver in one of several ways. For many studies, the patient will log onto a server at the central site (either over the Web or by direct dial-up) and then type in the data. Alternately, the patient may connect the measurement device to a personal computer or specialized modem and transfer the readings electronically.

More recently, a variety of monitoring devices have been developed that either connect directly to mobile telephones or transmit the data to the mobile phone using Bluetooth wireless. The mobile phone then transmits the data to a provider for review. A major advantage of direct electronic transfer is that it eliminates problems stemming from manual entry, including falsification, number preference and transcription errors. The role of mobile telephones in providing health services has grown so rapidly that a new term **mobile health** (or "mHealth") has been coined. The term appeared first, one time, in 2004 in PubMed. All of the other mentions have been since 2009.

Any condition that is evaluated by measuring a physiologic parameter is a candidate for remote monitoring. The parameter most measured in the remote setting is blood glucose for monitoring diabetes. A wide variety of research projects and commercial systems have been developed to monitor patients with diabetes. Patients with asthma can be monitored with peak-flow or full-loop **spirometers**. Patients with hypertension can be monitored with automated blood pressure cuffs. Patients with congestive heart failure (CHF) are monitored by measuring daily weights to detect fluid gain. Remote monitoring of pacemaker function has been available for a number of years and has recently been approved for reimbursement. Home coagulation meters have been developed that allows the monitoring of patients on chronic anticoagulation therapy. See Chap. 19 for more on patient monitoring systems.

Several factors limit the widespread use of remote monitoring. First is the question of efficacy. While these systems have proven acceptable to patients and beneficial in small studies, few large-scale controlled trials have been done. Second is the basic question of who will review the data. Research studies have utilized specially trained nurses at centralized offices but it is not clear that this will scale up. Third is money—for most conditions, remote monitoring is still not a reimbursed activity.

18.3.4 Remote Interpretation

Although Samuel was diagnosed with Type II diabetes over 20 years ago and realizes that visual loss can be a serious complication, he has only rarely received dilated eye exams for retinopathy screening. There is no eye doctor conveniently located near his home, and he feels that the appointments are always too long and that he has no problems such as blurred vision. However, his primary care doctor has recently implemented a new retinal screening machine in the office. During a routine medical examination, Samuel receives a retinal photograph from an office technician that is then interpreted by a remote ophthalmologist. Samuel is told that he has high-risk diabetic retinopathy that requires treatment to prevent visual loss. He is emergently referred to an ophthalmologist, who performs a successful laser procedure to treat the diabetic retinopathy.

Remote interpretation is a category of store-and-forward telehealth that involves the capture of images, or other data, at one site and their transmission to another site for interpretation. This may include radiographs (*teleradiology*), photographs (*teledermatology, teleophthalmology, telepathology*), wave forms such as ECGs (e.g. *telecardiology*), and text-based medical data.

The store-and-forward telehealth modalities have benefited most from the development of the **commodity Internet** and the increasing availability of affordable high bandwidth connections that is provides. The shared commodity Internet provides relatively high bandwidth, but the available bandwidth is continuously varying. This makes it much better suited for the transfer of text-based data and image files, rather than for streaming data or video connections. Although image files are often tens or hundreds of megabytes in size, the files are typically transferred to the interpretation site and cached there for later interpretation. From a logistical perspective, multiple remote interpretations may be batched and performed together, thereby providing important workflow and convenience advantages over traditional medical examinations or real-time video telehealth paradigms.

18.3.4.1 Teleradiology

By far, teleradiology is the largest category of remote interpretation, and probably the largest category of telehealth. Teleradiololgy (along with telepathology) represents the most mature clinical domain in telehealth. With the deployment of **picture archiving and communications systems** (PACS) that capture, store, transmit and displays digital radiology images, the line between teleradiology and conventional radiology is blurring. In fact, routine medical care in radiology and pathology is increasingly being delivered primarily through "telehealth" strategies (Radiology image management is discussed in more detail in Chap. 20).

Many factors have contributed to the more rapid adoption of telehealth in domains such as radiology and pathology. One important factor is the relationship between these specialists and their patients. In both domains, the professional role is often limited to the interpretation of images, and the specialist rarely interacts directly with the patient. To patients, there is therefore little perceived difference between a radiologist in the next building and one in the next state.

An important factor driving the growth of teleradiology is that it is reimbursable by insurance payers. Because image interpretation does not involve direct patient contact, few payers make any distinction about where the interpretation occurred. Rapid dissemination of teleradiology systems has also been supported by widespread adoption of vendor-neutral image storage and transmission standards such as **Digital Imaging and Communication in Medicine** (DICOM; discussed in more detail in Chaps. 7 and 20). Finally, numerous evaluation studies have demonstrated that digital image interpretation by through teleradiology has comparable, or potentially even better, accuracy and efficiency compared to traditional film-based radiological examination (Franken et al. 1992; Reiner et al. 2002; Mackinnon et al. 2008).

18.3.4.2 Teleophthalmology

Another area of remote interpretation that is growing rapidly is teleophthalmology, particularly for retinal disease screening. As one example, diabetic retinopathy (retinal disease) is a leading cause of blindness that can be treated if detected early. However, it has been found that nearly 50 % of diabetics are non-compliant with guidelines recommending annual screening eye examinations (Brechner et al. 1993). Systems have been developed that allow nurses or technicians in primary care offices to obtain high quality digital retinal photographs. These images are sent to regional centers for interpretation. If diabetic retinopathy is identified or suspected, the patient is referred for full ophthalmologic examination.

Large-scale operational systems have been implemented by the Veterans Health Administration and by other institutions, particularly in areas with limited accessibility to eye care specialists (Cavalleranno et al. 2005; Cuadros and Bresnick 2009). In fact, remote interpretation of retinal images by certified reading centers, when taken after dilation of the eyes using standard photographic protocols originally developed for clinical research trials, has been demonstrated to classify diabetic retinopathy more accurately than traditional dilated eye examination. This is likely because retinal abnormalities found on photographs may be reviewed in more detail than what is generally feasible during traditional eye examinations.

As another example of teleophthalmology, retinopathy of prematurity (ROP) is a leading cause of blindness in premature infants, and hospitalized infants are examined regularly to identify treatment-requiring disease. However, these examinations are logistically difficult and time consuming, and the number of ophthalmologists willing to perform them has decreased. As a result, systems have been developed in which trained nurses capture retinal photographs and transmit them to experts for remote interpretation (Fig. 18.2) (Richter et al. 2009).

18.3.5 Video-based Telehealth

To many people telehealth is videoconferencing. Whenever the words "telehealth" or "telemedicine" are mentioned, most people have a mental image of a patient talking to a doctor over some type of synchronous video connection. Indeed, most early telehealth research did

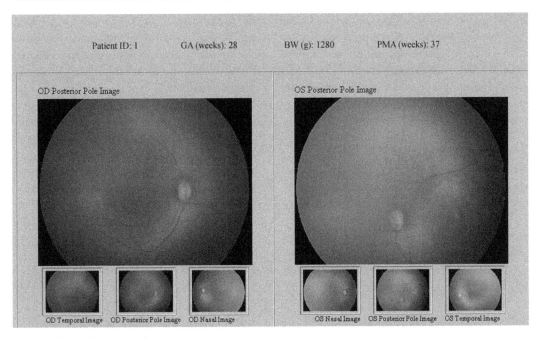

Patient ID: 1   GA (weeks): 28   BW (g): 1280   PMA (weeks): 37

OD Posterior Pole Image   OS Posterior Pole Image

OD Temporal Image   OD Posterior Pole Image   OD Nasal Image   OS Nasal Image   OS Posterior Pole Image   OS Temporal Image

Fig. 18.2 Store-and-forward telemedicine system for ophthalmic disease, in which a remote grader interprets retinal images, along with relevant clinical data, captured by a nurse. Three images from different areas of the patient's right eye (*OD*) and left eye (*OS*) are displayed. Diagnosis and recommendations are then sent back to the local site (Source: Chiang .2007. *Archives of Ophthalmology*, *125*(11), 1531. Copyright © (2007) American Medical Association. All rights reserved)

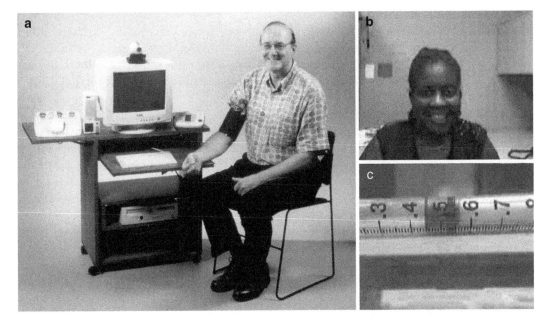

Fig. 18.3 Plain old telephone service (POTS)–based home telehealth. Panel (**a**) shows the IDEATel Home Telemedicine Unit. Panel (**b**) shows a typical full-motion video image transmitted over POTS. Because of frame-to-frame compression, images of nonmoving objects can be of even higher quality. Many home telehealth systems are also equipped with close-up lenses to allow providers to monitor medications or wounds. Panel (**c**) shows a close-up video image of a syringe indicating that the patient has drawn up 44 units of insulin. The small markings are roughly 0.6 mm apart (Source: Starren 2003, reproduced with permission)

focus on synchronous video connections. For many of the early studies, the goal was to provide access to specialists in remote or rural areas. Nearly all of the early systems utilized a hub-and-spoke topology where one hub, usually an academic medical center, was connected to many spokes, usually rural clinics.

Many of the early telehealth consults involved the patient and the primary care provider at one site conferring with a specialist at another site. Most of the state-wide telehealth networks operated on this model. This was so engrained in the telehealth culture, that the first legislation allowing Medicare reimbursement of telehealth consults required a "presenter" at the remote site.

This requirement for a "presenter" exacerbated the scheduling problem. Because synchronous video telehealth often uses specialized videoconferencing rooms, the televisits need to be scheduled at a specific time. Getting the patient and both clinicians (expert and presenter) at the right places at the right time has forced many telehealth programs to hire a full-time scheduler. The scheduling problem, combined with the advent of more user-friendly equipment, ultimately led Medicare to drop the presenter requirement. Even so, scheduling is often the single biggest obstacle to greater use of synchronous video consultations.

A second obstacle has been the availability of relevant clinical information. Because of the inability to interface between various EHRs, it was not unusual for staff to print out results from the EHR at one site and then to fax those to the other site prior to a synchronous video consultation.

Unlike store-and-forward telehealth, synchronous video requires a stable data stream. Although video connection can use conventional phone lines (commonly referred to as **plain old telephone service**, or POTS) that provide 64 bits-per-second (64 kbs) transmission speed, diagnostic quality video typically requires at least 128 Kbs and more commonly 384 Kbs (see Chap. 5). In order to guarantee stable data rates, synchronous video in clinically critical situations still relies heavily on dedicated circuits, either **Integrated Service Digital Network** (ISDN) connections or leased lines. Within single organizations, or in consultative or educational settings, Internet Protocol (IP) based video conferencing has become the dominant modality.

Synchronous video telehealth has been used in almost every conceivable situation. In addition to traditional consultations, the systems have been used to transmit grand rounds and other educational presentations. Video cameras have been placed in operating rooms at hub sites to transmit images of surgeries for educational purposes. Video cameras have been placed in emergency departments and operating rooms at spoke sites to allow experts to "telementor" less experienced physicians in the remote location. Video cameras have also been placed in ambulances to provide remote triage.

More recently, the growing popularity of mobile devices is creating potential for new strategies involving real-time video communication between patients and health care providers. This is especially promising because mobile networks are low-cost and widely-available for consumers, and because they are increasingly accessible even in developing countries. However, health information exchange using mobile networks raises concerns about privacy, security, and compliance with **Health Insurance Portability and Accountability Act** (HIPAA). With appropriate encryption settings, wireless video communication using mobile device applications may be HIPAA-compliant (e.g. FaceTime; Apple Computer, Cupertino, CA). In the future, these mobile technologies may provide opportunities for greater communication between patients and providers.

Prior to the adoption of IP-based videoconferencing, programs begun with grant funding ended soon after the grant funding ended. Even after the advent of IP-based conferencing, many programs have struggled. This is in spite of the fact that Medicare has begun reimbursing for synchronous video under limited circumstances.

Some rural health care providers, such as the Marshfield Clinic in Wisconsin, have integrated synchronous telehealth into their standard care model to provide routine specialist services to outlying location. Some categories of synchronous video telehealth have developed sustainable models: telepsychiatry, correctional telehealth; home telehealth, emergency telehealth, and remote intensive care.

18.3.5.1 Telepsychiatry

In many ways, psychiatry is the ideal clinical domain for synchronous video consultation. Diagnosis is based primarily on observing and talking to the patient. The interactive nature of the dialog means that store-and-forward video is rarely adequate. Physical examination is relatively unimportant, so that the lack of physical contact is not limiting. There are very few diagnostic studies or procedures, so that interfacing to other clinical systems is less important. In addition, state offices of mental health deliver a significant fraction of psychiatric services, minimizing reimbursement issues. This is illustrated by two projects. In 1995, the South Carolina Department of Mental Health established a telepsychiatry network to allow a single clinician to provide psychiatric services to deaf patients throughout the state (Afrin and Critchfield 1997). The system allowed clinicians, who had previously driven all over the state, to spend more time in patient care and less time traveling.

The system was so successful that it was expanded to multiple providers and roughly 20 sites. The second example comes from the New York State Psychiatric Institute (NYSPI), which is responsible for providing expert consultation to mental health facilities and prisons throughout the state. As in South Carolina, travel time was a significant factor in providing this service. To address the problem, the NYSPI created a videoconference network among the various state mental health centers. The system allows specialists at NYSPI in New York City to provide consultations in a timelier manner, improving care and increasing satisfaction at the remote sites.

18.3.5.2 Correctional Telehealth

Prisons tend to be located far from major metropolitan centers. Consequently, they are also located far from the specialists in major medical centers. Transporting prisoners to medical centers is an expensive proposition, typically requiring two officers and a vehicle. Depending on the prisoner and the distance, costs for a single transfer range from hundreds to thousands of dollars. Because of the high cost of transportation, correctional telehealth was economically viable even before the advent of newer low cost systems.

Correctional telehealth also improves patient satisfaction. A fact surprising to many is that inmates typically do not want to leave a correctional institution to seek medical care. Many dislike the stigma of being paraded through a medical facility in prison garb. In addition, the social structure of prisons is such that any prisoner who leaves for more than a day risks losing privileges and social standing. Correctional telehealth follows the conventional model of providing specialist consultation to supplement to on-site primary care physicians. This has become increasingly important with the rising prevalence of AIDS in the prison population.

18.3.5.3 Home Telehealth

After Samuel misses two scheduled visits, the Diabetes Educator calls see what is the matter. Samuel explains that it is a 1-h drive from his home to the diabetes center, that his daughter had trouble taking time off from work to drive him, and that he would have difficulty leaving his wife home alone because she has been ill recently. The Diabetes Educator notes that Samuel lives in a rural area and is eligible to receive educational services via teleheath. She signs Samuel up to receive a Home Telehealth Unit and schedules delivery. The unit is initially difficult for him to use because he is not familiar with computer systems. However, after this initial learning process, Samuel rarely misses a video education session. At one visit, Samuel complains that his children and wife are always "on his case" about his injections. The nurse schedules the next video visit during an evening when Samuel's daughter can attend. She also schedules Samuel to have a video visit with the dietician.

Somewhat paradoxically, one of the most active areas of telehealth growth is at the lowest end of the bandwidth spectrum—telehealth activities into patients' homes. In the late 1990s, many believed that home broadband access would soon become ubiquitous and a number of vendors abandoned POTS-based systems in favor of IP-based video solutions. The broadband revolution was slower than expected, especially in rural and economically depressed areas most in need of home telehealth services. A few research projects paid to have broadband or ISDN installed in patients' homes. In response to this, the American Telemedicine Association released new guidelines for Home Telehealth in 2002 in which synchronous video is provided over POTS connections.

Most vendors have returned to POTS-based solutions and a number of new products have appeared in the past 3 years. In addition to video, the devices typically have data ports for connection of various peripheral devices, such as a digital stethoscope, glucose meter, blood pressure meter, or spirometer. Although the video quality would not be adequate for many diagnostic purposes, it is adequate for the management of existing conditions. Figure. 18.3 shows actual POTS video quality.

Home telehealth can be divided into two major categories. The first category, often called **telehome care**, is the telehealth equivalent of home nursing care. It involves frequent video visits between nurses and, often homebound, patients. With the advent of prospective payment for home nursing care, telehome care is viewed as a way for home care agencies to provide care at reduced costs. As with home nursing care, telehome care tends to have a finite duration, often focused on recovery from a specific disease or incident. Several studies have shown that telehome care can be especially valuable in the management of patients recently discharged from the hospital and can significantly reduce readmission rates.

The second category of home telehealth centers on the management of chronic diseases. Compared with telehome care, this type of home

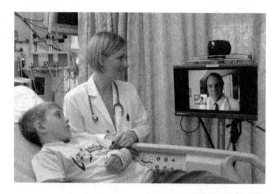

Fig. 18.4 Emergency telemedicine care system, in which a remote expert performs videoconsultation with a local physician or nurse (University of California, Davis Health System, 2010, reproduced with permission)

telehealth frequently involves a longer duration of care and less frequent interactions. Video interactions tend to focus on patient education, more than on evaluation of acute conditions.

The largest such project to date is the Informatics for Diabetes Education and Telemedicine (IDEATel) project (Starren et al. 2002). Started in 2000, the IDEATel project was an 8-year, $60 million demonstration project funded by the Center for Medicare and Medicaid Services (CMS, formerly the Health Care Financing Administration, or HCFA) involving 1665 diabetic Medicare patients in urban and rural New York State. In this randomized clinical trial, half of the patients received Home Telemedicine Units (HTU) (Fig. 18.3), and half continued to receive standard care.

At peak, 636 patients were actively using the HTU's. In addition to providing 2-way POTS-based video, the HTU allowed patients to interact in multiple ways with their online charts. When patients measure blood pressure or fingerstick glucose with devices connected directly to the HTU, the results were automatically encrypted and transmitted over the Internet into the Columbia University Web-based Clinical Information System (WebCIS; Hripcsak et al. 1999) at New York Presbyterian Hospital (NYPH) and to diabetes-specific case management software. Nurse case managers monitored patients by viewing the uploaded results, participating in bulletin board discussions, videoconferencing, and answering e-mailed questions daily. The case manager received an alert when a patient's transmitted values exceed set thresholds.

An important distinction between telehome care and disease management telehealth is that interactions in the former are initiated and managed by the nurse. Measurements, such as blood pressure, are typically collected during the video visit and uploaded as part of the video connection. For disease management, the HTU also needs to support remote monitoring, patient-initiated data uploads and, possibly, Web-based access to educational or disease management resources.

A project that reversed the conventional notion of home telehealth was the Baby CareLink project (Gray et al. 2000). This project focused on very low birth weight infants who typically spend months in neonatal intensive care units (NICU). The project used high-speed (ISDN) video connections to connect from the NICU into the parents' home. This allowed parents who could not visit the NICU regularly to maintain daily contact with their infants. The video connection was supplemented by communication and educational material on a project Web site.

18.3.5.4 Emergency Telemedicine

Samuel develops slurred speech and weakness on the right side of his body. His daughter, who is with him at the time, calls 911. The ambulance crew notifies the emergency room that they are in route with a possible stroke victim. On arrival, the rural emergency department (ED) physician does a quick evaluation and connects via telemedicine with a stroke neurologist at an academic health center. The neurologist talks with the Samuel and his daughter, and participates in the examination with the ED physician. Following laboratory work and a CT negative for hemorrhage, the ED physician again consults with the neurologist who confirms the diagnosis of ischemic stroke and institutes thrombolytic therapy via pre-arranged protocol. Samuel is transferred to the intensive care unit for close monitoring of his diabetes, hypertension, and evolving stroke.

"Just in time" consultation in the emergency setting potentially represents one of the most beneficial uses of telehealth (Fig. 18.4). Emergency telemedicine has been used in a variety of ways and has demonstrated significant benefits, including in such area as tele-trauma care, burn care, and critical care pediatric specialists consulting on critically ill or injured children (Ricci et al. 2003; Saffle et al. 2009; Heath et al 2009). Telehealth in the emergency setting is likely to have the greatest benefit when time-limited critical decision making by a specialist physician regarding a specific intervention is necessary.

An important and increasingly frequently used application demonstrating this is in the evaluation and treatment of the stroke patient. Best practice management of ischemic stroke in appropriate patients now includes the use of thrombolytic therapy such as tissue plasminogen activator (tPA), which has been shown to have statistically significant clinical and financial benefits. Recommendations and drug labeling limit the use of intravenous tPA to within 3 h of when the patient was last seen as well or had witnessed onset of symptoms.

This therapy, however, has significant complications, particularly in patients with hemorrhagic rather than ischemic events – requiring urgent specialty consultation, along with rapid expert interpretation of imaging and laboratory work. Many settings lack the specialty expertise to have on-site "stroke teams" to accomplish best practice. Telemedicine can bring specialty expertise to a remote location for emergency evaluation of the patient directly, while transmit images and laboratory work for immediate interpretation.

This model of care, first called "telestroke" care by Levine and Gorman, has been increasingly used throughout the country (Levine 1999). The efficacy of this model, compared to traditional telephone consultation, was evaluated by Meyer et al. (2008). These investigators found that telestroke care resulted in more accurate decision making than did telephone consultation.

Based on a comprehensive review of evidence, the American Heart Association and American Stroke Association have recommended that "whenever local or on-site acute expertise or resources are insufficient to provide around-the-clock coverage for a health care facility, telestroke systems should be deployed to supplement resources at participating sites" (Schwamm et al. 2009). This comprehensive and detailed report makes other recommendations in support of telemedicine in the area of stroke care.

18.3.5.5 Remote Intensive Care

Samuel was admitted to the intensive care unit (ICU) in his local hospital with the diagnosis of stroke, diabetes and hypertension. He is being treated with thrombolytic therapy. During the night, Samuel's blood pressure begins to rise significantly above the recommended level for patients under treatment with thrombolytic therapy. This is quickly recognized by a remote tele-ICU team that provides coverage for all of the ICU beds in Samuel's rural hospital. This remote intensive care team has complete access to Samuel's electronic health record and bedside monitors and they also have video and audio connectivity into the room. The remote critical care team is able to quickly connect to Samuel's room and do a neurological exam with the assistance of the on-site nursing team. They determine that the exam is unchanged from the emergency room. They are able to order appropriate medications, recommend more frequent neurological checks, and directly follow his blood pressure response.

Consultation models in the in-patient setting using telemedicine in a variety of specialties have been reported. including intensive care where timely consults are often essential (Assimacopoulos et al. 2008; Marcin et al. 2004). Although, these consultation models in critical care have shown benefit, a comprehensive multi-modality model has becomeh more common. This is often referred to as tele-ICU, and is defined as care provided to critically ill patients with at least some of the managing physicians and nurses in a remote location.

Some of the initial work in this area, done by Rosenfield and Bresslow in the Sentara Health System, demonstrated improved mortality, reduced lengths of stay and decreased costs (Rosenfeld et al. 2000). Remote intensive care has grown significantly over time with an estimated 10 % of all ICU beds in the U.S. covered under this model of care, in large part due to a shortage of critical care physicians Typically, a single "Command Center" can cover multiple intensive care units over a large geographic region creating significant efficiencies and economies of scale.

This model of care integrates several of the technologies discussed in this book and is primarily enabled using electronic health records, evidenced based decision support tools, connections to bedside monitoring systems and audio/video based telemedicine into patient rooms. Most commonly, critical care health professionals co-manage care from a Command Center led by board-certified critical care physicians. Protocols and treatments reviews for patient management are incorporated into the care process using data from the monitoring and alert systems that indicate when changes in care should take place. The goal is to assure adherence to best practice, achieve shorter response times to alarms, abnormal laboratory values and more rapid initiation of life saving interventions (Lilly et al. 2011).

Recent studies have shown mixed results in terms of the benefits of tele-ICU. Morrison and colleagues studied mortality, length of stay, and total cost in 4,088 patients admissions at two metropolitan hospitals. Age, gender, race/ethnicity, trauma status, **APACHE III** score, and physician utilization of the eICU were included as covariates. In this study, the investigators did not find a reduction in mortality, length of stay, or hospital cost attributable to the introduction of the eICU (Morrison 2009). In a study by Thomas in 2009, the investigators found that although remote monitoring of ICU patients was not associated with an overall improvement in mortality or LOS, there was a significant interaction between the tele-ICU intervention and severity of illness (P < .001), in which tele-ICU was associated with improved survival in sicker patients but with no improvement or worse outcomes in less sick patients (Thomas et al. 2009).

In a more recent study, Lilly et al. reported that in a single academic medical center, implementation of tele-ICU was associated with reduced mortality and LOS, as well as lower rates of preventable complications (Lilly et al. 2011). Further research is needed in this area to determine the benefits of tele-ICU and the specific components that account for these benefits.

18.3.6 Telepresence

Telepresence involves systems that allow clinicians to not only view remote situations, but also to act on them. The archetypal telepresence application is telesurgery. The most basic surgical telepresence systems simply permit two-way audio-video communications, by which remote surgeons can observe, teach, and collaborate with local surgeons while they operate on patients.

More advanced surgical telepresence systems allow procedures to actually be performed remotely. Although largely still experimental, a trans-Atlantic gall bladder operation was demonstrated in 2001 (Kent 2001). The military has funded considerable research in this area in the hope that surgical capabilities could be extended to the battlefield. Telepresence requires high bandwidth, low **latency** connections. Optimal telesurgery requires not only teleoperation of robotic surgical instruments, but also accurate **force feedback** (or **haptic feedback**) that requires extremely low network latencies.

Accurate millisecond force feedback has been historically limited to distances under 100 miles. The endoscopic gall bladder surgery mentioned above is an exception to this general principle because that specific procedure relied almost exclusively on visual information. It used a dedicated and custom configured 10 Mb/s fiberoptic network with a 155 ms latency.

Providing tactile feedback over large distances actually requires providing the surgeon with simulated feedback while awaiting transmission of the actual feedback data. Such simulation requires massive computing power and is an area of active research. Telesurgery also require extremely high-reliability connections. Loss of a connection is an annoyance during a consultation; it can be fatal during a surgical procedure.

Robotic surgery systems have been commercially available since the early 2000s. In these systems, surgical instruments and a camera are introduced into the patient through small incisions. The surgeon controls these instruments remotely, while he or she is viewing a magnified three-dimensional camera image of the patient's anatomical structures. These systems are currently being used in some medical centers for small-incision surgery, typically performed by surgeons seated adjacent to their patients. The increasing availability and use of these robotic surgery systems creates possibilities for an increasing number of telesurgery applications.

To date, robotically-assisted surgery has been most common in fields such as cardiothoracic surgery, gynecology, and urology. Potential advantages of remote robotically-assisted surgery may include smaller incisions, improved anatomic visualization, and finer control of surgical instrumentation. Several clinical studies comparing robotically-assisted surgery with traditional surgery have suggested that the outcomes are similar (Allemann et al. 2010; Ficarra et al. 2009). However, additional research is required to determine the optimal role of robot-assisted surgery and its applications to telesurgery.

A novel form of telepresence gives clinicians the ability to not only to see, but also to walk around. Since the early 2000s, a commercially-available system has combined conventional

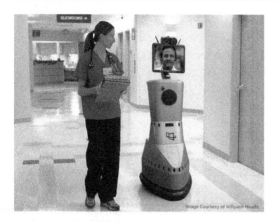

Fig. 18.5 Telehealth robot. This is controlled by a remote clinician, and includes videoconferencing and remote monitoring capabilities. In this example, physician is speaking with a nurse while conducting remote patient rounds (Source: InTouch Health, reproduced with permission)

video telehealth with a remote controlled robot (Fig. 18.5). It allows clinicians to literally make remote video rounds. A frequent problem with telehealth systems is having the equipment where it is needed. With this system, the telehealth equipment is literally able take itself to wherever it is needed. Remote monitoring may be also performed by interfacing digital devices such as stethoscopes or imaging systems to the remote-controlled robot. These remote-controlled systems are most often used by physicians and nurses to examine patients in nursing homes or other long-term facilities, improve health care access in rural areas, and perform post-operative examinations. It is too early to tell whether this model of telepresence will become widely adopted, but, like many earlier innovative systems, it raises many interesting questions.

18.4 Challenges and Future Directions

As telehealth evolves from research novelty to being a standard way that health care is delivered, many challenges must be overcome. Some of these challenges arise because the one patient, one doctor model no longer applies. Basic questions of identity and trust become paramount. At the same time, the shifting focus from treating illness to managing health and wellness requires that clinicians know not only the history of the individuals they treat but also information about the social and environmental context within which those individuals reside. In the diabetes example, knowledge of the family history of risk factors, diseases, and the appropriate diagnostic and interventional protocols, aid the clinical staff in providing timely and appropriate treatment.

18.4.1 Challenges to Using the Internet for Telehealth Applications

Because of the public, shared nature of the Internet, its resources are widely accessible by citizens and health care organizations. This public nature also presents challenges to the security of data transmitted along the Internet. The openness of the Internet leaves the transmitted data vulnerable to interception and inappropriate access. In spite of significant improvements in the security of Web browsing several areas, including protection against viruses, authentication of individuals and the security of email, remain problematic.

Ensuring every citizen access to the Internet represents a second important challenge to the ability to use it for public health purposes. Access to the Internet presently requires computer equipment that may be out of reach for persons with marginal income levels. Majority-language literacy and the physical capability to type and read present additional requirements for effective use of the Internet. Preventing inequalities in access to health care resources delivered via the Internet will require that health care agencies work with other social service and educational groups to make available the technology necessary to capitalize on this electronic environment for health care.

As health care becomes increasingly reliant on Internet-based telecommunications technology, the industry faces challenges in insuring the quality and integrity of many devices and network pathways. These challenges differ from previous medical device concerns, because the diversity and reliability of household equipment is under the control of the household, not the health care providers. There is an increased interdependency between the providers of health services, those who manage telecommunication infrastructure and the manufacturers of commercial electronics. Insuring effective use of telehealth for home and community based care requires that clinical services be supported by appropriate technical resources.

18.4.2 Licensure and Economics in Telehealth

Licensure is frequently cited as the single biggest problem facing telemedicine involving direct patient-provider interactions. This is because medical licensure in the United States is state-based, while telemedicine frequently crosses state or national boundaries. The debate revolves around the questions of whether the patient "travels" through the wire to the clinician, or the clinician "travels" through the wire to the patient. Several states have passed legislation regulating the manner in which clinicians may deliver care remotely or across state lines. Some states have enacted "full licensure models" that require practitioners to hold a full, unrestricted license in each state where a patient resides. Many of these laws have been enacted specifically to restrict the out-of-state practice of telemedicine. To limit Web-based prescribing and other types of asynchronous interactions, several states have enacted or are considering regulations that would require a face-to-face encounter before any electronically delivered care would be allowed. In contrast, some states are adopting regulations to facilitate telehealth by exempting out-of-state physicians from in-state licensure requirements provided that electronic care is provided on an irregular or episodic basis. Still other models would include states agreeing to either a mutual exchange of privileges, or some type of "registration" system whereby clinicians from out of state would register their intent to practice via electronic medium.

At the same time, national organizations representing a variety of health care professions (including nurses, physicians and physical therapists) have proposed a variety of approaches to these issues. While the existing system is built around individual state licensure, groups that favor telemedicine have proposed various interstate or national licensure schemes. The Federated State Board of Medical Examiners has proposed that physicians holding a full, unrestricted license in any state should be able to obtain a limited telemedicine consultation license using a streamlined application process. The American Medical Association is fighting to maintain the current state-based licensure model while encouraging some reciprocity. The American Telemedicine Association supports the position that—since patients are "transported" via telemedicine to the clinician—the practitioner need only be licensed in his or her home state. The National Council of State Boards of Nursing has promoted an Interstate Nurse Licensure Compact whereby licensed nurses in a given state are granted multi-state licensure privileges and are authorized to practice in any other state that has adopted the compact. As of 2002, 19 states had enacted the compact.

The second factor limiting the growth of telehealth is reimbursement. Prior to the mid-1990s there was virtually no reimbursement for telehealth outside of teleradiology. At present Medicare routinely reimburses for synchronous video only for rural patients. Nineteen states provide coverage for synchronous video for Medicaid recipients. Five states also mandate payments by private insurers. A few insurers have begun experimenting with reimbursement for electronic messaging and online consultation, although this has been limited to specific pilot projects. Although teleradiology is often reimbursed, payments for other types of store-and-forward telehealth or remote monitoring remain rare. Few groups have even considered reimbursement for telehealth services that do not involve patient-provider interaction. An expert system could provide triage services; tailored on-line educational material, or customized dosage calculations. Such systems are expensive to build and maintain, but only services provided directly by humans are currently reimbursed by insurance.

Historically, patients have been perceived as reluctant to pay directly for telehealth services, especially when face-to-face visits were covered by insurance. This may be changing. The Marshfield Clinic in Wisconsin has reported that many patients are willing to pay a small technology fee ($10–20) to avoid a several hour drive to see the specialist face-to-face. Private companies have begun providing direct-to-patient video consults utilizing normal Web browsers and Flash™ video at a charge of $45 for 10 min and have placed video stations in workplaces and pharmacies. Some insurers have begun reimbursing for such visits when a patient's primary clinician is not available.

Finally, home telehealth monitoring may reduce the health care costs associated with unreimbursed hospital readmissions. For example, some insurance payers do not reimburse for hospital readmissions that occur within 30 days of discharge, and there are anecdotal reports of health systems paying for 32 days of home monitoring post-discharge. Determining whether, and how much, to pay for telehealth services will likely be a topic of debate for years to come.

18.4.3 Logistical Requirements for Implementation of Telehealth Systems

Telehealth systems must be carefully evaluated before implementation for routine use in individual disease situations, to ensure that they have sufficient diagnostic accuracy and reproducibility for clinical application. Appropriate training and credentialing standards must be developed for personnel who capture clinical data and images from patients locally, as well as for physicians and nurses who perform remote interpretation and consultation. Clear rules and responsibilities must be developed for remote patient management, including the appropriate response for situations in which data are felt to be of insufficient quality for telehealth. Guidelines for medicolegal

liability must be established. Software that displays clinical information required for remote management, and that integrates into existing workflow patterns and maximizes efficiency through good usability principles will be required. Methods for providing added value from technology toward telehealth diagnostic systems through strategies such as links to consumer health resources or computer-based diagnosis may be explored (Koreen et al. 2007). Finally, studies have suggested that patient satisfaction with telehealth systems is high (Lee et al. 2010). However, the practitioner-patient relationship is fundamental to health care delivery, and mechanisms must be developed that this bond is not lost from telehealth.

18.4.4 Telehealth in Low Resource Environments

In many parts of the developing world, the density of both health care providers and of technology is quite low. Thus, the demand for telehealth is high, but the ability to deliver it is challenged. Many of these regions have largely skipped traditional land-line telephony and moved directly to cellular infrastructure (Foster 2010). This, combined with advances in low-cost laptop computers that do not depend on stable power-grids, has allowed the development of a wide variety of telehealth and tele-education applications. The majority of these are based on an asynchronous model. Transport media range from standard broadband in the urban areas, to satellite connections, to cellular data, to **SMS messaging**. The largest group of applications focuses on the provision of remote consultations for difficult cases using computer-based systems, while general health education and remote data collection have been the primary applications using cellular telephony applications. However, the development of smart mobile telephones with high-resolution cameras is rapidly blurring this distinction. The e-book by Wootton provides an overview of this domain (Wootton 2009) and Foster focuses on the role of mobile telephones (Foster 2010).

18.5 Future Directions

Telehealth validation studies across a range of clinical domains have demonstrated good diagnostic accuracy, reliability, and patient satisfaction. Based on these results, numerous real-world telehealth programs have been implemented throughout the world. In the long term, successful large-scale expansion of these programs will require addressing the above challenges.

Beyond these practical factors, traditional medical care uses a workflow model based on synchronous interactions between clinicians and individual patients. The workflow model is also a sequential one in that the clinician may deal with multiple clinical problems or data trends but only within the context of treating a single patient at a time. Medical records, both paper and electronic, as well as billing and administrative systems all rely on this sequential paradigm, in which the fundamental unit is the "visit." Advances in telehealth are disrupting this paradigm. Devices have been developed that allow remote electronic monitoring of diabetes, hypertension, asthma, congestive heart failure (CHF), and chronic anticoagulation. As a result, clinicians may become inundated by large volumes of electronic results. This may mean that clinicians will no longer function in an assembly-line fashion, but will become more like dispatchers or air-traffic controllers, electronically monitoring many processes simultaneously. Clinicians will no longer ask simply, "How is Mrs. X today?" They will also ask the computer "Among my 2,000 patients, which ones need my attention today?" Neither clinicians, nor EHRs, are prepared for this change.

Perhaps the greatest long-term effect of the information and communication revolution will be the breaking down of role, geographic, and social barriers. Medicine is already benefiting from this effect. Traditional "doctors and nurses" are collaborating with public health professionals, and anyone with computer access can potentially communicate with patients or experts around the world. The challenge will be to facilitate productive collaborations among patients, their caregivers, biomedical scientists, and information technology experts.

Suggested Readings

Bashshur, R.L., Shannon, G.W., Krupinski, E.A., Grigsby, J., Kvedar, J.C., Weinstein, R.S., et al. (2009). National telemedicine initiatives: Essential to healthcare reform. *Telemedicine and e-Health*, 15, 600–610. This paper discusses cost-benefit tradeoffs associated with telemedicine within the context of large-scale efforts promoting health care reform in the United States.

Gray, J.E., Safran, C., Davis, R.B., Pompilio-Weitzner, G., Stewart, J.E., Zaccagnini, L., et al. (2000). Baby CareLink: Using the internet and telemedicine to improve care for high-risk infants. *Pediatrics, 106*, 1318–1324. Families of very-low-birthweight babies use interactive television and the world-wide-web to monitor the babies' progess while in hospital and to receive professional coaching and support once the babies return home.

Richter, G.M., Williams, S.L., Starren, J., Flynn, J.T., & Chiang, M.F. (2009). Telemedicine for retinopathy of prematurity diagnosis: Evaluation and challenges. *Survey of Ophthalmology*, 54, 671–685. This article reviews the potential benefits and implementation challenges associated with the use of store-and-forward telemedicine for an ocular disease affecting infants hospitalized in neonatal intensive care units.

Schwamm, L.H., Holloway, R.G., Amarenco, P., Audebert, H.J., Bakas, T., Chumbler, N.R., et al. (2009). A review of the evidence for the use of telemedicine within stroke systems of care: A scientific statement from the American Heart Association/American Stroke Association. *Stroke*, 40, 2616–2634. This is a systematic evidence-based review of scientific data examining the use of telemedicine for stroke care delivery by two major medical organizations. Published studies are categorized according to their level of certainty and class of evidence.

Shea, S., Weinstock, R.S., Teresi, J.A., Palmas, W., Starren, J., Cimino, J.J., et al. (2009). A randomized trial comparing telemedicine case management with usual care in older, ethnically diverse, medically underserved patients with diabetes mellitus: 5 year results of the IDEATel study. *Journal of the American Medical Informatics Association: JAMIA, 16*, 446–456. This paper describes an evaluation study examining the effectiveness of home telemedicine for clinical case management in a group of over 1,600 medically-underserved patients with diabetes mellitus.

Questions for Discussion

1. Telehealth has evolved from systems designed primarily to support consultations between clinicians to systems that provide direct patient care. This has required changes in hardware, user

interfaces, software, and processes. Discuss some of the changes that must be made when a system designed for use by health care professionals is modified to be used directly by patients.

2. There are many controversies regarding reimbursement for telemedicine services. Imagine that you are negotiating with an insurance carrier to obtain reimbursement for a store-and-forward telemedicine service that you have developed. The medical director of the second insurance payer states: "Telemedicine seems like 'screening' rather than a mechanism for delivering health care. This is because you are simply using technology to identify patients who need to be referred to a real doctor, rather than providing true medical care. Therefore we should only reimburse a very small amount for these screening services." In your opinion, is this a legitimate argument? Explain.

3. Using telehealth systems, patients can now have interaction with a large number of health care providers, organizations and resources. As a result, coordination of care becomes increasingly difficult. Two solutions have been proposed. One is to develop better ways to transfer patient-related information among existing EHRs. The other is to give the give the patient control of the health record, either by giving them a smart card or placing the records on a central web site controlled by the patient. Assume and defend one of these perspectives.

Patient Monitoring Systems

19

Reed M. Gardner, Terry P. Clemmer, R. Scott Evans, and Roger G. Mark

After reading this chapter, you should be able to answer these questions

1. What is patient monitoring, and why is it used?
2. What patient parameters do bedside physiological monitors provide?
3. What are the major problems with acquisition and presentation of monitoring parameters?
4. In addition to bedside physiological parameters, what other information is fundamental to the care of acutely ill patients?
5. How are patient care protocols used to enhance the care of critically ill patients?
6. Why is real-time computerized decision support potentially more beneficial than monthly or quarterly quality of care reporting?
7. What technical and social factors must be considered when implementing real-time data acquisition and decision support systems?

R.M. Gardner, PhD (✉)
Department of Informatics, University of Utah,
Biomedical Informatics, 1745 Cornell Circle,
Salt Lake City, UT 84108, USA
e-mail: reed.gardner@hsc.utah.edu

T.P. Clemmer, MD
Pulmonary – Critical Care Medicine,
LDS Hospital, Intermountain Healthcare,
8th Avenue and "C" Street, Salt Lake City,
UT 84143, USA
e-mail: terry.clemmer@imail.org

R.S. Evans, BS, MS, PhD
Medical Informatics Department, LDS Hospital,
Intermountain Healthcare, 8th Ave and C Street,
Salt Lake City, UT 84143, USA
e-mail: rgmark@mit.edu, rscott.evans@imail.org

R.G. Mark, MD, PhD
Institute of Medical Engineering and Science,
Department of Electrical Engineering and Computer
Science (EECS), Massachusetts Institute of
Technology, Room E25-505, Cambridge,
MA 02139, USA
e-mail: scott.evans2@imail.org

19.1 What is Patient Monitoring?

Continuous measurement of patient physiologic parameters such as heart rate, heart rhythm, arterial blood pressure, respiratory rate, and blood-oxygen saturation, have become common during the care of the critically ill patient. When accurate and prompt decision making is crucial for effective patient care, bedside monitors are used to collect, display and store physiological data. Increasingly, such data are collected by non-invasive sensors connected to patients in intensive care units (ICUs), new-born intensive care units (NICUs), operating rooms (ORs), labor and delivery (L&D) suites, emergency rooms (ERs), and other hospital care units where patient acuity is increased.

We often think of a patient monitor as something that watches for – and warns about – serious or life-threatening events in patients, and

This chapter is adapted from an earlier version in the third edition authored by Reed M. Gardner and M. Michael Shabot

E.H. Shortliffe, J.J. Cimino (eds.), *Biomedical Informatics*,
DOI 10.1007/978-1-4471-4474-8_19, © Springer-Verlag London 2014

provides guidance for care of the critically ill. Such systems must include continuous observations of a patient's physiological measurements and the assessment of the function of attached life support equipment. Such monitoring is important in detecting life-threatening conditions and guiding management decision making – including when to make therapeutic interventions and to assess the effect of those interventions.

In this chapter, we discuss the use of computers in collecting, displaying, storing, and interpreting clinical data, making therapeutic recommendations, and alarming and alerting. In the past, most clinical data were in the form of heart and respiratory rates, blood pressures, and vital fluid flows. However, today's ICU monitoring systems integrate data from bedside monitors and devices as well as data from many sources outside the ICU. Although the presentation made here deals primarily with patients who are in ICUs, the general principles and techniques are also applicable to other hospitalized patients and electronic health records (EHR). For example, patient monitoring may be performed for diagnostic purposes in the ER or for therapeutic purposes in the OR. Techniques that just a few years ago were only used in the ICU such as bedside monitors are now used routinely on general hospital wards and in some situations even by patients in their homes.

19.1.1 Case Report

We will use a case report to provide a perspective on the problems faced by the team caring for a critically ill patient: a 27-year-old male is injured in an automobile accident. He has multiple chest and head injuries. His condition is stabilized at the scene of the accident by skilled paramedics using a portable computer-based electrocardiogram (ECG) and pulse oximeter, and he is quickly transported to a trauma center. Once in the trauma center, the young man is connected via non-invasive sensors to a computer-based bedside monitor that displays physiological signals, including his heart rate and rhythm, arterial oxygen saturation, and blood pressure. X-ray and magnetic resonance imaging provide further information for care.

Because of the head injury, the patient has difficulty breathing, so he is connected to a computer-controlled ventilator that has both therapeutic and monitoring functions and he is transferred to the ICU. A bolt is placed in a hole drilled through his skull and a fiber optic sensor is inserted to continuously measure intracranial pressure with another computer-controlled monitor. Blood is drawn and clinical chemistry and blood-gas tests are promptly performed by the hospital laboratory. Results of those tests are displayed to the ICU team as soon as they are available. With intensive treatment, the patient survives the initial threats to his life and now begins the long recovery process. Figure 19.1

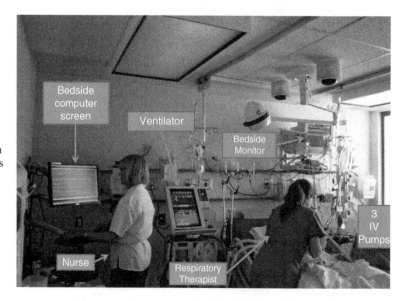

Fig. 19.1 Overall view of an ICU Patient's room. Shown is a nurse standing at the bedside computer screen a ventilator (*center*) with a respiratory therapist suctioning the patient. The patient is connected to the ventilator, bedside monitor (*upper right*) and to three IV pumps (*lower right*)

shows a nurse at the patient's bedside surrounded by a bedside monitor, infusion pumps, a ventilator and other devices.

Unfortunately, a few days later, the patient is beset with a problem common to multiple trauma victims—he has a major **nosocomial hospital-acquired infection**, develops sepsis, and acute respiratory distress syndrome (ARDS), which leads to multiple organ failure. As a result, antibiotics and electrolytes are required for treatment and are dispensed via intravenous (IV) pumps. The quantity of information required to care for the patient has increased dramatically.

Multiple patient monitoring computer systems that support this ICU patient are tightly integrated and data are automatically gathered and stored, primarily in a coded format so that real-time computerized decision support can be used. Figure 19.2 shows a schematic of the HELP system at

Intermountain Healthcare as an example of such a system. Based on the data available to the HELP system from these multiple data sources, its computerized decision support system makes and displays suggestions for optimum care for the specific problems such as sepsis and ARDS. The system provides audible and visual alerts for life-threatening situations. In addition, the system organizes and reports the large amount of data so that the medical team can make prompt and reliable treatment decisions. The patient's physicians are automatically alerted about life-threatening laboratory and other findings. The Infection Control Department automatically receives emails alerting them of any infections in sterile body sites, new nosocomial infections, and any antibiotic resistant pathogens. The patient's ARDS is managed with the assistance of standardized computer generated protocols. The sepsis is managed with a computer-

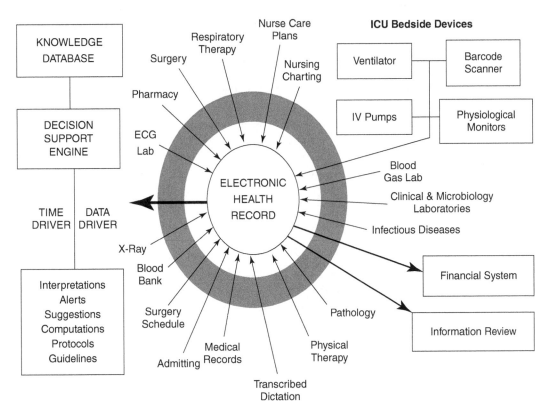

Fig. 19.2 Diagram of HELP the System used by Intermountain Healthcare's Hospitals (including LDS Hospital in Salt Lake City). At the *center* is the database for the electronic health record (*EHR*). Data from a wide variety of clinical and administrative sources flow into the EHR. As the data flows into the EHR, the Data-Driver

capabilities of the HELP Decision Support System (*red cylinder*) are activated. In addition Time Driven decisions are also made. Shown schematically, in the *upper right* hand corner of the diagram are blocks representing ICU bedside devices including the physiological monitor, ventilator, IV pumps and barcode scanner

ized "antibiotic assistant" that recommends the antibiotic to be given as well as the dose, route, and interval based on specific information in the patient's computerized record.

19.1.2 Patient Monitoring in Intensive Care Units

There are at least three categories of patients who need physiological monitoring:

1. Patients with compromised physiological regulatory systems; for example, a patient whose respiratory system is suppressed by a drug overdose or during anesthesia
2. Patients who are currently stable but with a condition that could suddenly change to become life threatening; for example, a patient who has findings indicating an acute myocardial infarction (heart attack) or immediately after open-heart surgery, or a fetus during labor and delivery
3. Patients in a critical physiological state; for example, patients with multiple trauma or septic shock like the one in our case study

Care of critically ill patients requires prompt and accurate decisions so that life-protecting and life-saving therapy can be appropriately applied. Because of these requirements, ICUs have become widely established in hospitals. Such units use computers almost universally for the following purposes:

1. To acquire physiological data frequently or continuously, such as blood pressure
2. To communicate information from data-producing systems to remote locations e.g., laboratory and radiology departments
3. To store, organize, and report patient information
4. To integrate, organize and correlate data from multiple sources
5. To provide clinical alerts and advisories based on multiple sources of data
6. To function as an automated decision support tool that health professionals may use in planning the care of critically ill patients
7. To measure the severity of illness for patient classification purposes
8. To analyze the outcomes of ICU care in terms of clinical effectiveness and cost effectiveness

19.2 Historical Perspective

19.2.1 The Measurement of Vital Signs

The earliest foundations for acquiring physiological data occurred at the end of the Renaissance period. In 1625, Santorio, who lived in Venice, published his methods for measuring body temperature with the spirit thermometer and for timing the pulse (heart) rate with a pendulum. The principles for both devices had been established by Galileo, a close friend. Galileo worked out the uniform periodicity of the pendulum by timing the movement of the swinging chandelier in the Cathedral of Pisa and comparing that to his own pulse rate. The results of this early biomedical-engineering collaboration, however, were ignored. The first scientific report of the pulse rate did not appear until Sir John Floyer published "Pulse-Watch" in 1707. The first published course of fever for a patient was plotted by Ludwig Taube in 1852. With subsequent improvements in the clock and the thermometer, the temperature, pulse rate, and respiratory rate became the standard vital signs.

In 1896, Scipione Riva-Rocci introduced the sphygmomanometer (blood pressure cuff), which permitted the fourth vital sign, systolic blood pressure, to be measured. A Russian physician, Nikolai Korotkoff, applied Riva-Rocci's cuff with a stethoscope developed by the French physician Rene Laennec which allowed the measurement of both systolic and diastolic arterial pressure. Harvey Cushing, a preeminent U.S. neurosurgeon of the early 1900s, predicted the need for and later insisted on routine arterial blood pressure monitoring in the operating room. At the same time Cushing also raised the following questions – that are still being asked today:

1. Are we collecting too much data?
2. Are the instruments used in clinical medicine too accurate?
3. Would not approximated values be just as good?

Cushing answered his own questions by stating that vital sign measurements should be made routinely and that their accuracy was important (Cushing 1903). More recently the

American College of Critical Care Medicine (Haupt et al. 2003) and the American Society of Anesthesiologists (ASA 2010) have made similar recommendations.

Since the 1920s, the four vital signs—temperature, respiratory rate, heart rate, and arterial blood pressure—have been recorded in all patient charts. In 1903, Willem Einthoven devised the string galvanometer for displaying and quantifying the electrocardiogram (ECG), for which he was awarded the 1924 Nobel Prize in physiology. The ECG has become an important adjunct to the clinician's inventory of tests for both acutely and chronically ill patients. Continuous measurement of physiological variables has become a routine part of the monitoring of critically ill patients.

At the same time that advances in monitoring were made, major changes in the therapy of life-threatening disorders were also occurring. Prompt quantitative evaluation of measured physiological and biochemical variables became essential in the decision-making process as physicians applied new therapeutic interventions. For example, it is now possible—and in many cases essential—to use ventilators when a patient cannot breathe independently, cardiopulmonary bypass equipment when a patient undergoes open-heart surgery, hemodialysis when a patient's kidneys fail, and IV nutritional and electrolyte support when a patient is unable to eat or drink.

19.2.2 Development of Intensive Care Units

Until about 1960, if patients had severe cardiac events, there were few treatment options for physicians to care for them. As a consequence, many patients who had life-threatening acute cardiac or pulmonary problems died. However, in the early 1960's two major medical care treatment modalities were developed that provided treatment for heretofore fatal situations. Development of closed chest cardiopulmonary resuscitation (CPR); (Kouwenhoven et al. 1960) and closed chest defibrillation (Zoll et al. 1956; Lown et al. 1962) provided means for delivering life-saving treatment. Because of availability of these treatments, the

demand for continuous monitoring of high risk patients escalated. Hospitals began to cluster patients with complex disorders together into new organizational units—called ICUs—beginning in the early 1960s. Some of the earliest units were coronary care units where patients were cared for after myocardial infarctions or other acute, life-threatening cardiac events.

Surgical intensive care units (SICUs) had their beginnings in the late 1950s when post-operative patients were kept in the recovery rooms for extended time periods after cardiac or other high risk surgery for close observation. Initially these recovery rooms did not have the benefit of cardiac monitoring. However, as more sophisticated monitoring became available, special units were created and designated as SICUs or thoracic intensive care units (TICUs).

Intensive care units proliferated rapidly during the late 1960s and early 1970s. The types of units included coronary, thoracic surgery, surgical, medical, shock-trauma, burn, pediatric, neonatal, respiratory, and other multipurpose medical-surgical units. Today there are more than six million patients admitted each year into adult, pediatric, and neonatal intensive care units in the United States alone. In the past three decades, the demand for ICU services in the United States has risen dramatically. The average life expectancy is rising and estimates of the U.S. Population over 65 (who use ICUs disproportionally more than the rest of the population) will increase by 50 % by 2020 and 100 % by 2030, continually increasing demand (Kelley et al. 2004; Groves et al. 2008).

19.2.3 Development of Bedside Monitors

A signature feature of each of these early ICUs was the bedside monitor. The original bedside monitors were used primarily to acquire and display the ECG. Soon it became possible to acquire and display arterial and venous blood pressure signals by inserting catheters directly into a patient's vein or artery and connecting them to transducers. In some cases these catheter-transducer systems were already in place when

Fig. 19.3 Waveforms on Two Types of Bedside Monitors. Displays from the Philips (**a**) and General Electric (**b**) show the real-time beat-by beat from a patient's bedside monitor with multiple channels of ECG with the arterial pressure and pulse oximeter signals along with other physiological signals and their derived variables

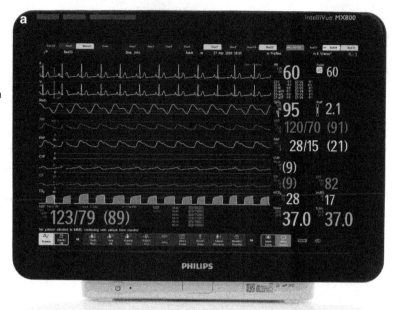

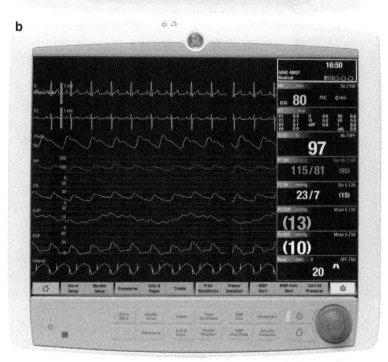

open-heart patients returned from surgery. The bedside monitor could also display the ECG and the arterial waveform (See Fig. 19.3a, b). Because of the complexity of care and the increased acuity of these patients, the need for specialized nursing care increased dramatically. In a typical acute patient care situation, one nurse may be responsi-

ble for the care of five or more patients. However, because of the observations and care that these acutely ill patients required, intensive care nurses typically are assigned one to three patients.

As a result of the detailed ECG information provided by the new patient monitors, treatment for serious cardiac arrhythmias (heart rhythm disturbances) and cardiac arrest (abrupt cessation of heartbeat)—major causes of death after myocardial infarctions (heart attack) —became possible. Mortality rates from 1960 to 1970 were about 35 %, dropped to about 23 % between 1970 and 1980 and to about 20 % between 1980 and 1990. During the 1990's reperfusion of the coronary arteries became common and mortality rate dropped to about 5 % (Braunwald 1988; Rogers et al. 2000).

In the 1960's bedside monitors were built using analog computer technologies. These systems amplified the electrocardiographic signal and displayed the results on an oscilloscope. Such systems required nurses or technicians to watch the oscilloscope to determine if there was a cardiac arrest or other life threatening cardiac rhythm. Soon after these analog systems were developed, methods for generating high- and low-heart-rate alarm thresholds were included. The alarms were usually audible and very annoying. Unfortunately, since the beginning of the use of these alarms, the false positive rate has far exceeded the true positive rate. As a result, many times alarm systems for bedside monitors are ignored or turned off.

19.2.4 Development of Computer-Based ICU Monitoring

Teams from several cities in the United States introduced computers into the ICU to assist in physiological monitoring, beginning in Los Angles with Shubin and Weil (Shubin and Weil 1966) followed by Warner and colleagues (Warner et al. 1968) in Salt Lake City. These investigators had several objectives:

1. To increase the availability and accuracy of the physiological data
2. To compute derived variables that could not be measured directly
3. To increase patient-care efficacy
4. To allow display of the time trends of the patient's physiological data, and
5. To assist in computer-aided decision making

Each of these teams developed their applications on large **mainframe computer systems**, which required large computer rooms and trained staff to keep the system operational 24 h a day. The computers used by these developers cost over $200,000 each in 1965 dollars. During that time, other researchers were attacking more specific challenges in patient monitoring. For example, Cox (Cox 1972) at Barnes Hospital in St. Louis, developed algorithms to analyze the ECG for heart rhythm disturbances in real-time. The arrhythmia-monitoring system, which was installed in the CCU in 1969, ran on a relatively inexpensive **mini-computer** rather than a mainframe computer. With the advent of **integrated circuits** and **microprocessors**, affordable computing power increased dramatically. What was considered computer-based patient monitoring by these pioneers in the late 1960s and early 1970s is now entirely built into bedside monitors and is considered simply a "bedside monitor." Clemmer provides an important overview of "where we started and where we are now" (Clemmer 2004) to summarize the four decades since the initiation of computers in the ICU.

19.3 Modern Bedside Monitors

The heart and lungs are crucial to normal body function. For example if the heart stops (cardiac arrest) there is a cessation of normal circulation of the blood. Likewise, if there is a pulmonary arrest there is a cessation of breathing. Each of these situations leads to a reduced delivery of oxygenated blood (hypoxia) to the body, with major physiological hazards. For example, brain injury will occur if hypoxia is untreated within 5 min. As a consequence, detection of either of these situations is required if life-saving treatments are to be administered. The treatment for cardiac arrest is CPR, which provides circulatory and pulmonary support. Following the application of CPR, if the patient does not regain a normal rhythm, they may have to be shocked with a defibrillator to reestablish a normal rhythm.

Although it is highly desirable to monitor critically ill patients to determine life-threatening events, the process of doing so is very demanding on information systems. For example if a patient in the ICU had a heart rate of 90 beats per minute, that patient would have 5,400 beats each hour and almost 130,000 heart beats each day. With the digitization of the ECG and other physiological signals, it is possible to determine the heart rate and other parameters for each heartbeat. Certainly a computerized monitor should be much better at monitoring such parameters than a human.

19.3.1 ECG Signal Acquisition and Processing

The ECG provides a representation of the electrical activity of the human heart and is a very important tool for the diagnosis of disturbances of heart rate and rhythm. The ECG is derived by placing electrical leads on a patient's chest and limbs and provided one of the first methods for automatically determining heart rate (HR) and detecting irregular rhythms of the heart. Original monitors allowed physicians and nurses the ability to watch the ECG trace on an oscilloscope. Since ECG signal measured on the skin is very small (1 mV), it is subject to artifacts (noise) caused by such things as patient movement, electrode movement, and electrical power interference. By using sophisticated analog and digital techniques and presenting data from multiple leads, the quality and reliability of the ECG signals monitored has improved dramatically over the past three decades (Weinfurt 1990; Gregg et al. 2008). At the same time, the demand for improved quality of the ECG signal and an increase in the number and types of parameters has increased. Initially, the ECG signal was processed to obtain HR and basic rhythm (periodicity of the beat) while today's monitors can detect signals from artificial heart pacemakers, complex arrhythmias, **myocardial ischemia** and disturbances in the conduction of electrical signals through the heart muscle.

Two types of computerized ECG analysis are in common use today:

1. The 12-lead ECG is typically performed in a physician's office or in the hospital. Usually a technician brings a recording device to the patient's bedside and attaches the leads, and records the signal acquisition during a short interval while the patient is lying quietly in a supine position. From this 12-lead ECG, a wide variety of ECG diagnoses are made. Computer processing of these ECG signals taken at that moment in time has become the definitive practical option for ECG interpretation. Automated ECG analysis has become widespread in clinical practice since the mid-1980s although, in most hospitals, cardiologists will also read them to confirm the automated findings. Automated ECG analysis is quite accurate, especially in normal individuals, but disagreements with cardiologists are seen and may be clinically important (Guglin 2006; Bogun et al. 2004). On the other hand, cardiologists are not perfect either (Clark et al. 2010)!

   Today, physicians expert in ECG interpretation from multiple professional organizations such as the American Heart Association and the Electrocardiographic Society have come to consensus and established standards designed to improve computerized ECG interpretation. In biomedical informatics terminology, these experts have developed the knowledge base for diagnostic ECG interpretation. The detailed pattern recognition and signal processing does not need to occur in real-time. Thus the 12-lead ECG processing can be more sophisticated than with the requirements of real time monitoring situations (Gregg et al. 2008).

2. Continuous, real-time monitoring is required while the patient is in the ICU. Because of patient movement, caregiver activities such as administering medications, bathing and the like, the amount of artifact generated poses important challenges to real-time monitoring. To minimize these effects, filtering of the acquired ECG signal is performed. This filtering slightly distorts the ECG but at the same time makes it possible to process the signals on a beat-by-beat basis. Although standards for interpretation of ECG monitoring are more recent than those for 12-lead monitoring, they are now becoming more common and

sophisticated (Drew and Funk 2006; Funk et al. 2010), The clinical experts who are establishing the knowledge base now include critical-care nurses, cardiologists, anesthesiologists, and thoracic surgeons (Crossley et al. 2011).

ECG processing in today's vendor-supplied bedside monitors continues to improve and become more reliable. Sophisticated pattern recognition and signal processing techniques are used to allow extraction of key parameters in real-time while adding the ability to measure the utility of new physiological parameters (Crossley et al. 2011). Recently, investigators have created publically available databases of ECG waveforms and other physiological signals as well as other important data from actual patients to allow validation of these monitoring systems (Saeed et al. 2011; Burykin et al. 2011).

19.3.2 Arterial Blood Pressure Signal Acquisition and Processing

Accurate and continuous monitoring of arterial pressure requires insertion of a catheter into an artery. Once the catheter is successfully inserted into an artery the catheter is connected, via a length of sterile fluid-filled tubing, to a stop-cock with a "continuous flush" device and a factory calibrated disposable blood pressure transducer (Gardner 1996). The blood pressure transducer is then connected to an amplifier and the pulsatile signal it detects is displayed on the screen of the bedside patient monitor. With the advent of inexpensive, disposable, accurate pressure transducers, the quality and accuracy of arterial pressure monitoring has improved dramatically. However, two sources of inaccuracy of the arterial pressure signal still depend on medical staff set-up and validation: (1) zeroing is the process by which the monitor is informed when a port on the stopcock is opened to the atmosphere at "mid-heart level" – thus becoming the point from which pressure is measured; (2) since the arterial pressure signal contains pulsatile characteristics with

frequencies up to 20 Hz that must be transmitted from the artery through the plumbing system to the transducer, the dynamic response characteristics must be optimized. Optimization is typically done by doing a "fast flush" test (by pushing sterile saline through the tubing) to optimize the system by removing blood and very tiny air bubbles that can dramatically distort the arterial pressure waveform and result in erroneous measures of systolic and diastolic pressure.

At least two types of artifacts in the arterial pressure signal are commonly observed. If a patient rapidly moves or a care giver bumps the tubing, a pressure artifact is generated and transmitted to the transducer and displayed. In addition, when the clinical staff draws arterial blood for laboratory tests, they typically turn off the stopcock connected to the transducer and draw blood through the tubing, causing an immediate loss of the pulsatile arterial pressure signal. The pressure sensed by the transducer then typically rises to that found in the pressurized flush solution. Thus, continuous vigilance on the part of nurses and other care givers is needed for the arterial catheter and monitoring systems to be properly maintained. As a historical note, the continuous flush device was developed over 40 years ago to prevent arterial catheters from clotting and to allow one of the pioneering computerized monitoring systems to become more reliable (Gardner et al. 1970). Since that time, investigators have developed computerized methods to minimize these "human caused artifacts" (Li et al. 2009; Gorges et al. 2009).Unfortunately, these strategies have seldom been implemented into commercially available bedside monitors.

Since the early 1900's, efforts have been made to estimate **cardiac output** from the pulsatile pressure in the arterial system by multiplying the HR with estimates of stroke volume (the volume of blood ejected from the heart during a single contraction) made from the pressure waveform. Warner and his colleagues at the Mayo clinic published some early work in 1953 (Warner et al. 1953) on the topic and followed up again in 1983 further substantiating the feasibility of the method. However, (Cundick and Gardner 1980) showed that the widely varying mean blood pressures found in critically ill patients adversely affected the reliability of the method. Since that early work, multiple publications and commercially available devices using the pulse-pressure method have appeared. The issue is still active, with such recent publications (Chen et al. 2009; Sun et al. 2009; Gardner and Beale 2009). Other estimates of stroke volume and cardiac output have been made from determining the "Bioreactance" – a measure of the degree of phase-shift in the electrical signal - across the chest. This method shows promise of being a rather simple, continuous and non-invasive method for measuring cardiac output (Keren et al. 2007).

More recently, several investigators have made assessments of delta pulse pressure (DPP), which measures the variability of the peak to peak arterial pressure pulse signal across the breathing cycle to make an estimate of a patient's fluid balance. The supposition is that if there is larger variability in this DPP marker the patient may require fluid administration (Deflandre et al. 2008).

It is clear that future methods that process available physiological signals will be applied to enhance and improve the availability of important measures of cardiac function – a key parameter for making treatment decisions used by critical caregivers.

19.3.3 Pulse Oximeter Signal Acquisition and Processing

One of the most common technological devices used in hospitals today is the pulse oximeter. The pulse oximeter sensing device is usually placed on a finger and measures oxygen saturation and pulse rate - HR (Clark et al. 2006). The device works by shining red and infrared light generated by two light emitting diodes through the tissue. With each arterial pulse there is a variation in the light as it passes through the tissue and is sensed by a light-sensitive photodiode on the opposite side. The more oxygenated the blood is, the more red light is transmitted, with less infrared light passing through. By calibrating these devices,

reasonably accurate estimates of arterial oxygen saturation (SpO_2) can be determined. Although the pulse oximeter is convenient and easy to use, it has several important limitations, including motion artifact, when the patient moves, and other physiological considerations such as anemia, low perfusion state and low peripheral skin temperature. If the blood flow to the hand gets disturbed, by perhaps squeezing the arm during blood pressure with a sphygmomanometer, the blood flow to the hand is interrupted and the pulsatile blood pressure signal required for the pulse oximeter is no longer available.

19.3.4 Bedside Data Display and Signal Integration

While colorful and dynamic, the displays on the bedside monitor can be complex – See Fig. 19.3a, b for typical bedside monitor displays from Philips and General Electric (GE) bedside monitor displays. Each vendor of bedside monitors has made a "best effort" at displaying the variety of physiological signals derived. In most cases this consists of three channels: ECG, arterial blood pressure, and pulse oximeter. Additional important physiologic parameters can be derived from these signals, as noted in Table 19.1.

Today's bedside monitors still present both waveforms and derived parameters in a "single-sensor-single-indicator" format. That is, for each individual sensor attached to the patient there is a single indicator – waveform with derived values presented on the screen (Drews et al. 2008). One of the simplistic consequences of this display strategy is that each indicator is treated as if it had come from a different patient. For example, if ECG, arterial blood pressure and pulse oximeter signals were displayed, they would each have the capability of determining heart rate. Thus, three different heart rate measures might be displayed. Although there are physiological reasons for such differences, the most common situation is that the heart rate should be an "integrated assessment" of the three signals since "artifact" is a far more common event than the unusual conditions that would cause the differences in heart rate. Drews

Table 19.1 Bedside physiological monitoring capabilities

Signals	Transducer	Frequency		Parameters		
ECG	Chest electrodes	Continuous	Heart rate	Heart rhythm	Complete ECG interpretation	Pacemaker signal
Arterial blood pressure invasive	Catheter & blood pressure transducer	Continuous	Heart rate	Systolic, diastolic & mean pressure	Estimates of cardiac output	Pulse pressure variation & fluid loading
Arterial blood pressure non-invasive	Inflatable cuff	Intermittent	Heart rate	Systolic diastolic pressure		
Pulse oximeter	Finger probe	Continuous	Arterial oxygen saturation	Heart rate		
Temperature	Skin sensor	Continuous	Temperature			
Respiration	Chest belt	Continuous	Respiratory rate			
Bioreactance	Electrodes	Continuous	Cardiac output	Heart rate	Stroke volume	

and his colleagues suggest that there are better methods for designing hemodynamic monitoring displays (Doig et al. 2011; Drews et al. 2008).

A more important problem relates to the integration of data from multiple bedside devices. Two examples will illustrate the problem:

1. The patient's pulse oximeter has shown a recent increase of SpO$_2$. However, the bedside monitor has no knowledge that the respiratory therapist has increased the FiO$_2$ from 30 to 40 % on the ventilator.
2. The patient's heart rate has recently increased from a dangerously low value of 45 beats per minute to 72 beats per minute. Unfortunately, the bedside monitor has no way of knowing that a nurse has increased the drip rate of a cardio-active medication.

Patients in today's ICUs can have 50 or more electronic devices attached (Mathews and Pronovost 2011). Many of these electronic devices were developed by independent companies and do not easily interface or communicate with each other. However, even though in recent years the larger monitoring companies have purchased several of the "specialty monitoring" companies, the problems still exist although it was understood more than three decades ago, and standards for bedside data interchange (CEN ISO/IEEE 11073) (Gardner et al. 1989, 1991) were developed. The **Medical Information Bus** (MIB) is the simple term used to designate CEN ISO/IEEE 11073. So, why has the MIB been a commercial failure to this point? There are multiple reasons; unfortunately, the MIB standard was designed during the time when serial communications via **RS-232** was the norm; there were no **Universal Serial Bus** (USB) interfaces or convenient wireless devices at the bedside. Furthermore, each vendor of bedside devices and ICU data management systems would like to be the "data integrator" (for a price) and thus has little incentive to adhere to standards that would allow other vendors to compete for the integrator role. The business model apparently has not worked (Kennelly and Gardner 1997; Mathews and Pronovost 2011).

In spite of the lack of interface standards, the group at Intermountain Healthcare has been actively interfacing ventilators, IV pumps and similar devices for almost three decades (Dalto et al. 1997; Vawdrey et al. 2007). Details of the importance of these interfaces and real-time clinical record capture are discussed later in, Sect. 19.4.2.

19.3.5 Challenges of Bedside Monitor Alarms

Care of the critically ill is complex and challenging. Most of these patients have medical problems or injuries that are life threatening. They might have heart problems that within minutes could result in sudden death, or they might have breathing problems that require mechanical ventilation to maintain life. As a consequence, each of these situations requires intense minute-by-minute observation with real-time, continuous physiologic monitoring. For those conditions, the requirement for record keeping, monitoring, and alarming is intense.

The requirements for record keeping are not unlike those found in a modern commercial airplane, with its sophisticated flight recorder. Each commercial aircraft has two pilots who serve the function of observers and data collectors; much as nurses, physicians and other care givers do for the critically ill. The modern airplane has sophisticated sensors and measurement systems and a multitude of displays. In addition there are complex alarm systems that warn pilots, and record those warnings about impending problems on the data and voice recorders. It would be ideal if such recording and alarming systems were available to those caring for the critically ill. However, we have not yet developed the capabilities to accomplish the level of care as is provided in a commercial airplane. As complex as flight recorder technology may be, it is not nearly as complex as understanding the systems of the human body – each being a bit different and changing over time.

We are able to record and process physiological signals with much greater capability than we did just a decade ago, but we are still learning about what data to collect, how to collect those data in a timely manner, and how to generate alerts and alarms that assist care givers to provide optimum patient care. Not only is the human body complex with its multiple internal control systems, but each individual is genetically programmed slightly differently and in many cases those control systems have been injured or rendered partially or completely inoperable by traumatic injury or medical malfunction. Thus, while we may have a few hundred models of commercial aircraft we have billions of models of human patients. Thus, although it is possible to record data minute-by-minute, and even second-by-second (and some have attempted that (Saeed et al. 2011; Burykin et al. 2011)), we are still not able to fully understand all the complex details.

A recent article in the *Boston Globe*, entitled "Patient alarms often unheard, unheeded" (Kowalczyk 2011), presents the clear expectation that bedside physiological monitors, ventilators,

IV pumps and similar devices attached to patients should provide "true and valid" alarms and that care givers will be promptly notified and provide the needed care immediately for those patients. On the other hand, a report from the New England Journal of Medicine outlines 24 electronic requirements for classification of a hospital as having a comprehensive electronic record system (Jha et al. 2009), yet recording of data from bedside physiological monitoring systems with their alarming systems and data gathering from other bedside devices such as ventilators and IV pumps were not even mentioned.

So, currently there is a curious and inexplicable set of expectations being generated for care of the critically ill patients. As a consequence there are "nitch" vendors who have built their own data gathering and recording systems and nurse charting systems; in some cases these systems include simple interfaces to allow them to acquire laboratory data and perhaps data from the administrative admissions process. They may even include bedside computers or displays to allow care givers to have access to such things as X-ray images, dictated reports and the like. But, these systems do not typically provide interfaces to *transmit* their physiological data to the hospital's EHR.

Over the past decade, the number of physiological signals that can and are being monitored has grown. With each signal and derived parameter that is added there is typically a "high" and "low" alarm added to warn the clinical staff of actual or impending patient crisis. Alarms may be highlighted on the bedside monitor's screen by using a color change or flashing indicators. Most alarms also generate a sound. Over the past 20 years, alarms have become more widespread because of a greater interest in and attention to safety, and also to litigation that may follow when an adverse incident occurs.

Figures 19.4 and 19.5 give examples of the complexity of determining whether an alarm is "true" or "false" based on two life-threatening conditions. Alarms for Ventricular Tachycardia are shown in Fig. 19.4. Figure 19.4a shows a true ventricular tachycardia (VT) alarm condition while Fig. 19.4b shows a false VT condition. Figure 19.4b has only a few seconds of ECG

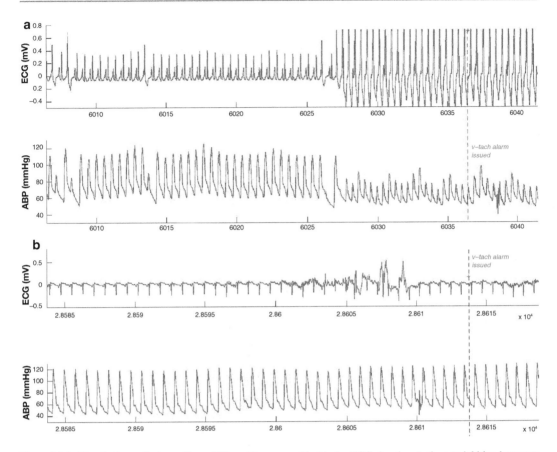

Fig. 19.4 Ventricular Tachycardia (*VT*) Alarm Conditions. (**a**) shows a true alarm; note that the ventricle is still pumping but that the arterial pulse pressure is dramatically reduced. (**b**) shows a false alarm caused by artifact in the ECG signal; note the arterial blood pressure waveform is stable during the same time interval. *ECG* Electrocardiogram, *ABP* Arterial Blood Pressure

artifact, which causes the bedside monitors' alarm detection system to issues an alarm.

Arterial hypotension alarms are shown in Fig. 19.5. Figure 19.5a shows a true arterial hypotension alarm condition while Fig. 19.5b shows a false condition. If the monitor or human observer only watches the arterial blood pressure (ABP) signal, the two conditions appear similar. However, by simultaneously following the ECG signal, the human observer will note that for some unknown reason the ABP signal displays a false representation of the patient's pulsatile blood pressure. The "unknown reason" is likely related to the catheter and tubing parts of the arterial monitoring system. Alerting the clinical staff to examine the catheter and transducer system is certainly appropriate.

Imhoff and colleagues (Imhoff and Kuhls 2006) noted from 1.6 to 14.6 alarms for each ICU patient each hour. Up to 90 % of those alarms were false! "Alarm overload" is clearly a significant issue in ICU monitoring; from clinical informatics professionals working in the ICU is needed to minimize the number of false alarms. Just noting the titles of several Editorials and articles should be informative:

1. Alarms in the intensive care unit: How can the number of false alarms be reduced? (Chambrin 2001)
2. Monitoring the monitors – beyond risk management (Thompson and Mahajan 2006)
3. Alarms and human behavior: Implications for medical alarms (Edworthy and Hellier 2006)

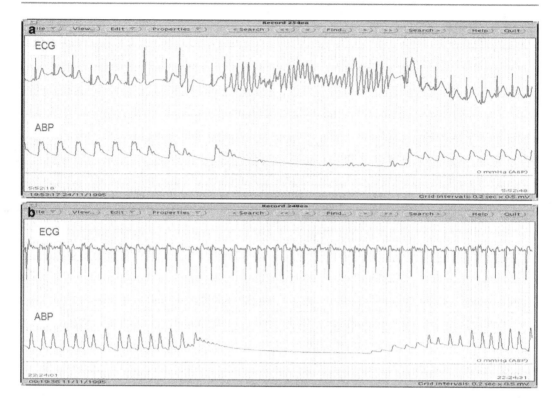

Fig. 19.5 Arterial Hypotension Alarm Conditions. (**a**) shows a true alarm; note the normal ventricular beats followed by ventricular fibrillation that renders the heart unable to generate an effective blood pressure. (**b**) shows a false alarm; note for some non-physiological reason the arterial pressure signal loses its pulsatile characteristics and then eventually it returns

4. Alarms in the intensive care unit: Too much of a good thing is dangerous: Is it time to add some intelligence to alarms? (Blum and Tremper 2010)
5. Intensive care unit alarms – How many do we need? (Siebig et al. 2010)

Biomedical informaticians, biomedical engineers and bedside monitor vendors have recently renewed their efforts to reduce false alarms and improve the relevance of existing alarms. Most of the false alarms are caused by noise or artifacts in the primary signals. To help minimize these problems, two examples are used to illustrate the challenges and opportunities to improve bedside alarms.

1. After observing over 200 h of alarms from bedside monitors and ventilators in an adult medical ICU, Gorges and his colleagues (Gorges et al. 2009) used the data recorded to recommend a two-step process that would

dramatically reduce the number of false alarms. The first step was to add a 19 s delay into the alarming system. That step by itself reduced the number of alarms by 67 %. They then noted that by having some method for automatically detecting when a patient was being suctioned, repositioned, given oral care or being washed, there would be a further 13 % reduction of ineffective alarms. By using these just these two methods, almost 80 % of the false alarms could be eliminated.

2. Using multiple signals to derive identical measures should be an effective method of reducing false alarms. As will be noted in Fig. 19.3a, b, there are five signals that can be used to derive heart rate: ECG 1, ECG 2, ECG 3, Arterial Blood Pressure, and Pulse Oximeter. Since the probability of all those signals having an artifact is smaller than any single physiological signal, "smart alarm"

algorithms that are more robust should be possible. Two investigators have developed and tested such algorithms (Zong et al. 2004; Poon 2005). The Zong pressure alarm algorithm reduced false alarms from 26.8 to 0.5 %. Poon found that the usual heart rate and rhythm alarm system produced 65.4 % false alarms, while an algorithm that integrated multiple signals generated only 31.5 % false alarms. Two other findings from the Poon study were also encouraging. By merely delaying the alarms by 10 s there was a 60 % reduction in false alarms. In addition, he found that default settings for high and low heart rate alarms were not optimized to prevent false alarms. For example, if a patient had an average heart rate of 65 beats per minute and the default low heart rate alarm was 60 beats per minute; there was an increased likelihood of false low heart rate alarms. Several bedside monitor vendors now provide these more sophisticated alarm algorithms in their newest monitors.

Still other informaticians have found different strategies to provide more accurate arterial blood pressure and cardiac arrhythmias alarm rates (Aboukhalil et al. 2008; Zhang and Szolovitz 2008). Having electronic archives of physiological waveforms that are publically available should permit development of even better smart alarm algorithms, which should lead to a reduced number of false alarms generated by bedside monitors (Saeed et al. 2011; Burykin et al. 2011).

19.3.6 Strategies for Incorporating Bedside Monitoring Data into an Integrated Hospital EHR

Three general strategies are currently used to transfer bedside monitoring data into the hospital's EHR. The first is the simplest: nurses observe data presented on the bedside monitor screen and manually "key-in" the observations into an integrated EHR. As simple as this may be to implement, such manual data collection strategy is inefficient and does not collect representative data gathered by the bedside monitor.

The second strategy used by ICU information systems, such as CareVue (Philips Healthcare) or MetaVision (iMDSoft), is to acquire vital sign data directly from the bedside monitoring system's network by using an HL7 feed (see Chap. 7). The information is automatically gathered by the ICU information system; nurses have the option of either accepting or modifying the data. In typical clinical settings, nurses perform the selection and transfer of bedside monitoring data from the ICU information system to the EHR about once an hour. These ICU information systems typically retain the high frequency bedside monitoring data and can achieve near-real-time computerized decision support. In many cases, the nurse's notes are also entered into the ICU information system – generally once per shift – and some summary vital sign information may find its way into those notes. Physician progress notes are also entered into ICU information systems in a similar fashion. Unfortunately, data in the ICU information system "EHR" may never find its way into the hospital's EHR. For these systems, the ICU data are usually archived separately. As a consequence, these data cannot be used for real-time decision making by the hospital's EHR.

The third strategy is to have the ICU information system or the hospital's EHR system automatically transfer vital sign data from the bedside monitoring system to the EHR. Most systems that automatically gather data with this strategy take a "median" of the vital sign data over a 15 min time interval to smooth the data (Warner et al 1968; Gardner et al. 1991; Vawdrey et al. 2007). This strategy provides real-time data for computations and computerized decision support for the hospital's EHR and is the preferred strategy.

There are opportunities to improve the automated data gathering from bedside monitors, especially if the false alarm rate can be minimized. In addition to acquiring 15 min median data, one may wish to detect bedside alarms and record data in the intervals just before and just after these alarms. Thus, there is still opportunity for informaticians to make major improvements in both data recording and bedside monitoring alarms.

19.4 Information Management in Intensive Care Units

19.4.1 Early Pioneering in ICU Systems

A good way to understand the implementation and use of computerized intensive care monitoring systems is to follow the development of a system that was begun 40 years ago at Intermountain Healthcare's LDS Hospital. There, a team of people developed what was known as the HELP System (Pryor et al. 1983; Kuperman et al. 1991; Gardner et al. 1999). Initially only physiological data were acquired from the bedside monitors. Nursing note charting promptly followed with ability to chart medications ordered and given, including IV drip rates. Soon, it became apparent that much of the data needed to care for these critically ill patients came from the clinical laboratory and other sites such as radiology (X-rays). As a consequence, multiple modules were added to the HELP system to support the ICUs.

About 5 years after this initial computerization of the ICUs, studies were made during structured "teaching rounds" where physicians, nurses, respiratory therapists, pharmacists and others evaluated each patient. Since the early motivation was to use the computer as a decision support system, observations were made on 63 patients during morning ICU rounds to determine what data were used by the critical care team to make clinical care decisions (Bradshaw et al. 1984). Table 19.2 outlines the data types evaluated with the percentage of time that each type of data was used to make a care decision. In addition, the source of each of the data elements was noted. Many of the data came from automated instruments in the laboratory, but a large number came from nurse observations and actions that were manually charted into the computerized record.

Finding that data from the physiological monitor accounted for only 13 % of the data was used to make treatment decisions was a surprise to the investigators. However, as described earlier, the physiological monitor serves a very crucial function during critical situations such as cardiac

Table 19.2 Data used for ICU decision making

Data types	%	Data source
Clinical & blood-gas laboratories	42	Laboratory interfaces
Drug I/O IV	22	Nurse charting & IV pump interface
Observations	21	Nurse charting & physician notes
Physiological data	13	Bedside monitor interface
Other	2	

Adapted from Bradshaw et al. 1984

arrest. The observations showed the crucial need for a fast and reliable laboratory interface *and* the importance of data that came from nurse charting. Knowing which drugs the patient was receiving, when those drugs were given, and the types and administration rates of IV medications were crucial to clinical decision making. In addition, the observations made by nurses and physicians were important for making many decisions.

As a consequence of these observations, obtaining real-time computerized nurse charting became a top priority. With paper charting systems, there is little ability to audit and improve the timeliness of nurse charting. To enhance the ease and timeliness of bedside charting, terminals were installed at each bedside. Studies were conducted and nurses were trained to chart in real-time – e.g., within 1 min of when a medication was given or a procedure was performed. As a result of these actions, the computer record became a more real-time representation of the patient's status (Oniki et al. 2003; Nelson et al. 2005). Thus, nurses, physicians, therapists, and the computerized decision support modules could reliably act on the data stored in the computer. It is surprising that even today, almost 30 years later; many computerized ICU systems do not store real-time physiological data and nurse charting information. Having made recent observations at several computerized ICUs it is surprising that the old standard of having the chart "up-to-date at the end of the shift" is still the norm. Clearly, with that philosophy and operational mode, computerized decision support and access to data by the clinical staff is sub-optimal and as a result, medical errors can and do occur.

19.4.2 Clinical Charting Systems (Nurses, Pharmacists, Physicians, Therapists)

Table 19.2 clearly shows that a major part (43 %) of the data used at LDS Hospital for decision-making during rounds came from data charted by nurses and other clinicians (Bradshaw et al. 1984). In a more recent study in the ICU at the Mayo Clinic, the team found that as they developed what they referred to as their "novel presentation" of ICU data, they required similar data content (Pickering et al. 2010).

At LDS Hospital the computerized nurse charting module allows nurses to enter patient care tasks, qualitative and quantitative data and a patient's response to therapy (Willson 1994; Willson et al. 1994; Nelson et al. 2005). In addition, nurses interact with a pharmacy module to chart all given medications including IV drip rates (Pryor 1989; Kuperman et al. 1991). Initial nurse charting at LDS Hospital was done at a central station, since at that time large cathode ray tubes were used as display devices making bedside installation of terminals inconvenient and expensive. Now, virtually all clinician charting is done at bedside terminals, primarily with a bar code scanner.

Soon after the nurse charting was implemented at LDS Hospital, respiratory therapists chose to enter their qualitative and quantitative ventilator data and care given to patients (Andrews et al. 1985; Gardner 2004). The motivation for the on-line charting was to provide clinicians with access to timely and accurate data to make patient care decisions. In addition, these data could be used to implement protocol-controlled ventilator weaning systems (East et al. 1992; Morris 2001).

To optimize the performance of routine care deemed essential for ICU patient recovery, computer "reminders" were generated (Oniki et al. 2003). For example, one of the goals of the reminders was to provide assistance in determining the required level of sedation while avoiding over-sedation. By providing the computerized reminders to nurses, charting deficiencies were reduced by 40 % and the number of deficiencies at the end of the shift was improved. To optimize care provided by the reminders, real-time charting

was required. However, during a quality improvement process, it was determined that 29 % of the medication errors that should have been prevented by on-line nurse charting were still present. A careful evaluation revealed that the actual nurse charting workflow was different than that envisioned by the system planners. Instead of charting the given medication using a bedside terminal, nurses administered the medication and then at some later time, at the central nursing station, charted that the medication had been given. As a consequence errors were occurring. After careful training and feedback with the nursing staff, the real-time charting rate increased from 40 to 75 % and remained at that level a year later. This example shows that having computerized decision support systems in place without having real-time data entry was ineffective. Conceptually, one could make the same logical observation if the ICU were operating as a tele-ICU as discussed later in this chapter.

For generations, nurses and other care givers who have used conventional paper records have had the notion that if their paper chart was up-to-date at the end of the shift then they had met their requirements for good patient care. Clearly, the above example shows that such a strategy is flawed. However, it is interesting that even today reports are being made about charting and use of data for end-of-shift nursing care exchanges and patient "handovers", suggesting that the EHR still may not be real-time (Hripcsak et al. 2011; Collins 2011). Collins and associates found that clinicians preferred oral communications compared to EHR documentation and stated that the perceptions that the EHR was a "shift behind" might have only been a manifestation of the lack of real-time charting by nurses and acquisition of real time data from bedside monitors in their ICU (Collins 2011).

An early survey of nurses and physicians use of the HELP clinical expert system was conducted in 1994 (Gardner and Lundsgaarde 1994). The investigators were encouraged by a positive response from both nurse and physician users who appreciated having the data available with interpretation and alerting features provided by the HELP system. At the time the survey was conducted, ICU charting and decision support was a major feature of the HELP system. It is exciting to note that recently, other institutions have begun to assess factors related to acceptance of an EHR in critical care (Carayon et al. 2011). The Carayon study showed that ease of use as well as data presentation strategies were major determinants of acceptability of their system.

19.4.3 Automated Data Acquisition from All Bedside Devices

As noted in Table 19.2 and from the HELP System Diagram shown in Fig. 19.2, much of the information required for patient care comes from laboratories and devices that automatically acquire data. In the upper right hand corner of the diagram, shown in block diagram format, data from the ventilator, IV pumps and the bedside monitor are noted. While most of the physiological bedside monitor vendors now acquire ECG, blood pressure, and pulse oximetry data, they do not provide access to data from ventilators or information from IV pumps. As a consequence data from these devices must be obtained by developing hardware and software interfaces (Gardner et al. 1991; Dalto et al 1997; Kennelly and Gardner 1997; Vawdrey et al. 2007).Based on studies by these investigators, it is clear that automatically collecting data from all of these devices in real-time is more timely and accurate than manually charted data collected by nurses or respiratory therapists. Although data from these devices can contain artifacts, methods for minimizing those artifacts have been implemented in operational systems.

It is unfortunate that the Medical Information Bus (MIB) standard (CEN ISO/IEEE 11073), designed to help gather data from bedside devices has not been more widely implemented (Mathews and Pronovost 2011). Section 19.3.4 gives the background of the issues. Fortunately, battery power and wireless communications with IV pumps are now widely available. By using wireless technology, interfaces with the IV pumps are fast, mobile and easy for nurses to implement and tangled wires are no longer an issue with the IV

pumps. In addition, communications with IV pumps can be carried throughout the hospital – in the operating room, while on transport and in the ICU.

Although early studies of nurses and therapists showed that computerized charting took longer than manual charting, it is almost certain with automated acquisition available today that charting takes less time and is more accurate. As a consequence, in institutions that have historically collected IV pump and ventilator data automatically, there is a commitment to collect data from every bedside monitoring device. These include, measures of urine output, fluid drainage and similar measures.

19.4.4 Establishing Collaborative Care Processes

The care of critically ill patients in the ICU requires collaboration among a diverse team of very competent care givers to achieve the best care (Clemmer et al. 1998). The teamwork and communications required in this complex care process are unusual. Establishing a collaborative "care society" does not occur without thoughtful effort, with appreciation and respect for every team member. In the early years of working with the collaborative teams of nurses, therapists, pharmacists, physicians, and informaticians and attempting to implement complex computerized charting with decision support in the ICUs, Dr. Gardner often said "this process is 80 % sociology and 20 % technology". Those observations are likely still true today – over 40 years later.

The rounds activity at LDS Hospital is an exemplar of the collaborative process. Figure 19.6 shows the clinical care team during rounds. There are physicians, house officers, advanced practice clinicians, nurses, pharmacists, respiratory therapists, dieticians, case managers, and others who gather each day to assess each patient and make key care decisions. The rounds leader is usually a physician, but each team member is considered an equal partner, providing key information (most of it stored in the computer record) and given the opportunity to discuss their interpretation and

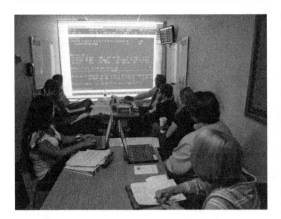

Fig. 19.6 ICU Rounds room at LDS Hospital in Salt Lake City. The compuerized ICU "rounds report" is displayed by a projector on the wall to physicians, a nurse practitioner, medical students, a respiratory therapist, a pharmacist, and a patient's family member. An important laboratory result is highlighted in red by the rounds director. Note several laptops *and* paper notes used by each of the participants

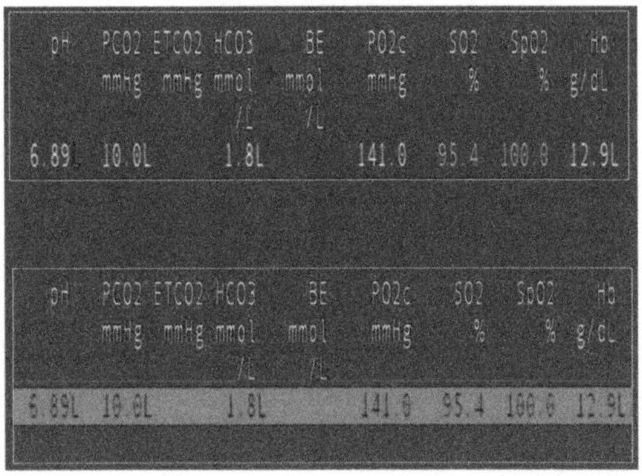

Fig. 19.7 Close-up of the Rounds Report. A set of laboratory tests is highlighted in *red* by the Rounds Director to draw attention to the abnormal findings. See Fig. 19.6 for the context of the "Rounds Room" configuration

make recommendations about the patient's care. Over decades, the social process of conducting these rounds has created a very open and cooperative environment. The purpose of rounds is to reduce errors from human factors, to give structure to the evaluation, and to make sure all sides of the decision process are considered as each member considers the decisions from their point of view. The information from the computer system is organized to support the process. The computerized record is *the* patient record. Information from other sources such as X-ray images and "free-text" reports are also readily available (Gurses and Xiao 2006).

19.4.5   ICU Change-of-Shift and Handover Issues

Recently, cognitive scientists have taken an interest in and studied the dynamic and distributed work environment in critical care medicine (Patel and Cohen 2008; Patel et al. 2008; Ahmed et al. 2011). They have studied issues such as provider task load, errors of cognition, and performance of clinicians involved in these complex tasks. The "change-of-shift" and "handover" times are especially critical and require complex exchanges of

information that must occur rapidly and efficiently. These investigators have found that errors can occur during this time because of corruption of information and a failure to transfer crucial care facts. Having the majority of the patient record in electronic form and having that data timely and accurate should allow optimization of computerized decision making tools and methods for sharing the patient data. The Rounds Report developed at LDS Hospital three decades ago (Figs. 19.7 and 19.8) and recent developments at the Mayo Clinic provide laboratory models for better understanding the issues and improving efficiency and eliminating medical errors for ICU patients during shift changes and patient handover times (Pickering et al. 2010; Ahmed et al. 2011).

19.5   Computerized Decision Support in Intensive Care

In addition to the alarms from bedside monitors, there are many other types of alerts and decision support tools that can be helpful for the care of hospitalized patients. A sampling of the types of decision support mechanism that have been reported is provided below to give the reader a sense for the breadth of capabilities that have been applied in intensive care as well as other care settings of hospitals. Key to the application of such computerized decision support tools is having access to an integrated, real-time, accurate and

Doe, Jane Q   000000000   T599   I   07/19/11   4   ADMT DIAGNOSIS: SEPSIS, PNA, ESRD   REPORT DATE: 07/29/11
DR. KRAFT, ADAM M.   SEX: F   AGE: 45   HEIGHT: 167   WEIGHT: 112.40   APACHE II: 18   MOF: 7   BSA: 2.18

CARDIOVASCULAR: 1
　LAST/MAX/MIN   SP: 96/110/ 79   DP: 47/ 55/ 22   MP: 59/ 65/ 44   HR:110/110/ 45 | CPK   60 (08:46) CPK-MB   3 (08:46)
　-- NO CARDIAC OUTPUT DATA AVAILABLE   CVP   6 (14:00) | LACT   5.4 (09:35) TRP-I   1.13 (08:46)

RENAL, FLUIDS, LYTES: 1
　IN 4271 CRYST 2996 COLLOID   BLOOD   NG/PO 1170 IRRIG   NA 139 (09:35) K   4.2 (09:35)
　OUT 5301 URINE 1650 NGOUT   DRAINS 3175   CRE 1.1 (03:09) CL 117 (09:35) CO2 19.0 (03:09)
　NET -1030 WT   WT-CHG   LOSS   476 STOOL   BUN 48 (03:09) OSM   UNA   AG   3 CAG 9.0

RESPIRATORY: 0   RR = 11;   FIO2 = 2.0; (28 22);   SPO2 = 94; (14:15);
-- BLOOD GASES --
Date/Time Samp pH PCO2 ETCO2 HCO3   BE PO2c SO2 SpO2 Hb COHb / MT O2Ct FIO2   P/F Temp AVO2 PK/PL/PP MR/SR
　　　　　　　mmHg mmHg mmol mmol mmHg   %   % g/dL % / % vol% L/M   C mL cmH2O bpm
　　　　　　　　/L /L   　　　 or %   /dl
29JUL 09:35 MIXV 7.31L 35.7   17.3L -7.8 57.7 86.7   11.4L 2.4H/0.4 13.9   2   36.0
28JUL 21:10 ART 7.38L 29.0   16.7L -7.0 110.0 95.8 98.0 11.6L 2.6H/0.6 15.8   2 5500.0 37.0
27JUL 11:55 ART   96.0   21   37.0
PO2c=Temperature corrected PO2

　-- NO SPONTANEOUS PARAMETERS WITHIN THE LAST 24 HOURS --

NEURO AND PSYCH: 0 SLEEP 6 07/29 06:00   LAST EYE OPENING 4   LAST MOTOR 6   LAST VERBAL 4   07/29 14:00
　　　　　　6   12   18   0   6
　　　　+---+---+---+----+---+---+---+---+---+---+---+---+---+---+---+---+---+---+---+---+---+
GCS   [3-15]   15   15 15   14   13   15   14
RASS [-5 to 4]
CAM-ICU[+/-/S]
PAIN   [0-10]   0   3 5 8 7   7   7   10   6
ICP   [0-99]

COAGULATION: 2
　PT 38.9 (03:09) INR   4.0 (03:09) PTT   75 (11:28) PLATELETS 30 (03:09) FIBR 172 (11:25) D-DIMER
B-TYPE NATRIURETIC PEPTIDE:
　BNP

METABOLIC --- NUTRITION: 0   BEE 1806
KCAL   0 GLU 165 (03:09) ALB   1.6 (03:09) CA 7.2 (03:09) TRG
KCAL/N2 0 UUN   I-CA   1.2 (09:35) PO4 4.3 (08:46) MG 3.1   (03:09) CHOL

GI, LIVER, AND PANCREAS: 3 / 0
　HCT 33.0 (03:09) TOT BILI 5.7 (03:09) ALT 65 (03:09) ALKPO4 102 (03:09) LDH   LIPASE   AMONIA
　GUAIAC   DIR BILI   AST 40 (03:09) GGT   AMYL   GAST Ph

INFECTION:
　WBC 13.0 (03:09) TEMP 36.7 (28 21)   DIFF: EARLY FORMS 0, P 88, L 3, M 4, E 5(03:09)
　Positive Micro Results, F10 for more information

SKIN AND EXTREMITIES: Braden Score 15 (28 22)

PALLIATIVE CARE:
　Symptom Rx: Last Family Conference: Goals of Care:

ICU ROUTINES:
　DVT Prophylaxis: Stress Ulcer Prophylaxis:PANTOPRAZOLE (ProT Activity / Fall Risk:

PROTOCOLS:
　Feed___ Vent___ Oxygenation___ Insulin___ Fever___ Sed___ Heparin___ K___ Brain___

MEDICATIONS:
　HYDROmorphOne (DILAUDID)   1.9 MG   LACTULOSE, SOLUTION   60 GM   URSODIOL (ACTIGALL), CAP 900 MG
　ASPIRIN, TABLET CHEWABLE 324 MG   SODIUM CHLORIDE 0.9%, IV 1300 ML   OMEPRAZOLE (PriloSEC), C 20 MG
　CefTAZIDime (FORTAZ), AD 6000 MG   POTASSIUM CHLORIDE (10%) 20 MEQ   INSULIN ASPART (NovoLOG) 3 UNITS
　LINEZOLID (ZYVOX), IV SO 1200 MG   SODIUM CHLORIDE 0.9% (SA   8 EA   **INJ** HydrocorTISone (50 MG
　RiFAXimin (XIFAXAN), TAB 1100 MG   LACTATED RINGERS, IV SOL 1000 ML   BIVALIRUDIN (ANGIOMAX), 32 MG
　SODIUM CHLORIDE 0.9%, IV 25.6 ML   MESALAMINE (PENTASA), CA 4000 MG
　POTASSIUM PHOSPHATE/NACL 10.1 MMOL ONDANSETRON (ZOFRAN), VI 4 MG

INVASIVE LINE: TYPE SITE/.../DAY   Central line: R/ 9;
　　　　　　　　--- End of Report ---

Fig. 19.8 Printed 24 h Rounds Report from Intermountain Healthcare's LDS Hospital

coded EHR. Most of the examples noted are from the HELP system (Gardner et al. 1999). A key function of the HELP system is that the computerized decision support system is activated when new patient data are added to the patient's database, the process is called "data-driven" decision making. An example would be when the pO_2 is put into the medical record an instruction is given to the respiratory therapist to modify the FiO_2 or PEEP accordingly. Some functions of the HELP system such as alerts require that computerized decision support be activated at specific times and that process is called "time driven" decision making. An example would be to remind the nurse the next glucose check is due when on an insulin drip, or instructing the computer to automatically calculate today's APACHE score and update all the reports at 06:00.

19.5.1 Laboratory Alerts

During the developmental period of the HELP system in the 1980's, it became apparent that on occasion life-threatening laboratory results were not being acted upon promptly. On acute care nursing floors, the initial alert response time averaged from 5.1 to 58.2 h (Bradshaw et al. 1989). By posting alerts on computer terminals on nursing floors, the average response time was reduced to 3.6 h. Then a flashing light, similar to those found on road maintenance vehicles, was installed on each nursing floor. The average response time then decreased to 6 min but the light was very annoying to the nursing staff (Bradshaw et al. 1989). Later, a sophisticated nurse paging system was set up that paged the particular nurse caring for the patient with the laboratory alert and required nurses to acknowledge the alerts (Tate et al. 1995). The new pager system was equally effective and less annoying. Similar work was done by Shabot and associates at Cedars-Sinai Hospital in Los Angeles using a Blackberry pager (Shabot 1995). Since that time, wireless communications technology has improved dramatically and a variety of even better feedback mechanisms are now available. As a result of the early computerized laboratory alerting experiences, it was surprising to find a 2011 review article on the topic which concluded "The existing evidence suggests that the problem of missed test results is considerable and reported negative impacts on patients warrants the exploration of solutions. Attention must be paid to integration of solutions, particularly those which involve information technology, into clinical work practices." (Callen et al. 2011)

19.5.2 Ventilator Weaning Management and Alarm System

Weaning patients from ventilators was one of the first applications of a computerized expert system to routine patient care at Intermountain Healthcare's LDS Hospital. As a result of the nurse and respiratory therapist charting described earlier, it was possible to develop and test computerized ventilator management protocols. Patient therapy was controlled by protocol 95 % of the time and 90 % of the protocol instructions were followed by clinicians. Several of the computerized instructions not followed were due to ventilator charting errors. Patients cared for with the computerized protocol had required less positive pressure in the ventilator system, and physiological measures were disturbed less. The investigators concluded that such protocols could make the ventilator weaning processes "less mystifying, simpler, and more systematic" (East et al. 1992). Since that early work, several other investigators have implemented similar ventilator weaning algorithms.

In the process of implementing automated charting of ventilator parameters at LDS Hospital (Vawdrey et al. 2007), it became clear that critical ventilator alarms were being missed. As discussed earlier, alarm sounds emitted from ventilators were blended with bedside monitor alarm sounds. As a consequence, when a patient became disconnected from a ventilator the alarms could be missed (Evans 2005). Once this situation was recognized, an enhanced notification system was implemented. Figure 19.9 illustrates a ventilator disconnect alarm presented on the patient's bedside display and on every other computer display in the same ICU. The efficacy and user acceptance of the new alarm system has enhanced patient safety and allowed documentation of this important clinical event.

19.5.3 Infectious Diseases Monitoring – Antibiotic Assistant

Early data available to the HELP system at LDS Hospital included microbiology culture results.

Several programs were developed to present these results and predict pathogens and list most likely empiric antibiotic regimens. Based on the physician use of and approval of computerized **antibiograms**, empiric antibiotic suggestions, and a therapeutic antibiotic monitor, an anti-infective agent management program known as the "antibiotic assistant" was developed (Evans

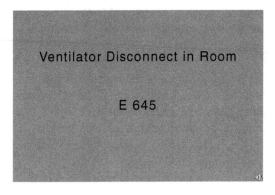

Ventilator Disconnect in Room

E 645

Fig. 19.9 Ventilator Disconnect Alarm. This is for the patient in Room E645, but it is displayed on every computer screen in that particular ICU

et al. 1998). Figure 19.10 shows an example screen display from the program. The screen display was designed by infectious disease and critical care physicians who wanted a one-screen display of relevant data and recommendations. The upper section displays pertinent patient data, the middle sections displays suggested anti-infective agents along with dose, route and interval, and the lower panel provides quick and easy access to other relevant patient information. Over the past decade this antibiotic assistant has been implemented in Intermountain Healthcare's Primary Children's Medical Center (Mullett et al. 2001) and ten other large hospitals operated by Intermountain Healthcare.

19.5.4 Adverse Drug Event Detection and Prevention

Detection and prevention of **adverse drug events** (ADEs) has been a long term goal of care givers, the World Health Organization (WHO), and

```
000000000 Doe, Jane Q      E606      67yr      F          Dx:ABD SEPSIS
» Max 24 hr WBC=21.0↓ (21.3)        Admit:07/27/11.14:55        Max 24hr    Temp=38.7↑ (38.2)
Patient's Diff shows a left shift, max 24hr bands = 22 ↑ (11)
» RENAL FUNCTION: Decreased,  CrCl = 50    Max 24hr  Cr= 1.0↓ (1.1)     IBWeight: 58kg
» ANTIBIOTIC ALLERGIES: Ampicillin,
» CURRENT ANTIBIOTICS:
1.  07/27/11      5DAYS   VANCOMYCIN (VANCOMYCIN),    VIAL 1500.        Q 12 hrs
2.  08/01/11      2DAYS   AMPHOTERICIN B (FUNGIZONE), VIAL 35 .        Q 24 hrs
    Total amphotericin given = 71mg   K= 3.6mg/dl 08/03/11   MAG= 2.5mg/dl   08/03/11 » »
» IDENTIFIED PATHOGENS                    SITE                  COLLECTED
p Gram negative Bacilli                  Peritoneal Fluid      07/27/11.17:12
  Yeast                                  Peritoneal Fluid      07/27/11.17:12
  Torulopsis glabrata                    Peritoneal Fluid      07/27/11.17:12
» THERAPEUTIC SUGGESTION     DOSAGE       ROUTE  INTERVAL
      Imipenem               500mg        IV     *q12h   (infuse over 1hr)
      Amphotericin B         35mg         IV     q24h    (infuse over 2-4hrs)
*Adjusted based on patient's renal function.
-- The therapeutic suggestion should not replace clinical judgment--
P=Prelim; Susceptibilities based on antibiogram or same pathogen w/ suscept.
<1>Micro  <2>OrganismSuscept,  <3>Drug Info,  <4>ExplainLogic,  <5>Empiric Abx,
<6>Abx Hx  <7>ID Rnds,  <8>Lab/Abx Levels,  <9>Xray,  <10>Data Input Screen,
<Esc>EXIT,  <F1>Help,  <0>UserInput,  <.>OutpatientModels,  <+orF12>Change Patient
↑↓,  ORDER:  <*>Suggested Abx,  <Enter>Other Abx,  </>D/C Abx,  <->Modify Abx,
```

Fig. 19.10 Screen Display of "Antibiotic Assistant". The display provides relevant patient data, current antibiotics, and antibiotic therapy suggestion for this particular patient as well, at the *bottom* of the screen is a list of sites for review of other important patient information

```
              INTERMOUNTAIN MEDICAL CENTER
            POSSIBLE ADVERSE DRUG EVENT REPORT
                     FOR 29 AUG 2011
                 FOR 2 DAYS BACK ON TICU
                  PRINT TIME:  8/29/11.10:51

***** 08/26/11.17:55   SBP < 90, DOWN 20 WITHIN 48HR & ON HYPOTENSIVE
DRUG
@PAT: 000000001 Doe, Roger Q.          82Y  M  S999  MR#: 111111
DOC: 00009  Jones, John L.
ADMITTED: 08/21/11.20:15  ADMIT DIAG: SYCOPE

***** 08/27/11.00:10   PATIENT W/ DOUBLING OF CR
@PAT: 000000002 Lake, Brent H.         64Y  M  S999  MR#: 111121
DOC: 00008  Smith, James Q.
ADMITTED: 08/13/11.00:40  ADMIT DIAG: VASCULAR INSUFFICIENCY

***** 08/27/11.01:25   GLUCOSE > 350 mg/dL
@PAT: 00000003 Wright, Ruth P.         73Y  F  S999  MR#:  111131
DOC: 00007  Young, Andrew R.
ADMITTED: 08/23/11.00:09  ADMIT DIAG: PULMONARY EDEMA
```

Fig. 19.11 Possible Adverse Drug Events (ADEs) for two days for the TICU at Intermountain Healthcare's Intermountain Medical Center

the U.S. Food and Drug Administration (FDA) (Classen et al. 1991). Physicians, pharmacists, and informaticians at Intermountain Healthcare's LDS Hospital developed a computer-based ADE monitor that detected a variety of "triggers" in the EHR that could indicate potential ADEs, such as sudden medication stop orders, medication antidote ordering, and specific abnormal laboratory and physiologic results. Pharmacists followed up on each ADE alert and each was verified and categorized. During an 18 month period, 36,653 hospitalized patients were monitored and 731 true ADEs occurred in 648 patients – 701 were classified as moderate or severe. Only 92 of the ADEs were identified by traditional voluntary reporting methods. Using this knowledge, the investigators developed methods for preventing ADEs. An example is the nurse charting work of Nelson (Nelson et al. 2005). Figure 19.11 shows a printout of "possible Adverse Drug Events ADE for 2 days in the Thoracic ICU (TICU) at Intermountain Healthcare's Intermountain Medical Center.

Classen and colleagues followed up their earlier surveillance system for adverse drug events. They found that the attributable length of stay and costs of hospitalization for ADEs were substantial. If a patient had an ADE there was an increased length of stay of 1.74 days, an increased cost of $2,013, and an increased risk of death of 1.88 (Classen et al. 1997).

Even with the enhanced computerized methods for detecting, preventing and monitoring adverse drug events, there is still room for improvement (Petratos et al. 2010). Critically ill patients are particularly susceptible to ADEs due to their unstable physiology, complex therapeutic medications, and the large percentage of IV medications (Hassan et al. 2010). Better systems must be developed and implemented to prevent ADEs.

19.5.5 IV Pump and Medications Monitoring

Intravenous medication administration occurs in 90 % of hospitalized patients; virtually every ICU patient is connected to an IV pump to receive fluids, nutrients, and medications. Although so-called "smart pumps" have been developed to minimize errors, those pumps are not yet integrated with the EHR and as a result are not capable of helping to prevent IV administration errors. Evans and associates at LDS Hospital have recently used cabled or wireless IV pumps integrated with the HELP system to enhance notification of IV pump programming errors (Evans et al. 2010). The medication charting system can detect and provide real-time alerts whenever an initial or potential pump rate programming error occurs. A set of 23 high-risk medications are monitored by the HELP system. Whenever IV pump flow rate for one of these medications is outside the acceptable range, a visual alert such as that shown in Fig. 19.12 is presented on the bedside display and on all other computer displays in the same ICU. Over a 2 year period, they found that there were alerts on 4 % of the initial or dose rate changes or about 1.4 alerts per day. Of those alerts, 14 % were found to have prevented potential patient harm.

Clearly the monitoring and alerting system for ICU patients involves quite a different process and strategy than the usual bedside monitoring alarms. However, by having the integrated clinical record and the computerized decision support system available, these investigators have made major advances in minimizing ADEs and providing higher quality patient care.

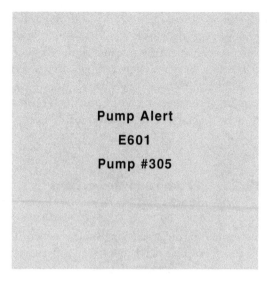

Pump Alert

E601

Pump #305

Fig. 19.12 IV Pump Alert. This is for Pump #305 located in Room E601, but it is displayed on every computer screen in that particular ICU

19.5.6 Predictive Alarms and Syndrome Surveillance

In recent years a series of **machine learning** and surveillance methods have been developed to assist clinician decision makers in the care of complex care situations (Lee and Mark 2010). The work of Lee and Mark at Harvard/MIT presents a methodology that has great promise (Lee et al. 2010). These investigators used machine learning to see if they could use pattern recognition approaches to predict impending hypotension in intensive care patients. Using the high-resolution vital sign trends from the **MIMIC II Database**, they trained their system to predict impending hypotension. Although the results were not perfect, they were able to identify patients at higher risk for developing hypotensive episodes within the subsequent 2 h, thus alerting busy clinicians to be vigilant to impending events. As of this writing, the system still needs to be tested in a clinical environment.

Herasevich and his associates at the Mayo Clinic have mined their Multidisciplinary Epidemiology and Translational Research in Intensive Care Data Mart to explore the ability to detect high-risk syndromes in the critically ill and to alert clinicians if therapy has not yet been started (Herasevich et al. 2009; 2010; 2011). These investigators have provided excellent recommendations for development and use of large databases to allow better understanding of the complexities of patients who are critically ill.

19.5.7 Protocols Versus Guidelines

Computerized decision support tools are intended to aid clinicians and enable them to deliver evidence-based care consistently. Several terms, including guidelines and protocols are used to describe these decision support tools. Protocols (also called algorithms) are detailed and provide explicit instructions for each clinical decision. In contrast, guidelines are more general statements of concepts and provide less instruction about specific clinical decisions (Morris 2003). Computerized protocols can be configured to contain much more detail than textual guidelines or paper-based flow diagrams. Several case studies of computerized protocols such as mechanical ventilation and management of intravenous fluid and hemodynamic factors in patients with acute respiratory distress syndrome have been studied. Protocols currently used at Intermountain Healthcare's Salt Lake City Hospitals are:

Computerized Protocols:

Insulin infusion for glucose control,

Ventilator management and weaning,

Blood ordering,

Antibiotic assistant,

Total Parenteral Nutritional,

Paper Based Protocols:

- Potassium replacement,
- Magnesium replacement,
- Phosphate replacement,
- Subcutaneous insulin correction factor,
- Heparin anticoagulation,
- Fluid optimization,
- Lasix Drip
- Intracranial pressure control,
- Sepsis treatment,
- Enteral Nutrition
- Pneumonia antibiotic selection

Although the paper based protocols could be computerized, most are very simple, consisting of one or two pages usually containing a simple look-up table. The reason they have not been computerized is for convenience: it is easier and faster for the nurse to have the protocol on their clipboard and use the table rather than log onto the computer to get the recommendation. When the protocols are more complicated and require following complex flow diagrams or performing a set of calculations, the computer does a better job with fewer errors.

19.6   Tele-ICU Development

Tele-ICU is defined as the provision of care to critically ill patients by health care professionals located remotely. Tele-ICU clinicians use audio, video, and electronic links to assist the bedside caregivers in monitoring patients to help provide best practice and to help with the execution of optimized patient care plans. These types of systems have the potential of improving patient outcomes by having shorter response times to bedside monitor alarms and to abnormal laboratory values, initiating life-saving therapies, providing best practice more frequently, and providing expertise to smaller or remote ICUs where subspecialists are not readily available (Lilly et al. 2011). Historically Tele-ICU concepts date back to the mid-1980s, but it was not until the early 2000's that there was a dramatic increase in the use of such systems (Breslow 2007).

19.6.1   What is Tele-ICU and How Does It Work?

Tele-ICU has built on the concepts of computerized patient monitoring discussed earlier in this chapter. The real-time, electronic patient record is fundamental to making Tele-ICU care practical. The clinical information system is one of the keys to allow clinicians not physically present in the ICU to be able to suggest appropriate care. The HELP system provides an example of such a clinical information system. Enhanced bedside data acquisition and alarm systems, as well as clinical decision support systems (such as those

Table 19.3 Comparison of typical ICU care processes with tele-ICU care processes

Typical current ICU	Tele-ICU
Bedside monitor alarms	Physiological trend alerts
	Abnormal laboratory value alerts
	Review of response to alerts
	Off-site team rounds
Daily goal sheet	Electronic detection of non-adherence
	Real-time auditing
	Nurse manager audits
	Team audits
Telephone case review initiated by house staff or affiliate practitioner	Workstation review initiated by intensivists including electronic medical record, imaging studies, interactive audio and video of patient, integrated with nurse and respiratory therapist and assessment of responses to therapy

Adapted from Lilly et al. 2011

described above) are required if remote clinicians are to provide practical and effective care for patients located in multiple remote ICUs (Rosenfeld et al. 2000; Celi et al. 2001; Breslow 2007, and Lilly et al. 2011). Table 19.3, gives an overview of the differences between a typical ICU with no electronic record compared with a Tele-ICU.

19.6.2   Future Informatics Impact on Tele-ICU Care

Recent findings of the impact of Tele-ICU are encouraging and exciting. Patients receiving such care have lower hospital and ICU mortality and shorter hospital and ICU lengths of stay. Measures of adherence to best care practices are increased and complication rates are decreased (Lilly et al. 2011). However, the investigators pointed out that they had to implement major process and culture changes in their "reengineering" activities to make their system work (Lilly et al. 2011). An editorial accompanying the Lilly article outlines challenges still to be studied and understood about Tele-ICU (Kahn 2011a). Since many changes were made from the typical ICU to the Tele-ICU intervention, simply adding better electronic data recording, electronic physiological surveillance and computerized decision support may have provided the same benefit – independent of the telemedicine feature. Informaticians clearly have exciting opportunities to improve care of critically ill patients and answer important process and intervention questions.

19.7 Implementation Strategies for ICU Systems with Computerized Decision Support

In the process of developing, testing, evaluating, and maintaining the HELP system for several decades, we have come to realize the complexity and challenges of implementing a sophisticated computerized medical decision support system (Gardner 2004). Five steps describe the primary issues and challenges. Those steps are illustrated in Table 19.4. A brief discussion of each of the steps is outlined below.

19.7.1 Acquiring the Data

A fundamental part of any computerized decision support system, just as with any human clinical decision support system, is the acquisition of data. Clinicians develop observational, interpersonal and technical skills as they collect accurate patient data. Likewise, a computerized decision support system depends on high-quality, timely data. In a typical ICU today, most medical data continue to be collected on paper flow sheets. Some of the data on those flow sheets are now being entered into computerized patient records in a structured and coded format while others (such as the progress note) are be stored in a free text format (either handwritten or typed) (Celi et al. 2001; Pickering et al. 2010; Ahmed et al. 2011; Hripcsak et al. 2011). As noted in Chap. 8, natural language processing of free text to obtain coded and structured information has seen dramatic improvement over the past decade; however, the process is still not perfect.

As system implementers look at acquiring and entering clinical data for computerized decision support they must decide:

- *Who* should enter the data: automated acquisition from electronic instruments (such as the bedside monitor) versus manual entry using a keyboard, bar code reader, touch screen, voice input or some similar method
- *When* to enter the data: accurate ICU decision making often requires data to be acquired in a timely manner, sometimes within 1 min of an event the decision about:

Table 19.4 Clinical Computerized Decision Making Strategies for ICU and Patient Monitoring Systems

#	Step	Activities & issues	Implementation time
1	Acquire the required clinical data	Decide WHAT data is required. Issues such as free-text with Natural Language Processing (NLP) vs. coded data. What coding system to use. Deciding WHO, WHEN, WHERE, HOW and HOW MUCH data will be entered.	5+ years & continuous update
2	Establishing the quality and timeliness of the required data	Is the data accurate? Is the data entered promptly? Is the data representative?	2+ years & continuous update
3	Decide how & where to present the data	Display media - Printer, terminal, hand held device (cell phone, iPhone, iPad) format, (e.g. numbers vs. graphics), who gets to see the data and how. (Patient, Insurer, etc.) How to handle life-threatening alert notifications?	6 months & continuous update
4	Decide on the decision rules	Who is the expert? Simple rule structure (IF, THEN, ELSE) vs. complex structures such as neural nets, Bayesian, logistic regression, etc. How to implement alerts, alarms and protocols?	6 months & continuous update
5	Executing the decision presenting the results	Decision support computer system executes the decision rules based on the data in the EHR and presents the decisions	Seconds

Adapted from Gardner 2004

- *Where to enter the data*: this automated data will naturally be acquired from the bedside monitor or instrument located at the bedside; manual data entry should optimally occur at the bedside as well
- *How* data should be collected: methods should take into account the occurrence of artifacts in the patient data; many EHR systems allow nurses to review and validate bedside vital sign data minutes to hours after they are collected, although this process does not meet the requirement for real-time data collection and can lead to "human" and computerized decision support errors (Nelson et al. 2005; Vawdrey et al. 2007)
- *How much* to collect: this is particularly an issue with systems such as bedside monitors that *can* generate a heart rate, systolic and diastolic blood pressure value for each heartbeat, resulting in hundreds of thousands of values per day; except for very special situations, the collection of such intensive data collection is inappropriate, but deciding on the appropriate amount to collect is not a trivial consideration and depends on the individual patient and the stage of their medical care

The process of developing and implementing the systems for acquiring data involves not only technology, but adapting that technology to the human users; training those users to properly use the system is complex and difficult. Consequently, developers and adopters of such systems should plan for and be prepared for challenges that may take 5 years to implement and optimize, with continuous monitoring and updating after the initial implementation required.

19.7.2 Establishing Quality and Timeliness of the Required Data

There are still major problems with acquiring ICU data either automatically or manually (Gardner et al. 1989, 1991; Dalto et al. 1997; Nelson et al. 2005; Vawdrey et al. 2007). Data from bedside monitors, ventilators and IV pumps should be acquired automatically with a real-time

technology such as the Medical Information Bus. Data thus acquired is timely and by appropriate signal processing methods can be validated (Dalto et al. 1997; Vawdrey et al. 2007; Ahmed et al. 2011; Lilly et al. 2011). Changes in ventilator settings such as FiO_2 may only be present for a few minutes, but blood-gas measurements taken during that time interval will be misinterpreted if only manual electronic charting is used. Similar interpretation errors were found to occur with IV pump drip rate charting when manual charting methods were compared to automated acquisition. Gathering accurate, representative and timely computerized ICU data requires attention to detail and careful planning to assure its quality. When transitioning from a manual, on-paper charting system to a computerized system, the processes of gathering and recording data must change dramatically. As a consequence, establishing mechanisms to gather appropriate data may take 2 or more years, with continuous effort directed at updating quality processes.

19.7.3 Presentation of Data

Once data have been collected, their quality verified, and the results stored, one must decide how the data should be presented. Currently, most data are presented on a colorful screen similar to that shown in Fig. 19.7. However, some care givers will still prefer a paper copy, so the Rounds Report shown in Fig. 19.8 might be required. Still others will prefer to view these reports on their iPhones, iPads or other mobile devices. For ICU patients, it is clear that specialized reports must be developed. The traditional method of segmented reporting (separate reports for laboratory data, vital signs reports, medication lists, etc.) has proven inadequate (Clemmer 2004; Ahmed et al. 2011). The ICU group at Mayo Clinic has recently presented their "ICU Summary Report" (Pickering et al. 2010), which they have sought to patent. Thus, one can see there is value in the integration of and presentation of data. As of this writing, there is probably not a single ICU summary report that will satisfy all ICU users. Thus, such reports will require special effort for each institution and perhaps even each ICU within that institution. For example, the report generated for a thoracic ICU is unlikely to be identical to that required by the neonatal ICU. Accomplishing such tasks typically requires 6 months or more, with continuous ongoing effort to update the report as new data are acquired and care givers needs evolve.

19.7.4 Establishing the Decision Rules and Knowledge Base

Deciding on the decision rules that should be installed in a computerized ICU decision support system is difficult. Health care is currently driven by implementing evidence-based protocols. However, few of these protocols have been computerized. The long-standing work with the HELP system and some recent exciting work being done at the Mayo Clinic and at the University of Massachusetts are exceptions (Clemmer 2004; Morris 2000; East et al. 1992; Ahmed et al. 2011; Lilly et al. 2011). Using a consensus process to develop treatment-decisions is essential. However, generating a consensus is a tedious, difficult and slow process. At the moment, the consensus process involving all the clinical care-givers in the ICU is the best approach, as rules developed by individuals are often not widely accepted or used. However, in some departments there may be trusted clinical leaders who become the "agreed to" local expert. Developing the rules for clinical decision support is complex and those rules are always subject to change. Development of appropriate rules can take up to 6 months and the rules will need to be continuously reviewed and updated (Gardner 2004; Ahmed et al. 2011; Lilly et al. 2011).

19.7.5 Execution of Computerized Decision Support Rules and Measuring Care Improvement

Once the four earlier steps have been completed, the rules must be included in the institution's ICU system. In the past, commercially available ICU EHRs and stand-alone ICU systems did not have convenient methods for programming and execution of computerized decision support rules. However, recent surveys by Sitting and Wright have shown that more and more commercial vendor systems have improved capability for providing clinical computerized decision support (Sittig et al. 2011; Wright et al. 2011).

Once computerized decisions are made, they must be used to notify clinicians so that the feedback can be used to more effectively care for patients. The most common notification method is presentation on the computer screen when a clinician is interacting with the computer in some task such as order entry or charting. However, as noted in some earlier examples such as laboratory alerting and ventilator disconnect alerts, the issues of *how* to notify and *who* to notify are much more challenging (Tate et al. 1995; Shabot 1995). Further, verifying that such feedback results in the appropriate care is becoming ever more important. Research continues on identifying the most efficient and effective notification methods. Just as with the false alarms generated by bedside monitors, alarm feedback from computer systems must present timely and accurate recommendations with a minimum number of false alarms.

19.8 Opportunities for Future Development

Throughout this chapter, we have discussed many challenges and opportunities that remain in the field of patient monitoring systems. There are still important opportunities in the development of better and more effective bedside monitoring systems, especially in the area of maximizing true alarms and minimizing false alarms. Integrating clinical data from a broad variety of hospital and personal records is still challenging and important. Being able to apply computerized decision support systems to warn of life-threatening situations or advise caregivers about optimum patient treatment strategies is still a relatively new aspect of health care. Development of patient care protocols and then having them be "executable" by computers, especially for ICU patients, is also a new and exciting field of endeavor. Below are other areas of opportunity for informaticians to enhance the field of patient monitoring. Enjoy the challenges and opportunities that these and similar tasks will give you. We still believe that applying informatics in the ICU is a "contact sport" – that is you must be involved at the patient care level and work with the incredibly talented clinical teams to maximize the benefits that biomedical informaticians can provide.

19.8.1 Evaluation of Value of Computerized ICU Care Processes

Challenges and opportunities lies in proving the value of health information systems. A recent review by Chaudhry and associates assessing the impact of health information technology on the quality, efficiency and cost of medical care is illustrative of the challenge (Chaudhry et al. 2006). An even more sobering report was presented by Karsh and associates (Karsh et al. 2010). These investigators suggest that not only is rate of adoption of health information technology low, but such technology may not improve quality of care or reduced costs.

19.8.2 Genomics Applied to the Critically Ill

The application of computational biology and new biomarker testing technologies to the critically ill and injured has exciting potential. The ability to detect the appropriate biomarkers of changes in gene expression induced by infection, shock, trauma or other inflammatory triggers is moving forward rapidly (Cobb et al. 2008). Today, the diagnosis of infections uses genomic data to detect bacterial DNA and rapidly assist in the selection of the most appropriate antibiotics.

19.8.3 Closed-Loop Therapy

Since the early 1950's, when physicians began to understand control system theory, there has been a fascination with having control systems that "closed the loop" without the need for any human intervention. Implantable defibrillators and pacemakers are examples closed-loop devices. The natural outcome of the remarkable developments discussed in this chapter would seem to lead to closed-loop control of physiological processes. While many of the problems discussed earlier in this chapter continue to hamper efforts to develop such systems, we believe that the opportunity to do so is drawing near (Gardner et al. 2009).

19.8.4 Sharing Decision Support Rules – Alerts, Alarms and Protocols

Once alerts, alarms and protocols are developed that are shown to be effective in improving patient care, it will be incumbent on care givers to use those tools. Unfortunately, many of these decision support rules being developed have not been designed to use computerized decision making systems. As a consequence, the biomedical informatics community will need to be much more active in the development and implementation process of sharable decision support rules for ICU patient care (see Chap. 22).

19.8.5 Commercialization of Patient Monitoring Systems

Initially patient monitoring systems such as the HELP System (Gardner et al. 1999) were "home grown" by informatics research centers. Later, several hardware and software vendors began to supply specialty systems designed to interface with bedside monitors and other bedside devices. More recently, vendors of large hospital information systems have begun to adapt their systems to allow automatic acquisition of data from bedside monitors and also provide the level of nursing charting that meets the needs of the ICU patient. Today, companies like Philips, General Electric, Siemens and others have not only developed bedside monitors, but have also developed primarily stand-alone charting systems.

At the moment, there are a variety of alternative options for critical care units as they seek to have Patient Monitoring Systems. These include the following:

1. Local Development – Home grown
2. Vendor developed ICU System – Stand-alone
3. Vendor developed ICU System – Integrated with laboratory and Hospital EHR
4. Software interface applications from bedside monitors to existing Hospital EHR
5. Mixture of existing Hospital EHR systems with planning to have an integrated ICU system

One of the opportunities for clinical informaticians will be to help their hospitals select systems that enhance patient monitoring by not only enabling automated and real time acquisition of data from bedside monitors and bedside care devices such as IV pumps, but that will also enable clinicians to chart in real time such that computerized decision support systems will be available to optimize patient care.

19.8.6 Establishment of the Subspecialty of Clinical Informatics

With the leadership of the American Medical Informatics Association (AMIA), recommendations for the content of and the "fellowship" education for the medical subspecialty of clinical informatics has been established (Gardner et al. 2009; Safran et al. 2009). Initially this subspecialty will only be for physicians. However, plans are under way to allow engineers, computer scientists and informaticians to eventually be able to achieve a clinical informatics certification. The opportunity to receive training and practice in the field of clinical informatics will provide a major boost to the profession and will have an energizing effect on advancing the implementation of and improvement of patient monitoring systems.

Suggested Readings

Greenes, R. A. (Ed.). (2007). *Clinical decision support: The road ahead*. Burlington: Elsevier Inc.

Shabot, M. M., & Gardner, R. M. (Eds.). (1994). *Decision support systems in critical care*. Boston: Springer.

Kuperman, G. J., Gardner, R. M., & Pryor, T. A. (1991). *HELP: A dynamic hospital information system*. New York: Springer.

Clemmer, T. P. (2004). Computers in the ICU: Where we started and where we are now. *J Crit Care, 19*, 204–207. PMID 15648035.

Gardner, R.M. (2009). Clinical decision support systems: The fascination with closed-loop control. *IMIA Yearbook of Medical Informatics*, 12–21. PMID 19855866

Morris, A. H. (2001). Rational use of computerized protocols in the intensive care unit. *Crit Care, 5*, 249–254. PMID 11737899.

Questions for Discussion

1. Describe how the integration of information from multiple bedside monitoring signals, the pharmacy and clinical laboratory data can help improve alarm systems used in an ICU.
2. How would you decide whether to buy a "stand-alone" ICU patient monitoring system versus an integrated EHR system?
3. How do care providers impact the installation and optimization of real-time data collection and real-time decision support?
4. Perhaps "real-time data collection" and "computerized decision support" are not necessary. How would you assess these issues? Is there sufficient literature to validate or disprove your supposition? If not, what is missing?

5. How would you go about selecting the optimum data for monitoring and improving the care of a critically ill patient?
6. How would you optimize a patient monitoring system that you were building or buying to provide the most accurate, timely and helpful computerized decision support capabilities? Be specific and give literature references to support your optimization plan.
7. If you were the Chief Clinical Information Officer of a large hospital without data from the ICU integrated into your EHR system, what factors would you have to consider to implement such a system AND to apply computerized clinical decision support to optimize such a system? How long do you think it would take to implement such a system?

Imaging Systems in Radiology

20

Bradley Erickson and Robert A. Greenes

After reading this chapter you should know the answers to these questions:

- What are the key components of Medical Image interpretation?
- What are the roles of the Radiology Information System (RIS), Picture Archiving and Communication System (PACS), Computer-Aided Diagnosis (CAD), and Advanced Visualization Systems in a typical medical imaging department?
- How does the DICOM standard differ from HL-7 in its information model structure?

20.1 Introduction

In Chap. 9, we introduce the concept of **digital images** as a fundamental data type that, because of its ubiquity, must be considered in many applications. We define biomedical **imaging informatics** as the study of methods for generating, manipulating, managing, extracting, and representing imaging information, plus integrating images in many biomedical applications.

In this chapter we continue the study of imaging informatics, begun in Chap. 9, by describing many of the methods for generating and manipulating images, particularly as applied to the brain, and discuss the relationship of these methods to structural informatics. We emphasize methods for managing and integrating images, focusing on how images are acquired from imaging equipment, stored, transmitted, and presented for interpretation. We also focus on how these processes and the image information are integrated with other clinical information and used in the health care enterprise, so as to have an optimal impact on patient care.

We discuss these issues in the context of Radiology, since imaging is the primary focus of that field.[1] Yet imaging is an important part of many other fields as well, including Pathology, Hematology, Dermatology, Ophthalmology, Gastroenterology, Cardiology, Surgery (for minimally invasive procedures especially) and

B. Erickson, MD, PhD (✉)
Department of Radiology and Medical Informatics, Mayo Clinic, Mayo Building, E2, 200 First St. SW, Rochester, MN 55905, USA
e-mail: bje@mayo.edu

R.A. Greenes, MD, PhD
Department of Biomedical Informatics, Arizona State University, Tempe, AZ, USA

Department of Biomedical Informatics, College of Medicine, Mayo Clinic, Samuel Johnson Research Bldg., 13212 East Shea Blvd, Scottsdale, AZ 85259, USA
e-mail: greenes@asu.edu

This chapter is adapted from an earlier version in the third edition authored by Robert A. Greenes and James F. Brinkley

[1] The name Radiology is itself a misnomer, since the field is involved in using ultrasound, magnetic resonance, optical, thermal, and other non-radiation imaging modalities when appropriate. Radiology departments in some institutions are thus referred to alternatively as Departments of Medical Imaging or Diagnostic Imaging.

E.H. Shortliffe, J.J. Cimino (eds.), *Biomedical Informatics*,
DOI 10.1007/978-1-4471-4474-8_20, © Springer-Verlag London 2014

Obstetrics, which often do their own imaging procedures; most other fields that use imaging rely on Radiology and Pathology for their imaging needs.

The distribution of imaging responsibility has given rise to the need of many departments to address issues of image acquisition, storage, transmission, and interpretation. As these modalities have gradually become largely digital in format, the development of electronic systems to support these tasks has been needed.

We begin by describing some of the roles of imaging across all of biomedicine, then concentrate on their management and integration in radiology systems, bringing in illustrative examples from other disciplines where appropriate. Many Radiology departments are becoming highly distributed enterprises, with acquisition sites in intensive care unit areas, regular patient floors, emergency departments, vascular services, screening centers, ambulatory clinics, and in affiliated community-based practice settings. Interpretation of images may be in those locations when dedicated onsite radiologists are needed. Increasingly, however, due to high-speed network availability, interpretation can be done at sites far from acquisition, either in a central location or in widely distributed locations according to the different methods of organization. This variation is possible because image acquisition and interpretation can be effectively decoupled. Independent imaging centers in a community face some of the same issues and opportunities, although to a lesser degree, so we focus primarily on the distributed medical center-based Radiology department in this chapter.

20.2   Basic Concepts and Issues

20.2.1   Roles for Imaging in Biomedicine

Imaging is a central part of the health care process for diagnosis, treatment planning, image-guided treatment, assessment of response to treatment, and estimation of prognosis. In addition, it plays important roles in medical communication and education, as well as in research.

20.2.1.1 Detection and Diagnosis

The primary uses of images are for the detection of medical abnormalities and for diagnostic purposes. Detection focuses on identifying the presence of an abnormality, but in the case in which the findings are not sufficiently specific to be characteristic of a particular disease, other information is required for actual diagnosis. This is the case, for example, with mammograms, which are often used for screening for breast cancer; once a suspicious abnormality is detected, a biopsy procedure is usually required for diagnosis. In other circumstances, the image finding is adequate to diagnose the abnormality, for example, the finding of focal stenosis or obstruction of a coronary artery during angiography is diagnostic in itself, and some tumors, congenital abnormalities, or other diseases have highly characteristic appearances. Most often there is a continuum between detection and diagnosis, with a test able not only to detect but also to narrow the range of possibilities, known as the **differential diagnosis** (see Chap. 2).

Diagnosis and detection can be done with a wide variety of imaging procedures. Images produced by visible light, as in ophthalmology, for example, can be used for retinal photography; in dermatology, to view skin lesions; and in pathology, for gross specimen viewing and for light microscopy. The visible-light spectrum is also responsible for producing images seen endoscopically, rendered typically as video images or sequences. Sound energy, in the form of echoes from internal structures, is used to form images in ultrasound, a modality used primarily in cardiac, abdominal, pelvic, breast, and obstetrical imaging, as well as in imaging of small parts, such as the thyroid and testes. In addition, **Doppler shifts** of sound frequency are used to evaluate blood flow in many organs and in major vessels. X-ray energy produces radiographic and **computed-tomography** (CT) images of most parts of the body: The differential absorption of X-rays by various tissues produces the varying densities that enable radiographic images to portray normal and abnormal structures. Isotope emissions of radioactive particles are used to produce nuclear-medicine images, which result from the differential concentration of radioactively tagged molecules in various tissues. **Magnetic-resonance imaging** (**MRI**) depicts energy fluctuations of certain atomic nuclei—primarily of hydrogen—when they are aligned in a magnetic field and then perturbed by a radiofrequency pulse. Parameters such as proton density, the rate at which the nuclei return to alignment, the rate of loss of phase coherence after the pulse, diffusion of water, and even the concentration of certain chemicals can be measured. These quantities differ in various tissues under normal conditions, with more variations due to disease, thus enabling MRI to distinguish among them. Figure 20.1 shows some example images.

20.2.1.2 Assessment and Planning

In addition to being used for detection and diagnosis, imaging is often used to assess a patient's health status in terms of progression of a disease process (such as determination of tumor stage), response to treatment, and estimation of prognosis. We can analyze cardiac status by assessing the heart's size and motion echocardiographically. Similarly, we can use ultrasound to assess fetal size and growth, as well as development. Computed tomography is used frequently to determine approaches for surgery or for radiation therapy. In the latter case, precise calculations of radiation-beam configuration can be optimized to maximize dose to the tumor while minimizing absorption of radiation by surrounding tissues. This calculation is often performed by simulating multiple radiation-beam configurations and iterating to a best treatment plan. For surgical planning, three-dimensional volumes of CT or MRI data can be constructed and presented for viewing from different perspectives to facilitate determination of the most appropriate surgical approach.

20.2.1.3 Image-Guided Procedures

Images can provide real-time guidance when virtual-reality methods are used to superimpose a surgeon's visual perspective on the appropriate image view in the projection that demonstrates the abnormality. With endoscopic and minimally invasive surgery, this kind of imaging can provide

a localizing context for visualizing and orienting the endoscopic findings, and can enable monitoring of results of interventions such as focused ultrasound, cryosurgery, or thermal ablation. It is also possible to use intra-operative imaging to update the position and appearance of pre-operative imaging used for procedural planning. Figure 20.2 shows an example of a CT-guided biopsy of a lesion in the neck. High quality imaging allows precise targeting of small targets even near important structures like the carotid artery.

Such minimally invasive surgery can be conducted at a distance (see Chap. 18), although it is practical to do so only in limited settings. Because the abnormality is viewed through a video monitor that displays the endoscopic field, the view can be physically remote, a technique called **telepresence**. Similarly, the manipulation of the endoscope itself can be controlled by a robotic device that reproduces the hand movements of a remote operator, and can provide **haptic feedback** reproducing the sensations of tissue textures, margins, and resistance.

20.2.1.4 Communication

Medical decision-making, including diagnosis and treatment planning, is often aided by allowing clinicians to visualize images concurrently with textual reports and discussions of interpretations. Thus, we consider imaging to be an important adjunct to communication and images to be a desirable component of a multimedia electronic medical record. Because medical imaging is an essential element of the practice of medicine, support for transmission and remote image viewing is also a critical component of telemedicine (Chap. 18). Medical images can also be helpful in doctor-patient communication, to enable the provider to illustrate an abnormality or explain a surgical procedure to a patient (Chap. 17).

20.2.1.5 Education and Training

Images (2D or static, 3D, 4D (e.g., 3D CT or ultrasound through time), and video) are an essential part of medical education and training because so much of medical diagnosis and treatment depends on imaging and on the skills

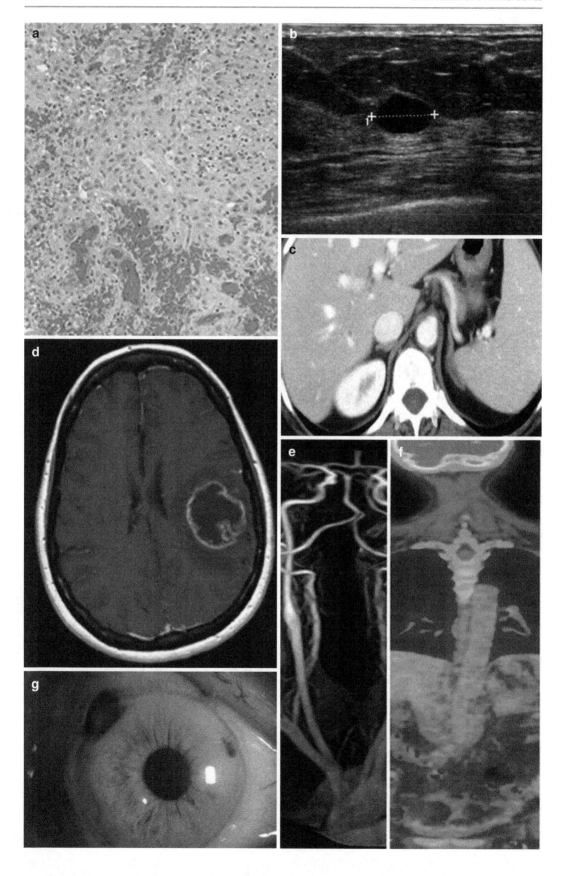

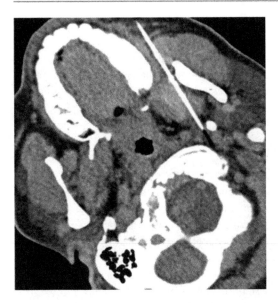

Fig. 20.2 An example of a CT-guided biopsy of a lesion in the neck. High quality imaging allows precise targeting of small targets even near important structures like the carotid artery

needed to interpret such images (see Chap. 22). Case libraries, tutorials, atlases, three-dimensional models, quiz libraries, and other resources using images can provide this kind of educational support.

Taking a history, performing a physical examination, and conducting medical procedures also demand appropriate visualization and observation skills. Training in these skills can be augmented by viewing images and video sequences, as well as through practice in simulated situations. An example of the latter is an approach to training individuals in endoscopy techniques by using a mannequin and video images in conjunction with tactile and visual feedback that correlate with the manipulations being carried out.

As noted in the previous section, patients increasingly expect to understand more about their disease, and patient communications can be more effective by including relevant images. Imaging also has a consumer/patient education benefit, since access to appropriate images can be included along with the provision of instructions and educational materials to patients—about their diseases, about procedures to be carried out, about follow-up care, and about healthy lifestyles.

20.2.1.6 Research

Imaging is, of course, also intimately involved in many aspects of research. An example is structural modeling of DNA and proteins, including their 3D and 4D configurations (see Chap. 24). Another is the images obtained in molecular or cellular biology to follow the distributions of fluorescent or radioactively tagged molecules. The study of **morphometrics**, which is literally the measurement of shape, depends on the use of imaging methods. Figure 20.3 shows an example of a detailed segmentation of the brain into various anatomic structures by the Free Surfer package.[2] It uses a combination of image intensities and expected shapes for the brain and substructures to produce its output. **Functional mapping**—for example, of the human brain—relates specific sites on images to particular functions. While such quantitative imaging efforts often begin in the laboratory, translation of such quantitative methods is increasingly important to the practice of medicine. Figure 20.4 provides an example of functional mapping of a patient with a brain tumor, where functional mapping is used to identify critical structures, and thus to guide surgical therapy.

20.2.1.7 The Radiologic Process and Its Interactions

As noted in the introduction, we concentrate in this chapter on the subset of imaging that falls under the purview of **Radiology**. Radiology departments are engaged in all aspects of the health care process, from detection and diagnosis to treatment, follow-up and prognosis assessment, and they illustrate well the many issues involved in acquiring and managing images, interpreting them, and communicating those interpretations.

---

[2] http://surfer.nmr.mgh.harvard.edu/ (Accessed 1/27/2013)

Fig. 20.1 Medical imaging leverages a variety of types of images to measure, diagnose and store information about a patient. Some examples are (**a**) Dermatopathology, (**b**) Ultrasound (US), (**c**) Computed Tomography (CT), (**d**) Magnetic Resonance Imaging (MRI), (**e**) magnetic resonance angiogram, (**f**) fused PET-CT image, and (**g**) photographic image of the eye

Space does not permit us to discuss the other disciplines that utilize imaging, but the processes involved and issues faced, which we discuss in the context of radiology, pertain to the other disciplines also. Additional examples are also provided in Chap. 9. Occasionally, we intersperse examples from other areas, where we wish to emphasize a

particular point, and imaging for educational purposes is discussed at length in Chap. 23.

The primary function of a Radiology department is the acquisition and analysis of medical images but also increasingly, the conduct of minimally invasive image-guided procedures. Through imaging, health care personnel obtain information that can help them to establish diagnoses, to plan or administer therapy, and to follow the courses of diseases or therapies.

Diagnostic studies in the Radiology department are typically performed at the request of referring clinicians, who then use the information for subsequent decision-making. The Radiology department produces the images, and the radiologist provides the primary analysis and interpretation of the radiologic findings. Thus, radiologists play a direct role in clinical problem-solving and in diagnostic-work-up planning. **Interventional radiology** and image-guided surgery (if done by the radiologist) are activities in which the radiologist plays a primary role in treatment.

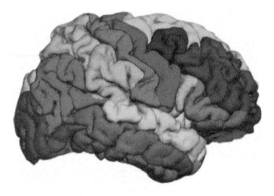

Fig. 20.3 Shows an example of a detailed segmentation of the brain into various anatomic structures by the FreeSurfer (http://surfer.nmr.mgh.harvard.edu/) package. It uses a compbination of image intensities and expected shapes for the brain and substructures to produce its output

The radiologic process (Greenes 1989) is characterized by seven kinds of tasks, each of

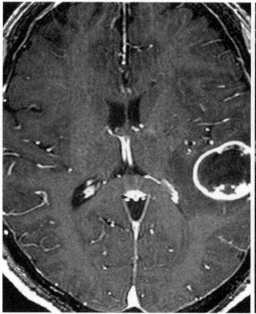
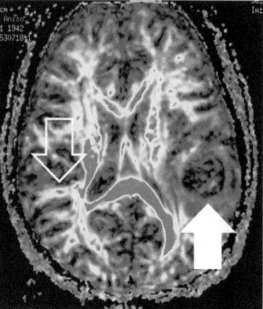

Fig. 20.4 Provides an example of diffusion tractography in a patient with a high grade brain tumor. In this case, one can see the replacement of the normal tracts (*open arrow*) with lack of tract signal in the region of the tumor suggest-

ing they are involved with tumor. *Closed arrow* points to a brain tumor which has displaced or replaced the normal white matter tracts

Fig. 20.5 The radiologic interpretation process

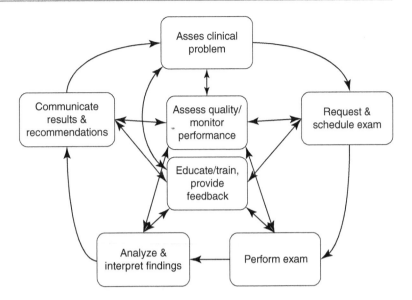

which involves information exchange and which can be augmented and enhanced by information technology, as illustrated in Fig. 20.5. The first five tasks occur in sequence, whereas the final two are ongoing and support the other five.

1. The process begins with an evaluation by a clinician of a clinical problem and determination of the need for an imaging procedure. Decision support tools (Chap. 22) are commonly used to help determine if, and what type of, testing should be performed.
2. The procedure is requested and scheduled, the indication for the procedure is stated, and relevant clinical history is made available.
3. The imaging procedure is carried out, and images are acquired. The procedure may be tailored for particular clinical questions or patient status considerations.
4. The radiologist reviews the images in the context of the clinical history and questions to be answered and may manipulate the images. This task actually involves interrelated subtasks: (a) detection of the relevant findings and (b) interpretation of those findings in terms of clinical meaning and significance.
5. The radiologist creates a report and may also directly communicate the results to the referring clinician, as well as making suggestions for further evaluation as needed. The anno-

tation and markup of images can be very helpful in communicating locations of findings, and serves as helpful landmarks for subsequent exams and for surgical or radiation procedures.

6. Quality control and monitoring are carried out, with the aim of improving the foregoing processes. Factors such as patient waiting times, workloads, numbers of exposures obtained per procedure, quality of images, radiation dose, yields of procedures, and incidence of complications are measured and adjusted.
7. Continuing education and training are carried out through a variety of methods, including access to atlases, review materials, teaching-file cases, and feedback of subsequently confirmed diagnoses to interpreting radiologists.

All these tasks are now, in a growing number of departments, computer-assisted, and most of them involve images in some way. In fact, radiology is one branch of medicine in which even the basic data are usually produced by computers and stored directly in computer memory. Radiology has also contributed strongly to advances in computer-aided instruction (see Chap. 23), in technology assessment (see Chap. 11), and in clinical decision support (see Chap. 22). Speech recognition is commonly used for report creation.

20.2.2 Electronic Imaging Systems

20.2.2.1 Image Acquisition

The first radiographs used an integrated detection, recording and display system—that is, the glass plate (and later, film) served both to detect the photons and to record them in a permanent form (after being 'developed') and also to display the data. This integrated arrangement survived for about a century. Today, most radiographs are either (a) recorded in a latent form (i.e., they are not directly visible, such as an electronic signal on a charged plate) and a 'reader' scans the plate to create a digital image (known as **computed radiography** or CR) or (b) the photons are directly converted to digital images (known as **digital radiography** or DR). The digital image can then be transmitted and stored like any digital data, using conventional networks and storage systems. They are displayed using conventional display systems. The matrix size of the images is variable, ranging from as low as 64×64 for some nuclear medicine images, up to $5,000 \times 4,000$ picture elements (pixels) for mammograms. The size of typical radiology images and examinations is shown in Table 20.1.

20.2.2.2 DICOM

The first medical devices to produce digital images routinely were CT scanners, and soon after, MRI scanners. The availability of digital data that represented a three-dimensional image stimulated the field of medical image processing, which had been a relatively quiescent, largely research endeavor until then. But an early challenge to such investigations was that the medical device vendors supported the then-common half-inch tape media, but each vendor (and usually model of scanner) had its own format. Such formats were considered proprietary, and required each investigator to reverse engineer the format of the tape just to gain access to the data. Although computer networks were used in hospitals at that time, few if any scanners supported network connections.

The need to write all data to tape, and then read it into a computer using software unique to each scanner resulted in significant unnecessary effort. The need to exchange images efficiently demanded that they be represented in a standard fashion. This need was recognized by the American College of Radiology (ACR) and the National Electrical Manufacturer's Association (NEMA), and led to the development of the ACR/NEMA standard for medical images in 1985. As other imaging devices started to produce digital images, and as the information about the images became richer, the second version was published in 1989. That standard described both standardized representations of the data, and prescribed a special connector for transferring image data between devices. This was demonstrated at the 1990 Radiological Society of North America (RSNA) conference. Soon after, **TCP/IP** became a widely accepted network standard, and while the ACR/NEMA standard did not describe a

Table 20.1 Typical sizes for radiology examinations

Modality	Image size (pixels/image)	Images/exam	Exam size (MB)
CR/DR	5,000,000	3	29
CT	262,144	500	250
MRI	65,536	500	63
US	262,144	50	25
Mammography	20,000,000	4	153
Interventional/Fluoro	1,048,576	50	100
Nuclear Medicine	16,384	25	1

CR computer radiography, *DR* digital radiography, *CT* computed tomography, *MRI* magnetic resonance imaging, *US* ultrasound

Note that there is variability in image size and images per examination, and these numbers should be viewed as very rough estimates. Furthermore, there is a strong trend for both increased image resolution (increasing image size) and more images per examination since the emergence of digital imaging

method for transferring data over TCP/IP, investigators fairly quickly implemented this, and it worked well. Continued improvements in the information model, as well as extension to medical specialties other than radiology, and standards for storage on physical media like optical disks demanded further revisions. The addition of non-radiology images also demanded a name change, and thus 'ACR/NEMA 3.0' was rebranded as **DICOM**, which stands for Digital Image Communications in Medicine.

The major adoption of DICOM by all image equipment providers was not until 1992–94. In 1992, the RSNA commissioned the creation of **Central Test Node** (**CTN**) software, for demonstrating the standard over a local area network in the info**RAD** section of RSNA '92, followed by increasingly sophisticated versions over the next 2 years. The RSNA then made it available for free public access as a model for understanding the standard and design of utilities and tools by developers. During those years, the RSNA annual meetings hosted a major digital image interoperability demonstration that became progressively more sophisticated and demanding. RSNA and its meetings accordingly facilitated demonstration of the interconnection of vendor products through the Internet, promoted DICOM compatibility as a feature that could be visualized at participating vendor exhibits, and created a model **RFP** for radiology practices and hospitals to use to craft a DICOM requirement as part of the procurement of imaging systems. These efforts turned out to be extremely successful in transforming the marketplace from one that was dominated by proprietary formats to one that was standards-based and interoperable.

DICOM continues to be updated and improved through an international committee process. While it is hard for any standard to be both widely accepted and perfectly up-to-date, the DICOM governance has done a remarkable job of adapting to rapid changes. The governance continues to reflect its roots of combining industry and medical experts who are interested in providing the best technology that can be put into commercial products.

20.2.2.3 Image Transmission, Storage, and Display

Digital imaging provides the opportunity to store the images in digital form. In the early days, the size of the images represented a challenge—the amount of data was quite large relative to the capacity of storage devices. As a consequence, there was intense interest in using compression methods that could reduce the amount of storage that was required–as well as increase the speed of network transmission of images. Even with compression, the amount of storage used for images is quite large relative to non-image data stored in a hospital. A hospital must therefore carefully consider how images are stored. In the early days of **Picture Archive and Communications Systems** (**PACS**), there was little choice, because the storage system was tightly integrated with the display and transmission. This was done because the high demands on storage, transmission, and display all required special hardware. As computer technology caught up, there was less need for specialized versions of networks, archives, and displays.

Early PACS utilized proprietary networking methods or other uncommon, even if standard, networks suited to high volume transmission. An example of the former is the PACS developed by LORAL, which leveraged technology developed for its defense applications. Its network was a hybrid of 10 Mbps **Ethernet**, which provided control signaling, and a unidirectional star configuration optical network that had lossless compression built into the network card. The optical network signaled at 100 Mbps, and because it was unidirectional, it routinely realized its theoretical speed. This speed was required to meet a design demand that any image be visible on the display screen within 2 s of the request. Even today, few PACS are able to meet this specification. Other vendors utilized **FDDI**, which also was an optical network that signaled at 100 Mbps. However, its handling of contention was much less effective, and its performance suffered. Today, standard Ethernet signaling at either 100 Mbps or 1 Gbps can provide adequate performance, as long as reasonable attention is paid to network layout and implementation.

The next part of the PACS concept to begin to separate was the archive. In the early PACS, updating the system to take advantage of new workstation or network technology meant that the whole archive needed to be updated or migrated. Because the data were not stored in a standard format, it was necessary to get the cooperation of the vendor to migrate the data to the new system. Because workstations rapidly change, but archive contents do not, there was perceived value in separating these two functions (Erickson and Hangiandreou 1998). Today, there are a number of vendors that sell 'vendor-neutral archives' which leverage the DICOM standard to allow a wide variety of image-producing and image-consuming systems to access the archive in a standard fashion.

Because the image datasets are quite large, there is interest in finding ways to reduce storage requirements. Image compression does exactly this, in one of two ways. There are **lossless compression** methods, which encode redundancy in the image in a way that allows the original to be *exactly* reproduced. **Lossy** (or irreversible) **compression** produces an image that is similar to the original. Exactly how similar depends on the algorithm and user-selectable settings that reflect the trade-off between fidelity and compression ratio (the ratio of original size to compressed size). The major challenge is that one cannot select a given setting, reliably get images that are not visibly altered, and also achieve a good compression ratio. While lossless compression methods can only get about 2.5:1 reductions in size, lossy compression can gain as much as 40:1 without a perceptible or diagnostic loss, *for certain types of images*. While the size of image examinations continues to increase, the decrease in storage cost is more rapid, lessening the demand for lossy compression. The use of lossy compression is more widely accepted in non-radiology specialties, such as cardiology and pathology, in part because of the greater uniformity of image characteristics, allowing easy specification of acceptable methods. A key goal of lossy compression is that it not have an adverse impact on diagnostic value to the human or to computer aided diagnostic algorithms at routinely applied compression levels (Zheng et al. 2000). Thus lossy methods are usually tuned to the diagnostic task at hand so as not to have adverse impacts.

Early PACS also required specialized display devices. At the time, standard computer displays were as high as 640×480, but commonly less. Images were more than 2,048 pixels in each direction. Liquid crystal technology for large displays was also not developed, meaning that the displays were large cathode ray tubes. These displays were large, heavy, produced much heat, and degraded rather rapidly. Nearly all were monochrome. Imaging also required a higher luminance for detection of subtle gray level distinctions than was possible with consumer-oriented displays, even more so with the focus in consumer devices on color displays which often did not have a bright white background. Expensive displays were accordingly needed to provide both the high resolution and high luminance. Today, flat panel technology that meets the demands of most radiological images is widely available. Some have advocated the use of consumer-grade displays (Hirschorn and Dreyer 2006), though the more common practice is to use medical grade devices (Langer et al. 2006). Another work of the DICOM committees was the establishment of display requirements for medical purposes—requirements that the device be able to show enough unique levels of gray to enable diagnosis, and that the scale be perceptually linear (ACR-NEMA 2006). Computer values sent to the display may range from 0 to 255 in intensity. However, the difference in perceived intensity when digital values change from 0 to 10 is not the same as the perceived intensity change when the digital values change from 100 to 110. That is because the eye's sensitivity to photons does not match the change in the number of photons produced by a display at different intensity levels, i.e., the eye's sensitivity to photons has a nonlinear response curve. Since this non-linear response is fairly consistent between humans, it is possible to adjust the digital values to create a perceptually linear display, which should be optimal for the human perceptual system.

20.2.3 Integration with Other Health Care Information

20.2.3.1 Radiology Information Systems (RIS)

A **Radiology Information System**, or RIS, is responsible for much of the textual information in a radiology department. There are some core functions that all RISs must be able to perform, including the capture of the interpretation for a given examination, and the recording of the status of an imaging examination. Most RISs also do more, depending on what other systems are available and preferred for a given situation. Most examinations must be ordered (there may be exceptions in cases like an emergency department). Once ordered, the examination must be scheduled—the time and imaging device must be known and coordinated with the schedule of the patient, and inclusion of patient demographics. These functions may be performed by the hospital information system (HIS) or electronic health record (EHR) system. Similarly, the report must be provided to the ordering physician, and a bill must be issued. These functions may also be provided by the HIS or EHR system, but must be provided by the RIS in cases where there is no HIS or EHR (such as many outpatient imaging centers). Early RISs needed to provide a mechanism for entering reports, usually by a transcriptionist typing into the RIS. Once transcribed, the RIS would usually also provide a way for the radiologist to review the transcription to assure it was correct, and then electronically sign it, at which time the examination was considered final. In cases where the transcription occurred substantially after the dictation, some RISs provided a mechanism to access the audio file. At institutions with residents or fellows, the RIS would usually also provide a preliminary interpretation provided by the resident/fellow, but before the staff person approved the report as final.

20.2.3.2 Speech Recognition

We noted that the RIS previously would provide a means for a transcriptionist to type the text of the report into the RIS. Today, the vast majority of radiologists use speech recognition to convert their speech into text. In some cases the text is immediately reviewed by the radiologist and approved as final. This model has the advantages of rapid **turn-around time**—the time from the examination being ready to be reported to the time it has a final report available. In this model, a separate application (the speech recognition system) converts the audio to an HL-7 message, which is sent to the RIS along with the final (or other appropriate status). In other cases, a 'correctionist' reviews the text created by the speech recognition system, and corrects it based on listening to the audio file. In this case, the radiologist must then review the text again to make it final.

There are two major advantages to using speech recognition: First, it enables rapid turn-around time. Before speech recognition, turn-around times of 1 week were common, but now, turn-around times of less than 2 h are common (Hart et al. 2010; Krishnaral et al. 2010; Mattern et al. 1999). This improvement in turn-around time undoubtedly improves the quality of care provided to patients. Second, it reduces staffing for radiology departments or hospitals by eliminating or reducing the number of transcriptionists/correctionists needed. Of course, some decrease in productivity is commonly observed for radiologists, which reduces the economic benefit (Langer 2002; Strahan and Schneider-Kolsky 2010).

Over the years, there have been multiple research efforts aimed at enabling radiologists to generate structured reports from selection of choices in forms, and through use of drop-down menus, macros that produce predetermined text phrases, and other techniques. Some of these are now used in specific situations, especially where reports have a largely anticipated format and structure, e.g., mammography and obstetrical ultrasound, and macros are used in conjunction with speech recognition approaches for certain "canned" sections or reports. However, there is not yet widespread adoption of structured reporting in radiology.

20.2.3.3 Computer-Aided Diagnosis (CAD)

The interpretation task consists of detection, description, and diagnosis. In some cases, the detection task can be quite challenging, particularly

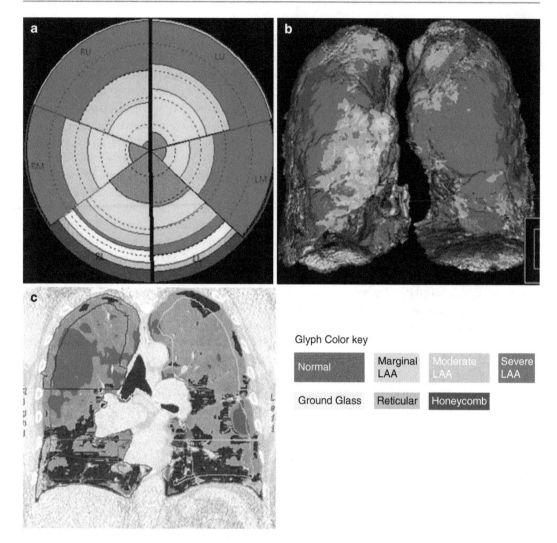

Fig. 20.6 (**a–c**) shows the output of the experimental algorithm CALIPER, rendered as a 3D image, to show the distribution and change of different degrees of interstitial lung disease in a patient (Courtesy Brian J. Bartholmai, MD)

for screening tasks involving mammography and chest X-rays because the incidence is rather low, and the volume is high. Particularly at the end of a long shift, human observers probably have decreased performance due to fatigue. For these cases, computer algorithms that highlight suspicious regions of an image may be useful to assure that important findings aren't missed. Some have called this role 'computer-aided diligence'.

In most studies of the value of **computer-aided diagnosis (CAD)**, the value is either minimal, or provides benefit mostly to non-expert readers (Gur and Sumkin 2006). It is not clear that

CAD adds value for radiologists that subspecialize in the body part being imaged (e.g., mammographers do not benefit from current CAD algorithms for mammograms). However, just as it was unimaginable that a computer could beat the best chess players in the early days, it is likely that over time, CAD will become better than humans.

Another role for CAD is in assisting with diagnosis. This has been most commonly used for high resolution CT images of the chest with findings of interstitial lung disease, though it has been described for other findings, including mammography (Elter and Horsch 2009). The

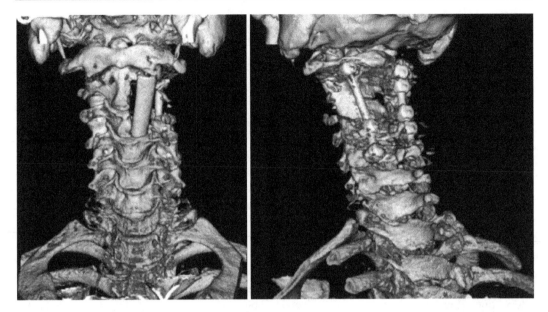

Fig. 20.7 Provides an example advanced visualization of the cervical spine after resection of a tumor, distributed via a web client. This allows the surgeon to review findings and discuss them in their own office

CAD algorithm can assist in differentiating the various types of lung disease. Again, this is probably most useful to radiologists who do not do a large volume of lung imaging, and may have less experience with various interstitial lung diseases and their appearance. Figure 20.6 shows an image of the output of the experimental algorithm CALIPER, rendered as a 3D image, to show the distribution and change of different degrees of interstitial lung disease in a patient.

20.2.3.4 Advanced Visualization

CT and MR scanners provide images that can be thought of as 3D images, even if they are not always truly acquired as 3D, but rather, as a series (or stack) of 2D images. In fact, some imaging devices can acquire a series of 3D images through time, thus representing a 4D image (time becomes the fourth dimension in these cases). In particular, cardiac imaging benefits from 4D capability so that the beating heart can be examined throughout the cardiac cycle. Such data sets are quite large, and proper demonstration of the important findings requires visualization of the data as specially processed images. For instance, if one wishes to see a skeletal finding using CT, one can set a threshold to select bony structures, and then render it using traditional computer rendering methods. This can be done on multiple time points to produce movies of moving structures.

The great challenge in medical visualization is **segmentation**—deciding whether a volume element (voxel) is a part of the structure of interest or not. In the case of a CT image of bone, segmentation is quite easy. If intravascular contrast is administered during the examination, that can make it fairly straightforward to select vessels (arteries and/or veins depending on the timing). Soft tissue organs like livers, kidneys, and muscles are more challenging, but very feasible. A description of the rendering algorithms and their trade-offs is provided in Chap. 9.

A recent advance in visualization tools is to have the computation done on a central server, with interactive segmentation and rendering capability available via web browsers. This provides access to a much larger population of physicians, and can be valuable for surgeons contemplating surgery, as well as for patient education. Figure 20.7 provides an example advanced visualization of the spine, distributed via a web client, which allows surgeons to better plan and review treatment options in their own office, with the patient.

20.2.3.5 Advanced Reporting

While textual reports have served medical practice fairly well for the past century, there are opportunities to improve reporting. Multimedia reports provide a richer representation of the information present in the examination, and might include links from portions of the text report to specific images and locations on the images, moving images ('video'), or audio files such as the heart sounds. In some diseases, it can be important to have specific measurements made, and possibly tracked over time. If these measurements are encoded in a specific way, it will be easier to extract and use that information elsewhere in the medical record, and for other purposes like research. **Lexicons**, such as RadLex, can be helpful in conveying some of the information. There is great interest in routinely collecting more quantitative information from images, because it appears that for an increasing number of diseases, quantitation is receiving increased attention in clinical realms.

A structured report is produced when all of the concepts are represented using coded terminology. There is a DICOM specification for structured reporting, though adoption has been poor as noted in Chap. 9. This is because there are currently not efficient user interfaces for creation of structured reports in most areas of radiology. The best example of structured reporting is the use of BIRADS in breast imaging. Because the possible disease findings are limited in mammography, the list of anatomic structures and associated pathologies are limited. BIRADS assumes the organ of interest is the breast, and offers a targeted coding system for the type of lesion that is seen and the recommended clinical approach to that lesion.

20.2.3.6 Workflow Management (Including Dashboards)

The ability to monitor and control events in an imaging department is critical to efficient and effective operation. **Dashboards** have been applied in many business arenas as tools that give quick visual displays of **Key Performance Indicators** (**KPIs**) for a particular business. Such dashboard technology is now becoming widely used within imaging departments for monitoring

such KPIs as report turn-around time, patient waiting time, number of days out to schedule certain types of examinations, and revenue days-outstanding. The dashboards give people a quick view of what is happening, and can alert them to problem areas. Figure 20.8 is an example of a radiology dashboard that shows important departmental metrics, including report turn-around time, compliance with notification requirements, and patient waiting times.

Most dashboards provide a mechanism to 'drill down' on a particular problem area. For instance, if the patient waiting time monitor goes 'red', clicking on that indicator light could show the waiting time by location (maybe just one facility is causing the problem), total patient volume (maybe the site is experiencing a spike in patient volume), or examination time (maybe the complexity of examinations is going up). Such information is critical to enabling a timely and effective response to sub-par performance.

20.2.3.7 Teleradiology

Teleradiology is the practice of interpreting images at a location that is physically distant from the place where the images are collected. Initially, this referred to transmitting images from the hospital to the radiologist's home in the middle of the night so that the physician did not need to drive in to see the image onsite. While this is still done, it is now common for a hospital to contract with a 'nighthawk' service that will provide these nighttime interpretations. A nighthawk service contracts with many hospitals—enough to keep a team of radiologists busy during the night. Having a team continuously operating is usually more efficient, and allows for specialization of image interpretation. Teleradiology is now also practiced during the day to balance clinical workload and to provide specialized interpretation on a routine basis. The technology to rapidly transmit images across large distances is widely available and inexpensive. The greatest challenges to teleradiology are licensing/credentialing issues, especially if films are read across state lines or internationally (radiologists may be licensed to practice where they review the films but not in the location where the patients were located when the images were acquired).

**University of Informatica
Department of Radiology Dashboard**

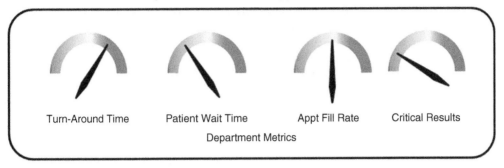

Turn-Around Time   Patient Wait Time   Appt Fill Rate   Critical Results

Department Metrics

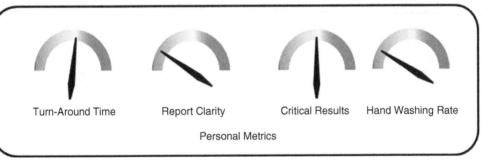

Turn-Around Time   Report Clarity   Critical Results   Hand Washing Rate

Personal Metrics

Fig. 20.8 is an example of a radiology dashboard that shows important departmental metrics, including report turn-around time, compliance with notification requirements, and patient waiting times

20.2.3.8 Enterprise Integration (Including HL7, CPOE)

Medicine is an information-rich business, and providing access to the relevant information in a timely fashion is critical to success. Integration of systems with the relevant pieces of information is necessary, and in hospitals is generally done with HL-7 messages (see Chap. 7). Referring physicians increasingly expect to view images and to see reports with rich information. HL-7 does not address these demands well. Similarly, many EHRs are not able to address these needs.

Because medical imaging has been a major component of increases in total health care costs, there has been much attention paid to assuring that only necessary examinations are performed. To help assure this, decision-support systems to guide proper ordering have been developed that have been shown to have an impact on utilization of imaging studies (Sistrom et al. 2009). Such systems have been shown to decrease the total

number of examinations performed, and in particular to decrease the number of examinations that appear to be unnecessary. In addition to alerting the user to a potentially improper order, educational materials are often provided to help the ordering physician understand when and what imaging examinations might be appropriate for the given indication. In addition, such systems can provide management reports to improve the understanding of ordering practices.

20.3 Imaging in Other Departments

20.3.1 Cardiology

Cardiac imaging has many similarities to radiological imaging, and in many cases is performed either by radiology departments or in conjunction with radiology. The primary imaging modalities for cardiology include echocardiography (ultrasound), catheterization (interventional/vascular, involving fluoroscopy and angiography, i.e., vessel visualization via contrast die administration), MR, CT, and PET. The workflow can be similar, but can be different in those cases where the imaging is performed by the same department and even by the same individual as the person who ordered it. In such cases, there can be less formal ordering, scheduling, and reporting. However, as the imaging is increasingly a part of the general enterprise, such informality will become a greater challenge.

Cardiology has been more aggressive in its use of lossy compression. This is primarily because the nature of cardiac imaging is much more stereotyped and there is less concern about fine resolution. There is primary focus on the heart, whereas in radiology many different organs with very different appearances can challenge compression methods. The echocardiographic and interventional images are also much more like video—usually being motion-oriented rather than focused on static capture. In fact, the major cardiovascular societies have published and supported the use of specific compression technologies and settings for cardiac imaging (Simon et al. 1994; ACC/ACR/NEMA Ad hoc Group 1995).

Because the focus is primarily on the heart and its function, cardiac imaging is more advanced in structured reporting. The primary variables that are of interest in cardiac imaging (left ventricular volumes, stroke volumes) are of interest in most cases, and are routinely measured. This has driven the acceptance of structured reporting for the common measurements in cardiac imaging—particularly echocardiography.

20.3.2 Obstretrics and Gynecology

Obstetrical and gynecological imaging is rather like cardiac imaging, except that it is much more focused on ultrasound. Much like cardiac imaging, there are a well-defined and accepted set of measurements and observations expected for the routine obstetric exam, and as such, structured reports for these findings are widely used.

Estimates of fetal gestational age and development are typically automatically assessed, on the basis of measurements using well-tested prediction models.

20.3.3 Intraoperative/Endoscopic Visible Light

It is increasingly common to capture still images and video of endoscopic procedures as well as traditional open surgical procedures. These images are valuable for documenting the important findings (or lack thereof) during a procedure. They are also useful for educational purposes, including informing the patient of the findings and procedures carried out. Some surgeons have suggested that medicolegal demands will require routine capture of entire surgical procedures.

Such images can be more graphic and revealing than radiological images, and in some cases have driven the expectation of need for an additional level of privacy protection. In one institution, for instance, all photographic images from the Plastic Surgery department are protected from access—only physician members of the Plastic Surgery department can routinely view those images, with a process for granting temporary access to other care providers (Erickson et al. 2007).

20.3.4 Pathology and Dermatology

Pathology and dermatology have similar needs, except that dermatology includes photographic visible light images of skin lesions. For these purposes, consumer-grade photographs can be sufficient, but transporting those images (usually in JPEG form) to a medical-grade imaging system will usually require an import process. This process will require confidence about the accuracy of patient and site location information. Often, the JPEG images are then 'wrapped' with DICOM information to assure that the connection between a photograph and a patient exists at the file level, rather than via a link to a filename. Image viewers require color capability, but otherwise are not substantially different from what is provided in most radiological image viewers. If images are converted to DICOM, the archive system is usually able to store them without difficulty.

Microscopic images represent a bigger challenge. At this point, there are two strategies for the capture of microscope images: the first is **whole slide digitization** in which the entire specimen is digitized; the other is capture of specific views that are of interest. In both cases, though more so in whole-slide imaging, there is a need for multi-resolution viewing. That is because the workflow is very different. Whole-slide scanning is usually done *prior* to the pathologist reviewing the images, while the spot-capture is done by the pathologist at the time of viewing. In the former case, the computer performs the pan-zoom function, while in the latter case the optical microscope performs that function. In the former, the computer is a diagnostic device, while in the latter, it is used mostly for documentation purposes.

Whole-slide scanning is of greater interest, because it has greater possibilities for improving health care delivery by allowing the slides to go to the pathologist. It also represents a much greater challenge, because much larger amounts of data must be stored and the associated computer-based viewing application requires the ability to display low resolution and high resolution images. Computing low resolution images from high resolution images can be computational expensive. Instead, the DICOM standard uses compression methods that start with low-resolution representations, and builds high-resolution views from the lower-resolution images. As such, it is both computationally efficient and data storage-efficient.

Another important issue differentiating pathology imaging from radiological imaging is that retrieval of old images is uncommon in digital pathology. This would usually only occur when there is a medicolegal issue, or possibly in case of disease recurrence or metastasis, where there is a need to compare the older sample with a newer one.

20.4 Cross-Enterprise Imaging

20.4.1 CD Image Exchange

When images were stored on film, sharing images with another hospital required that the films be either physically transferred or copied. Copying a film was labor-intensive and expensive. Therefore, it was standard practice to 'loan' films to other facilities when needed.

With digital images, it is much easier to copy the digital data onto media like a compact disc (CD) and give that to the patient. There are well-accepted standards (DICOM) for how to store the images on a CD. However, it is challenging for most hospitals to use the images on CDs. In some cases, the images can be imported into the PACS, but that can cause confusion about where the study was done, and can be challenging for the RIS to represent this (who ordered the CD exam, and where the report is located). On the other hand, if one does not import the study into the local viewing environment, there may not be viewing applications for the images on physicians' computers. Including the software for a viewer on the same CD means the physician must learn how to use that viewer if they are not already familiar with it.

In addition, there are important data integrity issues—as much as 0.1 % of CDs have been shown to include images for patients other than the intended patient (Erickson 2011), leading to important health delivery and legal risks.

20.4.2 Direct Network Image Exchange

The problems with CD image exchange noted above, as well as the time delays and costs, have driven many institutions to use internet transfer mechanisms. In cases where there is a high volume and a high level of trust, one can establish **virtual private networks** (**VPNs**) that allow secure transfer between two institutions. While this allows rapid and low-cost transfer, it still requires confident patient identification, and a method for importing the images into some form of clinical viewer.

For less frequent/ad hoc transfers, setting up a VPN is not practical. There is an attempt currently underway to leverage **Personal Health Records (PHRs)** (see Chap. 17) to allow transfer of images (RSNA 2009). This system 'gives' the images to a patient-controlled online health record. By giving it to the patient, issues of security and HIPAA are significantly reduced. Still, although the problem of how a 'receiving' institution will view or import the images from the patient need to be addressed, this option appears appealing. The major challenge to this model is lack of widespread adoption (see the health record bank discussion in Chap. 13).

20.5 Future Directions for Imaging Systems

The increasing capabilities of mobile devices and the increasing expectations of ready access to medical professionals have driven imaging onto mobile devices. At present, the FDA has limited the use of such devices for diagnosis. On the other hand, these devices can be extremely useful for consultation on specific areas of an image, or when therapeutic options are being considered, or for patient communication. As the bandwidth and display qualities improve, these devices will likely play an increasing role in both diagnosis and therapy planning.

Cloud technology (see Chap. 5) is also looming as an important technology in the future of medical imaging. The ability to leverage efficiencies of scale is an important economic driver that is pushing many smaller imaging providers to use cloud-based storage. Perhaps a greater medical need driving the use of cloud is the widespread access that cloud technology provides. As more images are transferred to cloud storage, we expect that greater computational capabilities in the cloud may drive more computer aided diagnosis and advanced visualization to cloud providers.

Phenome characterization (see Chap. 25) is becoming an important aspect of the move to individualizing medicine sometimes referred to as '**precision medicine**'. Data contributing to phenome characterization can certainly come from reports of imaging procedures, but it may also be true that image features themselves, e.g., parameters describing nodules or tissue characteristics, may contribute to this knowledge base. This will become especially true as advanced imaging methods such as specialized MRI techniques and imaging at the cellular level are used for biomarker characterization.

Suggested Readings

Branstetter, B. F. (2009). *Practical imaging informatics*. New York: Springer. As its title implies, this book is a practice-oriented book primarily aimed at those responsible for implementing and maintaining a digital imaging practice. The format of the book is an outline with many practical tips from a wide variety of experts.

Dreyer, K. J. (2006). *PACS: A guide to the digital revolution*. New York: Springer. This is also a book focused on the practical aspects of implementing and maintaining a digital imaging department. Its format is that of a traditional textbook, and covers a broad range of topics.

Geoff, D. (2009). *Digital image processing for medical applications*. Cambridge/New York: Cambridge University Press. This is an excellent, practical book on concepts of image processing algorithms used in medical imaging. ISBN 978-0521860857.

Liu, Y., & Jihong, W. (2011). *PACS and digital medicine*. Boca Raton: CRC Press. This book goes into greater detail of the technology of PACS, and to a lesser degree RIS and EMR. This is a very good resource for those interested in more details of DICOM and how a PACS can be configured to address specific needs.

Wolfgang, B. 2010. *Applied medical image processing*: A *basic course*. CRC Press. As the title says, this is an introductory book, with many excellent explanations and example code (mostly MatLab). ISBN 978-1439824443.

Questions for Discussion

1. What are the Pros and Cons of a highly structured technology like DICOM? DICOM has been highly successful in terms of adoption as a standard, and virtually all image communication utilizes it. This differs markedly from some other standards. What are factors that have contributed to this success, and what lessons can be drawn from this in terms of how to promote adoption of standards in the future?

2. If one were to design medical imaging systems today, would the optimal design continue to have PACS and RIS as separate systems, or would they be combined into one system? Should these be separate from the EHR?

3. What are the ways in which radiology reports of examination interpretations can be generated, and what are the advantages and disadvantages of each approach, in terms of ease and efficiency of report creation, timeliness of availability of report to clinicians, usefulness for retrieval of cases for research and education?

4. In these days of high bandwidth and low storage costs, is there still a good reason to use lossy compression in medical imaging? What kinds of trends are likely to affect image growth, as part of the patient's medical record?

5. What are the arguments for maintaining raw rather than compressed data (not only for imaging data but for compression or summarization of other types of data)?

6. Describe a classification of ways in which image data are used in medical decision making.

7. What are the data management implications of using a separate advanced visualization system for clinicians that is distinct from the PACS used by radiologists for interpretations? What if the radiologists use that system in addition to the PACS?

Information Retrieval and Digital Libraries

William R. Hersh

After reading this chapter, you should know the answers to these questions:

- What types of online knowledge-based information are available and useful to clinicians, biomedical researchers, and consumers?
- What are the major components of the information retrieval process?
- What are the major categories of available knowledge-based information?
- How do techniques differ for indexing various types of knowledge-based biomedical information?
- What are the major approaches to retrieval of knowledge-based biomedical information?
- How effectively do searchers use information retrieval systems?
- What are the important research directions in information retrieval?
- What are the major challenges to making digital libraries effective for health and biomedical users?

Information retrieval (IR), sometimes called **search**, is the field concerned with the acquisition, organization, and searching of knowledge-based information (Hersh 2009). Although biomedical IR has traditionally concentrated on the retrieval of text from the biomedical literature, the domain over which IR can be effectively applied has broadened considerably with the advent of multimedia publishing and vast storehouses of images, video, chemical structures, gene and protein sequences, and a wide range of other digital media of relevance to biomedical education, research, and patient care. With the proliferation of IR systems and online content, the notion of the library has changed substantially, and new digital libraries have emerged (Lindberg and Humphreys 2005).

IR systems and digital libraries store and disseminate knowledge-based information. What exactly does that mean? Although there are many ways to classify biomedical information and the informatics applications that use them, in this chapter we will broadly divide them into two categories. *Patient-specific information* applies to individual patients. Its purpose is to tell health care providers, administrators, and researchers about the health and disease of a patient. This information comprises the patient's medical record. The second category of biomedical information is *knowledge-based information*. This is information that has been derived and organized from observational or experimental research. In the case of clinical research, this information provides clinicians, administrators, and researchers with knowledge derived from experiments and observations, which can then be applied to

W.R. Hersh, MD, FACMI, FACP
Department of Medical Informatics and Clinical Epidemiology, Oregon Health and Science University, 3181 SW Sam Jackson Park Rd., Mail Code BICC, Portland 97239, OR, USA
e-mail: hersh@ohsu.edu

This chapter is adapted from an earlier version in the third edition authored by William R. Hersh, P. Zoë Stavri, and William M. Detmer.

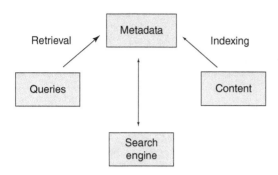

Fig. 21.1 Basic overview of the information retrieval process. Retrieval is made possible via metadata, which is produced via indexing and applied in queries by users. The metadata is used by the search engine, which directs the user to the content (Reproduced with permission of Springer (Hersh 2009))

individual patients. This information is most commonly provided in books and journals but can take a wide variety of other forms, including clinical practice guidelines, consumer health literature, Web sites, and so forth.

A basic overview of the IR process is shown in Fig. 21.1 and forms the basis for most of this chapter. The overall goal of IR or search is to find **content** that meets a person's information needs. This is done by posing a *query* to the IR system. A **search engine** matches the query to content items through **metadata**, which is "data about data" that describes the content items (Foulonneau and Riley 2008). There are two intellectual processes of IR. **Indexing** is the process of assigning metadata to content items, while **retrieval** is the process of the user entering his or her query and retrieving content items.

21.1 Evolution of Biomedical Information Retrieval

As with many chapters in this volume, this area has changed substantially over the four editions of this book. In the first edition, this chapter was titled "Bibliographic-Retrieval Systems," reflecting the type of knowledge that was accessible at the time. The second edition saw the emergence of the **World Wide Web** (**WWW** or **Web**) as a delivery mechanism for knowledge-based information. In the third edition, we added "Digital

Libraries" to the chapter name, reflecting that the entire biomedical library and beyond was now part of available online knowledge. This fourth edition reflects the fact that information is ubiquitous on computers, smartphones, tablets, and other devices.

Although this chapter focuses on the use of computers to facilitate IR, methods for finding and retrieving information from medical sources have been in existence for over a century. In 1879 Dr. John Shaw Billings created Index Medicus to help medical professionals find relevant journal articles (DeBakey 1991). Journal article citations were indexed by author name(s) and subject heading(s) and then aggregated in bound volumes. A scientist or practitioner seeking an article on a topic could manually search the index for the single best-matching subject heading and then be directed to citations of published articles.

The printed **Index Medicus** served as the main biomedical IR source but, in 1966, the National Library of Medicine (NLM) unveiled an electronic version, the **Medical Literature Analysis and Retrieval System** (**MEDLARS**) (Miles 1982). Because computing power and disk storage were very limited, MEDLARS and its follow-on **MEDLARS Online** (**MEDLINE**), stored only limited information for each article, such as author name(s), article title, journal source, and publication date. In addition, the NLM assigned to each article a number of terms from its **Medical Subject Headings** (**MeSH**) vocabulary (see Chap. 7). Searching was done by users having to mail a paper search form to the NLM and receiving results back a few weeks later. Only librarians who had completed a specialized course were allowed to submit searches.

As computing power grew and disk storage became more plentiful in the 1980s, full-text databases began to emerge. These new databases allowed searching of the entire text of medical documents. Although lacking graphics, images, and tables from the original source, these databases made it possible to retrieve the full text of important documents quickly from remote locations. Likewise, with the growth of **time-sharing networks**, end users were now allowed to search the databases directly, though at a substantial cost.

In the early 1990s, the pace of change in the IR field quickened. The advent of the Web and the exponentially increasing power of computers and networks brought a world where vast quantities of medical information from multiple sources with various media extensions were now available over the global Internet (Berners-Lee et al. 1994). In the late 1990s, the NLM made all of its databases available to the entire world for free. Also during this time, the notion of digital libraries developed, with the recognition that the entire array of knowledge-based information could be accessed using this technology (Borgman 1999).

Now in the twenty-first century, use of IR systems and digital libraries has become ubiquitous. Estimates vary, but among individuals who use the Internet in the United States, over 80 % have used it to search for information relevant to their own health or that of an acquaintance (Fox 2011; Taylor 2010). Virtually all physicians use the Internet (Davies 2010). Furthermore, access to systems has gone beyond the traditional personal computer and extended to new devices, such as smartphones and tablet devices.

21.2 Knowledge-Based Information in Health and Biomedicine

Knowledge-based information can be subdivided into two categories. **Primary knowledge–based information** (also called primary literature) is original research that appears in journals, books, reports, and other sources. This type of information reports the initial discovery of health knowledge, usually with either original data or reanalysis of data (e.g., systematic reviews and meta-analyses). **Secondary knowledge–based information** consists of the writing that reviews, condenses, and/or synthesizes the primary literature. The most common examples of this type of literature are books, monographs, and review articles. Secondary literature includes the growing quality of patient/consumer-oriented health information that is increasingly available via the Web. It also encompasses opinion-based writing (such as editorials and position or policy papers),

clinical practice guidelines, narrative reviews, and health information on Web pages. In addition, it includes the plethora of pocket-sized manuals that were formerly a staple for practitioners in many professional fields. As will be seen later, secondary literature is the most common type of literature used by physicians.

Libraries have been the historical place where knowledge-based information has been stored. Libraries actually perform a variety of functions, including the following:

- Acquisition and maintenance of collections
- Cataloging and classification of items in collections to make them more accessible to users
- Serving as a place where individuals can get assistance with seeking information, including information on computers
- Providing work or study space (particularly in universities)

Digital libraries provide some of the same services, but their focus tends to be on the digital aspects of content.

21.2.1 Information Needs and Information Seeking

Different users of knowledge-based information have differing needs based on the nature of their information need and available resources. The information needs and information seeking of physicians have been most extensively studied. Gorman and Helfand (1995) has defined four states of **information need** in the clinical context:

- Unrecognized need—clinician unaware of information need or knowledge deficit
- Recognized need—clinician aware of need but may or may not pursue it
- Pursued need—information seeking occurs but may or may not be successful
- Satisfied need—information seeking successful

There is a great deal of evidence that the majority of information needs are not being satisfied and that IR applications may help. Among the reasons that physicians do not adhere to the most up-to-date clinical practices is that they often do not recognize that their knowledge is incomplete. While this is not the only reason for such practices, the evidence is compelling. For example, physicians do not provide patients with most up-to-date care (McGlynn et al. 2003), do not adhere to established guidelines (Diamond and Kaul 2008), and vary widely in how they provide care (Wennberg 2010).

When physicians recognize an information need, they are likely to pursue only a minority of unanswered questions. A variety of studies over several decades have demonstrated that physicians in practice have unmet information on the order of two questions for every three patients seen and only pursue answers for about 30 % of these questions (Covell et al. 1985; Ely et al. 1999; Gorman and Helfand 1995). When answers to questions are actually pursued, these studies showed that the most frequent source for answers to questions was colleagues, followed by paper-based textbooks. Therefore, it is not surprising that barriers to satisfying information needs remain (Ely et al. 2002). Physicians use electronic sources more now than were measured in these earlier studies, with the widespread use of the **electronic health record** (**EHR**) as well as ubiquity of portable smartphones and tablets. One possible approach to lowering the barrier to knowledge-based information is to link it more directly with the context of the patient in the EHR (Cimino and delFiol 2007).

The information needs of other users are less well-studied. For consumers, ongoing surveys find about 80 % of all Internet users have searched for personal health information (Fox 2011; Taylor 2010). About 4.5 % of all queries to Web search engines are health-related (Eysenbach and Kohler 2004). The most common type of search focuses on a specific disease or medical problem (66 % of all who have searched), followed by a specific medical treatment or procedure (56 %). Consumers also use the Web to search for physicians, health care institutions, and health insurance. Less studied are the information needs of researchers, but one recurrent finding is the idiosyncratic nature of their use of IR and other systems (Bartlett and Toms 2005).

21.2.2 Changes in Publishing

The Internet and the Web have had a profound impact on the publishing of knowledge-based information. The technical impediments to electronic publishing of journals have been overcome, such that virtually all scientific journals are published electronically now. A modern Internet connection is sufficient to deliver most of the content of journals. Indeed, a near-turnkey solution is already offered through Highwire Press,[1] a spin-off from Stanford University, which has an infrastructure that supports the tasks of journal publishing, from content preparation to searching and archiving.

There is great enthusiasm for electronic availability of journals, as evidenced by the growing number of titles to which libraries provide access. When available in electronic form, journal content is easier and more convenient to access. Furthermore, since most scientists have the desire for widespread dissemination of their work, they have incentive for their papers to be available electronically. Not only is there the increased convenience of redistributing reprints, but research has found that freely available on the Web have a higher likelihood of being cited by other papers than those that are not (Eysenbach 2006; Lawrence 2001; Moed 2007). As citations are important to authors for academic promotion and grant funding, authors have incentive to maximize the accessibility of their published work.

The technical challenges to electronic scholarly publication have been replaced by economic and political ones (Hersh and Rindfleisch 2000; Sox 2009). Printing and mailing, tasks no longer needed in electronic publishing, comprised a significant part of the "added value" from publishers of journals. There is still however value added by publishers, such as hiring and managing editorial staff to produce the journals, and managing the peer review process. Even if publishing companies, as they currently exist today, were to vanish, there would still be some cost to the production of journals. Thus, while the cost of producing

---

[1] www.highwire.org

journals electronically is likely to be less, it is not zero, and even if journal content is distributed "free," someone has to pay the production costs. The economic issue in electronic publishing, then, is who is going to pay for the production of journals (Sox 2009). This introduces some political issues as well. One of them centers around the concern that much research is publicly funded through grants from federal agencies such as the National Institutes of Health (NIH) and the National Science Foundation (NSF). In the current system, especially in the biomedical sciences (and to a lesser extent in other sciences), researchers turn over the copyright of their publications to journal publishers. The political concern is that the public funds the research and the universities carry it out, but individuals and libraries then must buy it back from the publishers to whom they willingly cede the copyright. This problem is exacerbated by the general decline in funding for libraries.

Some proposed models of "open access" scholarly publishing keep the archive of science freely available (Albert 2006; Björk et al. 2010). The basic principle of open access publishing is that authors and/or their institutions pay the cost of production of manuscripts up front after they are accepted through a peer review process. After the paper is published, it becomes freely available on the Web. Since most research is usually funded by grants, the cost of open access publishing should be included in grant budgets. The uptake of publishers adhering to the open access model has been modest, with the most prominent being **Biomed Central (BMC)**[2] and the **Public Library of Science (PLoS)**[3].

Another model that has emerged is **PubMed Central (PMC**, pubmedcentral.gov). PMC is a repository of life science research that provides free access while allowing publishers to maintain copyright and even optionally keep the papers housed on their own servers. A lag time of up to 6 months is allowed so that journals can reap the revenue that comes with initial publication. The

National Institutes of Health (NIH)[4] now requires all research funded by its grants to be submitted to PMC, either in the form published by publishers or as a PDF of the last manuscript prior to journal acceptance.[5] Publishers have expressed concern that copyrights give journals more control over the integrity of the papers they publish (Drazen and Curfman 2004). An alternative approach, advocated by non-commercial (professional society) publishers is the **Washington DC Principles for Free Access to Science**,[6] which advocates:

- Reinvestment of revenues in support of science.
- Use of open archives such as PMC as allowed by business constraints.
- Commitment to some free publication, access by low-income countries, and no charges to publish.

21.2.3 Quality of Information

The growth of the Internet and the Web has led to another concern, which is the quality of information available. A large fraction of Web-based health information is aimed at nonprofessional audiences. Many laud this development as empowering those most directly affected by health care—those who consume it (Eysenbach et al. 1999). Others express concern about patients misunderstanding or being purposely misled by incorrect or inappropriately interpreted information (Jadad 1999). Some clinicians also lament the time required to go through stacks of printouts downloaded by patients and brought to the office. The Web is inherently democratic, allowing anyone to post information. This is an asset in a democratic society like that of the United States. However, it is potentially at odds with the operation of a professional field, particularly one like health care, where practitioners are ethically bound and legally required to adhere to the highest standard of

---

[2] www.biomedcentral.com
[3] www.plos.org

[4] www.nih.gov
[5] www.publicaccess.nih.gov
[6] www.dcprinciples.org

care. Thus, a major concern with health information on the Web is the presence of inaccurate or out-of-date information. Although research in this area has declined, one **systematic review** of studies assessing the quality of health information found that 55 of 79 studies came to the conclusion that quality of information was a problem (Eysenbach et al. 2002).

The impact of poor-quality information is unclear. People have been harmed by incorrect and misleading health information since time immemorial. One well-known self-help expert has argued that patients and consumers actually are savvy enough to understand the limits of quality of information on the Web. This view holds that patients and consumers should be trusted to discern quality using their own abilities to consult different sources of information and to communicate with health care practitioners and with others who share their condition(s) (Ferguson 2002). Indeed, the ideal situation may be a partnership among patients and their health care practitioners, as it has been shown that patients desire that their practitioners be the primary source of recommendations for online information (Tang et al. 1997).

This concern about quality of information has led a number of individuals and organizations to develop guidelines for assessing the quality of health information. These guidelines usually have explicit criteria for a Web page that a reader can apply to determine whether a potential source of information has attributes consistent with high quality. One of the earliest and most widely quoted set of criteria was published in JAMA (Silberg et al. 1997). These criteria stated that Web pages should contain the name, affiliation, and credentials of the author; references to the claims made; explicit listing of any perceived or real conflict of interest; and date of most recent update. Another early set of criteria was the **Health on the Net** (HON) codes,[7] a set of voluntary codes of conduct for health-related Web sites. Sites that adhere to the HON codes can display the HON logo. Another approach to insuring Web site quality is accreditation by a third party.

URAC (formerly, the Utilization Review Accreditation Commission) has a process for such accreditation.[8] The URAC standards cover six general issues: health content editorial process, disclosure of financial relationships, linking to other Web sites, privacy and security, consumer complaint mechanisms, and internal processes required to maintain quality over time.

21.2.4 Evidence-Based Medicine

The growing quantity of clinical information available in IR systems and digital libraries requires new approaches to select that which is best to use for clinical decisions. The philosophy guiding this approach is **evidence-based medicine** (EBM), which can be viewed a set of tools to inform clinical decision making. It allows clinical experience ("art") to be integrated with best clinical science (Haynes et al. 2002). Also, EBM makes the medical literature more clinically applicable and relevant. In addition, it requires the user to be facile with computers and IR systems. There are many well-known books and Web resources for EBM, with the original textbook now in a fourth edition (Straus et al. 2005). The process of EBM involves three general steps:

- Phrasing a clinical question that is pertinent and answerable.
- Identifying evidence (studies in articles) that address the question.
- Critically appraising the evidence to determine whether it applies to the patient.

The phrasing of the clinical question is an often-overlooked portion of the EBM process. There are two general types of clinical question: background questions and foreground questions (Straus et al. 2005). **Background questions** ask for general knowledge about a disorder, whereas **foreground questions** ask for knowledge about managing patients with a disorder. Background questions are generally best answered with textbooks and classical review articles, whereas foreground questions are answered using EBM

---

[7] www.hon.ch

[8] http://www.urac.org/consumers/overview.aspx

techniques. There are four major foreground question categories:

- Therapy (or intervention)—benefit of treatment or prevention.
- Diagnosis—test diagnosing disease.
- Harm—detrimental health effects of a disease, environmental exposure (natural or man-made), or medical intervention.
- Prognosis—outcome of disease course.

Identifying evidence involves selecting the best evidence for a given type of question. EBM proponents advocate, for example, that randomized controlled trials or a meta-analysis that combines multiple trials provide the best evidence for or against particular health care interventions. Likewise, diagnostic test accuracy is best assessed with comparison to a known gold standard in an appropriate spectrum of patients to whom the test will be applied (see Chap. 3). Questions of harm can be answered by randomized controlled trials when it is ethical to do so; otherwise they are best answered with observational case control or cohort studies. There are checklists of attributes for these different types of studies that allow their critical appraisal and applicability to a given patient in the EBM resources described above.

The original approach to EBM has evolved over time, with less emphasis on critically appraising original evidence and more on synthesized evidence being made readily available to clinicians, usually through electronic sources, including clinical decision support systems (see Chap. 22, DiCenso et al. 2009; Hersh 1999). There have also been a number of criticisms of EBM, as summarized by Cohen et al. (2004).

21.3 Content of Knowledge-Based Information Resources

The previous sections of this chapter have described some of the issues and concerns surrounding the production and use of knowledge-based information in biomedicine. It is useful to classify the information to gain a better understanding of its structure and function. In this section, we classify content into bibliographic, full-text, annotated, and aggregated categories, although some content does not neatly fit within them.

21.3.1 Bibliographic Content

The first category consists of **bibliographic content**. It includes what was for decades the mainstay of IR systems: **literature reference databases**. Also called **bibliographic databases**, this content consists of citations or pointers to the medical literature (i.e., journal articles). The best-known and most widely used biomedical bibliographic database is **MEDLINE**, which contains bibliographic references to all of the biomedical articles, editorials, and letters to the editors in approximately 5,000 scientific journals. The journals are chosen for inclusion by an advisory committee of subject experts convened by NIH. At present, about 700,000 references are added to MEDLINE yearly. It contained over 22 million references by the end of 2012.

The current MEDLINE record contains up to 49 fields. A clinician may be interested in just a handful of these fields, such as the title, abstract, and indexing terms. But other fields contain specific information that may be of great importance to other audiences. For example, a genome researcher might be highly interested in the Supplementary Information (SI) field to link to genomic databases. Even the clinician may, however, derive benefit from some of the other fields. For example, the Publication Type (PT) field can help in the application of EBM, such as when one is searching for a practice guideline or a randomized controlled trial. MEDLINE is accessible by many means and available without charge via the **PubMed** system (pubmed.gov), produced by the **National Center for Biotechnology Information** (**NCBI**,)[9] of the NLM. A number of other information vendors, such as Ovid Technologies[10] and Aries Systems,[11] license the content of MEDLINE and other databases and

---

[9] www.ncbi.nlm.nih.gov
[10] www.ovid.com
[11] www.ariessys.com

provide value-added services that can be accessed for a fee by individuals and institutions.

MEDLINE is only one of many databases produced by the NLM. Other more specialized databases are also available, covering topics from AIDS to space medicine and toxicology. There are several non-NLM bibliographic databases that tend to be more focused on subjects or resource types. The major non-NLM database for the nursing field is the **Cumulative Index to Nursing and Allied Health Literature** (CINAHL, CINAHL Information Systems),[12] which covers nursing and allied health literature, including physical therapy, occupational therapy, laboratory technology, health education, physician assistants, and medical records.

Another well-known bibliographic databases is **EMBASE**,[13] which is sometimes referred to as the "European MEDLINE." It contains over 24 million records and covers many of the same medical journals as MEDLINE but with a more international focus, including more non-English-language journals. These journals are often important for those carrying out meta-analyses and systematic reviews, which need access to all the studies done across the world.

A second, more modern type of bibliographic content is the **Web catalog**. There are increasing numbers of such catalogs, which consist of Web pages containing mainly links to other Web pages and sites. It should be noted that there is a blurry distinction between Web catalogs and aggregations (the fourth category; see Sects. 21.3 and 21.4, below). In general, the former contain only links to other pages and sites, while the latter include actual content that is highly integrated with other resources. Some well-known Web catalogs include:

- HealthFinder (healthfinder.gov)—consumer-oriented health information maintained by the Office of Disease Prevention and Health Promotion of the U.S. Department of Health and Human Services.
- HON Select[14] —a European catalog of quality-filtered, clinician-oriented Web content from the HON foundation.

- Translating Research into Practice (TRIP)[15]—a database of content deemed to meet high standards of EBM.
- Open Directory[16] —a general Web catalog that has significant health content.

Another more modern bibliographic resource is the **National Guidelines Clearinghouse (NGC)**[17]. Produced by the Agency for Health care Research and Quality (AHRQ), it contains exhaustive information about clinical practice guidelines. Some of the guidelines produced are freely available, published electronically and/or on paper. Others are proprietary, in which case a link is provided to a location at which the guideline can be ordered or purchased. The overall goal of the NGC is to make evidence-based clinical practice guidelines and related abstract, summary, and comparison materials widely available to health care and other professionals.

A final kind of bibliographic-like content consists of **RSS feeds** (originally RDF Site Summary, often dubbed "Really Simple Syndication"), which are short summaries of Web content, typically news, journal articles, blog postings, and other content. Users set up an RSS aggregator, which can be though a Web browser, email client, or standalone software, configured for the RSS feed desired, with an option to add a filter for specific content. There are two versions of RSS (1.0 and 2.0) but both provide:

- Title—name of item
- Link—URL to content
- Description—a brief description of the content

21.3.2 Full-text Content

The second type of content is **full-text content**. A large component of this content consists of the online versions of books and periodicals. As already noted, most traditionally paper-based medical literature, from textbooks to journals, is now available electronically. The electronic versions

---

[12] http://www.ebscohost.com/cinahl/

[13] www.embase.com

[14] www.hon.ch/HONselect

[15] www.tripdatabase.com

[16] www.dmoz.org

[17] www.guideline.gov

may be enhanced by measures ranging from the provision of supplemental data in a journal article to linkages and multimedia content in a textbook. The final component of this category is the Web site. Admittedly, the diversity of information on Web sites is enormous, and sites may include every other type of content described in this chapter. However, in the context of this category, "Web site" refers to the vast number of static and dynamic Web pages at a discrete Web location.

Electronic publication of journals allows additional features not possible in the print world. Journal editors often clash with authors over the length of published papers (editors want them short for readability whereas authors want them long to be able to present all ideas and results). To address this situation, the British Medical Journal (BMJ) initiated an **electronic-long, paper-short (ELPS)** system that provides on the Web site supplemental material that did not appear in the print version of the journal. Journal Web sites can provide supplementary data of results, images, and even raw data. A journal Web site also allows more dialog about articles than could be published in a "Letters to the Editor" section of a print journal. Electronic publication also allows true bibliographic linkages, both to other full-text articles and to the MEDLINE record.

The Web also allows linkage directly from bibliographic databases to full text. PubMed maintains a field for the Web address of the full-text paper. This linkage is active when the PubMed record is displayed, but users may be met by a password screen if the article is not available for free. Many sites allow both access to subscribers or a pay-per-view facility. Many academic organizations now maintain large numbers of subscriptions to journals available to faculty, staff, and students. Other publishers, such as Ovid and MD Consult,[18] provide access within their own password-protected interfaces to articles from journals that they have licensed for use in their systems.

The most common secondary literature source is traditional textbooks, an increasing number of which are available in computer form. A common approach with textbooks is bundling them,

sometimes with linkages across the bundled texts. An early bundler of textbooks was Stat!-Ref (Teton Data Systems)[19] that, like many, began as a CD-ROM product and then moved to the Web. Stat!-Ref offers over 30 textbooks. Most other publishers have similar aggregated their libraries of textbooks and other content. Another collection of textbooks is the NCBI Bookshelf, which contains many volumes on biomedical research topics.[20] A separate book on the NCBI Web site is Online Mendelian Inheritance in Man (OMIM)[21], which is continually updated with new information about the genomic causes of human disease.

Electronic textbooks offer additional features beyond text from the print version. While many print textbooks do feature high-quality images, electronic versions offer the ability to have more pictures and illustrations. They also have the ability to use sound and video, although few do at this time. As with full-text journals, electronic textbooks can link to other resources, including journal references and the full articles. Many Web-based textbook sites also provide access to continuing education self-assessment questions and medical news. Finally, electronic textbooks let authors and publishers provide more frequent updates of the information than is allowed by the usual cycle of print editions, where new versions come out only every 2–5 years.

As noted above, Web sites are another form of full-text information. Probably the most effective provider of Web-based health information is the U.S. government. Not only do they produce bibliographic databases, but the NLM, AHRQ, the National Cancer Institute (NCI), Centers for Disease Control (CDC), and others have also been innovative in providing comprehensive full-text information for health care providers and consumers. One example is the popular CDC Travel site.[22] Some of these will be described later as aggregations, since they provide many different types of resources.

---

[18] www.mdconsult.com

[19] www.statref.com

[20] http://www.ncbi.nlm.nih.gov/entrez/query.fcgi?db=Books

[21] http://www.ncbi.nlm.nih.gov/omim

[22] http://www.cdc.gov/travel/

A large number of commercial biomedical and health Web sites have emerged in recent years. On the consumer side, they include more than just collections of text; they also include interaction with experts, online stores, and catalogs of links to other sites. Among the best known of these are Intelihealth[23] and NetWellness.[24] There are also Web sites, either from medical societies or companies, that provide information geared toward health care providers, typically overviews of diseases, their diagnosis, and treatment; medical news and other resources for providers are often offered as well.

Other sources of on-line health-related content include encyclopedias, the so-called "**body of knowledge**" (BOK; the complete set of concepts, terms and activities that make up a professional domain), and **Weblogs** or **blogs**. A well-known online encyclopedia with a great deal of health-related information is Wikipedia,[25] which features a distributed authorship process whose content has been found to reliable (Giles 2005; Nicholson 2006) and frequently shows up near the top in health-related Web searches (Laurent and Vickers 2009). A growing number of organizations have a body of knowledge, such as the **American Health Information Management Association** (**AHIMA**).[26] Blogs tend to carry a stream of consciousness but often high-quality information is posted within them.

21.3.3 Annotated Content

The third category consists of **annotated content**. These resources are usually not stored as freestanding Web pages but instead are often housed in **database management systems**. This content can be further subcategorized into discrete information types:

- **Image databases**—collections of images from radiology, pathology, and other areas

- **Genomics databases**—information from gene sequencing, protein characterization, and other genomic research
- **Citation databases**—bibliographic linkages of scientific literature
- **EBM databases**—highly structured collections of clinical evidence
- **Other databases**—miscellaneous other collections

A great number of biomedical image databases are available on the Web. These include:

- Visible Human[27]
- BrighamRad[28]
- WebPath[29]
- Pathology Education Instructional Resource (PEIR)[30]
- DermIS[31]
- VisualDX[32]

Many genomics databases are available on the Web. The first issue each year of the journal *Nucleic Acids Research* (NAR) catalogs and describes these databases, and is now available by open access means (Galperin and Cochrane 2011). NAR also maintains an ongoing database of such databases, the Molecular Biology Database Collection.[33] Among the most important of these databases are those available from NCBI (Sayers et al. 2011). All their databases are linked among themselves, along with PubMed and OMIM, and are searchable via the **Entrez** system.[34] More details on the specific content of genomics databases is provided in Chap. 24.

Citation databases provide linkages to articles that cite others across the scientific literature. The earliest citation databases were the Science Citation Index (SCI, Thomspon-Reuters) and Social Science Citation Index (SSCI, Thomspon-Reuters), which are now part of the larger Web of

---

[23] www.intelihealth.com

[24] www.netwellness.com

[25] www.wikipedia.org

[26] http://library.ahima.org/bok

[27] http://www.nlm.nih.gov/research/visible/visible_human.html

[28] http://brighamrad.harvard.edu/

[29] http://library.med.utah.edu/WebPath/webpath.html

[30] www.peir.net

[31] www.dermis.net

[32] www.visualdx.com (requires a subscription fee)

[33] http://www.oxfordjournals.org/nar/database/a/

[34] www.ncbi.nlm.nih.gov/Entrez

Science. Two well-known bibliographic databases for biomedical and health topics that also have citation links include SCOPUS[35] and Google Scholar.[36] These three were recently compared for their features and coverage (Kulkarni et al. 2009). A final citation database of note is CiteSeer,[37] which focuses on computer and information science, including biomedical informatics.

EBM databases are devoted to providing annotated evidence-based information. Some examples (all available with through subscription fees) include:

- The Cochrane Database of Systematic Reviews—one of the original collections of systematic reviews[38]
- Clinical Evidence—an "evidence formulary"[39]
- Up-to-Date—content centered around clinical questions[40]
- InfoPOEMS—"patient-oriented evidence that matters"[41]
- Physicians' Information and Education Resource (PIER)—"practice guidance statements" for which every test and treatment has associated ratings of the evidence to support them[42]

There is a growing market for a related type of evidence-based content in the form of clinical decision support order sets, rules, and health/disease management templates. Publishers include EHR vendors whose systems employ this content as well as other vendors such as Zynx[43] and Thomson-Reuters.[44]

There are a variety of other annotated content. The ClinicalTrials.gov database began as a database of clinical trials sponsored by NIH. In recent years it has expanded its scope to be a registry of all clinical trials (DeAngelis et al. 2005; Laine et al. 2007) and to containing actual results of trials (Zarin et al. 2011). Another important database for researchers is NIH RePORTER,[45] which is a database of all research funded by NIH.

21.3.4 Aggregated Content

The final category consists of **aggregations** of content from the first three categories. The distinction between this category and some of the highly linked types of content described above is admittedly blurry, but aggregations typically have a wide variety of different types of information serving the diverse needs of users. Aggregated content has been developed for all types of users from consumers to clinicians to scientists.

Probably the largest aggregated consumer information resource is **MedlinePlus**[46] from the NLM. MedlinePlus includes all of the types of content previously described, aggregated for easy access to a given topic. MedlinePlus contains health topics, drug information, medical dictionaries, directories, and other resources. Each topic contains links to health information from the NIH and other sources deemed credible by its selectors. There are also links to current health news (updated daily), a medical encyclopedia, drug references, and directories, along with a preformed PubMed search related to the topic.

Aggregations of content have also been developed for clinicians. Most of the major publishers now aggregate all of their content in packages for clinicians. Another aggregated resource for clinicians is **Merck Medicus**,[47] developed by the well-known publisher and pharmaceutical house, is available for free to all licensed U.S. physicians, and includes such well-known resources as Harrison's Online, MDConsult, and DXplain.

---

[35] www.scopus.com

[36] scholar.google.com

[37] http://citeseerx.ist.psu.edu/

[38] www.cochrane.org

[39] www.clinicalevidence.com

[40] www.uptodate.com

[41] www.infopoems.com

[42] www.pier.acponline.org

[43] www.zynxhealth.com

[44] www.thomsonreuters.com

[45] http://projectreporter.nih.gov/reporter.cfm

[46] www.medlineplus.gov

[47] www.merckmedicus.com

Another well-known group of aggregations of content for genomics researchers is the **model organism databases**. These databases bring together bibliographic databases, full text, and databases of sequences, structure, and function for organisms whose genomic data have been highly characterized. One of the oldest and most developed model organism databases is the Mouse Genome Informatics resource.[48] More details are provided in Chap. 22.

21.4 Indexing

As noted at the beginning of the chapter, indexing is the process of assigning metadata to content to facilitate its retrieval. Most modern commercial content is indexed in two ways:

1. **Manual indexing**—where human indexers, usually using a controlled terminology, assign indexing terms and attributes to documents, often following a specific protocol.
2. **Automated indexing**—where computers make the indexing assignments, usually limited to breaking out each word in the document (or part of the document) as an indexing term.

Manual indexing is done most commonly with bibliographic databases and annotated content. In this age of proliferating electronic content, such as online textbooks, practice guidelines, and multimedia collections, manual indexing has become either too expensive or outright unfeasible for the quantity and diversity of material now available. Thus there are increasing numbers of databases that are indexed only by automated means. Before covering these types of indexing in detail, let us first discuss controlled terminologies.

21.4.1 Controlled Terminologies

A **controlled terminology** contains a set of terms that can be applied to a task, such as indexing. When the terminology defines the terms, it is usually called a **vocabulary**. When it contains

variants or synonyms of terms, it is also called a **thesaurus**. Before discussing actual terminologies, it is useful to define some terms. A **concept** is an idea or object that exists in the world, such as the condition under which human blood pressure is elevated. A **term** is the actual string of one or more words that represent a concept, such as "Hypertension" or "High Blood Pressure". One of these string forms is the preferred or **canonical form**, such as "Hypertension" in the present example. When one or more terms can represent a concept, the different terms are called **synonyms**.

A controlled terminology usually contains a list of terms that are the canonical representations of the concepts. If it is athesaurus, it contains relationships between terms, which typically fall into three categories:

- **Hierarchical**—terms that are broader or narrower. The hierarchical organization not only provides an overview of the structure of a thesaurus but also can be used to enhance searching (e.g., MeSH tree explosions that add terms from an entire portion of the hierarchy to augment a search).
- **Synonym**—terms that are synonyms, allowing the indexer or searcher to express a concept in different words.
- **Related**—terms that are not synonymous or hierarchical but are somehow otherwise related. These usually remind the searcher of different but related terms that may enhance a search.

The MeSH terminology is used to manually index most of the databases produced by the NLM (Coletti and Bleich 2001). The latest version contains over 26,000 subject headings (the word MeSH uses for the canonical representation of its concepts). It also contains over 170,000 synonyms to those terms, which in MeSH jargon are called **entry terms**. In addition, MeSH contains the three types of relationships described in the previous paragraph:

- Hierarchical—MeSH is organized hierarchically into 16 trees, such as Diseases, Organisms, and Chemicals and Drugs
- Synonym—MeSH contains a vast number of entry terms, which are synonyms of the headings

---

[48] www.informatics.jax.org

Fig. 21.2 A slice through the Medical Subject Headings (MeSH) hierarchy for "Hypertension" and related terms, showing the location of the term in the C. Diseases. The arrows show links to broader terms in the hierarchy, while the codes give the tree address used internally by the MeSH system (Reproduced with permission of Springer (Hersh 2009))

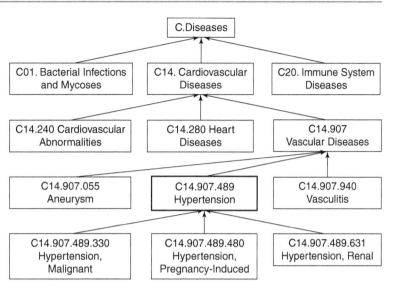

- Related—terms that may be useful for searchers to add to their searches when appropriate are suggested for many headings

The MeSH terminology files, their associated data, and their supporting documentation are available on the NLM's MeSH Web site.[49] There is also a browser that facilitates exploration of the terminology.[50] Figure 21.2 shows a slice through the MeSH hierarchy for "Hypertension" and related cardiovascular diseases in the C. Diseases tree.

There are features of MeSH designed to assist indexers in making documents more retrievable. One of these is **subheadings**, which are qualifiers of subject headings that narrow the focus of a term. In Hypertension, for example, the focus of an article may be on the diagnosis, epidemiology, or treatment of the condition. Another feature of MeSH that helps retrieval is **check tags**. These are MeSH terms that represent certain facets of medical studies, such as age, gender, human or nonhuman, and type of grant support. Related to check tags are the geographical locations in one particular part of the MeSH hierarchy (called the "Z tree", because their term codes start with "Z"). Indexers must also include these, like check tags, since the location of a study (e.g., Oregon) must

be indicated. Another feature gaining increasing importance for EBM and other purposes is the **publication type**, which describes the type of publication or the type of study. A searcher who wants a review of a topic may choose the publication type Review or Review Literature. Or, to find studies that provide the best evidence for a therapy, the publication type Meta-Analysis, Randomized Controlled Trial, or Controlled Clinical Trial would be used.

MeSH is not the only thesaurus used for indexing biomedical documents. A number of other thesauri are used to index non-NLM databases. CINAHL, for example, uses the **CINAHL Subject Headings**, which are based on MeSH but have additional domain-specific terms added. EMBASE has a terminology called **EMTREE**, which has many features similar to those of MeSH.[51]

One problem with controlled terminologies, not limited to IR systems, is their proliferation. As already described in Chap. 7, there is great need for linkage across these different terminologies. This was the primary motivation for the **Unified Medical Language System (UMLS) Project**, which was undertaken in the 1980s to address this problem (Humphreys et al. 1998).

---

[49] http://www.nlm.nih.gov/mesh/

[50] http://www.nlm.nih.gov/mesh/MBrowser.html

[51] http://www.embase.com/info/helpfiles/emtree-tool/emtree-thesaurus

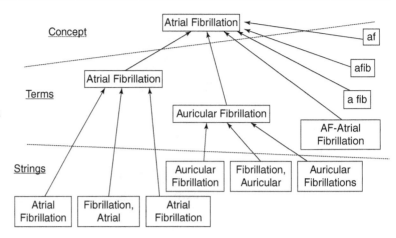

Fig. 21.3 Concepts, terms, and strings for the Metathesaurus concept atrial fibrillation. Each string may occur in more than one vocabulary, in which case each would be an atom (Reproduced with permission of Springer (Hersh 2009))

There are three components of the **UMLS Knowledge Sources**: the **Metathesaurus**, the **UMLS Semantic Network**, and the **Specialist Lexicon**. The Metathesaurus component of the UMLS links parts or all of over 100 terminologies (Bodenreider 2004).

In the Metathesaurus, all terms that are conceptually the same are linked together as a concept. Each concept may have one or more terms, each of which represents an expression of the concept from a source terminology that is not just a simple lexical variant (i.e., differs only in word ending or order). Each term may consist of one or more strings that represent all the lexical variants that are represented for that term in the source terminologies. One of each term's strings is designated as the preferred form, and the preferred string of the preferred term is known as the canonical form of the concept. There are rules of precedence for determining the canonical form, the main one being that the MeSH heading is used if one of the source terminologies for the concept is MeSH.

Each Metathesaurus concept has a single concept unique identifier (CUI). Each term has one term unique identifier (LUI), all of which are linked to the one (or more) CUIs with which they are associated. Likewise, each string has one string unique identifier (SUI), which is likewise linked to the LUIs in which they occur. In addition, each string has an atomic unique identifier (AUI) that represents information from each instance of the string in each vocabulary.

Figure 21.3 depicts the English-language concepts, terms, and strings for the Metathesaurus concept atrial fibrillation. (Each string may occur in more than one vocabulary, in which case each would be an atom.) The canonical form of the concept and one of its terms is atrial fibrillation. Within both terms are several strings that vary in word order and case.

The Metathesaurus contains a wealth of additional information. In addition to the synonym relationships between concepts, terms, and strings described earlier, there are also non-synonym relationships between concepts. There are a great many attributes for the concepts, terms, strings, and atoms, such as definitions, lexical types, and occurrence in various data sources. Also provided with the Metathesaurus is a word index that connects each word to all the strings it occurs in, along with its concept, term, string, and atomic identifiers.

21.4.2 Manual Indexing

Manual indexing is most commonly done for bibliographic and annotated content, although it is sometimes for other types of content as well. Manual indexing is usually done by means of a controlled terminology of terms and attributes. Most databases utilizing human indexing usually have a detailed protocol for assignment of indexing terms from the thesaurus. The MEDLINE database is no exception. The principles of

MEDLINE indexing were laid out in the two-volume MEDLARS Indexing Manual (Charen 1976, 1983). Subsequent modifications have occurred with changes to MEDLINE, other databases, and MeSH over the years. The major concepts of the article, usually from two to five headings, are designed as main headings, and designated in the MEDLINE record by an asterisk. The indexer is also required to assign appropriate subheadings. Finally, the indexer must also assign check tags, geographical locations, and publication types. Although MEDLINE indexing is still manual, indexers are aided by a variety of electronic tools for selecting and assigning MeSH terms.

Few full-text resources are manually indexed. One type of indexing that commonly takes place with full-text resources, especially in the print world, is that performed for the index at the back of the book. However, this information is rarely used in IR systems; instead, most online textbooks rely on automated indexing (see Sect. 21.4.3, below). One exception to this is MDConsult,[52] which uses back-of-book indexes to point to specific sections in its online books.

Manual indexing of Web content is challenging. With billions of pages of content, manual indexing of more than a fraction of it is not feasible. On the other hand, the lack of a coherent index makes searching much more difficult, especially when specific resource types are being sought. A simple form of manual indexing of the Web takes place in the development of the Web catalogs and aggregations as described earlier. These catalogs contain not only explicit indexing about subjects and other attributes, but also implicit indexing about the quality of a given resource by the decision of whether to include it in the catalog.

Two major approaches to manual indexing have emerged on the Web that are often complementary. The first approach, that of applying metadata to Web pages and sites, is exemplified by the **Dublin Core Metadata Initiative (DCMI,)**[53] (Weibel and Koch 2000). The second

approach, to build directories of content, was popularized initially by the Yahoo search engine.[54] A more open approach to building directories was taken up by the Open Directory Project,[55] which carries on the structuring of the directory and entry of content by volunteers across the world.

The goal of the DCMI has been to develop a set of standard data elements that creators of Web resources can use to apply metadata to their content. The specification has defined 15 elements, as shown in Table 21.1. The DCMI was recently approved as a standard by the **National Information Standards Organization (NISO)** with the designation Z39.85. It is also a standard with the **International Organization for Standards (ISO)**, ISO Standard 15836:2009.

There have been some medical adaptations of the DCMI. The most developed of these is the Catalogue et Index des Sites Médicaux Francophones (CISMeF).[56] (Darmoni et al. 2000). A catalog of French-language health resources on the Web, CISMeF has used DCMI to catalog over 40,000 Web pages, including information resources (e.g., practice guidelines, consensus development conferences), organizations (e.g., hospitals, medical schools, pharmaceutical companies), and databases. The Subject field uses the French translation of MeSH but also includes the English translation. For Type, a list of common Web resources has been enumerated.

While Dublin Core Metadata was originally envisioned to be included in **Hypertext Markup Language (HTML)** Web pages, it became apparent that many non-HTML resources exist on the Web and that there are reasons to store metadata external to Web pages. For example, authors of Web pages might not be the best people to index pages or other entities might wish to add value by their own indexing of content. An emerging standard for cataloging metadata is the **Resource Description Framework (RDF)** (Akerkar 2009). A framework for describing and

---

[52] www.mdconsult.com

[53] www.dublincore.org

[54] www.yahoo.com

[55] www.dmoz.org

[56] www.cismef.org

Table 21.1 Elements of Dublin Core Metadata

Element	Definition
DC.title	The name given to the resource
DC.creator	The person or organization primarily responsible for creating the intellectual content of the resource
DC.subject	The topic of the resource
DC.description	A textual description of the content of the resource
DC.publisher	The entity responsible for making the resource available in its present form
DC.date	A date associated with the creation or availability of the resource
DC.contributor	A person or organization not specified in a creator element who has made a significant intellectual contribution to the resource but whose contribution is secondary to any person or organization specified in a creator element
DC.type	The category of the resource
DC.format	The data format of the resource, used to identify the software and possibly hardware that might be needed to display or operate the resource
DC.identifier	A string or number used to uniquely identify the resource
DC.source	Information about a second resource from which the present resource is derived
DC.language	The language of the intellectual content of the resource
DC.relation	An identifier of a second resource and its relationship to the present resource
DC.coverage	The spatial or temporal characteristics of the intellectual content of the resource
DC.rights	A rights management statement, an identifier that links to a rights management statement, or an identifier that links to a service providing information about rights management for the resource

interchanging metadata, RDF is usually expressed in **Extensible Markup Language (XML)**, a standard for data interchange on the Web. RDF also forms the basis of what some call the future of the Web as a repository not only of content but also of knowledge, which is also referred to as the **Semantic Web** (Akerkar 2009). Dublin Core Metadata (or any type of metadata) can be represented in RDF.

Another approach to manually indexing content on the Web has been to create directories of content. The first major effort to create these was for use in the Yahoo! search engine, which created a subject hierarchy and assigned Web sites to elements within it. When concern began to emerge that the Yahoo directory was proprietary and not necessarily representative of the Web community at large, an alternative movement sprung up: the Open Directory Project.

Manual indexing has a number of limitations, the most significant of which is inconsistency. Funk and Reid (Funk and Reid 1983) evaluated indexing inconsistency in MEDLINE by identifying 760 articles that had been indexed twice by the NLM. The most consistent indexing occurred with check tags and central concept headings, which were only indexed with a consistency of 61–75 %. The least consistent indexing occurred with subheadings, especially those assigned to non-central-concept headings, which had a consistency of less than 35 %. A repeat of this study in more recent times found comparable results (Marcetich et al. 2004). Manual indexing also takes time. While it may be feasible with the large resources the NLM has to index MEDLINE, it is probably impossible with the growing amount of content on Web sites and in other full-text resources. Indeed, the NLM has recognized the challenge of continuing to have to index the growing body of biomedical literature and is investigating automated and semiautomated means of doing so (Aronson et al. 2004).

21.4.3 Automated Indexing

In automated indexing, the indexing is done by a computer. Although the mechanical running of the automated indexing process lacks cognitive input, considerable intellectual effort may have gone into development of the system for doing it, so this form of indexing still qualifies as an intellectual process. In this section, we will focus on the automated indexing used in operational IR systems, namely the indexing of documents by the words they contain.

Some might not think of extracting all the words in a document as "indexing," but from the standpoint of an IR system, words are descriptors of documents, just like human-assigned indexing terms. Most retrieval systems actually use a hybrid of human and word indexing, in that the human-assigned indexing terms become part of the document, which can then be searched by using the whole controlled term or individual words within it. As will be seen in the next chapter, most MEDLINE implementations have always allowed the combination of searching on human indexing terms and on words in the title and abstract of the reference. With the development of full-text resources in the 1980s and 1990s, systems that allowed only word indexing began to emerge. This trend increased with the advent of the Web.

Word indexing is typically done by defining all consecutive **alphanumeric** sequences between white space (which consists of spaces, punctuation, carriage returns, and other non-alphanumeric characters) as words. Systems must take particular care to apply the same process to documents and the user's query, especially with characters such as hyphens and apostrophes. Many systems go beyond simple identification of words and attempt to assign weights to words that represent their importance in the document (Salton 1991).

Many systems using word indexing employ processes to remove common words or conflate words to common forms. The former consists of filtering to remove **stop words**, which are common words that always occur with high frequency and are usually of little value in searching. The stop word list, also called a **negative dictionary**, varies in size from the seven words of the original MEDLARS stop list (and, an, by, from, of, the, with) to the list of 250–500 words more typically used. Examples of the latter are the 250-word list of van Rijsbergen (1979), the 471-word list of Fox (1992), and the PubMed stop list (Anonymous 2007). Conflation of words to common forms is done via **stemming**, the purpose of which is to ensure words with plurals and common suffixes (e.g., -ed, -ing, -er, -al) are always indexed by their stem form (Frakes 1992). For example, the words cough, coughs, and coughing are all indexed via their stem cough. Both stop word remove and stemming reduce the size of indexing files and lead to more efficient query processing.

A commonly used approach for **term weighting** is **TF*IDF weighting**, which combines the **inverse document frequency** (**IDF**) and **term frequency** (**TF**). The IDF is the logarithm of the ratio of the total number of documents to the number of documents in which the term occurs. It is assigned once for each term in the database, and it correlates inversely with the frequency of the term in the entire database. The usual formula used is:

$$IDF\left(term\right) = \log \frac{\text{number of documents in database}}{\text{number of documents with term}} + 1 \qquad (21.1)$$

The TF is a measure of the frequency with which a term occurs in a given document and is assigned to each term in each document, with the usual formula:

$$TF\left(term, document\right) = \text{frequency of term in document} \qquad (21.2)$$

In TF*IDF weighting, the two terms are combined to form the indexing weight, WEIGHT:

$$WEIGHT\left(term, document\right) = TF\left(term, document\right) * IDF\left(term\right) \qquad (21.3)$$

Another automated indexing approach generating increased interest is the use of **link-based** methods, fueled by the success of the **Google** search engine.[57] This approach gives weight to pages based on how often they are cited by other pages. The **PageRank (PR) algorithm** is mathematically complex, but can be viewed as giving more weight to a Web page based on the number of other pages that link to it (Brin and Page 1998). Thus, the home page of the NLM or a major medical journal is likely to have a very high PR, whereas a more obscure page will have a lower PR. Google has also had to develop new computer architectures and algorithms to maintain pace with indexing the Web, leading to a new paradigm for such large-scale processing called MapRecuce (Dean and Ghemawat 2008; Lin and Dyer 2010).

General-purpose search engines such as Google and Microsoft Bing use word-based approaches and variants of the PageRank algorithm for indexing. They amass the content in their search systems by "crawling" the Web, collecting and indexing every object they find on the Web. This includes not only HTML pages, but other files as well, including Microsoft Word, Portable Document Format (PDF), and images.

Word indexing has a number of limitations, including:

- Synonymy—different words may have the same meaning, such as high and elevated. This problem may extend to the level of phrases with no words in common, such as the synonyms hypertension and high blood pressure.
- Polysemy—the same word may have different meanings or senses. For example, the word lead can refer to an element or to a part of an electrocardiogram machine.
- Content—words in a document may not reflect its focus. For example, an article describing hypertension may make mention in passing to other concepts, such as congestive heart failure (CHF) that are not the focus of the article.
- Context—words take on meaning based on other words around them. For example, the relatively common words high, blood, and

pressure, take on added meaning when occurring together in the phrase high blood pressure.
- Morphology—words can have suffixes that do not change the underlying meaning, such as indicators of plurals, various participles, adjectival forms of nouns, and nominalized forms of adjectives.
- Granularity—queries and documents may describe concepts at different levels of a hierarchy. For example, a user might query for antibiotics in the treatment of a specific infection, but the documents might describe specific antibiotics themselves, such as penicillin.

Chapter 8 on Natural Language Processing (NLP) describes automated methods for addressing these limitations.

21.5 Retrieval

There are two broad approaches to retrieval. Exact-match searching allows the user precise control over the items retrieved. Partial-match searching, on the other hand, recognizes the inexact nature of both indexing and retrieval, and instead attempts to return to the user content ranked by how close it comes to the user's query. After general explanations of these approaches, we will describe actual systems that access the different types of biomedical content.

21.5.1 Exact-Match Retrieval

In exact-match searching, the IR system gives the user all documents that exactly match the criteria specified in the search statement(s). Since the **Boolean operators** AND, OR, and NOT are usually required to create a manageable set of documents, this type of searching is often called **Boolean searching**. Furthermore, since the user typically builds sets of documents that are manipulated with the Boolean operators, this approach is also called **set-based searching**. Most of the early operational IR systems in the 1950s through 1970s used the exact-match approach, even

---

[57] www.google.com

though Salton was developing the partial-match approach in research systems during that time (Salton and McGill 1983). Currently, exact-match searching tends to be associated with retrieval from bibliographic and annotated databases, while the partial-match approach tends to be used with full-text searching.

Typically the first step in exact-match retrieval is to select terms to build sets. Other attributes, such as the author name, publication type, or gene identifier (in the secondary source identifier field of MEDLINE), may be selected to build sets as well. Once the search term(s) and attribute(s) have been selected, they are combined with the Boolean operators. The Boolean AND operator is typically used to narrow a retrieval set to contain only documents with two or more concepts. The Boolean OR operator is usually used when there is more than one way to express a concept. The Boolean NOT operator is often employed as a subtraction operator that is applied to a pair of sets, with the result being the documents found in the first set but not in the second set. Some systems more accurately call this the ANDNOT operator.

Some systems allow terms in searches to be expanded by using the wild-card character, which adds all words to the search that begin with the letters up until the wild-card character. This approach is also called truncation. Unfortunately, there is no standard approach to using wild-card characters, so syntax for them varies from system to system. PubMed, for example, allows a single asterisk at the end of a word to signify a wild-card character. Thus the query word can* will lead to the words cancer and Candida, among others, being added to the search.

21.5.2 Partial-Match Retrieval

Although **partial-match searching** was conceptualized very early, it did not see widespread use

in IR systems until the advent of Web search engines in the 1990s. This is most likely because exact-match searching tends to be preferred by "power users" whereas partial-match searching is preferred by novice searchers. Whereas exact-match searching requires an understanding of Boolean operators and (often) the underlying structure of databases (e.g., the many fields in MEDLINE), partial-match searching allows a user to simply enter a few terms and start retrieving documents.

The development of partial-match searching is usually attributed to Salton and McGill (1983), who pioneered the approach in the 1960s. Although partial-match searching does not exclude the use of nonterm attributes of documents, and for that matter does not even exclude the use of Boolean operators (e.g., (Salton et al. 1983)), the most common use of this type of searching is with a query of a small number of words, also known as a **natural language query**. Because Salton's approach was based on **vector mathematics**, it is also referred to as the **vector-space model** of IR. In the partial-match approach, documents are typically ranked by their closeness of fit to the query. That is, documents containing more query terms will likely be ranked higher, since those with more query terms will in general be more likely to be relevant to the user. As a result this process is called **relevance ranking**. The entire approach has also been called **lexical–statistical retrieval**.

The most common approach to document ranking in partial-match searching is to give each a score based on the sum of the weights of terms common to the document and query. Terms in documents typically derive their weight from the TF*IDF calculation described above. Terms in queries are typically given a weight of one if the term is present and zero if it is absent. The following formula can then be used to calculate the document weight across all query terms:

$$Document\ weight = \sum_{all\ query\ terms} Weight\ of\ term\ in\ query * Weight\ of\ term\ in\ document \qquad (21.4)$$

This may be thought of as a giant OR of all query terms, with sorting of the matching documents by weight. The usual approach is for the system to then perform the same stop word removal and stemming of the query that was done in the indexing process. (The equivalent stemming operations must be performed on documents and queries so that complementary word stems will match.)

21.5.3 Retrieval Systems

This section describes searching systems used to retrieve content from the four categories previously described in Sect. 21.3.

As noted above, PubMed is the system at NLM that searches MEDLINE and other bibliographic databases. Although presenting the user with a simple text box, PubMed does a great deal of processing of the user's input to identify MeSH terms, author names, common phrases, and journal names (described in the on-line help system of PubMed). In this automatic term mapping, the system attempts to map user input, in succession, to MeSH terms, journals names, common phrases, and authors. Remaining text that PubMed cannot map is searched as text words (i.e., words that occur in any of the MEDLINE fields). A results screen on a search combining the angiotensin-converting (ACE) inhibitor class of drugs and the disease congestive heart failure (CHF) is shown in Fig. 21.4.

PubMed allows the use of wild-card characters. It also allows phrase searching whereby two or more words can be enclosed in quotation marks to indicate they must occur adjacent to each other. If the specified phrase is in PubMed's phrase index, then it will be searched as a phrase. Otherwise the individual words will be searched. PubMed allows specification of other indexing attributes via "Limits." These include publication

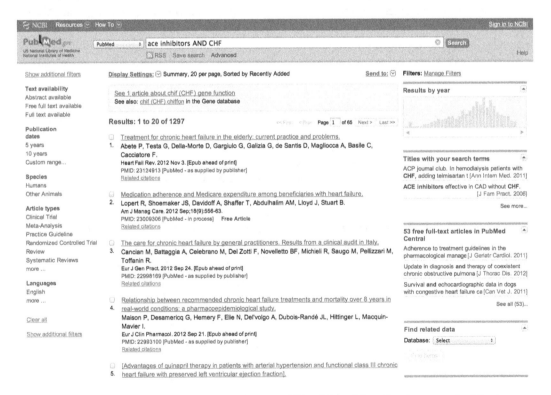

Fig. 21.4 Setting limits in PubMed. This screen shows some of the many limits that are available in PubMed, including article type, species type, subject subsets, availability of the article online, language of publication, gender, age group, and others (Courtesy of National Library of Medicine)

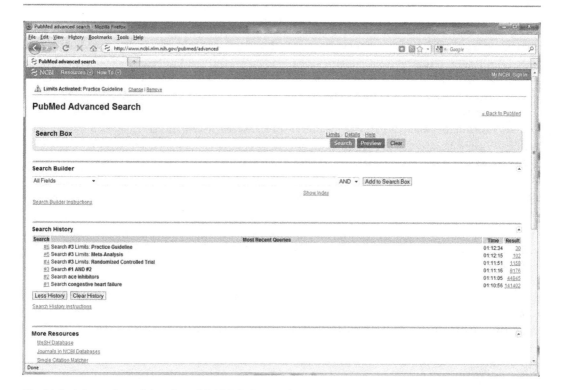

Fig. 21.5 Advanced search interface of PubMed, showing the use of sets and application of Boolean operators as well as limits. The user started with a search on the disease "congestive heart failure" and the drug class "ACE inhibitors." He or she subsequently narrowed the search by limited the output to "Randomized Controlled Trials," "Meta-Analysis," or "Practice Guidelines" (Courtesy of National Library of Medicine)

types, subsets, age ranges, and publication date ranges. These are accessed from the left-hand side of the results screen, with the most commonly used ones shown and the others accessible by additional mouse clicks.

As in most bibliographic systems, users can also search PubMed by building search sets and then combining them with Boolean operators to tailor the search. This is called the "advanced search" function of PubMed. Consider a user searching for studies assessing the reduction of mortality in patients with CHF through the use of ACE inhibitors. A simple approach to such a search might be to combine the terms ACE Inhibitors and CHF with an AND. The easiest way to do this is to enter the search string ace inhibitors AND CHF. Figure 21.5 shows the PubMed advanced search screen such a searcher might develop. This searcher has limited the output (using some of the limits listed in Fig. 21.4) with various publication types known to contain the best evidence for this question.

PubMed has another approach to finding the best evidence, which is through the use of its Clinical Queries function, where the subject terms are limited by search statements designed to retrieve the best evidence based on principles of EBM. There are two different approaches. The first uses strategies for retrieving the best evidence for the four major types of clinical questions. These strategies arise from research assessing the ability of MEDLINE search statements to identify the best studies for therapy, diagnosis, harm, and prognosis (Haynes et al. 1994). The second approach to retrieving the best evidence aims to retrieve evidence-based resources that are syntheses and synopses, in particular meta-analyses, systematic reviews, and practice guidelines. The strategy derives in part from research by Boynton et al. (1998). When the clinical queries interface is used, the search statement is processed by the usual automatic term mapping and the resulting output is limited (via AND) with the appropriate statement.

As noted already, a great number of biomedical journals use the Highwire system for online access to their full text. The Highwire system provides a retrieval interface that searches over the complete online contents of a given journal. Users can search for authors, words limited to the title and abstract, words in the entire article, and within a date range. The interface also allows searching by citation by entering volume number and page as well as searching over the entire collection of journals that use Highwire. Users can browse through specific issues as well as collected resources.

Once an article has been found, a wealth of additional features is available. First, the article is presented both in HTML and PDF form, with the latter providing a more readable and printable version. Links are also provided to related articles from the journal as well as the PubMed reference and its related articles. Also linked are all articles in the journal that cited this one, and the site can be configured to set up a notification e-mail when new articles cite the item selected. Finally, the Highwire software provides for "Rapid Responses," which are online letters to the editor. The online format allows a much larger number of responses than could be printed in the paper version of the journal. Other journal publishers use comparable approaches.

A growing number of search engines allow searching over many resources. The general search engines Google, Microsoft Bing, and others allow retrieval of any types of documents they have indexed via their Web crawling activities. Other search engines allow searching over aggregations of various sources, such as NLM Gateway,[58] which allows searching over all NLM databases and other resources in one simple interface.

21.6   Evaluation

There has been a great deal of research over the years devoted to evaluation of IR systems. As with many areas of research, there is controversy as to which approaches to evaluation best provide

results that can assess searching in the systems they are using. Many frameworks have been developed to put the results in context. One of those frameworks organized evaluation around six questions that someone advocating the use of IR systems might ask (Hersh and Hickam 1998):

1. Was the system used?
2. For what was the system used?
3. How well did they use the system?
4. Were the users satisfied?
5. What factors were associated with successful or unsuccessful use of the system?
6. Did the system have an impact?

A simpler means for organizing the results of evaluation, however, groups approaches and studies into those that are system-oriented, i.e., the focus of the evaluation is on the IR system, and those that are user-oriented, i.e., the focus is on the user.

21.6.1   System-Oriented Evaluation

There are many ways to evaluate the performance of IR systems, the most widely used of which are the relevance-based measures of **recall** and **precision**. These measures quantify the number of relevant documents retrieved by the user from the database and in his or her search. Recall is the proportion of relevant documents retrieved from the database:

$$\text{Recall} = \frac{\text{number of retrieved and relevant documents}}{\text{number of relevant documents in database}}$$

(21.5)

In other words, recall answers the question, for a given search, what fraction of all the relevant documents have been obtained from the database?

One problem with Equation (21.5) is that the denominator implies that the total number of relevant documents for a query is known. For all but the smallest of databases, however, it is unlikely, perhaps even impossible, for one to succeed in identifying all relevant documents in a database. Thus most studies use the measure of **relative recall**, where the denominator is redefined to be the total number of unique, relevant documents identified by one or more searches on the query topic.

Precision is the proportion of relevant documents retrieved in the search:

$$\text{Precision} = \frac{\text{number of retrieved and relevant documents}}{\text{number of documents retrieved}} \qquad (21.6)$$

This measure answers the question, for a search, what fraction of the retrieved documents is relevant?

One problem that arises when one is comparing systems that use ranking versus those that do not is that nonranking systems, typically using Boolean searching, tend to retrieve a fixed set of documents and as a result have fixed points of recall and precision. Systems with relevance ranking, on the other hand, have different values of recall and precision depending on the size of the retrieval set the system (or the user) has chosen to show. For this reason, many evaluators of systems featuring relevance ranking will create a recall precision table (or graph) that identifies precision at various levels of recall. The "standard" approach to this was defined by Salton and McGill (1983), who pioneered both relevance ranking and this method of evaluating such systems.

To generate a recall-precision table for a single query, one first must determine the intervals of recall that will be used. A typical approach is to use intervals of 0.1 (or 10 %), with a total of 11 intervals from a recall of 0.0–1.0. The table is built by determining the highest level of overall precision at any point in the output for a given interval of recall. Thus, for the recall interval 0.0, one would use the highest level of precision at which the recall is anywhere greater than or equal to zero and less than 0.1. An approach that has been used more frequently in recent times has been the **mean average precision (MAP)**, which is similar to precision at points of recall but does not use fixed recall intervals or interpolation. Instead, precision is measured at every point in the process in which a relevant document is obtained, and the MAP measure is found by averaging these points for the whole query.

A good deal of evaluation in IR is done via **challenge evaluations**, in which a common IR task is defined and a **test collection** of documents, topics, and **relevance judgments** are developed. The relevance judgments define which documents are relevant for each topic in the task, allowing different researchers to compare their systems with others on the same task and improve them. The longest running and best-known challenge evaluation in IR is the **Text REtrieval Conference** (**TREC**, trec.nist.gov), which is organized by the U.S. **National Institute for Standards and Technology** (**NIST**,).[59] Started in 1992, TREC has provided a testbed for evaluation and a forum for presentation of results. TREC is organized as an annual event at which the tasks are specified and queries and documents are provided to participants. Participating groups submit "runs" of their systems to NIST, which calculates the appropriate performance measure(s). TREC is organized into tracks geared to specific interests. A book summarizing the first decade of TREC provides more information on this important IR initiative that is still ongoing (Voorhees and Harman 2005).

While TREC has been focused on general IR, there was a track that ran for several years devoted to retrieval from genomics resources (Hersh et al. 2006; Hersh and Voorhees 2009). In addition, more recently TREC has added a track focused on medical records based on the use case of identifying patients as potential candidates for clinical studies (Voorhees and Tong 2011; Voorhees and Hersh 2012).

Some researchers have criticized or noted the limitations of relevance-based measures. While no one denies that users want systems to retrieve relevant articles, it is not clear that the quantity of relevant documents retrieved is the complete measure of how well a system performs (Harter 1992; Swanson 1988). Hersh (1994) has noted

---

[59] www.nist.gov

that clinical users are unlikely to be concerned about these measures when they simply seek an answer to a clinical question and are able to do so no matter how many other relevant documents they miss (lowering recall) or how many nonrelevant ones they retrieve (lowering precision).

21.6.2 User-Oriented Evaluation

What alternatives to relevance-based measures can be used for determining performance of individual searches? Harter admits that if measures using a more situational view of relevance cannot be developed for assessing user interaction, then recall and precision may be the only alternatives. Some alternatives have focused on users being able to perform various information tasks with IR systems, such as finding answers to questions (Egan et al. 1989; Hersh and Hickam 1995; Hersh et al. 1996; Mynatt et al. 1992; Wildemuth et al. 1995). For several years, TREC featured an Interactive Track that had participants carry out user experiments with the same documents and queries (Hersh 2001). A number of user-oriented evaluations have been performed over the years looking at users of biomedical information. Most of these studies have focused on clinicians.

One of the original studies measuring searching performance in clinical settings was performed by Haynes et al. (1990). This study also compared the capabilities of librarian and clinician searchers. In this study, 78 searches were randomly chosen for replication by both a clinician experienced in searching and a medical librarian. During this study, each original ("novice") user had been required to enter a brief statement of information need before entering the search program. This statement was given to the experienced clinician and librarian for searching on MEDLINE. All the retrievals for each search were given to a subject domain expert, blinded with respect to which searcher retrieved which reference. Recall and precision were calculated for each query and averaged. The results showed that the experienced clinicians and librarians achieved comparable recall in the range of 50 %, although the librarians had better precision. The

novice clinician searchers had lower recall and precision than either of the other groups. This study also assessed user satisfaction of the novice searchers, who despite their recall and precision results said that they were satisfied with their search outcomes. The investigators did not assess whether the novices obtained enough relevant articles to answer their questions, or whether they would have found additional value with the ones that were missed.

A follow-up study yielded some additional insights about the searchers (McKibbon et al. 1990). As was noted, different searchers tended to use different strategies on a given topic. The different approaches replicated a finding known from other searching studies in the past, namely, the lack of overlap across searchers of overall retrieved citations as well as relevant ones. Thus, even though the novice searchers had lower recall, they did obtain a great many relevant citations not retrieved by the two expert searchers. Furthermore, fewer than 4 % of all the relevant citations were retrieved by all three searchers. Despite the widely divergent search strategies and retrieval sets, overall recall and precision were quite similar among the three classes of users.

Recognizing the limitations of recall and precision for evaluating clinical users of IR systems, Hersh and coworkers have carried out a number of studies assessing the ability of systems to help students and clinicians answer clinical questions. The rationale for these studies is that the usual goal of using an IR system is to find an answer to a question. While the user must obviously find relevant documents to answer that question, the quantity of such documents is less important than whether the question is successfully answered. In fact, recall and precision can be placed among the many factors that may be associated with ability to complete the task successfully.

The first study by this group using the task-oriented approach compared Boolean versus natural language searching in the textbook Scientific American Medicine (Hersh and Hickam 1995). Thirteen medical students were asked to answer ten short-answer questions and rate their confidence in their answers. The students were then randomized to one or the other interface and asked to search on the five questions for which they had rated confidence the lowest. The study showed that both groups had low correct rates before searching (average 1.7 correct out of 10) but were mostly able to answer the questions with searching (average 4.0 out of 5). There was no difference in ability to answer questions with one interface or the other. Most answers were found on the first search to the textbook. For the questions that were incorrectly answered, the document with the correct answer was actually retrieved by the user two-thirds of the time and viewed more than half the time.

Another study compared Boolean and natural language searching of MEDLINE with two commercial products, CD Plus (now Ovid) and Knowledge Finder (KF; Hersh et al. 1996). These systems represented the ends of the spectrum in terms of using Boolean searching on human-indexed thesaurus terms (Ovid) versus natural language searching on words in the title, abstract, and indexing terms (KF). Sixteen medical students were recruited and randomized to one of the two systems and given three yes/no clinical questions to answer. The students were able to use each system successfully, answering 37.5 % correctly before searching and 85.4 % correctly after searching. There were no significant differences between the systems in time taken, relevant articles retrieved, or user satisfaction. This study demonstrated that both types of systems can be used equally well with minimal training.

A more comprehensive study looked at MEDLINE searching by medical and nurse practitioner (NP) students to answer clinical questions. A total of 66 medical and NP students searched five questions each (Hersh et al. 2002). This study used a multiple-choice format for answering questions that also included a judgment about the evidence for the answer. Subjects were asked to choose from one of three answers:

• Yes, with adequate evidence.
• Insufficient evidence to answer question.
• No, with adequate evidence.

Both groups achieved a presearching correctness on questions about equal to chance (32.3 % for medical students and 31.7 % for NP students). However, medical students improved their

correctness with searching (to 51.6 %), whereas NP students hardly did at all (to 34.7 %).

This study also attempted to measure what factors might influence searching. A multitude of factors, such as age, gender, computer experience, and time taken to search, were not associated with successful answering of questions. Successful answering was, however, associated with answering the question correctly before searching, spatial visualization ability (measured by a validated instrument), searching experience, and EBM question type (prognosis questions easiest, harm questions most difficult). An analysis of recall and precision for each question searched demonstrated a complete lack of association with ability to answer these questions.

Two studies have extended this approach in various ways. Westbook et al. (2005) assessed use of an online evidence systems and found that physicians answered 37 % of questions correctly before use of the system and 50 % afterwards, while nurse specialists answered 18 % of questions correctly and also 50 % afterwards. Those who had correct answers before searching had higher confidence in their answers, but those not initially knowing the answer had no difference in confidence whether their answer turned out to be right or wrong. McKibbon and Fridsma (2006) performed a comparable study of allowing physicians to seek answers to questions with resources they normally use employing the same questions as Hersh et al. (2002). This study found no difference in answer correctness before or after using the search system. Clearly these studies show a variety of effects with different IR systems, tasks, and users.

Pluye and Grad (2004) performed a qualitative study assessing impact of IR systems on physician practice. The study identified four themes mentioned by physicians:

• Recall—of forgotten knowledge
• Learning—new knowledge
• Confirmation—of existing knowledge
• Frustration—that system use not successful

The researchers also noted two additional themes:

• Reassurance—that system is available
• Practice improvement—of patient-physician relationship

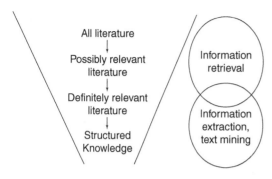

Fig. 21.6 Funnel of knowledge discovery, showing how an information need starts with a search (information retrieval) leading to a large possibly relevant set of literature that is winnowed down to a smaller definitely relevant set (usually by human inspection but with techniques like information extraction and text mining possibly automating the process in the future). Ultimately actionable knowledge is obtained that can be applied by a human or fashioned into, for example, rules for a computer-based decision support system (Reproduced with permission of Springer (Hersh 2009))

21.7   Research Directions

The above evaluation research shows that there is still plenty of room for IR systems to improve their abilities. In addition, there will be new challenges that arise from growing amounts of information, new devices, and other new technologies.

There are also other areas related to IR where research is ongoing in the larger quest to help all involved in biomedicine and health—including patients, clinicians and researchers—to better apply knowledge to improve health. Figure 21.6 shows this author's "funnel" by which the user searches all of the scientific literature using IR systems to obtain a set of possibly relevant literature. In the current state of the art, he/she reviews this literature by hand, selecting which articles are definitely relevant and may become "actionable knowledge" that can be acted upon to make better decisions.

Our ability to carry out the activities in the upper part of the funnel, i.e., IR, is much better than those in the lower part. These areas include:

- **Information extraction** and **text mining**—usually through the use of natural language processing (NLP, see Chap. 8) to extract facts and knowledge from text. These techniques

are often employed to extract information from the EHR, with a wide variety of accuracy as shown in a recent systematic review (Stanfill et al. 2010).

- **Summarization**—Providing automated extracts or abstracts summarizing the content of longer documents (Fiszman et al. 2004)
- **Question-answering**—Going beyond retrieval of documents to providing actual answers to questions, as exemplified by IBM's Watson system (Ferrucci et al. 2010).

21.8   Digital Libraries

Discussion of IR "systems" thus far has focused on the provision of retrieval mechanisms to access online content. Even with the expansive coverage of some IR systems, such as Web search engines, they are often part of a larger collection of services or activities. An alternative perspective, especially when communities and/or proprietary collections are involved, is the **digital library**. Digital libraries share many characteristics with "brick and mortar" libraries, but also take on some additional challenges. Borgman (1999) noted that libraries of both types elicited different definitions of what they actually are, with researchers tending to view libraries as content collected for specific communities and librarians alternatively viewing them as institutions or services. Lindberg and Humphreys (2005) laid out a vision in 2005 for libraries 10 years hence, noting that while collections would be virtual and accessed in many diverse ways, other elements of science would stay intact, including journals and the peer review process.

This section provides an overview of key issues of digital libraries, with an orientation toward biomedical libraries.

21.8.1   Functions and Definitions of Libraries

The central function of libraries is to maintain collections of published literature. They may also store unpublished literature in archives, such as letters, notes, and other documents. The general focus on published literature has implications. One of these is that, for the most part, quality control can be taken for granted. Until recently, most published literature came from commercial publishers and specialty societies that had processes such as peer review, which, although imperfect, allowed the library to devote minimal resources to assessing their quality. While libraries can still cede the judgment of quality to these information providers in the Internet era, they cannot ignore the myriad of information published only on the Internet, for which the quality cannot be presumed.

Other functions of libraries besides maintaining collections include cataloging and classification of items in those collections, being a place (even virtual) where individuals could go to get assistance with information seeking, and providing space for work or study, particularly in universities.

The paper-based nature of traditional libraries carrieda number of assumptions that are challenged in the digital era. For example, items were produced in multiple copies, freeing the individual library from excessive worry that an item could not be replaced. In addition, items were fairly static, simplifying their cataloging. With digital libraries, this status quo is challenged. There is a great deal of concern about archiving of content and managing its change when fewer "copies" of it exist on the file servers of publishers and other organizations. A related problem for digital libraries is that they do not own the "artifact" of the paper journal, book, or other item. This is exacerbated by the fact that when a subscription to an electronic journal is terminated, access to the entire journal is lost; that is, the subscriber does not retain accumulated back issues, as was taken for granted with paper journals.

21.8.2 Access

Probably every Web user is familiar with clicking on a Web link and receiving an error message that a page cannot found. Digital libraries and commercial publishing ventures need mechanisms to

ensure that documents have persistent identifiers so that when the document itself physically moves, it is still obtainable. The original architecture for the Web envisioned by the Internet Engineering Task Force was to have every **uniform resource locator** (**URL**), the address entered into a Web browser or used in a Web hyper-link, linked to a **uniform resource name** (**URN**) that would be persistent (Sollins and Masinter 1994). The combination of a URN and a URL, a **uniform resource identifier** (**URI**), would provide persistent access to digital objects. However, no publicly available resource for resolving URNs and URIs was ever implemented on a large scale.

One approach that has seen widespread adoption by publishers, especially scientific journal publishers, is the **digital object identifier** (**DOI**,)[60] (Paskin 2006). The DOI has recently been given the status of a standard by the NISO with the designation Z39.84. The DOI itself is relatively simple, consisting of a prefix that is assigned by the International DOI Foundation (IDF) to the publishing entity and a suffix that is assigned and maintained by the entity. For example, the DOI for articles from the Journal of the American Medical Informatics Association have the prefix 10.1197 and the suffix jamia. M####, where #### is a number assigned by the journal editors. Publishers are encouraged to facilitate resolution by encoding the DOI into their URLs in a standard way, e.g., http://dx.doi.org/10.1197/jamia.M0996 for a paper cited earlier in the chapter (Hersh et al. 2002).

21.8.3 Interoperability

As noted throughout this chapter, metadata is a key component for accessing content in IR systems. It takes on an additional value in the digital library, where there is desire to allow access to diverse but not necessarily exhaustive resources. One key concern of digital libraries is **interoperability** (Besser 2002). That is, how can resources with heterogeneous metadata be accessed? Arms

---

[60] www.doi.org

et al. note that three levels of agreement must be achieved in digital libraries:

1. Technical agreements over formats, protocols, and security procedures
2. Content agreement over the data and the semantic interpretation of its metadata
3. Organizational agreements over ground rules for access, preservation, payment, authentication, and so forth

21.8.4   Intellectual Property

Intellectual property issues are a major concern in digital libraries. Intellectual property is difficult to protect in the digital environment because although the cost of production is not insubstantial, the cost of replication is near nothing. Furthermore, in circumstances such as academic publishing, the desire for protection is situational. For example, individual researchers may want the widest dissemination of their research papers, but each one may want to protect revenues realized from synthesis works or educational products that are developed. The global reach of the Internet has required that intellectual property issues be considered on a global scale. The **World Intellectual Property Organization (WIPO,)**[61] is an agency of the United Nations devoted to developing worldwide policies, although understandably, there is considerable diversity about what such policies should be.

21.8.5   Preservation

Another function of libraries of all types is preservation of materials. In paper-based libraries, the goal of preservation was the survival of the physical object, i.e., the book, journal, image, etc. that could become lost, stolen, or deteriorated. Preservation issues in digital libraries are somewhat different. Digital libraries still do need to be concerned with physical survival of the information. Lesk (2005) compared the longevity of digital materials. He noted that the longevity for

magnetic materials was the least, with the expected lifetime of magnetic tape being 5–10 years. Optical storage has somewhat better longevity, with an expected lifetime of 30–100 years depending on the specific type. Ironically, paper has a life expectancy well beyond all these digital media. Rothenberg (1999) has noted that the Rosetta Stone, which provided help in interpreting ancient Egyptian hieroglyphics and has survived over 20 centuries. He reiterated Lesk's description of the reduced lifetime of digital media in comparison with traditional media, and to note another problem familiar to most long-time users of computers, namely, data can become obsolete not only owing to the medium, but also as a result of data format. Both authors noted that storage devices as well as computer applications, such as word processors, have seen their formats change significantly over the last couple of decades.

The US Library of Congress has devoted considerable effort to digital preservation, documenting its efforts on the Web site.[62] The largest preservation effort in the US is National Digital Information Infrastructure Preservation Program (NDIIPP)[63] of the Library of Congress. Other digital preservation efforts include Portico,[64] a collaboration of publishers, libraries, and government agencies to preserve electronic scholarly content and LOCKSS (Lots of Copies Keep Stuff Safe,[65] which provides libraries with digital preservation tools and support. An effort related to the latter is CLOCKSS,[66] which is a "trusted community-governed archive."

21.9   Future Directions for IR Systems and Digital Libraries

There is no doubt that considerable progress has been made in IR and digital libraries. Seeking online information is now done routinely not

---

[61] www.wipo.org

[62] www.digitalpreservation.gov

[63] www.digitalpreservation.gov

[64] www.portico.org

[65] www.lockss.org

[66] www.clockss.org

only by clinicians and researchers, but also by patients and consumers. There are still considerable challenges to make this activity more fruitful to users. They include:

- How do we lower the effort it takes for clinicians to get to the information they need rapidly in the busy clinical setting?
- How can researchers extract new knowledge from the vast quantity that is available to them?
- How can consumers and patients find high-quality information that is appropriate to their understanding of health and disease?
- Can the value added by the publishing process be protected and remunerated while making information more available?
- How can the indexing process become more accurate and efficient?
- Can retrieval interfaces be made simpler without giving up flexibility and power?
- Can we develop standards for digital libraries that will facilitate interoperability but maintain ease of use, protection of intellectual property, and long-term preservation of the archive of science?

Suggested Readings

Baeza-Yates, R., & Ribeiro-Neto, B. (2011). *Modern information retrieval: The concepts and technology behind search* (2nd ed.). Reading: Addison-Wesley. A book surveying most of the automated approaches to information retrieval.

Croft, W., Metzler, D., & Strohman, T. (2009). *Search engines: Information retrieval in practice*. Boston: Addison-Wesley. A book surveying most of the automated approaches to search engines.

Frakes, W., & Baeza-Yates, R. (Eds.). (1992). *Information retrieval: Data structures and algorithms*. Englewood Cliffs: Prentice-Hall. A textbook on implementation of information retrieval systems. Covers all of the major data structures and algorithms, including inverted files, ranking algorithms, stop word lists, and stemming. There are plentiful examples of code in the C programming language.

Hersh, W. (2009). *Information retrieval: A health and biomedical perspective* (3rd ed.). New York: Springer. A textbook on information retrieval systems in the health and biomedical domain that covers state-of-the-art as well as research systems.

Lindberg, D., & Humphreys, B. (2005). 2015 – The future of medical libraries. *New England Journal of Medicine, 352*, 1067–1070. A vision of the future of medical libraries from two leaders of the NLM.

Miles, W. (1982). *A history of the National Library of Medicine: The nation's treasury of medical knowledge*. Bethesda: U.S. Department of Health and Human Services. A comprehensive history of the National Library of Medicine and its forerunners, covering the story of Dr. John Shaw Billings and his founding of Index Medicus to the modern implementation of MEDLINE.

Straus, S. E., Glasziou, P., et al. (2010). *Evidence-Based Medicine: How to Practice and Teach it* (4th ed.). New York, NY, Churchill Livingstone.

Questions for Discussion

1. With the advent of full-text searching, should the National Library of Medicine abandon human indexing of citations in MEDLINE? Why or why not?

2. Explain why you think open-access publishing will succeed or not.

3. How would you aggregate the clinical evidence-based resources described in the chapter into the best digital library for clinicians?

4. Devise a curriculum for teaching clinicians and patients the most important points about searching for health-related information.

5. Find a consumer-oriented Web page and determine the quality of the information on it.

6. What are the limitations of recall and precision as evaluation measures and what alternatives would improve upon them?

7. Select a concept that appears in two or more clinical terminologies and demonstrate how it would be combined into a record in the UMLS Metathesaurus.

8. Describe how you might devise a system that achieves a happy medium between of intellectual property and barrier-free access to the archive of science.

Clinical Decision-Support Systems

22

Mark A. Musen, Blackford Middleton, and Robert A. Greenes

After reading this chapter, you should know the answers to these questions:
- What are the key motivations for clinical decision support?
- How is clinical decision support relevant to the concept of "meaningful use" of EHRs in the United States?
- What are typical design considerations when building a decision-support system?
- What are some ways in which developers of decision-support systems encode clinical knowledge?
- What are some current standards in the HIT industry that facilitate the construction of decision-support applications?
- Why has adoption been slow and what are prospects for broader use?

M.A. Musen, MD, PhD (✉)
Center for Biomedical Informatics Research,
Stanford University School of Medicine, 1265 Welch
Road, Room X-215, Stanford 94305-5479, CA, USA
e-mail: musen@stanford.edu

B. Middleton, MD, MPH, MSc
Informatics Center, Vanderbilt University Medical
Center, 3401 West End Ave., Suite 700,
Nashville 37203, TN, USA
e-mail: blackford.middleton@vanderbilt.edu

R.A. Greenes, MD, PhD
Department of Biomedical Informatics,
Arizona State University, Tempe, AZ, USA

Division of Health Sciences Research,
College of Medicine, Mayo Clinic, Samuel Johnson
Research Bldg, 13212 East Shea Boulevard,
Scottsdale 85259, AZ, USA
e-mail: greenes@asu.edu

- What are the key areas for research and development in clinical decision-support systems?

In this chapter, we discuss information technology that assists with **clinical decision support** (CDS) – the process that "provides clinicians, staff, patients, or other individuals with knowledge and person-specific information, intelligently filtered or presented at appropriate times, to enhance health and health care" (Osheroff et al. 2007). Systems that provide CDS do not simply assist with the retrieval of relevant information; they communicate information that takes into consideration the particular clinical context, offering situation-specific information and recommendations. At the same time, such systems do not themselves perform clinical decision making; they provide relevant knowledge and analyses that enable the ultimate decision makers—clinicians, patients, and health care organizations—to develop more informed judgments. Ideally, CDS systems may be described in terms of five *right* things that they do: they "provide the right information, to the right person, in the right format, through the right channel, at the right point in workflow to improve health and health care decisions and outcomes" (Osheroff et al. 2004).

Systems that provide CDS come in three basic varieties: (1) They may use information about the current clinical context to retrieve highly relevant

We are grateful to the co-authors of the chapter on this subject that appeared in the previous edition of this textbook, Drs. Yuval Shahar and Edward H. Shortliffe.

E.H. Shortliffe, J.J. Cimino (eds.), *Biomedical Informatics*,
DOI 10.1007/978-1-4471-4474-8_22, © Springer-Verlag London 2014

online documents, as with so-called "**infobuttons**" (introduced in Chap. 12); (2) they may provide patient-specific, situation-specific alerts, reminders, physician order sets, or other recommendations for direct action; or (3) they may organize and present information in a way that facilitates problem solving and decision making, as in **dashboards**, graphical displays, documentation templates, structured reports, and order sets. Order sets are a good example of the latter because they both may facilitate decision making by providing a mnemonic function and also may enhance workflow by providing a means to select a group of relevant activities quickly. As we discussed in Chap. 1, many observers consider knowledge resources that distill the medical literature and that facilitate manual selection of content relevant to the current situation to be simple decision-support systems.

This chapter provides a motivation for computer-based decision aids, emphasizing the current health care situation in the United States while keeping an eye on global trends. It offers some historical background regarding CDS systems, then provides a description of current implementation strategies and challenges, and closes with discussion of critical research questions that must be addressed to ensure optimal effectiveness of CDS in clinical practice.

22.1 The Nature of Clinical Decision-Making

If you ask people what the phrase "computers in medicine" means, they often describe a computer program that helps physicians to make diagnoses. Although computers play numerous important clinical roles, people have recognized, from the earliest days of computing, that computers might support health-care workers by helping these people to sift through the vast collections of possible diseases, findings, and treatments.

We can view the contents of this entire book as addressing clinical data and decision-making. In Chap. 2, we discussed the central role of accurate, complete, and relevant data in supporting the decisions that confront clinicians and other health-care workers. In Chap. 3, we described the nature of good decisions and the need for clinicians to understand the proper use of information if they are to be effective and efficient decision-makers. In Chap. 4 we introduced the cognitive issues that underlie clinical decision making and that influence the design of systems for decision support. Subsequent chapters have mentioned many real or potential uses of computers to assist with such decision-making. Medical practice *is* medical decision-making, so most applications of computers in health care are intended to have a direct or indirect effect on the quality of health care decisions. In this chapter, we bring together these themes by concentrating on methods and systems that have been developed specifically to assist health workers in making decisions.

By now, you are familiar with the range of clinical decisions. The classic problem of **diagnosis** (analyzing available data to determine the pathophysiologic explanation for a patient's symptoms) is only one of these. Equally challenging, as emphasized in Chaps. 3 and 4, is the **diagnostic process**—deciding which questions to ask, tests to order, or procedures to perform, and assessing the value of the results that can be obtained in relation to associated risks or financial costs. Thus, diagnosis involves not only deciding what is true about a patient but also what data are needed to determine what is true. Even when the diagnosis is known, there often are challenging **management** decisions that test the physician's knowledge and experience: Should I treat the patient or allow the process to resolve on its own? If treatment is indicated, what should it be? How should I use the patient's response to therapy to guide me in determining whether an alternate approach should be tried or, in some cases, to question whether my initial diagnosis was incorrect after all? (In that sense, the response to treatment is also a type of diagnostic test). Lastly, when a clinician and a patient are faced with alternative treatments, and they seek help to choose among them, the estimation of prognosis for cure or risk of death or complications is an important decision-making activity.

Biomedicine is also replete with decision tasks that do not involve specific patients or their diseases. Consider, for example, the biomedical scientist who is using laboratory data to help with the design of her next experiment or the hospital administrator who uses management data to guide decisions about resource allocation in his hospital. Although we focus on systems to assist with clinical decisions in this chapter, we emphasize that the concepts discussed generalize to many other problem areas as well. In Chap. 27, for example, we examine the need for formal decision techniques and tools in creating health policies. As we develop databases that can identify patients with specific diseases, with risks of complications, or in need of specific interventions such as screening tests or immunizations (see Chap. 16), so-called **population management** can be used to provide a form of decision support for groups of patients. Some clinical decision support is also aimed directly at patients, in terms of alerts, reminders, or aids to interpretation of information; techniques for assessing prognosis and risk of alternative strategies should involve shared decision making between providers and patients, which is also an important area of activity.

In this chapter, we focus on decision aids for the provider in particular. The requirements for excellent decision-making fall into three principal categories: (1) accurate data, (2) pertinent knowledge, and (3) appropriate problem-solving skills.

The data about a patient must be adequate for making an informed decision, but they must not be excessive (see Chap. 4). Indeed, a major challenge occurs when decision-makers are bombarded with so much information that they cannot process and synthesize the information intelligently and rapidly (see, for example, Chap. 19). Thus, it is important to know when additional data will confuse rather than clarify and when it is imperative to use tools (computational, visual, or otherwise) that permit data to be summarized for easier cognitive management (see Chap. 4). Operating rooms and intensive-care units are classic settings in which this problem arises; patients are monitored extensively, numerous data are collected, and decisions often have to be made on an emergent basis.

Equally important is the quality of the available data. In Chap. 2, we discussed imprecision in terminology, illegibility and inaccessibility of records, and other opportunities for misinterpretation of data. Similarly, measurement instruments or recorded data may simply be erroneous; use of faulty data can have serious adverse effects on patient-care decisions. Thus, clinical data often need to be validated.

Even good data are useless if we do not have the knowledge necessary to apply them properly. Decision-makers must have broad knowledge of medicine, in-depth familiarity with their area of expertise, and access to information resources that provide pertinent additional information. Their knowledge must be accurate, with areas of controversy well understood and questions of personal choice well distinguished from those where a more prescriptive approach is appropriate. Their knowledge must also be current; in the rapidly changing world of medicine, facts decay just as certainly as dead tissue does.

Good data and an extensive factual knowledge base still do not guarantee a good decision; good problem-solving skills are equally important. Decision-makers must know how to set appropriate goals for a task, how to reason about each goal, and how to make explicit the trade-offs between costs and benefits of diagnostic procedures or therapeutic maneuvers. The skilled clinician draws extensively on personal experience, and new physicians soon realize that good clinical judgment is based as much on an ability to reason effectively and appropriately about what to do as it is on formal knowledge of the field or access to high-quality patient data. Thus, clinicians must develop a strategic approach to test selection and interpretation, understand ideas of sensitivity and specificity, and be able to assess the urgency of a situation. Similar issues relating to test or treatment selection, in terms of costs, risks, and benefits, must be understood. Awareness of biases and of the ways that they can creep into problem-solving also are crucial (see Chap. 3). This brief review of issues central to clinical decision-making serves as a fitting introduction to the topic of *computer-assisted* decision-making: Precisely the same topics are pertinent when we develop a computational tool for CDS. The program must have access to good data, it must have extensive background knowledge encoded for the clinical domain in question, and it must embody an intelligent approach to problem-solving that is sensitive to requirements for proper analysis, appropriate cost–benefit trade-offs, and efficiency.

22.2 Motivation for Computer-Based CDS

Since the 1960s, workers in biomedical informatics have been interested in CDS systems both because of a desire to improve health care and to understand better the process of medical decision-making. Building a computer system that attempts to process data as a clinician does provides insight into the nature of medical problem solving and enables the creation of formal models of clinical reasoning. At the same time, construction of such systems offers obvious societal benefits if the computer programs can aid practitioners in their care of patients and lead to better clinical outcomes. Although the more academic considerations have provided strong motivation for work in the area of computer-based decision aids over several decades, the recognition of the importance of **clinical decision support systems** (CDSSs) as practical tools has increased markedly in recent years as a result of the inexorable growth in health care complexity and cost, as well as the introduction of health care legislation aimed at addressing these trends—which have made the development and broad adoption of CDS technology a priority.

The twenty-first century has seen changes in health care practices that make the development of CDS technology particularly necessary. Computer-based CDS has taken on increasing urgency for three reasons: (1) increasing challenges related to knowledge and information management in clinical practice, (2) the pressure to adopt and meaningfully use electronic medical records, and (3) the goal of delivering increasing personalized health care services – tailored to the patient's preferences for care and to his or her individual genome. We consider these three factors in turn.

22.2.1 Physician Information Needs and Clinical Data Management

Modern clinical practice is characterized by an ever-expanding knowledgebase in clinical medicine, and by a growing clinical data set describing every patient characteristic from phenotype to genotype (Kohn et al. 2002). Despite the growing amounts of data and knowledge with which physicians need to work, health care workers have seen the average time for a clinical encounter steadily decrease, particularly in the United States, where the pressures of the prevalent fee-for-service reimbursement system and a concomitant rise in the amount of paperwork required for administrative management and billing continue to squeeze practitioners (Baron 2010). Studies of information needs among physicians in clinical practice have long revealed that unanswered clinical questions are common in ambulatory clinical encounters, with as many as one or two unanswered clinical questions about diagnosis, therapy, or administrative issues arising in every visit (Covell et al. 1985). In as many as 81 % of clinical encounters in ambulatory care, clinicians may be missing critical information, with an average of four missing items per case (Tang et al. 1994b, 1996). Providers consequently face major challenges in accessing relevant information, acquiring a complete picture of the patient's clinical state and history, and knowing what further testing or therapeutic actions are best to take. Studies suggest that as many as 18 % of medical errors may be due to inadequate availability of patient information (Leape 1994). The demands for increased information management in the setting of an ever expanding clinical knowledge base are primary drivers for the adoption of CDS systems. (See Chap. 21 for a deeper discussion of physician information needs.)

22.2.2 EHR Adoption and Meaningful Use

These challenges, coupled with the seemingly inexorable rise in health care costs, have led to a variety of cost-containment and quality-improvement strategies in recent years. Health care delivery in the United States is in the midst of a profound transformation, in part due to Federal public policy efforts to encourage the adoption and use of health information technology (HIT). The American Recovery and Reinvestment Act (ARRA) of 2009, and the **HITECH regulations** within it, created incentives for the widespread adoption of health information technologies (Blumenthal 2009; see Chap. 27). These public policy efforts are often viewed as an essential adjunct to current health payment reform efforts in the United States, and a prelude to additional health care delivery redesign, payment reform, and cost containment. Even as recently as 2012, only 34.8 % of physicians in ambulatory practice in the United States used a basic or comprehensive electronic medical record (Decker et al. 2012), and 26.6 % of U.S. hospitals used health information technologies in inpatient care-delivery settings (DesRoches et al. 2012), although these numbers are on a rapid upward trajectory. The ARRA and HITECH policies, and the resulting technology adoption, are changing the practice of medicine and clinical care delivery in both beneficial and untoward ways (Sittig and Singh 2011). To achieve meaningful and effective use of HIT, the software must be viewed as one component of a complex sociotechnical system, in which all elements must work effectively (Institute of Medicine 2011a).

One of the principal motivations for EHR adoption is to provide an infrastructure with which to improve the quality, safety, and efficacy of health care delivery. In recent years, the U.S. government has placed considerable emphasis on the adoption of quality measures and quality-reporting requirements as part of meaningful use of HIT (Clancy et al. 2009; Institute of Medicine 2011a). Quality measures, despite their ability to provide feedback that stimulates improved performance by the clinician, are only part of the process needed to make the desired improvements. Prospective, proactive clinical decision support must also be in place. The U.S. government's rules for **meaningful use** of HIT have required only minimal CDS compliance at the time of this writing, but Phase III of the meaningful use regulations in 2016 is expected to increase the mandate for CDS in EHR systems substantially (Blumenthal and Tavenner 2010; see Chap. 27).

22.2.3 Personalized Medicine

The fundamental model for the practice of medicine has undergone dramatic change in the past century or so. The objectives of clinical care have shifted radically from the archaic goal of correcting putative imbalances of bodily humors to the scientific understanding of pathophysiology and of mechanisms for eliminating pathogens and for remedying biological aberrancies. The resulting view of medicine as the application of biological principles was at the core of the report produced by Abraham Flexner (1910) that upended medical education in the early twentieth century and that had led to the **reductionist biomedical model** that prevailed for the rest of that century. More recently, however, George Engel's **biopsychosocial model** (Engel 1977) brought to the fore of clinical care the need to address psychological and social factors in clinical treatment plans in addition to underlying biomedical problems. By the end of the twentieth century, it became increasingly accepted that CDS requires not only communication of scientific medical knowledge, but also adaptation of that knowledge to reflect the psychological and social situation that would temper the application of the knowledge. Added to this complexity is the aging of the population, owing in part to advances in health and health care, resulting in a much higher burden of chronic diseases, multiple diseases, and multiple testing and treatment options, with both their positive and negative consequences that must be balanced—all contributing to the increasing intricacy of care.

As a further extension of these trends, the genomic era in which we now live has further increased the need for clinical practice to reflect **personalized medicine** and the need to tailor care to individual factors in ways that never before were imaginable (Ginsburg and Willard 2009). Personalized medicine is characterized by decision making that takes into account and that is specific to patient personal history, family history, social and environmental factors, along with genomic data and patient preferences regarding their own care (see Chap. 25). In this approach, clinical decision making is explicitly patient-centered in new ways, bringing the best evidence at the genetic level to bear on many clinical scenarios, while incorporating patient preferences for acquiring and applying genetic information (Fargher et al. 2007). Personalized genetic medicine (Chan and Ginsburg 2011) is already generating data that outstrip the information and knowledge processing capabilities of practitioners, and many clinicians feel threatened by the impending tsunami of additional knowledge that they will need to master (Baars et al. 2005). As personalized medicine becomes the norm, primary-care and specialist practitioners alike will need to manage their patients by interpreting genomic tests along with myriad other data at the point of care. It is hard to imagine how clinicians will manage to perform such activities without substantial computer-based assistance. Informatics is well suited to support a personalized approach to clinical genetic medicine (Ullman-Cullere and Mathew 2011).

Another related change is growing recognition of the importance of promoting optimal health and wellness, not just by treating disease but by encouraging healthy lifestyles, fostering compliance with health and health care regimens, and carrying out periodic health-risk assessments. Key to personalized medicine will be tools to support such *prospective medicine* (Langheier and Snyderman 2004)—assisting the acquisition of a detailed family history, social history, and environmental history, providing health-risk assessments, and managing genomic information (Hoffman and Williams 2011; Overby et al. 2010).

22.2.4 Savings Potential with Health IT and CDS

CDS has been shown to influence physician behavior (Colombet et al. 2004; Lindgren 2008; Schedlbauer et al. 2009), diagnostic test ordering

and other care processes (Bates and Gawande 2003; Blumenthal and Glaser 2007), and the costs of care (Haynes et al. (2010)), and it may have a modest impact on clinical outcomes (Bright et al. 2012). While there is great promise with HIT and CDS, their implementation is not without potential peril: HIT poorly designed or implemented, or misused, can generate unintended consequences (Ash et al. 2007; Harrison et al. 2007; Bloomrosen et al. 2011), and introduce new types of medical errors (Institute of Medicine 2011a).

Only a handful of studies have examined the **return on investment** (ROI) for HIT, and even fewer have investigated that for decision-support specifically. The value of CDS in terms of ROI is difficult to measure. Isolated studies of various hand-crafted systems in academic centers have shown value, but adoption elsewhere has often been problematic. Broad adoption has not occurred, for many reasons discussed later in this chapter, including the proprietary nature of systems for CDS and for representation of knowledge, the lack of interoperability of data, the mismatch of CDS to workflow, and usability concerns.

Systematic reviews of the scientific literature, such as the one performed by Bright and colleagues (Bright et al. 2012), have not been able to demonstrate an effect of CDS on patient outcomes except in the short term. This finding is not surprising, however, because the time point at which CDS occurs is often long before a final outcome, and many intervening factors may have a greater effect. In the case of CDS for many chronic diseases whose complications ensue over years or decades, it simply may be impractical to continue longitudinal studies long enough to be able to measure meaningful differences in outcome.

Historically, the adoption of CDS technology has been motivated by a virtuous desire to enhance the performance of clinicians when dealing with complex situations. The recent advent of legal, regulatory, and financial drivers, as well as the increasing importance of personalizing medical decision making on the basis of genomic data, now make CDS an essential element of modern clinical practice.

22.3 Methods of CDS

As we have already noted, CDS systems (1) may use information about the current clinical context to retrieve pertinent online documents; or they (2) may provide patient-specific, situation-specific alerts, reminders, physician order sets, or other recommendations for direct action; or they (3) may organize information in ways that facilitate decision making and action. Category (2) largely consists of the various computer–based approaches ("classic" CDS systems) that have been the substrate for work in biomedical informatics since the advent of applied work in probabilistic reasoning and artificial intelligence in the 1960s and 1970s. Such systems provide custom-tailored assessments or advice based on sets of patient-specific data. They may follow simple logics (such as algorithms), they may be based on decision theory and cost–benefit analysis, or they may use probabilistic approaches only as an adjunct to symbolic problem solving. Some diagnostic assistants (such as DXplain Barnett et al. 1987) suggest differential diagnoses or indicate additional information that would help to narrow the range of etiologic possibilities. Other systems suggest a single best explanation for a patient's symptomatology. Other systems interpret and summarize the patient's record over time in a manner sensitive to the clinical context (Shahar and Musen 1996). Still other systems provide therapy advice rather than diagnostic assistance (Musen et al. 1996).

It is helpful to review some of the early work on such systems to get a sense of the scientific questions that need to be addressed in order to build CDS systems and to understand the challenges that currently confront the field.

Since the earliest days of computers, health professionals have anticipated the time when machines would assist them in the diagnostic process. The first article dealing with this possibility appeared in the late 1950s (Ledley and Lusted 1959), and experimental prototypes appeared within a few years (Warner et al. 1964). Many problems prevented the widespread introduction of such systems, however, ranging from the limitations of the scientific underpinnings to the lack of availability of needed data and to the logistical difficulties that developers encountered when encouraging clinicians to use and accept systems that were not well integrated into the practitioners' usual workflow.

Three advisory systems from the 1970s provide a useful overview of the origin of work on CDS systems and demonstrate paradigms for CDS implementation that still are prevalent today. These decision aids are de Dombal's system for diagnosis of abdominal pain (de Dombal et al. 1972), Shortliffe's MYCIN system for selection of antibiotic therapy (Shortliffe 1976), and the HELP system for delivery of inpatient medical alerts (Kuperman et al. 1991; Warner 1979). We emphasize these three artifacts not because any of them has had a durable effect on clinical practice, but because they each demonstrate very well defined principles for automated decision making that, in their own ways, continue to inspire modern CDS systems that are more complex and more eclectic in their computational architectures.

22.3.1 Leeds Abdominal Pain System

Starting in the late 1960s, F. T. de Dombal and his associates at the University of Leeds studied the diagnostic process and developed computer-based decision aids using Bayesian probability theory (see Chap. 3). Using surgical or pathologic diagnoses as the gold standard, they emphasized the importance of deriving the conditional probabilities used in Bayesian reasoning from high-quality data that they gathered by collecting information on thousands of patients (Adams et al. 1986). Their system, the Leeds abdominal pain system, used sensitivity, specificity, and disease-prevalence data for various signs, symptoms, and test results to calculate, using Bayes' theorem, the probability of seven possible explanations for acute abdominal pain (appendicitis, diverticulitis, perforated ulcer, cholecystitis, small-bowel obstruction, pancreatitis, and nonspecific abdominal pain). To keep the Bayesian computations manageable, the program made the assumptions of (1) conditional independence of the findings for the various diagnoses and of (2) mutual exclusivity and exhaustiveness of the seven diagnoses (see Chap. 3).

In one system evaluation (de Dombal et al. 1972), physicians filled out data sheets summarizing clinical and laboratory findings for 304 patients who came to the emergency room with abdominal pain of sudden onset. The data from these sheets provided the attributes that were analyzed using Bayes' rule. Thus, the Bayesian formulation assumed that each patient had one of the seven conditions and selected the most likely one on the basis of the recorded observations. Had the program been used directly by emergency-room physicians, results could have been available, on average, within 5 min after the data form was completed. During the study, however, the cases were run in batch mode; the computer-generated diagnoses were saved for later comparison (1) to the diagnoses reached by the attending clinicians and (2) to the ultimate diagnosis verified during surgery or through appropriate tests (the "gold standard"; see Chap. 2).

In contrast to the clinicians' diagnoses, which were correct in only 65–80 % of the 304 cases (with accuracy depending on the individual clinician's training and experience), the program's diagnoses were correct in 91.8 % of cases. Furthermore, in six of the seven disease categories, the computer was more likely to assign the patients to the correct disease category than was the senior clinician in charge of the case. Of particular interest was the program's accuracy regarding appendicitis—a diagnosis that is often made incorrectly (or, less often, is missed or at least delayed). In no cases of appendicitis did the computer fail to make the correct diagnosis, and in only six cases were patients with nonspecific abdominal pain incorrectly classified as having appendicitis. Based on the actual clinical decisions, however, more than 20 patients with nonspecific abdominal pain underwent unnecessary surgery for an incorrect diagnosis of appendicitis, and 6 patients who did have appendicitis were observed for more than 8 h before they were finally taken to the operating room.

With the introduction of personal computers, de Dombal's system began to achieve widespread use—from emergency departments in other countries to the British submarine fleet. Surprisingly, the system has never obtained the same degree of diagnostic accuracy in other settings that it did in Leeds—even when adjustments were made for differences in prior probabilities of disease. There are several reasons possible for this discrepancy. The most likely explanation is that there may be considerable variation in the way that clinicians interpret the data that must be entered into the computer. For example, physicians with different training or from different cultures may not agree on the criteria for identification of certain patient findings on physical examination, such as "rebound tenderness."[1] Another possible explanation is that there are different probabilistic relationships between findings and diagnoses in different patient populations.

22.3.2 MYCIN

A different approach to computer-assisted decision support was embodied in the MYCIN program, a rule-based consultation system that combined diagnosis with appropriate management of patients who have infections (Shortliffe 1976). MYCIN's developers believed that straightforward algorithms or statistical approaches were inadequate for this clinical problem in which the underlying knowledge was poorly understood and even the experts often disagreed about how best to manage specific patients, especially before definitive culture results became available. As a result, the researchers were drawn to the use of interacting rules to represent knowledge about organisms that might be causing a patient's infection and the antibiotics that might be used to treat it.

---

[1] *Rebound tenderness* is pain that is exacerbated when the physician presses down on the abdomen and then suddenly releases, generating a "rebound" when the abdomen returns to its baseline position.

Rule507

IF:

1) The infection that requires therapy is meningitis
2) Organisms were not seen on the stain of the culture
3) The type of infection is bacterial
4) The patient does not have a head injury defect, AND
5) The age of the patient is between 15 years and 55 years

THEN

The organisms that might be causing the infection are
Diplococcus-pneuominae and Neisseria-meningitidis

Fig. 22.1 A typical rule from the MYCIN system. Rules are conditional statements that indicate what conclusions can be reached or actions taken if a specified set of conditions is found to be true. In this rule, MYCIN is able to conclude probable bacterial causes of infection if the five conditions in the premise are all found to be true for a specific patient. Not shown are the measures of uncertainty that are also associated with inference in the MYCIN system

Knowledge of infectious diseases in MYCIN was represented as production rules (Fig. 22.1). A production rule is simply a conditional statement that relates observations to associated inferences that can be drawn. The conclusions drawn by one production rule may be considered as input observations by other rules when a system of rules is used for reasoning. MYCIN's power was derived from such rules in a variety of ways:

- The MYCIN program determined which rules to use and how to chain them together to make decisions about a specific case. The MYCIN reasoning program used an approach called **backward chaining**; whenever a rule was being considered such that the system did not know whether the condition on the left-hand side of the rule (i.e., the premise) was true, MYCIN would look backward to see whether the knowledge base contained any other rules that, when evaluated, could conclude information that might inform the evaluation of the current rule's premise. (Nearly all contemporary rule-based systems, on the other hand, use an inference method known as **forward chaining**: Whenever a production rule "fires" and the conclusion of that rule is proven to be true, the system looks forward for other rules in the rule base that could also might be able to fire now that the new conclusion is known to be true.)
- The rules often formed a coherent explanation of MYCIN's reasoning—those that applied to the current decision were displayed in response to a user's questions (Fig. 22.2). Although rules were stored in a machine-readable format, English translations could be displayed.
- By removing, altering, or adding rules, system developers could modify the program's knowledge structures rapidly, without explicitly reprogramming or restructuring other parts of the knowledge base. Making such changes, however, could lead to significant, unintended side effects.

The developers evaluated MYCIN's performance on therapy selection for patients with blood-borne bacterial infections (Yu et al. 1979b), and for those with meningitis (Yu et al. 1979a). In the latter study, MYCIN gave advice that compared favorably with that offered by experts in infectious diseases. MYCIN, however, is best viewed as an early exploration of methods for capturing and applying expert knowledge to solve important medical problems. Although the program was never used clinically, it paved the way for a great deal of research and development. Work on MYCIN helped to clarify how techniques known as **knowledge acquisition** could help developers to work with subject-matter experts to build new rule bases, how general-purpose rule interpreters could help offer decision support for new application areas when developers swapped in a new rule base, and why computer systems tailored to offer CDS are not always capable of offering their users compelling explanations of their decision logic.

In this series, how many of the cultures were positive for E.coli   *(typical system prompt)*
(ORGANISM-1)?

**WHY   *(request from user to determine motivation for question)*

[i.e. WHY is it important to determine the number of cultures which were   *(system's rephrasing of the WHY*
positive for the organism?]   *question, and answer)*

[1.0] This will help to determine whether there is significant disease
associated with this occurrence of the organism.
    It has already been established that
        [1.1] the culture was taken from a sterile source
        [1.2] the number of cultures in the series is greater than 2
    Therefore, if
        [1.3] the number of cultures which were positive for ORGANISM-1
            is greater than 2
    Then there is suggestive evidence (.5) that there is significant disease
           associated with this occurrence of the e.coli (ORGANISM-1).
        [RULE049]
        **WHY   *repeated WHY to determine relevance of previous explanation)*

[i.e. WHY is it important to determine if there is significant disease
associated with this occurrence of the organism?]

[2.0] This will help to determine a diagnosis for which the infection should
be treated.
    It has already been established that
        [2.1] the infection is not one of: primary bacteremia, meningitis
        [2.2] for some current culture of the patient it is true that the site
            of the culture is blood
    Therefore, if
        [2.3] there is significant disease associated with this occurrence of
            the organism
    Then
        It is definite (1.0) that the diagnosis for which the infection should
        be treated is secondary-bacteremia
        [RULE103]

Fig. 22.2 Two examples of MYCIN's explanation capabilities. User input is shown in boldface capital letters and follows the double asterisks. The system expands each ["WHY"] question (enclosed in square brackets) to ensure that the user is aware of its interpretation of the query

22.3.3   HELP

The HELP system, an integrated hospital information system at LDS Hospital in Salt Lake City that was built up locally during the 1970s and 1980s, provided one of the first demonstrations of the importance of integrating CDS capabilities with underlying information technology. HELP had the ability to generate automated alerts when abnormalities in the patient record were noted, and its impact on the development of the field was immense, with applications and methodologies that span nearly the full range of activities in biomedical informatics (Kuperman et al. 1991).

HELP added to a conventional medical-record system a monitoring program and a mechanism for storing decision logic in **HELP sectors** that could be viewed as rules that relate the values of data in the patient database to actions that health care workers might be reminded to take. HELP thus provided a mechanism for event-driven generation of specialized warnings, alerts, and reports. Beginning in the 1990s, workers at LDS Hospital, Columbia Presbyterian Medical Center, and elsewhere created and adopted a standard formalism for encoding decision rules known as the **Arden Syntax**—a programming language that provides a canonical means for writing rules that relate specific patient situations to appropriate actions for practitioners to follow (Hripcsak et al. 1994). In the Arden Syntax, each decision rule, or HELP sector, is called a **medical logic**

MAINTENANCE:

Title:	Diabetic Foot Exam Reminder;;
Mlmname:	Diabetic_Foot_Exam.mlm;;
Arden:	Version 2.8;;
Version:	1.00;;
Institution:	Intermountain Healthcare ;;
Author:	Peter Haug (Peter.Haug@imail.org) ;;
Specialist:	Peter Haug (Peter.Haug@imail.org) ;;
Date:	2011-11-28;;
Validation:	testing;;

LIBRARY:

Purpose:	Alert for Diabetic Foot Exam Yearly;;
Explanation:	This MLM will send an alert if the patient is a diabetic (diabetes in problem list or discharge diagnoses) and Foot Exam is recorded within the last 12 months.;;
Keywords:	diabetes; Foot Exam;;
Citations:	Boulton AJM, Armstrong DG, Albert SF, Frykberg RG,Richard Hellman, Kirkman MS, Lavery LA, LeMaster JW, Mills JL, Mueller MJ, Sheehan P,Dane K. Wukich DK. Comprehensive Foot Examination and Risk Assessment. Diabetes Care. 2008 August; 31(8): 1679–1685.;;
Links:	http://en.wikipedia.org/wiki/Diabetic_foot_ulcer;;

KNOWLEDGE:

Type:	data_driven;;
Data:	Problem_List_Problem := object [Problem, Recorder];
	Problem_List := read as Problem_List_Problem {select problem, recorded_by from Problem_List_Table};
	Patient_Dx_Object := object [Dx];
	Diabetic_Dx := read as Patient_Dx_Object {ICD_Discharge_Diagnoses};
	Foot_Examination := object [Recorder, Observation];
	Observation := object [Abnormatlity, Location, Size, Units];
	Foot_Exam := read as Foot_Examination latest {select Recorder, Observation.Abnormatlity, Observation.Location, Observation.Size, Observation.Units from PE_Table};
	Registration_Event := event { registration of patient };
	ICD_for_Diabetes := (250 , 250.0 , 250.1 , 250.2 , 250.3 , 250.4 , 250.5 , 250.6 , 250.7 , 250.8 , 250.9); ;;
Evoke:	Registration_Event;;
Logic:	if (Diabetic_Dx.Dx is in ICD_for_Diabetes or (exist Problem_List and "Diabetes" is in Problem_List.Problem)) then Diabetes_Present := true ; endif;
	if (Diabetes_Present and exist Foot_Exam and Foot_Exam occurred not within past 12 months) then conclude true ; endif; conclude false ; ;;
Action:	write "Patient is a diabetic with no Diabetic Foot Exam in last 12 months. Please order or perform one.";;

Fig. 22.3 This medical logic module (MLM), written in the Arden syntax, prints a warning for health care workers whenever a patient who has diabetes is registered for a clinic visit and has not had a documented foot examination in the past year. The *evoke* slot defines a situation that causes the rule to be triggered; the *logic* slot encodes the decision logic of the rule; the *action* slot defines the procedure to follow if the logic slot reaches a positive conclusion. The *data* slot defines the variables that are to be used by the MLM; the text between curly braces must be translated into queries on the local patient database when the MLM is deployed locally (Source: P. J. Haug, Intermountain Healthcare)

module (MLM). Figure 22.3 shows one such MLM and its representation in the Arden syntax. An MLM is a specialized form of what is known as an **Event-Condition-Action (ECA) rule**, in that evaluation of situation-specific conditional expression logic is triggered by an external event, and, if the condition evaluates to be "true", then an action is performed.

Whenever new data about a patient became available, regardless of the source, the HELP system checked to see whether the data matched the criteria for invoking an MLM. If they did, the system would evaluate the MLM to see whether that MLM was relevant for the specific patient. The logic in these MLMs was developed by clinical experts who collaborated with workers in informatics. The output generated by successful MLMs included, for example, alerts regarding untoward drug actions, interpretations of laboratory tests, or calculations of the likelihood of diseases. This output was communicated to the appropriate people through the hospital information system's workstations or on written reports, depending on the urgency of the output message and the location and functions of the person for whom the report was intended.

Another important extension of the idea of alerts is *clinical reminders*, in which the triggering event is usually time – such as the age of the patient, or an elapsed time since a previous event – coupled with other conditions, first popularized and implemented widely at Regenstrief Institute of Medicine in Indianapolis, Indiana (McDonald 1976). Like the HELP system implemented at LDS Hospital, the Regenstrief Medical Information System used MLMs encoded as rules to generate one-step decision logic (McDonald 1981).

22.3.4 Comparing the Early CDS Systems

The Leeds system, MYCIN, and HELP demonstrate the most fundamental issues that developers of computer-based decision aids face: (1) identifying the input data that will drive decision making, (2) determining how the output of the CDS system will be communicated, and (3) constructing a mechanism to reason about the inputs to generate appropriate output. We will address each of these issues in detail in the remainder of this chapter. First, however, it is useful to review how these elements were addressed in each of these classic systems.

The three historical systems differed radically in how the input data were collected. In the Leeds abdominal pain system, the input was derived from a simple checklist completed by the clinician that enumerated some of the findings that a patient with abdominal pain might have. Data collection was not burdensome, since the checklist was rather short, although the results did need to be transcribed into the computer. Some observers have suggested that the availability of the checklist itself could have been responsible for many of the benefits of the Leeds system, since it reminded the clinicians of key questions that they needed to ask their patients in the first place (see Gawande 2009). On the other hand, use of the MYCIN system required a potentially lengthy question-and-answer dialog with the computer that would have to take place outside of the usual clinical workflow. The barrier imposed by this style of interaction remains a major impediment to the adoption of MYCIN-style computer-based consultation systems (although with modern EHRs, some of the data could be obtained in such a system directly from the stored record instead of being entered manually by a user). With the HELP system, of course, there are no problems of human–computer interaction; the data are already available, provided by the health information system as a function of routine care. Although the ability to drive a CDS system based on data that require no manual entry has compelling advantages, HELP had the obvious disadvantage that any data that were not in the database—or that were in the database but not available in coded or numerical form—could not be brought to bear on the decision process. Nevertheless, the integration of CDS with EHR functionality in the HELP system was an important move away from the idea of standalone "consultation systems," such as MYCIN, which might provide comprehensive and complete patient advice for a particular problem, to more opportunistic CDS technology that could use readily available, but sometimes incomplete patient data to offer recommendations in a manner that did not require clinicians to step outside their usual workflow (Miller and Masarie 1990).

The output of the Leeds system was simply a posterior probability for each of the seven diagnoses for abdominal pain for which it had been programmed. MYCIN provided the user with an elaborate description of the infections that might be present in the patient, the antibiotics that should be administered, and the possible side effects of those antibiotics. More important, MYCIN supported a **mixed-initiative dialog** through which the user could investigate the chain of inference rules that supported some aspects of the program's output. With HELP, the output was a predefined text message (sometimes customized for the patient's particular clinical situation) that would appear on a line printer at the patient's nursing station or at some other appropriate location in the hospital. In subsequent versions of HELP, as with more contemporary systems that offer alerts or reminders, such messages appeared in the form of popup windows in the EHR or emails or text messages sent directly to the provider.

The three decision aids differ significantly in the manner in which they reached their conclusions. The Leeds system used a large database of case histories to calculate the conditional probabilities of a fixed number of diseases given a fixed number of possible patient findings, and applied Bayes' theorem to specific sets of input data. MYCIN, on the other hand, eschewed the use of formal probability theory and pioneered the use of chaining production rules that interacted at runtime to deduce the possible pathogens causing infection and to suggest a treatment regimen that could provide coverage for each of these germs. The developers of MYCIN did explore a heuristic method for dealing with uncertainty, called "certainty factors," that propagated uncertainty about the conclusions of rules when the rules were chained, and which did have a relationship to subjective probability estimations (Shortliffe and Buchanan 1975). HELP adopted a rule-based approach, but its rules typically did not "chain," and rule firing was totally deterministic if the condition part of the MLM evaluated to "true" based on the pattern of findings in the patient database.

22.4 Principles of CDS System Design

Modern CDS systems typically achieve their results using Bayesian reasoning, production rules, MLMs, knowledge-based groupings of physician orders, referred to as "order sets," and other templates, or by the use of prediction associations derived by mining and analysis of EHR data (or some combination of these approaches). Like the historical programs that we reviewed in Sect. 22.3, contemporary systems may acquire the data on which they base their recommendations interactively from users or directly from a health information system (or some combination of these approaches). We now discuss the issues that drive CDS system design, and we highlight how these issues are manifest in current clinical decision aids.

22.4.1 Acquisition and Validation of Patient Data

A prerequisite to any decision making process is having available all the data that are required to perform the required actions. As emphasized in Chap. 2, few problems are more challenging than the development of effective techniques for capturing patient data accurately, completely, and efficiently. You have read in this book about a wide variety of techniques for data acquisition, ranging from keyboard entry, to speech input, to methods that separate the clinician from the computer (such as scannable forms, real-time data monitoring, and intermediaries who transcribe written or dictated data for use by computers).

The problems of data acquisition go beyond entry or extraction from the EHR of the data themselves, however. A primary obstacle is that we lack standardized ways of expressing most clinical situations in a form that computers can interpret. As discussed in detail in Chap. 7, there are several controlled medical terminologies that health care workers use to specify precise diagnostic evaluations (e.g., the International Classification of Diseases and SNOMED-CT), clinical procedures (e.g., Current Procedural

Terminology and LOINC codes), and so on. Still, there is no controlled terminology that can capture all the nuances of a patient's history of present illness or findings on physical examination. There is no coding system that can reflect all the details of physicians' or nurses' progress notes. Given that much of the information in the medical record that we would like to use to drive decision support is not available in a structured, machine-understandable form, there are clear limitations on the data that can be used to assist clinician decision-making. The prose of progress notes, consultation notes, operation reports, discharge summaries, and other documents contains an enormous amount of information that never makes it to the coded part of the EHR. Nevertheless, even when computer-based patient records store substantial information only as free-text entries, those data that *are* available in coded form (typically, diagnosis codes and prescription data) can be used to significant advantage (van der Lei et al. 1991).

The desire to access information from the EHR that may be available only in free text has been a topic of great concern to the CDS community. Some information systems provide options for **structured data entry**, asking clinicians to use fill-in-the-blanks forms or templates on the computer screen to enter information that otherwise would be entered as part of a textual note. In general, providers have resisted such human–computer interfaces, often finding it restrictive and cumbersome to make selections from predefined menus when they would much rather express themselves more freely in prose. Fortunately, work in **natural language processing** has made major advances in recent years, making it increasingly possible to mine the textual notes of EHRs to identify information that might bear on the CDS process (see Chap. 8).

22.4.2 Decision-Making Process

When building CDS systems, most of the work is concentrated on the development of the reasoning system and the specification of the knowledge on which that reasoning system operates.

There is a wide range of strategies, each addressing different requirements that workers in biomedical informatics have adopted when building such computational resources.

22.4.2.1 Infobuttons

The simplest, and perhaps most common, form of CDS uses contextual information from an EHR to perform information retrieval from a database of information about online documents. A person viewing data in an EHR may see selectable icons (**infobuttons**) next to the names of drugs, laboratory tests, patient problems, or other elements of the patient record. Clicking on an infobutton causes the clinical information system to perform a query on the database, providing the user with one or more immediately accessible resources that can offer more information about the item in question. Alternatively, the system may automatically query one or more of those external resources and return the results of the queries for display (Cimino et al. 2002a). Clicking on an infobutton next to a drug, for example, might allow the user to access information about customary dosing, side effects, or alternative medications (see Fig. 12.8). The query that retrieves the links to the documents is tailored based on whatever is next to the infobutton icon on the screen. The query may also take into account contextual information, such as patient-related data, the activity in which the user is engaged, and the role of the user in the health care enterprise (physician, nurse, patient, and so on).

An **infobutton manager** mediates the queries between the clinical information system and the available information resources. HL7 has created a standard for "context-aware knowledge retrieval," leading to infobutton managers that have been adopted by many commercial EHR vendors. Infobutton managers need to anticipate how the clinical context might tailor the specific query performed by any given infobutton, so that the result of the query is highly precise and relevant to the situation at hand. Detailing specifically how contextual information might alter the queries performed by each infobutton type can be tedious, and requires developers to be adept at second-guessing all the reasons that might cause a user to click on a particular infobutton. Current research concentrates on the development of a Librarian Tailoring Infobutton Environment (LITE) that promises to aid the authoring of infobutton queries via "wizards" and other user-interface conveniences.

Although infobuttons are unquestionably important knowledge resources, many people would argue that they are not true CDS systems. Infobuttons retrieve relevant information for a user, but they do not explicitly address particular *decisions* that the user needs to make. The possible reasons that a user might click on an infobutton are folded into the query specification at the time that the infobutton is created; at runtime, of course, there is no way for the system to know exactly why the user selected the infobutton. Infobutton managers therefore require sophisticated query capabilities, but they do not need to reason from a clinical situation to a particular recommendation.

When the goal is to generate a situation-specific recommendation regarding diagnosis or therapy, developers need to turn to methods that can perform some kind of inference. The sophistication of the required technique is a function of the kind of inference that is necessary to render a result for the user.

22.4.2.2 Branching Logic

From a computational perspective, there is nothing simpler than encoding an algorithm directly. Numerous CDS systems have taken problem-specific flowcharts designed by clinicians and encoded them for use by a computer. Although such algorithms have been useful for the purpose of triaging patients in urgent-care situations and as a didactic technique used in journals and books where an overview for a problem's management has been appropriate, they have been largely rejected by physicians as too simplistic or generic for routine use (Grimm et al. 1975). In addition, the advantage of their implementation on computers has not been clear; the use of simple printed copies of the algorithms generally has proved adequate for clinical care (Komaroff et al. 1974). A noteworthy exception that gained enormous

attention in the early 1970s was a computer program deployed in Boston at what was then the Beth Israel Hospital (Bleich 1972); it used detailed algorithmic logic to provide advice regarding the diagnosis and management of acid–base and electrolyte disorders. More recently, such branching-logic approaches have been widely adopted in the administrative information systems that third-party payers use to process requests to pre-certify payment for expensive services such as MRI studies and elective surgery.

Although flowcharts alone often are inadequate for representing the decision making required for the execution of robust clinical-practice guidelines, the algorithmic representation of clinical procedures is extremely useful for clinicians when they think about the representation of preferred clinical workflows. It is therefore common to see a branching-logic representation of clinical protocols and guidelines as one component of the complex, heterogeneous knowledge representations needed to drive sophisticated CDSS systems, such as those described later in this section when we discuss ontology-driven decision support.

22.4.2.3 Probabilistic Systems

Because computers were traditionally viewed as numerical calculating machines, people recognized by the 1960s that they could be used to compute the posterior probability of diseases based on observations of patient-specific parameters. Large numbers of **Bayesian diagnosis programs** have been developed in the intervening years, many of which have been shown to be accurate in selecting among competing explanations of a patient's disease state. As we mentioned earlier, among the most significant experiments were those of de Dombal and associates (1972) in England, who adopted a **naïve Bayesian model** that assumed that there are no conditional dependencies among findings (i.e., a model that could make the inappropriate assumption that the presence of a finding such as fever never affects the likelihood of the presence of a finding such as chills).

Although a naïve Bayesian model may have limitations in accurately modeling a diagnostic problem, a major strength of this approach is computational efficiency. When the findings that bear on a hypothesis are assumed to be conditionally independent, then the order in which the findings are considered in the Bayesian analysis does not matter. The computer starts by considering a given finding, the prior probability of each possible diagnosis under consideration (generally the prevalence of each diagnosis in the population), and the conditional probabilities of the finding (or the absence of the finding) given each diagnosis (or the absence of the diagnosis)—the *sensitivity* and *specificity* of the finding (see the introduction of these concepts in Chap. 2). The computer then applies Bayes' rule to calculate the posterior probability of each diagnosis given the value of the finding. The computer now is poised to update the probability of each diagnosis given the value of a second finding. The prior probability for each diagnosis in this case is not the prevalence of the diagnosis in the population, however. Having applied Bayes' rule once, we have more information than we had at the start. We can treat the *posterior probability* of each diagnosis given the first finding as the *prior probability* of the diagnosis when we apply Bayes' rule a second time. When it is time to consider a third finding, the posterior probability for each diagnosis after processing the second finding serves as the prior probability for the next application of Bayes rule. The process continues until the value of each finding has been considered. This **sequential Bayes** approach was explored as early as the 1960s for the diagnosis of congenital heart disease (Gorry and Barnett 1968) and has been used in many CDS systems since.

Much of the early interest in the sequential Bayesian approach stemmed from a conviction that it simply was impractical to construct Bayesian systems in which the assumption of conditional independence was lifted: There would be too many probabilities to assess when building the system and the necessary computation could be intractable. Recent work on the use of **belief networks**, however, has demonstrated that it actually is realistic to develop more expressive Bayesian systems in which conditional dependencies are modeled explicitly—often by taking advantage of newer algorithms for

concluding the posterior probabilities that are computationally efficient in most cases. (Belief networks are described in detail in Chap. 3.) Currently, most modern CDS systems that make recommendations based on probabilistic relationships use belief networks as their primary representation of the underlying clinical situation, and then "solve" the belief network at runtime to calculate the posterior probabilities of the conditions represented in the graph. The use of belief networks is popular because the formalism makes probabilistic relationships perspicuous, overcomes the assumption of conditional independence, and enables the attendant probabilities to be learned from analysis of appropriate data sets (for example, EHR data). The approach has been demonstrated in numerous diagnostic systems, from belief networks that ascertain the status of newborns from data in the neonatal ICU (Saria et al. 2010) to belief networks that offer interpretations of biomedical image data (Kahn et al. 1997).

Because making most decisions in medicine requires weighing the costs and benefits of actions that could be taken in diagnosing or managing a patient's illness, researchers also have developed tools that draw on the methods of decision analysis (Sox et al. 1988; Weinstein and Fineberg 1980). **Decision analysis** adds to Bayesian reasoning the idea of explicit decisions and of **utilities** associated with the various outcomes that could occur in response to those decisions (see Chap. 3). One class of programs for decision-analysis is designed for use by the analysts themselves; such programs are of little use to the average clinician or patient (Pauker and Kassirer 1981). A second class of programs uses decision-analysis concepts within systems designed to advise physicians who are not trained in these techniques. In such programs, the underlying decision models generally have been prespecified—either as decision trees that enumerate all possible decisions and all possible ramifications of those decisions or as belief networks in which explicit decision and utility nodes are added, called **influence diagrams**.

There are a whole host of **supervised learning techniques** that can determine how data are associated with hypotheses, and that consequently can be trained on EHR data to infer conclusions based on some set of input data. For example, the decision-support capabilities of the patient monitoring systems discussed in Chap. 19 often apply statistical methods to the current data stream to infer corresponding classifications to inform care providers of the patient's current state. Regression analysis or more sophisticated techniques, such as artificial neural networks and support vector machines, when applied to routinely collected patient data, have enabled investigators to develop decision aids such as the APACHE III system (Knaus et al. 1991), which offers prediction models providing prognostic information regarding patients in the ICU (see Chap. 10).

22.4.2.4 Rule-Based Approaches

Since the 1970s, workers in medical AI have been exploring the use of methods that emphasize symbolic associations rather than purely probabilistic relationships to drive decision support (Clancey and Shortliffe 1984). This work has led to the construction of **knowledge-based systems**—programs that symbolically encode-concepts derived from experts in a field in a **knowledge base** and that use that knowledge base to provide the kind of problem analysis and advice that the expert might provide. If–then production rules, such as those in MYCIN (see Fig. 22.1), often have been used to build knowledge-based systems, as have more recent approaches that encode explicit models of the application area or of the reasoning methods required (David et al. 1993; Musen 1997). The knowledge in a knowledge-based system may include probabilistic relations, such as between symptoms and underlying diseases. Typically, such relations are augmented by additional qualitative relations, such as causality and temporal relations. When a knowledge-based system is encoded using production rules, it is referred to as a **rule-based system** (Buchanan and Shortliffe 1984).

Rule-based systems provide the dominant mechanism for developers to build CDS capabilities into modern information systems. From CDS systems that interpret ECG signals to those that

recommend guideline-based therapy, rules provide an extremely convenient means to encode the necessary knowledge. Rule-based systems require a formal language for encoding the rules, plus an interpreter (sometimes called an **inference engine**) that operates on the rules to generate the necessary behavior. MYCIN, for example, required the developer to encode rules in a predefined manner using the Lisp programming language (see Fig. 22.1), and had an inference engine that could interpret the rules, determine whether the rules led to conclusions that were true or false, and, if necessary, automatically evaluate other rules in the knowledge base to help determine the truth value of a given rule that might be under consideration. Although the developers of MYCIN had to construct their own syntax for encoding rules and had to program their own inference engine to evaluate the rules, there now are many open-source and proprietary "rule engines" that provide custom-tailored editors for writing rules and inference engines that can execute the rules at runtime. For example, JESS is a popular Java-based rules engine that can be licensed from Sandia National Laboratory and that currently is free for academic use; JESS is based on a rules engine programmed in C, called CLIPS, created by NASA in the 1980s. Drools is an open-source rules engine developed by the JBoss community that also has had substantial adoption.

Developers use JESS, Drools, and proprietary rules engines to create CDS systems that contain multiple rules that, as with MYCIN, chain together to generate conclusions based on a sequence of inference steps. Decision support sometimes requires multiple rules to execute at runtime, together generating a final recommendation that derives from the consequences of the rules chaining off one another.

In most installed information systems, however, rule-based decision support is much simpler and also more limited. As in the HELP system, most CDS systems have rules that generally do not chain together, but that are triggered individually, each time either there is a relevant change to the data in a patient database that should generate an alert or there is a time event that should trigger a reminder. Each rule, or MLM, examines the state of the database and generates a corresponding action, alert, or reminder that is usually sent to a particular clinician or to members of the health care team.

Arden Syntax became an international standard for MLMs endorsed by HL7 and ANSI in 1999 (see Fig. 22.3). Arden Syntax provides a standard mechanism for declaring the variables about whose values the system will perform its reasoning (values that derive from data in the clinical information system); the conditions that, if true, would predicate specific actions; and the actions that should be taken. The standard was created with the idea that the shared syntax would allow an MLM written in an idiosyncratic representation system (for example, the one adopted by HELP) to be translated into a canonical format for execution in other information systems. The hope was that the informatics community would develop whole libraries of MLMs, all written in Arden Syntax, which could operate in any clinical environment where an information system could interpret the standard format.

A significant obstacle to the sharing of MLMs is that Arden Syntax is, in fact, just a syntax. What is missing from the standard is any notion of the *semantics* of the data on which the MLMs operate. When an MLM executes, the variables that are used in the logic of the rule are bound to values that derive from the patient database of the information system in which the MLMs operate. Arden Syntax specifies that the individual database queries needed to determine the values of the variables should appear within the "curly braces" of variable definitions in the portion of the MLM known as the "data slot" (see Fig. 22.3). What a developer should include within the curly braces depends on the particular schema of the relevant patient database and mechanism for performing queries. EHR information models and the way in which elements are coded differ from system to system. Thus, all system-specific aspects of MLM integration need to be provided within the curly braces. To adapt an MLM for use in a new environment, a programmer needs to consider the variables on which the MLM operates, determine whether those variables have

counterparts in the local patient database, and write an appropriate query that will execute at runtime.

The problem is compounded because there may be assumptions regarding the semantics of the variables themselves that may not be obvious to the local implementer: If the MLM refers to serum potassium, should the logic be executed if the original specimen was grossly hemolyzed?[2] If a serum potassium value is not available in the database, but there is a value for a whole-blood potassium, should the MLM be executed using that value instead?[3] If there is no serum potassium value available for today, but there is one from last night, should the logic execute using the most recent value? MLMs cannot simply be dropped from one system into another and be shared effortlessly; rather, considerable thought, analysis, and computer skill needs to go into writing the appropriate database queries that go within the curly braces to make MLMs operational.

This obstacle to sharing MLMs that are written in the Arden Syntax is known, appropriately and whimsically, as the **curly braces problem**. The lack of standards for what goes between Arden's curly braces has been a major impediment both to the sharing of MLMs and to the creation of reference libraries of clinical decision rules. HL7 recognized this difficulty early on, and developed an abstract expression language for specifying database queries known as GELLO, which was adopted as a standard in 2005 (Sordo et al. 2004). The organization also advocated the use of a specification for canonical kinds of data that one might find in an EHR—a *virtual* EHR—so that MLMs written in terms of GELLO queries on the virtual EHR can be translated programmatically into actual queries on patient data as available at a local institution (Kawamoto et al. 2010). In 2012, HL7 approved a **draft standard for trial use** (DSTU)

---

[2] If the red blood cells in a specimen *hemolyze* (burst), they release potassium, which can cause an inaccurate elevation in the measured potassium value.

[3] The *serum* is the liquid that is left when the cells are removed from whole blood.

for a virtual EHR (known for historical reasons as a *virtual medial record*, or vMR; Johnson et al. 2001a). We discuss these standards further in Sect. 22.5.2. For the reasons described in that section, despite these HL7 standards, it is unlikely that the curly braces problem will be going away anytime soon.

In the case of Arden Syntax, developers write rules to deal with one clinical problem at a time. There may be one MLM to deal with the problem of administering a drug like penicillin to a patient with a history of penicillin allergy; another MLM may report that a patient has a dangerously low serum potassium value. Unlike the rules in MYCIN, MLMs are generally not intended to interact with one another or to be chained together to generate complex inferences. MLMs may be coerced to chain together when one MLM posts to the patient database a value that can trigger another MLM. This mechanism also allows one MLM to set up information in the database that might invoke another MLM in the case of some future event, thus enabling the recommendation of actions that unfold over time, as in the case of many clinical practice guidelines for chronic diseases. Although this approach allows developers to program complex problem-solving behavior, the technique has the same disadvantages that came to light with chaining rule-based systems such as MYCIN: When the rule base grows to a large size, interactions among rules may have unanticipated side effects. Furthermore, when rules are added to or deleted from a previously debugged knowledge base, there may be unexpected system behaviors that emerge as a result (Clancey 1984; Heckerman and Horvitz 1986).

For MLMs to work well in practice, moreover, the rules need to be tailored to the particular clinical environment—triggered by appropriate workflow events, interacting with particular kinds of participants, customizing logic to account for various business and workflow processes, and notifying the user in setting-specific ways. To customize an MLM to account for such considerations requires that it become less portable. Much of the effort required to introduce CDS systems into the health care enterprise involves precisely such adaptations. To accelerate porta-

bility, MLM developers must seek a balance between a generic specification of logic that is widely agreed upon, and site-specific customizations that will facilitate the use of that logic. Achieving the right balance will always remain an elusive target (see also Sect. 22.5.4).

22.4.2.5 Ontology-Driven CDS Systems

There is a class of CDS systems that use higher-level abstractions of clinical knowledge and problem-solving knowledge to overcome some of the limitations of the more prevalent CDS architectures. These systems make an explicit distinction between the *static knowledge* of the clinical domain (e.g., knowledge of the specifications entailed by a clinical practice guideline) and the *problem-solving knowledge* needed to apply the static knowledge to a particular patient (e.g., the means to generate specific prescriptions for medications based on the general guideline recommendations and the particular clinical situation that the patient is experiencing). This distinction makes it possible for system builders to address different elements of the knowledge needed to be represented in the computer using tailored approaches and tools (Musen 1998; DeClerq et al. 2004).

The ATHENA-CDS system exemplifies this component-oriented approach (Goldstein et al. 2000). ATHENA-CDS is a computer system that is integrated with the HIS used by the U.S. Department of Veterans Affairs (VA), known as VistA (see Chap. 12). ATHENA-CDS is installed at several VA medical centers and has been the subject of a number of evaluation experiments (Chan et al. 2004; Lin et al. 2006). ATHENA-CDS offers advice regarding patients who have certain chronic diseases, whose physicians would like to treat those patients in accordance with recognized evidence-based clinical practice guidelines (Fig. 22.4). Currently, ATHENA-CDS draws on several electronic knowledge bases, each one capturing the knowledge of a particular guideline (e.g., for hypertension, for hyperlipidemia, for diabetes, and so on). Each time that a patient with a relevant diagnosis (e.g., hypertension) is seen in the outpatient clinic, ATHENA-CDS takes as input the corresponding guideline

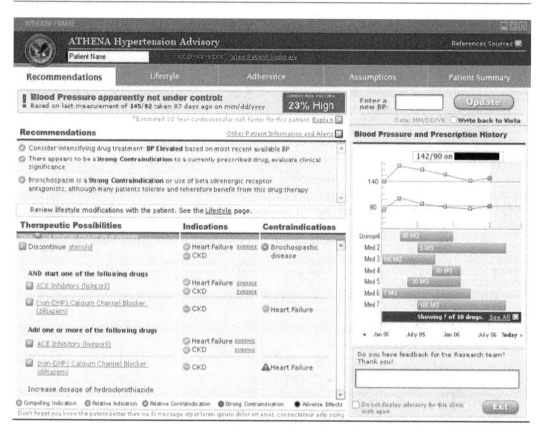

Fig. 22.4 An example of the ATHENA-CDS system interface. ATHENA-CDS provides decision-support for the management of hypertension and several other chronic diseases by using a declarative knowledge base created as an instantiation on a generic guideline ontology. In the screen capture, the provider has entered the patient's most recent blood pressure, and is offered advice about possible alterations in therapy based on the relevant clinical-practice guideline (Source: M. K. Goldstein, VA Palo Alto Healthcare System)

knowledge base and patient-specific data from the VistA EHR, and generates as output suggestions to the clinician for treating the patient to ensure that the treatment is consistent with the care that the guideline would recommend. Because the standard documents that define clinical practice guidelines can be long and complicated, it is extremely helpful for the computer to focus the clinician's attention on precisely which interventions should be considered to guarantee that the patient's care is consonant with the medical evidence captured by a given guideline (Fig. 22.5).

ATHENA-CDS was engineered using an approach that separates out static knowledge about the clinical application area from knowledge about problem solving (Musen et al. 1996).

The developers began by creating an **ontology** of clinical guidelines in general. An ontology is like a **controlled terminology** (see Chap. 7) that includes not only an enumeration of the important entities in some application area, but also—in machine-processable form—the relationships among those entities and, possibly, constraints on those entities. Thus, an ontology contains taxonomic relationships that indicate, for example, that *cholesterol* is a kind of *lipid* or that a *serum potassium* is a kind of *laboratory test*. An ontology may also contain partitive relationships that indicate, for example, that a *systolic blood pressure measurement* is part of a *blood pressure measurement*, or that the *guideline drugs* are part of a *guideline*. To construct ATHENA-CDS, it was necessary first to define an ontology of

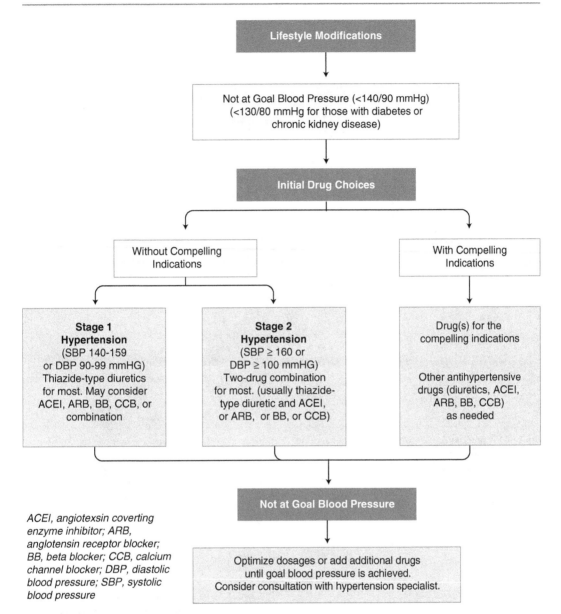

Fig. 22.5 Professional societies, health care practices, private foundations, and other organizations are all working to capture "best practices" for managing patients in accordance with scientific evidence in terms of clinical practice guidelines. Unfortunately, nearly all these guidelines are published initially as large paper documents. Here is a high-level, paper-based flowchart from the guideline developed by Joint National Commission on Hypertension. The flowchart summarizes detailed recommendations that the guideline document specifies in many pages of text. Synopses of such guidelines are available online at http://guidelines.gov

clinical practice guidelines (Fig. 22.6). The guideline ontology makes it clear that all guidelines must include *eligibility criteria* that indicate which patients should be treated in accordance with the guideline, a *clinical algorithm* that specifies the sequence of treatments recommended by the guideline, and *guideline drugs* that represent all the medications that patients might be given when their provider follows the guideline. Because the guideline ontology is general, it does not contain information about any *particular* clinical algorithm, any *particular* eligibility

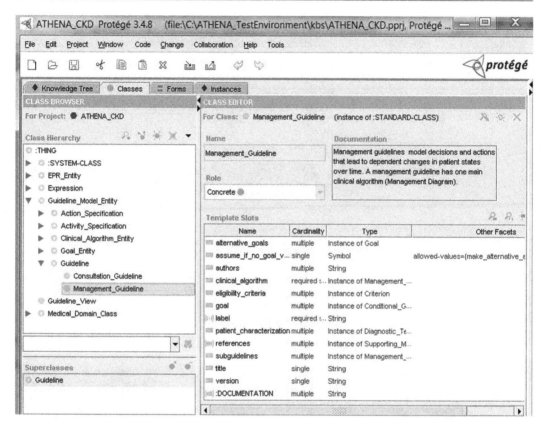

Fig. 22.6 A small portion of the ontology of clinical guidelines used by ATHENA-CDS as entered into the Protégé ontology-editing system. The hierarchy of entries on the left includes entities that constitute building blocks for constructing guideline descriptions. The panel on the right shows the attributes of whatever entity is highlighted on the left. Here, *goal*, *eligibility_criteria*, and *clinical_algorithm*, for example, are attributes of the entity known as *Mangement_Guideline*. The ontology entered into Protégé reflects concepts believed to be common to all guidelines, but does not include specifications for any guidelines in particular. The complete domain model is used to generate automatically a graphical knowledge-acquisition tool, such as the one shown in Fig. 22.7

criteria, and so on. The ontology merely states that all guidelines for management of chronic diseases have such characteristics.

Developers of ATHENA-CDS used the Protégé ontology-development system (Gennari et al. 2003) to create the ontology of clinical practice guidelines (see Fig. 22.6). They then used Protégé to allow the guideline ontology to structure **knowledge bases** that define how to manage patients in accordance with particular guidelines. The developers created a knowledge base for management of hypertension reflecting the guideline that is used by the VA and the Department of Defense (DOD), supplemented with recommendations from the Joint National Commission on Hypertension (National High Blood Pressure Education Program 2004;

Fig. 22.7). They instantiated the ATHENA-CDS guideline ontology to build a knowledge base for management of congestive heart failure based on the guideline developed by the American Heart Association and the American College of Cardiology. The developers built a knowledge base for management of chronic pain, based on the guideline promoted by the VA and the DOD (Trafton et al. 2010). Other knowledge bases for guideline-based care of diabetes, hyperlipidemia, and chronic kidney disease were created in a similar manner.

The ATHENA-CDS guideline ontology can be viewed as a hierarchy of classes in an object-oriented language. Each object defines an entity in the ontology (e.g., clinical algorithm, guideline drugs). To create a knowledge base (such as the

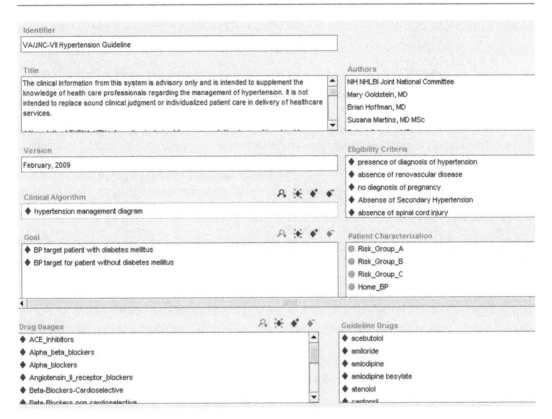

Fig. 22.7 A screen from a Protégé-generated knowledge-acquisition tool for entry of clinical-practice guidelines. The tool is generated automatically from domain ontology, shown in Fig. 22.6. The entries into the tool specify the knowledge required to treat patients in accordance with the guideline for chronic hypertension adopted by the Department of Veterans Affairs

one for hypertension management), the classes in the object hierarchy are instantiated to define the particular *clinical algorithm* mandated by the hypertension guideline, the particular *guideline drugs* required to treat hypertension, and so on. Similarly, creating the diabetes knowledge base for ATHENA-CDS required instantiating the *clinical algorithm* class with information about the sequence of events that take place in the management of diabetes, and so on. Although creating the ATHENA-CDS guideline ontology required careful analysis and modeling, it is a much easier task to use a knowledge-editing system such as Protégé to instantiate the ontology with the information required for individual guidelines. Indeed, editing and maintaining the ATHENA-CDS knowledge bases has been something that trained clinicians generally have done on their own without much assistance from workers in informatics.

In the approach demonstrated by ATHENA-CDS, software engineers create specialized computer programs that encode the procedures needed to perform different tasks using the knowledge base. For example, in ATHENA-CDS, a problem-solving program uses a guideline knowledge base (for example, the knowledge base that encodes the VA/DOD/JNC guideline for management of hypertension) in conjunction with data that the program queries from the VistA EHR to make situation-specific recommendations to providers regarding therapy for high blood pressure. The approach separates the static knowledge base from problem solvers that operate on that knowledge base. Thus, a different problem-solving program could use the knowledge base and available EHR data to determine whether a patient is eligible for treatment in accordance with the guideline. Another problem-solving program could perform **quality**

assurance to assess whether past patients have been treated in accordance with the guideline, when appropriate (Advani et al. 2003). Another program could estimate the cost of treating a patient in accordance with the guideline.

The ontology-driven approach makes it possible to start with a particular ontology (in this case, one for clinical practice guidelines for management of chronic disease) to create multiple knowledge bases, each one instantiating the ontology to specify the knowledge required for particular guidelines. Similarly, the different knowledge bases can be mapped to different problem-solving programs, such that each problem solver automates a different task associated with guideline-based care (therapy planning, eligibility determination, and so on). The ability to "mix and match" knowledge bases and problem solvers offers considerable flexibility, and enables developers to reuse elements of previous solutions to address new CDS problems that require different domain knowledge or different problem-solving procedures.

22.5 Translating CDS to the Clinical Enterprise

So far in this chapter, you have learned about the foundational elements of CDS systems. We have emphasized the research challenges that confront the informatics community to offer more useful CDS and to make it easier for developers to encode clinical knowledge in electronic form. Bringing CDS technology to the point of care, however, requires a parallel set of challenges that concern integration of CDS systems both within the information infrastructure available in real-world settings and within the workflows of their users. Deployment of CDS systems within the clinical enterprise requires an understanding of the complexities of existing HIT and of the processes by which the HIT vendor community adopts the standards that enable interoperation among different HIT components.

Over the past several decades, advanced CDS systems have been developed and deployed in a number of academic medical centers. The tech-

nology slowly has diffused into commercial EHR systems and into routine practice (Chaudhry et al. 2006). The uptake has been greater in medium-to-large hospitals and in medical-center–based networks, including affiliated practices, and has been much less in smaller hospitals, clinics, and independent practices. Although these trends have been sluggish, the recent advent of "meaningful use" regulations for HIT promises to accelerate the adoption of CDS technology dramatically.

In general, the CDS systems deployed to date in vendor EHR systems are relatively limited in scope. The greatest uptake has been in the form of simple alerts and reminders, standard physician order sets, CPOE-based prescription templates with dose checks, allergy checks, identification of drug–lab and drug–drug interactions, and some use of infobuttons or access to context-specific knowledge resources. In some specific settings, rule-based systems have been used to drive the intelligent collection of clinical information in a comprehensive, structured form (Schnipper et al. 2008b).

A few vendors have been successful at distributing knowledge resources, making available clinical knowledge in the form of drug-interaction databases, order sets for common indications, rule-based knowledge, documentation templates, and information resources for infobutton-based queries.

Nonetheless, even these kinds of resources have had relatively limited adoption to date. There are several reasons for the slow uptake of CDS, as enumerated in the sections that follow.

22.5.1 Lack of a Standard Patient Information Model

CDS rules and other knowledge forms need to operate on specific patient data. If those data are stored in a proprietary format and with non-standard encodings, then a set of rules needs to be customized to use data in that form, or the data need to be translated to a common information model. The former has been the usual process, and, as a result, vendor EHR systems tend to have libraries of rules that operate only in their own

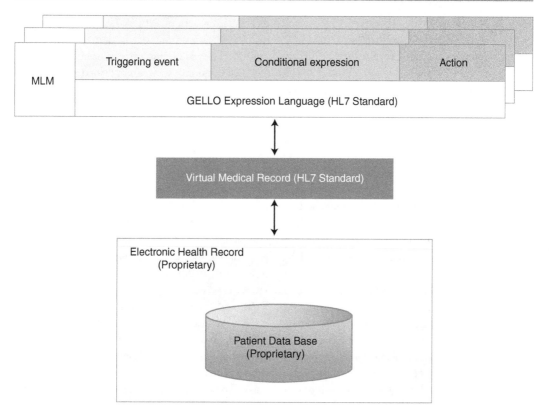

Fig. 22.8 HL7 Version 3 offers a solution to the "curly braces problem" that has to date impeded the sharing of MLMs. In Version 3, EHR vendors may adopt a standard *virtual medical record* (vMR) interface that provides a common framework (a "wrapper") for accessing patient data stored in diverse, proprietary EHR databases. In Version 3, developers of medical logic modules (MLMs) can use a standard object-oriented query language, GELLO, to access the vMR. Although it has been hoped that use of standards such as GELLO and the vMR will encourage widespread sharing of libraries of MLM decision rules, the vMR is based on the HL7 Reference Information Model (RIM), which to date has received limited adoption by the vendor community

systems, using their proprietary data dictionaries and data models; sharing across platforms and systems has been limited, and considerable work is required to integrate vendor HIT products with external CDS systems.

The informatics community is responding to this problem through the creation of new standards (see Chap. 7). For example, HL7 has developed an XML mark-up specification for the **Continuity of Care Document** (CCD), providing a standard mechanism for structuring in a static form the many data elements that are needed to record clinical encounters. Although industry adoption of the CCD specification has been slow, the use of the CCD standard offers considerable opportunity for CDS systems to interoperate across vendor platforms.

As discussed in Sect. 22.4.2, in 2012, a *virtual medical record* (vMR) based on the HL7 version 3.0 **Reference Information Model** (RIM) was approved by HL7 as a draft standard for trial use for linking dynamically at runtime the arbitrary data elements available in the patient database of an EHR to CDS systems that assume the standard vMR framework for data encoding (Kawamoto et al. 2010). The vMR thus acts as an interface between proprietary database formats and standards-based CDS systems that developers might plug into any EHR that can make its data available in a vMR-compliant manner (Fig. 22.8). HL7 is supporting ongoing work to map the vMR to standard terminologies and clinical data element definitions.

22.5.2 Lack of Adoption of Standard Knowledge Representation Models

Although Arden Syntax has been an HL7 and ANSI standard since 1999, only a few vendor systems manage their libraries of decision rules using Arden Syntax. Even doing so, of course, the rules still need to be customized for use with vendor-specific patient databases on a tedious, rule-by-rule basis to overcome the infamous curly-braces problem described in Sect. 22.4.2. As noted in that section, HL7 and ANSI adopted a query language called GELLO. GELLO can be used in rules written in Arden Syntax (and in other languages) as a standard approach for writing down the logical expressions and data queries needed for the rules to access patient-specific information stored in an EHR. GELLO assumes that the EHR data can be accessed in a manner that is consistent with the HL7 Version 3.0 RIM. GELLO itself is based on the **Object Constraint Language** (OCL) developed by the Object Management Group (OMG), and has the expressivity required both to compose complex references to clinical data elements and to construct queries. It has been hoped that GELLO will be incorporated into subsequent versions of Arden Syntax to obviate the need for curly braces. However, the HL7 Version 3 RIM has had limited uptake by vendors, who continue to rely mostly on the message-oriented HL7 Version 2 syntax for communication between systems. As a result, adoption of the GELLO query language also has been slow.

HL7 approved a standard for the Infobutton Manager in 2010 and a draft standard for order-set specification in 2012. In 2011, the organization approved a specification for a **service-oriented architecture** (SOA) to drive CDS, called the Decision Support Service (DSS).

Notably lacking from all this standards work is a shared ontology for representing clinical practice guidelines in a form suitable for execution at run time. The **Guideline Element Model** (GEM; Shiffman et al. 2000) is an XML mark-up specification that is an American National Standards Institute (ANSI) standard, now in its third revision, that guideline authors can use to annotate their narrative guidelines to identify key elements for both quality assessment and execution. GEM allows authors to demarcate the text that identifies guideline actions or eligibility criteria, and thus can serve an intermediary purpose in work to transform a prose guideline into a computable specification, but the standard does not itself provide a mechanism to translate a marked-up guideline document into a structure that a computer can interpret and execute.

A goal of some proponents is to have an ontology of clinical practice guidelines, such as the one adopted by ATHENA-CDS (see Fig. 22.6), that can inform the creation of computer-understandable knowledge bases that are able to capture knowledge about specific guidelines. Such knowledge bases then could allow a CDS system to use knowledge about the guideline, data from the EHR, and information concerning patient preferences and available resources to offer situation-specific, guideline-directed advice. An underlying infrastructure known as EON (Musen et al. 1996) drives the ATHENA-CDS system. Other ontology-based approaches have appeared over the years, including GLIF, GUIDE, PRODIGY, Pro*forma*, Asbru, and GLARE (deClerq et al. 2004). Peleg and colleagues (2003) compared many of these guideline models, and showed significant commonalities among them. Despite the large degree of agreement, however, work in this area has not yet led to anything near a standard. Part of the problem is that there is wide variation in the structure, granularity, and specificity of existing clinical practice guidelines, making it difficult to develop a single comprehensive and yet readily applicable guideline model. Analysis of the use of guidelines also indicates that guidelines themselves are rarely "executed" without considerable adaptation, except in situations such as protocol-driven care (for example, in clinical trials or in very specific procedures such as renal dialysis). ATHENA-CDS thus dispenses with offering specific guideline-based recommendations, and instead suggests to the clinicians when certain treatment options might be "compellingly indicated" or "relatively contraindicated." In highly regimented settings such as the administration of chemotherapy for cancer, however, a CDS system generally would need to be much more "prescriptive" in offering recommendations to clinicians.

22.5.3 Limited Modes of Deployment of CDS

One of the impediments to widespread adoption of CDS, particularly the use of rules and alerts, is clinician annoyance with popups, messages, emails, and other notifications that interrupt workflow. Ideally CDS systems should be integrated into the organization and presentation of information to facilitate workflow and decision making, by anticipating what information is needed for a decision, pre-fetching it, displaying it in ways that support visualization of trends or relationships, and tying these analyses to care plans or actions that can be offered immediately and quickly selected by the user. Order sets, as stated earlier, form a good example of use of CDS both to suggest appropriate actions in a given setting and to make it easy to accomplish those actions, by immediately enabling the orders in the set to be entered automatically into the EHR, perhaps with modification.

There is much ongoing research to develop methods for managing the processes of data capture, data presentation, data visualization, and selection of actions, but this work is usually being done outside of vendor EHRs. Given limited interoperability and access to the internals of proprietary systems, this kind of experimentation is now tending to take place in the form of "apps" and services that operate on externally extracted data (Mandl and Kohane 2012). Close interoperation with underlying EHRs is not currently feasible in most cases, and it remains to be seen whether the push to "apps" and services will become a force to change the industry.

22.5.4 Workflow and Setting-Specific Factors

As noted in Sect. 22.4.2, applications based on single-step situation–action rules are among the most prevalent and useful types of CDS systems. Such systems can be invoked in many contexts to provide either recommendations in real time or reminders or alerts that are processed in batch, based on time-oriented triggers or data-evaluation events. Rules can invoke other knowledge resources—providing new information content, triggering other rules, or offering order sets.

Rule content is ideally based on analysis of clinical evidence, such as recommendations or guidelines emanating from the U.S. Preventive Services Task Force, or from professional society studies of best practices for specific diseases. The job of formalizing these recommendations into executable logic requires that they be expressed in a formal way, but even having done so, such rules are not typically ready to execute in a particular environment, even if they are expressed in a rule execution language "understood" by an EHR system, and if they refer to the data elements in the EHR in its expected format. The reason they are not readily executable is also the reason that rules that work well in one environment are often not able to be successfully deployed elsewhere without substantial modification (even if in the same representation format and if using the same data model).

The reason for the failure is lack of adaptation to what we refer to as *setting-specific factors* (SSFs). To work effectively, rules need to integrate well with the clinical setting, workflow, users, application environment, and other factors. These requirements are reflected in how and when the rule should be triggered—on various events such as examination of some element of the EHR, on login to the system, or on the availability of laboratory test results. Rules may also be in developed in the form of reminders that are triggered when the CDSS evaluates on a batch basis a practice's list of patients to be seen on a given day, the patients who have a birthday in a given month, the passage of a specific interval of time since a previous comparison event, and so on. The rules additionally may vary based on the practice setting (the emergency department, an office practice, an inpatient unit); particular inclusion or exclusion criteria or threshold modifications that may be site-specific; how the recommendation should be transmitted (electronic mail, popup windows, sidebar messages); whether the recommendation requires acknowledgment by the recipient; whether it can be overridden; whether the alert should be escalated to supervising clinicians, and so on. Rules that have been custom tailored in such ways by means of executable code naturally are less sharable than are generic rules. Failure to capture the kinds of customizations that are needed, however, makes it time consuming for individual sites to adapt generic medical recommendations to their particular requirements or to capitalize on the experiences of others. What is needed is a way to represent useful experience in terms of SSF combinations that work, without needing to do so at the level of detailed code that is difficult for users to visualize and modify.

22.5.5   Lack of a Mode for Sharing Best-Practice Knowledge for CDS

There is no established mechanism for accessing reliable, vetted libraries of best-practice knowledge in computational form that are relevant to particular clinical problem areas—for example, management of diabetes. It generally falls on each health care organization, user group, or other entity to undertake its own process of identifying and managing the best-practice knowledge it wants to deploy in its CDS systems. Even having a national or international repository of such knowledge would not preclude the need for customization, but it would certainly make it easier for each health care entity to start with a trusted source. Where such a repository should be hosted, how it might integrate public and private knowledge sources, who would have oversight over it, how knowledge would be peer reviewed and quality-rated, and how it would be sustained are among the many questions that have not yet been answered. As a consequence, health care organizations continue to perform this kind of knowledge-curation work for their own constituencies, and pilot projects often have no clear pathway to becoming operational, sustainable activities.

22.6   Future Research and Development for CDS

Workers in biomedical informatics have studied problems in assisting with complex decision making for more than half a century. It seems that

it is only now, with the very recent adoption of HIT on a widespread basis, that the foundations are finally in place for the rapid advance of CDS technology in clinical settings. Although considerable logistical problems still must be surmounted as outlined in Sect. 22.5, this is an extremely exciting time in which to study CDS and its translation from the laboratory to the point of care.

22.6.1   Standards Harmonization for Knowledge Sharing and Implementation

Many implementation challenges remain for the broad adoption and effective use of CDS in EHR systems. As mentioned, one of the most active areas of current research focuses on development of standard approaches to knowledge sharing for CDS. Knowledge sharing may take the form of human-readable artifacts, machine-interpretable artifacts, or executable Web services (Osheroff et al. 2007). A capability for CDS sharing, as well as CDS functionality itself, would be substantially facilitated by the continued development and use of common standards designed to serve health care CDS needs. As noted, several standards currently exist that are aimed at specific areas of CDS and types of CDS artifacts, or that could be leveraged to benefit CDS. For example, the Clinical Decision Support Consortium, a large collaborative research and development group supported by the Agency for Healthcare Research and Quality has adopted an enhanced version of the Continuity of Care Document (CCD) to serve as the foundation for input data for multi-institutional trials of CDS technology (Middleton 2009). The CDS Consortium will soon leverage the HL7 vMR standard as the input patient information model. When taking advantage of most current standards, systems developers tend to adopt not only the standards but also particular implementation approaches, more as ad hoc solutions to specific problems than as integrated components to be used within a comprehensive framework for CDS.

To date, standards and related efforts addressing CDS overall have heavily emphasized specific

CDS execution methods and representation of the clinical context of the patient. For example, as we have noted previously, a variety of frameworks for working with rules, including Arden Syntax, Drools, JESS, and several proprietary formats, have worked their way into vendor offerings. This diversity has inhibited the exchange of best-practice knowledge. The unfortunate situation is that there are simply no repositories of clinical rules that are ready for "plug and play" adoption. Further work needs to be done to establish a common patient information model with a formal ontology, an event model for triggering events, an action model for CDS intervention recommendations, a workflow model for appropriately inserting CDS interventions into the clinical workflow, a knowledge-representation schema with a standard regular expression language, and, ideally, a measurement standard to assess CDS performance in use. In 2012, the US Office of the National Coordinator launched the Health e-Decisions initiative within its Standards and Interoperability Framework to promote coordinated community-based collaboration that would address this need. A goal of the Health eDecisions process is to create a model-driven framework for representing decision-support knowledge that can be translated among different implementation languages. As of the end of 2012, this work is being considered by HL7 as a possible standard.

22.6.2 Usability Research and CDS

The use of CDS within EHRs, and that of health IT in general, have been identified as double-edged swords: technology may provide benefit, but it also may cause considerable harm. Clinician error when using information systems that may result in untoward outcomes and unintended consequences (Karsh et al. 2010; Sittig and Singh 2009) may be an emerging property that is demonstrated only after system implementation or widespread use. Medical errors related to use of health IT are problematic, since they may represent a mismatch between the user's model of the task being performed and the actual outcome of a computation (National Research Council (US)

Committee on Engaging the Computer Science Research Community in Health Care Informatics et al. 2009), the application's intended functionality and the resulting action or event (Harrison et al. 2007), or a latent health IT-related error yet to happen (Ash et al. 2007). Excessive alert fatigue can undermine the efficacy of clinical decision support in CPOE (Isaac et al. 2009; Strom et al. 2010), and in other IT functions (Chused et al. 2008), and result in very high user override rates (Shah et al. 2006; van der Sijs et al. 2006; Weingart et al. 2003). Critical research questions need to focus on the potential mismatch between the user's mental model or intent and the application design and use case (Zhang and Walji 2011; Patel et al. 2010). Further attention needs to be given to basic principles of human-factors engineering, such as the use of colors and layout within the application interface. Additional questions remain regarding the ideal design of methods and controls with which a user might interact to choose a medication from a long list, or identify and encode patient problems. More advanced research will enable visualization and decision making by matching problems with care plans, and facilitation of continuity and coordination of care based on underlying CDS rules and guideline-based workflows. Especially challenging is addressing the need for structured data to support clinical decision support, and quality reporting, in a manner that is efficient for the end-user, perhaps combining structured documentation during data entry, and natural language processing for data abstraction from the clinical narrative. Most important, however, are methods to direct CDS to the right user, at the right time, with the right level of alerting.

22.6.3 Data-Driven CDS

A major area of research in informatics concerns methods for deriving knowledge from large data sets using a variety of techniques. With the adoption of health IT broadly, investigators are drawing on large-scale data-mining methods to provide CDS for population monitoring, public health surveillance, and even to offer patient-specific recommendations based on cohort data when there is no specific evidence that could otherwise guide therapy. With the increasing availability of data from diverse sources relevant to patient care, large data sets may be created and used for both discovery of previously unknown associations, and novel clinical predictions. Critical research questions here will include how to define like cohorts of patients, how to structure and frame the index decision, what methods to use to assess the likelihood of alternate prediction scenarios, and how to model and elicit the patient's preferences for each scenario. The Institute of Medicine (2011b) has articulated a long-term vision for a Learning Health System, in which clinical and administrative data of all kinds will begin to inform and enhance clinical practice on a national level in a wide variety of ways.

22.7 Conclusions

The future of CDS systems inherently depends on progress in developing useful computer programs and in reducing logistical barriers to implementation. Although ubiquitous computer-based decision aids that routinely assist physicians in most aspects of clinical practice are currently the stuff of science fiction, progress has been real and the potential remains inspiring. Early predictions about the effects that such innovations would have on medical education and practice have not yet come to pass (Schwartz 1970), but growing successes support an optimistic view of what technology will eventually do to assist practitioners with processing of complex data and knowledge. The research challenges have been identified much more clearly, legislative mandates are creating not only new financial incentives but also the practical substrate of increased EHR adoption and convergence toward data interoperability, and the implications for health-science education are much better understood. The basic computer literacy of health professional students can be generally assumed, but health-science educators now must teach the conceptual foundations of biomedical informatics if their graduates are to be prepared for the technologically sophisticated world that lies ahead.

Equally important, we have learned much about what is not likely to happen. The more that investigators understand the complex and changing nature of medical knowledge, the clearer it becomes that trained practitioners of biomedical informatics will always be required as participants in fostering a cooperative relationship between physicians and computer-based decision tools. There is no evidence that machine capabilities will ever equal the human's ability to deal with unexpected situations, to integrate visual and auditory data that reveal subtleties of a patient's problem, to work with patients to incorporate their values and priorities in care plans, or to deal with social and ethical issues that are often key determinants of proper medical decisions. Considerations such as these will always be important to the humane practice of medicine, and practitioners will always have access to information that is meaningless to the machine. Such observations argue cogently for the discretion of health care workers in the proper use of decision-support tools.

Suggested Readings

Bright, T. J., Wong, A., Dhurjati, R., Bristow, E., Bastian, L., Coeytaux, R. R., Samsa, G., Hasselblad, V., Williams, J. W., Musty, M. D., Wing, L., Kendrick, A. S., Sanders, G. D., & Lobach, D. (2012). Effect of clinical decision-support systems: A systematic review. *Annals of Internal Medicine, 157*(1), 29–43. This thorough analysis of studies of CDS systems demonstrates that there is good evidence that CDS technology can alter clinician behavior in positive ways, but that evidence that CDS systems can improve long-term patient outcomes is still inconclusive. The paper is also useful for its comprehensive bibliography.

Greenes, R. A. (Ed.). (2006). *Clinical decision support: The road ahead.* New York: Academic. This book offers a comprehensive discussion of the nature of medical knowledge and of information technology to assist with medical decision making. It provides detailed discussions of the computational, organizational, and strategic challenges in the design, development, and deployment of CDS systems.

Institute of Medicine. (2011). *Digital infrastructure for the learning health system: The foundation for continuous improvement in health and healthcare.*

Workshop series summary. Washington, DC: The National Academies Press. This monograph summarizes the vision for a national Learning Health System and offers the perspective of a wide range of thought leaders on the work required to achieve that vision.

Ledley, R., & Lusted, L. (1959). Reasoning foundations of medical diagnosis. *Science, 130*, 9–21. This is the paper that started it all. This classic article provided the first influential description of how computers might be used to assist with the process of diagnosis. The flurry of activity applying Bayesian methods to computer-assisted diagnosis in the 1960s was largely inspired by this provocative paper.

Sittig, D. F., Wright, A., Osheroff, J. A., Middelton, B., Teich, J. M., Ash, J. A., Campbell, E., & Bates, D. W. (2008). Grand challenges in clinical decision support. *Journal of Biomedical Informatics, 41*(2), 387–392. A rank-ordered list of some of the principal challenges for CDS technology development and implementation, intended "to educate and inspire researchers, developers, funders, and policy makers".

Questions for Discussion

1. Researchers in medical AI have argued that CDS systems should reason from clinical data in a way that closely matches the reasoning strategies of the very best clinical experts, as such experts are the most clever diagnosticians and the most experienced treatment specialists that there are. Other researchers maintain that expert reasoning, no matter how excellent, is at some level inherently flawed, and that CDS systems must be driven from the mining of large amounts of solid data. How do you account for the apparent difference between these views? Which view is valid? Explain your answer.

2. Transitioning CDS systems from one clinical setting to another has always been problematic. The Leeds Abdominal Pain System was installed in several major clinical settings, and yet the system never performed as well elsewhere as it had done in Leeds. The Arden Syntax, created expressly to facilitate knowledge sharing across institutions, has yet to meet this goal to a significant degree. Why kinds of setting-specific factors make it difficult to transplant decision-support technology from one environment to another? What kinds of research might lead to better methods for knowledge sharing in the future?

3. In one evaluation study, the decision-support system ONCOCIN provided advice concerning cancer therapy that was approved by experts in only 79 % of cases (Hickam et al. 1985). In another study, the HyperCritic CDS system for the management of hypertension offered the same comments that were generated by a panel of experts in only 45 % of cases (Van der Lei, et al. 1991). Such system performance is fairly typical for computer programs that suggest patient therapy. Do you believe that this performance is adequate for a computational tool that is designed to help physicians to make decisions regarding patient care? What problems might CDS systems encounter as their developers attempt to make the systems more comprehensive in the advice that they offer? Why might it be more difficult for computer systems to offer acceptable recommendations for patient therapy than seems to be the case for diagnosis? What safeguards, if any, would you suggest to ensure the proper use of such systems? Would you be willing to visit a particular physician if you knew in advance that she made decisions regarding treatment that were approved by expert colleagues less than 80 % of the time? If you would not, what level of performance would you consider adequate? Justify your answers.

4. A large international organization once proposed to establish an independent laboratory—much like

Underwriters Laboratory in the United States—that would test CDS systems from all vendors and research laboratories, certifying the effectiveness and accuracy of those systems before they might be put into clinical use. What are the possible dimensions along which such a laboratory might evaluate decision-support systems? What kinds of problems might such a laboratory encounter in attempting to institute such a certification process? In the absence of such a credentialing system for CDS systems, how can health-care workers feel confident in using a clinical decision aid?

5. Why did the United States federal government move to stimulate the adoption of EHRs in 2009? What mechanisms have been put in place to encourage adoption of EHRs and of CDS? What challenges remain to make CDS more pervasive in health care? Why might future clinicians be more or less attracted to CDS than is the case today?

6. There is considerable untapped potential for CDS to help in managing patients with multiple complex conditions. What are the challenges in dealing with such patients, and how can CDS be helpful? What are the features required of an algorithm that might integrate recommendations from the multiple clinical-practice guidelines that a CDS system could apply?

7. CDS is often implemented poorly, resulting in dissatisfaction, if not outright annoyance. What are the human factors that need to be taken into consideration in implementing CDS effectively? Discuss issues and approaches to enhancing usability. What are situations in which graphics and visualization might be used? How can CDS be used to enhance rather than to impede workflow? What are strategies to help avoid unintended consequences of poorly implemented CDS?

Computers in Health Care Education

23

Parvati Dev and Titus K.L. Schleyer

After reading this chapter, you should know the answers to these questions:

- How can computers improve the delivery of in-class and self-learning, as well as in-practice learning?
- How can constructivist approaches to learning be implemented using computers?
- How can simulations supplement students' exposure to clinical practice?
- What are the issues to be considered when developing computer-based educational programs?
- What are the significant barriers to widespread integration of computer-aided instruction into the medical curriculum?

23.1 Introduction

The current view of a desirable approach to health care education is one that acknowledges that medicine is practiced in a multi-disciplinary team environment in an information-rich world where constant learning is required to deliver high quality medical care. However, the actual practice of health care education remains primarily a **Flexnerian** one of science-based acquisition of medically relevant knowledge, followed by on-the-job apprentice-style acquisition of experience, and accompanied by evolution and expansion of the curriculum to add new fields of knowledge (Flexner 1910). The power of information technology today promises to transform the traditional Flexnerian learning model to a new one that applies information technology for successfully using the increasing volume of knowledge, learning evidence-based medical practice, collecting and critically analyzing data, collaborating through connectivity, distance learning and simulation-based learning, as well as team training.

This needed evolution of health care education is discussed by Frenk et al. (Frenk 2010) and is summarized in Table 23.1. Learning the scientific basis of medicine was an immensely important step that was driven by acceptance of the Flexner approach in the early twentieth century. An unfortunate corollary was the increasing use of lectures and, over the decades, reduced students' access to actual work with patients. It also led to ever-increasing specialization and loss of perspective of the health condition of the whole patient. In the 1960s, McMaster University in Canada pioneered a new approach, **problem-based learning**, where

P. Dev, PhD (✉)
Innovation in Learning Inc., 12600 Roble Ladera Road, Los Altos Hills, CA 94022, USA
e-mail: parvati@parvatidev.org

T.K.L. Schleyer, DMD, PhD
Center for Biomedical Informatics Regenstrief Institute, Inc., 410 West 10th Street, Suite 2000, IN 46202-3012, Indianapolis
e-mail: titus@pitt.ed

The authors gratefully acknowledge the co-authors of the previous chapter edition, Edward P. Hoffer, and G. Octo Barnett.

Table 23.1 Evolution of health care education systems

Basis of health care education	Science based	Problem based	Systems based
Instruction (can precede or be simultaneous with Training experience)	Scientific curriculum	Problem-based learning	Competency-based learning
Training experience	In-hospital basic training, then discipline-specific training	In-hospital and community-based basic training, then discipline-specific training	In-hospital and community-based basic training, multidisciplinary team experience, and discipline-specific training

Adapted from Frenk et al. 2010

small groups of students, supported by a facilitator, learned through discussion of individual case scenarios (Neville 2009). This problem-based approach was proposed as an alternative to didactic lectures, supporting individualized learning, and placing this learning in the context of the patient rather than the context of a single discipline. More recently, a renewed examination of the health care process, the sources of medical error and the need for higher quality of care, have highlighted the systems aspect of medical care (Kohn et al. 2000). From the systems perspective, learners need to be taught the linkages and complexity of the many hospital systems, as well as bodies of knowledge that are brought to bear on the treatment of a single patient, and how to use information technology to support them in the care of the patient.

23.2 Theories of Learning

Understanding how computers can support this evolution of education in the health sciences requires understanding how individuals learn, and how we can support this process through teaching. Educational software and other applications are tools for education, not education itself. In order to use a tool appropriately, one must understand how the tool and its design relate to the task, as well as the task's context, goals and outcomes. We therefore present a brief review of what we know about how people learn (see also Chap. 4).

Behaviorism, originating in the field of psychology in the early 1900s, stipulated that understanding the working of the mind could be reduced to the study of observable behaviors and the stimulus conditions that caused them. Behaviorists argued that learning mainly consists of making connections between stimuli and responses. However, not all mental processes, such as understanding, reasoning and thinking, can be observed or made observable. Behaviorism was thus not only limited in the degree to which it could explain the process of learning, but also in how it could help educators determine how to influence it.

Cognitive science (see Chap. 4), arising in the 1970s, began to model the mind as an information processing system. In the cognitive view, the mind perceives information from external stimuli, represents it internally, and transforms it through mental processes. The cognitive approach to learning posits that even though learning can be inferred from behavior, it is separate from the behavior itself. Rather, learning is a permanent change in cognition that is the result of experience. Cognitive science allowed educators to view the brain not as a black box, but as a dynamic, changeable system.

Today's view of learning is dominated by the constructivist view, epitomized by the problem-based learning approach described above. **Constructivism** argues that humans generate knowledge and meaning from an interaction between their experiences and their ideas. It does not consider the student's head to be an empty vessel to be filled with information and knowledge, but suggests that teachers must actively consider what students already know and think about a subject when educating them. Problem-based learning, in which students receive a problem and research potential answers/solutions in a group, is based on this constructivist approach to education. Instead of emphasizing the learning of a large and complete body of knowledge, problem-based learning is focused on the process of arriving at a solution through accessing and using a body of knowledge. Today, it is commonly used in health professional education.

Bransford et al. (2000) emphasize three key findings from educational research that are also highly important for health science education:

- *Students have preconceived notions about what they learn, regardless of whether they are aware of them or not. Teaching must take make these notions explicit and work actively to change them when necessary.* Numerous experiments show that pre-existing conceptions persist among older students even in the face of evidence refuting the validity of existing mental models. The process of education, therefore, must pay attention to a learner's pre-existing knowledge and beliefs, use this knowledge as a starting point for instruction, and monitor how students' conceptions change as instruction proceeds.
- *To become competent, students must have a deep foundation of factual knowledge that is embedded in an appropriate conceptual framework. They must be able to organize knowledge in ways that facilitate retrieval and application.* Research on medical cognition has shown that expert performance, for instance in diagnosis, requires a richly structured information base. Therefore, students should not only learn facts, but also be able to use and connect these facts in the right way. This "learning with understanding" implies that students transform facts into usable knowledge.
- *Students should not only be able to learn, but also assess what and how they learn. This "metacognitive" approach helps them define their own learning goals and monitor their progress in achieving them.* Health science education attempts to produce the "lifelong learner," i.e. the professional who can recognize and remedy knowledge deficits over

time. Reflecting this goal, many states in the US require physicians, dentists and nurses to complete a defined number of continuing education hours annually.

How can computers be used to help teachers implement these approaches to learning? We discuss computers as tools for teaching next.

23.3 Computers as Tools for Teaching

Various pedagogic designs can be implemented using computers, supporting any of the learning theories above. It is valuable, therefore, to understand how these pedagogic designs are implemented when one is determining how to use computers to support the objectives of the educational program. As examples, we discuss how to support seven different types of learning methods using computers: (1) drill and practice, (2) didactic learning in lectures, (3) exploration versus structured interaction, (4) scenario-, case- and problem-based learning, (5) learning through design, (6) simulation and, lastly, (7) intelligent tutoring systems, mentoring, feedback and guidance.

23.3.1 Drill and Practice

Drill and practice was the first widespread use of computer-based learning, developed almost as soon as computers became available. Teaching material is presented to the student, who is evaluated immediately via multiple-choice questions. The computer grades the selected answers and, based on the accuracy of the response, repeats the teaching material, or allows the student to progress to new material (Fig. 23.1).

Although it can be tedious, drill and practice still has a role in helping students learn factual material. It allows the educational system to manage the wide variation in ability of students to assimilate material and frees up instructors for more one-on-one interaction where that technique is most effective. It also allows the instructor to concentrate on more advanced material

Fig. 23.1 Drill and practice. In this image-based quiz, the student is presented with a dissected part and is asked to identify the structure marked with a flag. The question is presented in a multiple-choice format. If he or she wishes, the student can switch to the more difficult option of typing in a textual answer. In typical use, students will use the multiple-choice option while learning the material and the free-text option when evaluating themselves (Source: Parvati Dev with permission)

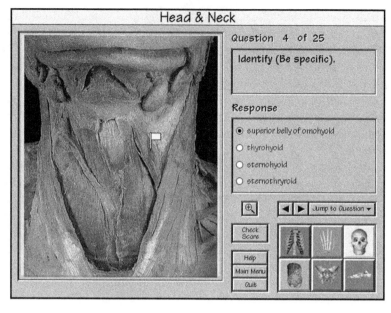

23.3.2 Digital Lectures

Although much of the focus of computer-based teaching is on the more innovative uses of computers to expand the range of available teaching formats, computers can be employed usefully to deliver didactic material, with the advantage of the removal of time and space limitations. A professor can choose to record a lecture and to store, on the computer, the digitized video of the lecture as well as the related slides or other teaching material. This approach has the advantage that relevant background or remedial material can also be made available through links at specific points in the lecture. The disadvantage, of course, is that the professor may not be available to answer questions when the student reviews the lecture (Fig. 23.2).

This approach is widely used for webinars and podcasts – essentially lectures that are available online with or without accompanying slides and video. Such content is available at iTunes University, through the iTunes application, as well as on popular Web video sites, such as YouTube, and slide sharing sites, such as SlideShare. The Open Course Ware movement, originating at the Massachusetts Institute of Technology in 2001, makes lectures and accompanying material freely available on the Web sites of member universities.[1]

23.3.3 Exploration Versus Structured Interaction

Teaching programs differ in the degree to which they impose structure on a teaching session. In general, drill-and-practice systems are highly structured. The system's responses to students' choices are specified in advance; students cannot control the course of an interaction directly. In contrast, other programs create an exploratory environment in which students can experiment without guidance or interference. For example, a neuroanatomy teaching program may provide a student with a fixed series of images and lessons

---

[1] http://www.ocwconsortium.org/. (Accessed 9/15/2013). A large collection of public health lecture slides are also available at http://www.pitt.edu/~super1/ (Accessed 9/15/2013).

Fig. 23.2 Didactic teaching. A digital video lecture is presented within a browser for the Web. The video image in the upper left is augmented with high-resolution images of the lecture slides on the right. Because the whole is presented within a Web browser, additional information, such as links to other Web sites or to study material, could have been added to the Web page (Source: Parvati Dev, with permission)

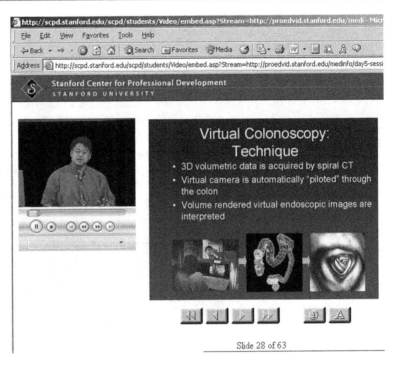

on the brainstem, or it may allow a student to select a brain structure of interest, such as a tract, and to follow the structure up and down the brainstem, moving from image to image, observing how the location and size of the structure changes.

Each of these approaches has advantages and disadvantages. Fixed path learning programs ensure that no important fact or concept is missed but they do not allow students to deviate from the prescribed course or to explore areas of special interest. Conversely, programs that provide an exploratory environment and that allow students to choose any actions in any order encourage experimentation and self-discovery. Without structure or guidance, however, students may waste time following unproductive paths and may fail to learn important material, the result being inefficient learning.

An example is the Tooth Atlas, used in dentistry (Fig. 23.3). Understanding tooth three-dimensional structure is important for clinical dentistry. The key instructional objective of the program is to help students learn the complex external and internal anatomy of the variety of teeth in three dimensions. The rich, interactive, 3D visualizations show teeth as they would be

visually perceived as well as through very high resolution computed tomography scans, radiographs and physical cross-sections. The learners rotate and section the computed models, and can control the transparency of each structure so as to study inter-relationships. While the visualization is highly exploratory, the embedded pedagogy is very structured, consisting of detailed textual quizzes with multiple-choice answers.

23.3.4   Scenario-, Case- and Problem-Based Learning

In this type of instruction, the computer presents the learner with a story that includes a problem. The presentation may be only in text, with text and graphics, or as an interactive movie in a near-realistic three-dimensional environment that replicates a space such as a clinic. The learner's role may be constrained such that the learner knows who they represent, what resources are available, and what the problem is that must be solved. Alternatively, the learner may be required to investigate the situation (examine the patient), define the problem, find any supporting resources

Fig. 23.3 The Tooth Atlas offers free exploration in the domain of dental anatomy. Each tooth is represented (from *left*) in a photograph, 3D model and radiograph that the student can rotate freely. In addition, cuts following the transversal plane are available on the *right* (Reproduced with permission of Eric Herbranson)

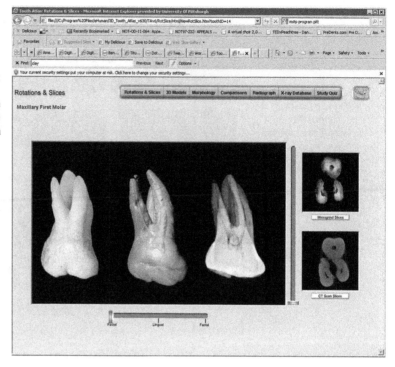

(what imaging and laboratory tests are available or what learning resources are at hand) and guide the scenario to an end goal. As the learner proceeds, the scenario evolves on the computer based on the actions taken and the progress of time.

Tales from the Heart, produced by McMaster University, is a case-based program for learning the basic concepts of cardiology. It illustrates principles of heart disease by presenting patient cases with different cardiologic conditions and explaining the physiological basis for the observed clinical phenomena. The major goal of the program is to enable the learner to link clinical reasoning to principles of applied physiology. Each module begins with a brief story of the clinical presentation. It then discusses the physiological basis for the clinical presentation (Fig. 23.4), and presents the student with periodic decision points to assess understanding. The student's responses, whether correct or not, are positively reinforced with feedback designed to illustrate how applied physiology facilitates the diagnosis and rationalizes an approach to management.

An approach that combines the benefits of exploration with the constraint of a linear path

through the material is one that breaks the evolving scenario into a series of short vignettes. A situation is presented, information and action options are available, and a decision must be made. Each decision triggers the presentation of the next vignette. This could lead to a branching story line but, usually, the next vignette presents the result of the best actions from the previous vignette. A scenario about a virtual patient could have vignettes that lead the learner through the steps of diagnosis, tests, and the course of treatment. This approach is commonly used in computer-based testing of clinical knowledge where assessment of learner performance would be extremely difficult if the interactions were completely unconstrained.

The ability of the computer to track and store the learner's actions allows post-processing and analysis of the tracked data. An interesting analytic capability is one that compares the performance of novice learners and experts to detect features that define expert information gathering or action sequences. Stevens et al. (1996) compared the information gathering and the conclusions of novices and experts on a set of

Fig. 23.4 In Tales from the Heart, students study the neurological and physiological basis of cardiology in the context of a patient case (Reproduced with permission of Anthony J. Levinson)

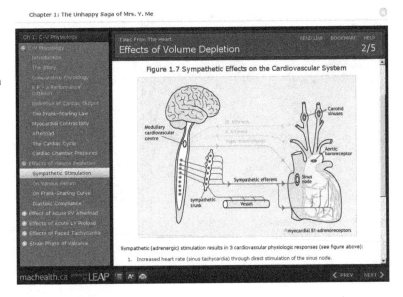

immunological cases. They analyzed the performance data using **artificial neural networks** and were able to detect consistent differences in the problem solving approach of novices compared to experts. In particular, novices exhibited considerably more searching and lack of recognition of relevant information while experts converged rapidly on a common set of information items. The potential of demonstrating such expert patterns of performance to learners as a new learning tool has not been widely explored in health sciences.

23.3.5 Learning Through Design

In learning through designing, students are required to construct something. The process of construction in itself is expected to teach the student new content. A simple example is when a student is asked to become the teacher. The act of preparing the material to be taught, and then teaching it to learners who each have a different grasp of the material, often results in excellent learning by the student teacher. Moving this concept to the computer, teachers have asked students to create Web sites, games, virtual patient simulations, and other constructs, as learning tools for other students. Learning through design can be a powerful learning tool but is not used

much in the health sciences because it is perceived to be too time-consuming for the benefit received. Lack of teacher understanding of this tool is another reason that the method is rarely used.

23.3.6 Simulation

Many advanced teaching programs use **simulations** to engage the learner (Gaba 2004). Learning takes place most effectively when the learner is engaged and actively involved in decision making. The use of a simulated patient presented by the computer can approximate the real-world experience of patient care and concentrates the learner's attention on the subject being presented.

Simulation programs may be either **static** or **dynamic**. Figure 23.5 illustrates an interaction between a student and a simulated patient. Under the static simulation model, each case presents a patient who has a predefined problem and set of characteristics. At any point in the interaction, the student can interrupt data collection to ask the computer-consultant to display the differential diagnosis (given the information that has been collected so far) or to recommend a data collection strategy. The underlying case, however, remains static. Dynamic simulation programs, in

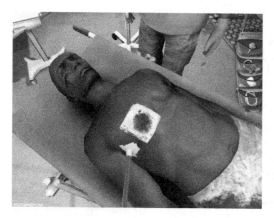

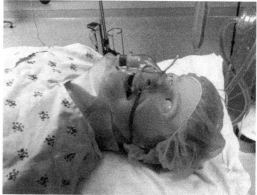

Fig. 23.5 The learner can select tools from the medical kit on the right, and drag them onto the simulated patient to clean and compress the wound or to listen to heart and lung sounds

Fig. 23.6 This plastic mannequin simulates many of the functions of a living patient, including eye opening and closing, breathing, heart rate and other vital signs. Gases, medications, and fluids can be administered to this mannequin, with resulting changes to its simulated vital signs

contrast, simulate changes in patient state over time and in response to students' therapeutic decisions. Thus, unlike those in static simulations, the clinical manifestations of a dynamic simulation can be programmed to evolve as the student works through them. These programs help students to understand the relationships between actions (or inactions) and patients' clinical outcomes. To simulate a patient's response to intervention, the programs may explicitly model underlying physiological processes and use mathematical models.

Immersive simulated environments, with a physical simulation of a patient in an authentic environment such as an operating room, have evolved into sophisticated learning environments. The patient is simulated by an artificial manikin with internal mechanisms that produce the effect of a breathing human with a pulse, respiration, and other vital signs (Fig. 23.6). In high-end simulators, the manikin can be given blood transfusions or medication, and its physiological response will change based on these treatments. These human patient simulators are now used around the world both for skills training and for cognitive training such as crisis management or leadership in a team environment (Fig. 23.7). The environment can represent an operating room, a neonatal intensive care unit, a trauma center, or a physician's office. Teams of learners play roles

such as surgeon, anesthetist, or nurse, and practice teamwork, crisis management, leadership, and other cognitive exercises. An extension of the physical human patient simulator is the virtual patient in a virtual operating room or emergency room. Learners are also present virtually, logging in from remote sites, to form a team to manage the virtual patient. Products such as Second Life[2] and CliniSpace[3] are being used to construct and deliver these virtual medical environments.

Procedure trainers or part task trainers have emerged as a new method of teaching, particularly in the teaching of surgical skills. This technology is still under development, and it is extremely demanding of computer and graphic performance. Early examples have focused on endoscopic surgery and laparoscopic surgery in which the surgeon manipulates tools and a camera inserted into the patient through a small incision. In the simulated environment, the surgeon manipulates the same tool controls, but these tools control simulated instruments that act on computer-graphic renderings of the operative field. Feedback systems inside the tools return pressure and other **haptic sensations** to the surgeon's hands, further increasing the realism of the surgical experience. Simulated environments

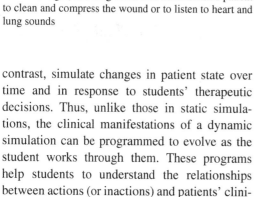

[2] http://secondlife.com/ (Accessed 9/15/2013)

[3] http://www.clinispace.com/ (Accessed 9/15/2013)

Fig. 23.7 Three-dimensional computer-generated virtual medical environments are used to present clinical scenarios to a team of learners. Each learner controls a character in the scenario and, through it, interacts with devices, the patient, and the other characters. Learning goals may include medical goals such as stabilization of the patient, communication goals such as learning to point out an error to more senior personnel, or team goals of leadership and delegation

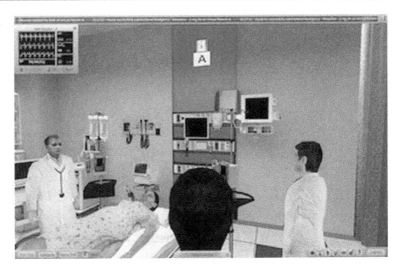

will become increasingly useful for all levels of surgery, beginning with training in the basic operations of incision and suturing and going all the way to complete surgical operations. Commercial trainers are now available for some basic surgical tasks and for training eye–hand coordination during laparoscopic procedures.

23.3.7 Intelligent Tutoring Systems, Mentoring, Feedback and Guidance

Closely related to the structure of an interaction is the degree to which a teaching program provides **feedback** and **guidance** to students. Virtually all systems provide some form of feedback—for example, they may supply short explanations of why answers are correct or incorrect, present summaries of important aspects of cases, or provide references to related materials. Many systems provide an interactive help facility that allows students to ask for hints and advice.

More sophisticated systems allow students to take independent action but may intervene if the student strays down an unproductive path or acts in a way that suggests a misconception of fact or inference. Such **mixed-initiative systems** allow students freedom but provide a framework that constrains the interaction and thus helps students to learn more efficiently. Some researchers make a distinction between **coaching** systems and **tutor-**

ing systems. The less proactive coaching systems monitor the session and intervene only when the student requests help or makes serious mistakes. Tutoring systems, on the other hand, guide a session aggressively by asking questions that test a student's understanding of the material and that expose errors and gaps in the student's knowledge. Mixed-initiative systems are difficult to create because they must have models both of the student and of the problem to be solved (Eliot et al. 1996).

Beginning health sciences students are building their fundamental knowledge. This knowledge is stored and is applied only to simple biomedical problems where they can identify basic symptoms and generate immediate diagnoses. As they progress to clinical problems, they acquire procedural knowledge, where they link basic knowledge to real situations. Ideally, they learn to develop hypotheses and establish or reject strategies, that is, they learn clinical reasoning. However, some students tend to learn the case as an entity without progressing to a problem solving approach. Experienced physicians continue to accumulate experience and learn to generalize from a set of cases to a set of rules that they can apply to circumstances that they have never encountered before. In health science education it is difficult to detect the cognitive level of the learner and thus apply an appropriate pedagogical strategy. The potential of intelligent tutoring systems to interrogate the learner and identify reasoning gaps is tantalizing but is yet to be realized.

Fig. 23.8 In this illustration from SlideTutor, the student has correctly identified the proliferation of melanocytes. However, SlideTutor provides the hint that the location of this finding is incorrect (Reproduced with permission of Rebecca Crowley)

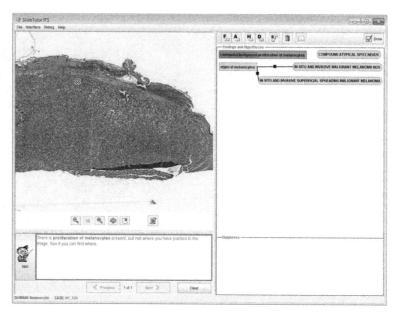

SlideTutor is an example of an intelligent tutoring assistant, supporting a "virtual apprenticeship" in pathology. It simulates a student sitting at a double-headed microscope across from an expert pathologist and working through clinical cases. As the student explores the histologic slide, the system records what parts of the digital slide the student has examined, which findings and diagnoses were reported, and continuously analyzes these data to see whether the student is on the right track. If necessary, it corrects the student's approach and provides hints (Fig. 23.8). It has other intelligent functions that model student progress and help students write correct reports with the help of natural language processing. Evaluation studies have shown that the intelligent tutoring system is highly effective. On average, students improve their diagnostic and reporting performance by a factor of four after as little as 4 h of use of the system (Crowley et al. 2007).

23.4 Uses of Technology to Support Learning

The ubiquity of technology-supported learning is apparent when one considers the many different ways in which it is used.

23.4.1 Medical, Nursing, Dental and Other Health Science Students

Basic science programs in medical schools were among the first in their implementation of technology-supported learning. Visually rich content in anatomy, neuroanatomy and pathology was much more accessible on the computer than through the microscope or via the cadaver dissection room. Excellent 3D learning programs for anatomy are available, including Netter Interactive 3D, Primal Pictures, eHuman, Visible Body, Osirix, and other companies, providing ever more accurate visualization of the 3D human. The use of microscopes among basic science students has virtually disappeared. Interestingly, in many schools, the use of cadavers has seen a resurgence, both as an important learning tool and as a rite of passage into the health care profession.

Nursing schools entered the use of technology later but have moved quickly to expand its use in education. One area in which they have a strong lead is the use of physical manikins for simulation of realistic nursing scenarios. Nursing schools that used to share a simulation center with a medical school have found their own demand high enough to require building their own simulation centers.

Dental schools often share parts of their curriculum with medical schools, and as a result use the same or similar learning content. However, they also need specialized anatomical and simulation content for dental and craniofacial topics. 3D software for dental anatomy is used widely in predoctoral dentistry. Historically, simulation of dental procedures was practiced using physical objects such as chalk or plastic teeth, a practice that is still widespread. More recently, high fidelity digital simulators have been developed.

For many years, teaching hospitals had patients with interesting diagnostic problems such as unexplained weight loss or fever of unknown origin. This environment allowed for thoughtful "visit rounds," at which the attending physician could tutor the students and house staff, who could then go to the library to research the subject. A patient might have been in the hospital for weeks, as testing was being pursued and the illness evolved. In the modern era of Medicare's system of lump-sum payment for **diagnosis-related groups** (DRGs) and of managed care, such a system appears as distant as professors in white lab coats. The typical patient in today's teaching hospital is very sick, usually elderly, and commonly acutely ill. The emphasis is on short stays, with diagnostic problems handled on an outpatient basis and diseases evolving at home or in chronic care facilities. Thus, the medical student is faced with fewer diagnostic challenges and has little opportunity to see the evolution of a patient's illness over time.

One response of medical educators has been to try to move teaching to the outpatient setting; another has been to use computer-modeled patients. Simulated patients allow rare diseases to be presented and allow the learner to follow the course of an illness over any appropriate time period. Faculty can decide what clinical material must be seen and can use the computer to ensure that this core curriculum is achieved. Moreover, with the use of an "indestructible patient," the learner can take full responsibility for decision making, without concern over harming an actual patient by making mistakes. Finally, cases developed at one institution

can be shared easily with other organizations. A well-known case library is MedEd PORTAL's Virtual Patients database from the Association of Medical Colleges (AAMC).[4]

23.4.2 The Practicing Professional, Continuing Education and Certification

Medical education does not stop after the completion of medical school and formal residency training. The science of medicine advances at such a rapid rate that much of what is taught becomes outmoded more or less rapidly, and it has become obligatory for physicians to be life-long learners both for their own satisfaction and, increasingly, as a formal government requirement to maintain licensure.

The practicing health care professional must maintain their certification through a prescribed number of hours of professional education. In addition, there is a need to have each person certified every few years in key clinical processes such as Advanced Trauma Life Support and Advanced Cardiac Life Support. While many do learn these in classroom courses, the availability of online courses that can be taken at one's convenience, have made these digital courses popular. An additional advantage of an online certification course is the automatic tracking of learner performance, and the accompanying automatic generation of institutional compliance reports.

23.4.3 Health Informatics Education

Health information technology (HIT) systems are considered key components in creating safer hospitals and in improving quality of care. Implementation of these HIT systems has required hospitals and clinics to purchase the requisite hardware and software. However, it has become clear that effective implementation and use of these systems will require that the

---

[4] https://www.mededportal.org/ (Accessed 9/15/2013)

average health care professional also be trained in the principles of health care informatics. Information management is a major activity of health care professionals and its effective use can lead to better decision making for patients as well as better management of the clinical practice.

The **American Medical Informatics Association** (AMIA) offers a program, "10×10 courses", for graduate-level training of health care professionals in the application of informatics.[5] The federal government sees a need for over 10,000 health IT professionals, and has invested in setting up informatics workforce development through training in community colleges and degree programs.[6]

23.4.4 Curriculum Inventory

Learning objectives or competency objectives are operationalized through the definition of a curriculum. These curricula differ between institutions based on the available teaching resources and specific local interests and needs. The AAMC has maintained an inventory of the curriculum at each medical school through its CURRMIT (curriculum information management tool) database, which has now evolved into the Curriculum Inventory Portal. The existence of this database supports some useful functions such as allowing a school to benchmark its curriculum against other schools with similar demographics, or allowing researchers to study curricular profiles across schools.

The Curriculum Inventory Portal uses the **Medbiquitous** standards (see Sect. 23.5.5, below) for competencies and learning objectives. It currently holds the curricula for basic medical education. The goal is to expand to incorporate graduate medical education and practicing professionals. At the graduate level, specification of curricula is determined by the specialty societies, and

implementation across schools is variable. Access to pooled information will be an impetus to improve the quality of the curriculum at each school.

23.4.5 Consumer Health Education

Today's patients are now repositioned as health care consumers; they often bring to the health care provider a mass of health-related information (and misinformation) gathered from the media. Medical topics are widely discussed in general interest magazines, in newspapers, on television, and on the Internet. Eighty percent of Internet users look for health care information (Pew 2011) online. Patients may use the Internet to join disease- or symptom-focused chat groups or to search for information about their own conditions. One in four Internet users with a chronic condition say that they have gone online to find others who share their health concerns (Pew 2011).

At the same time that patients have become more sophisticated in their requests for information, practitioners have become increasingly pressed for time under the demands of managed care. Shorter visits allow for less time to educate patients. Computers can be used to print information about medications, illnesses, and symptoms so that patients leave the office with a personalized handout that they can read at home. Personal risk profiling can be performed with widely available software, often provided for free by pharmaceutical firms. This type of software clearly illustrates for the patient how such factors as lack of exercise, smoking, or untreated hypertension or hyperlipidemia can reduce life expectation and how changing them can prolong it.

A torrent of consumer-oriented health sites has flooded the Web. As discussed in Chap. 15, one problem that complicates the use of any information site on the Internet is lack of control. Many consumers are not readily able to distinguish factual information from hype and snake oil. An important role for the health care provider today is to suggest high-quality Web sites that can be trusted to provide valid information. Many such sites are available from the various branches of the National Institutes of Health (NIH) and

[5] http://www.amia.org/education/10x10-courses (Accessed 9/15/2013)

[6] http://healthit.hhs.gov/portal/server.pt/community/healthit_hhs_gov__workforce_development_program/3659 (Accessed 1/8/2013)

from medical professional organizations. Good sources of qualified material in a wide variety of topics are available for consumers in National Library of Medicine's **Medline Plus**, the Centers for Disease Control and Prevention, and commercial sites such as **WebMD**. These sites provide additional links to numerous Web sites that have been evaluated for and found to meet a minimum level of quality. Most national disease-oriented organizations such as the American Heart Association and the American Diabetes Association also maintain Web sites that can be recommended with confidence.

23.5 The Ecosystem of Computers in Health Sciences Education

23.5.1 Accessing Learning Content: The Web

Eighty percent of Internet users look online for health information (Pew 2011). While this includes users of the Internet who are not health care professionals, it indicates the richness of available medical information. For the health science learner, there are numerous well-structured sources of learning content on the Internet. The federal agencies maintain portals such as the NLM's immense online library and bibliographic search facility as well as the other informational pages maintained by the various institutes and centers within the National Institutes of Health, the Agency for Health Care Research and Quality's content for team training and patient safety training, and the Centers for Disease Control and Prevention's health topics. The AAMC maintains the MedEd Portal, a peer-reviewed collection of medical and dental learning materials, including a rich collection of virtual patient cases (see Sect. 23.4.1). Medscape's professional site, emedicine, makes available detailed, professionally authored summaries of all major diseases and their management.[7] Collections such as Up-To-Date[8] and

Ovid[9] provide integrated access to a selection of journals and books to which the institution chooses to subscribe.

At many academic health centers, the medical library takes on the role of curating and making available Web portals for each subspecialty. For example, a portal for obstetrics and gynecology may include access to the key research and clinical journals in the field, digital versions of the key specialist textbooks, databases from national and global sources, evidence and consensus summaries, image collections and teaching videos, drug references and calculators, and information for patients.

The electronic medical record (EMR) has the potential to be a point-of-service learning tool for much of this information. The advantage of embedding access to this information in EMRs is that it supports "**just-in-time learning**" within the context of patient care. Educational research has shown that learning under these circumstances can be particularly effective. Decision support and alert tools built into the EMR can include information that teaches the clinical reasoning behind the alert or the suggested decision. Some EMR products support interfaces to third party knowledge products such that queries within the EMR can link to external knowledge bases. An example, **Infobuttons** (see Chap. 12), provide context-specific links from one information system, such as the EMR, to some other resource that provides relevant information.[10]

23.5.2 Accessing Learning Content: Learning Centers

Learning centers originally provided a location where students could access computers on campus. Now learning centers are distributed organizations that support all academic technology needs that are not part of the function of the library. Typically these include centralized computer centers as before, numerous locations with one or two computers for brief uses, management of the

---

[7] http://emedicine.medscape.com/ (Accessed 9/15/2013)

[8] http://www.uptodate.com/ (Accessed 9/15/2013)

[9] http://www.ovid.com/ (Accessed 9/15/2013)

[10] http://www.infobuttons.org/ (Accessed 9/15/2013)

technology within the classrooms to support smart boards, video recording, polling and other functions, authoring of content by local faculty and students, management of computerized test taking, and integration of all teaching functions with the local learning management system.

Learning centers also have the task of acquiring appropriate digital learning content for the institution. These may be recommended by faculty but often have to be reviewed and selected from the vast collection of content available commercially or for free. If the content is to be created by a local faculty member, the learning center provides the expertise for this development.

As in any other profession, the manager of the learning center is expected to be familiar with the state-of-the-art in support and delivery of computer-supported learning. The AAMC's Group on Educational Affairs maintains a subgroup that organizes conferences and workshops for the leaders of learning centers and others interested in learning technologies.

23.5.3 Accessing Learning Content: Simulation Centers

A **simulation center** is a specialized type of learning center, though its governance may reside in an academic department such as anesthesiology or surgery depending on the center's origin and history. Immersive, simulation-based learning is a bridge between classroom learning and real clinical experience. Simulation technologies are used to create realistic clinical experiences in which learners can practice in safety. They have the freedom to make mistakes and to learn from them. Another key value of simulation is that experiences can be provided that are difficult to provide in the daily life of hospitals, such as a terrorist-created emergency, or that are critical but rare, such as dealing with life-support equipment that fails while in use.

The components of a simulation center vary from site to site but include most of the following: a suite of examination rooms and associated support spaces for learning with standardized patients or patient actors; a wet/dry room for

practicing basic clinical procedures such as injections, catheterizations, suturing, and placing splints and casts; a simulated operating room, delivery room, ward room or examination room with one or more manikin-based patients; a room with computers for virtual worlds where students learn through role playing as physicians, nurses or other professionals; and a room for the use of task trainers such as laparoscopic surgery simulators or endoscopy/colonoscopy simulators.

Adequate support of a simulation center requires highly specialized staff. Technically skilled personnel are required to maintain the complex electro-mechanical systems that underlie manikin simulators or task trainers. Simulation programmers are needed to program scenarios for the manikins. Instructional designers are needed who understand how to create learning experiences using simulations, to achieve the desired learning objectives. Business managers maintain the fiscal soundness and stability of these expensive centers, determining the unique local potential for simulation-based learning and then making that need visible. Finally, trained faculty members are needed who understand how to teach with simulations and how to guide the activities and content development within the center.

23.5.4 Creating Learning Content

Technology-enabled learning content is now delivered across many platforms, ranging from the mobile phone and the tablet, through laptops and the Web, to physical manikins and game-like virtual worlds. However, the principles of such content development are unchanged and should use good instructional design principles. Instructional designers are specialists who can help formulate learning goals, offer suggestions for the design of instructional materials and tools to achieve those goals, design assessments and apply best practices from the educational research literature.

How to design efficient and effective educational software is the subject of a large number of books and other resources. Clark and Mayer (2011) provide practical application of e-learning principles, using findings from the educational research literature, and giving guidelines for selecting, designing, developing and evaluating educational software. They discuss important aspects of instructional design such as when and how to use media and text; how to facilitate collaborative learning with communication tools such as **chat** and **discussion boards**; how to help students build problem-solving skills; and how to use virtual coaches to improve learning. The design principles presented are also supported by research literature. Aldrich (2009) covers similar ground but with a focus on game and simulation-based learning. The ANSI/ADA Standard Guidelines for the Design of Educational Software (2006) from the **American National Standards Institute**'s (ANSI; see Chap. 7) Committee on Dental Informatics and the American Dental Association, offer a conceptual framework for quality assurance of educational software. As a framework, it is domain-neutral, does not restrict technical innovation, and leaves developers flexibility in design.

Creation of technology-enabled content can be labor intensive and time consuming and, hence, needs careful consideration. Three steps that should be considered are needs assessment, formative evaluation and summative evaluation, as described below.

Needs assessment: Defining the need for computer-based teaching in the curriculum is the first step. Are there difficult concepts that could be explained well through an interactive animated presentation? Is there a need for an image collection that exceeds that which is presented in the context of the lecture? Does the laboratory need support in the form of a guided tour through a library of digitized cross-section images? Could a quantitative concept be explained clearly through a simulation of the physiological or biochemical process, with the student being able to vary the important parameters? Is there a need for a discussion group to supplement the lectures or discussion sections? Would a central repository for course handouts reduce the load on departmental staff? This assumes that the necessary people and other resources are available. For example, are media of sufficient quality and comprehensiveness available, along with the necessary release of rights?

Formative evaluation: Prototyping, rapid iteration of development cycles, and formative evaluation are essential in creating a useful learning product. Because of the rich technology involved, frequently the intense focus on the technology brings a conviction that the resulting product will be useful. It is essential to test the early versions on real users and to listen carefully to their comments. Enthusiasm and positive feedback are not sufficient. The evaluation must answer the question whether users would actually use the product, as is, that same day on their own class. And if not, what is it that they would really use, and does this target keep moving each time they review the product.

Summative evaluation: Finally summative evaluation, after the product is in use, is valuable both to justify the completed project and to learn from one's mistakes. Table 23.2 provides an outline of the issues that can be considered in such an evaluation.

23.5.5   Standards for Learning Objects

The early interest in defining portions of learning modules as "learning objects" was to support reuse and repurposing of these components by institutions other than the developer institution, so as to justify the cost of content creation. For such sharing, standards had to be developed that allowed one object to be used by another software program. Groups active in such formalization include IMS Global Learning Consortium,[11] Advanced Distributed Learning,[12] and the IEEE Learning Technology Standards Committee.[13]

Even though a number of content collections and "education economies" developed, including some large collections such as MERLOT,[14] repurposing of individual learning objects did not develop into a major activity. On the other hand,

---

[11] http://www.imsglobal.org/background.html (Accessed 9/15/2013)

[12] http://www.adlnet.gov/overview (Accessed 9/15/2013)

[13] http://www.ieeeltsc.org:8080/Plone (Accessed 9/15/2013)

[14] taste.merlot.org (Accessed 9/15/13)

Table 23.2 Criteria for summative evaluation of a technology-enabled learning product

Criterion	Detail
System reliability	Does the system crash during the test? If yes, then measurement of usability or learning efficacy may be corrupted.
Content reviewed by subject matter experts	Content validity: Is the content appropriate for the target learner? Is it at the right level of complexity? Is it accurate?
Usability	Can the learner navigate through the content? Test this by setting tasks that require exercising all the interactive capabilities, and determine ease of use.
Validity	Face validity: Is the presentation of the material familiar and acceptable to the user? Construct validity: Does an expert perform better in this learning environment than a novice?
Learning efficacy	Does the user achieve the learning objective?
Curricular integration	The learning product may satisfy the criteria above, but is it embedded in the curriculum? If not, the likelihood of routine use is low.
Transfer to practice	Does use of this product cause measurable change in clinical practice?

it did become important to be able to manage the learner's use of diverse learning objects, and to capture information about the learner's performance for storage in a learning management system. Therefore, a major use of standards became the definition of communications between client side content and a host system, typically the learning management system. The Sharable Content Object Reference Model (SCORM) is a collection of standards and specifications that supports exchange of information between the client and the host. SCORM also specifies a Package Interchange Format that defines how to transfer or move content when packaging it in a transferable ZIP file. More sophisticated information exchange, such as a method for defining the sequencing of content presentation, has been less widely used than the learning management system communication and the package transfer described above. SCORM is developed and maintained by the federal government through Advanced Distributed Learning (ADL).[15]

A health care-specific standards group is **MedBiquitous**, a consortium lead by Johns Hopkins Medicine.[16] Standards for communicating about individual accomplishments have been developed for reporting professional education and certification, tracking a learner's educational trajectory, exchanging a professional profile including training and certification data. At the system level, standards are under development for specification of competencies, and communicating evaluation data in health care education. For learning object authoring, specifications have been developed for learning object metadata, a SCORM version of the same, and a format for sharing virtual patient scenarios. All these specifications are eventually submitted to ANSI for ratification.

23.6 Future Directions and Challenges

As this chapter has shown, computers have played, and will continue to play, an increasingly important role in health sciences education. How will the rapid change and fluid nature of innovation influence how we use technology in education in the future? As we increasingly "digitize" almost all aspects of our lives, we can expect information technology to continue to weave itself more and more into the essential fabric of how we teach and learn.

How can computers help *advance* teaching and learning? Most faculty, even many of those who would consider themselves Luddites, have embraced, or at least accepted, technology's growing role in education. Students often have higher expectations of technology use than most health sciences schools can fulfill. How computers can help improve education is a key question of interest

[15] http://www.adlnet.gov (Accessed 1/8/2013)

[16] http://www.medbiq.org/about_us/mission/index.html (Accessed 1/8/2013)

to faculty and students alike. Most faculty members are keenly interested in finding out how technology can help them become better teachers. Most students, on the other hand, want to know how computers can help them learn more efficiently and effectively. Answering these questions requires research and development in a number of areas. We briefly discuss a few of those below:

1. As a number of commentators have pointed out, attempting to prove the superiority of educational software over traditional teaching methods is not only the wrong question, it is also methodologically impossible. The media-comparative approach used to do so is confounded by too many variables to be meaningful. Instead, we need to determine which computer-based interventions in education are the most effective given a particular context, goal and learner. Cook (2005) has proposed comparing educational software at three increasingly granular levels: (1) configuration, i.e. the "big picture" of how the software is used, for instance as a tutorial or to support small group learning; (2) instructional method, i.e. the techniques that support learning processes, such as questions, simulations and interactive models; and (3) presentation, i.e. the detailed attributes of how a particular instructional method is presented to the learner.

2. As Friedman (1994) has suggested, we should continue to identify which unique types of learning outcomes educational software can support. The simulation and 3D environments discussed above offer the opportunity to show biologic structures and processes from fundamentally different vantage points than previously possible. For instance, we can now travel inside a tooth and look outward, or compress the duration of a pathophysiological process from decades to minutes. We need to understand the effects of these novel ways of representing content on learners and how they understand it.

3. As described above, educational software holds enormous potential for replicating and even enhancing the experience of personal tutoring. However, despite years of research on intelligent tutoring systems, user models and adaptive testing, we have not yet developed a generalizable approach to computer-based tutoring in biomedicine. Progress in more basic domains, such as K-12 algebra, has been promising. It is to be hoped that health care education can produce similar advances over time.

4. "Just-in-time" learning, or learning integrated with clinical practice, is a clear need in an age when clinicians are expected to use best practices in caring for their patients under time constraints. Learning in the context of clinical care can leverage the clinician's motivation in a real-life situation, increasing the likelihood of a positive learning outcome. However, what approaches should be used to ensure that just-in-time learning is systematic, quantifiable and effective? Answering questions such as these is crucial as continuing competence of health care providers increases in importance.

5. Last, we should consider the information infrastructure for learning and professional development from the learner's perspective. At present, the materials that learners either receive or produce during their education vary in content, format and platform. For instance, course syllabi, slide presentations, electronic books and papers, course discussion list and blogs, and list of references typically exist in different places, with different constraints on accessibility. The fact that most materials can be "tied together" through the Web interface of a learning management system is scant consolation. The simple fact is that it is difficult, if not impossible, for most learners to create and maintain a comprehensive and organized portfolio of their learning materials as it was possible in the paper world. With regard to education, we need to elevate the user-centered design philosophy discussed in Chap. 5 to the systems level. Doing so will help maintain learners create, maintain and enhance their personalized store of learning experiences in a systematic, easy-to-use and predictable way.

The listed research questions and considerations are only a small selection of the interesting challenges of educational research in biomedicine. Journals such as Academic

Medicine and the Journal of Educational Research periodically discuss these and other challenges in more depth.

23.7   Conclusion

Educational software has the potential to help students to master biomedical subject matter and to develop problem-solving skills. Properly integrated into the medical school curriculum, health science curricula and into the information systems that serve health care institutions and the greater medical community, computer-based learning can become part of a comprehensive system for lifelong education. The challenge to researchers in computer-based education is to develop this potential. The barriers to success are both technical and practical. To overcome them, we require dedication of support and resources within institutions and a commitment to cooperation among institutions.

Suggested Readings

AAMC Institute for Improving Medical Education. (2007, March). Washington, D. C.: American Association of Medical Colleges. https://members.aamc.org/eweb/upload/Effective%20Use%20of%20Educational.pdf *Effective use of educational technology in medical education. Colloquium on educational technology: Recommendations and guidelines for medical educators.* This report summarizes the discussion of an expert panel on the documented efficacy of educational technologies in the curriculum.

Bransford, J. D., Brown, A. L., & Cocking, R. R. (2000). *How people learn: Brain, mind experience and school.* Washington, D.C.: The National Academies Press. This National Research Council book synthesizes many findings on the science of learning, and explains how these insights can be applied to actual practice in teaching and learning.

Cook, D. A. (2005). The research we still are not doing: An agenda for the study of computer-based learning. *Acad Med, 80*(6), 541–548. Cook reviews the progress (or lack thereof) on Friedman's proposed directions for educational software research, and suggests strategies for meaningful comparisons in computer-based instructional design. He discusses additional research challenges, such as adaptation to individual learners, just-in time learning and simulation.

Crowley, R. S., Legowski, E., Medvedeva, O. M., Tseytlin, E., Roh, E., & Jukic, D. (2007). *Evaluation of an Intelligent Tutoring System in Pathology:* *Effects of External Representation on Performance JAMIA, 14*(2), 182–190. Crowley describes a study that evaluated SlideTutor with physicians in two academic pathology programs. On average, students improved their diagnostic and reporting performance by a factor of four after as little as four hours of use of the system.

Eliot C. R., Woolf B. P. (1996). An intelligent learning environment for advanced cardiac life support. Proceedings of the AMIA Annual Fall Symposium, Washington, DC, pp.7–11.

Gaba, D. M. (2004). The future vision of simulation in health care. *Qual Saf Health Care, 13*(Suppl 1), i2–i10. Gaba describes the range of technologies and methods available for simulation-based learning.

Kirkpatrick, D. L. (1994). *Evaluating training programs.* San Francisco: Berrett-Koehler. This book presents a multilevel system for evaluating training programs.

Rall, M., Gaba, D. M., Dieckmann, P., & Eich, C. (2010). Chapter 7: Patient simulation. In R. D. Miller (Ed.), *Anesthesia* (7th ed.). Philadelphia: Churchill Livingstone Elsevier. The authors summarize the history and current uses of manikin-based simulation, the most common type of simulation in use for clinical teaching.

Questions for Discussion

1. In developing effective educational interventions, you are often faced with a choice of instructional methods. Which of the instructional methods listed below would best match the instructional goals listed? Please justify your selection.

Instructional goal

1. Ability to intubate an unconscious patient
2. Memorize the terminology used in neuroanatomy
3. Recognize the symptoms of a patient with probable mental illness
4. Learn the pathophysiology of hypertension
5. Detect histopathologic variations on histology slides

Instructional method

1. Case-based scenarios that include video
2. Physical simulation with computer-based feedback
3. Didactic material that includes text, images and illustrations
4. Intelligent tutoring system
5. Drill-and-practice program

2. You have decided to write a computer-based simulation to teach students about the management of chest pain.

   (a) Discuss the relative advantages and disadvantages of the following styles of presentation:

      1. A sequence of multiple-choice questions,

      2. A simulation with a physical "mannequin" whose condition changes over time and in response to therapy; and

      3. A program that allows the student to enter free-text requests for information and that provides responses.

   (b) Discuss at least four problems that you would expect to arise during the process of developing and testing the program.

   (c) For each approach, discuss how you might develop a model that you could use to evaluate the student's performance in clinical problem solving.

3. Select a topic in physiology with which you are familiar, such as arterial blood–gas exchange or filtration in the kidney, and construct a representation of the domain in terms of the concepts and sub-concepts that should be taught for that topic. Using this representation, design a teaching program using one of the following methods: (1) a didactic approach, (2) a simulation approach, or (3) an exploration approach.

4. You are a junior faculty member at a major medical center and you just were appointed director for a course on clinical patient examinations. You decide to check out several sharing sites for curricular material, such as MedEdPortal, to try to find relevant teaching materials. What kind of issues/problems would you expect in integrating material from those sites in your course?

Bioinformatics

24

Sean D. Mooney, Jessica D. Tenenbaum,
and Russ B. Altman

After reading this chapter, you should know the answers to these questions:

- Why are sequence, structure, and biological pathway information relevant to medicine?
- Where on the Internet should you look for a DNA sequence, a protein sequence, or a protein structure?
- What are two problems encountered in analyzing biological sequence, structure, and function?
- How has the age of genomics changed the landscape of bioinformatics?
- What two changes should we anticipate in the medical record as a result of these new information sources?
- What are two computational challenges in bioinformatics for the future?

S.D. Mooney, PhD (✉)
Buck Institute for Research on Aging,
8001 Redwood Blvd, Novato, CA 94945-1400, USA
e-mail: smooney@buckinstitute.org

J.D. Tenenbaum, PhD
Duke Translational Medicine Institute, Duke University,
2424 Erwin Rd, Durham, NC 27705, USA
e-mail: jessie.tenenbaum@duke.edu

R.B. Altman, MD, PhD
Departments of Bioengineering,
Genetics and Medicine, Stanford University,
Clark Center, 318 Campus Drive, S172,
Stanford, CA 94305, USA
e-mail: russ.altman@stanford.edu

24.1 The Problem of Handling Biological Information

Bioinformatics is the study of how information is represented and analyzed in biological systems, especially information derived at the molecular level. Whereas clinical informatics deals with the management of information related to the delivery of health care, bioinformatics focuses on the management of information related to the underlying basic biological sciences. As such, the two disciplines are closely related—more so than generally appreciated (see Chap. 1). Bioinformatics and clinical informatics share a concentration on systems that are inherently uncertain, difficult to measure, and the result of complicated interactions among multiple complex components. Both deal with living systems that generally lack straight edges and right angles. Although **reductionist approaches** to studying these systems can provide valuable lessons, it is often necessary to analyze those systems using **integrative models** that are not based solely on first principles. Nonetheless, the two disciplines approach the patient from opposite directions. Whereas applications within clinical informatics usually are concerned with the social systems of medicine, the cognitive processes of medicine, and the technologies required to understand human physiology, bioinformatics is concerned with understanding how basic biological systems conspire to create molecules, organelles, living cells, organs, and entire organisms. Remarkably, however, the two disciplines share

E.H. Shortliffe, J.J. Cimino (eds.), *Biomedical Informatics*,
DOI 10.1007/978-1-4471-4474-8_24, © Springer-Verlag London 2014

significant methodological elements, so an understanding of the issues in bioinformatics can be valuable for the student of clinical informatics and vice versa.

The discipline of bioinformatics continues to be in a period of rapid growth, because the needs for information storage, retrieval, and analysis in biology—particularly in molecular biology and **genomics**—have increased dramatically over the past decade. History has shown that scientific developments within the basic sciences tend to have a delayed effect on clinical care and there is typically a lag of a decade before the influence of basic research on clinical medicine is realized. The types of information being gathered by biologists today will drastically alter the types of information and technologies available to the health care workers of tomorrow.

24.1.1   Many Sources of Biological Data

There are three sources of information that are revolutionizing our understanding of human biology and that are creating significant challenges for computational processing. The most dominant new type of information is the **sequence information** produced by genetic studies. This was enabled by the **Human Genome Project**, an international undertaking intended to determine the complete sequence of human DNA as it is encoded in each of the 23 human chromosomes. The first draft of the sequence was published in 2001 (Lander et al. 2001) and a final version was announced in 2003 coincident with the 50th anniversary of the solving of the Watson and Crick structure of the DNA double helix. The sequence continues to be revised and refined and efforts are underway to sequence the genomes of many different individuals (1,000 Genomes Consortium, 2010). Essentially, the entire set of genetically driven events from conception through embryonic development, childhood, adulthood, and aging are encoded by the DNA blueprints within most human cells. Given a complete knowledge of these DNA sequences, we are in a position to understand these processes at a

fundamental level and to consider the possible use of DNA sequences for diagnosing and treating disease.

While some scientists are studying the human genome, other researchers are studying the functions of the genomes of numerous other biological organisms, including important model organisms (such as mouse, rat, and yeast) as well as important human pathogens (such as *Mycobacterium tuberculosis* or *Haemophilus influenzae*). The genomes of these organisms have been determined, and efforts are underway to characterize them. These allow two important types of analysis: the analysis of mechanisms of pathogenicity and the analysis of animal models for human disease. In both cases, the functions encoded by genomes can be studied, classified, and categorized, allowing us to decipher how genomes affect human health and disease.

These ambitious scientific projects are not only proceeding at a furious pace, but also are accompanied in many cases by a new approach to biology, which produces a third source of biomedical information: **proteomics**, the study of the protein gene products of the genome – the proteome. Proteomics enables researchers to discover the state (quantity and configuration) of proteins within an organism. These protein states can be correlated with different physiological conditions, including disease states. Some of these protein states can be used as identifying markers of human disease.

Additionally, large-scale experimental methodologies are used to collect data on thousands or millions of molecules simultaneously. Scientists apply these methodologies longitudinally over time and across a wide variety of organisms or (within an organism) organs to observe the development of various physiological phenomena. Technologies give us the abilities to follow the production and degradation of molecules on **gene expression microarrays** (Lashkari et al. 1997), to study the expression of large numbers of genes with one another (Bai and Elledge 1997), and to create multiple variations on a genetic theme to explore the implications of changes in genome function on human disease. All these technologies, along with the genome-sequencing projects, are conspiring to produce a volume of biological information that at once contains secrets to age-old questions about health and disease and threatens to overwhelm our current capabilities of data analysis. Thus, bioinformatics is becoming critical for medicine in the twenty-first century.

24.1.2 Implications for Clinical Informatics

The effects of this new biological information on clinical medicine and clinical informatics are difficult to predict precisely. It is already clear, however, that some major changes to medicine will have to be accommodated.

1. *Genetic sequence information in the medical record.* With the first set of human genomes now available and prices for gene sequencing rapidly decreasing, it is now cost-effective to consider sequencing every patient genome or at least genotyping key sections of the genomes. The sequence of a gene involved in disease may provide the critical information that we need to select appropriate treatments. For example, the set of genes that produces essential hypertension may be understood at a level sufficient to allow us to target antihypertensive medications based on the precise configuration of these genes. Clinical trials now use information about genetic sequence to define precisely the population of patients who would benefit from a new therapeutic agent. Finally, clinicians may learn the sequences of infectious agents (such as of the *Escherichia coli* strain that causes recurrent urinary tract infections) and store them in a patient's record to record the precise pathogenicity and drug susceptibility observed during an episode of illness. In any case, it is likely that genetic information will need to be included in the medical record and will introduce special problems (see also Chap. 2 and Masys et al. 2012). Raw sequence information, whether from the patient or the pathogen, is meaningless without context and thus is not well suited to a printed medical record.

Like images (CAT scans, MRIs), sequence data can come in high information density and must be presented to the clinician in novel ways. As there are for laboratory tests, there may be a set of nondisease (or normal) values to use as comparisons, and there may be difficulties in interpreting abnormal values. Fortunately, most of the human genome is shared and identical among individuals; less than 1 % of the genome seems to be unique to individuals. Nonetheless, the effects of sequence information on clinical databases will be significant. As an example, Kaiser Permanente and UCSF recently completed identifying genome wide genetic variants in 100,000 individuals linked to their electronic health records.[1] The EMERGE research network is specifically focused on genetic discovery and replication using electronic medical records and genetics (McCarty et al. 2011).

2. *New diagnostic and prognostic information sources.* One of the main contributions of the genome-sequencing projects (and of the associated biological innovations) is that we are likely to have unprecedented access to new diagnostic and prognostic tools. **Single nucleotide polymorphisms** (**SNPs**) and other genetic markers are used to identify how a patient's genome differs from the draft genome. Diagnostically, the genetic markers from a patient with an autoimmune disease, or of an infectious pathogen within a patient, will be highly specific and sensitive indicators of the subtype of disease and of that subtype's probable responsiveness to different therapeutic agents. For example, the severe acute respiratory syndrome (SARS) virus was determined to be a corona virus using a gene expression array containing the genetic information from several common pathogenic viruses.[2] In general, diagnostic tools based on the gene sequences within a patient are likely

---

[1] http://www.ucsf.edu/news/2011/07/10305/ucsf-and-kaiser-permanente-complete-massive-genotyping-project (accessed November 30, 2012)

[2] http://www.cdc.gov/sars/index.html (accessed November 30, 2012)

to increase greatly the number and variety of tests available to the physician. Physicians will not be able to manage these tests without significant computational assistance. Moreover, genetic information will be available to provide more accurate prognostic information to patients. What is the standard course for this disease? How does it respond to these medications? Over time, we will be able to answer these questions with increasing precision, and will develop computational systems to manage this information.

Several **genotype**-based databases have been developed to identify markers that are associated with specific **phenotypes** and identify how genotype affects a patient's response to therapeutics. The Human Gene Mutation Database (HGMD) annotates mutations with disease phenotype.[3] This resource has become invaluable for genetic counselors, basic researchers, and clinicians. Additionally, the Pharmacogenomics Knowledge Base (PharmGKB) collects genetic information that is known to affect a patient's response to a drug (more on PharmGKB is described in Translational Bioinformatics, Chap. 25).[4] As these data sets, and others like them, continue to improve, the first clinical benefits from the genome projects will be realized.

3. *Ethical considerations*. One of the critical questions facing the genome-sequencing projects is "Can genetic information be misused?" The answer is certainly yes. With knowledge of a complete genome for an individual, it may be possible in the future to predict the types of disease for which that individual is at risk years before the disease actually develops. If this information fell into the hands of unscrupulous employers or insurance companies, the individual might be denied employment or coverage due to the likelihood of future disease, however distant. There is even debate about whether such information should

be released to a patient even if it could be kept confidential. Should a patient be informed that he or she is likely to get a disease for which there is no treatment? What about that patient's relatives, who share genetic information with the patient? This is a matter of intense debate, and such questions have significant implications for what information is collected and for how and to whom that information is disclosed (Durfy 1993; see Chap. 10). Passage of the Genetic Information Nondiscrimination Act in 2008 set initial federal guidelines on use of genetic information.[5] Additionally, the Personal Genome Project (PGP) has been working to define **open consent models** for releasing genetic information.[6]

24.2   The Rise of Bioinformatics

A brief review of the biological basis of medicine will bring into focus the magnitude of the revolution in molecular biology and the tasks that are created for the discipline of bioinformatics. The genetic material that we inherit from our parents, that we use for the structures and processes of life, and that we pass to our children is contained in a sequence of chemicals known as **deoxyribonucleic acid** (**DNA**).[7] The total collection of DNA for a single person or organism is referred to as the genome. DNA is a long polymer chemical made of four basic subunits. The sequence in which these subunits occur in the polymer distinguishes one DNA molecule from another, and the sequence of DNA subunits in turn directs a cell's production of proteins and all other basic cellular processes. **Genes** are discreet units encoded in DNA and they are transcribed into **ribonucleic acid** (**RNA**), which has a composition very similar to DNA. Genes are

---

[3] http://www.hgmd.org/ (accessed November 30, 2012)

[4] http://www.pharmgkb.org/ (accessed December 20, 2012)

[5] http://www.genome.gov/10002328 (accessed November 30, 2012)

[6] http://www.personalgenomes.org/ (accessed November 30, 2012)

[7] If you are not familiar with the basic terminology of molecular biology and genetics, reference to an introductory textbook in the area would be helpful before you read the rest of this chapter.

transcribed into messenger RNA (mRNA) and a majority of mRNA sequences are translated by ribosomes into protein. Not all RNAs are messengers for the translation of proteins. Ribosomal RNA, for example, is used in the construction of the ribosome, the huge molecular engine that translates mRNA sequences into protein sequences. Additionally, mRNAs can be modified through alternative splicing, degradation, and formation of secondary structures that influence transcriptions. Once expressed, proteins are frequently modified (such as phosphorylation), and these modifications can change the function of the protein.

Understanding the basic building blocks of life requires understanding the function of genomic sequences, genes, and proteins. When are genes expressed? Once genes are transcribed and translated into proteins, into what cellular compartment are the proteins directed? How do the proteins function once there? Do the proteins need to be modified in order for them to become active? How are the proteins turned off? Experimentation and bioinformatics have divided the research into several areas, and the largest are: (1) DNA and protein sequence analysis, (2) macromolecular structure–function analysis, (3) gene expression analysis, (4) proteomics, and (5) systems biology.

24.2.1 Roots of Modern Bioinformatics

Practitioners of bioinformatics have come from many backgrounds, including medicine, molecular biology, chemistry, physics, mathematics, engineering, and computer science. It is difficult to define precisely the ways in which this discipline emerged. There are, however, two main developments that have created opportunities for the use of information technologies in biology. The first is the progress in our understanding of how biological molecules are constructed and how they perform their functions. This dates back as far as the 1930s with the invention of electrophoresis, and then in the 1950s with the elucidation of the structure of DNA and the subsequent sequence of discoveries in the relationships

among DNA, RNA, and protein structure. The second development has been the parallel increase in the availability of computing power. Starting with mainframe computer applications in the 1950s and moving to modern workstations, there have been hosts of biological problems addressed with computational methods.

24.2.2 The Genomics Explosion

The benefit of the human genome sequence to medicine is both in the short and in the long term. The short-term benefits lie principally in diagnosis; the availability of sequences of normal and variant human genes will allow for the rapid identification of these genes in any patient (e.g., Babior and Matzner 1997). The long-term benefits will include a greater understanding of the proteins produced from the genome: how the proteins interact with drugs; how they malfunction in disease states; and how they participate in the control of development, aging, and responses to disease.

The effects of genomics on biology and medicine cannot be overstated. We now have the ability to measure the activity and function of genes within living cells. Genomics data and experiments have changed the way biologists think about questions fundamental to life. Whereas in the past, reductionist experiments probed the detailed workings of specific genes, we can now assemble those data together to build an accurate understanding of how cells work.

24.3 Biology Is Now Data-Driven

Twenty years ago, the use of computers was proving to be useful to the laboratory researcher. Today, computers are an essential component of modern research. This has led to a change in thinking about the role of computers in biology. Before, they were optional tools that could help provide insight to experienced and dedicated enthusiasts. Today, they are required by most investigators, and experimental approaches rely on them as critical elements. This is because advances in research methods such as **micro-array chips**, **drug screening robots**, **X-ray crystallography**, **nuclear magnetic resonance spectroscopy**, proteomic mass spectrometry and DNA sequencing experiments have resulted in experiments that generate massive amounts of data. These data pose new problems for basic researchers on how the data are properly stored, analyzed, and disseminated.

The volume of data being produced by genomics projects is staggering. There are now more than 135 million sequences in **GenBank** comprising more than 126 billion digits. Since 2008, sequencing has bested Moore's law (see Chap. 1).[8] But these data do not stop with sequence data: PubMed contains over 23 million literature citations, the **Protein Data Bank** (**PDB**) contains three-dimensional structural data for over 86,000 protein sequences, and the **Gene Expression Omnibus** (**GEO**) contains over 900,000 arrayed samples. These data are of incredible importance to biology, and in the following sections we introduce and summarize the importance of sequences, structures, gene expression experiments, systems biology, and their computational components to medicine.

24.3.1   Sequences in Biology

Sequence information (including DNA sequences, RNA sequences, and protein sequences) is critical in biology: DNA, RNA, and protein can be represented as a set of sequences of basic building blocks (bases for DNA and RNA, amino acids for proteins). Computer systems within bioinformatics thus must be able to handle biological sequence information effectively and efficiently.

One major difficulty within bioinformatics is that standard database models, such as relational database systems, are not well suited to sequence information. Any given position in a sequence can be important because of its own identity,

because it is part of a larger subsequence, or perhaps because it is part of a large set of overlapping subsequences, all of which have different significance. It is necessary to support queries such as, "What sequence motifs are present in this sequence?" It is often difficult to represent these multiple, nested relationships within standard relational database schema. In addition, the neighbors of a sequence element are also critical, and it is important to be able to perform queries such as, "What sequence elements are seen 20 elements to the left of this element?" For these reasons, researchers in bioinformatics are developing **object-oriented databases** (see Chap. 6) in which a sequence can be queried in different ways, depending on the needs of the user.

24.3.2   Structures in Biology

The sequence information mentioned in Sect. 24.3.1 is rapidly becoming inexpensive to obtain and easy to store. On the other hand, the **three-dimensional structure information** about the proteins, DNA, and RNA is much more difficult and expensive to obtain, and presents a separate set of analysis challenges. Currently, only about 75,000 three-dimensional structures of biological macromolecules are known.[9] These models are incredibly valuable resources, however, because an understanding of structure often yields detailed insights about biological function. As an example, the structure of the ribosome has been determined for several species and contains more atoms than any other structure to date. This structure, because of its size, took two decades to solve, and presents a formidable challenge for functional annotation (Cech 2000). Yet, the functional information for a single structure is dwarfed by the potential for comparative genomics analysis between the structures from several organisms and from varied forms of the functional complex. Since the ribosome is ubiquitously required for all forms of life these types of comparisons are possible. Thus a wealth of infor-

---

[8] http://www.genome.gov/sequencingcosts/ (accessed November 30, 2012)

[9] For more information see http://www.rcsb.org/pdb/ (accessed November 30, 2012)

mation comes from relatively few structures. To address the problem of limited structure information, the publicly funded structural genomics initiative aims to identify all of the common structural scaffolds found in nature and to increase the number of known structures considerably. In the end, it is the physical interactions between molecules that determine what happens within a cell; thus the more complete the picture, the better the functional understanding. In particular, understanding the physical properties of therapeutic agents is the key to understanding how agents interact with their targets within the cell (or within an invading organism). These are the key questions for structural biology within bioinformatics:

1. How can we analyze the structures of molecules to learn their associated function? Approaches range from detailed molecular simulations (Levitt 1983) to statistical analyses of the structural features that may be important for function (Wei and Altman 1998).

2. How can we extend the limited structural data by using information in the sequence databases about closely related proteins from different organisms (or within the same organism, but performing a slightly different function)? There are significant unanswered questions about how to extract maximal value from a relatively small set of examples.

3. How should structures be grouped for the purposes of classification? The choices range from purely functional criteria ("these proteins all digest proteins") to purely structural criteria ("these proteins all have a toroidal shape"), with mixed criteria in between. One interesting resource available today is the Structural Classification of Proteins (SCOP),[10] which classifies proteins based on shape and function.

24.3.3 Expression Data in Biology

The development of DNA microarrays has led to a wealth of data and unprecedented insight into

the fundamental biological machine. The traditional premise is relatively simple; tens of thousands of gene sequences derived from genomic data are fixed onto a glass slide or filter. The sequences for each spot are derived from a single gene sequence and the sequences are attached at only one end, creating a forest of sequences in each spot that are all identical. An experiment is performed where two groups of cells are grown in different conditions, one group is a control group and the other is the experimental group. The control group is grown normally, while the experimental group is grown under experimental conditions. For example, a researcher may be trying to understand how a cell compensates for a lack of sugar. The experimental cells will be grown with limited amounts of sugar. As the sugar depletes, some of the cells are removed at specific intervals of time. When the cells are removed, all of the mRNA from the cells is separated and converted back to DNA, using reverse transcriptase (a special enzyme that can create a DNA copy from an RNA template). This leaves a pool of cDNA molecules (DNA derived from mRNA is called complementary DNA or cDNA) that represent the genes that were expressed (turned on) in that group of cells. Using a chemical reaction, a red fluorescent molecule is attached to the experimental cDNA molecules (the "red group") and the cDNA from the control group is attached to green fluorescent molecules (the "green group"). These two samples are pooled together and then washed over the glass slide. The labeled cDNA in the pool sticks or hybridizes to the corresponding gene sequences in the spots on the glass slide. The molecules from the two groups will compete with each other to hybridize to the complementary sequences in the spots with the group that had more of a particular sequence binding more of the molecules stuck to the glass slide. Using a scanning confocal microscope and a laser to fluoresce the cDNA with their dye molecules, the amount of red and green fluorescence in each spot can be measured. The ratio of red to green fluorescence for a spot is a measure of the ratio of the expression of that gene product between the red and green groups. This ratio is a measure of whether a gene is being turned off (downregulated) in the

[10] http://scop.mrc-lmb.cam.ac.uk/scop/ (accessed November 30, 2012)

experimental group or whether the gene is being turned on (upregulated). As each glass slide can hold up to 40,000 spots each experiment has the potential of measuring the activity of all the genes in a cell due to some experimental change. Expressed genes can include genes that are translated into proteins (mRNA), ribosomal RNA (rRNA), regulatory microRNAs (miRNA) or other gene products. Although protein coding genes were initially the area most studied for disease, miRNAs have recently become increasingly important for disease associations because, unlike mRNA, miRNA's serve a regulatory role that determines how genes are expressed.

While is it possible for a researcher to measure the fluorescence of a spot on the gene expression glass slide, it is entirely impractical to measure the fluorescence of each of the 40,000 spots on each slide. Additionally, an experiment may be composed of several gene expression slides. Computers become critical for analyzing these data because it is impossible for a researcher to measure and analyze all of those red and green spots. Currently scientists are using gene expression experiments to study how cells from different organisms compensate for environmental changes, how pathogens fight antibiotics, and how cells grow uncontrollably (as is found in cancer). A challenge for biological computing is to develop methods to analyze these data, tools to store these data, and computer systems to collect the data automatically.

24.3.4 Genome Sequencing Data in Biology

Advances in sequencing technology are pivotal in enabling the practice of genomic medicine. Whereas the first human genome sequence was carried out over approximately 13 years at a cost of $2.7 billion (Davies 2010), whole human genomes can now be sequenced in a matter of days at a cost that is growing ever-closer to the magic, if somewhat arbitrary, $1000 price tag. This amount is commonly seen as the price at which it becomes feasible to sequence a patient in the course of clinical care, justifiable both clin-

ically and financially. In 2004, and again in 2011, the National Human Genome Research Institute (part of the National Institutes of Health) funded a number of efforts specifically aimed at increasing speed and decreasing the cost of genome scale sequencing. In addition, in 2006 the X Prize Foundation announced the genomics X PRIZE for sequencing ten high quality genomes in 10 days for under $10,000.

Traditional sequencing involves a method referred to as Sanger sequencing. This method typically is applied to sequences ranging from 300 to 1,000 nucleotides in a non-high throughput manner.[11] In the early to mid 2000s, several technologies were introduced to sequence large amounts of DNA in parallel. These technologies, including 454 Pyrosequencing, SOLiD or Solexa (now Illumina) sequencing typically determine much shorter sequences than Sanger based approaches, but can generate as many as 300 gigabases (300×10^9 bases) of sequence in short 75-base fragments at a cost well under $10,000.[12] These **next generation sequencing methods** are being used for many applications, including identification of genetic variants in clinical studies, characterizing genome function with specific experiments and sequencing novel species genomes. These studies have already discovered the genetic basis of rare genetic disorders by sequencing entire families (Ng et al. 2010), and we have seen a glimpse of the future of genome sequencing for routine health care in the analysis of both a single genome of a healthy man (Ashley et al. 2010) and a family of four (Dewey et al. 2011). Currently, we are seeing the introduction of third generation sequencing technologies that promise higher throughput, single molecule sequencing, higher accuracy, or lower cost. One emergent area of research is **metagenomics**, the study of microorganism ecosystems using DNA sequencing, including the association of human

---

[11] http://en.wikipedia.org/wiki/DNA_sequencing (accessed November 30, 2012)

[12] http://www3.appliedbiosystems.com/cms/groups/mcb_marketing/documents/generaldocuments/cms_061241.pdf ; (accessed November 30, 2012)

gut flora populations to disease phenotypes in humans (Qin et al. 2010).

24.3.5 Epigenetics Data

Epigenetics consists of heritable changes that are not encoded in the primary DNA sequence. Several types of epigenetic effects can now be studied in the laboratory, and they have been associated to disease and risks of disease (Goldberg et al. 2007). First, the regional structure of chromosomes affects which regions of the genome can be transcribed, that is which regions can be expressed. Large proteins, called histones, coordinate the structure of chromosomes and their structure and positions are regulated with protein posttranslational modifications to the histones bound to the DNA. These changes have been associated with spontaneous mutations in cancer, complex genetic diseases, and Mendelian inherited genetic diseases. Second, cytosine bases in the DNA can be methylated and this can affect gene expression. DNA methylation patterns can be passed on when DNA is replicated. Like chromosome structure, these modifications have been associated with human disease (Bird 2002).

24.3.6 Systems Biology

Recent advances in high throughput technologies have enabled a new, dynamic approach to studying biology, that of **systems biology**. In contrast to the historically reductionist approach to biology, studying one molecule at a time, systems biology looks at the entirety of a system including dynamic relationships between the different components. With that said, systems biology is still only in its infancy, and even within the field, researchers have not reached consensus on a single definition (Wishart 2008). As an analogy, consider an airplane. Having a "parts list" for a Boeing 747 does not enable us to understand how those parts work together to make the airplane operate. If the airplane breaks, the parts list alone does not tell us how to remedy the situation.

Rather, we need to understand how the parts interact, how one affects another, and how perturbations to one part of the system affect the rest of the system. Similarly, systems biology involves understanding not only the "parts list", i.e. the list of all genes, proteins, metabolites, etc., but also the dynamic networks of interactions among these parts. Recently an integrated simulation of an entire bacterial cell has shown the feasibility of accurate computational simulations of cell physiology (Karr et al. 2012).

Current research in -**omics technologies** have both enabled and catalyzed the advancement of systems biology. However, a systems biology approach goes beyond simply performing these high bandwidth methods for the purpose of biological discovery. Rather, systems biology implies a systematic, hypothesis-driven approach based on omic-scale (very large) hypotheses. Once the interactions in a biological network are understood, one can model that network to make predictions regarding the system's behavior, particularly in light of specific perturbations. Understanding how the system has evolved to work can also help us understand what goes wrong when the system breaks down, and how to intervene in order to restore the system to normal.

24.4 Key Bioinformatics Algorithms

There are a number of common computations that are performed in many contexts within bioinformatics. In general, these computations can be classified as sequence alignment, structure alignment, pattern analysis of sequence/structure, gene expression analysis, and pattern analysis of biochemical function.

24.4.1 Early Work in Sequence and Structure Analysis

As it became clear that the information from DNA and protein sequences would be voluminous and difficult to analyze manually, algorithms began to appear for automating the analysis of sequence information. The first requirement was to have a reliable way to align sequences so that their detailed similarities and distances could be examined directly. Needleman and Wunsch (1970) published an elegant method for using **dynamic programming** techniques to align sequences in time related to the cube of the number of elements in the sequences. Smith and Waterman (1981) published refinements of these algorithms that allowed for searching both the best global alignment of two sequences (aligning all the elements of the two sequences) and the best local alignment (searching for areas in which there are segments of high similarity surrounded by regions of low similarity). A key input for these algorithms is a matrix that encodes the similarity or substitutability of sequence elements: When there is an inexact match between two elements in an alignment of sequences, it specifies how much "partial credit" we should give to the overall alignment based on the similarity of the elements, even though they may not be identical. Looking at a set of evolutionarily related proteins, Dayhoff et al. (Dayhoff 1974) published one of the first matrices derived from a detailed analysis of which amino acids (elements) tend to substitute for others.

Within structural biology, the vast computational requirements of the experimental methods (such as X-ray crystallography and nuclear magnetic resonance) for determining the structure of biological molecules drove the development of powerful structural analysis tools. In addition to software for analyzing experimental data, graphical display algorithms allowed biologists to visualize these molecules in great detail and facilitated the manual analysis of structural principles (Langridge 1974; Richardson 1981). At the same time, methods were developed for simulating the forces within these molecules as they rotate and vibrate (Gibson and Scheraga 1967; Karplus and Weaver 1976; Levitt 1983).

The most important development to support the emergence of bioinformatics, however, has been the creation of databases with biological information. In the 1970s, structural biologists, using the techniques of X-ray crystallography,

set up the Protein Data Bank (PDB) specifying the Cartesian coordinates of the structures that they elucidated (as well as associated experimental details) and made PDB publicly available. The first release, in 1977, contained 77 structures. The growth of the database is chronicled on the Web: the PDB now has over 75,000 detailed atomic structures and is the primary source of information about the relationship between protein sequence and protein structure.[13] Similarly, as the ability to obtain the sequence of DNA molecules became widespread, the need for a database of these sequences arose. In the mid-1980s, the GENBANK database was formed as a repository of sequence information. Starting with 606 sequences and 680,000 bases in 1982, the GENBANK has grown by much more than 135 million sequences and 125 billion bases.[14] The GENBANK database of DNA sequence information supports the experimental reconstruction of genomes and acts as a focal point for experimental groups. Numerous other databases store the sequences of protein molecules[15] and information about human genetic diseases.[16]

Included among the databases that have accelerated the development of bioinformatics is the Medline database of the biomedical literature and its paper-based companion Index Medicus (see Chap. 21).[17] Including articles as far back as 1809 and brought online free on the Web in 1997, Medline provides the glue that relates many high-level biomedical concepts to the low-level molecule, disease, and experimental methods. In fact, this "glue" role was the basis for creating the Entrez and PubMed systems for integrating access to literature references and the associated databases.

---

[13] See http://www.rcsb.org/pdb/ (accessed April 26, 2013)

[14] http://www.ncbi.nlm.nih.gov/genbank/ (accessed November 30, 2012)

[15] http://www.uniprot.org/ (accessed November 30, 2012)

[16] http://www.ncbi.nlm.nih.gov/omim (accessed November 30, 2012)

[17] http://www.ncbi.nlm.nih.gov/pubmed (accessed November 30, 2012)

24.4.2 Sequence Alignment and Genome Analysis

Perhaps the most basic activity in computational biology is comparing two biological sequences to determine (1) whether they are similar and (2) how to align them. The problem of alignment is not trivial but is based on a simple idea. Sequences that perform a similar function should, in general, be descendants of a common ancestral sequence, with mutations over time. These mutations can be replacements of one amino acid with another, deletions of amino acids, or insertions of amino acids. The goal of **sequence alignment** is to align two sequences so that the evolutionary relationship between the sequences becomes clear. If two sequences are descended from the same ancestor and have not mutated too much, then it is often possible to find corresponding locations in each sequence that play the same role in the evolved proteins. The problem of solving correct biological alignments is difficult because it requires knowledge about the evolution of the molecules that we typically do not have. There are now, however, well-established algorithms for finding the mathematically optimal alignment of two sequences. These algorithms require the two sequences and a scoring system based on (1) exact matches between amino acids that have not mutated in the two sequences and can be aligned perfectly; (2) partial matches between amino acids that have mutated in ways that have preserved their overall biophysical properties; and (3) gaps in the alignment signifying places where one sequence or the other has undergone a deletion or insertion of amino acids. The algorithms for determining optimal sequence alignments are based on a technique in computer science known as **dynamic programming** and are at the heart of many computational biology applications (Gusfield 1997). Figure 24.1 shows an example of a Smith-Waterman matrix, the first described local alignment algorithm that utilizes a dynamic programming approach. The algorithm works by calculating a similarity matrix between two sequences, then finding optimal paths through the matrix that maximize a similarity score between the two sequences.

Unfortunately, the dynamic programming algorithms are computationally expensive to apply, so a number of faster, more heuristic methods have been developed. The most popular algorithm is the **Basic Local Alignment Search Tool** (**BLAST**) (Altschul et al. 1990). BLAST is based on the observation that sections of proteins are often conserved without gaps (so the gaps can be ignored—a critical simplification for speed) and that there are statistical analyses of the occurrence of small subsequences within larger sequences that can be used to prune the search for matching sequences in a large database. Another tool that has found wide use in mining genome sequences is BLAT (Kent 2003). BLAT is often used to search long genomic sequences with significant performance increases over BLAST. It achieves its 50-fold increase in speed over other tools by storing and indexing long sequences as short, non-overlapping sequences, allowing efficient storage, searching, and alignment on modest hardware.

24.4.3 Prediction of Structure and Function from Sequence

One of the primary challenges in bioinformatics is taking a newly determined DNA sequence (as well as its translation into a protein sequence) and predicting the structure of the associated molecules, as well as their function. Both problems are difficult, being fraught with all the dangers associated with making predictions without hard experimental data. Nonetheless, the available sequence data are starting to be sufficient to allow good predictions in a few cases. For example, there is a Web site devoted to the assessment of biological macromolecular structure prediction methods.[18] Recent results suggest that when two protein molecules have a high degree (more than 40 %) of sequence identity and one of the structures is known, a reliable model of the other can be built by analogy. In the case that sequence similarity is less than

---

[18] http://predictioncenter.org/. (accessed November 30, 2012)

Fig. 24.1 Example of sequence alignment using the Smith Waterman algorithm

a) Pairwise alignment between human chymotrypsin and human trypsin.

```
CTRB_HUMAN      MAFLWLLSCWALLGTTFPGCGVPAIHPVLSGLSRIVNGEDAVPGSWPWQVSLQDKTGFHFC
TRY1_HUMAN      MNPLLILTFVA---------AALAAPFDDDDKIVGGYNCEENSVPYQVSLN--SGYHFC

CTRB_HUMAN      GGSLISEDWVVTAAHCGVRTSDVVVAGEFDQGSDEENIQVLKIAKVFKNPKFSILTVNND
TRY1_HUMAN      GGSLINEQWVVSAGHC-YKSRIQVRLGEHNIEVLEGNEQFINAAKIIRHPQYDRKTLNND

CTRB_HUMAN      ITLLKLATPARFSQTVSAVCLPSADDDFPAGTLCATTGWGKTKYNANKTPDKLQQAALPL
TRY1_HUMAN      IMLIKLSSRAVINARVSTISLPTAPP--ATGTKCLISGWGNTASSGADYPDELQCLDAPV

CTRB_HUMAN      LSNAECKKSWGRRITDVMICAG--ASGVSSCMGDSGGPLVCQKDGAWTLVGIVSWGSDTC
TRY1_HUMAN      LSQAKCEASYPGKITSNMFCVGFLEGGKDSCQGDSGGPVVCNG----QLQGVVSWGDGCA

CTRB_HUMAN      STSSPGVYARVTKLIPWVQKILAAN-
TRY1_HUMAN      QKNKPGVYTKVYNYVKWIKNTIAANS
```

b) Smith Waterman matrix illustrating the aligned region in A, using the BLOSUM62 mutation matrix (Henikoff and Henikoff, 1994).

	G	F	L	E	G	G	K	D	S	C	Q	G	D	S	G	G	P	V	V	C	N	G	Q	L	Q
G	6	-3	-4	-2	6	6	-2	-1	0	-3	-2	6	-1	0	6	6	-2	-3	-3	-3	0	6	-2	-4	-2
A	0	-2	-1	-1	0	0	-1	-2	1	0	-1	0	-2	1	0	0	-1	0	0	0	-2	0	-1	-1	-1
S	0	-2	-2	0	0	0	0	0	4	-1	0	0	0	4	0	0	-1	-2	-2	-1	1	0	0	-2	0
G	6	-3	-4	-2	6	6	-2	-1	0	-3	-2	6	-1	0	6	6	-2	-3	-3	-3	0	6	-2	-4	-2
V	-3	-1	1	-2	-3	-3	-2	-3	-2	-1	-2	-3	-3	-2	-3	-3	-2	4	4	-1	-3	-3	-2	1	-2
S	0	-2	-2	0	0	0	0	0	4	-1	0	0	0	4	0	0	-1	-2	-2	-1	1	0	0	-2	0
S	0	-2	-2	0	0	0	0	0	4	-1	0	0	0	4	0	0	-1	-2	-2	-1	1	0	0	-2	0
C	-3	-2	-1	-4	-3	-3	-3	-3	-1	9	-3	-3	-3	-1	-3	-3	-3	-1	-1	9	-3	-3	-3	-1	-3
M	-3	0	2	-2	-3	-3	-1	-3	-1	-1	0	-3	-3	-1	-3	-3	-2	1	1	-1	-2	-3	0	2	0
G	6	-3	-4	-2	6	6	-2	-1	0	-3	-2	6	-1	0	6	6	-2	-3	-3	-3	0	6	-2	-4	-2
D	-1	-3	-4	2	-1	-1	-1	6	0	-3	0	-1	6	0	-1	-1	-1	-3	-3	-3	1	-1	0	-4	0
S	0	-2	-2	0	0	0	0	0	4	-1	0	0	0	4	0	0	-1	-2	-2	-1	1	0	0	-2	0
G	6	-3	-4	-2	6	6	-2	-1	0	-3	-2	6	-1	0	6	6	-2	-3	-3	-3	0	6	-2	-4	-2
G	6	-3	-4	-2	6	6	-2	-1	0	-3	-2	6	-1	0	6	6	-2	-3	-3	-3	0	6	-2	-4	-2
P	-2	-4	-3	-1	-2	-2	-1	-1	-1	-3	-1	-2	-1	-1	-2	-2	7	-2	-2	-3	-2	-2	-1	-3	-1
L	-4	0	4	-3	-4	-4	-2	-4	-2	-1	-2	-4	-4	-2	-4	-4	-3	1	1	-1	-3	-4	-2	4	-2
V	-3	-1	1	-2	-3	-3	-2	-3	-2	-1	-2	-3	-3	-2	-3	-3	-2	4	4	-1	-3	-3	-2	1	-2
C	-3	-2	-1	-4	-3	-3	-3	-3	-1	9	-3	-3	-3	-1	-3	-3	-3	-1	-1	9	-3	-3	-3	-1	-3
Q	-2	-3	-2	2	-2	-2	1	0	0	-3	5	-2	0	0	-2	-2	-1	-2	-2	-3	0	-2	5	-2	5
K	-2	-3	-2	1	-2	-2	5	-1	0	-3	1	-2	-1	0	-2	-2	-1	-2	-2	-3	0	-2	1	-2	1
D	-1	-3	-4	2	-1	-1	-1	6	0	-3	0	-1	6	0	-1	-1	-1	-3	-3	-3	1	-1	0	-4	0
G	6	-3	-4	-2	6	6	-2	-1	0	-3	-2	6	-1	0	6	6	-2	-3	-3	-3	0	6	-2	-4	-2
A	0	-2	-1	-1	0	0	-1	-2	1	0	-1	0	-2	1	0	0	-1	0	0	0	-2	0	-1	-1	-1
W	-2	1	-2	-3	-2	-2	-3	-4	-3	-2	-2	-2	-4	-3	-2	-2	-4	-3	-3	-2	-4	-2	-2	-2	-2
T	-2	-2	-1	-1	-2	-2	-1	-1	1	-1	-1	-2	-1	1	-2	-2	-1	0	0	-1	0	-2	-1	-1	-1
L	-4	0	4	-3	-4	-4	-2	-4	-2	-1	-2	-4	-4	-2	-4	-4	-3	1	1	-1	-3	-4	-2	4	-2
V	-3	-1	1	-2	-3	-3	-2	-3	-2	-1	-2	-3	-3	-2	-3	-3	-2	4	4	-1	-3	-3	-2	1	-2

25 %, however, performance of these methods is much less reliable.

When scientists investigate biological structure, they commonly perform a task analogous to sequence alignment, called **structural alignment**. Given two sets of three-dimensional coordinates for a set of atoms, what is the best way to superimpose them so that the similarities and differences between the two structures are clear? Such computations are useful for determining whether two structures share a common ancestry and for understanding how the structures' functions have subsequently been refined during evolution. There are numerous published algorithms for finding good structural alignments. We can apply these algorithms in an automated fashion whenever a new structure is determined, thereby classifying the new structure into one of the protein families (such as those that SCOP maintains).

One of these algorithms is MinRMS (Jewett et al. 2003).[19] MinRMS works by finding the minimal root-mean-squared-distance (RMSD) alignments of two protein structures as a function of matching residue pairs. MinRMS generates a

---

[19] http://www.cgl.ucsf.edu/Research/minrms/ (accessed November 30, 2012)

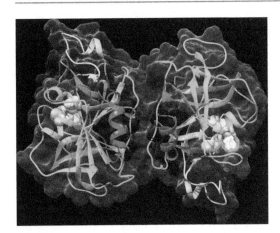

Fig. 24.2 Example of structural comparison. Comparison of the chymotrypsin and trypsin protein structures using Chimera and MinRMS (http://www.cgl.ucsf.edu/chimera; accessed 30 Nov 2012, with permission)

family of alignments, each with different number of residue position matches. This is useful for identifying local regions of similarity in a protein with multiple domains. MinRMS solves two problems. First, it determines which structural superpositions, or alignment, to evaluate. Then, given this superposition, it determines which residues should be considered "aligned" or matched. Computationally, this is a very difficult problem. MinRMS reduces the search space by limiting superpositions to be the best superposition among four atoms. It then exhaustively determines all potential four-atom matched superpositions and evaluates the alignment. Given this superposition, the number of aligned residues is determined, as any two residues with C-alpha carbons (the central atom in all amino acids) less than a certain threshold apart. The minimum average RMSD for all matched atoms is the overall score for the alignment. In Fig. 24.2, an example of such a comparison is shown.

A related problem is that of using the structure of a large biomolecule and the structure of a small organic molecule (such as a drug or cofactor) to try to predict the ways in which the molecules will interact. An understanding of the structural interaction between a drug and its target molecule often provides critical insight into the drug's mechanism of action. The most reliable way to assess this interaction is to use experimental methods to solve the structure of a drug–target complex. Once again, these experimental approaches are expensive, so computational methods play an important role. Typically, we can assess the physical and chemical features of the drug molecule and can use them to find complementary regions of the target. For example, a highly electronegative drug molecule will be most likely to bind in a pocket of the target that has electropositive features.

Prediction of function often relies on use of sequential or structural similarity metrics and subsequent assignment of function based on similarities to molecules of known function. These methods can guess at general function for roughly 60–80 % of all genes, but leave considerable uncertainty about the precise functional details even for those genes for which there are predictions, and have little to say about the remaining genes.

24.4.4 Clustering of Gene Expression Data

Analysis of gene expression data often begins by clustering the expression data. A typical experiment is represented as a large table, where the rows are the genes on each chip and the columns represent the different experiments, whether they be time points or different experimental conditions. Each row is then a vector of values that represent the results of the experiment with respect to a specific gene. Clustering can then be performed to determine which genes are being expressed similarly. Genes that are associated with similar expression profiles are often functionally associated. For example, when a cell is subjected to starvation (fasting), ribosomal genes are often downregulated in anticipation of lower protein production by the cell. It has similarly been shown that genes associated with neoplastic progression could be identified relatively easily with this method, making gene expression experiments a powerful assay in cancer research (see Yan and Gu 2009, for a review). In order to cluster expression data, a distance metric must be determined to compare a gene's profile with another gene's profile. If the vector data are a list

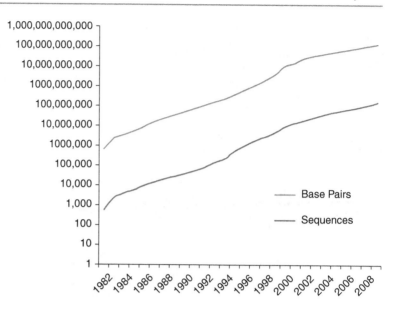

Fig. 24.3 The exponential growth of GENBANK. This plot shows that since 1982 the number of bases in GENBANK has grown by five full orders of magnitude and continues to grow by a factor of 10 every 4 years

of values, Euclidian distance or correlation distances can be used. If the data are more complicated, more sophisticated distance metrics may be employed. These methods fall into two categories: supervised and unsupervised. Supervised learning methods require some preconceived knowledge of the data at hand (discussed below). Usually, the method begins by selecting profiles that represent the different groups of data, e.g., genes that represent certain pathways, and then the clustering method associates each of the genes with the representative profile to which they are most similar. Unsupervised methods are more commonly applied because these methods require no knowledge of the data, and can be performed automatically.

Two such unsupervised learning methods are the hierarchical and K-means clustering methods. Hierarchical methods build a dendrogram, or a tree, of the genes based on their expression profiles. These methods are agglomerative and work by iteratively joining close neighbors into a cluster. The first step often involves connecting the closest profiles, building an average profile of the joined profiles, and repeating until the entire tree is built. K-means clustering builds k clusters or groups automatically. The algorithm begins by picking k representative profiles randomly. Then each gene is associated with the representative to which it is closest, as defined by the distance met-

ric being employed. Then the center of mass of each cluster is determined using all of the member gene's profiles. Depending on the implementation, either the center of mass or the nearest member to it becomes the new representative for that cluster. The algorithm then iterates until the new center of mass and the previous center of mass are within some threshold. The result is k groups of genes that are regulated similarly. One drawback of K-means is that one must chose the value for k. If k is too large, logical "true" clusters may be split into pieces and if k is too small, there will be clusters that are merged. One way to determine whether the chosen k is correct is to estimate the average distance from any member profile to the center of mass. By varying k, it is best to choose the lowest k where this average is minimized for each cluster. Another drawback of K-means is that different initial conditions can give different results, therefore it is often prudent to test the robustness of the results by running multiple runs with different starting configurations (Fig. 24.3).

The future clinical usefulness of these algorithms cannot be overstated. In 2002, van't Veer et al. (2002) found that a gene expression profile could predict the clinical outcome of breast cancer. The global analysis of gene expression showed that some cancers were associated with different prognosis, not detectable using traditional means. Another exciting advancement in this field is the potential use of microarray expression data to profile the molecular effects of known and potential therapeutic agents. This molecular understanding of a disease and its treatment will soon help clinicians make more informed and accurate treatment choices (for more, see Chap. 25 on Translational Bioinformatics).

24.4.4.1 Classification and Prediction

A high level description of some common approaches to classification or supervised learning are described below, but note that entire courses could be, and are, taught on each of these methods. For further details we refer readers to the suggested texts at the end of this chapter.

One of the simplest methods for classification is that of k-nearest-neighbor, or KNN. Essentially, KNN uses the classification of the k closest instances to a given input as a set of votes regarding how that instance should be classified. Unfortunately, KNN tends not to be useful for omics-based classification because it tends to break down in high-dimensional space. For high-dimensional data, KNN has difficulty in finding enough neighbors to make prediction, which will lead to large variation in the classification. This breakdown is one aspect of the "curse of dimensionality," described in more detail below (Hastie et al. 2009).

A more general statistical approach to supervised learning, and one which encompasses a number of popular methods, is that of function approximation. In this approach, one attempts to find a useful approximation of the function $f(x)$ that underlies the actual relation between the inputs and outputs. In this case, one chooses a metric by which to judge the accuracy of the approximation, for example the residual sum of squares, and uses this metric to optimize the model to fit the training data. Bayesian modeling, logistic regression, and Support Vector Machines all use variations on this approach.

Finally, there is the class of rule-based classifiers. This type of classifier may be thought of as a series of rules, each of which splits the set of instances based on a given characteristic. Details such as what criteria are used to choose the fea-

ture on which to base a rule, and whether the algorithm uses enhancements such ensemble learning (i.e., multiple models together) determine the specifics of the classifier type, for example decision trees, random forests, or covering rules.

Which approach to use depends both on the nature of the data and the question being asked. The question might prioritize sensitivity over specificity or vice versa. For example, for a test to detect a life-threatening infection that is easily treatable by readily available antibiotics, one might want to err on the side of sensitivity. In addition, data may be numeric or categorical or have differing degrees of noise, missing values, correlated features or non-linear interactions among features. These different qualities are better handled by different methods. In many cases the best approach is actually to try a number of different methods and to compare the results. Such comparative analysis is facilitated through freely available software packages such as R/Bioconductor[20] and Weka.[21]

24.4.5 The Curse of Dimensionality

In the post-genomic era, there is no shortage of data to analyze. Rather, many researchers have more data than they know what to do with. However this overabundance tends to be a factor of the dimensionality of the data, rather than the number of subjects. This mismatch can lead to challenges for experimental design and statistical analysis. Type 1 error, or the tendency to incorrectly reject the null hypothesis and say that indeed there is statistical significance to a pattern (see Chap. 11), is amplified by looking at high-dimensional data. This is one aspect of what is known as the "curse of dimensionality" (Hastie et al. 2009). Consider analysis of gene expression data for 20,000 genes, trying to detect a pattern that can predict outcome. In a sample of, say, 30 subjects—a reasonable number when

---

[20] http://bioconductor.org/ (accessed November 30, 2012)

[21] http://www.cs.waikato.ac.nz/ml/weka/ (accessed November 30, 2012)

testing a single hypothesis—by random chance, some number of genes will correlate with outcome. Essentially one is testing not one but 20,000 hypotheses simultaneously. One must therefore correct for multiple hypothesis testing. The Bonferroni method is a common and straightforward approach to correct for multiple hypothesis testing.[22] It entails dividing the threshold p-value one would use, traditionally 0.05, by the number of hypotheses. So, for a test of 20,000 genes, one would require a p-value of 2.5×10^{-6} to call a gene significant. Typically, analyses using high dimensional data such as gene expression are not sufficiently powered to pass this stringent test. One would need thousands of samples to be sufficiently powered. Another approach is to use q-value, or false discovery rate (Storey and Tibshirani 2003), rather than p-value. This approach relies on empirical permutation to determine the expected number of false positives if indeed the null hypothesis is correct, which enables approximation of the proportion of false positives among all reported positives. Consider again the microarray experiment above in which each array includes 20,000 genes. We want to know whether gene X was differentially expressed in cases versus controls. Choosing a threshold p-value, or false *positive* rate, of 0.05 means that 1 time in 20 we will erroneously reject the null hypothesis and predict a false positive. If a statistical test returns 2,000 positives, i.e. 2,000 genes appear to be significantly differentially expressed, we expect 1 in 20 of the genes being analyzed $(20,000 * (1/20) = 1,000)$ or approximately half of them to be false positives. A false *discovery* rate of 0.05, on the other hand, would mean that 5 % *of those called positive*, in this case 100 out of 2,000, are false positives. Q-value is thus less stringent than p-value, but may be of greater utility in a high-dimensional omics context than a traditional p-value or correction for multiple hypotheses.

Another approach to analysis of high dimensional data sets is to use dimensionality reduction methods such as feature selection or feature extraction. Feature selection entails extracting only a subset of the features at hand, in this case genes. This may be done in a number of ways, based on which genes vary the most, or on which genes seem to best predict the categorization at hand. In contrast, feature extraction creates a new smaller set of features that captures the essence of the original variation. As an example, imagine a plane flight from Seattle, WA to Key West, FL. One could use a 3-dimensional vector consisting of latitude and longitude to describe the plane's position at any given point along the way. In this case, one value would describe how far the plane had gone in the north/south direction, and one would indicate how far the plane had gone in the east/west direction. However, if we change the axis along which we are measuring to instead be the direct route along which the plane is flying, then we only need 1 dimension to describe where the plane is located. The distance flown tells us where the plane is located at any given time. This approach of changing the axes is the basis for principle components analysis (PCA), a common method for feature extraction. Instead of going from two dimensions to one, PCA on gene expression data typically goes from tens of thousands of features to just a few. Both for feature selection and feature extraction, it is important to replicate the findings in an independently generated data set in order to be sure the model is not over fitting the data on which it was trained.

24.5 Current Application Successes from Bioinformatics

Biologists have embraced the Web in a remarkable way and have made Internet access to data a normal and expected mode for doing business. Hundreds of databases curated by individual biologists create a valuable resource for the developers of computational methods who can use these data to test and refine their analysis algorithms. With standard Internet search engines, most biological databases can be found and accessed within moments. The large number of databases has led to the development of metadatabases that combine information from indi-

---

[22] http://en.wikipedia.org/wiki/Bonferroni_correction (accessed November 30, 2012)

vidual databases to shield the user from the complex array that exists. There are various approaches to this task.

The Entrez system from the National Center for Biotechnology Information (NCBI) gives integrated access to the biomedical literature, protein, and nucleic acid sequences, macromolecular and small molecular structures, and genome project links (including both the Human Genome Project and sequencing projects that are attempting to determine the genome sequences for organisms that are either human pathogens or important experimental model organisms) in a manner that takes advantages of either explicit or computed links between these data resources.[23] Newer technologies are being developed that will allow multiple heterogeneous databases to be accessed by search engines that can combine information automatically, thereby processing even more intricate queries requiring knowledge from numerous data sources. One example is the Bioconductor project, a toolbox for bioinformatics in the R programming language.[24]

24.5.1 Data Standards and Metadata

Chapter 7 on standards in biomedical informatics addresses standardized terminologies as well as standards for data exchange, and terminologies for translational research are discussed in Chap. 25 (Sect. 25.4.2). A number of specialized exchange formats are relevant to this space. The Human Proteome Organization (HUPO) Proteomics Standards Initiative (PSI), founded in 2002, has a family of **markup languages** (ML) for different aspects of proteomics: mzML for mass spectrometry, PSI-MI XML for molecular interactions, and mzIdentML for proteomics informatics. The FGED (Functional Genomics Data Society, formed in 1999 as MGED for Microarray Gene Expression Data Society) developed MAGE-ML (Microarray and Gene

Expression Markup Language) to enable sharing of microarray data. However, it was determined that MAGE-ML was too technical and cumbersome for labs without dedicated bioinformatics support, so FGED now recommends use of MAGE-TAB, a tab-delimited, spreadsheet-based format, instead.[25] The Metabolomics Standards Initiative was formed in 2005 to coordinate efforts among a number of existing groups and initiatives, though metabolomics standards have lagged somewhat behind the progress of their genomic and proteomic siblings (Sansone et al. 2007; Scalbert et al. 2009).

A third type of standard that has been emphasized in bioinformatics is the minimum information standard. The MIBBI (Minimum Information for Biological and Biomedical Investigations) consortium established the MIBBI project in 2008 to provide a freely accessible, web-based resource for minimum information standards and to enable owners of those standards to harmonize overlapping elements where applicable. The most well-known of these standards is MIAME, or Minimum Information About a Microarray Experiment, but the MIBBI portal lists over 30 minimum information reporting guidelines (Taylor et al. 2008). These guidelines identify only the types of information that must be included. They do not specify format or semantics. For example, MIAME enumerates six required pieces of information: (1) raw data, (2) processed data, (3) sample annotation, (4) experimental design including, e.g., which raw data file relates to which sample, which hybridizations are technical versus biological replicates, (5) array annotation, and (6) lab and data processing protocols. Array annotation could include a file that identifies the sequence of each individual spot on the array, or it could simply name a standard commercial microarray chip for which annotation is readily available from the manufacturer. Either of these methods would be MIAME compliant for the array annotation component in that it would enable someone looking at the data to understand what each spot represents. One could argue that these guidelines do not go

---

[23] http://www.ncbi.nlm.nih.gov/Entrez/ (accessed December 20, 2012)

[24] http://bioconductor.org/ (accessed November 30, 2012)

[25] http://www.mged.org/mage-tab/ (accessed November 30, 2012)

far enough—without specifying semantics or format, the information cannot be computed over and is therefore less useful than it could be. But some feel that the standards are already too onerous and represent a barrier to data sharing (Galbraith 2006).

Note that of the six facets included in the MIAME standard, only two apply directly to data generated through the experiment. The other four involve data *about* the data, or metadata. Without knowing what the data fields mean, and how the data was generated, the data itself are of no use. As discussed below, policies to ensure data sharing are becoming more common, but simply putting data on a server is not sufficient. The data must be annotated in a sufficiently complete and structured manner to enable data comprehension and reuse. To this end, a workshop was held in 2007 to explore the possibilities for a simple, common data format to describe data and metadata derived from biological, biomedical, and environmental studies involving omics data as well as more traditional data types (Sansone et al. 2008). The outcome from this workshop was the development of the ISA-Tab format for representation of experimental metadata, along with the open source ISA software suite of tools (Rocca-Serra et al. 2010).

24.5.2 Data Sharing Policies

In 1996, the First International Strategy Meeting on Human Genome Sequencing was held in Bermuda. In this meeting, a set of principles was agreed upon regarding sharing of human genome sequencing data. These principles came to be known as the Bermuda principles. They stipulated that (1) all sequence assemblies larger than 1 kb should be released as soon as possible, ideally within 24 h; (2) finished annotated sequences should be published immediately to public databases; and (3) that all human sequence data generated in large-scale sequencing centers should be made available in the public domain.[26]

Increasingly, journals and funders require that researchers deposit all types of research data in publicly available repositories (Fischer and Zigmond 2010). In 2009, President Obama announced an Open Government Directive that included plans to make federally funded research data available to the public.[27] This announcement describes the NIH's policy regarding published manuscripts in particular, but also notes that the results of government-funded research can take many forms, including data sets. Currently the NIH requires that proposals for funding of over $500,000 include a data sharing plan.[28]

24.5.2.1 Sequence and Genome Databases

The main types of sequence information that must be stored are DNA and protein. One of the largest DNA **sequence databases** is GENBANK, which is managed by the NCBI.[23] GENBANK is growing rapidly as genome-sequencing projects feed their data (often in an automated procedure) directly into the database. Figure 24.3 shows the logarithmic growth of data in GENBANK since 1982. Entrez Gene curates some of the many genes within GENBANK and presents the data in a way that is easy for the researcher to use (Fig. 24.4).

In addition to GENBANK, there are numerous special-purpose DNA databases for which the curators have taken special care to clean, validate, and annotate the data. The work required of such curators indicates the degree to which raw sequence data must be interpreted cautiously. GENBANK can be searched efficiently with a number of algorithms and is usually the first stop for a scientist with a new sequence who wonders "Has a sequence like this ever been observed before? If one has, what is known about it?" There are increasing numbers of stories about scientists using GENBANK to discover

---

[26] http://www.ornl.gov/sci/techresources/Human_Genome/research/bermuda.shtml (accessed November 30, 2012)

[27] http://edocket.access.gpo.gov/2009/E9-29322.htm (accessed November 30, 2012)

[28] http://grants.nih.gov/grants/guide/notice-files/NOT-OD-03-032.html (accessed November 30, 2012)

Fig. 24.4 The Entrez Gene entry for the digestive enzyme chymotrypsin. Basic information about the original report is provided, as well as some annotations of the key regions in the sequence and the complete sequence of DNA bases (a, g, t, and c) is provided as a link (Courtesy of NCBI)

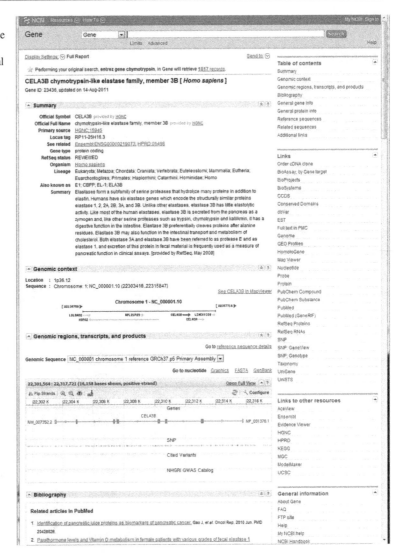

unanticipated relationships between DNA sequences, allowing their research programs to leap ahead while taking advantage of information collected on similar sequences.

A database that has become very useful recently is the University of California Santa Cruz Genome Browser[29] (Fig. 24.5). This data set allows users to search for specific sequences in the UCSC version of the human genome. Powered by the similarity search tool BLAT, users can quickly find annotations on the human genome that contain their sequence of interest. These

annotations include known variations (mutations and SNPs), genes, comparative maps with other organisms, and many other important data.

24.5.3 Structure Databases

Although sequence information is obtained relatively easily, structural information remains expensive on a per-entry basis. The experimental protocols used to determine precise molecular structural coordinates are expensive in time, materials, and human power. Therefore, we have only a small number of structures for all the molecules characterized in the sequence data-

---

[29] http://genome.ucsc.edu/ (accessed November 30, 2012)

Fig. 24.5 Screen from the
UC Santa Cruz genome
browser showing the
chymotrypsin C gene. The
rows in the browser show
annotations on the gene
sequence. The browser
window here shows a small
segment of human chromo-
some 15, as if the sequence of
a, g, c and t are represented
from left to right (5–3). The
annotations include gene
predictions and annotations as
well as an alignment of the
similarity of this region of the
genome when compared with
the mouse genome

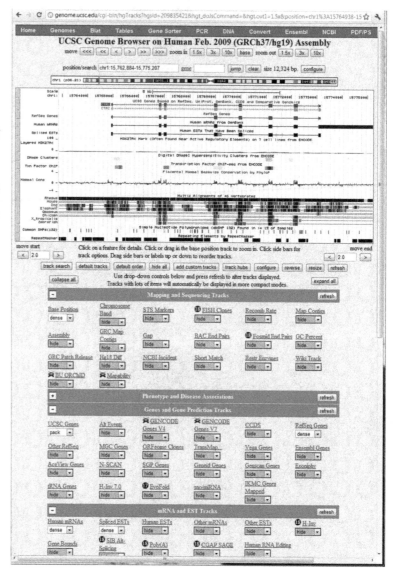

bases. The two main sources of structural information are the Cambridge Structural Database[30]
for small molecules (usually less than 100 atoms)
and the PDB[31] for macromolecules (see
Sect. 24.3.2), including proteins and nucleic
acids, and combinations of these macromolecules
with small molecules (such as drugs, cofactors,
and vitamins). The PDB has approximately
75,000 high-resolution structures, but this number is misleading because many of them are small
variants on the same structural architecture.
There are approximately 100,000 proteins in
humans; therefore many structures remain
unsolved (e.g., Burley and Bonanno 2002). In the
PDB, each structure is reported with its biological source, reference information, manual
annotations of interesting features, and the
Cartesian coordinates of each atom within the

[30] http://www.ccdc.cam.ac.uk/products/csd/ (accessed November
30, 2012)

[31] http://www.rcsb.org/pdb/ (accessed November 30, 2012)

molecule. Given knowledge of the three-dimensional structure of molecules, the function sometimes becomes clear. For example, the ways in which the medication methotrexate interacts with its biological target have been studied in detail for two decades. Methotrexate is used to treat cancer and rheumatologic diseases, and it is an inhibitor of the protein dihydrofolate reductase, an important molecule for cellular reproduction. The three-dimensional structure of dihydrofolate reductase has been known for many years and has thus allowed detailed studies of the ways in which small molecules, such as methotrexate, interact at an atomic level. As the PDB increases in size, it becomes important to have organizing principles for thinking about biological structure. SCOP[32] provides a classification based on the overall structural features of proteins. It is a useful method for accessing the entries of the PDB.

24.5.4 Analysis of Biological Pathways and Understanding of Disease Processes

The ECOCYC project is an example of a computational resource that has comprehensive information about biochemical pathways. ECOCYC is a knowledge base of the metabolic capabilities of E. coli; it has a representation of all the enzymes in the E. coli genome and of the chemical compounds those enzymes transform.[33] It also links these enzymes to their genes, and genes are mapped to the genome sequence.

EcoCyc also encodes the genetic regulatory network of E. coli, describing all protein and RNA regulators of E. coli genes. The network of pathways within ECOCYC provides an excellent substrate on which useful applications can be built. For example, they provide: (1) the ability to guess the function of a new protein by assessing its similarity to E. coli genes with a similar

sequence, (2) the ability to ask what the effect on an organism would be if a critical component of a pathway were removed (would other pathways be used to create the desired function, or would the organism lose a vital function and die?), and (3) the ability to provide a rich user interface to the literature on E. coli metabolism. Similarly, the Kyoto Encyclopedia of Genes and Genomes (KEGG) provides pathway datasets for organism genomes.[34]

24.5.5 Postgenomic Databases

A **postgenomic database** bridges the gap between molecular biological databases with those of clinical importance. One excellent example of a postgenomic database is the Online Mendelian Inheritance in Man (OMIM) database, which is a compilation of known human genes and genetic diseases, along with manual annotations describing the state of our understanding of individual genetic disorders.[35] Each entry contains links to special-purpose databases and thus provides links between clinical syndromes and basic molecular mechanisms (Fig. 24.6).

24.6 Future Challenges as Bioinformatics and Clinical Informatics Converge

Bioinformatics did solve all of its problems with the sequencing of the human genome. Indeed, if we can identify a set of challenges for the next generations of investigators, then we can more comfortably claim disciplinary status for the field. Fortunately, there is a series of challenges for which the completion of the first human genome sequence is only the beginning.

---

[32] http://scop.mrc-lmb.cam.ac.uk/scop/ (accessed November 30, 2012)

[33] http://ecocyc.org/ (accessed November 30, 2012)

[34] http://www.genome.jp/kegg/pathway.html (accessed November 30, 2012)

[35] http://www.ncbi.nlm.nih.gov/omim/ (accessed November 30, 2012)

Fig. 24.6 Screen from the Online Mendelian Inheritance in Man (*OMIM*) database showing an entry for pancreatic insufficiency, an autosomal recessive disease in which chymotrypsin (Entrez Gene entry shown in Fig. 24.2) is totally absent (as are some other key digestive enzymes) (Courtesy of NCBI)

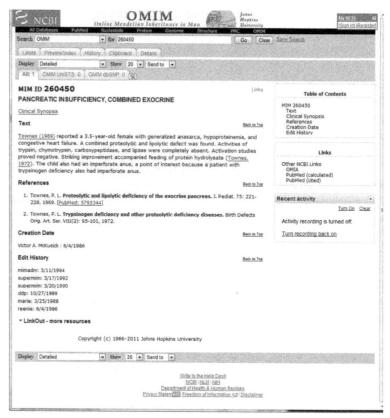

24.6.1 Completion of Multiple Human Genome Sequences

With the first human genome in hand, the possibilities for studying the role of genetics in human disease multiply. A new challenge immediately emerges, however: collecting individual sequence data from patients who have disease. Initial studies are promising for identification of the genetic cause of disease using individual or family based sequencing (Lupski et al. 2010). Currently, many researchers have chosen to sequence either entire genomes, or **exomes**, the regions of the genome that are transcribed into mRNA, and therefore the most likely to cause disease. Researchers now know that more than 99 % of the DNA sequences within humans are identical, but the remaining sequences are different and account for our variability in susceptibility to and development of disease states. It is not unreasonable to expect that for particular disease syndromes, the detailed genetic information for individual patients will provide valuable information that will allow us to tailor treatment protocols and perhaps let us make more accurate prognoses. There are significant problems associated with obtaining, organizing, analyzing, and using this information.

24.6.2 Linkage of Molecular Information with Symptoms, Signs, and Patients

There is currently a gap in our understanding of disease processes. Although we have a good understanding of the principles by which small groups of molecules interact, we are not able to explain fully how thousands of molecules interact within a cell to create both normal and abnormal physiological states. As the databases continue to accumulate information ranging from patient-specific data to fundamental genetic information, a major challenge is creating the conceptual links among these databases to create an audit trail from molecular-level information to macroscopic phenomena, as manifested in disease. The availability of these links will facilitate the identification of important targets for future research and will provide a scaffold for biomedical knowledge, ensuring that important literature is not lost within the increasing volume of published data.

24.6.3 Computational Representations of the Biomedical Literature

An important opportunity within bioinformatics is the linkage of biological experimental data with the published papers that report them. Electronic publication of the biological literature provides exciting opportunities for making data easily available to scientists. Already, certain types of simple data that are produced in large volumes are expected to be included in manuscripts submitted for publication, including new sequences that are required to be deposited in GENBANK and new structure coordinates that are deposited in the PDB. However, there are many other experimental data sources that are currently difficult to provide in a standardized way, either because the data are more intricate than those stored in GENBANK or PDB or they are not produced in a volume sufficient to fill a database devoted entirely to the relevant area. Knowledge base technology can be used, however, to represent multiple types of highly interrelated data.

Knowledge bases can be defined in many ways (see Chap. 22); for our purposes, we can think of them as databases in which (1) the ratio of the number of tables to the number of entries per table is high compared with usual databases, (2) the individual entries (or records) have unique names, and (3) the values of many fields for one record in the database are the names of other records, thus creating a highly interlinked network of concepts. The structure of knowledge bases often leads to unique strategies for storage

and retrieval of their content. To build a knowledge base for storing information from biological experiments, there are some requirements. First, the set of experiments to be modeled must be defined. Second, the key attributes of each experiment that should be recorded in the knowledge base must be specified. Third, the set of legal values for each attribute must be specified, usually by creating a controlled terminology for basic data or by specifying the types of knowledge-based entries that can serve as values within the knowledge base.

The development of such schemes necessitates the creation of terminology standards, just as in clinical informatics. There are now many controlled vocabularies (or ontologies) and metadata standards for annotation of genomic or proteomic data. For example, **Gene Ontology** (**GO**) is an ontology used for annotation of gene function, and arguably the most widely used ontology in basic research. Metadata standards help define information which should be collected and annotated upon various types of datasets. For example, the MIAME standard (Minimum Information About A Microarray Experiment) defines metadata one would annotate upon a microarray dataset. Recently, the Biosharing website[36] is providing links to terminologies and standards for a wide range of data types. Furthermore, a great many tools have been developed to help researchers access and analyze this data. For example, the previously mentioned Bioconductor project provides bioinformatic tools in the R language for solving common problems. Other commonly used tools include BioPerl, BioPython and MATLAB.[37]

24.6.4 Computational Challenges with an Increasing Deluge of Biomedical Data

An increasing challenge in biomedicine is storing, interpreting and integrating the massive amount

---

[36] http://biosharing.org/ (accessed November 30, 2012)

[37] http://www.open-bio.org/ (accessed November 30, 2012)

of datasets the biomedical community is generating, largely from modern technologies in high throughput experimentation. The amount of DNA sequence data being generated over time has dwarfed Moore's Law, for example. This issue is important for all areas of biomedical informatics, and is discussed in more detail in the Chapter on Translational Bioinformatics (Chap. 25).

24.7   Conclusion

Bioinformatics is closely allied to clinical informatics. It differs in its emphasis on a reductionist view of biological systems, starting with sequence information and moving to structural and functional information. The emergence of the genome sequencing projects and the new technologies for measuring metabolic processes within cells is beginning to allow bioinformaticians to construct a more synthetic view of biological processes, which will complement the whole-organism, top-down approach of clinical informatics. More importantly, there are technologies that can be shared between bioinformatics and clinical informatics because they both focus on representing, storing, and analyzing biological or biomedical data. These technologies include the creation and management of standard terminologies and data representations, the integration of heterogeneous databases, the organization and searching of the biomedical literature, the use of machine learning techniques to extract new knowledge, the simulation of biological processes, and the creation of knowledge-based systems to support advanced practitioners in the two fields.

Suggested Readings

Altman, R. B., Dunker, A. K., Hunter, L., & Klein, T. E. (2003). *Pacific symposium on Biocomputing'03*. Singapore: World Scientific Publishing. The proceedings of one of the principal meetings in bioinformatics, this is an excellent source for up-to-date research reports. Other important meetings include those sponsored by the International Society for Computational Biology (ISCB, http://www.iscb.org/), Intelligent

Systems for Molecular Biology (ISMB, http://iscb. org/conferences.shtml.35), and the RECOMB meetings on computational biology (http://www.ctw-congress.de/recomb/). ISMB and PSB have their proceedings indexed in PubMed.

Baldi, P., & Brunak, S. (2001). *Bioinformatics: The machine learning approach*. Cambridge, MA: MIT Press. This introduction to the field of bioinformatics focuses on the use of statistical and artificial intelligence techniques in machine learning.

Baldi, P., & Hatfield, G. W. (2002). *DNA microarrays and gene expression*. Cambridge: Cambridge University Press. Introduces the different microarray technologies and how they are analyzed.

Berg, J. M., Tymoczko, J. L., & Stryer, L. (2010). *Biochemistry*. New York: W.H. Freeman. The textbook by Stryer and colleagues is well written, and is illustrated and updated on a regular basis. It provides an excellent introduction to basic molecular biology and biochemistry.

Durbin, R., Eddy, S. R., Krogh, A., & Mitchison, G. (1998). *Biological sequence analysis: Probabilistic models of proteins and nucleic acids*. Cambridge: Cambridge University Press. This edited volume provides an excellent introduction to the use of probabilistic representations of sequences for the purposes of alignment, multiple alignment, and analysis.

Gusfield, D. (1997). *Algorithms on strings, trees and sequences: Computer science and computational biology*. Cambridge: Cambridge University Press. Gusfield's text provides an excellent introduction to the algorithmics of sequence and string analysis, with special attention paid to biological sequence analysis problems.

Malcolm, S., & Goodship, J. (Eds.). (2007). *Genotype to phenotype* (2nd ed.). Oxford: BIOS Scientific Publishers. This volume illustrates the different efforts to understand how diseases are linked to genes.

Pevsner, P. (2009). *Bioinformatics and functional genomics*. Hoboken, NJ: Wiley. A widely used excellent introduction to bioinformatics algorithms.

Questions for Discussion

1. How are DNA and protein sequence information changing the way that medical records are managed? Which types of systems are or will be most affected (laboratory, radiology, admission and discharge, financial, order entry)?

2. It has been postulated that clinical informatics and bioinformatics are working on the same problems, but in some areas one field has made more progress than the other. Identify three common

themes. Describe how the issues are approached by each subdiscipline.

3. Why should an awareness of bioinformatics be expected of clinical informatics professionals? Should a chapter on bioinformatics appear in a clinical informatics textbook? Explain your answers.

4. Why should an awareness of clinical informatics be expected of bioinformatics professionals? Should a chapter on clinical informatics appear in a bioinformatics textbook? Explain your answers.

5. One major problem with introducing computers into clinical medicine is the extreme time and resource pressure placed on physicians and other health care workers. Do you think that the same problems are arising in basic biomedical research?

6. Why have biologists and bioinformaticians embraced the Web as a vehicle for disseminating data so quickly, whereas clinicians and clinical informaticians have been more hesitant to put their primary data online?

7. If a patient's entire genome were present in their medical record how would one go about interpreting it clinically? Similarly, if we had an entire electronic health record database that included human genomes, how would a researcher go about finding new or novel genetic associations?

8. With the many high throughput experiments that are used in biomedical research, how are some ways to integrate those datasets using systems biology? For example, if you had a microarray dataset that annotated gene expression levels and a proteomics dataset that identified protein interactions, how could you jointly use both datasets to identify markers for a disease?

Translational Bioinformatics

25

Jessica D. Tenenbaum, Nigam H. Shah, and Russ B. Altman

After reading this chapter, you should know the answers to these questions:

- How does translational bioinformatics differ from the more general field of bioinformatics?
- What do T1 and T2 refer to in the context of translational research?
- What is a biomarker, and why is it important in medicine?
- What is personalized medicine, and how does it differ from traditional medical practice?
- What is the difference between pharmacokinetics and pharmacodynamics?
- What changes are needed from a clinical IT perspective to support personalized medicine?
- What is the difference between statistical significance and clinical significance?
- How are genomic data being used today in research, clinical care, and consumer health?

- What are some legal and ethical issues surrounding direct-to-consumer genetic testing?
- How are ontologies useful in translational bioinformatics?

25.1 What Is Translational Bioinformatics?

The preceding chapter described the field of bioinformatics, or the study of how information from biological systems is represented and analyzed. **Translational Bioinformatics** (**TBI**) is bioinformatics applied to human health and disease. It uses and extends the concepts and methods from bioinformatics to facilitate the practice of **translational medicine**, i.e. the translation of biological ("bench") discoveries into actual impact on clinical care ("bedside") and ultimately on population health (Fig. 25.1). The American Medical Informatics Association (AMIA) defines Translational Bioinformatics as "the development of storage, analytic, and interpretive methods to optimize the transformation of increasingly voluminous biomedical data, and genomic data, into proactive, predictive, preventive, and participatory health."[1] Those latter terms are often grouped together along with the more common descriptive of **personalized medicine**. The realization of personalized medicine will require methods for standards-based data

J.D. Tenenbaum, PhD (✉)
Duke Translational Medicine Institute,
Duke University, 2424 Erwin Rd,
Durham 27705, NC, USA
e-mail: jessie.tenenbaum@duke.edu

N.H. Shah, MBBS, PhD
Department of Medicine, Stanford University,
1265 Welch Road, X-229, Stanford 94305, CA, USA
e-mail: nigam@stanford.edu

R.B. Altman, MD, PhD
Departments of Bioengineering,
Genetics and Medicine, Stanford University,
Clark Center, 318 Campus Drive, S242,
Stanford 94305, CA, USA
e-mail: russ.altman@stanford.edu

---

[1] http://www.amia.org/applications-informatics/ translational-bioinformatics (Accessed 30/11/2012).

E.H. Shortliffe, J.J. Cimino (eds.), *Biomedical Informatics*,
DOI 10.1007/978-1-4471-4474-8_25, © Springer-Verlag London 2014

storage and retrieval, novel methods for analysis and interpretation, and aid to the clinician in decision support. In AMIA's description of TBI, they further state that it includes "...the evolution of clinical informatics methodology to encompass biological observations." That is, clinical informatics approaches will need to expand in scope to incorporate **omics** data (genomics, transcriptomics, metabolomics, and proteomics data) as it increasingly pertains to clinical care. In this chapter, we will discuss the three components of AMIA's definition—the novel methods, the voluminous data, and the personalized approach to health that TBI enables. We conclude with a discussion of challenges and future directions for the field.

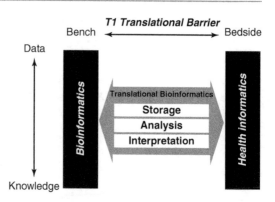

Fig. 25.1 TBI bridges the gap between bioinformatics on the "bench" side of the T1 barrier and health informatics on the "bedside" end of the spectrum. Novel methods for storage, analysis, and interpretation span the spectrum from data to knowledge (Adapted with permission from (Sarkar et al. 2011a, b))

25.1.1 Differences from "Traditional" Bioinformatics

TBI differs from the larger field of bioinformatics in a number of key ways. As described above, the focus of TBI is human health. As such, the discipline centers primarily, though not exclusively, around human data. This fact has a number of implications from an informatics perspective. First, one encounters a range of data management, regulatory, and privacy issues that do not arise in handling data from mice, yeast, *Escherichia coli*, or other model organisms. Laws such as the Health Information Portability and Accountability Act (HIPAA)[2] (see Chap. 10) dictate how patient data must be handled and safeguarded to protect patient privacy. Title 21 of the Code of Federal Regulations Part 11 (21 CFR part 11)[3] mandates how data must be managed if they are to be included as part of a submission to the Food and Drug Administration. In addition, institutional review boards (IRBs) typically require measures to ensure subject confidentiality before they will approve a research protocol. Making complete datasets publically accessible

for a mouse experiment is good scientific citizenship. Making the same type of data accessible for a human study would be a serious violation of privacy and confidentiality.

Another difference is that while experimental perturbation through small molecule agonists or antagonists, siRNA, or knock-out genes are straightforward and common in yeast or *E. coli*, such approaches would be neither feasible nor ethical in human subjects. This has significant implications for data generation and collection in translational research. **Phase I clinical trials** are the notable exception to this rule, but they are performed only on ostensibly therapeutic agents. They also require a number of preliminary steps, are very expensive, and are performed in a very small number of subjects. Other factors that differentiate research with human subjects include genetic and environmental heterogeneity, which can be controlled in model organisms. Instead, much translational data from human beings comes from *in vitro* experiments on cell lines and observational inquiries regarding factors such as genotype, environmental factors, and outcomes. With so much inherent noise, very large sample sizes are typically required for new discoveries. Novel approaches to data integration, mining, and reuse are thus particularly important in translational research.

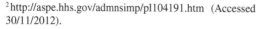

[2] http://aspe.hhs.gov/admnsimp/pl104191.htm (Accessed 30/11/2012).

[3] http://www.accessdata.fda.gov/scripts/cdrh/cfdocs/cfcfr/cfrsearch.cfm?cfrpart=11 (Accessed 30/11/2012).

25.1.2 A Few Words About Omics and Hamburgers

The word "genome" was coined in 1930 by a German Botanist named Hans Winkler, as a combination of the words "gene" and "chromosome."[4] The suffix "-ome" has subsequently come to be used in the context of biology to mean the totality of a thing, e.g. the *proteome* represents all proteins, and *proteomics*, the study of all proteins. Some use the term "genomics" to refer to information from genomes *and* their derivatives, i.e. RNA, proteins, and metabolites. Others use the more general term "omics" to refer to these different totalities. Here we shall adopt the more general *omics* neologism.

Omics technologies, then, are frequently referred to as "high-throughput" methods. This usage is not inaccurate in that many of these methods can be done in batch, for example in 384-well plates. However, focusing on the ability to run these assays *en masse* largely misses the point— the breadth or *bandwidth* of the technologies. A genetic assay measures one gene; a genomic assay measures thousands of genes. As an analogy, consider the food industry: McDonald's sells large quantities of food, quickly. In that respect, it is a high-throughput operation. But the breadth of their offerings is fairly narrow. A grocery store, on the other hand, sells thousands of types of food items, nearly every kind available. It is both high throughput (assuming cashiers are both plentiful and competent) and *high-bandwidth* (Butte 2009). This concept of bandwidth, the ability to observe thousands of types of molecules in a given assay, is the key attribute to these omic technologies.

25.2 The Rise of Translational Bioinformatics

25.2.1 Promise of the Human Genome Project

In January of 2000, two different groups announced that they had fully sequenced the human genome (see Chap. 24). The public project, published in *Nature*, was based on multiple individuals (Lander et al. 2001). The other genome, published in *Science*, was a private venture, performed on the DNA of biologist and entrepreneur Craig Venter (Venter et al. 2001). The vision for the human genome was that once all the genes were identified, they could be assigned functional annotations, and we would thus be able to understand what goes wrong when human beings succumb to disease. Additionally, this knowledge would help us to understand exactly which pathways and molecules needed to be targeted in order to prevent or cure disease. Of course, biological reality is not quite so straight forward. To begin with, the "central dogma" of biology (Crick 1970)— DNA is transcribed into mRNA, which is then translated into protein—is overly simplistic. Variations in regulatory regions can affect when the gene is turned on, and to what degree. Most genes have a number of different splice variants, producing a number of different proteins. In addition, proteins undergo post-translational modifications, which impact their structure and function. Finally, additional complexity is added through **epigenetics**, or heritable traits that are not coded for through DNA sequencing alone. An example is methylation of the DNA molecule, which has been shown to affect transcription (Cedar 1988). Despite this, the sequencing of the complete human genome marked a decisive turning point in biomedical research. The parts list had been assembled and researchers could move on to the more interesting aspects of the genome—what each part does, how the parts differ among individuals, and what it all means. The impact this would have on the field of clinical informatics was recognized immediately, reflected in the theme for the 2002 AMIA[5] Annual Symposium: "Bio*Medical Informatics: One Discipline" (Tarczy-Hornoch et al. 2007).

---

[4] http://dictionary.reference.com/browse/genome (Accessed 30/11/2012).

[5] AMIA is the American Medical Informatics Association, Bethesda, MD: http://www.amia.org

25.2.2 Translational Research and the CTSA Era

In the early 2000s, there was growing acknowledgement that the population at large, and patients in particular, were not reaping the full benefits of the considerable amount of research money being devoted to scientific discovery. It was recognized that researchers do not do a good job translating their discoveries "from bench to bedside," i.e. between biological discoveries in the lab and clinical application of the findings (Lenfant 2003). Two significant roadblocks were identified (Fig. 25.2)—one in translating discoveries into clinical care guidelines (dubbed T1 translation), and the other in translating clinical care guidelines into actual practice (T2 translation) (Sung et al. 2003). In 2004, the National Institutes of Health (NIH) launched the Roadmap for Medical Research, aimed at transforming life science research in the twenty-first century. Biomedical informatics plays a strong role across all three of the major Roadmap themes: New Pathways to Discovery, Research Teams of the Future, and Reengineering the Clinical Research Enterprise (Zerhouni 2006). As part of this Roadmap, the NIH embarked on a major initiative to break down translational barriers. The Clinical and Translational Science Award (CTSA) was a new funding mechanism established through the National Center for Research Resources within the NIH, with 12 awards in 2006 and approximately twelve each subsequent year until 2011, when the CTSA consortium comprised 60 institutions. As indicated in the NIH's request for applications, Biomedical Informatics was considered a key functional component of a Clinical and Translational Science Institution.[6] In fact, the word "informatics" appeared 38 times in the RFA itself, reflecting recognition by the NIH that informatics is crucial to addressing challenges in both T1 and T2 translational research (Butte 2008b).

It was in this context, with newfound attention to translational research, that Butte and Chen coined the term "translational bioinformatics" at

the AMIA annual symposium in 2006 in a paper entitled "Finding Disease-Related Genomic Experiments Within an International Repository: First Steps in Translational Bioinformatics" (Butte and Chen 2006). To assist in translating discoveries made using genomic technologies to medicine, they asserted, this emerging discipline "is focusing on the development of analytic, storage, and interpretive methods to optimize the transformation of increasingly voluminous genomic and biological data into diagnostics and therapeutics for the clinician." From there, the field became increasingly recognized by the larger informatics community. AMIA added TBI as one of its key supported domains and in 2008 held its first annual Summit on Translational Bioinformatics. (Although the "annual" qualifier was cautiously withheld until the event had proven to be a success.) Later that year, the *Journal of the American Medical Informatics Association* (JAMIA) published a perspective on TBI's "Coming of Age" that enumerated several reasons why the time was right for TBI to come into its own as a field (Butte 2008b). In 2009, the editors of the *Journal of Biomedical Informatics* published an explicit Editorial to announce a change in the journal's editorial policy to "focus its bioinformatics attention on innovations in the area of *translational bioinformatics*" (Shortliffe et al. 2009).

25.2.3 Personalized Medicine as a Driving Force

Personalized medicine is health care that is based on an individual's unique clinical, genetic, omic, and environmental profile, in addition to his or her specific values and preferences. The focus of personalized medicine is not only on diagnosis and therapeutic course, once a person falls ill. It also helps to guide health management based on individualized risk of disease in the future. Historically, guidelines for a healthy lifestyle have been presented as universal. Clinical care guidelines have been based primarily on macroscopic symptoms and qualities that can be observed in the course of a physical exam or reported by the patient. Personalized medicine aims to take advantage of all available modalities

---

[6] http://grants.nih.gov/grants/guide/rfa-files/ RFA-RM-06-002.html (Accessed 30/11/2012).

Fig. 25.2 Translational roadblocks along the continuum of biomedical research from scientific discoveries to changes in clinical practice and improvement of human health

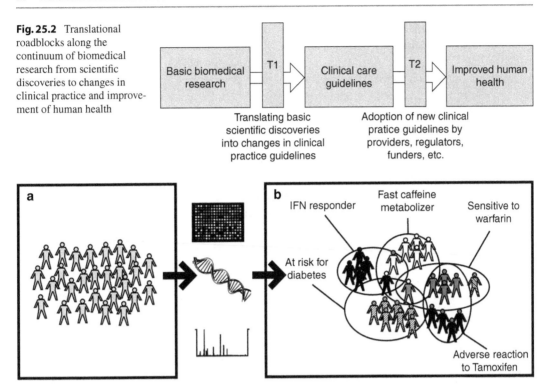

Fig. 25.3 Stratified or genomic medicine. A seemingly homogeneous group of people (**a**) can be divided into sub-groups (**b**) based on molecular fingerprints. This stratification can help to guide therapeutic decision

and sources of information regarding the individual. This may entail such non-traditional aspects as genotypic information or other molecular **biomarkers**, but also exposure to chemical cleaning agents, aversion to risk, a high threshold for pain, the impending birth of a first grandchild, etc. Of course, some of these variables have always been a part of clinical care to some extent, together with some degree of intangible qualitative judgment on the part of the clinician. Personalized medicine formalizes this integrated, patient-based approach, and incorporates the omics aspect. In 2004, Lee Hood coined the term "P4 medicine": predictive, personalized, preventive, and participatory (Weston and Hood 2004). Based on an individual's specific risk factors, interventions or changes in lifestyle could be adopted *before* the person falls ill, improving quality of life *and* saving significant costs in health care spending. Armed with this individualized knowledge, patients would be empowered to play an active role in their own health and medical care. Quality medical care has never been one-size-fits-all; personalized medicine acknowl-

edges this fact and seeks to change the practice of clinical care accordingly.

Many would agree that personalized medicine is the lodestar of medical practice; few would argue that we are close to achieving it. The same translational barriers that apply to clinical research more generally apply to personalized medicine in particular. Discoveries in the lab still take years to be incorporated into clinical care guidelines, and personalized clinical care guidelines take years to be widely adopted in practice. One stepping stone to truly personalized medicine that arguably *has* been achieved, and continues to evolve, is **genomic medicine**, also called **stratified medicine** (Trusheim et al. 2007; Ginsburg and Willard 2009). Stratified medicine involves clinical care that is based on specific qualities of an individual, often derived from molecular fingerprints. Subjects may be divided into different classes based on their genetics or some other high dimensional omic-scale biomarker (Fig. 25.3). This classification can then be used to guide clinical decision making.

25.3   Key Concepts for Translational Bioinformatics

As noted in the definition above, TBI involves the development of novel methods for data storage, analysis, and interpretation. In this section we elaborate on these different levels of informatics methodologies which can be framed as falling along a spectrum from data to knowledge (Fig. 25.1). *Data* represent specific values; at the simplest level, they can be reduced to ones and zeros. In the middle of the spectrum is *information*—ascribing new meaning to the data at hand through analysis. Finally, we arrive at *knowledge*—the ability to interpret information in a specific context, and for that interpretation to guide actions and behavior.

25.3.1   Data Storage

Data storage takes place at a number of different levels corresponding to different stages along the translational pipeline. At the "bench" end of bench-to-bedside, there is the need to store massive files of raw data generated through omics technologies (Stein 2010). In the case of genome sequencing, these files can be so large that is has been suggested (though not necessarily concluded) that for easily regenerated samples, it might be more cost-effective to discard the raw data and, if necessary, re-sequence at a later time (Hsi-Yang Fritz et al. 2011). For each raw data file type, one can generally choose among several different processing tools or algorithms. Thus, in addition to the raw data, a researcher or core facility may want to store one or more versions of processed data files, still frequently very large in size. In addition to the actual data, experimental **metadata** are needed in order to understand how the data were generated and how they were processed or analyzed. Annotation facilitates both comprehension and data provenance. Unfortunately, that information is rarely standardized, and frequently stored only in the researcher's head, paper notes, or hard drive. Increasingly, standards and tools such as the Ontology of Biomedical Investigations (OBI)

(Brinkman et al. 2010), Minimum Information lists (Taylor et al. 2008) and the Investigation/Study/Assay (ISA) infrastructure (Rocca-Serra et al. 2010) (see Chap. 24), are being developed to address this issue.

In the middle of the translational spectrum, there is an increasing need to store information related to subject consent. As DNA **Biobanks** (described below) become more common, researchers will have greater access to tissue samples of subjects they themselves did not recruit. It will no longer suffice to have consent information stored on a paper form, locked away in a file drawer. Even scanned images of the signed paper forms are insufficient for rapid and accurate information retrieval. Researchers and biobank administrators will need the ability to know to what each participant has consented, and to perform electronic queries to determine consent status on demand. Can John Doe's tissue be used for research beyond the study for which he was enrolled? Can the blood collected as a byproduct of care be used for **Genome-Wide Association Studies** (**GWAS**)? Can Jane Doe be contacted for enrollment in a follow-up study? In parallel with work being done to address issues of ethics and governance for this type of data capture and management, researchers are working to develop tools and terminologies to facilitate research permissions management (Obeid et al. 2010). To date, a clear solution has not emerged.

At the bedside end of the spectrum, clinicians do not have the time, nor usually the training, to analyze the underlying data. They need easy access to a patient's genotype, protein biomarker pattern, or metabolite profile without having to wade through volumes of sequence and biomarker data to learn the results of the test. They may also want to know some type of confidence or quality score for the data provided. HL7's Clinical Genomics Work Group is working to develop an HL7 standard in this area.[7] Just as important as the data itself, clinicians need to know what to do with that information.

---

[7] http://wiki.hl7.org/index.php?title=CG   (Accessed 12/3/2012).

Incorporating omic data into the EHR (Chap. 12) will not improve clinical care without the incorporation of these data types into clinical guidelines and tools for clinical decision support as discussed in Chap. 22 (Hoffman 2007).

25.3.2 Biomarkers

Fundamentally, the newfound ability to analyze and interpret high-throughput molecular datasets is about the discovery of biomarkers. The term **biomarker** has been used for decades, referring to any observation that could be used as an indication of an underlying physiological state. One commonly accepted definition is "a characteristic that is objectively measured and evaluated as an indicator of normal biological processes, pathogenic processes, or pharmacologic responses to a therapeutic intervention" (Atkinson et al. 2001). Exactly what constitutes a biomarker has historically depended in part on what types of observations could be made. Early biomarkers would have included fever, increased respiratory rate, or a rash. As our ability to probe living organisms increased, the domain of biomarkers expanded to the presence or concentration of specific molecules in the blood. For example, increased levels of glucose are indicative of diabetes, and an increase in PSA (prostate-specific antigen) suggests a risk for prostate cancer. Omics-era methodologies give us new types of data to which we can apply novel analytic methods to predict disease and progression. In the genomic era, biomarkers may consist of not just one but many different characteristics, which together give insight into underlying states or processes. Gene expression signatures are a common example of this type of multi-dimensional biomarker.

One important distinction to be made is that of predictive versus mechanistic biomarkers. Predictive biomarkers are essentially correlative markers of a given observation or outcome. They may or may not be causal for that outcome, but they can assist both clinicians and researchers through decision support by predicting outcomes or suggesting new focus areas for research.

Mechanistic biomarkers, on the other hand, can help shed light on what is happening at the molecular level that causes, for example, pathology, disease progression, or sensitivity to a given drug. Understanding a mechanism allows researchers to try to modify it through the activation or inhibition of specific molecules or pathways.

25.3.2.1 Predictive Biomarkers for Clinical Use

Predictive biomarkers can facilitate decision making in a number of ways. A biomarker indicating poor prognosis might suggest a more aggressive course of therapy than if that biomarker were not present. A signature indicating that lifestyle changes are likely to offer significant benefit to a patient could provide the motivation needed to follow through. For example, a signature indicating that weight loss is likely to improve insulin resistance could identify individuals for whom an intensive lifestyle changes is likely to have the most impact. Shah et al. were able to identify a **metabolomic** profile in subjects who had lost weight that, while independent of the amount of weight lost, was correlated with changes in insulin resistance (Shah et al. 2009b). On the flip side, a signature indicating that lifestyle changes alone are unlikely to confer the desired benefits may suggest that pharmaceutical intervention should be considered as well. Even if a biomarker is in no way actionable *yet*, it can be useful for biomedical research. As an example, osteoarthritis is a debilitating disease that is treated primarily through palliative measures to alleviate symptoms, but for which no disease-modifying therapeutic agents exist. One reason for this is the time and cost required to carry out a clinical trial. Gold standard radiographic methods for observing structural disease progression lack sensitivity and work best when the degeneration of a joint can be observed over time. Studies must therefore be carried out over of a period of several years. In addition, without knowledge of which subjects are likely to progress, studies must enroll large numbers of participants in order to be significantly powered (see Chap. 11). Identifying biomarkers to predict progression would enable cohort enrichment for individuals in whom disease progression is more likely, thus cutting the total number of subjects required and hence the cost of the trial (Kraus et al. 2011).

Biomarkers that are not clinically actionable may be personally actionable. As an example, relapsing-remitting multiple sclerosis (RRMS) is a form of multiple sclerosis in which the patient experiences exacerbations or relapses of neurologic symptoms, followed by periods of partial or complete recovery. If a test could be developed to enable RRMS patients to know in advance if relapses were likely to occur within an upcoming span of weeks or months, it could enable them to make more informed personal or professional decisions, such as when to plan a vacation, or whether to take a new job (Gregory 2011). Another example is the LRRK2 mutation that confers a significantly increased lifetime risk for Parkinson's disease. After learning of his carrier status for this mutation, Google co-founder Sergey Brin contributed tens of millions of dollars to Parkinson's research (Goetz 2010). A unique situation, to be sure, but it would be hard to argue that knowledge of a biomarker in this case was not actionable.

One major area for biomarker use is that of pharmacogenomics, described in Sect. 25.4.5 below. In many cases, a therapeutic gold standard exists, but only a fraction of patients respond to the given therapy. Knowing in advance who is likely not to respond to therapy, or who needs a higher or lower dose than the standard guidelines suggest, can be useful for tailoring therapeutic interventions. Interestingly, while the success of genetic biomarker discovery for common disease has been limited, genotypic biomarkers for response to drugs may be more promising because these variations would not have been selected against through evolution (Cirulli and Goldstein 2010). This may explain why, among published GWAS finding to date, the pharmacogenetic associations tend to have much higher odds ratios than those of genes associated with common diseases.

25.3.2.2 Molecular Mechanism for Therapeutic Targeting

Biomarkers may also be used for elucidation of disease mechanism which can then enable therapeutic targeting toward a specific molecule or pathway. Comparative analysis of high dimensional molecular signatures in patients versus healthy volunteers, tumors versus normal tissue, responders versus non-responders, etc., can reveal a set of molecules that are differentially expressed among these groups. One can then study those specific molecules more closely, or the pathways in which those molecules are involved, for example through gene ontology (GO) enrichment (see Sect. 25.4.2.2) or analysis using a curated pathway database such as Ingenuity's IPA, or Thomson Reuter's MetaCore (Chan et al. 2007). These types of tools also help to address a major challenge with pattern detection in high throughput data. Particularly in human data sets where differences are observational and not perturbed, it can be difficult, if not impossible, to know what is causal and what is simply correlated. Systems biology, described in Chap. 24, attempts to address this.

25.4 Computational Approaches to Biomarker Discovery

25.4.1 Classification and Prediction

One of the most common uses of biomarkers is to categorize samples or patients: cancerous samples versus normal tissues, good versus poor prognosis, bacterial versus viral infection. There are a number of ways to approach this problem, all of which fall under the heading of **supervised learning**. Fundamentally, supervised learning entails taking a set of inputs and corresponding outputs to try to learn a model that will enable one to predict output when faced with a previously unseen input. One is trying to predict one value, the *dependent variable*, based on some number of other values, also called *features* (in computer science), *independent variables* (in statistics), or *risk factors* (in clinical practice). If the dependent variable is categorical, typically one is actually predicting the probability of belonging to one class or the other. For example, one might want to predict whether a person will have a heart attack based on age, race, gender, weight, and cholesterol level. Or, in the context of TBI, one might want to predict the likelihood of a heart attack based on gene expression. Note that this latter approach is useful only if the gene expression signature increases the predictive capabilities beyond that offered by the clinical variables, which are typically easier to collect. Algorithmic approaches to classification and prediction are described in Chap. 24.

25.4.1.1 Clinical Relevance Versus Statistical Significance

Statistical significance is a measure of certainty that a test will give the right answer. Clinical relevance is a measure of how valuable this information is in guiding clinical care. It incorporates not only statistics, but also efficacy, safety, and cost. A test may be able to predict with 90 % accuracy whether, for example, a patient is likely to respond better to a treatment with unpleasant side effects over another, more innocuous therapy. However, if those side effects would significantly lower the patient's quality of life, then the test, while statistically significant, may not be clinically relevant. Similarly, if the cost of a false negative is very high, for example if a test predicts with 90 % accuracy that a patient will survive without a given intervention, that intervention will likely still be administered. On the other hand, if a test predicts with 90 %, or even 100 %, accuracy that a patient is likely to live 1 year longer with a given intervention but the intervention costs $1 million, this highly significant test is still not likely to affect clinical care.

Similarly, incorporation of molecular data or improvement upon an analytic method may increase a test's accuracy to a *statistically* significant degree while still not affecting clinical practice. Accuracy of a test is often measured by the area under the **receiver operating characteristic** (**ROC**) curve (AUC) (see Chap. 3), or the **C statistic**. The ideal ROC curve goes straight up the y-axis at x = 0, and then straight across the x-axis at y = 1, giving an AUC of 1. The more accurate a test, the closer it comes to that perfect path.

Figure 25.4 shows hypothetical ROC curves for two tests. Test 2 is a more accurate test in that it has a statistically significant higher C statistic, but as with the examples above, that may not change any clinical decisions. In light of this fact,

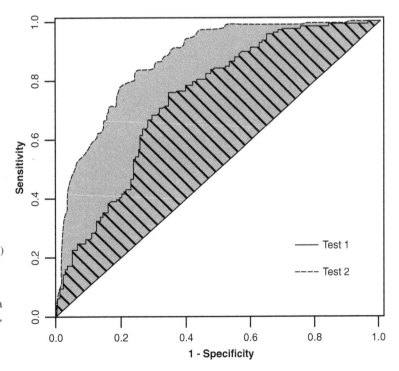

Fig. 25.4 A comparison between two Receiver Operator Characteristic (ROC) curves. The area under the curve (AUC) or C statistic is higher for Test 2 (*gray*) than for Test 1 (*diagonal lines*) to a statistically significant degree, but this increased accuracy does not necessarily imply clinical relevance

Table 25.1 Hypothetical reclassification of disease risk between two prognostic tests

| | Number of individuals (actual rate) | | |
| | Predicted 5-year risk for test 2 | | |
Predicted 5 year risk for Test 1	**0–5%**	**5–20%**	**> 20%**
0–5%	300 (3 %)	20 (2 %)	0
5–20%	30 (3 %)	300 (11 %)	40 (37 %)
> 20%	0	10 (35 %)	300 (42 %)

some have proposed that a better measure is needed for judging the incremental value of novel biomarkers and analytical approaches (Pencina et al. 2008). Alternative methods include **net reclassification improvement** (**NRI**), a measure of the net fraction of reclassifications made in the correct direction using the given biomarker or method over a method without the designated improvement (Steyerberg et al. 2011). This concept is illustrated in Table 25.1. Rows represent the risk level predicted by the hypothetical Test 1 for 1,000 subjects, columns represent the risk level predicted by Test 2. Values along the diagonal were predicted to have the same risk by both tests. Subjects in the black cells (30+40=70) were correctly reclassified by Test 2 (i.e., the actual rate in parentheses matches the appropriate risk category). Subjects in the light gray cells (10+20=30) were reclassified incorrectly. The resulting net reclassification improvement is (70–30)/1,000, or 4 %.

25.4.1.2 Biomarkers for Drug Repurposing

One very promising area for use of biomarkers is in **drug repurposing**, or drug repositioning. That is, identifying existing drugs that may be useful for indications other than those for which they were initially approved. Doing so allows circumvention of early clinical trials for toxicity as those have already been performed. A number of different approaches have typically been used to identify candidates for repositioning. In some cases, overlapping symptoms may suggest a potential match between one disease area and another. In other cases, empirical observation of unexpected positive effects may suggest alternative uses for a given drug. With omic-scale

biomarker discovery, it is possible to use underlying molecular pathway signatures to suggest new uses for existing drugs.

One of the prominent early examples of this approach came from the Broad Institute in the form of the "Connectivity Map," a resource intended to enable researchers to identify functional connections between drugs, genes, and diseases (Lamb 2007). The general idea was to identify a gene expression signature in a state of interest, e.g. a disease, and then compare that signature to the gene expression patterns observed upon exposure to a number of different compounds. Correlated signatures suggested pathways that were similarly perturbed between a disease state and an intervention. More importantly, anti-correlated signatures suggested potential utility for a given compound in trying to reverse the underlying molecular mechanisms of a given disease. A similar approach was used by Sirota et al. to identify the anti-ulcer drug cimetidine as a candidate agent to treat lung adenocarcinoma. They were then able to validate this alternate use *in vivo* using an animal model of the disease (Sirota et al. 2011). Their approach is illustrated in Fig. 25.5.

25.4.2 Ontologies for Translational Research

In order to apply computational methods for biomarker discovery, one needs a consistent way to refer to diseases, drugs, devices, etc. Several ontologies exist in the biomedical domain, many under active development, that provide the necessary terms for creating consistent annotations—preferably in an automated manner—for the various datasets that are at the core of conducting research in TBI. One primary need in TBI is to identify and refer unambiguously to disease using one or more disease ontologies. We use the term disease **ontology** to refer to artifacts—terminologies and vocabularies as well as true ontologies—that can provide a hierarchy of parent–child terms for disease conditions. Disease-specific and other clinically-oriented ontologies are discussed in detailed in Chap. 7.

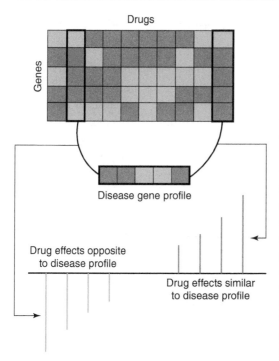

Fig. 25.5 A computational approach to candidate selection for drug repurposing. Sirota et al. first generated genomic signatures representing both diseases and drug exposure. For each disease signature, they compared it to the panel of drug signatures and assigned a drug-disease score based on profile similarity. Drugs whose pattern were most significantly *dis*similar to the disease state were ranked as lead candidates to treat the disease of interest

The Ontology for Biomedical Investigations (OBI) was developed as a collaboration among a number of experimental communities around the world in order to represent common aspects of biological and clinical investigations. It includes broadly applicable terms such as *assay*, as well as more specific terms, such as *transcription profiling by array assay*. It is particularly useful for annotation of experimental metadata, for example to record that a *protein expression profiling assay* was performed on a *blood specimen* (Brinkman et al. 2010).

25.4.2.1 Ontology-Related Resources for Translational Scientists

The use of ontology-based analyses for TBI, especially disease and drug ontologies as well as analyses using multiple ontologies, is a recent

development and the adoption and use of ontologies is likely to accelerate. Several resources are available for researchers who wish to use ontologies in making sense of large scale datasets. The UMLS, or Unified Medical Language System (see Chaps. 2 and 7), is a set of files and software that brings together many health and biomedical vocabularies and standards to enable interoperability among computer systems. One primary use of the UMLS is linking health information, medical terms, drug names, and billing codes across different computer systems, for example linking terms and codes among doctors' offices, pharmacies, and insurance companies. The UMLS has many other uses, including search engine retrieval, data mining, public health statistics reporting, and terminology research. The UMLS consists of three components, called the Knowledge Sources. These are: (1) The Metathesaurus, which provides terms and codes from many vocabularies, including RxNorm and SNOMED CT; (2) The Semantic Network, which provides broad categories (semantic types) such as 'Neoplastic process', 'Pharmacological Substance' and the relationships (semantic relations) among the categories; and (3) The SPECIALIST Lexicon and Lexical Tools, which provide natural language processing tools (see Chap. 8).

The National Library of Medicine provides Web based services called The UMLS Terminology Services (UTS), which provide comprehensive access to components of the Unified Medical Language System. UTS allows users to search and display content from the UMLS Metathesaurus, the Semantic Network and SNOMED CT. Users can also download content such as the UMLS knowledge sources, RxNorm monthly updates and SNOMED CT. UTS also provides an API for accessing the UMLS Metathesaurus content over the Web. In the field of TBI, the UMLS is a relatively underutilized resource, but that is changing quickly with the increase in the variety of access options (Aronson 2001; Bodenreider 2004; Aronson et al. 2008; Shah and Musen 2008; Aronson and Lang 2010; Mork et al. 2010) and heightened dissemination efforts by the National Library of Medicine.

The National Center for Biomedical Ontology maintains a repository of biomedical ontologies called BioPortal (Musen et al. 2011) which provides access through both Web pages and Web Services to more than 270 biomedical ontologies and controlled terminologies. Users go to the BioPortal Web site to browse biomedical ontologies and to search for specific ontologies relevant to their work. Using tools such as the Ontology Recommender, scientists who are unsure which of the dozens of ontologies in BioPortal provide the best coverage for capturing the entities in a particular application area can choose the right ontology. The NCBO Ontology Recommender Service (Jonquet et al. 2010) takes as input representative textual data relevant to a domain of interest and returns as output an ordered list of ontologies that would be most appropriate for annotating the corresponding text. By browsing ontologies on BioPortal and using tools such as the ontology recommender, a cancer biologist may find, for example, that although the Gene Ontology offers some terms for annotating her experimental data related to cell division, there are more precise terms in the NCIt. She may discover that the Foundational Model of Anatomy ontology provides terms for consistently naming body parts from which the experimental specimens were obtained, or that the National Drug File - Reference Terminology (NDF-RT) provides the properties of the drugs used in generating the experimental data. BioPortal allows users to navigate ontologies using a tree browser. Users also can visualize ontologies in BioPortal using special views that offer cognitive support for understanding the complexities of large ontologies (Fig. 25.6).

To provide the relationships between terms in two *different* ontologies, BioPortal provides mappings between the terms (Ghazvinian et al. 2009). The mappings can inform the user that the term *Melanoma* in the NCI Thesaurus is related to the term *Malignant, Melanoma* in SNOMEDCT and to *Melanoma* in the Human Disease Ontology. These mappings allow users to compare the use of related terms in different ontologies and to analyze how whole ontologies compare with one another (Ghazvinian et al. 2011). In addition to the curated mappings from the UMLS metathesaurus, Bioportal enables algorithmic and user-generated mappings as well.

25.4.2.2 Enrichment Analysis

Enrichment analysis is a statistical method to determine whether, for a set of items, a given concept or value is statistically over-represented compared to what one would expect at random. For example, informatics-related terms are over-represented in this book compared to what one would expect to find in a random sampling of words from all textbooks. The canonical example of enrichment analysis involves a list of genes differentially expressed in some condition. To determine the biological meaning of such a list, the usual solution is to perform enrichment analysis with the GO (Gene Ontology), which provides terms for consistent naming of the cellular component (CC) of gene products, the molecular functions (MF) they carry out, and the biological processes (BP) in which they participate. Several curation projects use the GO terms to annotate gene products from multiple organisms with terms from the three branches (CC, MF, BP) of the GO (Camon et al. 2003). These annotations form the basis for enrichment analysis in which we can aggregate the annotating GO concepts for each gene in this list, and arrive at a profile of the biological processes or mechanisms affected by the condition under study. This approach does have certain limitations, for example incomplete annotations for a number of genes, lack of conditional independence between annotations, and lack of a systematic mechanism to compensate for differing levels of depths in different branches of the ontology hierarchy (Khatri and Draghici 2005; Rhee et al. 2008). Despite this, such analysis is widely popular in the bioinformatics community and has resulted in over 100 tools listed on the GO website[8] and over 7,000 citations to the landmark paper on the Gene Ontology (Ashburner et al. 2000).

Disease and drug ontologies can be used to perform enrichment analysis in a manner simi-

---

[8] http://www.geneontology.org/GO.tools.shtml#alphabet (Accessed 12/3/2012).

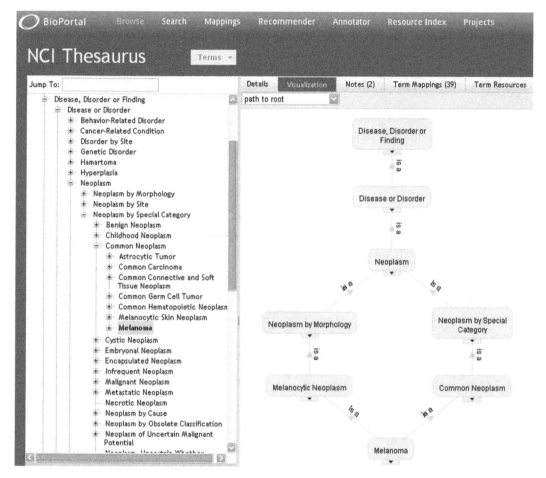

Fig. 25.6 A portion of the National Cancer Institute's thesaurus. The left pane shows a standard tree view for the term 'Melanoma'. The right pane shows a visualization that provides additional context by showing the parent classes of melanoma, all the way to the root node of 'Disease, Disorder or Finding'. The navigation bar just above the graphical visualization provides access to additional information, such as mappings which provide hooks into other disease ontologies that contain the concept Melanoma

lar to GO-based analyses for gene expression data (Subramanian et al. 2005; LePendu et al. 2011a). Just as scientists can ask *Which biological process is over-represented in my set of interesting genes or proteins*, we can also ask *Which disease (or class of diseases) is over-represented in my set of interesting genes or proteins?* For example, by annotating known protein mutations with disease terms, Mort et al. were able to identify a class of diseases—blood coagulation disorders—that were associated with a lower than expected rate of amino acid substitutions at O-linked glycosylation sites (Mort et al. 2010).

25.4.3 Natural Language Processing for Information Extraction

Ontologies are also useful in the context of extracting information from a body of text. In-depth methods for natural language processing are discussed in Chap. 8. Here we describe some applications in the context of translational research.

25.4.3.1 Mining Electronic Health Records

Researchers have shown that is possible to profile patient cohorts from EHRs using a variety of ontologies including SNOMED CT, MedDRA, and RxNorm (LePendu et al. 2011b). For example, LePendu et al. developed methods to annotate clinical text and methods for the mining of the resulting annotations to compute the risk of having a myocardial infarction on taking Vioxx (rofecoxib) for Rheumatoid arthritis. Their preliminary results show that it is possible to apply annotation analysis methods for detecting drug safety signals using electronic medical records (LePendu et al. 2011b).

Mining EHR data has also been proposed as a solution to the challenge of the large number of subjects that are needed for genome wide association studies (GWAS). Patients are increasingly able to consent to, or in some cases to opt out of, allowing excess biospecimens taken in the course of clinical care to be used in a de-identified fashion for genomic testing. Even for relatively strong genetic effects, GWAS requires thousands of individuals for sufficient statistical power (Chap. 11). For weaker effects, tens of thousands of subjects are likely to be needed. Although the cost of genotyping continues to decrease, recruitment and sample collection for these large numbers is both costly and labor-intensive. Leveraging the health care system and EHRs for subject recruitment offers a potential approach to circumvent this problem. Ritchie et al. demonstrated the feasibility of this approach by using EHR data and an associated biobank to replicate a number of previously discovered genotype-phenotype associations (Ritchie et al. 2010).

One major initiative in this area is the eMERGE (Electronic Medical Records and Genomics) Network, whose initial aim was to demonstrate that data captured through routine clinical care are sufficient to identify cases and controls accurately for GWAS (Thorisson et al. 2005). The eMERGE consortium includes five institutions with DNA repositories and associated electronic medical record systems. For each site, ontology-based data extraction and natural language processing algorithms are applied to the EHR in order to determine phenotypes such as dementia, cataracts, peripheral artery disease, type 2 diabetes, and cardiac conduction defects. This analysis is performed in a high-throughput, scalable fashion with results compared to a manually curated gold standard in order to determine positive and negative predictive values for cases and controls for the phenotypes in question (Kho et al. 2011). The consortium is also looking at cross-institutional algorithm application, ethical, legal, and social issues around DNA biobanks, and the potential for future incorporation of GWAS findings into clinical care.

These types of EMR-associated biobank resources enable a number of other approaches to data mining. For example, Denny et al. used BioVU at Vanderbilt University to perform what they called a "PheWAS," or a systematic, high-throughput **phenome-wide association scan** (Denny et al. 2010). Instead of measuring whole genomes across thousands of patients in order to find a gene associated with a phenotype in question, they measured only five alleles across thousands of patients and performed enrichment analysis for various diseases based on ICD9 codes. They then were able to reproduce known associations between those genes and certain diagnoses, *and* to generate new hypotheses for associations between these genes and other diagnoses that were statistically enriched for a given genotype. The ability to connect, at a molecular level, diseases that were not previously associated can have implications for therapeutic intervention.

25.4.3.2 Dataset Annotations

In addition to EHRs, public repositories for omics-scale datasets have been a heretofore underutilized resource for data mining. Upon submission, these datasets are typically annotated using only free-text descriptions. To address the lack of annotations, researchers have demonstrated that translational analyses are enabled by automatically annotating tissue and gene microarray datasets with ontology terms (Shah et al. 2009a). Researchers have also mapped the text annotations for records in databases such as the Stanford Tissue Microarray Database to terms from the NCI thesaurus to enable integrated analysis and query (Shah et al. 2007). Such automated annotation approaches have been generalized to create systems that process the free text metadata of diverse database elements such as gene expression data sets, descriptions of radiology images, clinical-trial reports, and PubMed article abstracts to annotate and index them with concepts from appropriate ontologies (Jonquet et al. 2011).

25.4.4 Network Analysis

Biology lends itself in various ways to modeling through networks or **graphs**. The term "graph" simply refers to a set of *nodes* or circles connected by a set of *edges* or lines. Typically, a node represents a molecular entity, and an edge represents some form of relationship between those molecular entities. This relationship may be a physical interaction (e.g., binds to), an influence (e.g., activates), or a similarity (e.g., is co-expressed with), among other possibilities. One frequently sees graphical models of gene regulatory networks, protein-protein interactions, and signaling cascades. The set of all of these sorts of physical interactions has been referred to as the *interactome* (Barabasi et al. 2011). Studying this **interactome** and its properties from a graph theory perspective enables useful insights regarding gene modules and pathways, and how these are disrupted in disease.

A number of researchers have attempted to develop gene association networks using gene expression data either alone or together with other sources of network data such as protein-protein interactions. The general idea is that co-expressed genes are likely to interact with each other or participate in the same pathway. But of course, correlation does not equal causality, and to be useful from a translational perspective, it is important to know the directionality of the influence between two molecules. Consider two genes, X and Y, whose expression is correlated (See Fig. 25.7). One can conclude that the genes interact in some way, whether directly or indirectly (i.e., through another molecule). However, without additional knowledge of any sort, we cannot know whether X influences Y (Fig. 25.7a), or Y influences X (Fig. 25.7b) or they share a third causal gene, Z (Fig. 25.7c). Which model

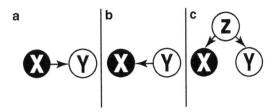

Fig. 25.7 Three possible causal relationships between two co-expressed genes. (**a**) Gene X affects Y. (**b**) Gene Y affects X. (**c**) Both X and Y are affected by a third causal gene Z

represents the true underlying relationship is important to know because if Y is involved in poor outcome, then targeting X will help to alleviate this condition in the first model, but not in the second or third.

One way to determine the actual underlying relationship, used frequently in model systems, is to actively perturb a specific variable in the system. If the other molecule changes accordingly, then we know that the perturbed variable was causal. This is the approach frequently used in a systems biology approach (see Chap. 24). Unfortunately, this is much harder to do in human beings than in *E. coli* or yeast. One clever approach to determination of causality in human biological networks is to integrate gene expression with genotypic information, in which case DNA sequence can be assumed to be the independent variable. If differential gene expression is correlated with differential genotype, one can conclude that the genotype caused the gene expression pattern and not the other way around. This is the basis for the approach taken by Eric Schadt et al. to develop **probabilistic causal networks** which can then be used to identify key drivers of disease (Zhu et al. 2008).

Network analysis in translational research need not be confined to concrete objects such as molecules. The Human Disease Network is a graphical model where nodes represent both known disease genes and disorders, linked by known associations between a given gene and disease (Goh et al. 2007). Figure 25.8 shows the "diseaseome" bipartite network, as well as the Human Disease Network, which connects diseases based on common genes, the and Disease

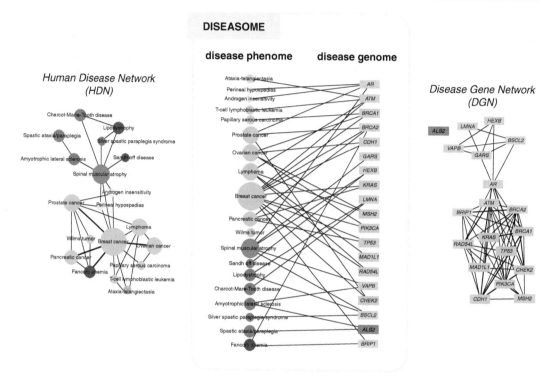

Fig. 25.8 The Human Disease Network. The *middle panel* shows a small subset of the bi-partite gene-disease network based on OMIM (Online Mendelian Inheritance in Man) gene-disease relationships. The Human Disease Network on the *left* shows diseases as nodes, with connec-tions representing common related genes. The Disease Gene Network on the *right* depicts genes as node, with connections indicating that they have been implicated in one or more of the same disorders (From Goh et al. (2007), ©2007 National Academy of Sciences, U.S.A.)

Gene Network, connecting genes based on diseases in common. Combining these disparate data types enables a graph theoretic approach to study the genetic basis for disease. Using this framework, one can analyze similarity between genes based not on co-expression or GO term annotation but based on the pathologies in which a gene is known to be involved. Such similarities could easily go undetected through gene expression analysis if, for example, the different diseases are caused by over-activation or inhibition of the gene respectively. A disease-gene network also enables the comparison of diseases not traditionally studied together, based on common underlying molecular mechanisms. Identifying disease similarities based on gene expression requires that one analyze expression data from those two diseases together in the first place, making it more difficult to discover novel, previously unsuspected relationships.

Building upon the Human Disease Network, Yildirim et al. created a network of drug-gene target interactions, thus enabling an additional layer of analysis regarding similarity between different drugs based on targeted genes, and between target molecules based on the drugs that target them (Yildirim et al. 2007). This type of network can be used as the basis for a number of different observations, including trends in drug development over time. For example, analysis of the structure of the graph revealed significant clustering of drug-gene interactions, suggesting a significant "me too" pattern to drug development (see Fig. 25.9). Inclusion of drugs still under investigation, i.e., not yet FDA approved at the time of analysis, demonstrated that the breadth of drug targets is expanding, suggesting a trend toward target diversity. Incorporating the cellular component of target proteins showed that the distribution of cellular location for target proteins,

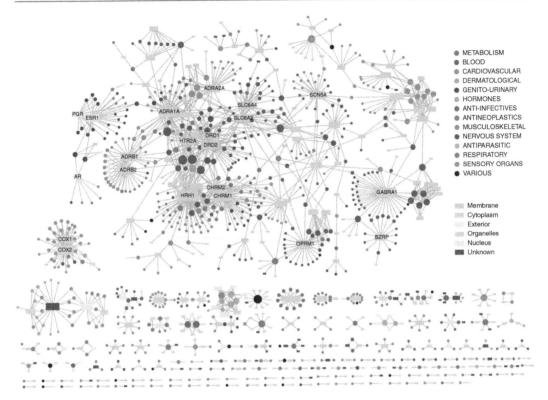

Fig. 25.9 Yildirim et al.'s Drug-Target network. Circles represent FDA-approved drugs and rectangles represent target proteins. Diseases are color-coded by anatomical system and protein targets according to their cellular location. Clusters of drugs associated with one target reflect the pharmaceutical industry's tendency to develop 'follow-on' drugs (Used with permission, Albert- Laszlo Barabasi)

previously nearly two-thirds membrane-associated, is becoming more diverse, better matching the known distribution for disease proteins. Finally, this group incorporated protein-protein interaction data to facilitate the study of network properties of drug target gene products. They looked for the shortest path between drug target genes and known disease genes for the disorder that drug was intended to treat and found that this number appears to be decreasing over time, suggesting that drugs are moving from a palliative approach (i.e. treating the symptoms and not the cause) to rational drug design (Yildirim et al. 2007).

25.4.5 Pharmacogenomics

Pharmacogenomics is the study of how genes and genetic variation influence drug response.

Drug response is a phenotype that can change in the context of genetic variation. The primary challenges for pharmacogenomics are to (1) identify the key genes that influence drug response, and (2) understand how specific variations in these genes modulate drug response. The term **pharmacogenetics** generally refers to drug-gene relationships that are dominated by a single gene, whereas the more general term refers to drug responses that result from a combination of interacting gene products. In this section, we use the word "gene" loosely to refer not only to the DNA coding regions for proteins and RNAs but also the protein and RNA products themselves. In many cases, the gene-drug relationship is really a relationship between the drug and the gene's protein product.

Pharmacogenomics is a prototypical TBI activity because it involves both clinical entities such as drugs, diseases, symptoms as well as molecular entities such as genes, proteins, DNA, RNA, small molecules and cellular processes. Because drug response is the key phenotype of interest, it is useful to review the basis for drug response. When a drug is administered, there are two distinct genetic "programs" that are relevant. The first is the **pharmacokinetic program** or PK, which describes the absorption, distribution, metabolism and excretion of the drug in the body. Genes implement this program (they encode transporter molecules that move the drug across membranes and the liver enzymes that transform the drug and prepare it for elimination via the kidney or liver) and variation in these genes can lead to a different blood level of drugs or a different timing of these levels. The second is the **pharmacodynamics program** or PD, which describes how the drug works, its protein target, and the mechanism by which it impacts cellular physiology in order to alleviate or cure disease. Genes are clearly also involved in this program (they encode the drug's primary targets, and the other proteins that interact with these targets to create the cellular response to the drug), and variation in these genes can lead to a different response to the drug. In short, PK is "what the body does to the drug", and PD is "what the drug does to the body." The goal of pharmacogenomics is to understand, for every drug, the key PK and PD genes, and which variation impacts their response. This will allow us to realize the vision of using the genome to choose drugs based on maximizing their likely efficacy and minimizing their likely toxicity.

25.4.5.1 Key Entities and Associated Data Resources

The key computational entities in pharmacogenomics are genes, drugs, and drug-related phenotypes (indications and effects, including side effects). There exist good informatics resources for all of these:

1. Genes. These are typically specified using the Human Genome Nomenclature Committee (HGNC) standard (Seal et al. 2011). They are typically situated within the genome as a series of exons that are spliced together to create a mature mRNA transcript that is then translated into a protein. This basic concept is made more complex because the strategy for splicing the exons may be variable (alternative splicing) thereby leading to several proteins, the RNA transcript may be degraded before it is translated, and the proteins may be modified after they are created. There are many resources on the web for gene information, and many aggregators of this information. These create a remarkably powerful network of associations that can be used creatively to make new associations. For example, Fig. 25.10 shows the links on a resource called PharmGKB (Pharmacogenomics Knowledge Base) for the drug VKORC1 and includes links to:

   - Entrez Gene: summarizes the sequence, variations, homologs across species
   - OMIM: provides information about rare genetic diseases involving this gene
   - UniProt: provides mapping information to relate this gene to its protein products
   - GeneCards: provides aggregated information about function, tissue localization, expression levels compound, literature references and more

2. Drugs and small molecules. The RxNorm standard for specifying drugs is a terminology standard (Parrish et al. 2006). DrugBank provides information about drugs, their targets, pharmacology, uses, and many other characteristics (Knox et al. 2011). There are only around 2,000 approved drugs in the United States, and so this list is relatively short. The list of small molecules that are not drugs is much larger and includes the contents of PubChem (Wang et al. 2009b, 2010), an NIH-built resource with basic information about the structure, function and literature on small molecules. The Zinc Database (Irwin and Shoichet 2005) lists 13 million commercially available compounds that can be purchased for use in research. Much drug information is contained within the "package insert" that is included in most drug packaging. This is information created by the drug company, but approved by the FDA. The FDA makes these available on a drug information

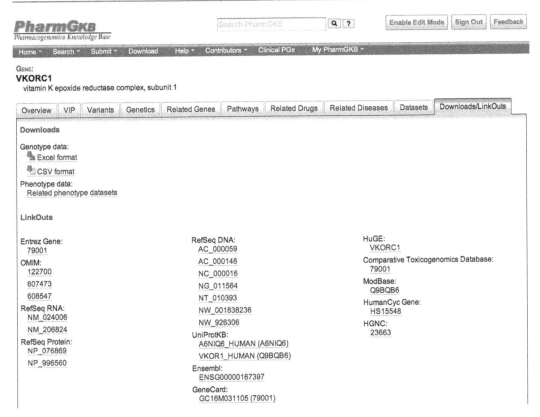

Fig. 25.10 PharmGKB gene pages are organized by tabs and the "Downloads/LinkOuts" tab shown here has links to many other sites with valuable information about human genes (Copyright PharmGKB, used with permission from PharmGKB and Stanford University)

site called DailyMed. For patients, the National Library of Medicine's MedlinePlus resource provides basic drug information as well.

3. <u>Drug indications and drug effects</u>. Drugs are used to treat particular diseases, and so controlled terminologies of drug indications and drug effects are useful for computational efforts. At the organism level, indications and effects are often diseases (diabetes is an indication) or side effects (hyperglycemia is a side effect). The UMLS and MeSH terminologies are often used to characterize such disease phenotypes (Bodenreider 2004). Of course, other disease terminologies such as SNOMED are also useful (Spackman et al. 1997a, b). For side effects, there are specialized terminologies, including the MedDRA terminology used by the FDA in adverse event reporting (MedDRA replaced a previous terminology

called COSTART), and the WHOART (World Health Organization Adverse Reactions Terminology) dictionary for adverse reactions (Brown et al. 1999; Alecu et al. 2006). The SIDER database (Kuhn et al. 2010) provides information mined from drug package inserts about drug indications and side effects. The Anatomic Therapeutic Chemical classification (ATC) from the World Health Organization provides a high level classification of drugs organized hierarchically by the anatomical location of target, the therapeutic category, the pharmacological subgroup, chemical subgroup and precise chemical substance (Miller and Britt 1995).

4. <u>Pharmacological properties of drugs</u>. There are resources on the web that provide molecular level assay data related to small molecules, including many drugs. The ChEMBLdb resource provides the ability to find targets,

binding affinities, inhibition concentrations and information about other drug-oriented assays (Overington 2009). BindingDB also provides binding affinities for small molecules and proteins (Liu et al. 2007).

5. Population-based data on drug effects. The FDA maintains information about all reports of adverse events in the FDA Adverse Event Reporting System (FDA AERS). These reports include demographic information, indications for treatment, drugs administered, side effects experienced and a summary of clinical outcomes. They are freely available at the FDA website. The Canadian equivalent system, also making data freely available, is available through the Health Canada website. These data are very noisy and have many confounding variables, but nonetheless can be useful for discovering "signals" suggesting dangerous side effects or drug-drug interactions (Tatonetti et al. 2011a).

6. Genomic data resources. Fundamental to understanding complex gene-drug interactions are high-throughput genomic measurements that provide information about these interactions. The primary sources of genomic data include:

   • Information about genetic variation. These are available through the HapMap projects which catalog variation over a wide variety of ethnic populations, in order to define the occurrence and frequency of common genetic variations (Rusk 2010). The 1,000 Genomes project is taking HapMap further to categorize the occurrence of more rare variations (changes in single DNA bases, as well as insertions/deletions, segmental duplications, and larger scale inversions and translocations) (Via et al. 2010). There are also resources about copy number variations.[9] dbSNP—**d**ata**b**ase of **S**ingle **N**ucleotide **P**olymorphisms is a publicly available catalog of genome variation. Contents primarily represent single nucleotide substitutions, but also include a small

number of other types of variation, for example microsatellite repeats and small insertions and deletions (Homerova et al. 2002). The PharmGKB resource specifically annotates genetic variations relevant to drug response (Altman 2007).

   • Gene expression information. The Gene Expression Omnibus contains an extremely large and diverse collection of high throughput gene expression experiments which allow one to evaluate whether a disease (or drug exposure) leads to up- or down-regulation of gene expression (Edgar et al. 2002). Particularly useful examples of gene expression for drug response are the Connectivity Map data set in which gene expression in response to 164 drugs was measured (Lamb et al. 2006). Similarly, the NCI 60 is a set of 60 cancer cell lines that have been exposed to hundreds of drugs in order to determine their sensitivity (Ross et al. 2000). Other efforts have looked at genetic variations that correlate with gene expression in order to associate these genomic regions with the function of the correlated genes (Gamazon et al. 2010; Nicolae et al. 2010).

   • Gene associations. The Genetic Association Database (Becker et al. 2004) provides curated information about the results of genetic association studies, including those studies that relate genetic variation to variation in drug response. The Human Genome Mutation Database (HGMD) also provides this information in a highly curated form (Stenson et al. 2009). dbGaP—**d**atabase of **G**enotypes **a**nd **P**henotypes is a resource to archive and distribute information about the interaction between genotype and phenotype (Mailman et al. 2007). The PharmGKB resource is devoted entirely to providing information about associations between human genetic variation and drug response phenotypes (Altman 2007).

   • Genetic pathways. Understanding drug action requires understanding the pathways and networks of drug action and drug

---

[9] http://humanparalogy.gs.washington.edu/structuralvariation/general/intro.html (Accessed 12/3/2012).

metabolism. The PharmGKB provides curated drug pathways for both drug action and drug metabolism, and has links to relevant external pathways created by the National Cancer Institute Pathway Interaction Database (Schaefer et al. 2009), Reactome (Joshi-Tope et al. 2005), and others.

25.4.5.2 TBI Applications in Pharmacogenomics

The network of data described above is a rich potential source of hypotheses about how genes combine to create drug response, as well as for predicting the particular consequences of genetic variation. This is still a new field, and there remain many opportunities for innovative use of these data. We highlight a few here to illustrate how integration of data can lead to novel discoveries.

GWAS to Discover Drug Response Genes

The most straightforward way to associate genes with drug response is to perform a genome-wide association study (GWAS) in which two groups are compared. One group (cases) has a drug response of interest (e.g., an adverse event in response to the drug or a particularly good response to it) and the other group (controls) does not have the drug response of interest. It is critical to ensure that the phenotype or response is carefully defined and measured. With each group, DNA is collected and typically 500,000 or 1,000,000 **SNPs** (single nucleotide polymorphisms) are measured using microarray technology. Then, for each SNP, an association is measured between the genotypes in cases and controls and the response of interest using a simple statistical test such as the chi-squared test. The SNPs that are most highly associated may represent regions of the genome that are involved in the response. These must be carefully vetted statistically, as there are many potential confounding variables. For example, it is important that the cases and controls are drawn from populations with similar ethnic origin, and that the significance remains after correcting for multiple testing. When one tests 500,000 or 1,000,000

hypotheses, adjustments such as Bonferoni correction (see Chap. 24) must be made in order to take into account the chance that an association is spurious. If the result is real, then the SNP may be used to identify nearby genes in the region that may be important for the drug response. For example, Shuldiner and colleagues were interested in the ability of the drug clopidogrel to protect patients from cardiovascular events. They found that a polymorphism RS12777823 was associated with a high-likelihood of having a cardiovascular event. They noted that this SNP was very close to the metabolizing enzyme CYP2C19, and in particular the "risk" allele for this SNP co-occurred with the CYP2C19*2 variant. Thus, they showed that CYP2C19 is important for the desired effect of clopidogrel, and found a variation of this gene that predicted poor response to the drug in affected patients (Shuldiner et al. 2009).

Mining the FDA AERS to Find Drug-drug Interactions

The FDA Adverse Events database associates multiple drugs with multiple diseases as indications as well as side effects. This database shows promise as a way to find new associations between single drugs and their side effects, as well as multiple drugs and their side effects. As mentioned above, the SIDER database is a "top down" database of side effects derived from the package label of drugs. Another approach to getting good lists of side effects is a more data-driven approach. One way to do this is to look for patterns of side effects associated with certain types of drugs using machine learning. For example, one may analyze the side effects of drugs that alter glucose in order to create a signature of the "typical" profile of side effects associated with a glucose-altering drug. Then, one can search a database of side effects (such as FDA AERS) for other drugs that match this profile. This was done by Tatonetti et al., who created a profile for glucose-altering drugs and found a set of 10 side effects either enriched or deficient (compared to background) in these drugs: hyperglycemia, diarrhea, hypoglycemia, and pain were higher than others, and paresthesia, nausea, pyrexia, abdominal pain, and anorexia were less likely than others (Tatonetti et al. 2011b). Using this pattern, more than 93 % of drugs that are known to alter glucose could be recovered. More interestingly, however, this pattern could be applied to patients on pairs of drugs to search for pairs that altered glucose. A highly correlated combination was the antidepressant paroxetine and the cholesterol medication pravastatin (Tatonetti et al. 2011b). In subsequent validation in three independent EHR systems, large increases in glucose were observed in patients on these two drugs, and in mouse studies of these two drugs, glucose was substantially increased. Thus, the adverse event patterns could be used to create patterns and detect new signals, not specifically reported in the database, but implied by the pattern of other side effects observed.

Mining the Literature to Build a Database of Gene-Drug Associations

Biomedical text can also be an important source of high quality information about the relationships among genes, drugs, and diseases (Garten et al. 2010). High fidelity natural language processing techniques (Chap. 8) can be used to extract information about gene-drug interactions. In some cases, the association between genes and drugs can be inferred simply by their co-occurrence in sentences (Garten and Altman 2009). In these cases, however, there can be many false positives due to sentences in which genes and drugs are mentioned, but are not actually interacting. A more precise method is based on careful parsing of sentences to find subjects and objects that are genes and drugs, and which are related by verbs that connect them (e.g. "CYP2D metabolizes codeine" has CYP2D as the subject, codeine as the object, and the verb "metabolizes" establishes their relationship) (Coulet et al. 2010). The rate of false positives is reduced in this case because more strict criteria are applied before claiming a relationship. These high quality interactions can be chained together to infer new knowledge. For example, drug-drug interactions often occur because two drugs share a common metabolizing gene and that gene becomes saturated in the presence of both drugs,

and cannot adequately metabolize both of them. Thus, the observations that "CYP2D metabolizes codeine" and "CYP2D metabolizes metoprolol" might be combined to infer that codeine and metoprolol have a potential drug-drug interaction. There are a large number of similar inferences that could be drawn about the relationships between genes, drugs and diseases given a high quality database of pairwise interactions drawn from the published literature. Of course, some pairwise interactions may be incorrect, and so evidence for interactions should be combined from several sources (including EMR validation, for example) and once predictions are made, they should be embraced only with skepticism.

Using Drug-Target Interactions to Predict New Ones

Another way to find new uses for old drugs is to predict interactions between drugs and new potential targets. Many drugs are designed to interact with a single target based on a detailed understanding of disease pathology. Once the drugs are administered, however, they may not bind only the original target, but they may unexpectedly have effects based on their binding to other targets. Most commonly, these "off target" effects are considered side effects and are avoided. In some cases, however, the "off target" effect may be beneficial in the setting of some other disease. Thus, both for explaining the molecular basis of side effects and for finding new molecular evidence for beneficial novel effects, it is useful to connect drugs to proteins. One way to do this is to build computational and visualization methods for docking a 3D representation of a small molecule into the 3D structure of a target protein. This can be very successful, and has led to the hypothesis that a Parkinson's disease drug may treat tuberculosis (Kinnings et al. 2009)! In that case, the 3D structure of a tuberculosis protein had a pocket that appeared to have high binding potential to a known Parkinson's disease drug, and thus the hypothesis arose that the Parkinson's drug might inhibit TB growth. These structure-based methods are powerful but limited because we have the 3D structure of only a subset of human proteins. Another approach, therefore, is based on looking for similarities in the list of drugs that have been shown experimentally to bind a protein. In this case, all that is needed are data from chemical assays showing which drugs bind which proteins. These are routinely collected in large screening experiments, and are available at the ChEMBL resource (Heikamp and Bajorath 2011), for example. Given two proteins with two lists of interacting drugs, we can compare the list of drugs to look for commonalities. If there are many commonalities between protein A and protein B, then one might conclude that the drugs that bind protein A may also bind protein B. This was the approach taken in the Similarity Ensemble Approach (SEA) where the list of drugs binding two proteins are compared using a measure of chemical similarity (Keiser et al. 2009). When the chemicals on the two lists are statistically similar (more than would be expected by chance), then the SEA method predicts cross-binding of ligands for the two structures. When this was applied to a large set of proteins, the authors found that the antidepressant fluoxetine (Prozac) had high potential binding to the beta-adrenergic receptor, and this was found experimentally to block the beta-1 receptor—demonstrating that Prozac is a type of beta-blocker!

Identifying Drug Targets Using Side-Effect Similarity

A critical goal in pharmacogenomics is to associate drugs with their target proteins (and thus their coding genes) in order to know where to look for variation that may affect drug response. Determining drug targets can involve a difficult and lengthy experimental program. Thus, it would be very useful to have computational methods for determining targets. One way to do this is to associate drugs to their side effects, and to look for side effect profiles that are similar across drugs. If one drug has a known target, and if another drug has a similar pattern of side effects, then the two drugs may share that target. This is based on the assumption that side effects arise from a few common mechanisms, and so genes involved in this mechanism may be targeted by multiple drugs or drug classes. In one study, Campillos et al. showed that they could create 1,018 drug-drug relationships based on shared side effects (Campillos et al. 2008). The side effects were taken from the SIDER database, and the drugs came from a list of 746 marketed drugs. Twenty of these drug-drug relationships were tested experimentally, and 13 of them were shown to bind common targets. Thus, a relatively straightforward association of drugs based on side effects allowed the definition of molecular targets. In related work, Hansen et al. showed that genes could be ranked by their likelihood of interacting with a drug based on looking at the degree of similarity between chemical structure and indications-of-use between the query drugs, and small molecules known to interact with the gene products and their close protein interaction neighbors (Hansen et al. 2009).

The examples we have discussed have several common features: they deal with the basic objects of diseases, drugs, and disease or adverse-event phenotypes; they integrate at least two sources of data to establish new relationships between these basic objects; and they connect clinical entities (drugs and diseases or adverse events) to molecular entities. Such examples represent only a small subset of the types of questions that can be asked with these valuable datasets. The key technical challenges are typically (1) finding adequate gold standards (Chap. 2) to evaluate the success of methods before applying them for novel discoveries; (2) understanding the sources of error and bias so that predictions are as reliable as possible; (3) designing careful statistical tests to ensure that the scoring and estimates of significance are accurate and useful (minimizing false positives, in particular); and (4) identifying and engaging experimental collaborators who can, when appropriate, test the predictions that are made in human or model systems. Recently, it has become clear that despite their shortcomings, EHRs can be extremely useful for initial validation of hypotheses about connections between drugs and adverse events (Tatonetti et al. 2011a). Gene-drug associations are typically tested in model systems with genes altered in order to reduce or eliminate their normal function, or by looking for covariation in human subjects.

25.4.5.3 Challenges for Pharmacogenomics

Target Expansion: Molecules to Networks

The emerging field of systems pharmacology is abandoning the view of "one drug, one target" and moving instead toward a view that "the network is the target." That is, the larger network of interacting genes is targeted by a drug at several points, and thus the systemic effects of drugs needs to be evaluated in order to understand better the molecular underpinnings of drug response. The challenges to systems pharmacology are similar to the challenges to the more general systems biology: defining the network topology and key players, creating ways to measure parameters, modeling nonlinear responses, and understanding how variation in the basic molecular players impacts the resulting phenotype—in this case drug response phenotypes.

Rare Variants

As whole genome sequencing increasingly provides data about rare variants, the paradigm of looking for common genetic variation that explains variation in drug response will need to be modified. There may be cases when variation in drug response is explained by multiple rare variants rather than one or a few common variants. This is particularly challenging because there will often be insufficient statistics to evaluate rare variants. In some cases, huge population-based studies may provide enough samples, but in other cases even these large cohorts will not have sufficient examples of any rare variant to allow statistical validation. In those cases, we will have to rely on computational techniques to assess the significance of very rare variations.

Computational Methods to Leverage Stem Cell-Based Model Systems

The rise in the use of stem cells will create opportunities for combining direct measurements of cellular response to drugs with systems models of response, whole genome variation, and epigenetic information. As we perfect methods for creating induced pluripotent stem cells and differentiating them into the target tissues, we will be in a position to measure the response to drugs directly on these cells, with identical genetic and perhaps epigenetic backgrounds. Computational methods for analyzing these responses and relating them to the expected response in the patients from whom these cells are derived will be a major challenge in the years ahead.

25.5 Basepairs to Bedside

Although the sequenced human genome has not been a panacea for human disease, it has enabled the beginnings of a new approach to human health and to the practice of **P4 (personalized, predictive, preventive and participatory) medicine** (Hood and Friend 2011). As the price of genomic sequencing falls and as our knowledge regarding the meaning of genomic variation increases, genotypic data is poised to become a standard component of a person's medical record. In this section we describe the translational path of genomics, from sequencing in the lab to clinical relevance for individuals.

25.5.1 Whole Genome Sequencing

25.5.1.1 Technologic Advances

The DNA-probe approach to genotyping, described in Chap. 24, may be compared to looking for one's car keys under the proverbial street lamp. That is, the technology shines the light on a certain portion of the genetic landscape, and that is where we look. Which SNPs are included on a chip is determined in large part by which SNPs have been detected in the past, for example through the HapMap project (Kang et al. 2006). A number of new associations have been found in this way, whether because the SNPs themselves were of interest, or due to genetic linkage—the tendency for alleles located close to one another on a chromosome to be inherited together. However, more recent findings have demonstrated that the concept of "common disease-common variant" is flawed (Zhu et al. 2011). Indeed, there has been some disappointment in the extent to which GWAS has been able to explain common diseases with known genetic components

(Manolio et al. 2009). Whole genome or, in some cases, whole exome sequencing allows researchers to identify rare variants (i.e., those with a minor allele frequency of <1 %) that account for genetic disease. Advances in sequencing technologies (e.g., "**nextgen**" **sequencing**, see Chap. 24) and the corresponding decrease in cost, make genome-scale sequencing increasingly feasible in translational research and even in clinical care.

25.5.1.2 Whole Genome Versus Exome

Even with recent advances in genome sequencing technology, the cost to sequence a full genome at a rate of coverage that enables the identification of novel SNPs is still significant, on the order of thousands of dollars. However, recall that only about 1 % of the genome actually codes for proteins and 85 % of known disease-causing mutations with large effects occur in proteins (Choi et al. 2009). One way to further decrease the time and cost of sequencing is to look at only those stretches that code for actual proteins. This can be justified because most variants known to underlie Mendelian disorders disrupt protein-coding sequences. Of course, this approach will miss causal variations if they exist in the other 99 % of the genome. Moreover, a recent cluster of publications from the ENCODE (**Enc**yclopedia **of DNA E**lements) Consortium asserts assignment of biochemical function for 80 % of the genome (Dunham et al. 2012). Some additional components, such as regulatory regions or splice acceptor and donor sites may be included as well to increase sensitivity without incurring significant additional cost. Exome sequencing in a small number of individuals has been used to identify the causal variant for rare diseases such as Miller's syndrome, a multiple malformation disorder (Ng et al. 2010), and Proteus syndrome, a disorder causing the overgrowth of tissues and organs, thought to have afflicted the 19th century Englishman known as *The Elephant Man* (Lindhurst et al. 2011).

25.5.1.3 Publicly Available Resources

The genomics community has generally been ahead of the curve with respect to data sharing. According to the *Policy for Sharing of Data*

Obtained in NIH Supported or Conducted Genome-Wide Association Studies (GWAS),[10] genotypic data must be deposited to the NIH database of Genotypes and Phenotypes (dbGaP). Genomic variation data is also available through a number of other online resources—see Sect. 24.4.5 and (Sherry et al. 2001; WTCCC 2007; Altshuler et al. 2010a). In 2008, researchers demonstrated that the presence of a single genome within a complex mixture of DNA samples could be ascertained (Homer et al. 2008). This caused both NIH and the Wellcome Trust[11] to limit access not only to individual genomes, but to aggregate genomic information as well. (Note that the ability to determine the presence or absence of an individual's DNA in a heterogeneous sample presupposes the availability of detailed genomic information about the individual in question.) These actions prompted responses that ranged from "too little, too late" to "a heavy-handed bureaucratic response to a practically minimal risk that will unnecessarily inhibit scientific research" (Church et al. 2009). Current NIH policy allows investigators to submit a data access request to be reviewed by an NIH Data Access Committee. Access to data is granted once a Data Use Certification is co-signed both by the investigator and the appropriate official[s] at the investigator's affiliated institution.[12] Additional online genomic resources include TCGA (**T**he **C**ancer **G**enome **A**tlas) and WTCCC (**W**ellcome **T**rust **C**ase **C**ontrol **C**onsortium). TCGA is a joint effort of the National Cancer Institute (NCI) and the National Human Genome Research Institute (NHGRI) to accelerate understanding of the molecular basis for cancer through application of genomic technologies, including genome sequencing.[13] The WTCCC, established in 2005, comprises 50 research groups across the UK who have performed a series of genome-wide

---

[10] http://grants.nih.gov/grants/guide/notice-files/NOT-OD-07-088.html (Accessed 12/6/2012).

[11] http://www.wellcome.ac.uk/ (Accessed 12/6/2012).

[12] http://grants.nih.gov/grants/guide/notice-files/NOT-OD-07-088.html (Accessed 12/6/2012).

[13] http://cancergenome.nih.gov/ (Accessed 12/6/2012).

association studies and made the data available through application to a Consortium Data Access Committee.[14]

25.5.2 Here Are Some Human Beings

Promising though genomic medicine may be, much remains to be worked out technically, scientifically, and from the ELSI (ethical, legal, and social implications) perspective (see Chap. 10). Some notable pilot projects have been embarked upon in order to catalyze progress in all of these areas. Craig Venter was the first person to have his complete genome published in 2007. Since then, a number of human genomes have been sequenced, and some of those have been made available in the public domain. The question becomes: now what? What can any given individual learn from his or her complete genomic sequence? What does an individual *want* to learn, or not want to learn, as the case may be? The only reliable way to answer these questions is with empirical input.

George Church is a pioneer in genomic sequencing, inventor of the Polonator sequencer, and founder of personal genome sequencing company Knome. In 2005, Church started the Personal Genome Project (PGP), ultimately aiming to sequence 100,000 individuals in order to advance understanding of how genes contribute, along with environment, to human traits. The project "hopes to make personal genome sequencing more affordable, accessible, and useful for humankind."[15] A vanguard of ten volunteers—the PGP-10—were selected to have their genomes sequenced. This endeavor differs from other projects in one crucial way: in addition to making the sequence data publicly available, complete phenotypic data, including personal and health information, family history, and even name and photographs would be shared as well. This was a departure for the type of projects the NIH

typically funds and supports. Generally, informed consent includes information on how the research team plans to secure privacy and confidentiality for the subject. In this case, sharing of personal data was part of the protocol itself. The first set of integrated data from this group was made available in October 2008.

Making this type of data both publicly available and personally identifiable was stepping out into socio-scientific *terra incognita*, generating some worry that it could affect health care, employment, insurance, and more. In 2008, the Genetic Information Nondiscrimination Act (GINA) was signed into law, but its scope is limited to employment and health care insurance. It does not address life, disability, or long term care insurance (Hudson et al. 2008). Though rare, there are a few notorious examples of lawsuits where employers performed genetic and health-related testing on employees without their consent (Angrist 2010), and though unlikely, the PGP warns prospective participants that their DNA could be artificially synthesized and planted at a crime scene (Lunshof et al. 2010). As much as the PGP has pushed the boundaries and helped to advance the technology, data management, and clinical issues involved with personal genomes, and will continue to do so, it also serves as a weather balloon from the ELSI perspective, generating empirical data on sociological atmosphere, ethical pressures, and legal winds of change (see Chap. 10 for additional discussion on these points).

Misha Angrist, a bioethicist at Duke University, is PGP Participant #4. As documented in his book *Here Is a Human Being: At the Dawn of Personal Genomics*, the early sequencing was slow going, the technology took time to work out the kinks, and the preliminary results were underwhelming even to the individuals who had been sequenced (Angrist 2010). The infrastructure is not yet in place to empower someone with his complete genomic profile to do much with that information. Angrist describes his own attempts to make use of tools for genomic interpretation—SNPedia,[16] Sequence Variant Analyzer (Ge et al.

---

[14] https://www.wtccc.org.uk/index.shtml (Accessed 12/6/2012).

[15] http://www.personalgenomes.org/ (Accessed 12/6/2012).

[16] http://www.snpedia.com/index.php/SNPedia (Accessed 12/6/2012).

2011), and the Church lab's open source Trait-o-Matic[17]—which he compares to the dial-up days of the internet. Out of all of the variants carried by the PGP10, only one was deemed serious. Steven Pinker carried a mutation for MYL2, which had been shown in some cases to cause hypertrophic cardiomyopathy (Angrist 2010). More importantly, however, the project has created a publicly available, integrated resource for genomic, environmental, and trait (GET) data (Lunshof et al. 2010) and an empirical test bed for tackling the ELSI issues brought to bear by such a resource.

As another proof of concept, collaborators at Stanford and Harvard did a complete sequencing, analysis, and genetic counseling for a 40-year-old male with family history of sudden death from cardiac arrest (Ashley et al. 2010). The goal was to determine how whole genome sequencing would translate to clinical application. The patient was found to have increased risk for myocardial infarction, type 2 diabetes, and some cancers. While most of the findings were not actionable, the patient had both increased risk for cardiovascular disease and genetic disposition to benefit from the use of statins and aspirin. Despite this, just over a year after publication, the patient maintained that he had "not been convinced that statins or aspirin would have enough beneficial effect relative to their risks," and had not therefore changed his pharmaceutical behavior (Quake 2011).

Just over a year after the Quake profile, the same group published their findings from performing whole exome sequencing on the first healthy nuclear family (Dewey et al. 2011). They generated an ethnically concordant reference sequence (i.e. a reference sequence based on a European population, reflecting the European background of the family in question), which enabled increased accuracy for rare mutations. Findings included high resolution inference of sites of recombination (i.e., where the parents' chromosomes "cross over" during meiosis), and a novel approach to HLA (Human Leukocyte Antigen) typing—important for risk in a number of diseases, particularly autoimmune disorders. For the family in question, they were able to determine that the father had passed down to his daughter a mutation for Factor V Leiden that poses increased risk for blood clotting. This is actionable information for women as the Factor V mutation is a contraindication for estrogen-based birth control pills (Singer 2011), and inherited thrombophilia is a known risk factor for pregnancy outcomes (Tenenbaum et al. 2012). (Note that Factor V mutations are also included in chip-based genotyping services, so whole genome sequencing was not the key enabling technology in this case.)

One key item reported in the paper by Ashley et al. was the fact that, in the absence of a centrally curated resource of all rare and disease-associated variants, the authors spent *hundreds of hours* reviewing databases. Moreover, the work was a collaborative effort among a number of highly trained experts in clinical genetics, genetic counseling, bioinformatics, internal medicine, pharmacogenomics, etc. (Ormond et al. 2010). Clearly new tools, automation, and infrastructure, as well as a whole new paradigm in genetic counseling, will be required to make incorporation of genomic data into health care feasible for the population at large.

25.5.2.1 Sequencing Early in Life

One crucial complication in the search for genomic explanations for any given disease or phenotype is the impact of environmental interactions. Over time, every person on earth is exposed to environmental factors that may differ based not only on a factory that disposes of industrial waste near a drinking water supply or the traffic on the street they grew up on, but also by the foods they eat, the climates in which they live, and the infections they have harbored. Those external variables, hard to control for and sometimes even to know, can have major effects on the downstream products and activities of one's genomic fingerprint. Early in life, however, those effects are less pronounced. Of course, the impact of the *in-utero* environment on the well-being of the developing fetus is well established. But a

---

[17] https://github.com/xwu/trait-o-matic/wiki (Accessed 12/19/2012).

genetic defect is much more likely to be the cause in a newborn with an unidentified disease than in an adult patient who has undergone a lifetime of environmental insults. In this vein, a number of initiatives have been established across the US to offer clinical sequencing services for young patients, including programs at Children's Hospital of Philadelphia, Duke University, Partners Health care, and the Baylor College of Medicine, and the Medical College of Wisconsin. More controversial on paper, and not yet being performed in practice, is pre-natal genome sequencing. Ethicists are just beginning to explore the potential implications of this possible direction (Donley et al. 2012).

Addressing the time and resources needed to perform genome interpretation, one striking success story was achieved at Children's Mercy Hospitals and Clinics in Kansas City, MO (Saunders et al. 2012). Investigators used an Illumina HiSeq 2500 machine and an internally-developed automated analysis pipeline to perform whole-genome sequencing and make a differential diagnosis for genetic disorders in under 50 h. The diagnoses in question are among the ~3,500 known monogenetic disorders that have been characterized. In this case, WGS is not being used to identify novel, previously unknown mutations. Rather, it is shortening to just over 2 days the family's agonizing waiting time that would traditionally take 4–6 weeks as a battery of tests were performed sequentially.

We offer one final example in which genome sequencing was used as a last resort in a medical odyssey to identify the cause of a mysterious bowel condition in a 4-year-old boy named Nicholas Volker (Worthey et al. 2011). Having ruled out every diagnosis they could conceive of, doctors resorted to exome sequencing, leading to the identification of 16,124 mutations, of which 1,527 were novel. A causal mutation was discovered in the gene XIAP. This gene was already known to play a role in XLP, or X-linked lymphoproliferative syndrome and retrospective review showed that colitis had been observed in 2 XLP patients in the past. Based on these findings, a cord blood transplant was performed, and 2 years later, Nic's intestinal issues have not

returned. News coverage of this story by the Milwaukee Journal Sentinel was awarded a Pulitzer Prize for explanatory reporting.[18]

25.5.3   Direct to Consumer Genetics

In the wake of the human genome project and the commoditization of genotypic data, a number of companies were founded to provide consumers with their own genetic information directly. These direct-to-consumer (DTC) genomic companies began making the services broadly available when deCODE genetics launched the deCODEme service in November 2007, followed a few days later by 23andMe, with the slogan "Genetics just got personal. Don't worry. We're here to help" (Davies 2008). Navigenics was launched the following spring. These companies offered consumers the opportunity to provide a saliva specimen or buccal swab through the mail, and in exchange to receive genotypic information for a range of known genetic markers. Different companies emphasized different aspects of genetic testing. Navigenics focused on known disease risk markers, while 23andMe was much broader, including disease markers but also ancestry information and "recreational" genetic information, for example earwax type and the ability to smell a distinct odor in urine after eating asparagus. Navigenics offered free genetic counseling as part of their service, while 23andMe and deCODEme provided referrals to genetic counselors. A study of concordance between these three services found >99.6 % agreement among them, but in some cases the predicted relative risks differed in magnitude or even direction (Imai et al. 2011). This disagreement is likely due to differences in the specific SNPs and the reference population used to calculate risk.

From the companies' perspectives, their customers offer a rich resource of genomic data for potential research and data mining. 23andMe created a research initiative called 23andWe through which they enlist customers as "collaborators,

---

[18] http://www.jsonline.com/news/milwaukee/120091754. html (Accessed 12/21/12).

advisers and participants."[19] They invite users to fill out questionnaires and then use the phenotypic information to perform genome-wide analysis studies. This approach enabled researchers at the company to replicate a number of known associations, and to discover a number of novel associations, recreational though they may be, for curly hair, freckling, sunlight-induced sneezing, and the ability to smell a metabolite in urine after eating asparagus (Sobradillo et al. 2011). deCODE, purchased by Amgen in 2012, boasts a large number of medically significant genetic discoveries to have come out of their volunteer registry of 140,000 Icelanders, more than half of the adult population of the country.[20] Navigenics was purchased by Life Technologies in 2012 and no longer offers their Health Compass genetic testing service.

25.5.3.1 Ethical, Legal, and Social Issues (ELSI)

Unknown Unknowns

In a companion article to the Quake profile, it was asserted that consent for a process in which the risks of knowledge gained are not wholly understood is more complex than for simple genetic testing. People have trouble interpreting probabilities. Patients must be advised that they may find out things they did not want to know about. The eminent scientist James Watson made a point of requesting that his ApoE status be redacted from the release of his full genome because he did not want to know if he was at risk. His grandmother had died of Alzheimer's at 83, and he did not want to worry that every subsequent memory lapse marked the onset of dementia (Angrist 2010). Statistics predict that any given patient will find out he is a carrier for *some* lethal autosomal recessive disease. Illness aside, the average global non-paternity rate has, astoundingly, been estimated to be as high as 10 % (Olson 2007). All of this information could

also have implications for the patient's children, present or future, and for other family members. Patients, this group concluded, must have access to trained professionals to provide answers to their questions, where answers exist. This will be difficult, lengthy, and expensive, but not to do it would undermine the consent process (Ormond et al. 2010).

ELSI and the Genomic Consumer

Direct to consumer genetic testing, and pursuit of genomic medicine more generally, raise a number of ethical, legal, and social issues (see also Chap. 10). Some worry that people are ill-equipped to process the results of these tests. But it is not clear that a paternalistic approach is a better alternative; there was a time when it was considered acceptable for a doctor not to disclose a cancer diagnosis to the patient himself (Novack et al. 1979). In addition, new discoveries are being made all the time—what are the obligations to follow up if something new (and dire? and actionable?) is discovered about a given subject? Other questions include whether enough is known for the results to be of any practical use, whether the service should be provided outside of the context of a relationship with a clinical caregiver, and whether results could have detrimental effects on a person's ability to secure health insurance. Some states have banned the services, others have made stipulations requiring clinician involvement and **CLIA certification** for the labs that handle the samples and process the results.[21]

Although knowing the "parts list" for the human genome is an important step, much remains to be understood about how genes factor into human health and disease. For most diseases, the environment plays as much, if not more, of a role as a person's DNA. Aside from some notable, deterministic exceptions such as Huntington's disease, most known risk alleles confer fairly low odds ratios unto themselves (see Chap. 3), making an individual, for example, approximately 1.1

[19] http://spittoon.23andme.com/2008/12/17/turning-research-participants-into-research-partners/ (Accessed 12/6/2012).

[20] http://www.decode.com/research/ (Accessed 12/6/2012).

[21] http://www.genomeweb.com/dxpgx/will-other-states-follow-ny-calif-taking-dtc-genetic-testing-firms (Accessed 12/6/2012).

times as likely as the average individual to develop a given condition. Even when ratios are as high as, say, twofold, it is of dubious actual utility to know that based on one's genotype, the odds of being diagnosed with Crohn's disease went from 0.5 in 100 to 1 in 100.

For certain disease markers, such as Alzheimer's or BRCA1 and BRCA2, it was, and largely still is, unknown what impact negative results might have on a customer's mental and emotion well-being. Some studies have shown that while a person experiences negative emotions immediately in the wake of learning the bad news, over a time period of months there is no significant difference in anxiety, depression, or test-related distress (Green et al. 2009). In any case, DTC genetics companies' websites must provide the ability to view sensitive results while protecting the customer from stumbling on these findings unintentionally. 23andMe, as an example, has spent considerable resources on the design of a user-friendly interface through which to present an individual's "health reports," or their individual genotype for markers that have been characterized through reliable, established research methods. Along with a text explanation, these health reports give a graphical depiction of a person's relative risk. Figure 25.11 shows one such graphic for an individual's risk of venous thromboembolism based on three specific clotting markers as well as the individual's sex and ethnicity. For sensitive results such as BRCA1 and 2, and markers for Alzheimer's and Parkinson's disease, the information is initially "locked." Users must explicitly click through an additional screen to confirm that they truly want to know genotype and relative risk for that trait.

Rulings and Regulations

From a regulatory perspective, it was not (and to some degree is still not) clear whether these services qualify as medical devices as defined by the FDA, and are therefore subject to regulation by the Agency. The DTC testing landscape is still rapidly evolving, and will continue to do so for the foreseeable future. Logistically, a prospective customer typically registers on the DTC compa-

ny's website and a sample collection kit is sent in the mail, though 23andMe's kit is also available for purchase through Amazon.com. In May 2010, Pathway Genomics and Walgreens announced a plan to sell these kits in Walgreens drugstores, but the FDA sent a letter to Pathway Genomics indicating their belief that the company's genomic report qualified as medical device (Bradley et al. 2011) and as such required FDA approval. Plans to sell the saliva collection container in brick-and-mortar stores were put on hold until the regulatory issues could be resolved, or at least addressed.

Another high profile legal issue is the case of *Assoc. for Molecular Pathology v. Myriad Genetics, Inc.*, et al., regarding Myriad's patent on the BRCA1 and BRCA2 genes, which are included in 23 and Me's offerings,[22] and more generally whether genes should be patentable at all. In 2011, a federal appeals court overturned a lower court in the case of and found that genes can, in fact, be patented (Pollack 2011). This ruling was upheld in a court of appeals in 2012, however, in 2013, the Supreme Court partially overturned that ruling and found that isolated genomic DNA (gDNA) is not patent-eligible, but cDNA is. Disappointingly, this ruling did not do much to reduce ambiguity around these issues.

Clinical Training

Another group that is affected by DTC genetic testing is primary care physicians. Most doctors have only a basic level of training in genetics, and are ill-equipped to answer in-depth questions from patients who bring to an appointment printouts of their results from these services (Frueh and Gurwitz 2004). More knowledge is required, in addition to training and tools, before family care providers, internists, and even specialists, are prepared to incorporate genomic information into their clinical practice (Chan and Ginsburg 2011; Ormond et al. 2010).

---

[22] https://www.23andme.com/health/BRCA-Cancer/ (Accessed 12/19/12).

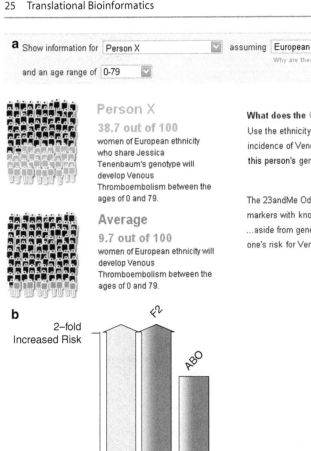

(**a**) *Colored figures* represent the number of people on average out of 100 who are likely to develop venous thromboembolism over the course of a lifetime. *Green figures* represent the individual's personal reported risk; *blue*

figures represent the average risk for females of European descent. (Accompanying text has been shortened for clarity.) (**b**) The individual's relative risk for each of three reported markers: factor V, factor 2, and ABO. (Specific values are displayed on the website when the user hovers the mouse over the *colored bars*)

25.6   Challenges and Future Directions

TBI as a discipline is in an exciting and dynamic phase—so much so that a number of items included in this chapter were announced or published during its writing and it is inevitable that new developments will have occurred by the time it is being read. Though challenges remain, the field is poised to become an increasingly crucial element of biomedical research and clinical practice. We conclude this chapter with a discussion of future directions and key challenges for this burgeoning discipline.

25.6.1   Expansion of Data Types

Genomic data are already being used to guide clinical care. Genomic data themselves are relatively straightforward in that an individual's genome is relatively static, and through the intrinsic physical properties of ribonucleic acids and the transcriptional process, DNA and RNA are relatively easy to capture, observe, and quantify. Proteins and metabolites are more challenging in this regard. Proteomic and metabolomic methodologies have primarily centered around isotopic labeling, but more recent approaches enable unbiased label-free identification and even quantification (Du et al. 2008; Wishart 2011). Identification of metabolites associated with disease has already enabled enzymatic drug targeting in diabetes, obesity, cardiovascular disease, and cancer, among other conditions (Chan and Ginsburg 2011). We expect that as proteomics and metabolomics standards and technologies continue to mature, they will play an increasingly significant role in translational research and practice.

The role of epigenetics needs to be understood more fully. It is clear that the environment can induce changes in the packaging and labeling of DNA. These environmental cues can include lifetime exposures to toxins, viruses, bacteria and nutritional compounds as well as drug exposures. Understanding the ways in which these epigenetic modifications affect phenotype is in its infancy, and so we must understand how to measure these effects, and then compute with them. The human microbiome is also an active area for translational research. **Metagenomics**, or genomics across organisms derived from an environmental sample, may be applied to the hundreds of bacterial species that make up the gut flora of every human being (Bruls and Weissenbach 2011). Finally, as standards are developed and clinicians and researchers see the value to be gained from structured data collection through studies such as The National Children's Study (Landrigan et al. 2006), structured environmental data is likely to be increasingly available to complete the picture for gene-environment interactions (Schwartz and Collins 2007).

25.6.2   Changes for Medical Training, Practice, and Support

Clinicians will need enhanced training in genetics and other areas described above. Curricular components relating to genetics, pharmacogenomics, statistics, and data standards will be increasingly important. Expertise in these fields will also need to be supplemented by an expanded workforce of genetic counselors. Increasingly, therapies will require accompanying diagnostic tests. As the opportunities for use of genomic data in clinical care continue to advance, it will become increasingly important to incorporate this information into both the electronic health record and into machine readable clinical care guidelines for clinical decision support. This in turn will require new standards to capture genomic findings, and new decision support tools to enable clinicians to incorporate this ever-increasing amount of information into their therapeutic decision making processes (Hoffman 2007). Clearly a number of standards exist in this space. The key will be in educating prospective users and in enforcing adoption. This applies to the full translational spectrum, from annotation of experimentally generated datasets to a common format for the exchange of clinically relevant omic data between EHR systems.

25.7 Conclusions

As the cost of data generation and storage continues to decrease, and the methods for data analysis and interpretation continue to advance, TBI is poised to be a key enabler of the vision for P4 medicine. One can imagine a day when every newborn has his or her genome sequenced and this information becomes a part of the medical record, much as blood type is recorded today. The biggest challenges to achieving this vision are likely not to be technical ones, but rather ethical, legal, and economic in nature (Schadt 2012). Society must strike a balance between privacy protection and facilitating progress in biomedical research. Legal issues will need to be worked out around direct-to-consumer genetic testing, preventing genetic discrimination, gene patenting, and many other such issues. Return on investment will need to be established through economic analysis combined with comparative effectiveness research (see Chaps. 11 and 26). Ultimately, someone will have to pay for these accompanying diagnostic tests. Major change is unlikely until an organization like the Center for Medicare and Medicaid Services (CMS) changes its policies. For example, CMS coverage for the genetic test to guide warfarin dosing is currently conditional upon it being ordered as part of a research protocol (Meckley and Neumann 2010). TBI will continue to play a key role in transforming these types of scientific discoveries into improvements in human health.

Suggested Readings

Altman, R. B., & Miller, K. S. (2011). 2010 translational bioinformatics year in review. *Journal of the American Medical Informatics Association, 18*, 358–366. This article summarizes Dr. Altman's third annual "year in review" presentation delivered at the 2010 AMIA Joint Summits on Translational Science in San Francisco.

Angrist, M. (2010). *Here is a human being: at the dawn of personal genomics*. New York: Harper. This text is written by one of the Personal Genome Project's first subjects, describing the project, the cohort, and the experience. It also gives a good overview of the background of the project and a number of ethical, legal, and social issues that it raises.

Capriotti, E., Nehrt, N. L., Kann, M. G., & Bromberg, Y. (2012 July). Bioinformatics for personal genome interpretation. *Briefings in Bioinformatics, 13*(4), 495–512. The authors of this review summarize key databases and bioinformatics tools that have been developed in recent years to aid in the intepretation of genomic variance. Resources covered include databases of variants, genotype/phenotype annotation databases, tools for gene prioritization and tools for interpretation of single nucleotide variants.

Davies, K. (2010). *The $1000 genome: The revolution in DNA sequencing and the new era of personalized medicine*. New York: Free Press. This text, written by the editor of BioIT World magazine, documents the characters, events, and issues in the race to achieve the $1000 Genome.

Hastie, T., Tibshirani, R., & Friedman, J. H. (2009). *The elements of statistical learning : data mining, inference, and prediction*. New York: Springer. A useful primer on the statistical concepts underlying machine learning approaches to biomarker discovery.

Kann, M.G, & Lewitter, F., (Eds.). (2012). *Translational bioinformatics*. PLOS Computational Biology Collections eBook. This eBook represents both the first "textbook" devoted entirely to TBI, and the first online, open access textbook from PLOS. In addition to many of the topics covered in this chapter, the collection includes chapters on related topics such as cancer genome analysis, micribiome analysis, structural variation, and protein interactions in disease.

Masys, D. R., Jarvik, G. P., Abernethy, N. F., Anderson, N. R., Papanicolaou, G. J., Paltoo, D. N., Hoffman, M. A., Kohane, I. S., & Levy, H. P. (2012). Technical desiderata for the integration of genomic data into electronic health records. *Journal of Biomedical Informatics, 45*(3), 419–422. The authors describe the characteristics of biomolecular data that differentiate it from other EHR data, enumerate a set of technical desiderata for management of biomolecular data in clinical settings (e.g., separation of molecular data observations from clinical interpretation, lossless data compression, support for readability by both humans and machines), and propose a technical approach to its representation.

Payne P.R.O., Sarkar, I.N., Embi, P.J., & Kahn M. (2011, December). *Journal of Biomedical Informatics, 44*(Suppl 1), S1–S108. This supplement to JBI's 44th volume highlights the top papers from the 2011 AMIA Joint Summits on Translational Science. An editorial by N. Sarkar, 2011 TBI scientific program committee chair, gives an overview of the conference contents, and provides context for the papers selected to appear in this issue.

Sarkar, I. N., & Payne, P. R. O. (2011, December). The joint summits on translational science: crossing the translational chasm. *Journal of Biomedical Informatics, 44*(Suppl 1), S1–2. This editorial discusses the spectrum of biomedical informatics, from biology to medicine, in the context of the NIH Roadmap and the Clinical and Translational Science Award program. It gives the history of the AMIA Joint Summits on Translational Science, and explains the emergence of TBI and CRI as disciplines unto themselves, intended to address the same issues that motivated those initiatives- namely translating scientific discoveries into meaningful changes in health care delivery.

Sarkar, I. N., Butte, A. J., Lussier, Y. A., Tarczy-Hornoch, P., & Ohno-Machado, L. (2011). Translational bioinformatics: linking knowledge across biological and clinical realms. *Journal of the American Medical Informatics Association, 18*, 354–357. The authors present the field of TBI in the context of successes from bioinformatics and health informatics.

Questions for Discussion

1. Should DTC genetic testing be regulated by the FDA?
2. Should genes be patentable?
3. Are there sufficient legal protections in place to prevent discrimination based on genomic information? If not, what regulations are needed?
4. Are we headed toward full disclosure of genomic information?
5. What are some reasons a researcher might not want to share research data? Should they be required to share? If so, under what circumstances (e.g., 6 months after first publication)?
6. For novel analyses applied to complex, high-dimensional datasets, should there be new guidelines in place to prevent reporting erroneous results through user error or data fraud? Why or why not?
7. What are the major barriers to incorporating the benefits of personalized medicine fully into standard practice?

Clinical Research Informatics

26

Philip R.O. Payne, Peter J. Embi, and James J. Cimino

After reading this chapter, you should know the answers to these questions:

- What is clinical research and what factors influence the design of clinical studies?
- What are the types of information needs inherent to clinical research and how can those information needs be stratified by research project phase or activity?
- What types of information systems can be used to address or satisfy the information needs of clinical research teams?
- How can multi-purpose platforms, such as electronic health record (EHR) systems (see Chap. 12), be leveraged to enable clinical research programs?
- What is the role of a clinical trial management system (CTMS) for supporting and enabling clinical research, and what types of functionality are common to such systems?
- What is the role of standards in supporting interoperability across and between actors and entities involved in clinical research activities?
- What are current and future CRI research "grand challenges" and how will they optimize or otherwise alter the conduct of clinical research?
- How does clinical research informatics relate to the field of Biomedical Informatics and the broader clinical and translational science continuum?

26.1 Introduction

The conduct of clinical research is fundamental to the generation of evidence that can in turn facilitate improvements in human health. However, the design, execution, and analysis of clinical research is an inherently complex information- and resource-intensive endeavor, involving a broad variety of stakeholders, workflows, processes, data types, and computational resources. At the intersection point between biomedical informatics and clinical research, a robust and growing sub-discipline of informatics has emerged, which for the remainder of this chapter we will refer to as **clinical research informatics (CRI)** (Embi and Payne 2009; Payne et al. 2005). Numerous reports have shown that innovations and best practices generated by

P.R.O. Payne, PhD, FACMI (✉)
Department of Biomedical Informatics,
The Ohio State University Wexner Medical Center,
3190 Graves Hall, 333 West 10th Avenue, Columbus,
OH, 43210, USA
e-mail: philip.payne@osumc.edu

P.J. Embi, MD, MS
Departments of Biomedical Informatics and Internal
Medicine, The Ohio State University Wexner Medical
Center, 3190 Graves Hall, 333 West 10th Avenue,
Columbus, OH, 43210, USA
e-mail: peter.embi@osumc.edu

J.J. Cimino, MD
Laboratory for Informatics Development, NIH
Clinical Center, 10 Center Drive, Room 6-2551,
Bethesda, MA, 20892, USA
e-mail: ciminoj@mail.nih.gov

E.H. Shortliffe, J.J. Cimino (eds.), *Biomedical Informatics*,
DOI 10.1007/978-1-4471-4474-8_26, © Springer-Verlag London 2014

the CRI community have contributed to improvements in the quality, efficiency, and expediency of clinical research (Chung et al. 2006; Payne et al. 2005; Sung et al. 2003). Such benefits can be situated in a full spectrum of contexts that extends from the activities of individual clinical investigators to the operations of multi-center research consortia that involve geographically and temporally distributed participants.

Given the recognition of CRI as a distinct and increasingly important sub-discipline of biomedical informatics, it is imperative that a common basis for defining and understanding CRI science and practice be established. Such a foundation must by necessity include explicit linkages to the major challenges and opportunities associated with the planning, conduct, and evaluation of clinical research programs. To provide a common frame of reference for the remainder of this chapter, we will use the National Institutes of Health (NIH) definition of clinical research :[1]

> *Clinical Research* involves, "*the range of studies and trials in human subjects that fall into the three sub-categories*: (1) *Patient-oriented research*: *Research conducted with human subjects (or on material of human origin such as tissues, specimens and cognitive phenomena) for which an investigator (or colleague) directly interacts with human subjects. Patient-oriented research includes*: (*a*) *mechanisms of human disease*; (*b*) *therapeutic interventions*; (*c*) *clinical trial*; *and* (*d*) *development of new technologies*. (2) *Epidemiologic and behavioral studies*. (3) *Outcomes research and health services research*."

A lack of sufficient information technology (IT) and applied biomedical informatics tools, expertise and methods, as well as a reliance on

workflows largely defined by historical precedent rather than optimal operational strategies, account for significant impediments to the rapid, effective, and resource-efficient conduct of clinical research projects (Payne et al. 2005). Compounding these challenges is the rapid pace of advancement in biomedical science and the resulting need for advances in diagnostics and therapeutics that can be validated and disseminated quickly and cost effectively (Butte 2008a, b; Embi and Payne 2009; Payne et al. 2005, 2009). The confluence of these factors has led to a number of major challenges and opportunities related to current and future CRI research and practice. For example, the importance of making clinical phenotype data available for the secondary use in support of clinical research has become a competitive requirement for research enterprises of all sizes (Chung et al. 2006; Embi and Payne 2009). Similarly, the increasing complexity of clinical research programs and the difficulty of recruiting sufficiently large patient cohorts, when combined with the regulatory overhead of conducting studies in large academic institutions, has led to an increase in the conduct of clinical studies in community practice settings. Such community-based research paradigms introduce new levels of complexity to the technical and policy aspects of data capture, management, and sharing plans (Embi and Payne 2009). This rapid evolution and the realities of an increasingly expansive clinical research landscape has led investigators and other decision makers in the health care and life sciences communities to call for increased investments in and delivery of innovative solutions to such information needs (Ash et al. 2008; Chung et al. 2006; Embi and Payne 2009; Payne et al. 2005; Sung et al. 2003). At the highest level, clinical research is a domain faced with significant information management challenges. At the same time, clinical research is an area of scientific endeavor that is at the forefront of attention for the governmental, academic, and private sectors, all of whom have significant scientific and financial interests in the conduct and outcomes of such efforts. These challenges and opportunities, when viewed collectively, have called, and continue to call, for

---

[1] NIH. (2011). Glossary & Acronym List Retrieved June 20, 2011, from http://grants.nih.gov/grants/glossary.htm (Accessed December 12, 2012)

the development and validation of innovative biomedical informatics methods and tools specifically designed to address clinical research information needs. It is this overall context that has motivated an increasing focus on the both basic and applied Clinical Research Informatics (CRI), which can be defined broadly as follows (Embi and Payne 2009):

> *Clinical Research Informatics (CRI) is the sub-domain of biomedical informatics concerned with the development, evaluation and application of informatics theory, methods and systems to improve the design and conduct of clinical research and to disseminate the knowledge gained.*

Examples of focus areas in which CRI researchers and practitioners apply biomedical informatics theories and methods can include the following:

- Evaluation and modeling of clinical research workflow
- Social and behavioral studies involving clinical research professionals and participants
- Designing optimal human-computer interaction models for clinical research applications
- Improving information capture and data flow in clinical research
- Leveraging data collected in EHRs
- Optimizing site selection, investigator and patient recruitment
- Improving reporting to regulatory agencies
- Enhancing clinical and research data mining, integration, and analysis
- Phenomic characterization of patients for cohort discovery and analytical purposes
- Integrating research findings into individual and population level health care

- Defining and promoting ethical standards in CRI practice
- Educating researchers, informaticians, and organizational leaders about CRI
- Driving public policy around clinical and translational research informatics

Building upon the preceding definitions and overarching challenges and opportunities relevant to CRI, in the remainder of this chapter we will provide an overview of the types of activities commonly undertaken as part of a variety of representative clinical research use cases, introduce the role of major classes and types of information system that enable or facilitate such activities, and conclude with a set analyses regarding the future directions of the field. The overall objective of this chapter is to provide the reader with the ability to evaluate critically the current and anticipated roles of biomedical informatics knowledge and practice as applied to clinical research.

26.2 A Primer on Clinical Research

In the following section, we will briefly introduce the characteristics of the modern clinical research environment (Sect. 26.2.1), including the design and execution of an exemplary class of clinical studies that were introduced in Chap. 11 and are known as randomized controlled trials (Sect. 26.2.2). This primer on clinical research will serve as the context for the remainder of the chapter, in which we will introduce major information needs and their relationships to a variety of basic and applied biomedical informatics practice areas and IT applications.

26.2.1 The Modern Clinical Research Environment

Clinical research comes in many forms and may include a variety of specific activities. All forms, however, share a common set of requirements related to the comprehensive management of study data – specifically, collection of data on human research subjects – and analysis of those data. As clinical research designs traverse the spectrum from passive or observational studies to interventional trials, the acuity of activities and associated data-management needs increases commensurately. For example, as introduced in Chap. 11, in a retrospective study subjects are selected based on the presence or absence of a particular condition and retrospective or pre-existing data are obtained from historical records (such as EHRs), whereas in natural history studies, subjects are recruited and followed in prospective manner, with additional collection of data performed solely for the purposes of research, rather than the normal process of patient care.

Further along the spectrum are clinical trials, in which research subjects participate in some additional activity, or *intervention*, that is intended either to induce a change in the subject or to prevent the occurrence of some change that would otherwise be expected. The intervention might be as simple as administering a substance already found in the human body (such as a vitamin) to measuring a change in that substance (such as a the amount of the vitamin found in the blood or urine). More complex studies involve interventions that have an impact on human disease, such as the administration of a preventive vaccine, the administration a curative drug, or a surgical procedure to remove, insert, repair or replace a structure or device in the subject's body. As with passive studies, data collection is critical to the proper performance of research and may become intense, with the collection of clinical information occurring more frequently and involving data describing the intervention materials (such as the purity of a drug or the performance of a device) in addition to data related to the human subject and their response to the intervention under study.

Although not an intrinsic requirement of clinical research, the inclusion of comparison groups is generally considered an important part of good scientific method. In some cases, **historical controls** can be used for comparison with a group of subjects under study. For example, if a disease is known to have a particular fatality rate, subjects could be given a potentially life-saving treatment and their fatality rate can be measured and compared to past experience. In **quasi-experiments**, comparison subject groups can also be selected for based on some known characteristic that distinguishes the two groups, such as gender or race, or their willingness to undergo a particular intervention.

A more rigorous method of establishing comparison groups is through randomization (Chap. 11), in which prospective subjects are assigned to different groups (often referred to as **study arms**) and undergo different interventions. Typically, randomization might take into account observable characteristics (such as gender and race) to create balanced groups, especially where the characteristics are known to have some influence on the effect of the intended intervention. Randomization also serves to distribute subjects based on unobserved characteristics, for example, unknown genetic traits, in order to reduce differences in the groups that might bias the results of the study. In a randomized controlled trial (RCT), one subject group will often receive a **control intervention** (for example, the usual treatment for a condition or even no treatment) while one or more other groups receive an **experimental intervention**.

Although intended to reduce bias, the randomization process itself must be carefully executed such that it does not introduce new sources of bias. For example, randomization can include **blinding**, in which the subject, the investigator, or both (as in **double-blinded** studies), are kept unaware of group assignment until after all assessments have been made. This might include the use of a **placebo** for a group receiving no treatment, in order to avoid the possibility that subjective improvement in a prior condition or the occurrence of random events (such as normally occurring illnesses) or are not ascribed to the intervention. This also may prevent subjects from deciding not to participate after randomization in a way that might unbalance the study groups (for example, if subjects prefer not to

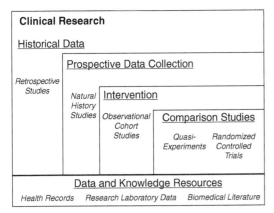

Clinical Research

Historical Data

Retrospective Studies	Prospective Data Collection		
	Natural History Studies	Intervention	
		Observational Cohort Studies	Comparison Studies
			Quasi-Experiments / Randomized Controlled Trials

Data and Knowledge Resources

Health Records   Research Laboratory Data   Biomedical Literature

Fig. 26.1 Overview of clinical study designs and associated information and data management needs. Underlying such design patterns are a common thread of systematic data management, leveraging resources such as health records, research-specific laboratory data, as well as broader knowledge collections such as the published biomedical literature

participate if they know they are not getting the experimental intervention) or even bias the assignments (for example, people less prone to take care of themselves might drop out if they find they are assigned to an intervention that requires a great deal of effort on their part).

The gold standard of clinical studies (introduced in Chap. 2) is generally considered to be the double-blinded, randomized, placebo-controlled trial (Cimino et al. 2000). However, such studies may not always be practical. For example, the use of a placebo when an effective therapy is known may be unethical, the blinding of a surgical repair may not be practical, or the condition under study may be so rare that only historical controls are available.

While different study designs have unique and differentiated information needs, they uniformly involve some form of systematic data management, as noted previously. Such data management activities usually include initial data collection, aggregation, analysis, and results dissemination, to name a few of many such tasks. As shown in Fig. 26.1, different study methods introduce new issues as successively more complex interventions and study design patterns are employed. For the remainder of this chapter, we will focus our discussion on RCTs as our proto-

typical study design, since they tend to involve most if not all of the informatics issues and information needs encountered in other study designs. Further information on the design characteristics, data management needs, and associated best practices related to various types of clinical trials can be found in a number of excellent textbooks on the subject (Gallin and Ognibene 2012), and further discussion is beyond the scope of this chapter.

26.2.2 Phased Randomized Controlled Trials

Most clinical studies begin with the identification of a set of driving or motivating hypotheses. The research questions that serve to define such hypotheses might be raised through an analysis of gaps in knowledge as found in the published biomedical literature or be informed by the results of a previous study. It is important to note that clinical research endeavors exist on a spectrum of scientific activity that is commonly referred to as **clinical and translational research**. A particular type of translational research, often referred to as T1-type translation (see Chap. 25), is a process by which basic science discoveries are used to design novel therapies. Such discoveries are then evaluated during clinical research studies, first pre-clinical and subsequent clinical trial phases (Payne et al. 2005). A second type of translational research, often referred to as T2 translation, involves methods such as those borrowed from **implementation science** and clinical informatics, and focus on translating the findings of such clinical research studies into common practice. A common colloquialism for this process of translating a novel basic science discovery through clinical research and into clinical practice is "bench to bedside" science.

Individual and distinct RCTs are often conducted for different purposes, most often motivated by the need to fill fundamental knowledge gaps about a particular intervention under study. By combining such knowledge gaps with the underlying biomedical mechanisms of physiology

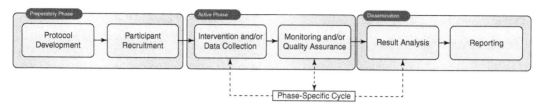

Fig. 26.2 Overview of the clinical research process for Phase I-III trials, divided into three major phases (preparatory, active, dissemination)

and disease, a motivating hypothesis or collections of hypotheses are established as to why a given intervention might lead to a given result or finding. Such hypotheses result in a natural sequence of research questions that can be asked relative to a novel intervention. Usually, an individual research study is designed to address one specific research question and hypothesis. In the case of the development and evaluation of a new therapeutic intervention, like a new drug, an individual research study is designed to address each **phase** in a line of research inquiry that will determine the efficacy and effectiveness of such a therapy (Spilker 1991). In most cases, this adheres to the following model:

- **Phase I**: Investigators evaluate the novel therapy in a small group of participants in order to assess overall safety. This safety assessment includes dosing levels in the case of non-interventional therapeutic trials, and potential side effects or adverse effects of the therapy. Often, Phase I trials of non-interventional therapies involve the use of normal volunteers who do not have the disease state targeted by the novel therapy.
- **Phase II**: Investigators evaluate the novel therapy in a larger group of participants in order to assess the efficacy of the treatment in the targeted disease state. During this phase, assessment of overall safety is continued.
- **Phase III**: Investigators evaluate the novel therapy in an even larger group of participants and compare its performance to a reference standard which is usually the current standard of care for the targeted disease state. This phase typically employs an RCT design, and often a multi-center RCT given the numbers of variation of subjects that must be recruited

to adequately test the hypothesis. In general, this is the final study phase to be performed before seeking regulatory approval for the novel therapy and broader use in standard-of-care environments.

- **Phase IV**: Investigators study the performance and safety of the novel therapy after it has been approved and marketed. This type of study is performed in order to detect long-term outcomes and effects of the therapy. It is often called "post-market surveillance" and is, in fact, not an RCT at all, but a less formal, observational study.

The phase of an RCT has implications for the kinds of questions being asked and the kinds of processes carried out to answer them. From an informatics perspective, however, the tasks are usually very similar. At a high level, the conduct of a Phase I, II or III clinical trial can be thought of in an operational sense as consisting of three major stages: preparatory, active, and dissemination (Fig. 26.2).

During these three stages, a specific temporal series of processes is executed. First, during the **preparatory phase**, a protocol document is generated as part of the project development process. The protocol document usually contains background information, scientific goals, aims, hypotheses and research questions to be addressed by the trial. In addition, the protocol describes policies, procedures, and data collection or analysis requirements. A critical aspect of the protocol document is the definition of a protocol schema, which defines at a highly granular level the temporal sequence of tasks and events required to both deliver the intervention under study and to ensure that data are collected and managed in a systematic manner commensurate

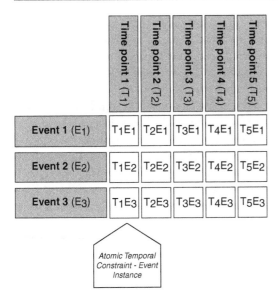

Fig. 26.3 Generic layout of a clinical trial protocol schema, composed of atomic temporal constraints. Event instances are shown as Time Point (T) – Event (E), using the notation: T_xE_y, where x is the Time Point descriptor, and y is the Event descriptor. In some instances, a transposed version of this grid is used

with the study hypotheses and aims. Such protocol schemata are often represented as a temporal grid (Fig. 26.3).

Once a protocol is deemed ready for execution, the feasibility of the study design (e.g., addressing questions such as "are there enough participants available in the targeted population to satisfy the study design defined in the protocol document?") is assessed either quantitatively (e.g., using historical data) and/or heuristically. Throughout the preparatory phase, a concurrent process of seeking regulatory approval from local and national bodies (e.g., local Institutional Review Boards ((Bernstam et al.), the Food and Drug Administration (FDA), etc.) occurs. Once a protocol plan is complete, deemed feasible, and regulatory approval has been received, potential participants are recruited and screened to determine if they meet the inclusion and exclusion criteria for the study (e.g., specific demographic and/or clinical parameters required for subjects to be eligible for the study). Once a potential participant has been deemed eligible for the study, they are provided with an informed consent document, which must be signed prior to pro-

ceeding with the enrollment process. **Enrollment** in the context of clinical trials means officially registering as a study subject, and is normally associated with the assignment of a study-specific identifier. Once a person agrees to become a participant, they are enrolled, and in the case of studies with multiple study groups or arms, randomized into one of those arms.

The preceding activities lead to the initiation of the next step in the research process, which we refer to as the **active phase**. During the active phase, the participant receives the therapeutic intervention indicated by their study arm and is actively monitored to enable the collection of study-specific data. This therapeutic intervention and active monitoring process is often iterative, involving multiple cycles of interventions and active monitoring. Follow-up activities begin once a participant has completed the interventional stage of a study. During this stage, subjects are contacted on a specified temporal basis in order to collect additional data of interest, such as long-term treatment effects, disease status or survival status (Spilker 1991).

Finally, during the **dissemination phase**, the results of the study are evaluated and formalized in publications or other knowledge dissemination media, for translation into the next phase of an RCT or into clinical practice. In some cases, such as adaptive study designs, this dissemination phase feeds back into the planning and active phases to allow for rapid revisions to a study design and iterative participant enrollment and data collection in support of such revised hypotheses and designs.

The quality of data produced by a clinical trial is assessed using multi-dimensional metrics that take into account the design, execution, analysis and dissemination of the study results. The quality of a clinical trial is also judged with respect to the significance or relevance of the reported study results within a clinical context (Juni et al. 2001). One key metric used to assess clinical trial quality is validity, which can be defined both internally and externally. **Internal validity** is defined as the minimization of potential biases during the design and execution of the trial, while **external validity** is the ability to generalize study results into clinical care (Juni et al. 2001).

It is important to note in a discussion of the role of biomedical informatics relative to clinical research that a large number of both basic and applied informatics practice areas concerning this domain focus upon platforms, interventions, and methods intended to reduce or mitigate such sources of bias, thus enhancing the validity and generalizability of study results.

26.3 Information Needs and Systems in the Clinical Research Environment

As can be inferred by the preceding section and its introduction to the definitional aspects of clinical research, such activities regularly involve a variety of data, information, and knowledge sources, as well a complicated set of complementary and over-lapping workflows. At the highest level, these characteristics of the clinical research environment can be related to a number of critical information needs, as summarized in Table 26.1. This representation of the information needs inherent to clinical research is presented using the specific context of a prototypical RCT, but the basic types of needs and example solutions provided can be extended to apply to the broader spectrum of research designs and patterns introduced in Sect. 26.2.

Building upon this broad definition of the information needs inherent to clinical research, in the following sub-sections we: (1) review the types of information systems that can support the phases that comprise a clinical study (Sect. 26.3.1); (2) explore the functional components that make up a clinical trials management system (Sect. 26.3.2); and (3) discuss the role of standards in enabling interoperability between such information systems (Sect. 26.3.3).

26.3.1 Information Systems Supporting Clinical Research Programs

It is helpful to conceptualize the conduct of clinical trials as a multiple-stage sequential model, as was introduced in Sect. 26.2.2 and is expanded upon in this section (Payne et al. 2005) (Fig. 26.4). At each stage in such a model, a combination of research-specific and general technologies can be employed to support or address related information needs.

There are numerous examples of general-purpose and clinical systems that are able to support the conduct of clinical research:

- **Bibliographic databases** and **information retrieval tools** such as PubMed and OVID (see Chap. 21) can be used to assist in conducting the background research necessary for the preparation of protocol documents (Briggs 2002; Ebbert et al. 2003; Eveillard 2000; Eysenbach et al. 2001; Eysenbach and Wyatt 2002).
- **Electronic health records** (EHRs, see Chap. 12) can be used to collect clinical data on research participants in a structured form that can reduce redundant data entry (Bates et al. 2003; Clark et al. 2001; Marks et al. 2001; McDonald 1997; McDonald et al. 1999; Padkin et al. 2001).
- **Data warehouses and associated data or text mining tools** can be used in multiple capacities, including: (1) determining if participant cohorts who meet the study inclusion or exclusion criteria can be practically recruited given historical trends, and (2) identifying specific participants and related data within existing databases (Butler 2001; Evans 2002; Marks and Power 2002).
- **Clinical decision-support systems** (CDSS, see Chap. 22) can be used to alert providers at the point-of-care that an individual may be eligible for a clinical trial (Bates et al. 1998; Butte et al. 2000; Embi et al. 2005; Marks and Power 2002).

In addition to the preceding general technologies, a number of research-specific technologies have been developed:

- **Feasibility analysis applications and data simulation and visualization tools** can streamline the pre-clinical research process (e.g., disease models) and assist in the analysis of complex data sets in order to assess the feasibility of a given study design (Holford et al. 2000; Kim et al. 2002).

Table 26.1 Overview of definitional information needs in the clinical research environment

Information needs	Major sub-components	Description
Support for research planning and conduct	Collaborative document and knowledge management Data sources and tools for feasibility analyses Regulatory approval workflows	*Study teams often involve geographically and temporally distributed participants, who need to engage in iterative protocol development and approval processes. Such activities by necessity incorporate document versioning, annotation, and associated metadata management tasks. Once a protocol has been developed, access to data sets for the purposes of assessing the feasibility of a given study design is critical, and often involves the use of de-identified data sets drawn from a data warehouse or research registry. Finally, the submission, tracking, and documentation of regulatory approvals often necessitate the coordination and management of complex, document-oriented workflows and record keeping tasks.*
Facilitation of data management, access, and integration	Secondary-use of EHR-derived data for research purposes Research project specific data capture, management, and reporting Distributed data management (spanning traditional organizational boundaries) Syntactic and semantic interoperability	*The ability to use primary clinical data from EHR or equivalent platforms to support secondary use in a research program has the potential to reduce redundancy and potential errors while increasing data quality. However, using such data in a secondary capacity also requires that appropriately structured data be captured and codified in clinical systems, and then be made available to research teams and research data management systems in a timely and resource efficient manner. In addition to such secondary use of clinical data, most clinical studies require the regular capture and management of study-specific data elements, a task that is usually accomplished via the use of Electronic Data Capture (EDC) or Clinical Trial Management Systems (CTMS). Finally, given the propensity to conduct studies that span traditional organizational boundaries in order to realize economies of scale and/or access sufficiently large patient populations, it is often necessary to query, integrate, and manage distributed data sets, and ensure their syntactic and semantic interoperability. Such a need is usually addressed through the use of Service Oriented Architectures, Cloud Computing, Data Warehousing, and Metadata Management technologies.*
Workforce training and support	Dissemination of study, methodological, and technical training materials Support for team collaboration and knowledge sharing	*A central need when conducting clinical studies is the ability to ensure that individuals involved in the execution of a protocol share common methods, data management practices, and workflows (thus reducing potential sources of study bias). Ensuring such shared knowledge and practices, particularly in distributed or multi-site settings, requires the use of distance education and team-science tools and platforms to enable knowledge sharing and distance learning paradigms.*
Management information capture and reporting	Support for research billing Operational instrumentation and reporting Regulatory monitoring Data quality assurance	*The business and management aspects of the conduct of clinical studies is complex, often requiring the disambiguation of standard-of-care and research specific charges as part of billing operations, as well as the tracking of key performance and data quality metrics that may be required to satisfy contractual commitments to the entities funding such studies. Furthermore, the monitoring of study data for critical or sentinel events that should or must be reported for regulatory purposes is both necessary and of extreme importance. All of the aforementioned activities require the application of a variety of management information system, business intelligence, and reporting tools, leveraging a broad variety of enterprise, administrative, and study-specific data sources.*

(Continued)

Table 26.1 (continued)

Information needs	Major sub-components	Description
Participant recruitment tools and methods	Cohort discovery Eligibility determination and alerting Participant registration, consent, and enrollment execution and tracking	*The identification of participant cohorts that satisfy key study design criteria, such as inclusion and exclusion criteria, is frequently a major barrier to the timely and efficient execution of clinical studies. A variety of information needs, related to the identification and engagement of such cohorts, to point-of-care alerting regarding potential study eligibility, to the management of registration, consent, and enrollment records is inherent to this information need. Such requirements are usually satisfied through a multi-modal approach, leveraging both clinical and research-specific information systems.*
Data standards	Standards for interoperability between research systems Standards for interoperability between research, enterprise (e.g. EHR), and administrative systems	*As has been noted relative to several of the preceding information needs, there is a frequent and reoccurring requirement for both syntactic and semantic interoperability between research-specific information systems, as well as between research-specific and clinical or administrative systems. Such a need necessitates the design, selection, and application of a variety of data standards, as well as the ability to map and harmonize between shared information models to support interactions between systems using a variety of standards.*
Workflow support	Integration of tools for combined standard-of-care and research visits Data, information, and knowledge transfer between stakeholders, project phases, activities, and associated information systems or tools.	*Much as was the case related to data standards, a closely aligned information need exists relative to the ability to support complex workflows between information systems and actors involved in the conduct of clinical research. Such workflow support requires both computational and application-level workflow orchestration, as well as the ability to define and apply reusable data analytic "pipelines."*
Data, information and knowledge dissemination	Knowledge management for clinical evidence generated during trials Guidelines and CDSS delivery mechanisms Publication mechanisms Data registries	*The ultimate objective of clinical research is to generate and apply new evidence in support of improvements in clinical care and human health. In order to do so, it is necessary to disseminate the findings generated during such studies in a variety of formats, including reusable/actionable knowledge resources, clinical guidelines, decision support rules, and/or publications and reports. In addition, increasing emphasis is being placed on the transparency and reproducibility of study designs, which is largely being accomplished through the creation of public registries via which study data sets can be shared and made available to the broader biomedical community.*

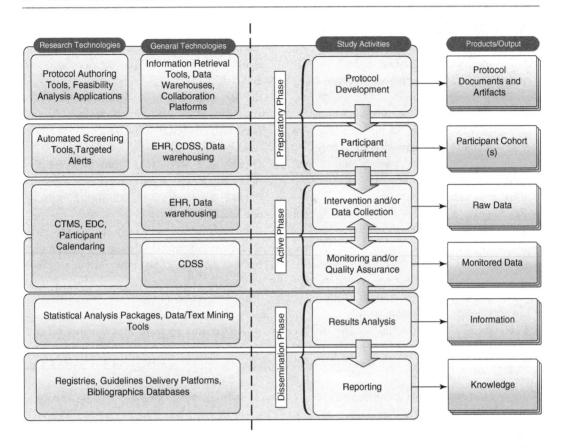

Fig. 26.4 Overview of study activities, and related research-specific and general information technologies, as well as targeted products or outputs associated with the sequential clinical research workflow paradigm

- **Protocol authoring tools** can allow geographically distributed authors to collaborate on complex protocol documents (Fazi et al. 2000, 2002; Goodman 2000; Rubin et al. 2000; Tai and Seldrup 2000).
- **Automated screening tools and targeted alerts** can assist in the identification and registration of research participants (Butte et al. 2000; Lutz and Henkind 2000; Marks and Power 2002; Pressler et al. 2012).
- **Electronic data capture (EDC) and Clinical Trial Management Systems (CTMS)** can be used to collect research-specific data in a structured form, and reduce the need for redundant and potentially error-prone paper-based data collection techniques (Harris et al. 2009; Kuchenbecker et al. 2001; Marks et al. 2001; Merzweiler et al. 2001; Wubbelt et al. 2000).

- **Research-specific decision support systems such as participant calendaring tools** provide protocol-specific guidelines and alerts to researchers, for example tracking the status of participants to ensure protocol compliance (Marks et al. 2001; Tai and Seldrup 2000).

26.3.2 Clinical Research Management Systems

One of the most widely used technology platforms in the clinical research domain is the **clinical research management system (CRMS)**. Such platforms were historically referred to as clinical *trials* management systems (CTMS), but the term CRMS is gaining popularity as such systems are increasingly used to manage the conduct of studies including but not limited to trials.

CRMS platforms are usually architected as composite systems that incorporates a number of task and role-specific modules intended to address core research-related information needs (Chung et al. 2006; Payne et al. 2005, 2009). Exemplary instances of such modules include the following:

- **Protocol Management** components that support document management functionality to enable the submission, version control, and dissemination of protocol related artifacts and associated metadata annotations.
- **Participant Screening and Registration** tools that allow for the application of electronic eligibility "check lists" to individual patients or cohorts in order to assess study eligibility, and when appropriate, record the registration and associated "baseline" data that are required per the study protocol.
- **Participant Calendaring** functionality allows for the instantiation of general protocol schemas (e.g., a definition of a protocols temporal series of tasks, events, and associated data collection tasks) in a participant specific manner, accounting for complex reasoning tasks including the dynamic recalculation of temporal intervals between evens based on actual completion dates/times, as well as the "windowing" of events in which a given task or event is allowed to fall within a range of dates rather a specific, atomic temporal specification.
- **Electronic Data Capture (EDC)** components allow for the definition, instantiation, and use of electronic case report forms (e.g., forms that define study and task/event specific data elements to be collected in support of a given trial or research program). Such **electronic case report forms (eCRFs)** are the basic instrument by which the majority of study-specific data are collected, and are usually populated via a combination of: (1) manual data entry (including abstraction from source documentation such as medical records); (2) the importation of secondary use data from clinical systems; or (3) a hybrid of the two preceding approaches.
- **Monitoring tools** enable the application of logical rules and conditions (e.g., range-checking, enforcement of data completion, etc.) using a rules engine or equivalent technology, in order to ensure the completeness and quality of research related data. Such tools may also be used to monitor patient compliance with study schemas, as reflected in the previously described patient calendar functionality.
- **Query and Reporting Tools** support the planned and ad-hoc extraction and aggregation of data sets from multiple eCRFs or equivalent data capture instruments as used with the CTMS. These types of tools are commonly used by biostatisticians and other quantitative scientists to perform interim and final analyses of study results, outcomes, and to enable higher-order safety analyses. In addition, such tools may be employed to comply with a broad variety of data submission and reporting standard set by both public- and private-sector entities, as described in Sect. 3.3.
- **Security and Auditing** functionality enables site, role, and study-specific access controls and end-user authentication/authorization relative to all of the preceding functionality, as well as the ability to track and report upon end-user interaction with and modifications to data contained in the CRMS. Such functionality is critical to enabling compliance with a broad variety of regulatory and privacy/confidentiality frameworks that apply to the use of protected health information (PHI) for research purposes.

In most CRMS platforms, the aforementioned functional modules share one or more common research databases or in the case of service-oriented architectures (SOA), common data services (See Chap. 5 for more details on SOA technologies). In more advanced platforms, these common data structures are populated with research-specific and/or clinical data from enterprise systems and sources (such as electronic health records, personal health records, and data warehousing platforms) via either a SOA paradigm (e.g., data service publication and consumption) or an **extract, transform, and load (ETL) approach** (See Chaps. 2 and 6 for further

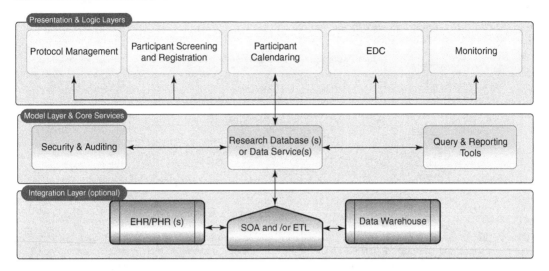

Fig. 26.5 Overview of the prototypical architecture of a clinical trial management system, divided into: (1) presentation and logic layers; (2) model layer and core services; and (3) an optional integration layer

details concerning architectural and methodological approaches to secondary use of clinical data). This overall architecture is illustrated in Fig. 26.5.

26.3.3 Data Standards in Clinical Research

The use of standards to represent clinical research information provides the same challenges and benefits found in other informatics application areas (see Chap. 7). Data may be captured with standard terminologies or translated into standards to support data reporting and sharing which, in turn, require agreed-upon standard frameworks to support such exchanges. Standards are even being developed for the representation of clinical trial protocols themselves. Figure 26.6 depicts how the various kinds of standards fit into the overall schema of clinical research, ranging from data models that define how data are to be represented, through standards for terminologies to actually represent the data and structures for exchanging them, out to standards for reporting and sharing. The standards described here are some of the current and most prevalent ones, but they continue to evolve and new standards relevant to the CRI domain are constantly emerging.

26.3.3.1 Emerging Standards and Domain Modeling in Clinical Research

Formats for data sharing typically include a data model for the information to be shared, leaving to individual contributors the later task of mapping local data into the exchange model. An alternative approach is the model-driven architecture, in which an underlying data model is created for the express purpose of representing all aspects of an information design, including data representation. Previously, the models used for clinical research management systems have been those required to support system functionality. New efforts are underway to create standards for modeling the actual research protocols, to enable a logical representation that includes the semantic aspects of the protocol (for example, the relationships between specific interventions and observations intended to measure their effects). While use of such models may make the research process somewhat more complicated, the mapping to standards used for exchanging data becomes greatly simplified.

For example, the National Cancer Institute (NCI) sponsors the *Cancer Biomedical Informatics Grid* (caBIG) program (Buetow 2009) which, among its many activities, has established a Clinical Trials Management

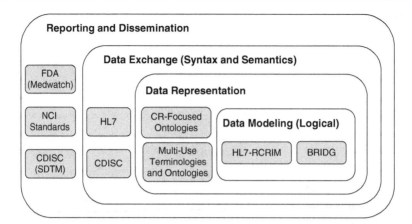

Fig. 26.6 Relationships of among various CRI standards. Data modeling, at the core, determines how terms from terminologies and ontologies will be recorded in clinical research databases. Exchange standards determine how data will map from the model to the messages used for interchanging the data. The use of messages is determined by the requirements of regulatory agencies and collaborating research groups. See text and Chap. 7 for explanation of acronyms

Systems Workspace (CTMS WS) that is developing standards to enable the design and execution of computable clinical trials. These efforts include the development of domain-specific workflow models and use cases to inform the design of CTMS's in a manner consistent with the "real-world" needs of clinical trials investigators, staff and sponsors. For example, a set of Life Science Business Architecture Models (Boyd et al. 2011) have been created to describe the vocabulary, goals and processes that are common in the business of life science research, including the actors, activities and data involved, using use cases described with the **Unified Modeling Language** (**UML**).

Similarly, Health-Level 7 (HL7; see Chap. 7) is an open standards development organization that develops consensus standards for all manner of clinical and administrative data, and is also working on clinical research-specific standards, such as the **Regulated Clinical Research Information Management** (**RCRIM**) model (Ohmann and Kuchinke 2009) in order to define messages, document structures, terminology and semantics related to the collection, storage, distribution, integration and analysis of research information. The main focus of the work is on data related to studies involving US Food and Drug Administration (FDA) regulated products (drugs and devices).

A key component of the previously described CTMS WS effort is the development of a data model known as the Biomedical Research Integrated Domain Group (BRIDG) Model.[2] BRIDG is designed to harmonize models from the HL7 RCRIM, the *Clinical Data Interchange Standards Consortium* (CDISC; see discussion of sharing and reuse later in this section) (Kuchinke et al. 2009), and models being developed by the CTMS WS itself. The modeling components of this project have focused primarily on logical abstractions of classes and data types, rather than domain-specific concepts, and are being put to practical use in a number of caBIG programs and resultant IT applications (Ohmann and Kuchinke 2009).

26.3.3.2 Using Standard Controlled Terminologies for Clinical Research Data

As described previously, the design of clinical protocols includes rigorous attention to the types of data to be collected and the format of those data. This often involves the use of controlled terminologies to capture categorical data. The terminology may be as small as "yes/no" or a

---

[2] hftp://www.cdisc.org/bridg (Accessed December 12, 2012)

ten-point pain scale for capturing subjects' symptoms, or it may be as vast as a list of all possible drugs or diseases in a subject's medical history. In many cases, researchers will simply compose sets of terms that meet their immediate needs and then require all investigators participating in the study to apply them consistently.

Because the terms used in clinical research are often identical to those used in clinical care, standard multi-use terminologies (such as those described in Chap. 7) are often appropriate for use in capturing clinical research data. However, there are some aspects of clinical research that are not well represented in mainstream terminologies; and in these cases, terminologies and their richer forms, ontologies, that are more focused on clinical research, are required. In particular, clinical research data and workflow models require controlled terminologies and ontologies that define domain-specific concepts and standard **common data elements (CDEs)**. Collections of standard terms for CDEs can be found in the NCI's Cancer Data Standards Repository (caDSR) and Enterprise Vocabulary Service (EVS).[3] In a similar manner, the Ontology for Biomedical Investigations (OBI) (Kong et al. 2011) is being developed by a consortium of representatives from across the spectrum of biomedical research, and includes terms to represent the design of protocols and data collection methods, as well as the types of data obtained and the analyses performed on them.

There are several reasons for considering the use of *standard* controlled terminologies in the capture of clinical research data. One reason is to take advantage of clinical data that are already being collected on research subjects for other purposes. A common example is the use of data on morbidity and mortality that are collected using one of the various versions and derivatives of the *International Classification of Diseases* (ICD; see Chap. 7). In the US, for example, patient diagnoses are reported for billing purposes using the *Clinical Modifications* of the ninth edition of ICD (ICD-9-CM). While such coded information is readily available, researchers repeatedly find that ICD-9-CM codes assigned to patient records have an undesired level of reliability or granularity, especially when compared to with the actual content of the records (Iezzoni 1990). Thus the convenience of using such standard codes may be outweighed by the imprecision, which can adversely affect study design and analytical results.

A second reason for adopting a standard controlled terminology is simply to avoid "reinventing the wheel." As is described in Chap. 7, a great deal of effort has been expended in the creation of domain-specific terminologies that are comprehensive, unambiguous, and maintained over time. Designating such terminologies for use in a protocol design can relieve researchers of having to worry about the quality of the terminology. For example, a researcher is unlikely to encounter novel concepts when recording subjects' demographic data, such as gender, marital status, religion and race. Specifying, for example, that an ISO standards should be used for these data elements greatly simplifies the protocol-design process.

A third reason for choosing standard terminologies relates to the ability to compare data collected in one study with those collected in others. For example, the use of a standard scale for recording a subject's pain will allow comparison of results from a study of one treatment with those from a second study of another treatment. The selection of an appropriate standard for a particular purpose is not straightforward (for example, by 2012 the NIH Pain Consortium was listing six different scales[4]). The choice may be

---

[3] http://ncicb.nci.nih.gov/NCICB/infrastructure/cacore_overview/cadsr (Accessed December 12, 2012)

[4] http://painconsortium.nih.gov/pain_scales/NumericRatingScale.pdf (Accessed December 12, 2012) http://painconsortium.nih.gov/pain_scales/COMFORT_Scale.pdf (Accessed December 12, 2012) http://painconsortium.nih.gov/pain_scales/FLACCScale.pdf (Accessed December 12, 2012)

http://painconsortium.nih.gov/pain_scales/CRIESPainScale.pdf (Accessed December 12, 2012)

http://painconsortium.nih.gov/pain_scales/ChecklistofNonverbal.pdf (Accessed December 12, 2012)

http://painconsortium.nih.gov/pain_scales/Wong-Baker_Faces.pdf (Accessed December 12, 2012)

determined simply based on the emerging popularity of one terminology over another in a wide community of those investigating similar problems.

A fourth use of standard terminologies relates to reporting requirements. Government agencies sometimes require the reporting of clinical research data and, when they do, often require certain data to be reported using a particular standard. For example, the FDA requires the use of the *Medical Dictionary for Regulatory Activities* (MedRA) for reporting all adverse events occurring in drug trials (Brown et al. 1999), while the Cancer Therapy Evaluation Program (CTEP) at the National Cancer Institute (NCI) requires the use of *Common Terminology Criteria for Adverse Events* (CTCAE) (Trotti et al. 2003). In an analogous manner, at the international level, the World Health Organization requires the use of the Adverse Reactions Terminology (WHO-ART).[5] Faced with such reporting requirements, researchers sometimes choose to record data in these terminologies as they are being captured. In those cases where the clinical questions being answered require more detailed data, however, researchers must resort to recording data with some other standard (such as SNOMED; see Chaps. 7 and 25), or a controlled terminology of their own creation, and then translating them to the terminology or terminologies required for reporting purposes. See Fig. 26.7 for a comparison of how similar clinical concepts are represented in various standard terminologies.

26.3.3.3 Sharing or Reusing Multi-modal Data to Support Clinical Research

Standards also exist for organizing clinical research data to enable sharing, reuse, and aggregation. CDISC, introduced previously and in Chap. 7, is a standards group motivated by the needs of the pharmaceutical and bio-technology industry entities that sponsor or otherwise support many clinical studies. CDISC is creating a standard for submitting regulatory information to

the FDA, while in a similar manner, HL7 has created a standard *Clinical Document Architecture* (CDA; see Chap. 7).

The caBIG project provides a variety tools to allow researchers, clinicians and patients to share, integrate and analyze data (Buetow and Niederhuber 2009). These tools are distributed as open-source software that is made freely available to a consortium of individuals and organizations who contribute to the common goal of advancing translational research (see Chap. 25). Although the work centers around cancer research, few aspects of the models or tools are specific to that domain, and researchers from other specialties are finding caBIG resources to be valuable for their own research.

Informatics for Integrating Biology and the Bedside (i2b2) is a project being developed under a National Center for Biomedical Computing grant from NIH. Originating from the research and development activities of Partners HealthCare System and Harvard University, i2b2 is developing an information system framework to allow clinical researchers to use existing clinical data for discovery research (Murphy et al. 2006). The i2b2 platform includes a workflow framework and a data repository, as well as tools for terminology management and natural language processing. Of note, many of the over 60 institutions receiving Centers for Translational Science Awards (CTSA) from the National Center for Advanced Translational Science (NCATS) are adopting i2b2 technologies to support research and collaboration.

For those seeking to share data, and to avail themselves of data shared by others, the National Center for Biotechnology Information (NCBI) at the NIH's National Library of Medicine is creating a public repository of individual-level data, including exposure history, signs, symptoms, diagnostic test results, and genetic data. Called the *Database of Genome and Phenome* (dbGAP), this project provides stable data sets that allow multiple researchers to reference the same samples in their publications of secondary analyses of the data (Mailman et al. 2007). Additional data from

---

[5] http://www.umc-products.com (Accessed 12/12/2012)

ICD-9-CM:
Symptoms
   787 Symptoms involving digestive system
     787.0 Nausea and vomiting
      787.01 Nausea with vomiting
      787.02 Nausea alone
      787.03 Vomiting alone

CTCAE:
Gastrointestinal Disorders
  Nausea
     Grade 1: Loss of appetite without alteration in eating habits
     Grade 2: Oral intake decreased without significant weight loss, dehydration
              or malnutrition
     Grade 3: Inadequate oral caloric or fluid intake; tube feeding, TPN, or
              hospitalization indicated
     Grade 4: Life-threatening consequences (version 3.0 only)
     Grade 5: Death (version 3.0 only)

MedDRA (partial):
  10017947 - Gastrointestinal disorders
    10018012 - Gastrointestinal signs and symptoms
      10028813 - Nausea
        10028815 - Nausea alone
        10066962 - Procedural nausea
          10036285 - Postoperative nausea
          10028818 - Nausea postoperative

SNOMED-CT (partial):
404684003 - Clinical finding
  118234003 - Finding by site
    386617003 - Digestive system finding
      386618008 - Gastrointestinal tract finding
        422587007 - Nausea
          51885006 - Morning sickness
            37031009 - Motion sickness
              33902006 - Air sickness
                21162009 - Outerspace sickness
              17783003 - Car sickness
              18530007 - Sea sickness
              249502005 - Train sickness
          16932000 - Nausea and vomiting
        64581007 - Postoperative nausea
          1488000 - Postoperative nausea and vomiting

Fig. 26.7 Examples of terms used to represent research subjects' report of nausea, taken from *ICD-9-CM*, *CTCAE*, *MedDRA*, and *SNOMED*. See text for explanation of acronyms

clinical trials, currently limited to summary results, are also being made available by the NLM through the *ClinicalTrials.gov* resource, which is a repository of descriptive metadata related to historical and actively recruiting clinical trials (Zarin et al. 2011).

26.3.3.4 Clinical Research Reporting Requirements

Requirements for reporting research data, particularly those related to outcomes and adverse events, are generally accompanied by specifications for the format of the data being reported. For example, the FDA's Center for Drug Evaluation and Research (CDER) accepts reports using the HL7 Individual Case Safety Report, while the NCI's CTEP allows submission of adverse event information to its Adverse Event Expedited Reporting System (AdEERS[6]) either manually, using a Web-based application, or electronically via a web-services API. As mentioned earlier in this section, these agencies require that data be coded with standard terminologies, such as MedDRA and CTCAE, respectively.

Several reporting requirements have emerged for the purpose of making clinical trial results publicly available, both to support reuse of the data by researchers and as information sources for patients and their families. In 2000, the US National Library of Medicine launched ClinicalTrials.gov to provide a mechanism for researchers to voluntarily register their trials so that those interested in participating as research subjects can identify, via the World Wide Web, studies relevant to their condition. ClinicalTrials.gov currently includes information from over 100,000 trials from over 170 countries. In 2004, the European Union initiated as similar effort, called the European Union Drug Regulating Authorities Clinical Trials (EudraCT). ClinicalTrials.gov and EudraCT also support the reporting of the clinical trials results. While the submissions are nominally voluntary, federal agencies often mandate the reporting as a requirement for obtaining research funds or to obtain approval for regulated drugs and devices. In the US, for example, the Food and Drug Administration Amendments Act of 2007 (FDAAA) strongly reinforced these requirements. In addition, the over 900 peer-reviewed biomedical journals that participate in the

International Consortium of Medical Journal Editors (ICJME) now require public, prospective registration in ClincialTrials.gov or similar databases of clinical trials of all interventions (including devices) in order for resultant manuscripts to be considered for publication.

Each repository has defined its own mechanisms for transmitting protocol data. ClinicalTrials.gov, for example, allows investigators to enter their data through an interactive Web site or to upload data in a defined XML (**eXtensible Markup Language**) format (see Chap. 5). Figure 26.8 shows an example of outcomes and adverse event data in this format. Clinical research data management systems that can export their study in this format can save the research much manual effort and assure accurate data entry (Zarin 2011).

26.4 Future Directions for CRI

As the preceding sections illustrate, significant progress has been made to advance the state of the CRI domain, and such advances have already begun to enable significant improvements in the quality and efficiency of clinical research (Chung et al. 2006; Murphy et al. 2012; Payne et al. 2005, 2010). These advances can be viewed as having been achieved at the individual investigator level (e.g., improvements in protocol development, study design, participant recruitment, etc.), through approaches and resources developed and implemented at the institutional level (e.g., development of methods and resources in data warehousing that enable storage and retrieval of clinical data for research, development of novel clinical trials management systems, etc.), and through mechanisms that have enabled and facilitated the endeavors multi-center research consortia to drive team science (e.g., innovations that enable data management and interchange for multi-center studies, etc.).

Many of these advances have been motivated by national and international funding and policy efforts that span the research and clinical-care enterprises. Among these are research funding

---

[6] http://ctep.cancer.gov/protocolDevelopment/electronic_applications/adeers.htm (Accessed December 12, 2012)

```
<clinical_results>
  <study_identifiers>
    <nct_id>NCT00687609</nct_id>
    <brief_title>Pilot Evaluation of Atomoxetine on Attention Deficit.... </brief_title>
    <results_first_received_date>July 22, 2010</results_first_received_date>
  </study_identifiers>
  <participant_flow>
    <group group_id="P1"><title>Atomoxetine</title>
      <description>0.5 milligrams per kilogram (mg/kg) daily ...</description>
    </group>
    <period><title>Overall Study</title>
      <milestone><title>STARTED</title></milestone>
  </participant_flow>
  <baseline>
    <measure><title>Age</title><units>Years</units>
      <param>Mean</param><dispersion>Standard Deviation</dispersion>
      <measurement group_id="B1" value="16.3" spread="0.95"/>
    </measure>
  </baseline>
  <outcome>
    <type>Primary</type>
    <title>Attention Deficit Hyperactivity Disorder (ADHD) Rating Scale...</title>
    <description>Measures the 18 symptoms contained in the....</description>
    <time_frame>12 weeks</time_frame>
    <group group_id="O1"></group>
    <measure><title>Number of Participants</title><units>participants</units></measure>
  </outcome>
  <reported_events>
    <other_events>
      <event><sub_title>Nausea</sub_title>
        <counts group_id="E1" events="8" subjects_affected="5" subjects_at_risk="7"/>
      </event>
    </other_events>
  </reported_events>
</clinical_results>
```

Fig. 26.8 Example of XML representation of a clinical trial, including outcomes data, from Clinical Trials.gov. For clarity, some sections of the document have been omitted

efforts like those we have mentioned (e.g., the NCI's caBIG initiative programs (Buetow 2009; Oster et al. 2008; Saltz et al. 2008), and the CTSA initiative). In addition, investments being made to accelerate the adoption and "meaningful-use" of health IT for clinical practice (see Chaps. 12 and 27) are laying the groundwork for grand opportunities to accelerate the research and discovery enterprise. Examples of this include initiatives by the US Office of the National Coordinator for Health IT (ONC) and the US Centers for Medicare and Medicaid services (CMS), that anticipate the health IT infrastructure in the US will ultimately be able to support information management and exchange in a manner that will

enable the reuse of data and information from clinical care for improvements in public health and research. As described by the ONC-based leaders of this initiative, this should greatly enable the creation of the so-called **learning health system** (Friedman et al. 2010).

As such efforts progress, and the demand for more evidence-based health care increases, the methods, theories and tools of CRI will be essential complements to those of clinical informatics in order to realize the potential of increasingly interconnected systems and ever-growing databases that can enable discovery and advance human health. While most of the efforts to date have appropriately focused on the development of technological solutions to the issues of data capture, storage and retrieval, future advances will increasingly require effort not just to advance the development and management of technologies and platforms, but also to enhance the foundational science of CRI in an increasingly electronic world (Payne et al. 2010). By facilitating an understanding of the information-dense aspects of clinical research, CRI methods and resources will increasingly drive hypothesis generation as well as facilitate the conduct of research programs to generate new and meaningful knowledge. CRI approaches and theories will enable the meaningful use of EHRs and other biomedical information systems that extend beyond the early definitions of meaningful use limited to the systematic capture of key data elements solely for clinical care. Ultimately, systems will drive not only adherence to current guidelines and increasingly the translation of scientific discoveries into practice via evidence-based-medicine, but also will feed back data from routine practice to generate evidence by informing hypotheses and driving future research based on real-world clinical experiences, thereby completing the translational cycle.

Even as progress continues toward such a goal, the landscape of research continues to change, thereby motivating ongoing developments in the CRI domain. For example, research efforts are expanding beyond the traditional environments of single academic medical centers to multi-center, community-based and global locations of research. While there are a variety of reasons for this, cost-effectiveness and efficiency are often cited among them. Given the information intensive nature of research and these fundamental changes to the nature and location of research activities, new CRI solutions and methods will be needed to enable efficient and effective research across geographical and institutional boundaries. To address this, new funding for research into such CRI solutions and methods is emerging from agencies including NIH, the Agency for Healthcare Quality and Research, and the Patient Centered Outcomes Research Institute (Lauer and Collins 2010; Slutsky and Clancy 2010).

Even with all of the progress in CRI over the past several years, as a 2009 study of self-identified CRI professionals documented, there exists a range of fundamental challenges and opportunities facing the domain. These were sorted into 13 distinct categories that spanned multiple stakeholder groups (Fig. 26.9). In addition to helping to define the current state of the domain, the challenges and opportunities identified offer a view of the work that will face CRI professionals in the coming years (Embi and Payne 2009).

One key element that will need to be addressed in order to achieve the advances envisioned for CRI is the growth of a dedicated workforce of experts focused in the CRI domain. Currently, most CRI professionals come to the field from many different disciplines and professional communities, including computer science, information technology, clinical research and various health care domains. Recent initiatives by consortia like the CTSA institutions as well as those of professional associations like AMIA have begun to provide professional communities and venues, such as the AMIA Summits on Translational Science[7], for scientific information sharing among those working in the CRI discipline. In addition, while there is as yet no dedicated scientific journal focused on the CRI domain, CRI-focused publications are increasingly found in major peer-reviewed journals, including a number of recent special issues published in both the Journal of the American Medical Informatics Association (JAMIA) and Journal of Biomedical Informatics (JBI) highlighting distinguished papers from the AMIA Joint Summits on Translational Science (Sarkar and Payne 2011).

Despite such progress, there remains a need to address the shortage of professionals dedicated to advancing the CRI domain. While formal programs specifically for training professionals in CRI are limited, National Library of Medicine supported fellowship programs focused on CRI

---

[7] http://www.amia.org/meetings-and-events   (Accessed 12/7/2012)

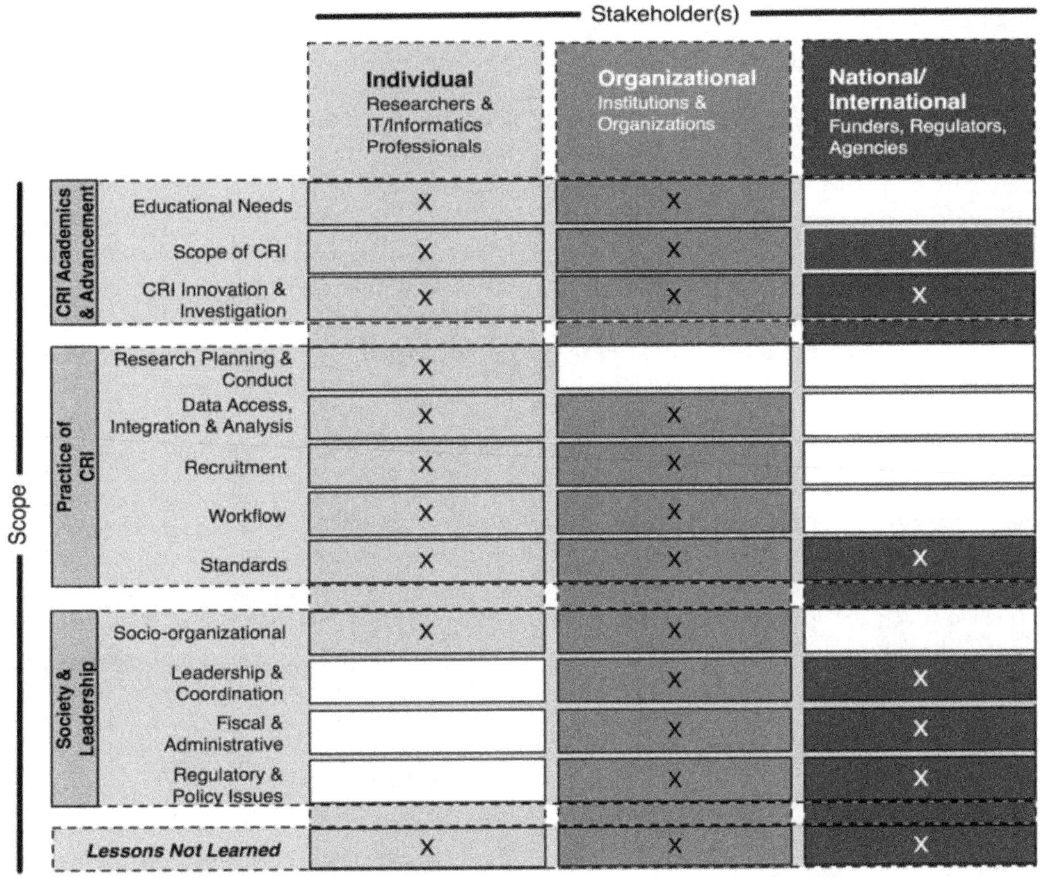

Scope		Stakeholder(s)		
		Individual Researchers & IT/Informatics Professionals	**Organizational** Institutions & Organizations	**National/ International** Funders, Regulators, Agencies
CRI Academics & Advancement	Educational Needs	X	X	
	Scope of CRI	X	X	X
	CRI Innovation & Investigation	X	X	X
Practice of CRI	Research Planning & Conduct	X		
	Data Access, Integration & Analysis	X	X	
	Recruitment	X	X	
	Workflow	X	X	
	Standards	X	X	X
Society & Leadership	Socio-organizational	X	X	
	Leadership & Coordination		X	X
	Fiscal & Administrative		X	X
	Regulatory & Policy Issues		X	X
	Lessons Not Learned	X	X	X

Fig. 26.9 Major challenges and opportunities facing CRI: This figure provides an overview of identified challenges and opportunities facing CRI, organized into higher-level groupings by scope, and applied across the groups of stakeholders to which they apply (Reproduced with permission, Embi and Payne 2009)

are emerging[8] and are expected to grow in the coming years. As with many biomedical informatics sub-disciplines, CRI curricula can be expected to be interdisciplinary, requiring the study of topics ranging from research methods and biostatistics, to regulatory and ethical issues in CRI, to the fundamental informatics and IT topics essential to data management in biomedical science. In addition, given the expectation that clinical information systems and environments will increasingly be sources of data and subjects for research, there is also a need to train not only technicians conversant in both clinical research and biomedical informatics to work in the CRI space, but also to educate clinical informaticians, clinical research investigators and staff, and institutional leaders concerning the theory and practice of CRI. Programs like AMIA's 10×10 initiative[9] and tutorials at professional meetings offer examples of what can be expected to grow. For example, The Ohio State University currently offers a distance education program focusing on CRI via the aforementioned 10×10 initiative[10].

As CRI continues to mature as a discipline, the current efforts focused on the relative "low

[8] http://www.nlm.nih.gov/ep/GrantTrainInstitute.html (Accessed 12/20/2012)

[9] http://www.amia.org/education/10x10-courses (Accessed 12/7/2012)

[10] http://medicine.osu.edu/bmi/education/distance/10x10/pages/index.aspx (Accessed 12/18/2012)

hanging fruit" of overcoming the significant day-to-day IT challenges that plague our traditionally low-tech research enterprise can be expected to give way to fundamental and systematic advances. In this way, CRI progress can be expected to mirror that seen years ago in the now-relatively more mature clinical informatics domain. Future years can be expected to see CRI not only instrument, facilitate and improve current clinical research processes, but it will generate advances that can be expected to change fundamentally the pace, direction, and effectiveness of the clinical research enterprise and discovery. Through CRI biomedical advances, discovery, health care quality improvement, and the systematic generation of evidence will become as routine and expected as advances in clinical informatics have already become in fostering the systematic application of evidence into health care practice.

26.5   Conclusion

This chapter has sought to introduce the following major themes: (1) design characteristics that serve to define contemporary clinical studies; (2) foundational information needs inherent to clinical research programs and the types of information systems can be used to address or satisfy such requirements; (3) the role of multi-purpose platforms, such as Electronic Health Record (EHR) systems, that can be leveraged to enable clinical research programs; (4) the role of standards in supporting interoperability across and between actors and entities involved in clinical research activities; and (5) future directions for the CRI domain and how such endeavors they may alter or optimize the conduct of clinical research. As we have explained, the clinical research environment is faced with significant workflow and information management challenges, and it is therefore increasingly garnering attention from the governmental, academic, and private-sectors. This progress explains CRI's emergence as a distinct and highly valued sub-discipline of biomedical informatics. Part of the evolution of CRI can be attributed to the extraor-

dinary increase in the scope and pace of clinical and translational science research and development that has been catalyzed by a variety of funding and policy initiatives that seek to re-engineer the way in which governmental, public, and private entities advance basic science discoveries into practical therapies. CRI has accordingly become a dynamic and relevant sub-domain of biomedical informatics knowledge and practice, providing a broad spectrum of research and development opportunities in context of both basic and applied informatics science.

Discussion Questions
1. How do the foundational information needs of clinical research differ depending on the type and phase of study being undertaken? Do study phases have an impact on the primacy of such information needs?
2. What is the role of biomedical informatics with regard to decreasing bias in RCTs and thus enhancing the internal validity, external validity, and generalizability of study results?
3. How can clinical or general purpose information systems and research-specific tools be employed synergistically to address clinical research-specific information needs, such as participant recruitment or the population of study-specific data capture instruments?
4. How do the core functional components of common clinical trial management systems (CTMS) overlap with or otherwise replicate the functionality of electronic health record (EHR) systems? To what extent does this similarity or difference inform the need for syntactic and/or semantic interoperability among such systems?
5. In what situations is the use of clinical research-specific terminologies or ontologies appropriate? In such situations, what challenges exists relative to

the selection, use, and maintenance of appropriate standards?

6. What is the role of data standards in enabling the dissemination and reuse of study-generated data sets? How can the use of such standards enable the cross-linkage or integrative analysis of data sets derived from multiple but independent studies?

7. Compare and contrast the future directions of CRI with those of other BMI sub-disciplines and focus areas described in this book. To what extent are they similar and different, and what are the implications of such findings relative to the role of common informatics theories and methods and their applicability to the clinical research domain?

Suggested Readings

Ash, J. S., Anderson, N. R., & Tarczy-Hornoch, P. (2008). People and organizational issues in research systems implementation. *Journal of the American Medical Informatics Association, 15*(3), 283–289. This paper summarizes critical people-centric issues, including cultural norms, policies, and perceptions, that influence the adoption and optimal use of informatics approaches intended to facilitate clinical research.

Chung, T. K., Kukafka, R., & Johnson, S. B. (2006). Reengineering clinical research with informatics. *Journal of Neurocytology, 54*(6), 327–333. This paper describes an exploration of socio-technical factors to be addressed in order to realize the benefits of integrating Biomedical Informatics theories and methods with the design, conduct, and dissemination of clinical studies.

Embi, P. J., & Payne, P. R. (2009). Clinical research informatics: challenges, opportunities and definition for an emerging domain. *Journal of the American Medical Informatics Association, 16*(3), 316–327. This manuscript summarizes a multi-modal study that serves to both define the field of clinical research informatics, as well as critical opportunities and challenges associated with the field.

Gallin, J. I., & Ognibene, F. (2012). *Principles and practice of clinical research* (3rd ed.). London: Academic Press. This book provides a broad overview of various aspects of clinical research with particular attention to data capture and quality.

Kush, R. D., Helton, E., Rockhold, F. W., & Hardison, C. D. (2008). Electronic health records, medical research, and the tower of Babel. *The New England Journal of Medicine, 358*(16), 1738–1740. This report provides a broad overview of critical standards commonly encountered in the clinical research domain.

Payne, P. R., Johnson, S. B., Starren, J. B., Tilson, H. H., & Dowdy, D. (2005). Breaking the translational barriers: the value of integrating biomedical informatics and translational research. *Journal of Neurocytology, 53*(4), 192–200. This report provides a targeted review of literature and supporting survey data highlighting informatics-specific issues related to the delivery and support of technologies and services capable of supporting and facilitating clinical research in academic health centers.

Richesson, R. L., & Krischer, J. (2007). Data standards in clinical research: gaps, overlaps, challenges and future directions. *Journal of the American Medical Informatics Association, 14*(6), 687–696. This paper provides an in-depth look at the current roles of the various terminology and data modeling standards that are relevant to clinical research informatics.

Sung, N. S., Crowley, W. F., Jr., Genel, M., Salber, P., Sandy, L., Sherwood, L. M., et al. (2003). Central challenges facing the national clinical research enterprise. *JAMA : The Journal of the American Medical Association, 289*(10), 1278–1287. This paper provides summary of critical cultural, policy, methodological, and technical challenges that serve as impediments to the efficient and timely conduct of clinical research in the United States. This report is the result, in part, of seminal work in this area conducted by the IOM.

Part III

Biomedical Informatics in the Years Ahead

Health Information Technology Policy

27

Robert S. Rudin, Paul C. Tang, and David W. Bates

After reading this chapter, you should know the answers to these questions:

- Why have health care professionals in the U.S. been slow to adopt electronic health records and other forms of health IT?
- How can public policy promote the adoption and use of health IT?
- How does health IT support national agendas and priorities for health and health care?
- Why it is important to measure the value of health IT in terms of improvements in care quality and savings in costs?
- How can public policies safeguard patient privacy in an era of electronic health information?
- What are the main policy issues related to exchanging health information among health care organizations?
- What are the major tradeoffs for regulating electronic health records in the same way that

other medical devices are regulated to ensure patient safety?
- What policies are needed to encourage clinicians to redesign their care practices to exploit better the capabilities of health IT?
- How does the U.S. approach to health IT policy compare with those of other countries?

27.1 Public Policy and Health Informatics

In the year 2000, an international survey in 20 of the world's most developed countries asked physicians about their use of electronic health records (EHRs; see Chap. 12). The survey found that in many of these countries, EHR penetration was high, especially for primary care physicians. Some countries such as Sweden and the Netherlands achieved near universal adoption with almost every physician using some form of EHR (Fig. 27.1). However, in other countries such as France and Portugal, only a few percent of physicians used them. The United States ranked 16th with only 17 % of physicians adopting EHRs.

Why would there be such variation in the levels of EHR adoption? And why would the U.S., which spends far more money per person on health care than any other country, be so far behind? The reason is not lack of interest among medical leaders. Since 1991, the U.S.-based Institute of Medicine (IOM)[1] has published

R.S. Rudin, BS, SM, PhD (✉)
Health Unit, Rand Corporation,
20 Park Plaza Suite 920, Boston 02116, MA, USA
e-mail: rrudin@rand.org

P.C. Tang, MD, MS
David Druker Center for Health Systems Innovation,
Palo Alto Medical Foundation, 2350 W. El Camino
Real, Mountain View 94040, CA, USA
e-mail: paultang@stanford.edu

D.W. Bates, MD, MSc
Division of General Internal Medicine and Primary
Care, Department of Medicine, Brigham and
Women's Hospital, 1620 Tremont St., Boston 02120,
MA, USA
e-mail: dbates@partners.org

[1] http://www.iom.edu (Accessed 12/9/2012)

E.H. Shortliffe, J.J. Cimino (eds.), *Biomedical Informatics*,
DOI 10.1007/978-1-4471-4474-8_27, © Springer-Verlag London 2014

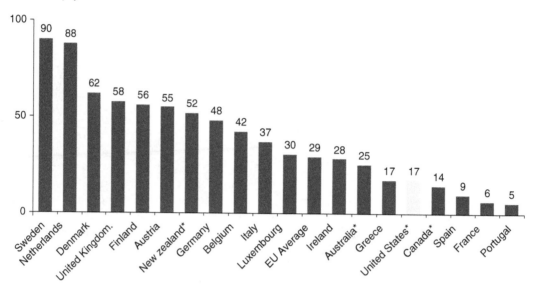

Fig. 27.1 Physicians Use of Electronic Medical Records in Developed Countries. Source: Commonwealth Fund National Scorecard on U.S. Health System Performance, 2006; European Union EuroBarometer (2001); Commonwealth Fund International Health Policy Survey of Physicians (Harris Interactive 2002); * data is from the year 2000

several widely cited reports extolling the potential benefits of health IT, calling for greater use of EHRs, and making the case that computers are critical for modernizing and improving health care systems. The reason for low adoption is likely not a lack of availability of EHR technology either. EHR vendor companies that have succeeded in Sweden or the Netherlands, for example, would undoubtedly try to expand into larger and more lucrative markets, especially in the U.S. Yet in 2013, many U.S. physicians still use paper charts.

To understand these low adoption rates of EHRs and how to accelerate adoption, one must look to public policy. The influence of policy can be found throughout a health care system. Policies shape the structure of health care delivery organizations and the markets for medical products. Directly or indirectly, policies influence the behaviors of all health care stakeholders including patients, providers, health plans and researchers. Much of the effectiveness or dysfunction in a health care system can be attributed to public policies.

In recent years, policymakers have taken a strong interest in fostering health IT. In 2004, U.S. President George W. Bush issued an executive order to establish the Office of the National Coordinator for Health IT.[2] In 2009, the U.S. Congress allocated approximately $30 billion to support providers' **meaningful use** of health IT. Governments of many other countries are also spending significant public funds on health IT and paying close attention to related policy issues.

In this chapter, we review some of the key policy goals relevant to informatics and discuss how researchers and policymakers are trying to address them. Accelerating adoption of health IT is one policy goal. Others include fostering interoperability of health IT products, protecting privacy of patients' health information, ensuring health IT products are safe for patients, and improving medical practice workflows.

---

[2] http://www.healthit.gov/newsroom/about-onc (Accessed 12/9/2012)

While informatics research has been occurring for several decades, research in health IT policy is still in its infancy. As stakeholders look to health IT to solve the major cost and quality problems in national health care systems, we expect the issues discussed in this chapter to become more important to policymakers and researchers in the fields of health policy and informatics.

27.2 How Health IT Supports National Health Goals: Promise and Evidence

Health IT is not an end in itself. Like all technology, it is simply a tool for achieving larger clinical, social and policy goals, such as improving health outcomes, improving the quality of care, and reducing costs. Health IT promises to have a tremendous impact on these goals.

Policymakers, however, are interested not only in the promise of health IT but also the reality. Like most software products, early versions of health IT products tend to have many problems, such as bugs, poor usability, and difficulties integrating with other products. Only after the technology matures is it possible for a larger portion of the promised benefits to be realized. Policymakers are reluctant to invest public funds, which are raised primarily in the form of taxes, on technologies that have not been proven in empirical studies to produce benefits.

Indeed, many studies have been able to detect empirical benefits of health IT (Buntin et al. 2011). However, a large portion of these studies come from a handful of academic medical centers (Linder et al. 2007; Chaudhry et al. 2006). It is not clear how well the benefits from academic centers will generalize to other care settings. Why haven't researchers been able to demonstrate the benefits of health IT more broadly (Jones et al. 2012)? We have already mentioned one possible reason: the technology used by most clinicians may not be mature. Another reason might be that users are not taking advantage of the technology's potential. Finally, it may be that the technology is actually producing benefits but

the benefits are inherently difficult to detect (see Chap. 11). It will be challenging to determine which of these reasons plays the greatest role.

Despite the limits of the empirical evidence, policymakers are currently investing substantial sums in health IT hoping that the technology will realize its promised benefits and support national health goals. However, they would potentially invest even more in technologies that are proven effective in empirical studies. This section presents an overview of both the promise and the evidence of how health IT supports policy goals.

27.2.1 Improving Care Quality and Health Outcomes

As informatics professionals understand intuitively, health IT has enormous potential to improve care quality and health outcomes, which is, of course, a central policy goal (Table 27.1). Just as computers have revolutionized many other industries, from banking to baseball, information technology has the potential to revolutionize health care through the creation of innovative applications. Policymakers in the U.S. appear to recognize this potential as demonstrated by the emphasis on health IT in the U.S. National Quality Strategy[3] and regulations related to **Accountable Care Organizations** (**ACOs**) (AHRQ 2011; Berwick 2011). Many other countries also specifically encourage adoption and use of health IT in order to improve health care quality.

Electronic health records (EHRs; Chap. 12) probably represent the form of health IT that has been evaluated most extensively. Several studies have demonstrated the benefits of EHRs in real clinical settings. For example, studies have found that EHRs with clinical decision support (Chap. 22) will reduce the number of adverse drug events from 30 to 84 % (Ammenwerth et al. 2008). In addition, physicians using EHRs with clinical decision support have been shown to make more appropriate medical decisions

---

[3] http://www.ahrq.gov/workingforquality/ (Accessed 12/9/2012).

Table 27.1 The promise of health IT (selected functionality)

Health IT functionality	Expected effect on care quality	Expected effect on cost
Electronic health record (EHR) with clinical decisions support (CDS)	Improved clinical decisions, fewer errors	Fewer unnecessary tests
Health information exchange (HIE)	Improved clinical decisions	Reduced burden of information gathering, reduced duplicate testing
Patient decision aids	More personalized treatment	Fewer procedures
Telehealth and personal health records (PHR)	More interaction with clinicians	Fewer office visits
E-prescribing	Fewer errors	Reduced costs from errors

(Tang et al. 1999a). One study that examines EHR use in several hospitals in Texas found that there are reduced rates of inpatient mortality, complications, and length of stay when EHRs are used (Amarasingham et al. 2009). Not all the benefits of EHRs have been demonstrated in empirical studies, but enough of the benefits have been proven so that policymakers are keenly interested in promoting widespread adoption.

Another component of health IT that may substantially improve quality of care is clinical data exchange, which is the ability to exchange health information among health care organizations and patients (see Chap. 13). There is a great need for this kind of capability. In the U.S., the typical Medicare beneficiary visits seven different physicians in four different offices per year on average, and many patients with chronic conditions see more than 16 physicians per year (Pham et al. 2007). Not surprisingly, in such a fragmented system, information is often missing. One study shows that primary care doctors reported missing information in more than 13 % of visits and other studies suggest much higher rates of missing data, affecting as much as 81 % of visits (Smith et al. 2005; van Walraven et al. 2008; Tang et al. 1994b). A study in one community found that

there may be a need to exchange data among local medical groups in as many as 50 % of patient visits (Rudin et al. 2011). However, few empirical studies have been able to show that real-world implementations of electronic clinical data exchange systems result in improvements in care quality or health outcomes.

Researchers and policymakers agree that improving the quality of health care must involve making it more patient-centric, and health IT will likely be crucial to achieving that goal on a large scale (Kaelber and Pan 2008). For example, **personal health records (PHRs)** and patient portals would give patients access to their clinical data (see Chap. 17), facilitate communication between patients and providers, and provide relevant and customized educational materials so that patients could take a more active role in their care (Tang et al. 2006; Halamka et al. 2008). PHRs may also incorporate patient decision-aids to help them to make critical health care decisions, taking into account their personal preferences (Fowler et al. 2011). **Telehealth** technologies, which enable patients to interact with clinicians over the Internet (see Chap. 18), would make health care more patient-centric by allowing patients to receive some of their care without having to go physically to the doctor's office. Few empirical studies have shown that these technologies result in improvements in care quality or health outcomes. However, studies have reported high levels of patient satisfaction with PHRs and many patients use them extensively in certain hospitals and medical centers.

One concern of policymakers is that there may be an emerging digital divide in health IT. One study found that minority groups were less likely to access web-based PHRs and, in general, minorities and disadvantaged groups have less web access than other groups (Yamin et al. 2011). On the other hand, adoption rates of mobile platforms do not show as much of a divide and it is likely that PHRs will soon be accessible via these platforms. Policies may be necessary to fund special approaches targeting minorities to prevent disparities in health care from getting worse and to ensure that the improvements in care quality enabled by health IT are enjoyed by all.

Unfortunately, health IT also has the potential to facilitate harmful unintended side effects (Bloomrosen et al. 2011). In one study involving a pediatric intensive care unit in Pittsburgh, patient mortality actually increased after computerized physician order entry (CPOE) was installed (Han et al. 2005). The study found that certain aspects of the ordering system they implemented and some of the implementation decisions they made, restricted clinicians' ability to work efficiently, causing delays in treatment, which was especially deleterious because of the urgent nature of the children's conditions. Implementation decisions involving configuration of the system and changes in workflows appear to have been the major contributors to the increase in mortality–the same EHR product was installed in another hospital without such adverse impacts on mortality (Beccaro et al. 2006). Nonetheless, questions about the need to regulate the safety of EHRs are being debated. Balancing the need to protect patients from unintended harm is the concern, further discussed later in this chapter, that over-regulation may impede innovation. Most researchers tend to believe that if health IT systems are well-designed and implemented with close attention to the needs of the users, these kinds of unintended consequences can be avoided and health IT systems will result in tremendous improvements in quality of care (Berg 1999).

27.2.2 Reducing Costs

In addition to improving quality, health IT is expected to reduce costs of care substantially (Table 27.1). Projections based on models show huge potential savings for many forms of health IT. One study by the RAND Corporation estimated that EHRs could save more than $81 billion per year (Hillestad et al. 2005). Another study estimated that electronic clinical data exchange has the potential to save $77.8 billion per year (Walker et al. 2005). Many of these savings are expected to come from reductions in redundant tests and use of generic drugs, as well as reductions in adverse drug events and other errors that EHRs might prevent (Bates et al.

1998; Wang et al. 2003). Telehealth and PHRs have also been projected to result in billions of dollars in savings (Kaelber and Pan 2008; Cusack et al. 2008).

One weakness of these projections is that they relied on expert opinions for some point estimates because, other than a number of studies showing that EHRs reduce costs by reducing medical errors, few studies have tried to examine empirically the effect of health IT on costs. Also, some of the projections have been criticized because they estimate potential savings rather than actual measured savings (Congressional Budget Office 2008). However, the projections do not include a number of types of savings that may result from providing better preventive care and care coordination which would reduce the need for patients' use of high cost procedures in hospitals and emergency rooms. They also do not include potential reductions in costs that may result from decision aids for patients, which may, for example, reduce the number of unnecessary surgeries (O'Connor et al. 2009). The actual savings therefore may be much greater than the projections suggest.

27.2.3 Using Health IT to Measure Quality of Care

All health care stakeholders agree that a health care system should deliver high quality care. But how does one measure care quality? Current methods of quality measurement rely largely on administrative claims submitted by providers to insurers. These data may be useful for certain quality measurements such as for assessing a primary care physician's mammography screening rates, but they lack important clinical details, such as the results of laboratory tests. They also do not represent a comprehensive picture of the care that is delivered, assess the appropriateness of most medical procedures, or determine if a patient's quality of life has improved after treatment. Also, most patients in the U.S. switch insurance companies every few years, limiting the ability of any one insurer to measure quality improvements over longer periods of time, which is required to assess accurately the treatment of many medical conditions. Clinical data are much more comprehensive than administrative claims, but only a minority of existing quality measures uses clinical data from EHRs. The lack of robust methods for measuring clinical quality represents a major impediment to making substantial improvements in quality. More attention should be paid to developing clinical quality measures, especially now that payments systems are moving from fee-for-service payments to ones based on quality (Tang et al. 2007). We discuss some of the issues surrounding paying providers based on quality measures later in the next section.

Health IT has the potential to improve **quality measurements** greatly by allowing clinical data automatically to produce standardized quality measures. In the U.S., there is growing policy interest in creating such measures as shown in the National Quality Strategy and other reports (AHRQ 2011). This approach has been highly successful in the United Kingdom (U.K.) where nearly 200 quality measures have regularly been assessed, with up to 40 % of payment for general practitioners based on performance on these measures. In addition, there is growing support for developing patient-reported **outcome measurements** which may be integrated in PHRs, or obtained through other mechanisms and integrated with the patient's clinical data (Cella et al. 2010).

However, using electronic clinical data to generate quality measures is also associated with a number of problems. Studies have found that clinical data in EHRs are often incomplete, inaccurate and may not be comparable across different EHRs (Chan et al. 2010). More research is needed to develop and standardize meaningful quality measures that would be worth the burden of reporting them.

27.2.4 Holding Providers Accountable for Cost and Quality

Currently, in the U.S., most care is delivered using a fee-for-service payment system, in which providers are paid for every procedure or patient visit. Under this payment method, providers have incentives to provide more care rather than less, which may lead to overtreatment. It is therefore not surprising to find that in the U.S., costs are high and rising, nearly double those of many other industrial nations, and quality of care is mixed (Fuchs and Milstein 2011). As Fig. 27.2 shows, the U.S. spends more money per capita on health care than any other country by a wide margin. Yet, several studies suggest that the U.S. is far the from the world's leader in overall care quality (Nolte and McKee 2008). A seminal study by McGlynn et al. found that patients in the U.S. received recommended care only about half of the time across a broad array of quality measures (McGlynn et al. 2003).

Policymakers are trying to replace the fee-for-service payment method with other methods that would hold providers accountable for the care they deliver. For these attempts, health IT systems are essential. In the U.S., one of the proposed mechanisms for accomplishing this is through Accountable Care Organizations (ACOs). As specified in the Affordable Care Act of 2010,[4] an ACO is a group of providers who are held accountable, to some extent, for both the cost and the quality of a designated group of patients (Berwick 2011; McClellan et al. 2010). Only a few pilot ACOs currently exist, but early indications suggest that they may be effective, and there is strong interest among medical professionals to form them. The concept of ACOs depends on having an electronic health information infrastructure in place, including widespread use of EHRs, because health IT would enable ACOs to improve quality, reduce costs, and measure their performance.

Many other countries have experimented with paying providers for quality and outcomes, or holding providers responsible for costs, although few have done both at the same time to a high degree. Health IT systems are critical for many of these efforts. For example, in the U.K. 40 % of general practitioner funding has been based on more than 170 quality measures for which the

---

[4] http://www.healthcare.gov/law/index.html (Accessed 12/9/2012)

Fig. 27.2 Health care expenditures and life expectancy in the United States and ten other developed countries (Fuchs and Milstein 2011, with permission)

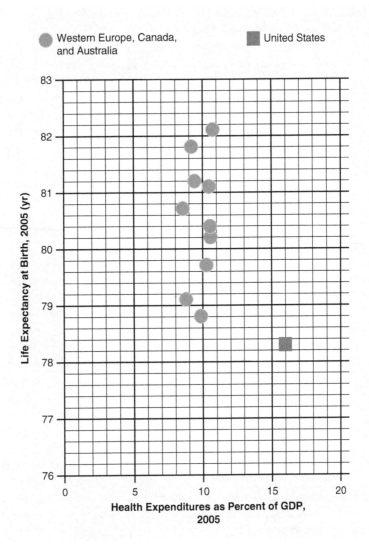

data are extracted directly from clinicians' computing systems. Few policymakers or researchers believe providers can be held accountable to a substantial degree for the care they delivery without a robust health IT infrastructure.

27.2.5 Informatics Research

As we mention above, many health IT capabilities are still emerging, or standards have not yet been defined. With health data just beginning to become widely accessible, new applications will still require additional research and development.

For example, we are still in the early stages of understanding how to design applications for team care (Chap. 15), remote patient monitoring (Chaps. 18 and 19), online disease management (Chaps. 17 and 18), clinical decision-making (Chap. 22), alerts and reminders (Chap. 22), public health and disease surveillance (Chap. 16), clinical trial recruiting (Chap. 26), and evaluations of the impact of technologies on care and costs (Chap. 11). One concern is that most provider organizations, and increasingly even academic medical centers, are now using software applications made by private vendors, and innovating with them has been challenging. Private vendors are not investing enough resources in research to produce transformational innovations (Shortliffe 2012). It will be essential to identify "sandboxes" in which new and innovative IT approaches can be developed and tested. More interactions between industry and academia may be a good way to accelerate progress.

Federal funding plays a major role in supporting this kind of upstream informatics research to help to incubate these new technologies. Because the benefits of such research will be enjoyed by everyone who uses the health care system, the investment of public funds is justified. Few private companies have taken the risk of doing this kind of experimental research to date because most health IT companies have been relatively small, and they are currently focused on adding the functionality that is needed to meet **meaningful use**. Much of the innovation in health informatics has occurred at universities and other government-funded research organizations affiliated with academic medical centers and that will likely continue.

27.3 Policy for Accelerating the Adoption of Health IT Infrastructure

Many governments around the world are actively developing and implementing policies to accelerate the adoption of health IT. Some countries have had more success than others. As we describe in the opening of this chapter, the U.S. has had a much lower adoption rate of EHRs compared with most other developed countries, although the current CMS meaningful use incentive program is starting to improve the statistics. It is likely that the new payment models, such as ACOs, and increased payment for practices involved in patient-centered medical home pilots, will accelerate health IT adoption even further because providers will see EHRs and other health IT, as necessary tools for achieving their cost and quality goals. However, there is no guarantee these new payment models will succeed. Also, they may take many years to become widespread, and they may require that health IT be adopted

first because health IT will allow the creation of the improved quality measures that new payment approaches will need in order to hold providers accountable. To overcome this chicken-or-the-egg problem, the U.S. is attempting to accelerate the adoption of health IT through direct incentives mentioned above. Other counties have taken different approaches. This section describes some of these efforts.

27.3.1 The U.S. Approach: Paying for 'Meaningful Use' of Health IT

The first published interest in promoting health IT directly through public policy and leadership in the U.S. dates back to at least 1989. For the next 15 years several informatics leaders published reports calling for the federal involvement and oversight. However, serious government activity in health IT promotion did not begin until the establishment of the Office of the National Coordinator for Health IT (ONC) in 2004. This office, which was later made permanent by an act of Congress, is located within the U.S. Department of Health and Human Services and tasked with "promoting development of a nationwide Health IT infrastructure that allows for electronic use and exchange of information."

The importance of this office grew considerably in 2009 when Congress passed legislation that is considered a major landmark in the history of health IT policy: the Health Information Technology for Economic and Clinical Health (HITECH) Act.[5] This legislation authorized $27 billion in stimulus funds to be paid to health care providers who demonstrate meaningful use of electronic health records. These incentive funds were made available to individual physicians and hospitals to help them implement and become meaningful users of health information technology to improve health outcomes of patients and

---

[5] http://en.wikipedia.org/wiki/Health_Information_Technology_for_Economic_and_Clinical_Health_Act (Accessed 12/9/2012)

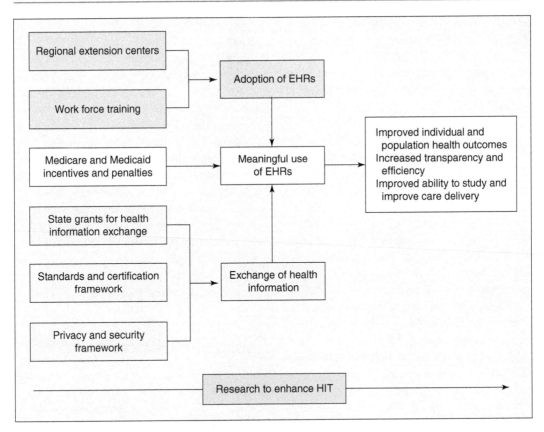

Fig. 27.3 The HITECH act's framework for meaningful use of Electronic Health Records (EHRs) (Blumenthal 2010, with permission)

populations. The criteria for qualifying for the incentive payments are based on demonstrated use of health IT to achieve health and efficiency benefits, and these criteria are to become more stringent over time. In addition to the incentive payments to providers to accelerate adoption of health IT, an additional $2 billion was allocated to provide workforce and infrastructure support needed to deploy the health IT systems nationwide and to facilitate clinical data exchange (Fig. 27.3). (Blumenthal 2010). The HITECH legislation also created two federal advisory committees, the Health IT Policy Committee,[6] which makes health IT-related policy recommendations to the U.S. Department of Health and Human Services, and the Health IT Standards

Committee,[7] which identifies or recommends standards to be used for certification of health IT products.

These incentives payments and related HITECH programs are important enablers for broader health systems reforms. As we describe earlier, policymakers in the U.S. hope to hold health care providers accountable for improvements in care quality, such as via ACOs, rather than for use of technology. The current policy approach of paying for use and then gradually raising the bar so that the government is paying for quality, with the eventual aim of moving to pay for actual outcomes, is probably wise because it will take time to realize quality benefits and it is important to get providers started on

---

[6] http://www.healthit.gov/policy-researchers-implementers/health-it-policy-committee (Accessed 12/9/2012)

[7] http://www.healthit.gov/policy-researchers-implementers/health-it-standards-committee (Accessed 12/9/2012)

the right path before expecting too much of them (Bates 2009). In the long run, it is likely that payments for both use of health IT and health outcomes may be necessary to ensure providers are fully realizing the potential of their health IT systems.

27.3.2 Electronic Health Records

Dr. David Blumenthal, the first national coordinator appointed after HITECH was enacted, described the purpose of HITECH as "creating a market." A market involves both buyers and sellers. Therefore, ONC has intended to influence both the buyers (physicians and hospitals) and the sellers (health IT product vendors). On the seller side, ONC has established a certification program for EHRs. Only EHR products that include specific features and adhere to standards can be certified, and only certified EHRs will allow providers to be eligible to receive meaningful use incentive payments. The intention of the certification program is to improve transparency in the marketplace for EHR products and ensure that physicians and hospitals will be able to use a minimum set of critical functionalities, such as clinician decision support and **e-prescribing**.

On the buyer side of the market, policies are trying to encourage clinicians to adopt EHRs by offering them direct payments if they can meet the meaningful use criteria. Many clinicians are reluctant to purchase EHRs, with good reason. The barriers to adoption include: initial capital costs, operating costs, downtime during installation and training, limited availability of knowledgeable trainers, limited number of proven EHR vendors, lack of technical standards, and privacy and security concerns. In the U.S. the lack of a solid business case is probably the most important barrier and the meaningful use payments may help with that considerably (Kleinke 2005). Initial signs suggest that the meaningful use program is working to enhance the functionality of commercial EHRs and accelerating their adoption. In fact, recent surveys (2012) report that more than 55 % of physicians are now using EHRs.

Other countries have taken very different approaches to encourage or require health IT use by providers. For example, the U.K. has been able to achieve near universal adoption of EHRs because it devoted substantial resources to the effort early on, and has a national health care system which directly manages most of the health care providers in the country (Cresswell and Sheikh 2009; Ashworth and Millett 2008). Most other industrialized nations have achieved fairly high levels of adoption in primary care (Jha et al. 2008). Levels of adoption in secondary care such as hospitals, however, lag behind. Countries that have particularly high levels of adoption in non-hospital settings include Denmark, the Netherlands, Sweden, Hong Kong, Singapore, Australia, and New Zealand.

27.3.3 Clinical Data Exchange

The U.S. is trying several approaches to promote clinical data exchange (See Chap. 13). ONC is working with state governments to establish regional health information exchanges (HIEs) around the country. These organizations integrate the EHRs of local health care providers to create aggregate longitudinal patient records. Many HIEs will also provide services for automating the delivery of laboratory results, integrating with pharmacies to facilitate e-prescribing, and facilitating public health and quality reporting.

As was discussed in Chap. 13, every state in the U.S. is actively building at least one HIE and the latest survey counts more than 150 of them (Adler-Milstein et al. 2011). However, the same survey found that only 13 HIEs were operational and supported basic data exchange functionality and none of them supported the kinds of HIE that would be needed to realize their potential value as estimated by projections. Most HIEs rely on public grants for support and few are financially sustainable. In the long term, it is not clear if HIEs will need to be supported as a public utility or if they will be able to find sustainable business models.

Why is it so difficult to establish an HIE? Part of the problem is that current EHR products are not using the same technical standards and are not interoperable. To address this problem, ONC is actively developing technical and semantic standards (See Chap. 7). However, many of the available standards may not be specific enough to make the integration much easier (Halamka 2010). Standards may require many more years of development before EHRs and HIEs become "plug and play."

Even if the technical aspects of integrating health IT systems were easier, vendors have few incentives to develop functionality that allows easy export of patient data into their competitors' systems. They may be "locking-in" patients and providers with their proprietary systems by not creating functionality that allows clinical data to be exported easily. ONC has indicated that, in subsequent stages of the meaningful use program, providers will be required have their EHRs integrated with HIEs. This policy effort might change the vendors' incentives considerably so that they may begin to compete for customers based on how effectively their products integrate with other products (Rudin 2010). Vendors may then also become more interested in agreeing to standards to ease their integration issues.

HIEs may have many other challenges including: recruiting providers who are reluctant to share data with competing medical groups, privacy and security concerns, legal issues, HIE-related fees, training clinicians to use the HIE, and the lack of a business case (Chap. 13). ONC as well as state government programs are trying to address every one of these issues. Creating the business case for providers may be the most difficult. Who will pay for the HIEs? The meaningful use payments may help in the short term by requiring providers to exchange data electronically with other providers who treat the same patients. Patients may also begin to demand that providers join HIEs to better coordinate their care, which may make providers more willing to pay for HIE services (Rudin 2010). Payers may be willing to subsidize HIEs if HIEs reduced their costs by reducing the number of redundant laboratory tests for example, but projections of these savings are not based on the experience of real-world HIEs and there has been little empirical

proof that HIEs save costs. In the long run, policy-makers believe that other programs such as ACOs will motivate providers to engage in HIEs to improve their quality metrics and to reduce their costs.

In a separate project, the U.S. is also trying to develop protocols that would allow secure point-to-point data exchange of medical information, essentially a system for secure email among medical professionals and health care organizations. Called the Direct Project,[8] these protocols may be useful for many situations in which data exchange is important, but they cannot support an aggregate longitudinal record of a patient's data, so they will not replace HIEs.

Some have proposed a different approach to data exchange in which an independent organization provides a secure electronic repository for storing and maintaining an individual's lifetime health records and allows the individual to have control of who accesses their data.[9] The history and details of this model are explained in Chap. 13. There has been an increase in interest in this approach recently. However, it is too early to tell if it will become widely adopted.

No country in the world has solved the problem of clinical data exchange, although some have made considerable progress. In every country that attempts to foster data exchange, the hardest issues appear to be political rather than technical, and there is clear agreement that health IT policy is particularly important to address these problems, especially in establishing standards. The U.K. has set up a "spine" which allows summary care documents to be widely exchanged (Greenhalgh et al. 2010). However, the overall program has encountered major political difficulties, and has been largely dismantled. Canada has established a program called Canada Health Infoway, which has emphasized setting up an infrastructure for data exchange (Rozenblum et al. 2011). While that effort has been somewhat successful, relatively little in the way of clinical data is being exchanged to date, in part because

---

[8] http://directproject.org/content.php?key=overview (Accessed 12/9/2012)

[9] http://www.healthbanking.org/ (Accessed 12/12/2012)

the adoption rate of electronic health records remains low. In Scandinavia, there has been substantial concern about the privacy aspects of data exchange, especially in Sweden, though data exchange is taking place in Denmark and its use is growing.

27.3.4 Personal Health Records and Telehealth

To encourage more patient-centric care, many countries are trying to foster the adoption of PHRs and Telehealth (see Chaps. 17 and 18), although adoption rates are modest. In the U.S., the meaningful use requirements strongly encourage deployment of patient portals in support of PHRs. However, policymakers have not yet decided what criteria will be used to determine that clinicians are indeed "meaningful" users of them. Federal efforts are also developing standards for improving PHR-EHR interoperability. To promote telehealth, policymakers are exploring the possibility of reimbursing for telehealth care, which would probably improve adoption of this technology considerably (Tang et al. 2007).

27.4 Policies to Support Medical Practice Redesign

Clinical workflows are inherently complex. Clinicians must manage huge amounts of medical information that may originate from patients, other clinicians, laboratories, imaging centers, and insurers. Well-designed EHRs and other forms of health IT have the potential to make their workflows easier. However, health IT systems themselves may also introduce new forms of complexity. For example, clinicians may find that actions that they could have carried out by simply scribbling a note on a slip of paper will demand several mouse clicks in their EHR. Health IT will also offer many capabilities that were not available to them in a paper world, such as medication management, reminders, and alerts that indicate when they are about to prescribe medications that could have adverse reactions. If these software tools are going to improve care, clinicians will

need to know how to use them and how to integrate them effectively into their workflows.

Even after the typical 1–3 months of training, clinicians often do not use EHRs to their fullest potential (Torda et al. 2010). Studies have shown that even experienced clinicians working with well-established health IT systems, such as those in the Veterans Affairs, will use "workarounds" for many clinical tasks which will involve ad hoc paper processes (Saleem et al. 2009a, 2011).

To address this problem, policies are funding efforts to train clinicians to integrate EHRs into their practice workflows. Regional health IT extension centers are being established around the U.S. that are responsible for training and educating clinicians to use health IT.

Another policy effort for improving clinical workflows is called the **patient-centered medical home** (**PCMH**) (American Academy of Family Physicians 2008). This effort focuses on the primary care clinician as coordinator of patients' medical care and will entail extensive use of health IT including telehealth, clinical data exchange, and clinical decision support (Bates and Bitton 2010; Kilo and Wasson 2010).

In the future, medical practices may have to change even more to exploit all the capabilities of health IT including: monitoring patient health status remotely, preventive health, and use of patient decision aids (Fowler et al. 2011). Clinical workflows will increasingly rely on health IT.

27.4.1 Informatics Workforce

Training and redesigning hundreds of thousands of medical practices in the U.S. will require a new pool of skilled workers. These workers will need expertise in both software and clinical workflows, which is rare to find in one person. In addition, to realize the full potential of the new health IT systems, these workers will need training in quality improvement, performance measurement, team dynamics, and medical practice culture (Torda et al. 2010). Policies have begun funding new training programs to build up this new professional workforce. Initial efforts have focused mostly on increasing training in community colleges. These efforts will need to be expanded to address the growing need for health IT and workflow expertise, and new policies may be needed to make sure clinical workflows continue improving.[10]

27.5   Policies to Ensure Safety of Health IT

As adoption of health IT accelerates, it is important to be vigilant about, and to reduce, the risk of unintended harmful side effects related to health IT use (Bloomrosen et al. 2011). Harm could arise from deficiencies in a number of areas when designing and deploying complex systems, including poor system design, inadequate testing and quality assurance, software flaws, poor implementation decisions, inattention to workflow design, or inadequate training. Policymakers are exploring various options to improve the safety of health IT design, deployment, and use, including direct regulations of products and dissemination of best practices.

27.5.1   Should Health IT be Regulated as Medical Devices?

One policy option for reducing the likelihood of health IT-related medical errors is to create regulations that require health IT product to adhere to strict principles of safe design, and be tested and certified (see also Chap. 10). This is how many medical devices are regulated by the U.S. Food and Drug Administration.[11] While this approach may ensure some degree of patient safety, the regulatory burden will increase the price of health IT systems, raise barriers of entry for new companies, and could stifle innovation. Also, even with regulations, health IT products might still have safety issues because software products can be used in many different ways, unlike other medical devices that have more limited utility. Also, principles

of safe design are not well developed in health IT and it is not clear how they would be applied by regulatory bodies. Thus, intensive regulation by the Food and Drug Administration is probably not the most effective approach, although some oversight of vendors may be appropriate (Miller et al. 2005a).

27.5.2   Alternative Ways to Improve Patient Safety

There are many other policy options to support patient safety. Policies may fund training programs to educate clinicians in how to use health IT safely and alert them to common mistakes. Policies might encourage providers to report problems with software, including usability issues and bugs, so that vendors can fix them quickly. Policies might also help to establish programs in which users can rate health IT products, an approach that vendors have so far resisted. Finally, funding research into the science of patient safety would improve our knowledge of how to design better products and identify risks of errors (Shekelle et al. 2011).

27.6   Policies to Ensure Privacy of Electronic Health Information

It is almost impossible to have a conversation about digital medical records without discussing issues of privacy. Although this topic arose in the discussion of ethics in Chap. 10, it also has policy implications and warrants mention here. In some ways, health IT offers the ability to have greater privacy protection compared to paper records because electronic accesses can be tracked and audited, whereas if someone inappropriately views a paper record, there is no audit trail. However, if an electronic record system is breached, the scale of the privacy violation may be enormous. If patient data are not kept private, patients may not trust their health care providers and they may forgo necessary treatment. Protecting privacy is clearly an important policy goal.

---

[10] http://www.healthit.gov/policy-researchers-implementers/workforce-development-program (Accessed 12/9/2012)

[11] http://www.fda.gov/ (Accessed 12/10/12)

27.6.1 Regulating Privacy

The Health Insurance Portability and Accountability Act (HIPAA) of 1996[12] and subsequent regulations created a legal category of "protected health information" which was defined to encompass most forms of clinical data. **Covered entities** which include providers and insurers are legally required under this law to safeguard electronic health information and would face fines if they did not.

Many states have additional privacy laws regarding data exchange (e.g., mental health and HIV status). The effectiveness of these privacy-protective laws has not been rigorously evaluated. They can inadvertently reduce privacy protection, particularly when exchanging data across state lines, and have been showed to slow the adoption of EHRs (Miller and Tucker 2009; Harmonizing State Privacy Law Collaborative 2009).

In other countries, privacy also has received a good deal of debate. In 2007, medical data on approximately 160,000 children in the U.K. were put on a compact disc that was lost in transit. Fortunately, the data were encrypted (EHI Primary Care 2007). There has also been substantial debate about privacy in Sweden, which has slowed down the development of data exchange. Governments are still trying to find the best policies to protect privacy of medical records without slowing the adoption of health IT.

27.6.2 Unique Health Identifiers

Many countries have adopted a **unique health identifier** (UHI). The advantage of such an identifier is to simplify the matching of health data to an individual. Without a unique identifier, organizations have to expend substantial resources disambiguating individuals. Although there are very good algorithms for doing this using data such as names and dates of birth, they sometimes results in incorrect matches or fail to find patient record that should be linked. Having a UHI could reduce

the frequency these errors and save the costs of purchasing the patient matching software.

Many privacy advocates in the U.S. vehemently oppose UHIs. Although some states are experimenting with voluntary health identifiers, Congress defunded any use of federal dollars to support development of a UHI. Despite these concerns, there is little evidence that suggest UHIs pose an increased a risk of privacy violations and, in fact, not having a UHI may be even more risky because other kinds of personal data such as social security numbers may be used instead (Greenberg et al. 2009).

27.7 The Growing Importance of Public Policy in Informatics

Public policy is becoming increasingly important to the field of informatics. Policies have an effect on everything from what research projects receive funding to whether a physician in a solo practice adopts an electronic health record. Many of the health IT policy issues we discuss in this chapter are just beginning to attract attention from policymakers, and further research is needed just to frame the issues.

Traditionally, most informatics research has focused on the development of new technologies and how they integrate into clinical practice. Relatively few studies provide advice to policymakers on health IT policy issues, even though policies have enormous consequences for informatics research and practice. We hope that researchers and policymakers will recognize that technology and policy issues affect each other, and it is necessary to use both perspectives to understand how information technology can be used to improve health care.

Suggested Readings

Bates, D. W., & Bitton, A. (2010). The future of health information technology in the patient-centered medical home. *Health Affairs (Project Hope)*, *29*(4), 614–621. This visionary paper supplies a comprehensive distillation of IT needs for the patient-centered medical home. It provides a reference for anyone wishing

---

[12] http://www.hhs.gov/ocr/privacy/index.html (Accessed 12/9/2012)

to implement a medical home and for anyone interested in the next phase of health IT innovation.

Chan, K. S., Fowles, J. B., & Weiner, J. P. (2010). Review: electronic health records and the reliability and validity of quality measures: a review of the literature. *Medical Care Research and Review, 67*(5), 503–527. This comprehensive review should be required reading for anyone thinking about using electronic data for quality measurement. It shows that making accurate, reliable, and comparable quality measures from disparate electronic sources may not be easy.

Institute of Medicine. (2001). *Crossing the quality chasm.* Washington, DC: National Academy Press. This classic report makes an urgent call for a fundamental redesign of the U.S. health care system and a "renewed national commitment to building an information infrastructure to support health care delivery, consumer health, quality measurement and improvement, public accountability, clinical and health services research, and clinical education." Optimistically, it opined that "this commitment should lead to the elimination of most handwritten clinical data by the end of the decade."

Hillestad, R., Bigelow, J., Bower, A., Girosi, F., Meili, R., Scoville, R., et al. (2005). Can electronic medical record systems transform health care? Potential health benefits, savings, and costs. *Health Affairs (Project Hope), 24*(5), 1103–1117. etc. One of the most widely read studies in health policy, this paper by the RAND Corporation estimated a potential cost savings of $81 billion per year due to health IT. It was often cited by politicians as justification for investing in health IT, and likely helped persuade the U.S. Congress to pass the HITECH law, which committed more than $27 billion in meaningful use incentive payments for providers to purchase electronic health records.

Jones, S. S., Heaton, P. S., Rudin, R. S., & Schneider, E. C. (2012). Unraveling the IT productivity paradox — Lessons for health care. *New England Journal of Medicine, 366*(24), 2243–2245. This brief perspective addresses the contentious issue of why few studies have been able to show that health IT produces an improvement in economic productivity. It makes its case by pointing out that the IT industry had the same problem in the 1980s and 1990s but managed to overcome these difficulties through better measurement of productivity, improved management of technology, and better usability.

Kleinke, J. D. (2005). Dot-gov: Market failure and the creation of a national health information technology system. *Health Affairs (Project Hope), 24*(5), 1246–1262. This widely read perspective piece rails against the market inefficiencies in the current health care system and the lack of health IT adoption. It makes the case for "aggressive government intervention."

Agency for Healthcare Research and Quality. (2011). *National strategy for quality improvement in health care.*http://www.healthcare.gov/law/resources/reports/quality03212011a.html (Accessed 12/10/12). This document provides a blueprint for improving quality in the U.S. health care systems, and includes discussion of the role of health IT in that effort.

Institute of Medicine. (1997). *The computer-based patient record: An essential technology for health care,* revised edition. Washington, DC: *National Academy Press*; This landmark report brought many health IT policy issues to public attention, including the importance of assessing the value of health IT products, development of standards, legal constraints of health IT adoption, and the nettlesome question that has always plagued health IT: who will pay for it?

Walker, J., Pan, E., Johnston, D., Adler-Milstein, J., Bates, D. W., & Middleton, B. (2005). The value of health care information exchange and interoperability. *Health Affairs (Project Hope),* Suppl Web Exclusives: W5–10–W5–18. This interesting study by the Center for Information Technology Leadership at Partners Healthcare in Boston provides a point of comparison with the RAND study regarding the value of electronic health records. This study focused only on clinical data exchange and estimated its potential value to be $77.8 billion per year.

Questions for Discussion

1. What are the key barriers to widespread implementation of EHRs and effective exchange of health information? Which of these challenges are amenable to public policy decisions?

2. What might be some of the tradeoffs of using administrative claims data compared with using clinical data from health IT systems for care quality analysis?

3. What might be some of tradeoffs of promoting health IT by paying for use compared with paying for quality?

4. Should health IT be regulated the same way as devices are regulated to protect patient safety? Why or why not?

5. If research finds strong evidence of a digital divide in health IT, what policy actions should be taken?

6. What kinds of health IT functionality are needed to support accountable care organizations and patient-centered medical homes?

7. Compare the U.K.'s approach to clinical data exchange with the U.S.'s approach. What are the advantages, disadvantages and risks of each?

The Future of Informatics in Biomedicine

28

Mark E. Frisse, Valerie Florance, Kenneth D. Mandl, and Isaac S. Kohane

After reading this chapter you should know the answers to these questions:

1. Which current trends will most influence the progress of biomedical informatics research and practice over the next decade?
2. What critical imperatives emerge from these trends?
3. How does the emerging massive, hyper-connected, and pervasive information technology infrastructure affect patients and other consumers?

4. What biomedical informatics "grand challenges" should be pursued over the next decade?

28.1 Goals

Each of this book's previous chapters emphasizes the state of the art while implying future courses of activity; but the primary focus of previous chapters is to summarize what has already been accomplished. This chapter addresses the future. Peter Drucker urges us to identify and prepare for the future by examining the trends and imperatives that define, liberate or constrain the actions individuals take to assure the health and well being of one another. Everyone – physicians, patients, scientists, policy makers, and citizens – must make decisions in the here and now based on the future they want (Drucker 1959). Our approach is to look toward the future by identifying present compelling trends, suggesting some challenge areas for biomedical informatics, and identifying building block areas that will lead to the future we want.

More than a decade ago, scientists at Xerox PARC described a future in which computers were pervasive – woven throughout the daily lives and activities of individuals (Weiser 1993b). Today, there is a massive, global, and ever more pervasive information network that connects people and computers all over the world, in real-time, in many commercial and non-commercial activities. Processing

M.E. Frisse, MD, MS, MBA (✉)
Department of Biomedical Informatics,
Vanderbilt University Medical Center,
432 Eskind Biomedical Library,
2209 Garland Avenue,
Nashville 37232-8340, TN, USA
e-mail: mark.frisse@vanderbilt.edu

V. Florance, PhD
Division of Extramural Programs, National Library
of Medicine, National Institutes of Health, DHHS,
6705 Rockledge Drive, Rockledge 1, Suite 301,
Bethesda 20892, MD, USA
e-mail: florancev@mail.nih.gov

K.D. Mandl, MD, MPH
Children's Hospital Informatics Program,
Boston Children's Hospital, Harvard Medical School,
300 Longwood Avenue, Boston 02446, MA, USA
e-mail: kenneth_mandlh@arvard.edu

I.S. Kohane, MD, PhD
Harvard Medical School Center for Biomedical
Informatics and Children's Hospital Informatics
Program, Boston 02115, MA, USA
e-mail: isaac_kohane@harvard.edu

E.H. Shortliffe, J.J. Cimino (eds.), *Biomedical Informatics*,
DOI 10.1007/978-1-4471-4474-8_28, © Springer-Verlag London 2014

power, input and output devices, bandwidth, storage, and even many common software services have become commoditized and make available to a global society an array of complex information and knowledge resources once afforded only to the elite (AAMC Task Force on Information Technology Infrastructure Requirements for Cross-Institutional Research 2010; Cairncross 2001; National Science Foundation (U.S.), Cyberinfrastructure Council (National Science Foundation) (2007)). For professionals and the public at large, internet-enabled decentralized, globalized and mobilized information sharing, when combined with the capabilities of common consumer technologies (e.g., smart phones) both broaden the availability of knowledge and expertise and lower participation costs. The proliferation of sensors and inexpensive local wireless connectivity and wearable computers creates new opportunities for ambient data collection and more thorough disease monitoring while at the same time posing threats to anonymity and personal privacy (Avancha et al. 2011; Chui et al. 2010; Nissenbaum 2010; Mandl and Kohane 2009).

Never has the need for coordinated innovation been more acute. Many nations are confronting costly increases in health care expenditures as a result of an aging populace, an increase in life expectancy, higher aggregate demand for health care services, and advanced but very expensive new approaches to caring for the very young and the critically ill. Health care costs are deemed unsustainable and pose a growing threat to the economies of nations. Facing massive costs for health care, retirement benefits, and other social programs, governments are increasingly forced to reexamine the funds they can invest in education, research, and vital technology infrastructures. Coordinated innovation is essential to find more efficient and effective means of lower health are expenditures and, at the same time, identifying new an innovative means of educating and conducting research. Without innovation, biomedical informatics may be the victim of a vicious circle in which insufficient support for research and care delivery only raises health care costs and consequently decreases informatics research support even more. This is the soil in which the seeds of the future are germinating.

28.2 Compelling Trends and Critical Imperatives

28.2.1 Trend One. Biomedical Research and Clinical Care Are Linked Through Computation

Laboratory research techniques are evolving rapidly as computational means for data collection, analysis, and simulation have become integral to traditional and novel experimental methods. The inexpensive and widespread use of genetic sequencing, candidate drug target identification, and related technologies creates data sets that exceed current capacities to analyze and interpret, and yet scientists face enormous difficulties in merging data sets to explore new hypotheses. The rate limiting step often is no longer availability of data but instead the ability to address the computational challenges around data integration, data analysis, and new means of visualizing and modeling multidimensional data that may include genotypes, phenotypes, physiological phenomena, and clinical data (Hey et al. 2009). New and innovative approaches to these challenges are emerging (Green and Guyer 2011; National Science Foundation (U.S.) and Cyberinfrastructure Council (National Science Foundation) 2007; President's Council of Advisors on Science and Technology 2010; Multiple Authors 2011b). More direct and immediate linkages among observational data captured in electronic health records and biological investigation research activities represent a new and dramatic collective research frontier. New notions of clinical trials emerge from the research laboratory. New insights derived *in silico* contribute to the prevention of adverse drug interactions and to compare the effectiveness of treatment alternatives. Biological hypotheses, in turn, are refined through more comprehensive and rapid integration of data produced in the routine delivery of health care. Collectively, these trends create, strengthen and refine real-time pipelines between observation in the laboratory and the clinic, and, in so doing, accelerate both the interpretation of data and the dissemination of new knowledge.

New formal or emergent organizational forms are evolving to capitalize more completely on the potential arising from public need and scientific capability (Collins 2011). Greater efforts are being made to strengthen the linkages between basic biomedical research activities and the health care system, within and across organizational, geographic and cultural boundaries (Olsen et al. 2011). Retaining and building upon new knowledge foster new approaches to traditional means of archiving data, knowledge artifacts, and scientific publications (Corn 2009; Luce 2008; National Science and Technology Council (U.S.). Interagency Working Group on Digital Data 2009).

28.2.2 Trend Two: Information Services Are Tailored to the Individual

Mass marketing and communication – be it in commercial or scientific arena – has been replaced by mass customization. In every information activity, users and purveyors of information benefit from decisions tailored to individual need. Internet commerce sites welcome people back by name and suggest a range of readings, music, or other services based on past buying and browsing history. Integrating information across sites allows for highly detailed demographic and preference information that is used to specify on-line advertisements highly tailored to the individual. Health care, while lagging behind the commercial sector for many reasons, has nonetheless recognized the potential of these phenomena both through the adverse impact of incomplete or impersonal information as well as through the growing number of domains in which care is improved through individualized application of highly personalized knowledge (Chan and Ginsburg 2011).

Every part in health care and biomedical research seeks to capitalize on the benefits of personalization while avoiding threats to privacy and other legitimate concerns. Enabled by online access to medical knowledge and data about health services quality and outcomes, consumers, patients, and their informal network of family and caregivers are playing a more active role in their personal health. These same underlying technologies are enabling individuals to filter information and seek answers to questions highly specific to their information needs, scientific questions, or care delivery issues. Common informatics techniques and problem-solving approaches are uniting consumers, clinicians, and biomedical scientists to the benefit of all concerned.

Customization is no longer a luxury; it is becoming a necessity. One can no longer find answers from a data flood unfiltered by knowledge and need. Information overload impedes our individual and collective abilities to perform at our best. Finding the right answers to important questions must be simple and easily understood in context of need, language, culture, and cognitive frameworks.

The explosion of research data in genomics exemplifies the sheer magnitude of the challenge. With next generation technologies, each of the 10–20 major genome sequencing laboratories is estimated to produce at least 400 GB of data daily. The size and complexity of data sets grows when comparison and analysis is conducted. A comparative study of 629 individuals consists of 7.9 TB of data (Kahn 2011b). Clinicians share the same concerns. Clinicians, researchers, and the public also experience information overload. The size of the bibliome is growing exponentially. By 2010, there were over 20 million citations indexed through PubMed alone (Lu 2011). EHR systems are developing capabilities of incorporating data from remote sensors, personal health records, and genotype determination, but the capabilities of EHRs to translate this information into meaningful knowledge lags. Despite powerful computational infrastructure, finding answers somehow seems more difficult – not simpler – as our technologies improve.

28.2.3 Trend Three. Society's Activities Are Increasingly Online and Collaborative

The majority of Americans say they use an online social network. Worldwide, the number of individuals using social networks at the time of this writing is near one billion. Crowd sourcing, flash mobs, blogs and virtual gatherings minimize the geographic and cultural boundaries between people and provide a sense of group action. Information is treated as a free good and a tool for social change (Shirky 2010).

This desire for free and spontaneous access runs counter to past conventions for intellectual property and privacy. Widespread deployment of sensor technologies, data collection, aggregation, and dissemination are changing the balance between open collaboration and protection of personal or proprietary interests. For the researcher, recognition and advancement could be hindered or enhanced. Commercial concerns expect that expensive investments will be recouped. For the individual, rights to privacy and desire to control access to personal information may not be well aligned with societal goals or group priorities (Nissenbaum 2010).

The potential of collaboration technology affords great new opportunities for accelerating scientific research, enabling new forms of collaborative learning at every educational level, adding to society's true health care status, and fostering new means of meeting health care and social needs. These technologies allow both informal conversation and decisive action. They provide the opportunity to broaden collective understanding and bring the right people together at the right time when important decisions or scientific interpretations must be made. The byproducts of these conversations and analyses become a part of the scientific or clinical record. Captured and integrated appropriately this record clarifies the context and evidentiary base for interpretations and decisions.

28.2.4 Trend Four: Electronic Health Records Are Changing Health Care

The use of electronic medical records in health care settings is growing. The use of health information technology has improved safety and efficiency within institutions, although such benefits have not been uniformly realized as individual

seek care across institutional or state or regional boundaries. Incentives for adoption of electronic medical records in the US, for the use of health data to improve patient outcomes and for regional health information exchange were created through the HITECH Act of 2009 (Blumenthal 2010; Buntin et al. 2010). Such initiatives can improve patient outcomes and lower costs if interoperability is assured and focus is shifted from individual encounters to individual and population health.

The sources and magnitude of data relevant to the care of the individual are growing. Clinicians are increasingly required to integrate their traditional EHR data with information from personal health records, family health histories, personal genotypes, and an array of data from glucometers, pedometers, heart monitors, and other body sensors. Environmental hazard information and location history are also relevant to direct patient care, epidemiology, and research. To make complete and reliable decisions, health care professionals will require more sophisticated tools for visualizing and analyzing data so that the important items can be identified and acted on in a timely fashion (Stead and Lin 2009). The communication capabilities of these systems (e.g., secure messaging, health information exchange) could support the development of distributed networks of care providers and coordinators tightly linked through advanced information technologies and focused on improving both efficiency and quality while supporting research and public health if policy and economic barriers are addressed.

Biomedical informatics is playing a critical role in shaping our emerging information technology infrastructure into a learning health care system – a system that is capable both of assuring that every decision is made with complete information and ensuring that every care instance can contribute a deeper understanding of care for individuals and populations. Efforts are underway to provide individuals, families, and clinicians with decision-making support that can adapt to great differences in health literacy levels and cultural context. Collectively, these efforts should realize dramatic improvements in care access, care quality, and care costs.

28.2.5 Trend Five: Data Sets Are Massive, Heterogeneous, and Interconnected

Data once stored in and used by only a single organization are becoming more accessible for use by others. Federal and private sector initiatives are increasingly releasing data in controlled ways to foster innovation in consumer health, care delivery, and scientific investigation (Park 2011). Health information exchange – one means by which more information can be made available to support individual care – has become an essential means by which both the quality and care of individuals and populations may be improved (Frisse et al. 2011). Surveys designed to collect data about personal behavior and preferences now include biological data and connect nature with nurture. Environmental data streams are continuous and plentiful and are available in real time as a factor in public health surveillance. The potential for effective use of information often exceeds the imagination of scientists unaware of impact that linking these new data sets affords.

Traditional approaches to computer-based knowledge representation and analysis appear inadequate to handle the emerging information environment. Informaticians, engineers and computer scientists, among others, are working hard to develop new approaches for managing complexity, minimizing fragmentation, improving data accuracy and completeness, and establishing meaningful linkages among data sets. Our emerging massive data sets contain 'chunks' of distinct but related data, not collected from the same sources or for the same purpose, but linked by the implications for human health.

Despite stunning progress in data collection and storage, the true potential of richer and more inter-connected data sets has not yet been realized. Computable data sets have untapped potential to provide new insights into clinical care, fundamental research, public health activities, educational efforts, and health care administration – in short, reaching into every aspect of health and biomedicine. The enormous range of expression of molecular and organism-level data routinely used by the laboratory-based biomedi-

cal scientist will be matched in complexity and diversity by the emergence of systems that combine genotype, phenotype, environmental data, lifestyle data, location, personal preferences and detailed analysis of inferences derived from ambient data collection.

Addressing critical imperatives will require unprecedented and consequential improvements to the efficiency and effectiveness in every aspect of research, education and care delivery. Most economically advanced nations are confronting costly increases in health care expenditures. These cost increases are the result of an aging society, an increase in life expectancy, higher aggregate demand for health care services, and new means for caring for the very young, the very old, and those at the end of life. By all accounts, these factors contribute significantly to an unsustainable increase in health care costs and a massive drain on national economies. If left unattended, the consequences will be dire. Escalating costs and weak economies force individuals and governments to make difficult choices between paying more to meet this generation's rising health care demands or investing more in the research necessary to meet the needs of the next generation.

28.3 Biomedical Informatics Grand Challenges

The science and practice of biomedical informatics are evolving in a world where computation is ubiquitous, data are heavily interlinked, people collaborate in new ways, economic needs and constraints increase, and the nature of biomedical research and discovery has changed. Grand Challenges require innovative breakthroughs across a range of disciplines, not just in a single field. Successful solutions to a Grand Challenge will transform the way people think, they way they work, and the way they care for themselves and one another (Omenn 2006; Sittig 1994; Sittig et al. 2008; van Bemmel 1997; Wild 2009). We frame five such Grand Challenges in terms of Drucker's questions: what futurity do we have to factor into our present thinking and doing, what time spans do we have to consider, and how do we converge them to a simultaneous decision in the present"? (Drucker 1959). Each Grand Challenge requires innovation and collaboration. Each is directed towards long-term goals but suggests identifiable immediate and intermediate milestones.

We present each Grand Challenge, describe possible outcomes if the Challenge is met, and place the Challenge in the context of critical scientific or societal imperatives. We suggest possible starting points by identifying some "building blocks" that, when developed, will contribute to successful outcomes. By virtue of the interdependencies among informatics foundations, technology, policy, and action, a building block elaborated under one Grand Challenge may very well be a critical component of other Challenges described.

28.3.1 Grand Challenge One. Comprehensive and Dynamic Information Resources for Research, Education, and Health Care Delivery

When this challenge is addressed, our ability to characterize and understand complex biomedical phenomena will increase as a result of new capacity to analyze and interpret data from ambient information, from deftly engineered vehicles for collecting research data or patient-reported observation, and from social networks and an array of intelligent medical devices.

Biomedical researchers, clinicians, and patients will benefit from extensive and tightly-linked data resources that improve understanding of disease mechanisms through deeper insights into relationships among genes, behavior and environment. New opportunities to improve health care delivery and biomedical research arise when more integrated and manageable systems are brought to bear at the very moment clinical or personal health decisions should be made.

Biomedical informatics professionals must ensure that the potential of a hyper-connected informatics infrastructure is realized. Data from disparate sources must be linked and integrated with sufficient precision to assure safe and effective use across a range of scientific, clinical, and

administrative actions that are increasingly reliant on large data sets and accurate machine interpretation. Data standards, ontologies, representation formalisms, pattern recognition, systems and many other techniques must be coordinated seamlessly to ensure efforts will scale and be applicable broadly to a wider array of researchers, teachers, clinicians, and individuals seeking answers to health questions. Standardized, open, and modular software architectures will be essential to ensure that development of and access to systems is affordable to all with needs.

28.3.1.1 Intelligent, Learning Machines

Both data mining and text mining can be used to markup data sets so scientists can identify trends and make discoveries. Real-time collection of reliable data must be more tightly linked with resources that present evidence and enable better clinical decision support. Linkages among full-text biomedical journals can guide ontology development and experimentation (Bada and Hunter 2011). Machine learning techniques should also be directed towards systems that can determine when and how new data suggest reconsideration of published research and care guidelines. The impact of quantifying data and embedded reasoning aids must be more thoroughly studied and understood.

28.3.1.2 Linkages, Multi-Scale Models, and Testing Environments

Integrating disparate systems will require both multidisciplinary collaboration and new data environments in which novel approaches may be tested. In clinical care, progress can be accelerated through more pilot programs designed to evaluate and improve large-scale computable phenotypes from disparate clinical data sources (Kullo et al. 2010). A wide array of open-source software systems, communications standards, natural language processing technologies, data mapping systems, and ontology resources must remain available to foster the broad collaborations necessary for substantive work (Multiple Authors 2011a). Using similar approaches, technologies, test beds, complex multidisciplinary collaborations, and other novel methods should be employed to transform increasingly voluminous bio molecular data into proactive, predictive, preventive and participatory health techniques (Kohane et al. 2011; Multiple Authors 2010).

28.3.1.3 Informative Interfaces

Sensors and other devices will deliver live data streams from homes, test labs and patients for analysis and knowledge management. Better approaches must be developed to present data to clinicians, researchers and consumers in ways that foster and enhance both understanding and use of the data. Each tool, from the most sophisticated systems used to plan surgery to the consumer-oriented gaming systems for health care promotion, must be tailored to the capabilities and needs of the individual using it at the moment. Each must evolve as the skills of the user grow. Systems are needed that can adapt to various needs and levels of literacy without requiring customized programming for each encounter.

28.3.1.4 New Models for Biology and Health

Collectively, linkage and analysis techniques can be used to formalize interdependencies between genotypic and phenotype data, drawing data from populations with multiple conditions to complement current clinical trials. Analysis of the value, investment and impact of different components in this cycle requires new statistical models as well as systems that can track or predict the elements taken into account in a decision. New forms of simulations must be developed to accelerate understanding in scientific and clinical settings.

28.3.2 Grand Challenge Two. Decision Support Is Fully Informed by Evidence and Personalized to the Individual

When this challenge is addressed, it will be far simpler to gather and personalize many types of evidence about an individual's health and information needs in ways that support personal decisions made alone or with the assistance of family members, clinicians or friends. Personal health information, medical records data, and published clinical trial results would be complemented by broader array of genetic information, environmental context, and ongoing clinical trial data that are presented at an appropriate level for the user.

The sophistication and reach of intelligent tools already embedded in the health information infrastructure makes this scenario possible, even likely. The seeds for receiving guidance this way are already planted – in software 'wizards', in e-commerce recommender systems, and in retrieval aids supporting consumer health information sites (Ricci et al. 2011). New efforts focused on health care and biomedical research should tailor plentiful and rich sources of data, information and knowledge to meet the individual needs in any context at any moment in time. Efforts may create more helpful dashboards summarizing health status summaries, recommending consumer health actions or even monitoring critical care delivery. They can also be directed to highly sophisticated treatment planning systems supporting the complex treatment protocols in modern oncology, critical care, and other disciplines in which lives depend on the results (Stead 2010). There is an opportunity to ensure that every appropriate health data item and every entry in a person's care record contribute appropriately to a sound health decision.

Once personalized diagnoses can be reached through integration of comprehensive information, the next step can be highly personalized care plans that are shaped by social, economic and cultural knowledge. Every health decision can be based on information that is made meaningful for the decision maker, delivered at the right time and place, in a usable form. For example, every decision to prescribe a medication could be made on the basis of a computer-generated synthesis (of current medications, past medication history, allergies, health status, phenotype, physiology, and full genetic profiles) that is delivered quickly to the clinician, saving hours of valuable time.

28.3.2.1 Personalized Choices

Each decision support application, from the most sophisticated systems used to plan surgery to the consumer-oriented gaming systems for health promotion, must be able to tailor itself to the capabilities and needs of the individual using it at the moment. Decision support applications based on ever-improving user modeling systems will afford greater adaptation to changes in needs and user sophistication. Decision support application research and practice can lead to systems that assess levels of literacy without needing specialized programming for each encounter. Through contextual analysis, these new systems can allow their users to focus on the decision at hand rather than the mechanics of software interfaces.

28.3.2.2 Personalized Health Libraries

In the current information-rich culture, information seeking and management are routine for everyone. Individuals increasingly expect all useful information to be available on the Internet in real time. Individuals expect continuing improvements in access to and management of personal health information collections drawn from health records, personal notes, correspondence, Internet sites, and health publications. Efforts to transform data collections into useful, self-managing, and usable personal libraries are promising research and application directions. Equally valuable will be health-library applications capable of searching through the universe of health information for possibly pertinent new data, assessing it, asking advice and making recommendations to the library owner about updates. Research is also needed to foster patient discussion with knowledgeable peers or professionals when advice and recommendations are sought about the relevance of a new piece of information.

28.3.2.3 Personalized Translators

Inevitably, clinicians, scientists and patients use technical jargon or culturally determined language that is clear to the members of their group, but not to others. They speak in phrases and not sentences, inject humor, scramble many ideas into a single thought, and make mistakes. Efforts that improve processing the spoken and written language of health care and biomedical research will increasingly be foundational components of far more sophisticated knowledge management

systems. Language applications capable of 'translating' across and among different cultural or technical domains may be as valued as those that translate among foreign languages.

28.3.2.4 Personalized Health Curricula

Efforts focusing on patient education are often situational, such as instructions for wound care. But longitudinal health records support a new approach, the ability to formalize a "learning curriculum" tailored to the needs of individual who receives care and to professionals and informal caregivers who support this care. Pilot programs should be developed linking the educational agenda of patients and doctors with the care plan. Social/behavioral research on health literacy, language barriers, culture and demographic factors that influence learning should be exploited in delivery of this curriculum (Woods and Kemper 2009). Similar efforts could apply to providing clinicians with continuous education about new types of information (e.g., genetic tests) feeding into the electronic health record and their utility in health decisions.

These efforts complement the use of collaborative models, individualization, and simulation in more traditional health science education. With few exceptions, our professional schools remain fixed on nineteenth century models of education, segregated by professional class, and certainly ill-suited to the collaborative nature of care essential for today's economy. Personalized education services are a part of a more systematic study of the transformation of traditional education through distance learning, computer-supported collaboration, team-based education, experiential knowledge gathering, and simulation. Much can be learned remotely – whether from the other side of a state or the other side of the world. Teams can be brought together sooner and exposed both to real world clinical and laboratory settings or simulations of critical complex problems. Teaching of surgical techniques must be developed to support widespread and routine pre-operative simulation and robotic surgery when such techniques yield cost-effective improvements. These same techniques can be applied to create far more customized case-based teaching technologies foster a greater reliance on three-dimensional interactive exploration over traditional anatomical dissection (Satava 2007).

28.3.2.5 Personalized Health Records

Clinicians, patients and their families need access to similar information whether in their homes, in care settings, in offices or other public settings. Information must flow between care-center based electronic health records and personalized health records maintained by patients and their families. Techniques for self-monitoring by an electronic health record, whether corporate or personal, can be improved through the addition of synchronized updates, gap identification, error avoidance, and a range of alerting applications. The integration of two (or more) views of a person's health history can help foster dialogue efficiently about new research findings, relevant changes in family health, or possible changes to a care plan suggested by data from sensor readings. Opportunities abound to create systems that allow individuals to use health information to link data, make personal discoveries, find others like themselves, and promote positive collaborative dialogue to extend the notion of the self-managing individual to the notion of the self-managing group (Kohane and Altman 2005).

28.3.3 Grand Challenge Three. Learning from Every Experiment and Health Care Decision

When this challenge is addressed, individuals and groups will be able to more readily exploit the virtuous circle of evidence creation, critical analysis, rapid application, rigorous evaluation and effective use (Frenk 2010). Research and practice become continually informed by new findings and the evidence supporting fairly limited situations becomes relevant to a broader and more complex population. Through this virtuous circle, research is transformed from a static set of activities to a continuous and never-ending process of advancement and transformation.

To optimize care, practitioners of evidence-based medicine use scientific information largely gleaned from the published literature, often based on randomized clinical trials. The challenge is to bring about a new paradigm in which evidence-based medical decisions include not only traditional published medical knowledge, but also evidence from highly processed clinical, environmental and epidemiological information.

Electronic medical record systems contain both structured and unstructured health data. These systems may hold more longitudinal data than a paper patient record held, but identifying all pertinent information for the problem at hand is not yet routine. The promise of this large data repository lies in the clinician's ability to quickly see outcomes for a given patient based on the experience of many similar patients. To use stored health data in this care paradigm requires novel probabilistic modeling paradigms and machine learning techniques.

The Institute of Medicine has called for a learning health care system that generates and applies "the best evidence for the collaborative health care choices of each patient and provider; to drive the process of discovery as a natural outgrowth of patient care; and to ensure innovation, quality, safety, and value in health care" (Etheredge 2007; Olsen et al. 2011). A recently shifting emphasis from clinical trials to post marketing surveillance creates one clear example. Withdrawals of major drugs such as cerivastatin and rofecoxib have highlighted the importance of post-marketing surveillance where pre-launch clinical trials often fail to detect adverse drug effects due to limits in sample size and demographic diversity, and in the diversity of co-morbidities and drug interactions represented in trials (McGettigan and Henry 2006; Staffa et al. 2002; Strom 2006; Wadman 2007). Hence, the data to support a complementary system of evidence, based on observational data about large numbers of patients, can be delivered. While there are inherent selection and confounding biases in evaluating outcomes in observational datasets, there are also advantages to measuring the impact of therapeutic trajectories in real world contexts.

To date, the term personalized medicine has denoted use of a patient's genotypes to define whom the patient most closely resembles, in order to target and tailor therapeutic options. In fact, genotype is only one variable that can be used to personalize therapies or to predict trajectories and outcomes. Another approach would be personalization based on clinical and quality outcomes across a similar population. For example, a given patient or her doctor considering a new medication might predict rates of adverse events and hospitalizations based on the experience of a cohort of individuals similar to the patient with respect to age, gender, genetic makeup, and underlying conditions (Polifka and Friedman 2002). The predictions may differ from those made by extrapolating the results of often small clinical studies and applying them to the patient at hand. More often than not, a patient differs from the population studied in traditional clinical trials in terms of age, race, ethnicity, co-morbidities, duration of exposure to the therapeutic and even indication.

With personalization of therapy based on contextualization of a patient among those with similar characteristics, clinical decisions are made not only on generic knowledge and the traditional medical history but also on a worldwide collective knowledge of how such decisions have affected the care of others with similar highly specific characteristics (Feero et al. 2010; Hamburg and Collins 2010; Kemper et al. 2010; Kho et al. 2011).

This contextualized information has a role in supporting decisions by patients and doctors. There is already a grassroots movement to share information among patients with similar diseases through online social networks. This movement is predicated on the belief that patients should be able to use their own information to find appropriate others with whom they can exchange ideas, share data, make discoveries on their own, and develop new collaboratively created knowledge resources (Kohane and Altman 2005; Weitzman et al. 2011a; Wicks et al. 2011).

28.3.3.1 Comprehensive, Self-Updating Data Sets

The generation of self-updating pan-health care datasets will be advanced through additional research and policy efforts directed towards data governance, de-identification, aggregation, and use policies. Data may come from EHRs, from public health documents, or from patients themselves (Fine et al. 2011). Meta-level representation is essential for simplifying integration, supporting new uses of data, and enforcing privacy. The 2010 report from the President's Council of Advisors on Science and Technology represents one general approach (President's Council of Advisors on Science and Technology 2010). Efforts to apply on a systematic basis meta-level representations to all forms of health care information will be vital both to support tractable machine-interpretation and to ensure data privacy and security policies are maintained.

28.3.3.2 Personalization Information Meeting Individual Needs

The precise synergy and complementarity of observational studies and traditional study designs (e.g., randomized controlled trials) must be established. Providing personalized decision-support services will require more systematic research and evaluation of methods that will find the cohort of patients similar to a given patient, identify the treatment paths taken for that cohort, and quantify outcomes as a function of treatment paths.

28.3.3.3 New Channels for Distribution and Discovery

Health information exchanges should allow processed clinical information to flow across boundaries among various clinical and public health environments, allowing a new awareness of epidemiologic context. But many technical, cultural, and policy challenges impede realizing the full potential of data exchange. Additional research, implementation, and evaluation in operational settings of means by which EHRs and PHRs can communicate with one another afford promising opportunities. Fruitful research directions include the adaptation of these principles to formal care coordination, virtual medical homes, and custom-tailored information services.

28.3.3.4 Personalization Information Meeting Group Needs

Through more widespread access to a range of information, new opportunities arise for under-standing the role of the individual within their environment. By "lifting one's head up" and looking at broader social needs, one can gain a broader perspective of the context in which systems are used. Research that helps prioritize what must be done and for whom will help assure that developers do not so much create software as they create societal value. These activities require a range of skills to assess needs and markets, to implement rapid and iterative user-centered systems, and to evaluate critically the extent to which their efforts help others do their work more effectively and efficiently.

28.3.3.5 Effective Support for Cognitive Work

In clinical settings, far greater attention must be paid to systems that will allow emphasis to shift from the administrative coordination of clin-ical and financial transactions to support for the cognitive work of teams (Gooch and Roudsari 2011; Stead et al. 2008). Research activities iden-tifying more effective means of supporting col-laborative work will be highly valued; systems that accomplish this goal while also supporting financial transaction management and other administrative tasks will be valued to an even greater degree.

28.3.4 Grand Challenge Four. Access to Information is Ubiquitous

Responding to this challenge will advance the coordination of care delivery and decision-making across the health care ecosystem. Individuals making health care decisions will no longer be burdened by seeking information but

instead can concentrate on effectively managing and applying biomedical knowledge. This will require the advancement of a comprehensive, modular, secure, sustainable, and transparent information infrastructure that automatically integrates data from disparate systems, maintains appropriate policy, privacy, and intellectual prop-erty controls, and ensures reliable and standard-ized access by individuals and organizations authorized to access and use the data and knowl-edge within.

28.3.4.1 All Relevant Information Available

Access ideally should conform to the A^7 princi-ple: Anywhere Anytime, Affordable Access to Anything by Anyone Authorized (Wing and Barr 2011). Whether viewed as part of an electronic health record or located by searching Google, MedlinePlus or another online health information source, optimal decisions can only be made effi-ciently if new means are developed to integrate disparate data sources in standardized ways. More consistent means can be developed to transform and integrate into decision-making contexts a wider range of audio, graphic and printed information. Many research avenues can be explored to develop support software that can be embedded in ways that enhance ability to mark-up and explain any item in the information at hand. These systems can confer a greater "intelligence" to information by demonstrably incorporating in appropriate ways and on a "real time" basis all relevant new information.

28.3.4.2 Modular, Open-Source Software

Novel methods for developing and evaluating the creation and distribution of open-source soft-ware are essential to afford interoperability, economy, and scalability. Affordable access to software systems that improve productivity and growth is every bit as important as the equally open and affordable "big data" systems that drive innovation. Modular and open-source sys-tems are vital to every topic discussed in this chapter. Through systematic study of foundation systems, developer intuition can be complemented by far-reaching and more formal needs assessments.

28.3.4.3 Leveraging the Promise of Emerging Technologies

In some contexts, sophisticated software systems can complement or replace human decision-making. As has been the case in the computer interpretation of electrocardiograms, efforts should be made to determine the circumstances in which pattern recognition and other techniques can confer the same accuracy and efficiencies in other areas such as radiology and histopathology (Burnside et al. 2006; Gabril and Yousef 2010; Noble et al. 2009; Rubin and Napel 2010). More broadly, new means of analysis can be applied to leverage genome-wide association studies and to personalize medical care. The former requires particular attention to the curation of massive data sets; the latter requires study of how mobile devices can be integrated into systems of care.

28.3.4.4 Compelling Demonstration of Value

Further work is needed to study the effectiveness and efficiency of interconnected systems and of the decision tools and other intelligent aids built into them. First, automated approaches associated with incorporating and integrating data from outside sources (e.g., environmental data, monitoring device information) must be studied. Second, widespread data exchange among mobile devices, personal health systems, electronic health records, and other technologies necessitates new analytic approaches derived from the perspective of individuals and systems (Friedman and Wyatt 2006). Of necessity, these analyses will include measuring impact on patients, families, providers, researchers, and those responsible for the financing of research and care. These analyses will require collaborative approaches across a range of technical, social, and economic disciplines. Finally, these same systems will provide new capabilities for knowledge discovery, post-market surveillance of drugs and medical devices, emergency preparedness, Biosurveillance, and public health.

28.3.5 Challenge Five. Policies that Ensure an Accessible, Secure, Reliable, Effective, and Sustainable Global Computational Infrastructure

Our hyper-connected global information infrastructure continually changes science, commerce, collaboration, education, migration, politics, government, and almost every other aspect of work and life (Friedman 2007). As demands for this infrastructure grow, it will in the aggregate become increasingly costly and will require some degree of continuous management and governance. The impact of this infrastructure upon biomedical informatics, scientific collaboration, education, clinical care and related disciplines is apparent (American Medical Informatics Association 2011; Breslow 2007; Christensen et al. 2009; National Research Council of the National Academies 2011). But at both a global and a local level, disagreements arise on the benefits to individuals and groups of both specific short- and long-term investments and, correspondingly, differences in opinions concerning financial support, governance, and management. Like transportation, utilities, education, and other public goods, the debate about global infrastructure is not about whether it is needed, it is about the value models, regulations for use, governance, and the equitable payment essential for long-term sustainability.

Through effective governance, individuals contributing information to a large and heavily connected system must be assured that their expectations for use and for recognition are reasonably met. Infrastructure governance structures – at any level from local to global – must be studied to validate their ability to maintain data provenance, protect intellectual property, and to ensure data are not disclosed or used in ways contrary to the consent provisions of the individuals or researchers who served as the primary contributors to any data item or collection. Starting from classic management theory, these new systems afford new and necessary opportunities to study of relationships between strategy, governance, operations, sustainability and growth (Evans 2011).

28.3.5.1 Data Privacy and Security

Data use must be consistent with policies and the expectations of those who contribute data (Avancha et al. 2011; Evans 2011; Markle Foundation 2006; Nissenbaum 2010). As data become more integrated, the challenge of enforcing policies and preferences becomes more problematic. Fruitful and significant efforts focus around the modeling of privacy policies and preferences, the discovery of policies and violations through audit log analysis, methods to anonymize data, and the creation of methods to ensure the protection of everything from massive distributed databases to individual wearable medical devices. As is the case with other biomedical corpora, privacy and security policies defy comprehensive translation into computable forms. Practical means of representing policies and developing policy enforcement mechanisms present major opportunities made even more challenging by the need to ensure these policies are operable in systems composed of mobile devices and other large-scale computing systems, multiple users, and multiple intentions for use (Avancha et al. 2011; Markle Foundation 2006; Nissenbaum 2010).

28.3.5.2 Sustainable Preservation

Pilots designed to study the preservation of new data sources and collections are essential components of a health care technology infrastructure. These collections may originate from machines, scientific research, care provision, patients, family members, social networks, ambient environmental sensors, formal and informal scientific or social publications, and many other sources. Derived artifacts may represent complex biological models, disease processes, health status of individuals or populations, or evidence for advancing research and clinical care. They may be relatively static or they may be generated

dynamically as needs arise. Approaches can be evaluated by the extent to which the collection and support of such artifacts are sustainable and by the extent to which they facilitate subsequent inquiry through exploration across a broad topic at a high level or through deep immersion into detail. Methods can be developed that are applicable across organizations, regions, and countries. Ideally, these methods can encompass the various representations and use intentions for clinical and administrative data. Current approaches to assessing sustainability models for digital data will benefit from a fusion of relevant techniques applicable to large-scale challenges in other domains.

28.4 Summary

This chapter summarizes some of the major, compelling trends in technology, society, economics, and science that serve as the context in which biomedical informatics research is conducted. Collectively these resources constitute an infrastructure that is pervasive, computationally powerful, and capable of providing dramatic scientific and clinical progress. These technologies are changing the way every person lives, works, and learns. Self-evident and irrevocable trends suggest a number of imperatives critical to social and scientific progress. Each imperative challenges the biomedical informatics community to build upon the momentum of technical and social change to address unresolved problems in the creation, management, mining, dissemination and use of biomedical data, information, and knowledge. Some future possibilities are apparent today; some are suggested in the Grand Challenges. Substantive and lasting engagement of the biomedical informatics community can make this possible future a reality.

Suggested Readings

Chan, I. S., & Ginsburg, G. S. (2011). Personalized medicine: progress and promise. *Annual Review of Genomics and Human Genetics, 12,* 217–244. This paper provides a comprehensive review of the full spectrum of personalized medicine, from laboratory discoveries to their application at the bedside.

Christensen, C. M., Grossman, J. H., & Hwang, J. (2009). *The innovator's prescription: a disruptive solution for health care*. New York: McGraw-Hill. This book provides background information on the notion of "disruptive technology" across a wide range of application and policy areas in health care. Based on observations in many industries, it describes the various ways in which innovation can emerge.

Chui, M., Loffler, M., & Roberts, R. (2010). The internet of things. McKinsey Quarterly, 2, 1–9. This book looks at the emerging technology of network-enabled sensors being embedded in everyday objects, from roadways to pacemakers. The pervasive nature of computing blurs boundaries between health care and broader consumer software systems.

Friedman, T. L. (2007). *The world is flat: a brief history of the twenty-first century* (1st further updated and expanded hardcover ed.). New York: Farrar, Straus and Giroux. This book provides a perspective on globalization of economies and technology and how they are "leveling the playing field" for international business competition. The combination of inexpensive computing, global networks, and liquid data change the very nature of collaboration in every setting.

Green, E. D., & Guyer, M. S. (2011). Charting a course for genomic medicine from base pairs to bedside. *Nature, 470*(7333), 204–213. This paper by the Director of the National Human Genome Research Institute offers predictions about how our increasing understanding of the genetic contributions to human health and disease will alter the way medical care is practiced.

Kohane, I. S. (2011). Using electronic health records to drive discovery in disease genomics. *Nature Reviews Genetics, 12*(6), 417–428. This paper provides a review of methods used to entrain EHR data into genomics research, makes comparisons with analogous aspects of conventional cohort-driven research, and summaries current major projects.

National Science Foundation (U.S.), & Cyberinfrastructure Council (National Science Foundation). (2007). *Cyberinfrastructure vision for 21st century discovery* (pp. iii, 58 p.). Retrieved from http://www.nsf.gov/pubs/2007/nsf0728/index.jsp. This publication from the NSF lays out its vision of the future of a culture of peer-to-peer collaboration that is emerging to support distributed communities focused on education, science and development.

President's Council of Advisors on Science and Technology. (2010). *Realizing the full potential of health information technology to improve healthcare for Americans: The path forward*. Washington, DC: Executive Office of the President. The "PCAST Report" reviews the state of health information technology, in particular, those aspects influenced by US federal efforts. The report argues for meta-data standards, mapping of sematic taxonomies onto tagged data elements connected through a common infrastructure. It describes how these features can promote privacy, increase data security, and broaden use of health care information.

Stead, W. W., & Lin, H. S. (Eds.). (2009). *Computational technology for effective health care: Intermediate steps and strategic directions*. Washington, DC: The National Academies Press. This report from the Computer Science and Telecommunications Board of the National Science Foundation describes the current status of transaction-based health care information systems and promotes the adoption of systems more focused on knowledge management and effective clinical use. It serves as a foundation for future research directions in health care informatics.

Questions for Discussion

1. Describe a hypothetical 3-year informatics research proposal that would enable you to address a specific grand challenge. What critical imperatives would your effort address?

2. Identify three organizations that support such research. Provide links and a rationale.

3. Identify research funded by these organizations that provides a methodological foundation for your proposed research.

4. Describe your specific aims, your methods, environmental dependencies, timelines, and a budget represented in terms of your time and financial resources required.

5. If working as a team, specify the specific roles and responsibilities each team member would assume.

6. If working independently, create a list of three informatics researchers from other institutions who pursue similar lines of inquiry. Explain the rationale for your choices by describing their hypothetical contributions to your effort and how you would contribute to their ongoing research.

7. If your interest is in health care delivery or public health, identify a hypothetical project that recognizes a critical imperative, responds to a grand challenge, and advances your organization's mission. Describe your approach, your requirements, and your resource commitments, and your expected results. Whenever possible, extend your personal efforts to encompass teams across the wide spectrum of health are activities from research, administration, care delivery, public health, individuals, and society.

Glossary

Key chapters in which a term is used are indicated in square brackets.

Accountability Security function that ensures users are responsible for their access to and use of information based on a documented need and right to know [5].

Accountable Care Organizations (ACOs) An organization of health care providers that agrees to be accountable for the quality, cost, and overall care of their patients. An ACO will be reimbursed on the basis of managing the care of a population of patients and are determined by quality scores and reductions in total costs of care [14,27].

Accountable care A descendant of managed care, accountable care is an approach to improving care and reducing costs. See: **AccountableCare Organizations** [10].

ACO See: Accountable Care Organizations [14, 27].

Active failures Errors that occur in an acute situation, the effects of which are immediately felt [4].

Active phase The phase of a clinical research study during which investigators collect data from participants receiving an intervention or interventions under study. It is also common to monitor study participants for adverse events during this phase [26].

Active storage In a hierarchical data-storage scheme, the devices used to store data that have long-term validity and that must be accessed rapidly [5].

Acute Physiology and Chronic Health Evaluation, Version III [APACHE III] A scoring system for rating the disease severity for particular use in intensive care units [18].

Address An indicator of location; typically a number that refers to a specific position in a computer's memory or storage device; see also: **Internet Address** [5].

ADE See: Adverse Drug Events [19].

Admission-discharge-transfer (ADT) The core component of a hospital information system that maintains and updates the hospital census, including bed assignments of patients [14].

ADT See: Admission-discharge-transfer [14].

Advanced Research Projects Agency Network (ARPANET) A large wide-area network created in the 1960s by the U.S. Department of Defense Advanced Research Projects Agency (DARPA) for the free exchange of information among universities and research organizations; the precursor to today's Internet [1,5].

Adverse drug events (ADEs) Undesired patient events, whether expected or unexpected, that are attributed to administration of a drug [19].

Aggregations In the context of information retrieval, collections of content from a variety of content types, including bibliographic, full-text, and annotated material [21].

AHIMA See: American Health Information Management Association [21].

Alert message A computer-generated warning that is generated when a record meets pre-specified criteria, often referring to a potentially dangerous situation that may require action; e.g., receipt of a new laboratory test result with an abnormal value [12].

Algorithmic process An algorithm is a well-defined procedure or sequence of steps for solving a problem. A process that follows prescribed steps is accordingly an algorithmic process [1].

Alphanumeric Descriptor of data that are represented as a string of letters and numeric digits, without spaces or punctuation [21].

E.H. Shortliffe, J.J. Cimino (eds.), *Biomedical Informatics*,
DOI 10.1007/978-1-4471-4474-8, © Springer-Verlag London 2014

Ambulatory medical record systems (AMRS)
A clinical information system designed to support all information requirements of an outpatient clinic, including registration, appointment scheduling, billing, order entry, results reporting, and clinical documentation [14].

American Health Information Management Association (AHIMA) Professional association devoted to the discipline of health information management (HIM) [21].

American Medical Informatics Association (AMIA) Professional association dedicated to biomedical and health informatics [15, 23].

American National Standards Institute [ANSI] A private organization that oversees voluntary consensus standards [7,23].

American Recovery and Reinvestment Act of 2009 Public Law 111–5, commonly referred to as the Stimulus or Recovery Act, this legislation was designed to create jobs quickly and to invest in the nation's infrastructure, education and healthcare capabilities [14].

American Standard Code for Information Interchange (ASCII) A 7-bit code for representing alphanumeric characters and other symbols [5].

AMIA See: American Medical Informatics Association [15, 23].

AMRS See: Ambulatory medical record systems [14].

Analog signal A signal that takes on a continuous range of values [5].

Analog-to-digital conversion (ADC) Conversion of sampled values from a continuous-valued signal to a discrete-valued digital representation [5].

Anchoring and adjustment A heuristic used when estimating probability, in which a person first makes a rough approximation (the anchor), then adjusts this estimate to account for additional information [3].

Annotated content In the context of information retrieval, content that has been annotated to describe its type, subject matter, and other attributes [21].

Anonymize Applied to health data and information about a unique individual, the act of de-identifying or stripping away any and all data which could be used to identify that individual [10].

ANSI See: American National Standards Institute [23].

Antibiogram Pattern of sensitivity of a microorganism to various antibiotics [19].

APACHE III See Acute Physiology and Chronic Health Evaluation, Version III [18].

Apache Open source web server software that was significant in facilitating the initial growth of the World Wide Web [6].

Applets Small computer programs that can be embedded in an HTML document and that will execute on the user's computer when referenced [5,6].

Application programming interface (API) A specification that enables distinct software modules or components to communicate with each other [6].

Application program A computer program that automates routine operations that store and organize data, perform analyses, facilitate the integration and communication of information, perform bookkeeping functions, monitor patient status, aid in education [5].

Applications (applied) research Systematic investigation or experimentation with the goal of applying knowledge to achieve practical ends [1].

Archival storage In a hierarchical data-storage scheme, the devices used to store data for long-term backup, documentary, or legal purposes [5].

Arden Syntax for Medical Logic Module A coding scheme or language that provides a canonical means for writing rules that relate specific patient situations to appropriate actions for practitioners to follow. The Arden Syntax standard is maintained by HL7 [6, 22].

Argument A word or phrase that helps complete the meaning of a **predicate** [8].

ARPANET See Advanced Research Projects Agency Network [1,5].

Artificial intelligence(AI) The branch of computer science concerned with endowing computers with the ability to simulate intelligent human behavior [1].

Artificial neural network A computer program that performs classification by taking as input a set of findings that describe a given situation, propagating calculated weights through a network of several layers of interconnected nodes, and generating as output a set of numbers, where each output corresponds to the likelihood of a particular classification that could explain the findings [23].

ASCII See: American Standard Code for Information Interchange [5].

Assembler A computer program that translates assembly-language programs into machine-language instructions [5].

Assembly language A low-level language for writing computer programs using symbolic names and addresses within the computer's memory [5].

Asynchronous Transfer Mode (ATM) A network protocol designed for sending streams of small, fixed length cells of information over very high-speed, dedicated connections, often digital optical circuits [5].

Audit trail A chronological record of all accesses and changes to data records, often used to promote accountability for use of, and access to, medical data [5].

Authenticated A process for positive and unique identification of users, implemented to control system access [5].

Authorized Within a system, a process for limiting user activities only to actions defined as appropriate based on the user's role [5].

Automated indexing The most common method of full-text indexing; words in a document are stripped of common suffixes, entered as items in the index, then assigned weights based on their ability to discriminate among documents (see vector-space model) [21].

Availability In decision making, a heuristic method by which a person estimates the probability of an event based on the ease with which he can recall similar events [3]. In security systems, a function that ensures delivery of accurate and up-to-date information to authorized users when needed [5].

Averaging out at chance nodes The process by which each chance node of a decision tree is replaced in the tree by the expected value of the event that it represents [3].

Backbone links Sections of high-capacity trunk (backbone) network that interconnect regional and local networks [5].

Backbone Network A high-speed communication network that carries major traffic between smaller networks [1].

Background question A question that asks for general information on a topic (see also: **foreground question**) [21].

Backward chaining Also known as goal-directed reasoning. A form of inference used in **rule-based systems** in which the **inference engine** determines whether the premise (left-hand side) of a given rule is true by invoking other rules that can conclude the values of variables that currently are unknown and that are referenced in the premise of the given rule. The process continues recursively until all rules that can supply the required values have been considered [22].

Bag-of-words A language model where text is represented as a collection of words, independent of each other and disregarding word order [8].

Bandwidth The capacity for information transmission; the number of bits that can be transmitted per unit of time [5].

Baseline rate:population The prevalence of the condition under consideration in the population from which the subject was selected; **individual**: The frequency, rate, or degree of a condition before an intervention or other perturbation [2].

Basic Local Alignment Search Tool (BLAST) An algorithm for determining optimal genetic sequence alignments based on the observations that sections of proteins are often conserved without gaps and that there are statistical analyses of the occurrence of small subsequences within larger sequences that can be used to prune the search for matching sequences in a large database [24].

Basic research Systematic investigation or experimentation with the goal of discovering new knowledge, often by proposing new generalizations from the results of several experiments [1].

Basic science The enterprise of performing basic research [1].

Bayes' theorem An algebraic expression often used in clinical diagnosis for calculating post-test probability of a condition (a disease, for example) if the pretest probability (prevalence) of the condition, as well as the sensitivity and specificity of the test, are known (also called Bayes' rule). Bayes' theorem also has broad applicability in other areas of biomedical informatics where probabilistic inference is pertinent, including the interpretation of data in bioinformatics [2,3].

Bayesian diagnosis program A computer-based system that uses Bayes' theorem to assist a user in developing and refining a differential diagnosis [22].

Before-after study (aka Historically controlled study) A study in which the evaluator attempts to draw conclusions by comparing measures made during a baseline period prior to the information resource being available and measures made after it has been implemented [11].

Behaviorism A social science framework for analyzing and modifying behavior [4,23]

Belief network A diagrammatic representation used to perform probabilistic inference; an influence diagram that has only chance nodes [3, 22].

Best of breed An information technology strategy that favors the selection of individual applications based on their specific functionality rather than a single application that integrates a variety of functions [14].

Best of cluster Best of cluster became a variant of the "best of breed" strategy by selecting a single vendor for a group of similar departmental systems, such laboratory, pharmacy and radiology [14].

Bibliographic content In information retrieval, information abstracted from the original source [21].

Bibliographic database A collection of citations or pointers to the published literature [21, 26].

Binary The condition of having only two values or alternatives [5].

Biobank A repository for biological materials that collects, processes, stores, and distributes biospecimens (usually human) for use in research [25].

Biocomputation The field encompassing the modeling and simulation of tissue, cell, and genetic behavior; see **biomedical computing** [1].

Bioinformatics The study of how information is represented and transmitted in biological systems, starting at the molecular level [1,10,24]

Biomarker A characteristic that is objectively measured and evaluated as an indicator of normal biological processes, pathogenic processes, or pharmacologic responses to a therapeutic intervention [25].

Biomed Central An independent publishing house specializing in the publication of electronic journals in biomedicine (see www.biomedcentral.com) [21].

Biomedical computing The use of computers in biology or medicine [1].

Biomedical engineering An area of engineering concerned primarily with the research and development of biomedical instrumentation and biomedical devices [1].

Biomedical informatics The interdisciplinary field that studies and pursues the effective uses of biomedical data, information, and knowledge for scientific inquiry, problem solving, and decision making, driven by efforts to improve human health [1].

Biomedical Information Science and Technology Initiative (BISTI) An initiative launched by the NIH in 2000 to make optimal use of computer science, mathematics, and technology to address problems in biology and medicine. It includes a consortium of senior-level representatives from each of the NIH institutes and centers plus representatives of other Federal agencies concerned with biocomputing. See: http://www.bisti.nih.gov [1]

Biomedical taxonomy A formal system for naming entities in biomedicine [4].

Biomolecular imaging A discipline at the intersection of molecular biology and *in vivo* imaging, it enables the visualisation of cellular function and the follow-up of the molecular processes in living organisms without perturbing them [1].

Biopsychosocial model A model of medical care that emphasizes not only an understanding of disease processes, but also the psychological and social conditions of the patient that affect both the disease and its therapy [22].

Biosurveillance A public health activity that monitors a population for occurrence of a rare disease of increased occurrence of a common one [8].

Bit depth The number of bits that represent an individual pixel in an image; the more bits, the more intensities or colors can be represented [5].

Bit rate The rate of information transfer; a function of the rate at which signals can be transmitted and the efficacy with which digital information is encoded in the signal [5].

Bit The logical atomic element for all digital computers [5]

BLAST See: Basic Local Alignment Search Tool [24].

Blinding In the context of clinical research, blinding refers to the process of obfuscating from the participant and/or investigator what study intervention a given participant is receiving. This is commonly done to reduce study biases [26].

Blue Button A feature of the Veteran Administration's VistA system that exports an entire patient's record in electronic form [17].

Body of knowledge An information resource that encapsulates the knowledge of a field or discipline [21].

Body The portion of a simple electronic mail message that contains the free-text content of the message [5].

Boolean operators The mathematical operators and, or, and not, which are used to combine index terms in information retrieval searching [21].

Boolean searching A search method in which search criteria are logically combined using and, or, and not operators [21].

Bootstrap A small set of initial instructions that is stored in read-only memory and executed each time a computer is turned on. Execution of the bootstrap is called booting the computer. By analogy, the process of starting larger computer systems [5].

Bottom-up An algorithm for analyzing small pieces of a problem and building them up into larger components [8].

Bound morpheme A morpheme that creates a different form of a word but must always occur with another morpheme (*e.g.*, *–ed*, *-s*) [8].

Bridge A device that links or routes signals from one network to another [5].

Broadband A data-transmission technique in which multiple signals may be transmitted simultaneously, each modulated within an assigned frequency range [5].

Browsing Scanning a database, a list of files, or the Internet, either for a particular item or for anything that seems to be of interest [5].

Bundled payments In the healthcare context, refers to the practice of reimbursing providers based on the total expected costs of a particular episode of care. Generally occupies a "middle ground" between fee-for-service and capitation mechanisms [14].

Business logic layer A conceptual level of system architecture that insulates the applications and processing components from the underlying data and the user interfaces that access the data [14].

Buttons Graphic elements within a dialog box or user-selectable areas within an HTML document that, when activated, perform a specified function (such as invoking other HTML documents and services) [5].

C statistic The area under an receiver operating characteristic (ROC) curve [25].

CAD See: Computer-aided diagnosis [20].

Canonical form A preferred string or name for a term or collection of names; the canonical form may be determined by a set of rules (e.g., "all capital letters with words sorted in alphabetical order") or may be simply chosen arbitrarily [21].

Capitated payments System of health-care reimbursement in which providers are paid a fixed amount per patient to take care of all the health-needs of a population of patients [14].

Capitation Payments to providers, typically on an annual basis, in return for which the clinicians provide all necessary care for the patient and do not submit additional fee-for-service bills [1].

Cardiac output A measure of blood volume pumped out of the left or right ventricle of the heart, expressed as liters per minute [19].

Care coordinator See: Case Manager [15].

Cascading finite state automata (FSA) A tagging method in natural language processing in which as series of finite state automata are employed such that the output of one FSA becomes the input for another [8].

Case Refers to the capitalization of letters in a word [8].

Case manager A person in charge of coordinating all aspects of a patient's care [15].

CCD See: Continuity of Care Document [22].

CCOW See: Clinical Context Object Workgroup [6].

CDC See Centers for Disease Control [7].

CDE See Common Data Element [26].

CDR See: Clinical data repository [8,14].

CDSS See: Clinical decision-support system [14, 22, 26].

CDW See: Clinical data warehouse [8].

Cellular imaging Imaging methods that visualize cells [9].

Centering theory A theory that attempts to explain what entities are indicated by referential expressions (such as pronouns) by noting how the center (focus of attention) of each sentence changes across the text [8].

Centers for Disease Control and Prevention (CDC) An agency within the US Department of Health and Human Services that provides the public with health information and promotes health through partnerships with state health departments and other organizations [7].

Central computer system A single system that handles all computer applications in an institution using a common set of databases and interfaces [14].

Central processing unit (CPU) The "brain" of the computer. The CPU executes a program stored in main memory by fetching and executing instructions in the program [5].

Central Test Node (CTN) DICOM software to foster cooperative demonstrations by the medical imaging vendors [20].

Certificate Coded authorization information that can be verified by a certification authority to grant system access [5].

Challenge evaluation An evaluation of information systems, often in the field of information retrieval or related areas, that provides a public test collection or gold standard data collection for various researchers to compare and analyze results [21].

Chance node A symbol that represents a chance event. By convention, a chance node is indicated in a decision tree by a circle [3].

Character sets and encodings Tables of numeric values that correspond to sets of printable or displayable characters. ASCII is one example of such an encoding [8].

Chart parsing A dynamic programming algorithm for structuring a sentence according to grammar by saving and reusing segments of the sentence that have been parsed [8].

Chat A synchronous mode of text-based communication [23].

Check tags In MeSH, terms that represent certain facets of medical studies, such as age, gender, human or nonhuman, and type of grant support; check tags provide additional indexing of bibliographic citations in databases such as Medline [21].

CHI See: Consumer health informatics [1, 10, 17, 18].

CHIN See: Community Health Information Network [13].

Chunking A natural language processing method for determining non-recursive phrases where each phrase corresponds to a specific part of speech [8].

CINAHL (or CINHL) See: Cumulative Index to Nursing and Allied Health Literature [21].

CINAHL Subject Headings A set of terms based on MeSH, with additional domain-specific terms added, used for indexing the Cumulative Index to Nursing and Allied Health Literature (CINAHL) [21].

CIS See: Clinical information system [14].

Citation database A database of citations found in scientific articles, showing the linkages among articles in the scientific literature [21].

Classification In image processing, the categorization of segmented regions of an image based on the values of measured parameters, such as area and intensity [7].

CLIA certification See: Clinical Laboratory Improvement Amendments of 1988 Certification [25].

Client–server Information processing interaction that distributes application processing between a local computer (the client) and a remote computer resource (the server) [5].

Clinical and translational research A broad spectrum of research activities involving the translation of findings from initial laboratory-based studies into early-stage clinical studies, and subsequently, from the findings of those studies in clinical and/or population-level practice. This broad area incorporates multiple Biomedical Informatics sub-domains, including both translational bioinformatics and clinical research informatics [26].

Clinical Context Object Workgroup (CCOW) A common protocol for single sign-on implementations in health care. It allows multiple applications to be linked together, so the end user only logs in and selects a patient in one application, and those actions propagate to the other applications [6].

Clinical data repository (CDR) Clinical database optimized for storage and retrieval for individual patients and used to support patient care and daily operations [8,14].

Clinical data warehouse (CDW) A database of clinical data obtained from primary sources such as electron health records, organized for re-use for secondary purposes [8].

Clinical datum Replaces medical datum with same definition [2]

Clinical decision support Any process that provides health-care workers and patients with situation-specific knowledge that can inform their decisions regarding health and health care [22].

Clinical decision-support system (CDSS) A computer-based system that assists physicians in making decisions about patient care [14, 22, 26].

Clinical Document Architecture An HL7 standard for naming and structuring clinical documents, such as reports [8].

Clinical expert system A computer program designed to provide decision support for diagnosis or therapy planning at a level of sophistication that an expert physician might provide [10].

Clinical guidelines Systematically developed statements to assist practitioner and patient decisions about appropriate health care for specific clinical circumstances [1, 13].

Clinical informatics The application of biomedical informatics methods in the patient-care domain; a combination of computer science, information science, and clinical science designed to assist in the management and processing of clinical data, information, and knowledge to support clinical practice [1].

Clinical information system (CIS) The components of a health-care information system designed to support the delivery of patient care, including order communications, results reporting, care planning, and clinical documentation [14].

Clinical judgment Decision making by clinicians that incorporates professional experience and social, ethical, psychological, financial, and other factors in addition to the objective medical data [10].

Clinical Laboratory Improvement Amendments of 1988 certification Clinical Laboratory Improvement Amendments of 1988, establishing laboratory testing quality standards to ensure the accuracy, reliability and timeliness of patient test results, regardless of where the test was performed [25].

Clinical modifications A published set of changes to the International Classification of Diseases (ICD) that provides additional levels of detail necessary for statistical reporting in the United States [7].

Clinical pathway Disease-specific plan that identifies clinical goals, interventions, and expected outcomes by time period [1, 14].

Clinical prediction rule A rule, derived from statistical analysis of clinical observations that is used to assign a patient to a clinical subgroup with a known probability of disease [3].

Clinical research informatics (CRI) The application of biomedical informatics methods in the clinical research domain to support all aspects of clinical research, from hypothesis generation, through study design, study execution and data collection, data analysis, and dissemination of results [26].

Clinical Research Management System (CRMS) A clinical research management system is a technology platform that supports and enables the conduct of clinical research, including clinical trials, usually through a combination of functional modules targeting the preparatory, enrollment, active, and dissemination phases of such research programs. CRMS systems are often also referred to as Clinical Trials Management Systems (CTMS), particularly when they are used to manage only clinical trials rather than various types of clinical research [26].

Clinical research The range of studies and trials in human subjects that fall into the three sub-categories: (1) Patient-oriented research:

Research conducted with human subjects (or on material of human origin such as tissues, specimens and cognitive phenomena) for which an investigator (or colleague) directly interacts with human subjects. Patient-oriented research includes: (a) mechanisms of human disease; (b) therapeutic interventions; (c) clinical trial; and (d) development of new technologies. (2) Epidemiologic and behavioral studies. (3) Outcomes research and health services research." [10, 26]

Clinical subgroup A subset of a population in which the members have similar characteristics and symptoms, and therefore similar likelihood of disease [3].

Clinical trials Research projects that involve the direct management of patients and are generally aimed at determining optimal modes of therapy, evaluation, or other interventions [1].

Clinical-event monitors Systems that electronically and automatically record the occurrence or changes of specific clinical events, such as blood pressure, respiratory capability, or heart rhythms [14].

Clinically relevant population The population of patients that is seen in actual practice. In the context of estimating the sensitivity and specificity of a diagnostic test, that group of patients in whom the test actually will be used [3].

Closed loop medication management system A workflow process (typically supported electronically) through which medications are ordered electronically by a physician, filled by the pharmacy, delivered to the patient, administered by a nurse, and subsequently monitored for effectiveness by the physician [14].

Closed loop Regulation of a physiological variable, such as blood pressure, by monitoring the value of the variable and altering therapy without human intervention [15].

Cloud technology or computing Cloud computing is using computing resources located in a remote location. Typically, cloud computing is provided by a separate business, and the user pays for it on per usage basis. There are variations such as private clouds,

where the 'cloud' is provided by the same business, but leverages methods that permit easier virtualization and expandability than traditional methods. Private clouds are popular with healthcare because of security concerns with public cloud computing [20].

Clustering algorithms A method which assigns a set of objects into groups (called clusters) so that the objects in the same cluster are more similar (in some sense or another) to each other than to those in other clusters [9].

Coaching system An intelligent tutoring system that monitors the session and intervenes only when the student requests help or makes serious mistakes [23]

Cocke-Younger-Kasami (CYK) A dynamic programming method that uses bottom-up rules for parsing grammar-free text; used only in conjunction with a grammar written in Chomsky normal form [8].

Code See Machine Language [5].

Cognitive artifacts human-made materials, devices, and systems that extend people's abilities in perceiving objects, encoding and retrieving information from memory, and problem-solving [4].

Cognitive engineering An interdisciplinary approach to the development of principles, methods and tools to assess and guide the design of computerized systems to support human performance[4]

Cognitive heuristics Mental processes by which we learn, recall, or process information; rules of thumb [3].

Cognitive load An excess of information that competes for few cognitive resources, creating a burden on working memory [4].

Cognitive science Area of research concerned with studying the processes by which people think and behave [1, 4, 23]

Cognitive task analysis The analysis of both the information-processing demands of a task and the kinds of domain-specific knowledge required performing it, used to study human performance [4].

Cognitive walkthrough (CW) An analytic method for characterizing the cognitive processes of users performing a task. The method is performed by an analyst or group of analysts "walking through" the sequence of actions necessary to achieve a goal, thereby seeking to identify potential usability problems that may impede the successful completion of a task or introduce complexity in a way that may frustrate users [4].

Collaborative workspace A virtual environment in which multiple participants can interact, synchronously or asynchronously, to perform a collaborative task [4].

Color resolution A measure of the ability to distinguish among different colors (indicated in a digital image by the number of bits per pixel). Three sets of multiple bits are required to specify the intensity of red, green, and blue components of each pixel color [5].

Commodity internet A general-purpose connection to the Internet, not configured for any particular purpose [18].

Common Data Elements (CDEs) Standards for data that stipulate the methods by which the data are collected and the controlled terminologies used to represent them. Many standard sets of CDEs have been developed, often overlapping in nature [26].

Communication Data transmission and information exchange between computers using accepted protocols via an exchange medium such as a telephone line or fiber optic cable [5].

Community Health Information Network (CHIN) A computer network developed for exchange of sharable health information among independent participant organizations in a geographic area (or community) [13].

Comparative effectiveness research A form of clinical research that compares examines outcomes of two or more interventions to determine if one is statistically superior to another [8].

Compiler A program that translates a program written in a high-level programming language to a machine-language program, which can then be executed [5].

Comprehensibility and control Security function that ensures that data owners and data stewards have effective control over information confidentiality and access [5].

Computational biology The science of computer-based mathematical and statistical techniques to analyze biological systems. See also **bioinformatics** [10].

Computed check A procedure applied to entered data that detects errors based on whether values have the correct mathematical relationship; (e.g., white blood cell differential counts, reported as percentages, must sum to 100 [12].

Computed tomography (CT) An imaging modality in which X rays are projected through the body from multiple angles and the resultant absorption values are analyzed by a computer to produce cross-sectional slices [9, 20].

Computer architecture The basic structure of a computer, including memory organization, a scheme for encoding data and instructions, and control mechanisms for performing computing operations [5].

Computer memories Store programs and data that are being used actively by a CPU [5].

Computer program A set of instructions that tells a computer which mathematical and logical operations to perform [5].

Computer-aided diagnosis (CAD) Any form of diagnosis in which a computer program helps suggest or rank diagnostic considerations [20].

Computer-based (or computerized) physician order entry (CPOE) A clinical information system that allows physicians and other clinicians to record patient-specific orders for communication to other patient care team members and to other information systems (such as test orders to laboratory systems or medication orders to pharmacy systems). Sometimes called **provider order entry** or **practitioner order entry** to emphasize such systems' uses by clinicians other than physicians [13,14].

Computer-based patient records (CPRs) An early name for **electronic health records (EHRs)** dating to the early 1990s [1].

Concept A unit of thought made explicit through the representation of propterties of an object or a set of common objects [7]. An abstract idea generalized from specific instances of objects that occur in the world [21].

Conceptual graph A formal notation in which knowledge is represented through explicit relationships between concepts. Graphs can be depicted with diagrams consisting of shapes and arrows, or in a text format [8].

Conceptual knowledge Knowledge about concepts [4].

Concordant test results Test results that reflect the true patient state (true-positive and true-negative results) [3].

Conditional probability The probability of an event, contingent on the occurrence of another event [3].

Conditionally independent Two events, A and B, are conditionally independent if the occurrence of one does not influence the probability of the occurrence of the other, when both events are conditioned on a third event C. Thus, $p[A \mid B,C] = p[A \mid C]$ and $p[B \mid A,C] = p[B \mid C]$. The conditional probability of two conditionally independent events both occurring is the product of the individual conditional probabilities: $p[A,B \mid C] = p[A \mid C] \times p[B \mid C]$. For example, two tests for a disease are conditionally independent when the probability of the result of the second test does not depend on the result of the first test, given the disease state. For the case in which disease is present, $p[$second test positive | first test positive and disease present$] = p[$second test positive | first test negative and disease present$] = p[$second test positive | disease present$]$. More succinctly, the tests are conditionally independent if the sensitivity and specificity of one test do not depend on the result of the other test (See **independent**) [3].

Conditioned event A chance event, the probability of which is affected by another chance event (the **conditioning event**) [3].

Conditioning event A chance event that affects the probability of occurrence of another chance event (the conditioned event) [3].

Confidentiality The ability of data owners and data stewards to control access to or release of private information [5].

Consistency check A procedure applied to entered data that detects errors based on internal inconsistencies; e.g., recognizing a problem with the recording of cancer of the prostate as the diagnosis for a female patient [12].

Constructivism Argues that humans generate knowledge and meaning from an interaction between their experiences and their ideas [23].

Consumer health informatics (CHI) Applications of medical informatics technologies that focus on patients or healthy individuals as the primary users [1, 10, 17, 18].

Content based image retrieval Also known as query by image content (QBIC) and content-based visual information retrieval (CBVIR) is the application of computer vision techniques to the image retrieval problem, that is, the problem of searching for digital images in large databases [9].

Content In information retrieval, media developed to communicate information or knowledge [21].

Context free grammar A mathematical model of a set of strings whose members are defined as capable of being generated from a starting symbol, using rules in which a single symbol is expanded into one or more symbols [8].

Contingency table A 2×2 table that shows the relative frequencies of true-positive, true-negative, false-positive, and false-negative results [3].

Continuity of Care Document (CCD) An HL7 standard that enables specification of the patient data that relate to one or more encounters with the healthcare system. The CCD is used for interchange of patient information (e.g., within Health Information Exchanges). The format enables all the electronic information about a patient to be aggregated within a standardized data structure that can be parsed and interpreted by a variety of information systems [22].

Continuity of care The coordination of care received by a patient over time and across multiple healthcare providers [2].

Continuum of care The full spectrum of health services provided to patients, including health maintenance, primary care, acute care, critical care, rehabilitation, home care, skilled nursing care, and hospice care [15].

Contract-management system A computer system used to support managed-care contracting by estimating the costs and payments associated with potential contract terms and by comparing actual with expected payments based on contract terms [14].

Contrast resolution A metric for how well an imaging modality can distinguish small differences in signal intensity in different regions of the image [9].

Contrast The difference in light intensity between dark and light areas of an image [5].

Control intervention In the context of clinical research, a control intervention represents the intervention (e.g. placebo, standard care, etc.) given to the group of study participants assigned to the control or comparator arm of a study. Depending on the study type, the goal is to generate data as the basis of comparison with the experimental intervention of interest in order to determine the safety, efficacy, or benefits of an experimental intervention [26].

Controlled terminology A finite, enumerated set of terms intended to convey information unambiguously [21, 22].

Copyright law Protection of written materials and intellectual property from being copied verbatim [10].

Coreference chains Provide a compact representation for encoding the words and phrases in a text that all refer to the same entity [8].

Coreference resolution In natural language processing, the assignment of specific meaning to some indirect reference [8].

Correctional Telehealth The application of telehealth to the care of prison inmates, where physical delivery of the patient to the practitioner is impractical [18].

Covered entities Under the HIPAA Privacy Rule, a covered entity is an organization or individual that handles personal health information. Covered entities include providers, health plans, and clearinghouses [27].

CPOE See: Computer-based (or Computerized) Physician (or Provider) Order Entry [13,14].

CPR (or CPRS) See: Computer-based patient records [1].

CPU See: Central processing unit [5].

CRI See: Clinical research informatics [26].

CRMS (or CRDMS) See: Clinical Research Management System [26].

Cryptographic encoding Scheme for protecting data through authentication and authorization controls based on use of keys for encrypting and decrypting information [5].

CT (or CAT) See: Computed tomography [9, 20].

Cumulative Index to Nursing and Allied Health Literature (CINHL) A non-NLM bibliographic database the covers nursing and allied health literature, including physical therapy, occupational therapy, laboratory technology, health education, physician assistants, and medical records [21].

Curly Braces Problem The situation that arises in **Arden Syntax** where the code used to enumerate the variables required by a **medical logic module** (MLM) cannot describe how the variables actually derive their values from data in the EHR database. Each variable definition in an MLM has {curly braces} that enclose words in natural language that indicate the meaning of the corresponding variable. The particular database query required to supply a value for the variable must be specified by the local implementer, however. The curly braces problem makes it impossible for an MLM developed at one institution to operate at another without local modification [22].

Cursor A blinking region of a display monitor, or a symbol such as an arrow, that indicates the currently active position on the screen [5].

CYK See: Cocke-Younger-Kasami [8].

Dashboard A user-interface element that displays data produced by several computer programs simultaneously and that allows users to interact with those programs in standardized ways [20,22].

Data buses An electronic pathway for transferring data—for instance, between a CPU and memory [5].

Data capture The process of collecting data to be stored in an information system; it includes entry by a person using a keyboard and collection of data from sensors [12].

Data Encryption Standard (DES) A widely-used method of for securing encryption that uses a private (secret) key for encryption and requires the same key for decryption (see also, public key cryptography) [5]

Data independence The insulation of applications programs from changes in data-storage structures and data-access strategies [5]

Data-interchange standards Adopted formats and protocols for exchange of data between independent computer systems [7]

Data layer A conceptual level of system architecture that isolates the data collected and stored in the enterprise from the applications and user interfaces used to access those data [14].

Data Recording The documentation of information for archival or future use through mechanisms such as handwritten text, drawings, machine-generated traces, or photographic images [2].

Database management system (DBMS) An integrated set of programs that manages access to databases [5, 21].

Database A collection of stored data—typically organized into fields, records, and files—and an associated description (schema) [2, 5].

Datum Any single observation of fact. A medical datum generally can be regarded as the value of a specific parameter (for example, *red-blood-cell count*) for a particular object (for example, a patient) at a given point in time [2].

DBMIS See: Database Management System [5].

DCMI See: Dublin Core Metadata Initiative [21].

Debugger A system program that provides traces, memory dumps, and other tools to assist programmers in locating and eliminating errors in their programs [5].

Decision analysis A methodology for making decisions by identifying alternatives and assessing them with regard to both the likelihood of possible outcomes and the costs and benefits of those outcomes [22].

Decision node A symbol that represents a choice among actions. By convention, a decision node is represented in a decision tree by a square [3].

Decision support The process of assisting humans in making decisions, such as interpreting clinical information or choosing a diagnostic or therapeutic action. See; **Clinical Decision Support** [4]

Decision tree A diagrammatic representation of the outcomes associated with chance events and voluntary actions [3].

Deduplication The process that matches, links, and or merges data to eliminate redundancies [16].

De-identified aggregate data Data reports that are summarized or altered slightly in a way that makes the discernment of the identity of any of the individuals whose data was used for the report impossible or so difficult as to be extremely improbable. The process of de-identifying aggregate data is known as statistical disclosure control [13].

Delta check A procedure applied to entered data that detects large and unlikely differences between the values of a new result and of the previous observations; e.g., a recorded weight that changes by 100 lb in 2 weeks [12].

Demonstration study Study that establishes a relation—which may be associational or causal—between a set of measured variables [11].

Dental informatics The application of biomedical informatics methods and techniques to problems derived from the field of dentistry. Viewed as a subarea of clinical informatics [1].

Deoxyribonucleic acid (DNA) The genetic material that is the basis for heredity. DNA is a long polymer chemical made of four basic subunits. The sequence in which these subunits occur in the polymer distinguishes one DNA molecule from another and in turn directs a cell's production of proteins and all other basic cellular processes [24].

Departmental system A system that focus on a specific niche area in the healthcare setting, such as a laboratory, pharmacy, radiology department, etc. [14]

Dependency grammar A linguistic theory of syntax that is based on dependency relations between words, where one word in the sentence is independent and other words are dependent on that word. Generally, the verb of a sentence is independent and other words are directly or indirectly dependent on the verb [8].

Dependent variable (also called outcome variable) In a correlational or experimental study, the main variable of interest or outcome variable, which is thought to be affected by or associated with the independent variables (q.v.) [11].

Derivational morphemes A morpheme that changes the meaning or part of the speech of a word (e.g., *–ful* as in painful, converting a noun to an adjective) [8].

DES See: Data Encryption Standard [5].

Descriptive study One-group study that seeks to measure the value of a variable in a sample of subjects. Study with no independent variable [11].

Design validation A study conducted to inform the design of an information resource, e.g. a user survey [11].

Diagnosis The process of analyzing available data to determine the pathophysiologic explanation for a patient's symptoms [1, 10, 22].

Diagnosis-based reimbursement Payments to providers (typically hospitals) based on the diagnosis made by a physician at the time of admission [14].

Diagnosis-related group(DRG) One of almost 500 categories based on major diagnosis, length of stay, secondary diagnosis, surgical procedure, age, and types of services required. Used to determine the fixed payment per case that Medicare will reimburse hospitals for providing care to elderly patients [13, 23].

Diagnostic decision-support system A computer-based system that assists physicians in rendering diagnoses; a subset of clinical decision-support systems. **See clinical decision-support system** [10].

Diagnostic process The activity of deciding which questions to ask, which tests to order, or which procedures to perform, and determining the value of the results relative to associated risks or financial costs [22].

DICOM See: Digital Image Communications in Medicine [18,20].

Dictionary A set of terms representing the system of concepts of a particular subject field [7].

Differential diagnosis The set of active hypotheses (possible diagnoses) that a physician develops when determining the source of a patient's problem [2, 20].

Digital computer A computer that processes discrete values based on the binary digit or bit. Essentially all modern computers are digital, but analog computers also existed in the past [5].

Digital Image Communications in Medicine (DICOM) A standard for electronic exchanging digital health images, such as x-rays and CT scans [18,20].

Digital image An image that is stored as a grid of numbers, where each picture element (pixel) in the grid represents the intensity, and possibly color, of a small area [20].

Digital library Organized collections of electronic content, intended for specific communities or domains [21].

Digital object identifier (DOI) A system for providing unique identifiers for published digital objects, consisting of a prefix that is assigned by the International DOI Foundation to the publishing entity and a suffix that is assigned and maintained by the entity [21].

Digital radiography (DR) The process of producing X-ray images that are stored in digital form in computer memory, rather than on film [9, 20].

Digital signal processing (DSP) An integrated circuit designed for high-speed data manipulation and used in audio communications, image manipulation, and other data acquisition and control applications [5].

Digital signal A signal that takes on discrete values from a specified range of values [5].

Digital subscriber line (DSL) A digital telephone service that allows high-speed network communication using conventional (twisted pair) telephone wiring [5]

Digital subtraction angiography (DSA) A radiologic technique for imaging blood vessels in which a digital image acquired before injection of contrast material is subtracted pixel by pixel from an image acquired after injection. The resulting image shows only the differences in the two images, highlighting those areas where the contrast material has accumulated [9].

Direct entry The entry of data into a computer system by the individual who personally made the observations [12].

Discourse Large portions of text forming a narrative, such as paragraphs and documents [8].

Discrete event simulation model A modeling approach that assesses interactions between people, typically composed of patients that have attributes and that experience events [3].

Discussion board An on-line [23]

Disease Any condition in an organism that is other than the healthy state [8].

Dissemination phase during the dissemination phase of a clinical research study, investigators analyze and report upon the data generated during the active phase [26].

Distributed cognition A view of cognition that considers groups, material artifacts, and cultures and that emphasizes the inherently social and collaborative nature of cognition [4]

Distributed computer systems A collection of independent computers that share data, programs, and other resources [14].

DNA See: Deoxyribonucleic Acid [24].

DNS See: Domain name system [5, 12].

Document structure The organization of text into sections [8].

DOI See: Digital object identifier [21].

Domain name system (DNS) A hierarchical name-management system used to translate computer names to Internet protocol (IP) addresses [5, 12].

Doppler shift A perceived change in frequency of a signal as the signal source moves toward or away from a signal receiver [20].

Double blind A clinical study methodology in which neither the researchers nor the subjects know to which study group a subject has been assigned [2].

Double-blinded study In the context of clinical research, a double blinded study is a study in which both the investigator and participant are blinded from the assignment of an intervention. In this scenario, a trusted third party must maintain records of such study arm assignments to inform later data analyses [26].

Draft standard for trial use A proposal for a standard developed by HL7 that is sufficiently well defined that early adopters can use the specification in the development of HIT. Ultimately, the draft standard may be refined and put to a ballot for endorsement by the members of the organization, thus creating an official standard [22].

DRG See Diagnosis-Related Groups [13, 23].

Drug repurposing Identifying existing drugs that may be useful for indications other than those for which they were initially approved [25].

Drug screening robots A scientific instrument that can perform assays with potential drugs in a highly parallel and high throughput manner [24].

DSA See: Digital subtraction angiography [9].

DSL See: Digital subscriber line [5].

DSP See: Digital signal processing [5].

Dublin Core Metadata Initiative (DCMI) A standard metadata model for indexing published documents [21].

Dynamic A simulation program that models changes in patient state over time and in response to students' therapeutic decisions [23].

Dynamic programming A computationally intensive computer-science technique used, for example, to determine optimal sequence alignments in many computational biology applications [24].

Dynamic transmission model A model that divides a population into compartments (for example, uninfected, infected, recovered, dead), and for transitions between compartments are governed by differential or difference equations [3].

Earley parsing A dynamic programming method for parsing context-free grammar [8].

EBM See Evidence-Based Medicine [21].

EBM database For **Evidence-Based Medicine database**, a highly organized collection of clinical evidence to support medical decisions based on the results of controlled clinical trials [21].

eCRF See: Electronic Case Report Form [26].

EDC See: Electronic Data Capture [26].

EDI See: Electronic data interchange [14].

EEG See: Electroencephalography [9].

EHR See: Electronic health record [6,10,12,13,21,26].

EIW See: Enterprise information warehouse [14].

Electroencephalography (EEG) A method for measuring the electromagnetic fields generated by the electrical activity of the neurons using a large arrays of scalp sensors, the output of which are processed to localize the source of the electrical activity inside the brain [9].

Electronic Case Report Form (eCRF) A computational representation of paper case report forms (CRFs) used to enable EDC [26].

Electronic Data Capture (EDC) EDC is the process of capturing study-related data elements via computational mechanisms [26].

Electronic data interchange (EDI) Electronic exchange of standard data transactions, such as claims submission and electronic funds transfer [14].

Electronic Health Record (EHR) A repository of electronically maintained information about an individual's lifetime health status and health care, stored such that it can serve the multiple legitimate users of the record. See also **EMR** and **CPR** [6,10,12,13,21,26].

Electronic health record system An electronic health record and the tools used to manage the information; also referred to as a computer-based patient-record system and often shortened to electronic health record [12].

Electronic Medical Record (EMR) The electronic record documenting a patient's care in a provider organization such as a hospital or a physician's office. Often used interchangeably with **Electronic Health Record(EHR)**, although EHRs refer more typically to an individual's lifetime health status and care rather than the set of particular organizationally-based experiences [14].

Electronic-long, paper-short (ELPS) A publication method which provides on the Web site supplemental material that did not appear in the print version of the journal [21].

ELPS See: Electronic-long, paper-short [21].

EMBASE A commercial biomedical and pharmacological database from ExcerptaMedica, which provides information about medical and drug-related subjects [21].

Emergent design Study where the design or plan of research can and does change as the study progresses. Characteristic of subjectivist studies [11].

EMPI See: Enterprise master patient index [14].

Emotion detection A natural language technique for determining the mental state of the author of a text document [8].

EMTREE A hierarchically structured, controlled vocabulary used for subject indexing, used to index **EMBASE** [21].

EMR (or EMRS) See: Electronic Medical Record [14].

Enabling technology Any technology that improves organizational processes through its use rather than on its own. Computers, for example, are useless unless "enabled" by operation systems and applications or implemented in support of work flows that might not otherwise be possible [14].

Encryption The process of transforming information such that its meaning is hidden, with the intent of keeping it secret, such that only those who know how to decrypt it can read it; see decryption [5].

Enrichment analysis A statistical method to determine whether an a priori defined set of concepts shows statistically significant over-representation in descriptions of a set of items (such as genes) compared to what one would expect based on their frequency in a reference distribution [25].

Enrollment during enrollment of a clinical research study, potential participants are identified and research staff determine their eligibility for participation in a study, based upon the eligibility criteria described in the study protocol. If a participant is deemed eligible to participate, there are then officially "registered" for the study. It is during this phase that in some trial designs, a process of randomization and assignment to study arms occurs [26].

Enterprise information warehouse (EIW) A data base in which data from clinical, financial and other operational sources are collected in order to be compared and contrasted across the enterprise [14].

Enterprise master patient index (EMPI) An architectural component that serves as the name authority in a health-care information system composed of multiple independent systems; the EMPI provides an index of patient names and identification numbers used by the connected information systems [14].

Entrez A search engine from the National Center for Biotechnology Information (NCBI), at the National Library of Medicine; Entrez can be used to search a variety of life sciences databases, including PubMed [21].

Entry term A synonym form for a subject heading in the Medical Subject Headings (MeSH) controlled, hierarchical vocabulary [21].

Epidemiologic Related to the field of epidemiology [1].

Epidemiology The study of the patterns, causes, and effects of health and disease conditions in defined populations [16].

Epigenetics Heritable phenotypes that are not encoded in DNA sequence [24, 25].

e-prescribing The electronic process of generating, transmitting and filling a medical prescription [27].

Error analysis In natural language processing, a process for determining the reasons for false-positive and false-negative errors [8].

Escrow Use of a trusted third party to hold cryptographic keys, computer source code, or other valuable information to protect against loss or inappropriate access [5]

Ethernet A network standard that uses a bus or star topology and regulates communication traffic using the Carrier Sense Multiple Access with Collision Detection (CSMA/CD) approach [20].

Ethnography Set of research methodologies derived primarily from social anthropology. The basis of much of the subjectivist, qualitative evaluation approaches [11].

ETL See: Extract, Transform, and Load [26].

Evaluation contract A document describing the aims of a study, the methods to be used and resources made available, usually agreed between the evaluator and key stakeholders before the study begins [11].

Event-Condition-Action (ECA) rule A rule that requires some *event* (such as the availability of a new data value in the database) to cause the *condition* (premise, or left-hand side) of the rule to be evaluated. If the condition is determined to be true, then some *action* is performed. Such rules are commonly found in active database systems, and form the basis of **medical logic modules** [22].

Evidence-based guidelines(EBM) An approach to medical practice whereby the best possible evidence from the medical literature is incorporated in decision making. Generally such evidence is derived from controlled clinical trials [1, 10, 21].

Exabyte 10^{18} **bytes** [5].

Exome The entire sequence of all genes within a genome, approximately 1–3 % of the entire genome [24].

Expected value The value that is expected on average for a specified chance event or decision [3].

Experimental intervention In the context of clinical research, an experimental intervention represents the treatment or other intervention delivered to a participant assigned to the experimental arm of the study in order to determine the safety, efficacy, or benefits of that intervention [26].

Experimental science Systematic study characterized by posing hypotheses, designing experiments, performing analyses, and interpreting results to validate or disprove hypotheses and to suggest new hypotheses for study [1].

Extensible markup language (XML) A subset of the **Standard Generalized Markup Language (SGML)** from the World Wide Web Consortium (W3C), designed especially for Web documents. It allows designers to create their own custom-tailored tags, enabling the definition, transmission, validation, and interpretation of data between applications and between organizations [5, 6, 8, 21,26].

External router A computer that resides on multiple networks and that can forward and translate message packets sent from a local or enterprise network to a regional network beyond the bounds of the organization [5].

External validity In the context of clinical research, external validity refers to the ability to generalize study results into clinical care [26].

Extract, Transform, and Load (ETL) ETL is the process by which source data is collected and manipulated so as to adhere to the structure and semantics of a receiving data construct, such as a data warehouse [26].

Extrinsic evaluation An evaluation of a component of a system based on an evaluation of the performance of the entire sytem [8].

F measure A measure of overall accuracy that is a combination of precision and recall [8].

Factual knowledge Knowledge of facts without necessarily having any in-depth understanding of their origin or implications [4].

False negative A negative result that occurs in a true situation. Examples include a desired entity that is missed by a search routine or a test result that appears normal when it should be abnormal [8].

False-negative rate (FNR) The probability of a negative result, given that the condition under consideration is true—for example, the probability of a negative test result in a patient who has the disease under consideration [3].

False-negative result (FN) A negative result when the condition under consideration is true—for example, a negative test result in a patient who has the disease under consideration [3].

False positive A positive result that occurs in a false situation. Examples include an inappropriate entity that is returned by a search routine or a test result that appears abnormal when it should be normal [8].

False-positive rate (FPR) The probability of a positive result, given that the condition under consideration is false—for example, the probability of a positive test result in a patient who does not have the disease under consideration [3].

False-positive result (FP) A positive result when the condition under consideration is false—for example, a positive test result in a patient who does not have the disease under consideration [3].

FDDI See: Fiber Distributed Data Interface [20].

Fiber Distributed Data Interface [FDDI] A transmission standard for local area networks operating on fiberoptic cable, providing a transmission rate of 100 Mbit/s [20].

Feedback In a computer-based education program, system-generated responses, such as explanations, summaries, and references, provided to further a student's progress in learning [23].

Fee-for-service Unrestricted system of health-care reimbursement in which payers pay provider for those services the provider has deemed necessary [14].

Fiberoptic cable A communication medium that uses light waves to transmit information signals [5].

Fiducial An object used in the field of view of an imaging system which appears in the image produced, for use as a point of reference or a measure [9].

Field function study Study of an information resource where the system is used in the context of ongoing health care. Study of a deployed system (cf. Laboratory study) [11].

Field In science, the setting, which may be multiple physical locations, where the work under study is carried out [11]. In database design, the smallest named unit of data in a database. Fields are grouped together to form records [5].

Field user effect study A study of the actual actions or decisions of the users of the resource [11].

File In a database, a collection of similar records [5].

File format Representation of data within a file; can refer to the method for individual characters and values (for example, **ASCII** or **binary**) or thei organization within the file (for example, **XML** or text) [8].

File server A computer that is dedicated to storing shared or private data files [5].

File system An organization of files within a database or on a mass storage device [5].

Filtering algorithms A defined procedure applied to input data to reduce the effect of noise [5].

Finite state automaton An abstract, computer-based representation of the state of some entity together with a set of actions that can transform the state. Collections of finite state automata can be used to model complex systems [8].

Fire-wall A security system intended to protect an organization's network against external threats by preventing computers in the organization's network from communicating directly with computers external to the network, and vice versa [5].

Flash memory card A portable electronic storage medium that uses a semiconductor chip with a standard physical interface; a convenient method for moving data between computers [5].

Flexnerian one of science-based acquisition of medically relevant knowledge, followed by on-the-job apprentice-style acquisition of experience, and accompanied by evolution and expansion of the curriculum to add new fields of knowledge [23].

Floppy disk An inexpensive magnetic disk that can be removed from the disk-drive unit and thereby used to transfer or archive files [5].

FM See: Frequency modulation [5].

fMRI See: Functional magnetic resonance imaging [9].

FN See: False-negative result [3].

Force feedback A user interface feature in which physical sensations are transmitted to the user to provide a tactile sensation as part of a simulated activity. See also **Haptic feedback** [18].

Foreground question Question that asks for general information related to a specific patient (see also **background question**) [21].

Form factor Typically refers to the physical dimensions of a product. With computing devices, refers to the physical size of the device, often with specific reference to the display. For example, we would observe that the form factor of a desktop monitor is significantly larger than that of a tablet or smart phone, and therefore able to display more characters and larger graphics on the screen [14].

Formative evaluation An assessment of a system's behavior and capabilities conducted during the development process and used to guide future development of the system [23]

Forward chaining Also known as data-driven reasoning. A form of inference used in **rule-based systems** in which the **inference engine** uses newly acquired (or concluded) values of variables to invoke all rules that may reference one or more of those variables in their premises (left-hand side), thereby concluding new values for variables in the conclusions (right-hand side) of those rules. The process continues recursively until all rules whose premises may reference the variables whose values become known have been considered [22].

FP See: False-positive result [3].

FPR See: False-positive rate [3].

Frame Relay A high-speed network protocol designed for sending digital information over shared wide-area networks using variable length packets of information [5].

Frame An abstract representation of a concept or entity that consists of a set of attributes, called slots, each of which can have one or more values to represent knowledge about the entity or concept [8].

Free morpheme A morpheme that is a word and that does not contain another morpheme (*e.g.*, *arm*, *pain*) [8].

Frequency modulation(FM) A signal representation in which signal values are represented as changes in frequency rather than amplitude [5].

Front-end application A computer program that interacts with a database-management system to retrieve and save data and to accomplish user-level tasks [5].

Full-text content The complete textual information contained in a bibliographic source [21].

Functional magnetic resonance imaging (fMRI) A **magnetic resonance imaging** method that reveals changes in blood oxygenation that occur following neural activity [9].

Functional mapping An imaging method that relates specific sites on images to particular physiologic functions [20].

Gateway A computer that resides on multiple networks and that can forward and translate message packets sent between nodes in networks running different protocols [5].

Gbps See: Gigabits per second [5].

GEM See: Guideline Element Model [22].

GenBank A centralized repository of protein, RNA, and DNA sequences in all species, currently maintained by the National Institutes of Health [24].

Gene expression microarray Study the expression of large numbers of genes with one another and create multiple variations on a genetic theme to explore the implications of changes in genome function on human disease [24].

Gene Expression Omnibus (GEO) A centralized database of gene expression microarray datasets [24].

Gene Ontology(GO) A structured controlled vocabulary used for annotating genes and proteins with molecular function. The vocabulary contains three distinct ontologies, Molecular Function, Biological Process and Cellular Component [24].

Genes units encoded in DNA and they are transcribed into ribonucleic acid (RNA) [24].

Genetic data An overarching term used to label various collections of facts about the genomes of individuals, groups or species [10].

Genome-Wide Association Studies (GWAS) An examination of many common genetic variants in different individuals to see if any variant is associated with a given trait, e.g. a disease [25].

Genomic medicine (also known as stratified-medicine) The management of groups of patients with shared biological characteristics, determined through molecular diagnostic testing, to select the best therapy in order to achieve the best possible outcome for a given group [25].

Genomics database An organized collection of information from gene sequencing, protein characterization, and other genomic research [21].

Genomics The study of all of the nucleotide sequences, including structural genes, regulatory sequences, and noncoding DNA segments, in the chromosomes of an organism [24].

Genotype The genetic makeup, as distinguished from the physical appearance, of an organism or a group of organisms [24].

Genotypic Refers to the genetic makeup of an organism [1].

GEO See: Gene Expression Omnibus [24].

Geographic Information System (GIS) A system designed to capture, store, manipulate, analyze, manage, and visually present all types of location-specific data [16].

Gigabits per second (Gbps) A common unit of measure for data transmission over high-speed networks [5].

Gigabyte 2^{30} or 1,073,741,824 bytes [5].

GIS See: Geographic Information System [16].

Global processing Computations on the entire image, without regard to specific regional content [9].

GO See: Gene Ontology [24].

Gold-standard test The test or procedure whose result is used to determine the true state of the subject—for example, a pathology test such as a biopsy used to determine a patient's true disease state [3].

Google A commercial search engine that provides free searching of documents on the World Wide Web [21].

GPU See: Graphics processing unit [5].

Grammar A mathematical model of a potentially infinite set of strings [8].

Graphical user interface (GUI) A type of environment that represents programs, files, and options by means of icons, menus, and dialog boxes on the screen [5].

Graphics processing unit (GPU) A computer hardware component that performs graphic displays and other highly parallel computations [5].

Graph In computer science, a set of *nodes* or circles connected by a set of *edges* or lines [25].

Gray scale A scheme for representing intensity in a black-and-white image. Multiple bits per pixel are used to represent intermediate levels of gray [5].

Guardian Angel Proposal A proposed structure for a lifetime, patient-centered health information system [17].

GUI See: Graphical user interface [5].

Guidance In a computer-based education program, proactive feedback, help facilities, and other tools designed to assist a student in learning the covered material [23].

Guideline Element Model (GEM) An XML specification for marking up textual documents that describe clinical practice guidelines. The guideline-related XML tags make it possible for information systems to determine the nature of the text that has been marked up and its role in the guideline specification [22].

GWAS See: Genome-Wide Association Studies [25].

Haptic feedback A user interface feature in which physical sensations are transmitted to the user to provide a tactile sensation as part of a simulated activity [18, 20].

Hard disk A magnetic disk used for data storage and typically fixed in the disk-drive unit [5].

Hardware The physical equipment of a computer system, including the central processing unit, memory, data-storage devices, workstations, terminals, and printers [5].

Harmonic mean An average of a set of weighted values in which the weights are determined by the relative importance of the contribution to the average [8].

HCI See: Human-computer interaction [4].

HCO See: Healthcare organization [14].

Head word The key word in a multi-word phrase that conveys the central meaning of the phrase. For example, a phrase containing adjectives and a noun, the noun is typically the head word [8].

Header (of email) The portion of a simple electronic mail message that contains information about the date and time of the message, the address of the sender, the addresses of the recipients, the subject, and other optional information [5].

Health Evaluation and Logical Processing [HELP] On of the first electronic health record systems, developed at LDS Hospital in Sal Lake City, Utah. Still in use today, it was innovative for its introduction of automated alerts [19].

Health informatics Used by some as a synonym for biomedical informatics, this term is increasingly used solely to refer to applied research and practice in clinical and public health informatics [1].

Health information and communication technology (HICT) The broad spectrum of hardware and software used to capture, store and transmit health information [18].

Health Information exchange (HIE) The process of moving health information electronically among disparate health care organizations for clinical care and other purposes; or an organization that is dedicated to providing health information exchange [6,12,13].

Health Information Infrastructure (HII) The set of public and private resources, including networks, databases, and policies, for collecting, storing, and transmitting health information [13, 16].

Health Information Technology (HIT) The use of computers and communications technology in healthcare and public health settings [1].

Health Information Technology for Economic and Clinical Health (HITECH) Also referred to as HITECH Act. Passed by the Congress as Title IV of the American Recovery and Reinvestment Act of 2009 (ARRA) in 2009, established four major goals that promote the use of health information technology: (1) Develop standards for the nationwide electronic exchange and use of health information; (2) Invest $20B in incentives to encourage doctors and hospitals to use HIT to electronically exchange patients' health information; (3) Generate $10B in savings through improvements in quality of care and care coordination, and reductions in medical errors and duplicative care and (4) Strengthen Federal privacy and security law to protect identifiable health information from misuse. Also codified the Office of the

National Coordinator for Health Information Technology (ONC) within the Department of Health and Human Services [14, 17].

Health Insurance Portability and Accountability Act (HIPAA) A law enacted in 1996 to protect health insurance coverage for workers and their families when they change or lose their jobs. An "administrative simplification" provision requires the Department of Health and Human Services to establish national standards for electronic healthcare transactions and national identifiers for providers, health plans, and employers. It also addresses the security and privacy of health data [1, 5, 8, 14, 18].

Health Level Seven (HL7) An ad hoc standards group formed to develop standards for exchange of health care data between independent computer applications; more specifically, the health care data messaging standard developed and adopted by the HL7 standards group [6, 8, 12, 14].

Health literacy A constellation of skills, including the ability to perform basic reading, math, and everyday health tasks like comprehending prescription bottles and appointment slips, required to function in the health care environment [4].

Health maintenance organization (HMO) A group practice or affiliation of independent practitioners that contracts with patients to provide comprehensive health care for a fixed periodic payment specified in advance [14].

Health on the Net[HON] A private organization establishing ethical standards for health information published on the World Wide Web [21].

Health Record Bank (HRB) An independent organization that provides a secure electronic repository for storing and maintaining an individual's lifetime health and medical records from multiple sources and assuring that the individual always has complete control over who accesses their information [13].

Healthcare organization (HCO) Any health-related organization that is involved in direct patient care [14].

Healthcare team A coordinated group of health professionals including physicians, nurses, case managers, dieticians, pharmacists, therapists, and other practitioners who collaborate in caring for a patient [2].

HELP See Health Evaluation and Logical Processing [19].

HELP sector A decision rule encoded in the HELP system, a clinical information system that was developed by researchers at LDS Hospital in Salt Lake City [22].

Helper (plug- in) An application that are launched by a Web browser when the browser downloads a file that the browser is not able to process itself [5].

Heuristic evaluation (HE) A usability inspection method, in which the system is evaluated on the basis of a small set of well-tested design principles such as visibility of system status, user control and freedom, consistency and standards, flexibility and efficiency of use [4].

Heuristic A mental "trick" or rule of thumb; a cognitive process used in learning or problem solving [2].

HICT See: Health information and communication technology [18].

HIE See: Health Information Exchange [6,12,13].

Hierarchical An arrangement between entities that conveys some superior-inferior relationship, such as parent–child, whole-part etc. [21]

High-bandwidth An information channel that is capable of carrying delivering data at a relatively high rate [18].

Higher-level process A complex process comprising multiple lower-level processes [1].

HII See: Health Information Infrastructure [13, 16].

Hindsight bias The tendency to over-estimate the prior predictability of an event, once the events has already taken place. For example, if event A occurs before event B, there may be a an assumption that A predicted B [4].

HIPAA See: Health Insurance Portability and Accountability Act [1, 5, 8, 14, 18].

HIS See: Hospital information system [1,14].

Historical control In the context of clinical research, historical controls are subjects who represent the targeted population of interest for a study. Typically, their data are derived from existing resources in a retrospective manner and that represent targeted outcomes in a non-interventional state (often resulting

from standard of care practices), so as to provide the basis for comparison to data sets derived from participants who have received an experimental intervention under study [26].

Historically controlled study See: **before-after study** [11].

HIT See: Health Information Technology [1].

HITECH See: Health Information Technology for Economic and Clinical Health [14, 17].

HITECH regulations The components of the Health Information Technology for Economic and Clinical Health Act, passed by the Congress in 2009, which authorized financial incentives to be paid to eligible physicians and hospitals for the adoption of "meaningful use" of EHRs in the United States. The law also called for the certification of EHR technology and for educational programs to enhance its dissemination and adoption [22].

HIV See: Human immunodeficiency virus [5].

HL7 See: Health Level 7 [6,7,8,12,14].

HMO See: Health maintenance organization [14].

Home Telehealth The extension of telehealth services in to the home setting to support activities such as home nursing care and chronic disease management [18].

HON See: Health on the Net [21].

Hospital information system (HIS) Computer system designed to support the comprehensive information requirements of hospitals and medical centers, including patient, clinical, ancillary, and financial management [1,14].

Hot fail over A secondary computer system that is kept in constant synchronization with the primary system and that can take over as soon as the primary fails for any reason [12].

Hounsfield number The numeric information contained in each pixel of a CT image. It is related to the composition and nature of the tissue imaged and is used to represent the density of tissue [9].

HRB See: Health Record Bank [13].

HTML See HyperText [5, 8, 21].

HTTP See: HyperText Transfer Protocol [5, 6].

Human-computer interaction (HCI) Formal methods for addressing the ways in which human beings and computer programs exchange information [4].

Human factors The scientific discipline concerned with the understanding of interactions among humans and other elements of a system, and the profession that applies theory, principles, data, and other methods to design in order to optimize human well-being and overall system performance [4].

Human Genome Project An international undertaking, the goal of which is to determine the complete sequence of human deoxyribonucleic acid (DNA), as it is encoded in each of the 23 chromosomes [2, 24].

Human immunodeficiency virus (HIV) A retrovirus that invades and inactivates helper T cells of the immune system and is a cause of AIDS and AIDS-related complex [5].

HyperText markup language (HTML) The document specification language used for documents on the World Wide Web [5, 8, 21].

HyperText Transfer Protocol (HTTP) The client–server protocol used to access information on the World Wide Web [5, 6].

Hypertext Text linked together in a nonsequential web of associations. Users can traverse highlighted portions of text to retrieve additional related information [5].

Hypothesis generation The process of proposing a hypothesis, usually driven by some unexplained phenomenon and the derivation of a suspected underlying mechanism [8].

Hypothetico-deductive approach A method of reasoning made up of four stages (cue acquisition, hypothesis generation, cue interpretation, and hypothesis evaluation) which is used to generate and test hypotheses. In clinical medicine, an iterative approach to diagnosis in which physicians perform sequential, staged data collection, data interpretation, and hypothesis generation to determine and refine a differential diagnosis [2,4].

Hypothetico-deductive reasoning reasoning by first generating and then testing a set of hypotheses to account for clinical data (i.e., reasoning from hypothesis to data) [4].

ICANN See: Internet Corporation for Assigned Names and Numbers [5].

ICD-9-CM See: International Classification of Diseases, 9th Edition, Clinical Modifications [7, 8, 14].

ICMP See: Internet Control Message Protocol [5].

Icon In a graphical interface, a pictorial representation of an object or function [5].

ICT See: Information and communications technology [12].

IDF See: Inverse document frequency [21].

IDN See: Integrated delivery network [10, 14, 15].

Image acquisition The process of generating images from the modality and converting them to digital form if they are not intrinsically digital [9].

Image compression A mathematical process for removing redundant or relatively unimportant information from an electronic image such that the resulting file appears the same (lossless compression) or similar (lossycompression) when compared to the original [18].

Image content representation Makes the information in images accessible to machines for processing [9].

Image database An organized collection of clinical image files, such as x-rays, photographs, and microscopic images [21].

Image enhancement The use of global processing to improve the appearance of the image either for human use or for subsequent processing by computer [9].

Image interpretation/computer reasoning The process by which the individual viewing the image renders an impression of the medical significance of the results of imaging study, potentially aided by computer methods [9].

Image management/storage Methods for storing, transmitting, displaying, retrieving, and organizing images [9]. The application of methods for storing, transmitting, displaying, retrieving, and organizing images.

Image metadata Data about images, such as the type of image (e.g., modality), patient that was imaged, date of imaging, image features (quantitative or qualitative), and other information pertaining to the image and its contents [9].

Image processing The transformation of one or more input images, either into one or more output images, or into an abstract representation of the contents of the input images [9].

Image quantitation The process of extracting useful numerical parameters or deriving calculations from the image or from ROIs in the image [9].

Image reasoning Computerized methods that use images to formulate conclusions or answer questions that require knowledge and logical inference [9].

Image rendering/visualization A variety of techniques for creating image displays, diagrams, or animations to display images more in a different perspective from the raw images [9]

Imaging informatics A subdiscipline of medical informatics concerned with the common issues that arise in all image modalities and applications once the images are converted to digital form [1, 20].

IMIA See: International Medical Informatics Association [15].

Immersive environment A computer-based set of sensory inputs and outputs that can give the illusion of being in a different physical environment; see; **Virtual Reality** [4].

Immersive simulated environment A teaching environment in which a student manipulates tools to control simulated instruments, producing visual, pressure, and other feedback to the tool controls and instruments [23].

Immunization Information System (IIS) Confidential, population based, computerized databases that record all immunization doses administered by participating providers to persons residing within a given geopolitical area. Also known as **Immunization Registries** [16].

Immunization Registry Confidential, population based, computerized databases that record all immunization doses administered by participating providers to persons residing within a given geopolitical area. Also known as **Immunization Information Systems** [16].

Implementation science Implementation science refers to the study of socio-cultural, operational, and behavioral norms and processes surrounding the dissemination and adoption of new systems, approaches and/or knowledge [26].

Inaccessibility A property of paper records that describes the inability to access the record by more than one person or in more than one place at a time [12].

Incrementalist An approach to evaluation that tolerates ambiguity and uncertainty and allows changes from day-to-day [11].

Independent variable In a correlational or experimental study, a variable thought to determine or be associated with the value of the dependent variable (q.v.) [11].

Independent Two events, A and B, are considered independent if the occurrence of one does not influence the probability of the occurrence of the other. Thus, p[A | B] = p[A]. The probability of two independent events A and B both occurring is given by the product of the individual probabilities: p[A,B] = p[A] × p[B]. (See conditional independence.) [3]

Index In information retrieval, a shorthand guide to the content that allows users to find relevant content quickly [8].

Index Medicus The printed index used to catalog the medical literature. Journal articles are indexed by author name and subject heading, then aggregated in bound volumes. The Medline database was originally constructed as an online version of the Index Medicus [21].

Index test The diagnostic test whose performance is being measured [3].

Indexing In information retrieval, the assignment to each document of specific terms that indicate the subject matter of the document and that are used in searching [21].

Indirect-care Activities of health professionals that are not directly related to patient care, such as teaching and supervising students, continuing education, and attending staff meetings [15].

Inference engine A computer program that reasons about a **knowledge base**. In the case of **rule-based systems**, the inference engine may perform **forward chaining** or **backward chaining** to enable the rules to infer new information about the current situation [22].

Inflectional morpheme A morpheme that creates a different form of a word without changing the meaning of the word or the part of speech (e.g., –ed, -s, -ing as in activated, activates, activating.) [8]

Influence diagram A belief network in which explicit decision and utility nodes are also incorporated [3, 22].

Infobutton manager **Middleware** that provides a standard software interface between **infobuttons** in an EHR and the documents and other information resources that the infobuttons may display for the user [22].

Infobutton A context-specific link from health care application to some information resource that anticipates users' needs and provides targeted information [6,12, 22, 23].

*info***RAD** The information technology and computing oriented component of the very large exhibition hall at the annual meeting of the Radiological Society of North America [20].

Information Organized data from which knowledge can be derived and that accordingly provide a basis for decision making [2].

Information and communications technology (ICT) The use of computers and communications devices to accept, store, transmit, and manipulate data; the term is roughly a synonym for information technology, but it is used more often outside the United States [12].

Information extraction Methods that process text to capture and organize specific information in the text and also to capture and organize specific relations between the pieces of information [8, 21].

Information model A representation of concepts, relationships, constraints, rules, and operations to specify data semantics for a chosen domain of discourse. It can provide sharable, stable, and organized structure of information requirements for the domain context [9].

Information need In information retrieval, the searchers' expression, in their own language, of the information that they desire [21].

Information resource Generic term for a computer-based system that seeks to enhance health care by providing patient-specific information directly to care providers (often used equivalently with "system") [11].

Information retrieval (IR) Methods that efficiently and effectively search and obtain data, particularly text, from very large collections or databases. It is also the science and practice of identification and efficient use of recorded media. See also **Search** [4, 8, 21, 26].

Information science The field of study concerned with issues related to the management of both paper-based and electronically stored information [1].

Information theory The theory and mathematics underlying the processes of communication [1].

Information visualization The use of computer-supported, interactive, visual representations of abstract data to amplify cognition [4].

Ink-jet printer Output device that uses a moveable head to spray liquid ink on paper; the head moves back and forth for each line of pixels [5].

Input and Output Devices, such as keyboards, pointing devices, video displays, and laser printers, that facilitate user interaction and storage [5] or just **Input**: The data that represent state information, to be stored and processed to produce results – (output).

Institute of Medicine The health arm of the National Academy of Sciences, which provides unbiases, authoritative advice to decision makers and the public [17].

Institutional Review Board (IRB) A committee responsible for reviewing an institution's research projects involving human subjects in order to protect their safety, rights, and welfare [5, 10].

Integrated circuit A circuit of transistors, resistors, and capacitors constructed on a single chip and interconnected to perform a specific function [5, 19].

Integrated delivery network (IDN) A large conglomerate health-care organization developed to provide and manage comprehensive health-care services [10, 14, 15].

Integrated Service Digital Network (ISDN) A digital telephone service that allows high-speed network communications using conventional (twisted pair) telephone wiring [5, 18].

Integrative model Model for understanding a phenomenon that draws from multiple disciplines and is not necessarily based on first principles [24].

Intellectual property Software programs, knowledge bases, Internet pages, and other creative assets that require protection against copying and other unauthorized use [10, 21].

Interactome The set of all molecular interactions in a cell [25].

Interface engine Software that mediates the exchange of information among two or more systems. Typically, each system must know how to communicate with the interface engine, but not need to know the information format of the other systems [14].

Intermediate effect process of continually learning, re-learning, and exercising new knowledge, punctuated by periods of apparent decrease in mastery and declines in performance, which may be necessary for learning to take place. People at intermediate levels of expertise may perform more poorly than those at lower level of expertise on some tasks, due to the challenges of assimilating new knowledge or skills over the course of the learning process [4].

Internal validity in the context of clinical research, internal validity refers to the minimization of potential biases during the design and execution of the trial [26].

International Classification of Diseases, 9th Edition, Clinical Modifications A US extension of the World Health Organization's International Classification of Diseases, 9th Edition [7, 8, 14].

International Medical Informatics Association (IMIA) An international organization dedicated to advancing biomedical and health informatics; an "organization of organizations", it's members are national informatics societies and organizations, such as **AMIA** [15].

International Organization for Standards (ISO) The international body for information and other standards [21].

Internet address See Internet Protocol Address [5]

Internet Protocol address A 32-bit number that uniquely identifies a computer connected to the Internet. Also called "Internet address" or "IP address" [5]

Internet Control Message Protocol (ICMP) A network-level Internet protocol that provides error correction and other information relevant to processing data packets [5].

Internet Corporation for Assigned Names and Numbers (ICANN) The organization responsible for managing Internet domain name and IP address assignments [5].

Internet protocol The protocol within TCP/IP that governs the creation and routing of data packets and their reassembly into data messages [5].

Internet service provider (ISP) A commercial communications company that supplies fee-for-service Internet connectivity to individuals and organizations [5].

Internet standards The set of conventions and protocols all Internet participants use to enable effective data communications [5].

Internet Support Group (ISG) An on-line forum for people with similar problems, challenges or conditions to share supportive resources [17].

Internet A worldwide collection of gateways and networks that communicate with each other using the TCP/IP protocol, collectively providing a range of services including electronic mail and World Wide Web access [5].

Interoperability The ability for systems to exchange data and operate in a coordinated, seamless manner [14, 21].

Interpreter A program that converts each statement in a high-level program to a machine-language representation and then executes the binary instruction(s) [5].

Interventional radiology A subspecialty of radiology that uses imaging to guide invasive diagnostic or therapeutic procedures [20].

Intrinsic evaluation An evaluation of a component of a system that focuses only on the performance of the component. See also **Extrinsic Evaluation** [8].

Intuitionist–pluralist or de-constructivist A philosophical position that holds that there is no truth and that there are as many legitimate interpretations of observed phenomena as there are observers [11].

Inverse document frequency (IDF) A measure of how infrequently a term occurs in a document collection [21].

$$IDFi = \log\left(\frac{\text{number of documents}}{\text{number of documents with term i}}\right) + 1$$

IOM See: Institute of Medicine [17]

IP address See: Internet Protocol Address [5]

IR See: Information retrieval [4, 8, 21, 26]

IRB See: Institutional Review Board [5, 10].

ISDN See: Integrated Service Digital Network [5, 18].

ISG See: Internet Support Group [17].

ISO See: InternationalOrganization for Standards [21].

ISP See: Internet service provider [5].

Job A set of tasks submitted by a user for processing by a computer system [5].

Joint Commission (JC) An independent, not-for-profit organization, The Joint Commission accredits and certifies more than 19,000 health care organizations and programs in the United States. Joint Commission accreditation and certification is recognized nationwide as a symbol of quality that reflects an organization's commitment to meeting certain performance standards. The Joint Commission was formerly known as JCAHO (the Joint Commission for the Accreditation of Healthcare Organizations) [7,14].

Just-in-time learning An approach to providing necessary information to a user at the moment it is needed, usually through anticipation of the need [23].

Kernel The core of the operating system that resides in memory and runs in the background to supervise and control the execution of all other programs and direct operation of the hardware [5].

Key field A field in the record of a file that uniquely identifies the record within the file [5].

Key Performance Indicator (KPI) A metric defined to be an important factor in the success of an organization. Typically, several Key Performance indicators are displayed on a Dashboard [20].

Keyboard A data-input device used to enter alphanumeric characters through typing [5].

Keyword A word or phrase that conveys special meaning or to refer to information that is relevant to such a meaning (as in an index) [8].

Kilobyte 2^{10} or 1024 bytes [5].

Knowledge acquisition The information-elicitation and modeling process by which developers interact with subject-matter experts to create electronic **knowledge bases** [22].

Knowledge base A collection of stored facts, heuristics, and models that can be used for problem solving [2, 22].

Knowledge Relationships, facts, assumptions, heuristics, and models derived through the formal or informal analysis (or interpretation) of observations and resulting information [2].

Knowledge-based system A program that symbolically encodes, in a knowledge base, facts, heuristics, and models derived from experts in a field and uses that knowledge to provide problem analysis or advice that the expert might have provided if asked the same question [22].

KPI See: Key Performance Indicator [20].

Laboratory function study Study that explores important properties of an information resource in isolation from the clinical setting [11].

Laboratory user effect study An evaluation technique in which a user is observed when given a simulated task to perform [11].

LAN See: Local-area network [5, 14].

Laser printer Output device that uses an electromechanically controlled laser beam to generate an image on a xerographic surface, which then is used to produce paper copies [5].

Latency The time required for a signal to travel between two points in a network [18]

Latent failures Enduring systemic problems that make errors possible but are less visible or not evident for some time [4].

Law of proximity Principle from Gestalt psychology that states that visual entities that are close together are perceptually grouped [4].

Law of symmetry Principle from Gestalt psychology that states that symmetric objects are more readily perceived [4].

LCD See: Liquid crystal display [5].

Lean A management strategy that focuses only on those process that are able to contribute specific and measurable value for the end customer. The LEAN concept originated with Toyota's focus on efficient manufacturing processes [14].

Learning health system A proposed model for health care in which outcomes from past and current patient care provide are systematically collected, analyzed and then fed back into decision making about best practices for future patient care [26].

Learning healthcare system The cycle related to turning healthcare data into knowledge, translating that knowledge into practice, and creating new data, typically through the use of advanced information technology [1].

LED See: Light-emitting diode [5].

Lexemes A minimal lexical unit in a language that represents different forms of the same word [8].

Lexical-statistical retrieval Retrieval based on a combination of word matching and relevance ranking [21].

Lexicon A catalogue of the words in a language, usually containing syntactic information such as parts of speech, pluralization rules, etc. [8, 20]

Light-emitting diode (LED) A semiconductor device that emits a particular frequency of light when a current is passed through it; typically used for indicator lights and computer screens because low power requirement, minimal heat generated, and durability [5].

Likelihood ratio (LR) A measure of the discriminatory power of a test. The LR is the ratio of the probability of a result when the condition under consideration is true to the probability of a result when the condition under consideration is false (for example, the probability of a result in a diseased patient to the probability of a result in a nondiseased patient). The LR for a positive test is the ratio of true-positive rate (TPR) to false-positive rate (FPR) [3].

Link-based An indexing approach that gives relevance weight to web pages based on how often they are cited by other pages [21].

Linux An **open source** operating system based on principles of Unix and first developed by Linus Torvalds in 1991 [6].

Liquid crystal display(LCD) A display technology that uses rod-shaped molecules to bend light and alter contrast and viewing angle to produce images [5].

Listserver A distribution list for electronic mail messages [5].

Literature reference database See: bibliographic database [21]

Local-area network (LAN) A network for data communication that connects multiple nodes, all typically owned by a single institution and located within a small geographic area [5, 14].

Logical Observations, Identifiers, Names and Codes [LOINC] A controlled terminology created for providing coded terms for observational procedures. Originally focused on laboratory tests, it has expanded to include many other diagnostic procedures [17].

Logical positivist A philosophical position that holds that there is a single truth that can be inferred from the right combination of studies [11].

Logic-based A knowledge representation method based on the use of predicates [8].

LOINC See: Logical Observations, Identifiers, Names and Codes [17].

Long-term memory The part of memory that acquires information from short-term memory and retains it for long periods of time [4].

Long-term storage A medium for storing information that can persist over long periods without the need for a power supply to maintain data integrity [5].

Lossless compression A mathematical technique for reducing the number of bits needed to store data while still allowing for the recreation of the original data [20].

Lossy compression A mathematical technique for reducing the number of bits needed to store data but that results in loss of information [20].

Low-level processes An elementary process that has its basis in the physical world of chemistry or physics [1].

LR See: Likelihood ratio [3].

Machine code The set of primitive instructions to a computer represented in binary code (machine language) [5].

Machine language The set of primitive instructions represented in binary code (machine code) [5].

Machine learning A computing technique in which information learned from data is used to improve system performance [8,19].

Machine translation Automatic mapping of text written in one natural language into text of another language [8].

Macros A reusable set of computer instructions, generally for a repetitive task [5].

Magnetic disk A round, flat plate of material that can accept and store magnetic charge. Data are encoded on magnetic disk as sequences of charges on concentric tracks [5].

Magnetic resonance imaging (MRI) A modality that produces images by evaluating the differential response of atomic nuclei in the body when the patient is placed in an intense magnetic field [9, 20].

Magnetic resonance spectroscopy A noninvasive technique that is similar to magnetic resonance imaging but uses a stronger field and is used to monitor body chemistry (as in metabolism or blood flow) rather than anatomical structures[9]

Magnetic tape A long ribbon of material that can accept and store magnetic charge. Data are encoded on magnetic tape as sequences of charges along longitudinal tracks [5].

Magnetoencephalography (MEG) A method for measuring the electromagnetic fields generated by the electrical activity of the neurons using a large arrays of scalp sensors, the output of which are processed in a similar way to CT in order to localize the source of the electromagnetic and metabolic shifts occurring in the brain during trauma [9].

Mailing list A set of mailing addresses used for bulk distribution of electronic or physical mail [5].

Mainframe computer system A large, expensive, multi-user computer, typically operated and maintained by professional computing personnel. Often referred to as a "mainframe" for short [5,19].

Malpractice Class of litigation in health care based on negligence theory; failure of a health professional to render proper services in keeping with the standards of the community [10].

Management The process of treating a patient (or allowing the condition to resolve on its own) once the medical diagnosis has been determined [22].

Manual indexing The process by which human indexers, usually using standardized terminology, assign indexing terms and attributes to documents, often following a specific protocol [21].

Markov cycle The period of time specified for a transition probability within a Markov model [3].

Markov model A mathematical model of a set of strings in which the probability of a given symbol occurring depends on the identity of the immediately preceding symbol or the two immediately preceding symbols. Processes modeled in this way are often called **Markov processes** [3].

Markov process A mathematical model of a set of strings in which the probability of a given symbol occurring depends on the identity of the immediately preceding symbol or the two immediately preceding symbols [8].

Markup language A document specification language that identifies and labels the components of the document's contents [24].

Master patient index (MPI) A database that is used across a healthcare organization to maintain consistent, accurate, and current demographic and essential clinical data on the patients seen and managed within its various departments [14].

Mean average precision (MAP) A method for measuring overall retrieval precisionin which precision is measured at every point at which a relevant document is obtained, and the MAP measure is found by averaging these points for the whole query [21].

Mean time between failures (MTBF) The average predicted time interval between anticipated operational malfunctions of a system, based on long-term observations [13].

Meaningful use The set of standards defined by the Centers for Medicare & Medicaid Services (CMS) Incentive Programs that governs the use of electronic health records and allows eligible providers and hospitals to earn incentive payments by meeting specific criteria. The term refers to the belief that health care providers using electronic health records in a meaningful, or effective, way will be able to improve health care quality and efficiency [1, 6, 12, 14, 16, 17, 22, 27].

Measurement study Study to determine the extent and nature of the errors with which a measurement is made using a specific instrument (cf. Demonstration study) [11].

Measures of concordance Measures of agreement in test performance: the true-positive and true-negative rates [3].

MedBiquitous A healthcare-specific standards consortium led by Johns Hopkins Medicine [23].

Medical computer science The subdivision of computer science that applies the methods of computing to medical topics [1].

Medical computing The application of methods of computing to medical topics (see **medical computer science**) [1].

Medical entities dictionary (MED) A compendium of terms found in electronic medical record systems. Among the best known MEDs is that developed and maintained by the Columbia University Medical Center and Columbia University. Contains in excess of 100,000 terms [14].

Medical errors Errors or mistakes, committed by health professionals, that hold the potential to result in harm to the patient [4].

Medical home A primary care practice that will maintain a comprehensive problem list to make fully informed decisions in coordinating their care [15].

Medical informatics An earlier term for the **biomedical informatics** discipline, medical informatics is now viewed as the subfield of clinical informatics that deals with the management of disease and the role of physicians [1].

Medical Information Bus (MIB) A data-communication system that supports data acquisition from a variety of independent devices [19].

Medical information science The field of study concerned with issues related to the management and use of biomedical information (see also **biomedical informatics**) [1].

Medical Literature Analysis and Retrieval System (MEDLARS) The initial electronic version of Index Medicus developed by the National Library of Medicine [21].

Medical Logic Module (MLM) A single chunk of medical reasoning or decision rule, typically encoded using the **Arden Syntax** [6, 22].

Medical record committees An institutional panel charged with ensuring appropriate use of medical records within the organization [10].

Medical Subject Headings (MeSH) Some 18,000 terms used to identify the subject content of the biomedical literature. The National Library of Medicine's MeSH vocabulary has emerged as the de facto standard for biomedical indexing [21].

Medication A substance used for medical treatment, typically a medicine or drug [8].

MEDLARS Online (MEDLINE) The National Library of Medicine's electronic catalog of the biomedical literature, which includes information abstracted from journal articles, including author names, article title, journal source, publication date, abstract, and medical subject headings [21].

Medline Plus An online resource from the National Library of Medicine that contains health topics, drug information, medical dictionaries, directories, and other resources, organized for use by health care consumers [21, 23].

Megabits per second (Mbps) A common unit of measure for specifying a rate of data transmission [5].

Megabyte 2^{20} or 1,048,576 bytes [5].

Member checking In subjectivist research, the process of reflecting preliminary findings back to individuals in the setting under study, one way of confirming that the findings are truthful [11].

Memorandum of understanding A document describing a bilateral or multilateral agreement between two or more parties. It expresses a convergence of will between the parties, indicating an intended common line of action [11].

Memory sticks A portable device that typically plugs into a computer's USB port and is capable of storing data. Also called a "thumb drive" or a "USB drive" [14].

Memory Areas that are used to store programs and data. The computer's working memory comprises read-only memory (ROM) and random-access memory (RAM) [5].

Mental images A form of internal representation that captures perceptual information recovered from the environment [4].

Mental models A construct for describing how individuals form internal models of systems. They are designed to answer questions such as "how does it work?" or "what will happen if I take the following action?" [4]

Mental representations internal cognitive states that have a certain correspondence with the external world [4].

Menu In a user interface, a displayed list of valid commands or options from which a user may choose [5].

Merck Medicus An aggregated set of resources, including Harrison's Online, MDConsult, and DXplain [21].

Meta-analysis A summary study that combines quantitatively the estimates from individual studies [3].

Metabolomic Pertaining to the study of small-molecule metabolites created as the end-products of specific cellular processes [25].

Metadata Literally, data about data, describing the format and meaning of a set of data [5, 21, 25].

Metagenomics Using DNA sequencing technology to characterize complex samples derived from an environmental sample, e.g., microbial populations. For example, the gut 'microbiome' can be characterized by applying next generation sequencing of stool samples [24, 25].

Metathesaurus One component of the Unified Medical Language System, the Metathesaurus contains linkages between terms in Medical Subject Headings (MeSH) and in dozens of controlled vocabularies [14, 21].

MIB See Medical Information Bus [7].

Microarray chips A microchip that holds DNA probes that can recognize DNA from samples being tested [24].

Microprocessor An integrated circuit that contains all the functions of a central processing unit of a computer [19].

Microsimulation models Individual-level health state transition models that provide a means to model very complex events flexibly over time [3].

MIMIC II Database See Multiparameter Intelligent Monitoring in Intensive Care [19].

Minicomputers A class of computers that were introduced in the 1960s as a smaller alternative to mainframe computers. Minicomputers enabled smaller companies and departments within organizations (like HCOs) to implement software applications at significantly less cost than was required by mainframe computers [14, 19].

Mistake Occurs when an inappropriate course of action reflects erroneous judgment or inference [4].

Mixed-initiative dialog A mode of interaction with a computer system in which the computer may pose questions for the user to answer, and vice versa [22].

Mixed-initiative systems An educational program in which user and program share control of the interaction. Usually, the program guides the interaction, but the student can assume control and digress when new questions arise during a study session [23].

Mobile health The practice of medicine and public health supported by mobile devices. Also referred to as mHealth or m-health [18].

Model organism databases Organized reference databases the combine bibliographic databases, full text, and databases of sequences, structure, and function for organisms whose genomic data has been highly characterized, such as the mouse, fruit fly, and Sarcchomyces yeast [21].

Modem A device used to modulate and demodulate digital signals for transmission to a remote computer over telephone lines; converts digital data to audible analog signals, and vice versa [5].

Modifiers of interest In natural language processing, a term that is used to describe or otherwise modify a named-entity that has been recognized [8].

Molecular imaging A technique for capturing images at the cellular and subcellular level by marking particular chemicals in ways that can be detected with image or radiodetection [9].

Monitoring tool The application of logical rules and conditions (e.g., range-checking, enforcement of data completion, etc.) to ensure the completeness and quality of research-related data [26].

Monotonic Describes a function that consistently increases or decreases, rather than oscillates [4].

Morpheme The smallest unit in the grammar of a language which has a meaning or a linguistic function; it can be a root of a word (e.g., –arm), a prefix (e.g., re-), or a suffix (e.g., –it is) [8].

Morphology The study of meaningful units in language and how they combine to form words [8].

Morphometrics The quantitative study of growth and development, a research area that depends on the use of imaging methods [20].

Mosaic The first graphical web browser credited with popularizing the World Wide Web and developed at the National Center for Supercomputing Applications (NCSA) at the University of Illinois [6].

Motion artifact Visual interference caused by the difference between the frame rate of an imaging device and the motion of the object being imaged [18].

Mouse A small boxlike device that is moved on a flat surface to position a cursor on the screen of a display monitor. A user can select and mark data for entry by depressing buttons on the mouse [5].

Multi-axial A terminology system composed of several distinct, mutually exclusive term subsets that care combined to support **postcoordination** [7].

Multimodal interface A design concept which allows users to interact with computers using multiple modes of communication or tools, including speaking, clicking, or touchscreen input [4].

Multiparameter Intelligent Monitoring in Intensive Care (MIMIC-II) A publicly and freely available research database that encompasses a diverse and very large population of ICU patients. It contains high temporal resolution data including lab results, electronic documentation, and bedside monitor trends and waveforms [19].

Multiprocessing The use of multiple processors in a single computer system to increase the power of the system (see parallel processing) [5].

Multiprogramming A scheme by which multiple programs simultaneously reside in the main memory of a single central processing unit [5].

Multiprotocol label switching (MPLS) A mechanism in high-performance telecommunications networks that directs data from one network node to the next based on short path labels rather than long network addresses, avoiding complex lookups in a routing table [18].

Multiuser system A computer system that shares its resources among multiple simultaneous users [5].

Mutually exclusive State in which one, and only one, of the possible conditions is true; for example, either A or not A is true, and one of the statements is false. When using Bayes' theorem to perform medical diagnosis, we generally assume that diseases are mutually exclusive, meaning that the patient has exactly one of the diseases under consideration and not more [3].

Myocardial ischemia Reversible damage to cardiac muscle caused by decreased blood flow and resulting poor oxygenation. Such ischemia may cause chest pain or other symptoms [19].

Naïve Bayesian model The use of **Bayes Theorem** in a way that assumes conditional independence of variables that may in fact be linked statistically [22].

Name Designation of an object by a linguistic expression [7].

Name authority An entity or mechanism for controlling the identification and formulation of unique identifiers for names. In the Internet, a name authority is required to associate common domain names with their IP addresses [14].

Named-entity normalization The natural language processing method, after finding a named entity in a document, for linking (normalizing) that mention to appropriate database identifiers [8].

Named-entity recognition In language processing, a subtask of information extraction that seeks to locate and classify atomic elements in text into predefined categories [8].

Name-server In networked environments such as the Internet, a computer that converts a host name into an IP address before the message is placed on the network [5].

National Center for Biotechnology Information (NCBI) Established in 1988 as a national resource for molecular biology information, the NCBI is a component of the National Library of Medicine that creates public databases, conducts research in computational biology, develops software tools for analyzing genome data, and disseminates biomedical information [21].

National Guidelines Clearinghouse A public resource, coordinated by the Agency for Health Research and Quality, that collects and distributes evidence-based clinical practice guidelines (see www.guideline.gov) [21].

National Health Information Infra–structure (NHII) A comprehensive knowledge-based network of interoperable systems of clinical, public health, and personal health information that is intended to improve decision-making by making health information available when and where it is needed [17].

National Information Standards Organization (NISO) A non-profit association accredited by the American National Standards Institute (ANSI), that identifies, develops, maintains, and publishes technical standards to manage information (see www.niso.org) [21].

National institute for Standards and Technology (NIST) A non-regulatory federal agency within the U.S. Commerce Department's Technology Administration; its mission is to develop and promote measurement, standards, and technology to enhance productivity, facilitate trade, and improve the quality of life (see www.nist.gov) [21].

National Quality Forum A not-for-profit organization that develops and implements national strategies for health care quality measurement and reporting [7].

Nationwide Health Information Network (NwHIN) A set of standards, services, and policies that have been shepherded by the Office of the National Coordinator of Health Information Technology to enable secure health information exchange over the Internet [12].

Natural language processing (NLP) facilitates tasks by enabling use of automated methods that represent the relevant information in the text with high validity and reliability [8, 22].

Natural language query A question expressed in unconstrained text, from which meaning must somehow be extracted or inferred so that a suitable response can be generated [21].

Natural language Unfettered spoken or written language. Free text [8].

Naturalistic Describes a study in which little if anything is done by the evaluator to alter the setting in which the study is carried out [11].

Needs assessment A study carried out to help understand the users, their context and their needs and skills, to inform the design of the information resource [11, 23].

Negative dictionary A list of **stop words** used in information retrieval [21].

Negative predictive value (PV–) The probability that the condition of interest is absent if the result is negative—for example, the probability that specific a disease is absent given a negative test result [3].

Negligence theory A concept from tort law that states that providers of goods and services are expected to uphold the standards of the community, thereby facing claims of negligence if individuals are harmed by substandard goods or services [10].

Nested structures In natural language processing, a phrase or phrases that are used in place of simple words within other phrases [8].

Net reclassification improvement (NRI) in classification methods, a measure of the net fraction of reclassifications made in the correct direction, using one method over another method without the designated improvement [25].

Network access provider A company that builds and maintains high speed networks to which customers can connect, generally to access the Internet (see also Internet service provider) [5].

Network Operations Center (NOC) A centralized monitoring facility for physically distributed computer and/or telecommunications facilities that allows continuous real-time reporting of the status of the connected components [13].

Network protocol The set of rules or conventions that specifies how data are prepared and transmitted over a network and that governs data communication among the nodes of a network [5].

Network stack The method within a single machine by which the responsibilities for network communications are divided into different levels, with clear interfaces between the levels, thereby making network software more modular [5].

Neuroinformatics An emerging subarea of applied biomedical informatics in which the discipline's methods are applied to the management of neurological data sets and the modeling of neural structures and function [9].

Next Generation Internet Initiative A federally funded research program in the late 1990s and early in the current decade that sought to provide technical enhancements to the Internet to support future applications that currently are infeasible or are incapable of scaling for routine use [17].

Next generation sequencing methods Technologies for performing high throughput sequencing of large quantities of DNA or RNA. Typically, these technologies determine the sequences of many millions of short segments of DNA that need to be reassembled and interpreted using bioinformatics [24].

Noise The component of acquired data that is attributable to factors other than the underlying phenomenon being measured (for example, electromagnetic interference, inaccuracy in sensors, or poor contact between sensor and source) [5].

Nomenclature A system of terms used in a scientific discipline to denote classifications and relationships among objects and processes [2, 4, 7].

Nosocomial hospital-acquired infection An infection acquired by a patient after admission to a hospital for a different reason [19].

NQF See: National Quality Forum [7].

Nuclear magnetic resonance (NMR) spectroscopy A spectral technique used in chemistry to characterize chemical compounds by measuring magnetic characteristics of their atomic nuclei [9, 24].

Nuclear medicine imaging A modality for producing images by measuring the radiation emitted by a radioactive isotope that has been attached to a biologically active compound and injected into the body [9].

Nursing informatics The application of biomedical informatics methods and techniques to problems derived from the field of nursing. Viewed as a subarea of clinical informatics [1].

NwHIN Direct A set of standards and services to enable the simple, direct, and secure transport of health information between pairs of health care providers; it is a component of the Nationwide Health Information Network and it complements the Network's more sophisticated components.

Nyquist frequency The minimum sampling rate necessary to achieve reasonable signal quality. In general, it is twice the frequency of the highest-frequency component of interest in a signal [5].

Object Any part of the perceivable or conceivable world [5].

Object Constraint Language (OCL) A textual language for describing rules that apply to the elements a model created in the Uniform Modeling Language. OLC specifies constraints on allowable values in the model. OCL also supports queries of UML models (and of models constructed in similar languages). OCL is a standard of the Object Modeling Group (OMG), and forms the basis of the GELLO query language that may be used in conjunction with the **Arden Syntax** [22].

Objectivist approaches Class of evaluation approaches that make use of experimental designs and statistical analyses of quantitative data [11].

Object-oriented database A database that is structured around individual objects (concepts) that generally include relationships among those objects and, in some cases, executable code that is relevant to the management and or understanding of that object [24].

Odds-ratio form An algebraic expression for calculating the posttest odds of a disease, or other condition of interest, if the pretest odds and **likelihood ratio** are known (an alternative formulation of **Bayes' theorem**, also called the odds-likelihood form) [3].

Office of the National Coordinator for Health Information Technology (ONC) An agency within the US Department of Health and Human Services that is charged with supporting the adoption of health information technology and promoting nationwide health information exchange to improve health care [1, 12].

Omics A set of areas of study in biology that use the suffix "-ome", used to connote breadth or completeness of the objects being studied, for example genomics or proteomics [25].

-omics technologies High throughput experimentation that exhaustively queries a certain biochemical aspect of the state of an organism. Such technologies include proteomics (protein), genomics (gene expression), metabolomics (metabolites), etc. [24]

On line analytic processing (OLAP) A system that focuses on querying across multiple patients simultaneously, typically by few users for infrequent, but very complex queries, often research [5].

On line transaction processing (OLTP) A system designed for use by thousands of simultaneous users doing repetitive queries [5].

Ontology A description (like a formal specification of a program) of the concepts and relationships that can exist for an agent or a community of agents. In biomedicine, such ontologies typically specify the meanings and hierarchical relationships among terms and concepts in a domain[8, 22, 25]

Open consent model A legal mechanism by which an individual can disclose their own private health information or genetic information for research use. This mechanism is used by the Personal Genome Project to enable release of entire genomes of identified individuals [24].

Open source An approach to software development in which programmers can read, redistribute, and modify the source code for a piece of software, resulting in community development of a shared product [6, 12].

Open standards development policy In standards group, a policy that allows anyone to become involved in discussing and defining the standard [7].

Operating system (OS) A program that allocates computer hardware resources to user programs and that supervises and controls the execution of all other programs [5].

Optical Character Recognition (OCR) The conversion of typed text within scanned documents to computer understandable text [12].

Optical coherence tomography (OCT) An optical signal acquisition and processing method. It captures micrometer-resolution, three-dimensional images from within optical scattering media (e.g., biological tissue) [9].

Optical disk A round, flat plate of plastic or metal that is used to store information. Data are encoded through the use of a laser that marks the surface of the disc [5].

Order entry The use of a computer system for entering treatments, requests for lab tests or radiologic studies, or other interventions that the attending clinician wishes to have performed for the benefit of a patient [14].

Orienting issues/questions The initial questions or issues that evaluators seek to answer in a subjectivist study, the answers to which often in turn prompt further questions [11].

Outcome data Formal information regarding the results of interventions [10].

Outcome measurements Using metrics that assess the end result of an intervention rather than an intervening process. For example, remembering to check a patient's Hemoglobin A1C is a process measure, whereas reducing the complications of diabetes is an outcome measure [27].

Outcome variable Similar to "dependent variable," a variable that captures the end result of a health care or educational process; for example, long-term operative complication rate or mastery of a subject area [11].

Output The results produced when a process is applied to input. Some forms of output are hardcopy documents, images displayed on video display terminals, and calculated values of variables [5].

P4 medicine P4 medicine: a term coined by Dr. Leroy Hood for healthcare that strives to be personalized, predictive, preventive and participatory [25].

Packets In networking, a variable-length message containing data plus the network addresses of the sending and receiving nodes, and other control information [5].

PageRank (PR) algorithm In indexing for information retrieval on the Internet, an algorithmic scheme for giving more weight to a Web page when a large number of other pages link to it [21].

Pager One of the first mobile devices for electronic communication between a base station (typically a telephone, but later a computer) and an individual person. Initially restricted to receiving only numeric data (e.g., a telephone number), pagers later incorporated the ability to transmit a response (referred to as "two way pagers") as well as alpha characters so that a message of limited length could be transmitted from a small keyboard. Pagers have been gradually replaced by cellular phones because of their greater flexibility and broader geographical coverage [14].

Page A partitioned component of a computer users' programs and data that can be kept in temporary storage and brought into main memory by the operating system as needed [5].

Parallel processing The use of multiple processing units running in parallel to solve a single problem (see multiprocessing) [5].

Parse tree The representation of structural relationships that results when using a grammar (usually context free) to analyze a given sentence [8].

Partial parsing The analysis of structural relationships that results when using a grammar to analyze a segment of a given sentence [8].

Partial-match searching An approach to information retrieval that recognizes the inexact nature of both indexing and retrieval, and attempts to return the user content ranked by how close it comes to the user's query [21].

Participant calendaring Participant calendaring refers to the capability of a CRMS to support the tracking of participant compliance with a study schema, usually represented as a calendar of temporal events [26].

Participant screening and registration participant screening and registration refers to the capability of a CTMS to support the enrollment phase of a clinical study [26].

Participants The people or organizations who provide data for the study. According to the role of the information resource, these may include patients, friends and family, formal and informal carers, the general public, health professionals, system developers, guideline developers, students, health service managers, etc. [11].

Part-of-speech tags Assignment of syntactic classes to a given sequence of words, e.g., determiner, adjective, noun and verb [8].

Parts of speech The categories to which words in a sentence are assigned in accordance with their syntactic function [8].

Patent A specific legal approach for protecting methods used in implementing or instantiating ideas (see **intellectual property**) [10].

Pathognomonic Distinctively characteristic, and thus, uniquely identifying a condition or object (100 % specific) [2].

Patient centered care Clinical care that is based on personal characteristics of the patient in addition to his or her disease. Such characteristics include cultural traditions, preferences and values, family situations and lifestyles [15].

Patient centered medical home A team-based health care delivery model led by a physician, physician's assistant, or nurse practitioner that provides comprehensive, coordinated, and continuous medical care to patients with the goal of obtaining maximized health outcomes [15, 27].

Patient portal An online application that allows individuals to view health information and otherwise interact with their physicians and hospitals [6, 17, 18].

Patient record The collection of information traditionally kept by a health care provider or organization about an individual's health status and health care; also referred to as the patient's chart, medical record, or health record, and originally called the "unit record." [12]

Patient safety The reduction in the risk of unnecessary harm associated with health care to an acceptable minimum; also the name of a movement and specific research area [4].

Patient triage The process of allocating patients to different levels or urgency of care depending upon the complaints or symptoms displayed [14].

Patient-tracking applications Monitor patient movement in multistep processes [14].

Pattern check A procedure applied to entered data to verify that the entered data have a required pattern; e.g., the three digits, hyphen, and four digits of a local telephone number [12]

Pay for performance Payments to providers that are based on meeting pre-defined expectations for quality [14].

Per diem Payments to providers (typically hospitals) based on a single day of care [14].

Perimeter definition Specification of the boundaries of trusted access to an information system, both physically and logically [5].

Personal clinical electronic communication Web-based messaging solutions that avoid the limitations of email by keeping all interactions within a secure, online environment [18].

Personal computers A small, relatively inexpensive, single-user computer [5].

Personal health application Software for computers, tablet computers, or smart phones that are intended to allow individual patients to monitor their own health or to stimulate their own personal health activities [17].

Personal health record (PHR) A collection of information about an individual's health status and health care that is maintained by the individual (rather than by a health care provider); the data may be entered directly by the patient, captured from a sensing device, or transferred from a laboratory or health care provider. It may include medical information from several independent provider organizations, and may also have health and well-being information [10, 12, 15, 17, 20, 27].

Personal Internetworked Notary and Guardian (PING) An early personally controlled health record, later known as Indivo [17].

Personalized medicine Also often call individualized medicine, refers to a medical model in which decisions are custom-tailored to the patient based on that individual's genomic data, preferences, or other considerations. Such decisions may involve diagnosis, treatment, or assessments of prognosis. Also known as **precision medicine** [2, 22, 25].

Personally controlled health record (PCHR) Similar to a **PHR**, the PCHR differs in the nature of the control offered to the patient, with such features as semantic tags on data elements that can be used to determine the subsets of information that can be shared with specific providers [17].

Petabyte A unit of information equal to 1000 terabytes or 10^{15} bytes [5].

Pharmacodynamics program (PD) The study of how a drug works, it's mechanism of action and pathway of achieving its affect, or "what the drug does to the body." [25]

Pharmacogenetics The study of drug-gene relationships that are dominated by a single gene [25].

Pharmacogenomics The study of how genes and genetic variation influence drug response [1,25].

Pharmacokinetic program Pharmacokinetics or PK is the study of how a drug is absorbed, distributed, metabolized and excreted by the body, or "what the body does to the drug." [25]

Pharmacovigilance The pharmacologicalscience relating to the collection, detection, assessment,

monitoring, and prevention of adverse effects with pharmaceutical products [8].

Phase I (clinical trial) Investigators evaluate a novel therapy in a small group of participants in order to assess overall safety. This safety assessment includes dosing levels in the case of non-interventional therapeutic trials, and potential side effects or adverse effects of the therapy. Often, Phase I trials of non-interventional therapies involve the use of normal volunteers who do not have the disease state targeted by the novel therapy [25, 26].

Phase II (clinical trial) Investigators evaluate a novel therapy in a larger group of participants in order to assess the efficacy of the treatment in the targeted disease state. During this phase, assessment of overall safety is continued [26].

Phase III (clinical trial) Investigators evaluate a novel therapy in an even larger group of participants and compare its performance to a reference standard which is usually the current standard of care for the targeted disease state. This phase typically employs anrandomized controlled design, and often a multi-center RCT given the numbers of variation of subjects that must be recruited to adequately test the hypothesis. In general, this is the final study phase to be performed before seeking regulatory approval for the novel therapy and broader use in standard-of-care environments [26].

Phase IV (clinical trial) Investigators study the performance and safety of a novel therapy after it has been approved and marketed. This type of study is performed in order to detect long-term outcomes and effects of the therapy. It is often called "post-market surveillance" and is, in fact, not an RCT at all, but a less formal, observational study [26].

Phase In the context of clinical research, study phases are used to indicate the scientific aim of a given clinical trial. There are 4 phases (**Phase I**, **Phase II**, **Phase III**, and **Phase IV**) [26].

Phenome characterization Identification of the individual traits of an organism that characterize its phenotype [20].

Phenome-wide association scan A study that derives case and controls populations using the EMR to define clinical phenotypes and then examines the association of those phenotypes with specific genotypes [25].

Phenotype definition The process of determining the set of observable descriptors that characterize an organism's phenotype [8].

Phenotype The observable physical characteristics of an organism, produced by the interaction of genotype with environment[24]

Phenotypic Refers to the physical characteristics or appearance of an organism [1].

Picture Archive and Communication Systems (PACS) An integrated computer system that acquires, stores, retrieves, and displays digital images [9, 18, 20].

Pixel One of the small picture elements that makes up a digital image. The number of pixels per square inch determines the spatial resolution. Pixels can be associated with a single bit to indicate black and white or with multiple bits to indicate color or gray scale [5, 9].

Placebo In the context of clinical research, a placebo is a false intervention (e.g. a mock intervention given to a participant that resembles the intervention experienced by individuals receiving the experimental intervention, except that it has no anticipated impact on the individual's health or other indicated status), usually used in the context of a control group or intervention [26].

Plain old telephone service (POTS) The standard low speed, analog telephone service that is still used by many homes and businesses [18].

Plug-in A software component that is added to web browsers or other programs to allow them a special functionality, such as an ability to deal with certain kinds of media (e.g., video or audio) [5].

Pointing device A manual device, such as a mouse, light pen, or joy stick, that can be used to specify an area of interest on a computer screen [5].

Population management Health care practices that assist with a large group of people, including preventive medicine and immunization, screening for disease, and prioritization of interventions based on community needs [22].

Positive predictive value (PV+) The probability that the condition of interest is true if the result is positive—for example, the probability that a disease is present given a positive test result [3].

Positron emission tomography A tomographic imaging method that measures the uptake of various metabolic products (generally a combination of a positron-emitting tracer with a chemical such as glucose), e.g., by the functioning brain, heart, or lung [9].

Postcoordination The combination of two or more terms from one or more terminologies to create a phrase used for coding data; for example, "Acute Inflammation" and "Appendix" combined to code a patient with appendicitis. See also, **precoordination** [7].

Posterior probability The updated probability that the condition of interest is present after additional information has been acquired [3].

Postgenomic database A database that combines molecular and genetic information with data of clinical importance or relevance. *Online Mendelian Inheritance in Man* (OMIM) is a frequently cited example of such a database [24].

Post-test probability The updated probability that the disease or other condition under consideration is present after the test result is known (more generally, the **posterior probability**) [3].

Practice management system The software used by physicians for scheduling, registration, billing, and receivables management in their offices. May increasingly be linked to an EHR [14].

Pragmatics The study of how contextual information affects the interpretation of the underlying meaning of the language [8].

Precision Medicine The application of specific diagnostic and therapeutic methods matched to an individual based on highly unique information about the individual, such as their genetic profile or properties of their tumor [20].

Precision The degree of accuracy with which the value of a sampled observation matches the value of the underlying condition, or the exactness with which an operation is performed. In information retrieval, a measure of a system's performance in retrieving relevant information (expressed as the fraction of relevant records among total records retrieved in a search) [5, 8, 21].

Precoordination A complex phrase in a terminology that can be constructed from multiple terms but is, itself, assigned a unique identifier within the terminology; for example, "Acute Inflammation of the Appendix". See also, **postcoordination** [7].

Predicate The part of a sentence or clause containing a verb and stating something about the subject [8].

Predicate logic In mathematical logic, the generic term for symbolic formal systems like first-order logic, second-order logic, etc. [8]

Predictive value (PV) The posttest probability that a condition is present based on the results of a test (see positive predictive value and negative predictive value) [2].

Preparatory phase In the preparatory phase of a clinical research study, investigators are involved in the initial design and documentation of a study (developing a protocol document), prior to the identification and enrollment of study participants [26].

Pretest probability The probability that the disease or other condition under consideration is present before the test result is known (more generally, the **prior probability**) [3].

Prevalence The frequency of the condition under consideration in the population. For example, we calculate the prevalence of disease by dividing the number of diseased individuals by the number of individuals in the population. Prevalence is the prior probability of a specific condition (or diagnosis), before any other information is available [2, 3].

Primary knowledge-based information The original source of knowledge, generally in a peer reviewed journal article that reports on a research project's results [21].

Prior probability The probability that the condition of interest is present before additional information has been acquired. In a population, the prior probability also is called the prevalence [3].

Privacy A concept that applies to people, rather than documents, in which there is a presumed right to protect that individual from unauthorized divulging of personal data of any kind [5].

Probabilistic context free grammar A context free grammar in which the possible ways to expand a given symbol have varying probabilities rather than equal weight [8].

Probabilistic relationship Exists when the occurrence of one chance event affects the probability of the occurrence of another chance event [3].

Probabilistic sensitivity analysis An approach for understanding how the uncertainty in all (or a large number of) model parameters affects the conclusion of a decision analysis [3].

Probability Informally, a means of expressing belief in the likelihood of an event. Probability is more precisely defined mathematically in terms of its essential properties [3].

Probalistic causal network Also known as a Bayesian network, a statistical model built of directed acyclic graph structures (nodes) that are connected through relationships (edges). The strength of each of the relationships is defined through conditional probabilities [25].

Problem impact study A study carried out in the field with real users as participants and real tasks to assess the impact of the information resource on the original problem it was designed to resolve [11].

Problem space The range of possible solutions to a problem [4].

Problem-based learning small groups of students, supported by a facilitator, learned through discussion of individual case scenarios [23].

Procedural knowledge Knowledge of how to perform a task (as opposed to factual knowledge about the world) [4].

Procedure An action or intervention undertaken during the management of a patient (e.g., starting an IV line, performing surgery). Procedures may also be cognitive [8].

Process integration An organizational analysis methodology in which a series of tasks are reviewed in terms of their impact on each other rather than being reviewed separately. In a hospital setting, for example, a process integration view would look at patient registration and scheduling as an integrated workflow rather than as separate task areas. The goal is to achieve greater efficiency and effectiveness by focusing on how tasks can better work together rather than optimizing specific areas [14].

Product An object that goes through the processes of design, manufacture, distribution, and sale [10].

Prognostic scoring system An approach to prediction of patient outcomes based on formal analysis of current variables, generally through methods that compare the patient in some way with large numbers of similar patients from the past [10].

Progressive caution The idea that reason, caution and attention to ethical issues must govern research and expanding applications in the field of biomedical informatics [10].

Propositions An expression, generally in language or other symbolic form, that can be believed, doubted, or denied or is either true or false [4].

Prospective study An experiment in which researchers, before collecting data for analysis, define study questions and hypotheses, the study population, and data to be collected [2,12].

Prosthesis A device that replaces a body part—e.g., artificial hip or heart [1].

Protected memory An segment of computer memory that cannot be over-written by the usual means [5].

Protein Data Bank (PDB) A centralized repository of experimentally determined three dimensional protein and nucleic acid structures [24].

Proteomics The study of the protein products produced by genes in the genome [24].

Protocol analysis In cognitive psychology, methods for gathering and interpreting data that are presumed to reveal the mental processes used during problem solving (e.g., analysis of "think-aloud" protocols) [4].

Protocol authoring tools A software product used by researchers to construct a description of a study's rationale, guidelines, endpoints, and the like. Such descriptions may be structured formally so that they can be manipulated by trial management software [26].

Protocol management Protocol management refers to the capability of a CRMS to support the preparatory phase of a clinical study [26].

Protocol A standardized method or approach [5].

Provider-profiling system Software that utilizes available data sources to report on patterns of care by one or several providers [14].

Pseudo-identifier A unique identifier substituted for the real identifier to mask the identify but can under certain circumstances allow linking back to the original person identifier if needed [16].

Public health informatics An application area of biomedical informatics in which the field's methods and techniques are applied to problems drawn from the domain of public health [1].

Public health The field that deals with monitoring and influencing trends in habits and disease in an effort to protect or enhance the health of a population, from small communities to entire countries [10, 16].

Public Library of Science (PLoS) A family of scientific journals that is published under the open-access model [21].

Publication type One of several classes of articles or books into which a new publication will fall (e.g., review articles, case reports, original research, textbook, etc.) [21].

Public-key cryptography In data encryption, a method whereby two keys are used, one to encrypt the information and a second to decrypt it. Because two keys are involved, only one needs be kept secret [5].

Public-private keys A pair of sequences of characters or digits used in data encryption in which one is kept private and the other is made public. A message encrypted with the public key can only be opened by the holder of the private key, and a message signed with the private key can be verified as authentic by anyone with the public key [12].

PubMed A software environment for searching the Medline database, developed as part of the suite of search packages, known as **Entrez**, by the NLM's **National Center for Biotechnology Information** (**NCBI**) [21].

PubMed Central (**PMC**) An effort by the National Library of Medicine to gather the full-text of scientific articles in a freely accessible database, enhancing the value of Medline by providing the full articles in addition to titles, authors, and abstracts [21].

QRS wave In an electrocardiogram (ECG), the portion of the wave form that represents the time it takes for depolarization of the ventricles [5].

Quality assurance A means for monitoring and maintaining the goodness of a service, product, or process [22].

Quality management A specific effort to let quality of care be the goal that determines changes in processes, staffing, or investments [15].

Quality measurements Numeric metrics that assess the quality of health care services. Examples of quality measures include the portion of a physician's patients who are screened for breast cancer and 30-day hospital readmission rates. These measurements have traditionally been derived from administrative claims data or paper charts but there is increasing interest in using clinical data form electronic sources [27].

Quality-adjusted life year (QALY) A measure of the value of a health outcome that reflects both longevity and morbidity; it is the expected length of life in years, adjusted to account for diminished quality of life due to physical or mental disability, pain, and so on [3].

Quasi-experiments A quasi-experiment is a non-randomized, observational study design in which conclusions are drawn from the evaluation of naturally occurring and non-controlled events or cases [26].

Query and Reporting Tool Software that supports both the planned and ad-hoc extraction and aggregation of data sets from multiple data forms or equivalent data capture instruments used within a clinical trials management system [26].

Query The ability to extract information from an EHR based on a set of criteria; e.g., one could query for all patients with diabetes who have missed their follow-up appointments [12].

Query-response cycle For a database system, the process of submitting a single request for information and receiving the results [13].

Question answering (QA) A computer-based process whereby a user submits a natural language question that is then automatically answered by returning a specific response (as opposed to returning documents) [8, 21].

Question understanding A form of natural language understanding that supports computer-based **question answering** [8].

Radiology Information System (RIS) Computer-based information system that supports radiology department operations; includes management of the film library, scheduling of patient examinations, reporting of results, and billing [20].

Radiology The medical field that deals with the definition of health conditions through the use of visual images that reflect information from within the human body [20].

Random-access memory (RAM) The portion of a computer's working memory that can be both read and written into. It is used to store the results of intermediate computation, and the programs and data that are currently in use (also called variable memory or core memory) [5].

Randomized clinical trial (RCT) A prospective experiment in which subjects are randomly assigned to study subgroups to compare the effects of alternate treatments [2].

Randomly Without bias [2].

Range check A procedure applied to entered data that detects or prevents entry of values that are out of range; e.g., a serum potassium level of 50.0 mmol/L—the normal range for healthy individuals is 3.5–5.0 mol/L [12].

Read-only memory (ROM) The portion of a computer's working memory that can be read, but not written into [5].

Really simple syndication (RSS) A form of **XML** that publishes a list of headlines, article titles or events encoded in a way that can be easily read by another program called a news aggregator or news reader [8].

Real-time acquisition The continuous measurement and recording of electronic signals through a direct connection with the signal source [5].

Recall In information retrieval, the ability of a system to retrieve relevant information (expressed as the ratio of relevant records retrieved to all relevant records in the database) [8,21].

Receiver In data interchange, the program or system that receives a transmitted message [7].

Receiver operating characteristic (ROC) A graphical plot that depicts the performance of a binary classifier system as its discrimination threshold is varied [3, 25].

Records In a data file, a group of data fields that collectively represent information about a single entity [5].

Reductionist approaches An attempt to explain phenomena by reducing them to common, and often simple, first principles [24].

Reductionist biomedical model A model of medical care that emphasizes pathophysiology and biological principles. The model assumes that diseases can be understood purely in terms of the component biological processes that are altered as a consequence of illness [22].

Reference Information Model (RIM) The data model for HL7 Version 3.0. The RIM describes the kinds of information that may be transmitted within health-care organizations, and includes *acts* that may take place (procedures, observations, interventions, and so on), relationships among acts, the manner in which health-care personnel, patients, and other entities may participate in such acts, and the roles that can be assumed by the participants (patient, provider, specimen, and so on) [7, 22].

Reference resolution In **NLP**, recognizing that two mentions in two different textual locations refer to the same entity [8].

Reference standard See gold standard test [8].

Referential expression A sequence of one or more words that refers to a particular person, object or event, e.g., "she," "Dr. Jones, "or "that procedure."[8]

Referral bias In evaluation studies, a bias that is introduced when the patients entering a study are in some way atypical of the total population, generally because they have been referred to the study based on criteria that reflect some kind of bias by the referring physicians [3].

Region of interest (ROI) A selected subset of pixels within an image identified for a particular purpose [9].

Regional Extension Centers (RECs) In the context of health information technology, the 60+ state and local organizations (initially funded by ONC) to help primary care providers in their designated area adopt and use EHRs through outreach, education, and technical assistance [13].

Regional Health Information Organization (RHIO) A community-wide, multi-stakeholder organization that utilizes information technology to make more complete patient information and decision support available to authorized users when and where needed [13].

Regional network A network that provides regional access from local organizations and individuals to the major backbone networks that interconnect regions [5].

Registers In a computer, a group of electronic switches used to store and manipulate numbers or text [5].

Regular expression A mathematical model of a set of strings, defined using characters of an alphabet and the operators concatenation, union and closure (zero or more occurrences of an expression) [8].

Regulated Clinical Research Information Management (RCRIM) An HL7 workgroup that is developing standards to improve information management for preclinical and clinical research [26].

Relations among named entities The characterization of two entities in **NLP** with respect to the semantic nature of the relationship between them [8].

Relative recall An approach to measuring recall when it is unrealistic to enumerate all the relevant documents in a database. Thus the denominator in the calculation of recall is redefined to represent the number of relevant documents identified by multiple searches on the query topic [21].

Relevance judgment In the context of information retrieval, a judgment of which documents should be retrieved by which topics in a test collection [21].

Relevance ranking The degree to which the results are relevant to the information need specified in a query [21].

Reminder message A computer-generated warning that is generated when a record meets prespecified criteria, often referring to an action that is expected but is frequently forgotten; e.g., a message that a patient is due for an immunization [12].

Remote access Access to a system or to information therein, typically by telephone or communications network, by a user who is physically removed from the system [5].

Remote Intensive Care Use of networked communications methods to monitor patients in an intensive care unit from a distance far removed from the patients themselves. See **remote monitoring** [18].

Remote interpretation Evaluating tests (especially imaging studies) by having them delivered digitally to a location that may be far removed from the patient [18].

Remote monitoring The use of electronic devices to monitor the condition of a patient from a distant location. Typically used to refer to the ability to record and review patient data (such as vital signs) by a physician located in his/her office or a hospital while the patient remains at home. See also **remote intensive care** [14, 18].

Remote-presence health care The use of video teleconferencing, image transmission, and other technologies that allow clinicians to evaluate and treat patients in other than face-to-face situations [10].

Report generation A mechanism by which users specify their data requests on the input screen of a program that then produces the actual query, using information stored in a database schema, often at predetermined intervals [5].

Representation A level of medical data encoding, the process by which as much detail as possible is coded [7].

Representational effect The phenomenon by whichdifferent representations of a common abstract structure can have a significant effect on reasoning and decision making [4].

Representational state A particular configuration of an information-bearing structure, such as a monitor display, a verbal utterance, or a printed label, that plays some functional role in a process within the system [4].

Representativeness A heuristic by which a person judges the chance that a condition is true based on the degree of similarity between the current situation and the stereotypical situation in which the condition is true. For example, a physician might estimate the probability that a patient has a particular disease based on the degree to which the patient's symptoms matches the classic disease profile [3].

Request for Proposals A formal notification of a funding opportunity, requiring application through submission of a grant proposal [20].

Research protocol In clinical research, a prescribed plan for managing subjects that describes what actions to take under specific conditions [2].

Resource Description Framework (RDF) An emerging standard for cataloging metadata about information resources (such as Web pages) using the Extensible Markup Language (XML) [21].

Results reporting A software system or subsystem used to allow clinicians to access the results of laboratory, radiology, and other tests for a patient [14].

Retrieval A process by which queries are compared against an index to create results for the user who specified the query [21].

Retrospective chart review The use of past data from clinical charts (classically paper records) of selected patients in order to perform research regarding a clinical question. See also **retrospective study** [2].

Retrospective study A research study performed by analyzing data that were previously gathered for another purpose, such as patient care. See also **retrospective chart review** [2, 12].

Return on investment A metric for the benefits of an investment, equal to the net benefits of an investment divided by its cost [22].

Review of systems The component of a typical history and physical examination in which the physician asks general questions about each of the body's major organ systems to discover problems that may not have been suggested by the patient's chief complaint [2].

RFP See: Request for Proposals [20].

Ribonucleic acid (RNA) Ribonucleic acid, a nucleic acid present in all living cells. Its principal role is to act as a messenger carrying instructions from DNA in the production of proteins [24].

Rich text format (RTF) A format developed to allow the transfer of graphics and formatted text between different applications and operating systems [8].

RIM See Reference Information Model [7].

Risk attitude A person's willingness to take risks [3].

Risk-neutral Having the characteristic of being indifferent between the expected value of a gamble and the gamble itself [3].

Role-limited access The mechanism by which an individual's access to information in a database, such as a medical record, is limited depending upon that user's job characteristics and their need to have access to the information [5].

Router/switch In networking, a device that sits on the network, receives messages, and forwards them accordingly to their intended destination [5].

RS-232 A commonly used standard for serial data communication that defines the number and type of the wire connections, the voltage, and the characteristics of the signal, and thus allows data communication among electronic devices produced by different manufacturers [19].

RSS feed A bliographicmessage stream that provides content from Internet sources [21].

Rule-based system A kind of **knowledge-based system** that performs inference using production rules [22].

Sampling rate The rate at which the continuously varying values of an analog signal are measured and recorded [5].

Schema In a database-management system, a machine-readable definition of the contents and organization of a database [5].

Schemata higher-level kinds of knowledge structures [4].

Script In software systems, a keystroke-by-keystroke record of the actions performed for later reuse [5].

SDO See: Standards development organizations [7].

Search engine A computer system that returns content from a search statement entered by a user [21].

Search See Information retrieval [21].

Secondary knowledge–based information Writing that reviews, condenses, and/or synthesizes the primary literature (see**primary knowledge-based information**) [21].

Secret-key cryptography In data encryption, a method whereby the same key is used to encrypt and to decrypt information. Thus, the key must be kept secret, known to only the sender and intended receiver of information [5].

Secure Sockets Layer (SSL) A protocol for transmitting private documents via the Internet. It has been replaced by Transport Layer Security. By convention, URLs that require an SSL connection start with https: instead of http: [5, 12]

Security The process of protecting information from destruction or misuse, including both physical and computer-based mechanisms [5].

Segmentation In image processing, the extraction of selected regions of interest from an image using automated or manual techniques [20].

Selectivity In data collection and recording, the process that accounts for individual styles, reflecting an ongoing decision-making process, and often reflecting marked distinctions among clinicians [2].

Semantic analysis The study of how symbols or signs are used to designate the meaning of words and the study of how words combine to form or fail to form meaning [8].

Semantic class in **NLP**, a broad class that is associated with a specific domain and includes many instances [8].

Semantic grammar A mathematical model of a set of sentences based on patterns of semantic categories, e.g., patient, doctor, medication, treatment, and diagnosis [8].

Semantic patterns The study of the patterns formed by the co-occurrence of individual words in a phrase of the co-occurrence of the associated semantic types of the words [8].

Semantic relations A classification of the meaning of a linguistic relationship, e.g., "treated in 1995" signifies time while "treated in ER" signifies location [8].

Semantic sense In **NLP**, the distinction between individual word meaning of terms that may be in the same **semantic class** [8].

Semantic types The categorization of words into semantic classes according to meaning. Usually, the classes that are formed are relevant to specific domains [8].

Semantic Web A future view which envisions the Internet not only as a source of content but also as a source of intelligently linked, agent-driven, structured collections of machine-readable information [21].

Semantics The meaning of individual words and the meaning of phrases or sentences consisting of combinations of words [5].

Semi structured interview Where the investigator specifies in advance a set of topics that he would like to address but is flexible about the order in which these topics are addressed, and is open to discussion of topics not on the pre-specified list [11].

Sender In data interchange, the program or system that sends a transmitted message [7].

Sensitivity (of a test) The probability of a positive result, given that the condition under consideration is present—for example, the probability of a positive test result in a person who has the disease under consideration (also called the **true-positive rate**) [2, 3].

Sentence boundary In **NLP**, distinguishing the end of one sentence and the beginning of the next [8].

Sentiment analysis The study of how symbols or signs are used to designate the meaning of words and the study of how words combine to form or fail to form meaning [8].

Sequence alignment An arrangement of two or more sequences (usually of DNA or RNA), highlighting their similarity. The sequences are padded with gaps (usually denoted by dashes) so that wherever possible, columns contain identical or similar characters from the sequences involved [24].

Sequence database A database that stores the nucleotide or amino acid sequences of genes (or genetic markers) and proteins respectively [24].

Sequence information Information from a database that captures the sequence of component elements in a biological structure (e.g., the sequence of amino acids in a protein or of nucleotides in a DNA segment) [24].

Sequential Bayes A reasoning method based on a **naïve Bayesian model**, where Bayes' rule is applied sequentially for each new piece of evidence that is provided to the system. With each application of Bayes' rule, the **posterior probability** of each diagnostic possibility is used as the new **prior probability** for that diagnosis the next time Bayes' rule is invoked [22].

Server A computer that shares its resources with other computers and supports the activities of many users simultaneously within an enterprise [5].

Service oriented architectures (SOA) A software design framework that allows specific processing or information functions (services) to run on an independent computing platform that can be called by simple messages from another computer application. Often considered to be more flexible and efficient than more traditional data base architectures. Best known example is the Internet which is based largely on SOA design principles [6, 14, 22].

Service An intangible activity provided to consumers, generally at a price, by a (presumably) qualified individual or system [10].

Set-based searching Constraining a search to include only documents in a given class or set (e.g., from a given institution or journal) [21].

Shallow parsing See partial parsing [8].

Shielding In cabling, refers to an outer layer of insulation covering an innerlayer of conducting material. Shielded cable is used to reduce electronic noise and voltage spikes [5].

Short-term/working memory An emergent property of interaction with the environment; refers to the resources needed to maintain information active during cognitive activity [4].

Signal processing An area of systems engineering, electrical engineering and applied mathematics that deals with operations on or analysis of signals, or measurements of time-varying or spatially-varying physical quantities [9].

Simple Mail Transport Protocol (SMTP) The standard protocol used by networked systems, including the Internet, for packaging and distributing email so that it can be processed by a wide variety of software systems [5, 17].

Simple Object Access Protocol (SOAP) A protocol for information exchange through the HTTP/HTTPS or SMTP transport protocol using web services and utilizing Extensible Markup Language (XML) as the format for messages [6].

Simulation A system that behaves according to a model of a process or another system; for example, simulation of a patient's response to therapeutic interventions allows a student to learn which techniques are effective without risking human life [23].

Simultaneous access Access to shared, computer-stored information by multiple concurrent users [5].

Simultaneous controls Use of participants in a comparative study who are not exposed to the information resource. They can be randomly allocated to access to the information resource or in some other way [11].

Single nucleotide polymorphism (SNP) A DNA sequence variation, occurring when a single nucleotide in the genome is altered. For example, a SNP might change the nucleotide sequence AAGCCTA to AAGCTTA. A variation must occur in at least 1 % of the population to be considered a SNP [24].

Single-photon emission computed tomography A nuclear medicine tomographic imaging technique using gamma rays. It is very similar to conventional nuclear medicine planar imaging using a gamma camera. However, it is able to provide true 3D information. This information is typically presented as cross-sectional slices through the patient, but can be freely reformatted or manipulated as required [9].

Single-user systems Computers designed for use by single individuals, such as personal computers, as opposed to servers or other resources that are designed to be shared by multiple people at the same time [5].

Six sigma A management strategy that seeks to improve the quality of work processes by identifying and removing the causes of defects and minimizing the variability of those processes. Statistically, a six sigma process is one that is free of defects or errors 99.99966 %, which equates to operating a process that fits six standard deviations between the mean value of the process and the specification limit of that process [14].

Slip A type of medical error that occurs when the actor selects the appropriate course of action, but it was executed inappropriately [4]

Slots In a frame-based representation, the elements that are used to define the semantic characteristics of the frame [8].

Smart phones A mobile telephone that typically integrates voice calls with access to the Internet to enable both access to web sites and the ability to download email and applications that then reside on the device [14].

SMS messaging The sending of messages using the text communication service component of phone, web or mobile communication systemsShort Message Service[18]

SNOMED Systematized Nomenclature of Medicine - A set of standardized medical terms that can be processed electronically; useful for enhancing the standardized use of medical terms in clinical systems [14].

SNOMED-CT The result of the merger of an earlier version of SNOMED with the Read Clinical Terms [8].

SNP See Single nucleotide polymorphism [25].

Social networking The use of a dedicated Web site to communicate informally (on the site, by email, or via SMS messages) with other members of the site, typically by posting messages, photographs, etc. [17]

Software development life cycle (SDLC) or software development process A framework imposed over software development in order to better ensure a repeatable, predictable process that controls cost and improves quality of a software product [6].

Software oversight committee A groups within organizations that is constituted to oversee computer programs and to assess their safety and efficacy in the local setting [10].

Software psychology A behavioral approach to understanding and furthering software design, specifically studying human beings' interactions with systems and software. It is the intellectual predecessor to the discipline of Human-Computer interaction [4].

Software Computer programs that direct the hardware how to carry out specific automated processes [5].

Solid state drive (SSD) A data storage device using integrated circuit assemblies as memory to store data persistently. SSDs have no moving mechanical components, which distinguish them from traditional electromechanicalmagnetic disks such as hard disk drives (HDDs) or floppy disks, which contain spinning disks and movable read/write heads [5].

Spamming The process of sending unsolicited email to large numbers of unwilling recipients, typically to sell a product or make a political statement [5].

Spatial resolution A measure of the ability to distinguish among points that are close to each other (indicated in a digital image by the number of **pixels** per square inch) [5, 9].

Specialist Lexicon One of three UMLS Knowledge Sources, this lexicon is intended to be a general English lexicon that includes many biomedical terms and supports natural language processing [21].

Specificity (of a test) The probability of a negative result, given that the condition under consideration is absent—for example, the probability of a negative test result in a person who does not have a disease under consideration (also called the **true-negative rate**) [2, 3].

Spectrum bias Systematic error in the estimate of a study parameter that results when the study population includes only selected subgroups of the clinically relevant population—for example, the systematic error in the estimates of sensitivity and specificity that results when test performance is measured in a study population consisting of only healthy volunteers and patients with advanced disease [3].

Speech recognition Translation by computer of voice input, spoken using a natural vocabulary and cadence, into appropriate natural language text, codes, and commands [5, 12].

Spelling check A procedure that checks the spelling of individual words in entered data [12].

Spirometer An instrument for measuring the air capacity of the lungs [18].

Standard of care The community-accepted norm for management of a specified clinical problem [10].

Standard order sets Predefined lists of steps that should be taken to deal with certain recurring situations in the care of patients, typically in hospitals; e.g., orders to be followed routinely when a patient is in the post-surgical recovery room [1].

Standard-gamble A technique for utility assessment that enables an analyst to determine the utility of an outcome by comparing an individual's preference for a chance event when compared with a situation of certain outcome [3].

Standards development organizations An organization charged with developing a standard that is accepted by the community of affected individuals [7].

Static In patient simulations, a program that presents a predefined case in detail but which does not vary in its response depending on the actions taken by the learner [23].

Stemming The process of converting a word to its root form by removing common suffixes from the end [21].

Stop words In full-text indexing, a list of words that are low in semantic content (e.g., "the", "a", "an") and are generally not useful as mechanisms for retrieving documents [21].

Storage devices A piece of computer equipment on which information can be stored [5].

Store-and-forward A telecommunications technique in which information is sent to an intermediate station where it is kept and sent at a later time to the final destination or to another intermediate station [18].

Strict product liability The principle that states that a product must not be harmful [10].

Structural alignment The study of methods for organizing and managing diverse sources of information about the physical organization of the body and other physical structures [24].

Structural informatics The study of methods for organizing and managing diverse sources of information about the physical organization of the body and other physical structures. Often used synonymously with "imaging informatics." [1]

Structure validation A study carried out to help understand the needs for an information resource, and demonstrate that its proposed structure makes sense to key stakeholders [11].

Structured data entry A method of human–computer interaction in which users fill in missing values by making selections from predefined menus. The approach discretizes user input and makes it possible for a computer system to reason directly with the data that are provided [22].

Structured encounter form A form for collecting and recording specific information during a patient visit [12].

Structured interview An interview with a schedule of questions that are always presented in the same words and in the same order [11].

Structured Query Language (SQL) A commonly used syntax for retrieving information from relational databases [5]

Study arm in the context of clinical research, a study arm represents a specific modality of an experimental intervention to which a participant is assigned, usually through a process of randomization (e.g., random assigned in a balanced manner to such an arm). Arms are used in clinical study designs where multiple variants of a given experimental intervention are under study, for example, varying the timing or dose of a given medication between arms to determine an optimal therapeutic strategy [26].

Study population The population of subjects—usually a subset of the clinically relevant population—in whom experimental outcomes (for example, the performance of a diagnostic test) are measured [3].

Subheadings In MeSH, qualifiers of subject headings that narrow the focus of a term [21].

Subjectivist approaches Class of approaches to evaluation that rely primarily on qualitative data derived from observation, interview, and analysis of documents and other artifacts. Studies under this rubric focus on description and explanation; they tend to evolve rather than be prescribed in advance [11].

Sublanguage Language of a specialized domain, such as medicine, biology, or law [8].

Summarization A computer system that attempts to automatically summarize a larger body of content [21]

Summary ROC curve A composite **ROC curve** developed by using estimates from many studies [3]

Summative evaluation after the product is in use, is valuable both to justify the completed project and to learn from one's mistakes [23]

Supervised learning technique A method for determining how data values may suggest classifications, where the possible classifications are enumerated in advance, and the performance of a system is enhanced by evaluating how well the system classifies a training set of data. Statistical regression, neural networks, and support vector machines are forms supervised learning [22]

Supervised learning An approach to machine learning in which an algorithm uses a set of inputs and corresponding outputs to try to learn a model that will enable prediction of an output when faced with a previously unseen input [25]

Surveillance The ongoing collection, analysis, interpretation, and dissemination of data on health conditions (e.g., breast cancer) and threats to health (e.g., smoking prevalence). In a computer-based medical record system, systematic review of patients' clinical data to detect and flag conditions that merit attention. [12, 13, 16]

Symbolic-programming language A programming language in which the program can treat itself, or material like itself, as data. Such programs can write programs (not just as charac-ter strings or texts, but as the actual data structures that the program is made of). The best known and most influential of these languages is LISP [5].

Syndromic surveillance An ongoing process for monitoring of clinical data, generally from public health, hospital, or outpatient resources, whereby the goal is early identification of outbreaks, epidemics, new diseases, or, in recent years, bioterrorist events [8, 10].

Synonyms Multiple ways of expressing the same concept [21].

Syntax The grammatical structure of language describing the relations among words in a sentence [5, 8].

System programs The operating system, compilers, and other software that are included with a computer system and that allow users to operate the hardware [5].

Systematic review A type of journal article that reviews the literature related to a specific clinical question, analyzing the data in accordance with formal methods to assure that data are suitably compared and pooled [21].

Systems biology Research on biological networks or biochemical pathways. Often, systems biology analyses take a comprehensive approach to model biological function by taking the interactions (physical, regulatory, similarity, etc.) of a set of genes as a whole [24].

Tablet Generally refers to a personal computing device that resembles a paper tablet in size and incorporates features such as a touch screen to facilitate data entry [14].

Tactile feedback In virtual or telepresence environments, the process of providing (through technology) a sensation of touching an object that is imaginary or otherwise beyond the user's reach. (see also haptic feedback) [5].

TCP/IP Transmission Control Protocol/Internet Protocol – A set of standard communications protocols used for the Internet and for networks within organizations as well [14, 20].

Teleconsultation The use of telemedicine techniques to support the interaction between two (or more) clinicians where one is providing advice to the other, typically about a specific patient's care [18].

Telegraphic In **NLP**, describes language that does not follow the usual rules of grammar but is compact and efficient. Clinical notes written by hand often demonstrate a "telegraphic style" [8].

Telehealth The use of electronic information and telecommunications technologies to support long-distance clinical health care, patient and professional health-related education, public health and health administration. See **telemedicine** [18, 27].

Telehome care The use of communications and information technology to deliver health services and to exchange health information to and from the home (or community) when distance separates the participants [18].

Tele-ICU See remote intensive care [19].

Telemedicine A broad term used to describe the delivery of health care at a distance, increasingly but not exclusively by means of the Internet [1, 10, 18].

Teleophthalmology The use of telemedicine methods to deliver ophthalmology services [18].

Telepresence A technique of telemedicine in which a viewer can be physically removed from an actual surgery, viewing the abnormality through a video monitor that displays the operative field and allows the observer to participate in the procedure [18, 20].

Telepsychiatry The use of telemedicine methods to deliver psychiatric services [18].

Teleradiology The provision of remote interpretations, increasing as a mode of delivery of radiology services [1, 18,20].

Telesurgery The use of advanced telemedicine methods to allow a doctor to perform surgery on a patient even though he or she is not physically in the operating room [18].

Temporal resolution A metric for how well an imaging modality can distinguish points in time that are very close together [9].

Terabyte A unit of information equal to one million million (10^{12}) or strictly, 2^{40} bytes [5].

Term frequency (TF) In information retrieval, a measurement of how frequently a term occurs in a document [21].

Term weighting The assignment of metrics to terms so as to help specify their utility in retrieving documents well matched to a query [21].

Term Designation of a defined concept by a linguistic expression in a special language [7]. In information retrieval, a word or phrase which forms part of the basis for a search request [21].

Terminal A simple device that has no processing capability of its own but allows a user to access a server [5].

Terminology A set of terms representing the system of concepts of a particular subject field [7].

Terminology authority An entity or mechanism that determines the acceptable term to use for a specific entity, descriptor, or other concept [14].

Terminology services Software methods, typically based on computer-based dictionaries or language systems, that allow other systems to determine the locally acceptable term to use for a given purpose [14].

Test collection In the context of information retrieval, a collection of real-world content, a sampling of user queries, and relevance judgments that allow system-based evaluation of search systems [21].

Test-interpretation bias Systematic error in the estimates of sensitivity and specificity that results when the index and gold-standard test are not interpreted independently [3].

Test-referral bias Systematic error in the estimates of **sensitivity** and **specificity** that results when subjects with a positive index test are more likely to receive the **gold-standard test** [3].

Tethered personal health record An EHR portal that is provided to patients by an institution and can typically be used to manage information only from that provider organization [15].

Text-comprehension A process in which text can be described at multiple levels of realization from surface codes (e.g., words and syntax) to deeper level of semantics [4].

Text generation Methods that create coherent natural language text from structured data or from textual documents in order to satisfy a communication goal [8].

Text mining The use of large text collections (e.g., medical histories, consultation reports, articles from the literature, web-based resources) and natural language processing to allow inferences to be drawn, often in the form of associations or knowledge that were not previously apparent. See also **data mining** [21].

Text processing The analysis of text by computer [8].

Text readability assessment and simplification An application of **NLP** in which computational methods are used to assess the clarity of writing for a certain audience or to revise the exposition using simpler terminology and sentence construction [8].

Text REtrieval Conference (TREC) Organized by NIST, an annual conference on text retrieval that has provided a testbed for evaluation and a forum for presentation of results. (see trec. nist.gov) [21].

Text summarization Takes one or several documents as input and produces a single, coherent text that synthesizes the main points of the input documents [8].

TF*IDF weighting A specific approach to term weighting which combines **the inverse document frequency** (**IDF**) and **term frequency** (**TF**) [21].

Thesaurus A set of subject headings or descriptors, usually with a cross-reference system for use in the organization of a collection of documents for reference and retrieval [21].

Thick-client A computer node in a network or client–server architecture that provides rich functionality independent of the central server. See also **thin client** [6].

Thin client A program on a local computer system that mostly provides connectivity to a larger resource over a computer network, thereby providing access to computational power that is not provided by the machine, which is local to the user [6, 14].

Think-aloud protocol In cognitive science, the generation of a description of what a person is thinking or considering as they solve a problem [4].

Thread The smallest sequence of programmed instructions that can be managed independently by an operating systemscheduler [5].

Three-dimensional structure information In a biological database, information regarding the three-dimensional relationships among elements in a molecular structure [24].

Time-sharing networks An historical term describing some of the earliest computer networks allowing remote access to systems. (*BH: might we want to exclude this term?*) [21]

Time-trade-off A common approach to utility assessment, comparing a better state of health lasting a shorter time, with a lesser state of health lasting a longer time. The time-tradeoff technique provides a convenient method for valuing outcomes that accounts for gains (or losses) in both length and quality of life [3].

Tokenization The process of breaking an unstructured sequence of characters into larger units called "token," e.g., words, numbers, dates and punctuation [8].

Tokens In language processing, the composite entities constructed from individual characters, typically words, numbers, dates, or punctuation [8].

Top-down In search or analysis, the breaking down of a system to gain insight into its compositional sub-systems [8].

Topology In networking, the overall connectivity of the nodes in a network [5].

Touch screen A display screen that allows users to select items by touching them on the screen [5].

Track pad A computer input device for controlling the pointer on a display screen by sliding the finger along a *touch*-sensitive surface: used chiefly in laptop computers. Also called a touchpad [5].

Transaction set In data transfer, the full set of information exchanged between a sender and a receiver [7].

Transcription The conversion of a recording of dictated notes into electronic text by a typist [12].

Transition matrix A table of numbers giving the probability of moving from one state in a **Markov model** into another state or the state that is reached in a finite-state machine depending on the current character of the alphabet [8].

Transition probability The probability that a person will transit from one health state to another during a specified time period [3].

Translational Bioinformatics (TBI) According to the AMIA: the development of storage, analytic, and interpretive methods to optimize the transformation of increasingly voluminous biomedical data, and genomic data, into proactive, predictive, preventive, and participatory health [25].

Translational medicine Translational medicine: the process of transferring scientific discoveries into preventive practice and clinical care [25].

Transmission control protocol/internet protocol (TCP/IP) The standard protocols used for data transmission on the Internet and other common local and wide-area networks [5].

Transport Layer Security (TLS) A protocol that ensures the privacy of data transmitted over the Internet. It grew out of Secure Sockets Layer [12].

Treatment threshold probability The probability of disease at which the expected values of withholding or giving treatment are equal. Above the threshold treatment is recommended; below the threshold, treatment is not recommended and further testing may be warranted [3].

Trigger event In monitoring, events that cause a set of transactions to be generated [7].

True negative In assessing a situation, an instance that is classified negatively and is subsequently shown to have been correctly classified [8].

True positive In assessing a situation, an instances that is classified positively and is subsequently shown to have been correctly classified [8].

True-negative rate (TNR) The probability of a negative result, given that the condition under consideration is false—for example, the probability of a negative test result in a patient who does not have the disease under consideration (also called **specificity**) [3].

True-negative result (TN) A negative result when the condition under consideration is false—for example, a negative test result in a patient who does not have the disease under consideration [3].

True-positive rate (TPR) The probability of a positive result, given that the condition under consideration is true—for example, the probability of a positive test result in a patient who has the disease under consideration (also called **sensitivity**) [3].

True-positive result (TP) A positive result when the condition under consideration is true—for example, a positive test result in a patient who has the disease under consideration [3].

Turn-around-time The period for completing a process cycle, commonly expressed as an average of previous such periods [20].

Tutoring A computer program designed to provide self-directed education to a student or trainee [23].

Twisted-pair wires The typical copper wiring used for routine telephone service but adaptable for newer communication technologies [5].

Type-checking In computer programming, the act of checking that the types of values, such as integers, decimal numbers, and strings of characters, match throughout their use [5].

Typology A way of classifying things to make sense of them, for a certain purpose [11].

Ubiquitous computing A form of computing and human-computerinteraction that seeks to embed computing power invisibly in all facets of life [4].

Ultrasound A common energy source derived from high-frequency sound waves [9].

UMLS See: Unified Medical Language System [21].

UMLS Knowledge Sources Components of the **Unified Medical Language System** that support its use and semantic breadth [21].

UMLS Semantic Network A knowledge source in the UMLS that provides a consistent categorization of all concepts represented in the Metathesaurus. Each Metathesaurus concept is assigned at least one semantic type from the Semantic Network [21].

Unicode Represents characters needed for foreign languages using up to 16 bits [5].

Unified Medical Language System (UMLS) Project A terminology system, developed under the direction of the National Library of Medicine, to produce a common structure that ties together the various vocabularies that have been created for biomedical domains [8, 21].

Unified Modeling Language (UML) A standardized general-purpose modeling language developed for object-oriented software engineering that provides a set of graphic notation techniques to create visual models that depict the relationships between actors and activities in the program or process being modeled [26].

Uniform resource identifier (URI) The combination of a URN and URL, intended to provide persistent access to digital objects [21].

Uniform resource locator (URL) The address of an information resource on the World Wide Web [5, 21].

Uniform resource name (URN) A name for a Web page, intended to be more persistent than a

URL, which often changes over time as domains evolve or Web sites are reorganized [21].

Unique health identifier (UHI) A government-provided number that is assigned to an individual for purposes of keeping track of their health information [27].

Universal Serial Bus(USB) A connection technology for attaching peripheral devices to a computer, providing fast data exchange [19].

Unobtrusive measures Measures made using the records accrued as part of the routine use of the information resource, including, for example, user log files [11].

Unstructured interview an interviewwhere there are no predetermined questions [11].

URAC An organization that accredits the quality of information from various sources, including health-related Web sites [21].

Usability The quality of being able to provide good service to one who wishes to use a product [4].

Usability testing A class of methods for collecting empirical data of representative users performing representative tasks; considered the gold standard in usability evaluation methods [4, 11].

User authentication The process of identifying a user of an information resource, and verifying that the user is allowed to access the services of that resource. A standard user authentication method is to collect and verify a username and password [6].

User-interface layer The architectural layer of a software environment that handles the interface with users [14].

Utility In decision making, a number that represents the value of a specific outcome to a decision maker (see, for example, quality-adjusted life-years) [3, 22].

Validity check A set of procedures applied to data entered into an EHR intended to detect or prevent the entry of erroneous data; e.g., range checks and pattern checks [12].

Variable Quantity measured in a study. Variables can be measured at the nominal, ordinal, interval, or ratio levels [11].

Vector mathematics In the context of information retrieval, mathematical systems for measuring and comparing vector representations of documents and their contents [21].

Vector-space model A method of full-text indexing in which documents can be conceptualized as vectors of terms, with retrieval based on the cosine similarity of the angle between the query and document vectors [21].

Vertically integrated Refers to an organizational structure in which a variety of products or services are offered within a single chain of command; contrasted with horizontal integration in which a single type of product is offered in different geographical markets. A hospital which offers a variety of services from obstetrics to geriatrics would be "vertically integrated". A diagnostic imaging organization with multiple sites would be "horizontally integrated" [14].

Veterinary informatics The application of biomedical informatics methods and techniques to problems derived from the field of veterinary medicine. Viewed as a subarea of clinical informatics [1].

Video-display terminal (VDT) A device for displaying input signals as characters on a screen, typically a computer monitor [14].

View schemas An application-specific description of a view that supports that program's activities with respect to some general database for which there are multiple views [5].

View In a database-management system, a logical submodel of the contents and structure of a database used to support one or a subset of applications [5].

Virtual address A technique in memory management such that each address referenced by the CPU goes through an address mapping from the virtual address of the program to a physical address in main memory [5].

Virtual memory A scheme by which users can access information stored in auxiliary memory as though it were in main memory. Virtual memory addresses are automatically translated into actual addresses by the hardware [5].

Virtual Private Network (VPN) A private communications network, usually used within a company or organization, or by several different companies or organizations, communicating over a public network. VPN message traffic is carried on public networking infrastructure (e.g., the Internet) using standard (often insecure) protocols [5, 20].

Virtual reality A collection of interface methods that simulate reality more closely than does the standard display monitor, generally with a response to user maneuvers that heighten the sense of being connected to the simulation [4].

Virus/worm A software program that is written for malicious purposes to spread from one machine to another and to do some kind of damage. Such programs are generally self-replicating, which has led to the comparison with biological viruses [5].

Visual-analog scale A method for valuing health outcomes, wherein a person simply rates the quality of life with a health outcome on a scale from 0 to 100 [3].

Vocabulary A dictionary containing the terminology of a subject field [4, 7, 21].

Volatile A characteristic of a computer's memory, in that contents are changed when the next program runs and are not retained when power is turned off [5].

Volume rendering A method whereby a computer program projects a two-dimensional image directly from a three-dimensional **voxel** array by casting rays from the eye of the observer through the volume array to the image plane [9].

vonNeuman machine A computer architecture that comprises a single processing unit, computer memory, and a memory bus [5]

Voxel A volume element, or small cubic area of a three-dimensional digital image (see pixel) [9]

WashingtonDC Principles for Free Access to Science An organization of non-profit publishers that aims to balance wide access with the need to maintain sustainable revenue models [21].

Web browser A computer program used to access and display information resources on the World Wide Web [5].

Web catalog Web pages containing mainly links to other Web pages and sites [21].

Web Services Discovery Language (WSDL) An XML-based language used to describe the attributes of a web service, such as a SOAP service [6].

Web-based technologies Computer capabilities that rely on the architecture principles of the Internet for accessing data from remote servers [14].

Weblogs/blogs A type of Web site that provides discussion or information on various topics [21].

WebMD An American company that provides web-based health information services [23].

Whole Slide Digitization The process of capturing an entire specimen on a slide into a digital image. Compared with capturing images of a single field of view from a microscope, this captures the entire specimen, and can be millions of pixels on a side. This allows subsequent or remote review of the specimen without requiring capture of individual fields [20].

Wide-area networks (WANs) A network that connects computers owned by independent institutions and distributed over long distances [5].

Word senses The possible meanings of a term [8].

Word size The number of bits that define a word in a given computer [5].

Word In computer memory, a sequence of bits that can be accessed as a unit [5].

Word sense disambiguation (WSD) The process of determining the correct sense of a word in a given context [8].

Workstation A powerful desktop computer system designed to support a single user. Workstations provide specialized hardware and software to facilitate the problem-solving and information-processing tasks of professionals in their domains of expertise [5].

World Intellectual Property Organization (WIPO) An international organization, headquartered in Geneva and dedicated to promoting the use and protection of intellectual property [21].

World Wide Web (WWW or Web) An application implemented on the Internet in which multimedia information resources are made accessible by any of a number of protocols, the most common of which is the **HyperText Transfer Protocol** (**HTTP**) [1, 5, 21].

Worm A self-replicating computer program, similar to a computer virus; a worm is self-contained and does not need to be part of another program to propagate itself [5].

XML A metalanguage that allows users to define their own customized markup languages. See **Extensible Markup Language** [14].

X-ray crystallography A technique in crystallography in which the pattern produced by the diffraction of x-rays through the closely spaced lattice of atoms in a crystal is recorded and then analyzed to reveal the nature of that lattice, generally leading to an understanding of the material and molecular structure of a substance [24].

Bibliography

AAMC Task Force on Information Technology Infrastructure Requirements for Cross-Institutional Research. (2010). *Challenges and opportunities for new collaborative science models:* Association of American Medical Colleges, Washington, DC.

Abbey, L. M., & Zimmerman, J. (Eds.). (1991). *Dental informatics: Integrating technology into the dental environment.* New York: Springer.

Aboukhalil, A., Nielsen, L., Saeed, M., Mark, R. G., & Clifford, G. D. (2008). Reducing false alarm rates for critical arrhythmias using the arterial blood pressure waveform. *Journal of Biomedical Informatics, 41,* 442–451. PMID 18440873.

ACC/ACR/NEMA Ad Hoc Group. (1995). American College of Cardiology, American College of Radiology and industry develop standard for digital transfer of angiographic images. *Journal of the American College of Cardiology, 25,* 800–802.

ACR-NEMA. (2006). *Digital imaging and communications in medicine (DICOM) part 14: Grayscale standard display function.* Rosslyn: National Electrical Manufacturers Association.

Adams, K., & Corrigan, J. (Eds.). (2003). *Priority areas for national action: Transforming health care quality. A report of the Institute of Medicine.* Washington, DC: National Academy Press.

Adams, I. D., Chan, M., Clifford, P. C., Cooke, W. M., Dallos, V., de Dombal, F. T., Edwards, M. H., Hancock, D. M., Hewett, D. J., & McIntyre, N. (1986). Computer aided diagnosis of acute abdominal pain: A multicenter study. *British Medical Journal, 293*(6550), 800–804.

Adler-Milstein, J., McAfee, A. P., Bates, D. W., & Jha, A. K. (2008). The state of regional health information organizations: Current activities and financing. *Health Affairs, 27,* w60–w69.

Adler-Milstein, J., Bates, D. W., & Jha, A. K. (2009). U.S. Regional health information organizations: Progress and challenges. *Health Affairs, 28,* 483–492.

Adler-Milstein, J., Bates, D. W., & Jha, A. K. (2011). A survey of health information exchange organizations in the United States: Implications for meaningful use. *Annals of Internal Medicine, 154*(10), 666–671.

Advani, A., Goldstein, M.A., Shahar, Y., Musen, M.A. (2003). Developing quality indicators and auditing protocols from formal guideline models: knowledge representation and transformations. *AMIA Annual Symposium Proceedings,* 11–15.

Afrin, J. N., & Critchfield, A. B. (1997). Low-cost telepsychiatry for the deaf in South Carolina. *Proceeding of the AMIA Fall Symposium,* 901.

Agency for Healthcare Research and Quality. (2006). *Costs and benefits of health information technology. Evidence report/technology assessment* 132, publication 06-E006. Available at http://www.ahrq.gov/clinic/tp/hitsystp.htm. Accessed 12 Aug 2011.

Agrawal, M., Harwood, D., et al. (2000). Three-dimensional ultrastructure from transmission electron micropscope tilt series. In *Proceedings, Second Indian Conference on Vision, Graphics and Image Processing,* Bangalore.

Ahern, D. K., Woods, S. S., Lightowler, M. C., Finley, S. W., & Houston, T. K. (2011). Promise of and potential for patient-facing technologies to enable meaningful use. *American Journal of Preventative Medicine, 40*(5 Suppl 2), S162–S172.

Ahmed, A., Chandra, S., Herasevich, V., Gajic, O., & Pickering, B. W. (2011). The effect of two different electronic health record user interfaces on intensive care provider task load, errors of cognition, and performance. *Critical Care Medicine, 39,* 1626–1634. PMID 21478739.

AHRQ. (2011). *National strategy for quality improvement in health care.* Agency for Healthcare Research and Quality. Rockville, MD.

Aine, C. J. (1995). A conceptual overview and critique of functional neuroimaging techniques in humans I. MRI/fMRI and PET. *Critical Reviews in Neurobiology, 9,* 229–309.

Ajzen, I. (1985). From intentions to actions: A theory of planned behavior. In J. Kuhl & J. Beckmann (Eds.), *Action control: From cognition to behavior.* Berlin/Heidelberg/New York: Springer.

Akerkar, R. (2009). *Foundations of the semantic Web: XML, RDF & ontology.* Oxford: Alpha Science International Ltd.

Akin, O. (1982). *The psychology of architecture design.* London: Pion.

Alberini, J. L., Edeline, V., et al. (2011). Single photon emission tomography/computed tomography (SPET/CT) and positron emission tomography/computed tomography (PET/CT) to image cancer. *Journal of Surgical Oncology, 103*(6), 602–606.

Albert, K. (2006). Open access: Implications for scholarly publishing and medical libraries. *Journal of the Medical Library Association, 94*, 253–262.

Aldrich, C. (2009). *Learning online with games, simulations and virtual worlds: Strategies for online instruction.* San Francisco: Jossey-Bass.

Alecu, I., Bousquet, C., Mougin, F., & Jaulent, M. C. (2006). Mapping of the WHO-ART terminology on Snomed CT to improve grouping of related adverse drug reactions. *Studies in Health Technology and Informatics, 124*, 833–838.

Allard, F., & Starkes, J. L. (1991). Motor-skill experts in sports, dance, and other domains. In K. A. Ericsson & J. Smith (Eds.), *Toward a general theory of expertise: Prospects and limits* (pp. 126–150). New York: Cambridge University Press.

Allemann, P., Leroy, J., Asakuma, M., Al Abeidl, F., Dallemagne, B., & Marescaux, J. (2010). *Archives of Surgery, 145*, 267–271.

Alpert, S. A. (1998). Health care information: Access, confidentiality, and good practice. In K. W. Goodman (Ed.), *Ethics, computing, and medicine: Informatics and the transformation of health care* (pp. 75–101). Cambridge: Cambridge University Press.

Altman, R. B. (2007). PharmGKB: A logical home for knowledge relating genotype to drug response phenotype. *Nature Genetics, 39*, 426.

Altman, R. B., Dunker, A. K., Hunter, L., & Klein, T. E. (2003). *Pacific Symposium on Biocomputing '03.* Singapore: World Scientific Publishing.

Altschul, S. F., Gish, W., Mille, W., Myers, E. W., & Lipman, D. J. (1990). Basic local alignment search tool. *Journal of Molecular Biology, 215*(3), 403–410.

Altshuler, D. M., Durbin, R. M., & Genomes Project Consortium. (2010a). A map of human genome variation from population-scale sequencing. *Nature, 467*, 1061–1073.

Altshuler, D. M., Gibbs, R. A., Peltonen, L., et al. (2010b). Integrating common and rare genetic variation in diverse human populations. *Nature, 467*, 52–58.

Amarasingham, R., Plantinga, L., Diener-West, M., Gaskin, D. J., & Powe, N. R. (2009). Clinical information technologies and inpatient outcomes: A multiple hospital study. *Archives of Internal Medicine, 169*(2), 108–114.

American Academy of Family Physicians. (2008). Joint principles of the patient-centered medical home. *Delaware Medical Journal, 80*(1), 21–22.

American College of Pathologists (1982). SNOMED. Skokie, IL: College of American Pathology.

American Medical Informatics Association. (2011). *AMIA 10 x 10 Courses: Training Health Care Professionals to serve as local informatics leaders and champions.* Retrieved September 1, 2011, from http://www.amia.org/education/10x10-courses

American Psychiatric Association. (1994). *Diagnostic and statistical manual of mental disorders (DSM-IV)*

(4th ed.). Washington, DC: American Psychiatric Association.

American Psychiatric Association. (2000). *Diagnostic and statistical manual of mental disorders (DSM-IV-TR)*. Washington, DC: American Psychiatric Association.

American Society for Testing and Materials. (1999). *Standard guide for properties of a universal healthcare identifier (UHID) (E1714-95.)*. West Conshohocken: American Society for Testing and Materials.

American Society of Anesthesiologist (ASA). (2010). *Standards for basic anesthetic monitoring.* Last amended on October 20, 2010.

Ammenwerth, E., Schnell-Inderst, P., Machan, C., & Siebert, U. (2008). The effect of electronic prescribing on medication errors and adverse drug events: A systematic review. *Journal of the American Medical Informatics Association: JAMIA, 15*(5), 585–600.

Ancker, J. S., & Kaufman, D. (2007). Rethinking health numeracy: A multidisciplinary literature review. *Journal of the American Medical Informatics Association: JAMIA, 14*(6), 713–721.

Anderson, J. R. (1983). Acquisition of proof skills in geometry. In R. S. Michalski, J. G. Carbonell, & T. M. Mitchell (Eds.), *Machine learning: An artificial intelligence approach* (pp. 191–219). Palo Alto: Tioga Publishing Company.

Anderson, J. R. (1985). *Cognitive psychology and its implications* (2nd ed.). New York: Freeman.

Anderson, J. G., & Aydin, C. E. (1994). Overview: Theoretical perspectives and methodologies for the evaluation of health care information systems. In J. G. Anderson, C. E. Aydin, & S. J. Jay (Eds.), *Evaluating health care information systems: Methods and applications* (pp. 346–354). Thousand Oaks: Sage.

Anderson, J. G., & Aydin, C. E. (1998). Evaluating medical information systems: Social contexts and ethical challenges. In K. W. Goodman (Ed.), *Ethics, computing, and medicine: Informatics and the transformation of health care* (pp. 57–74). Cambridge: Cambridge University Press.

Anderson, J. G., Aydin, C. E., & Jay, S. J. (Eds.). (1994). *Evaluating health care information systems.* Thousand Oaks: Sage Publications Inc.

André, B., Vercauteren, T., et al. (2009). Introducing space and time in local feature-based endomicroscopic image retrieval. Medical content-based retrieval for clinical decision support. In B. Caputo, H. Mller, T. Syeda-Mahmood, et al. (Eds.), *Lecture notes in computer science* (Vol. 5853, pp. 18–30). Berlin/Heidelberg: Springer.

Andrews, R. D., Gardner, R. M., Metcalf, S. M., & Simmons, D. (1985). Computer charting: An evaluation of a respiratory care computer system. *Respiratory Care, 30*, 695–707. PMID 10315682.

Angrist, M. (2010). *Here is a human being: At the dawn of personal genomics.* New York: Harper.

Anonymous. (1879). Practice by Telephone. Lancet 2, 819.

Anonymous. (2007). Stopwords. In Anonymous (Ed.), *PubMed Help*. Bethesda: National Library of Medicine.

ANSI/ADA Specification No. 1001. (2002). *Guidelines for the design of educational software* (reaffirmed 2006). Accessed at http://www.ada.org/805.aspx#1001, 21 Nov 2011.

Appel, B. (2001). Nomenclature and classification of lumbar disc pathology. *Neuroradiology, 43*(12), 1124–1125.

Armstrong, R. A. (2010). Review paper. Quantitative methods in neuropathology. *Folia Neuropathologica, 48*(4), 217–230.

Arocha, J. F., Wang, D. W., & Patel, V. L. (2005). Identifying reasoning strategies in medical decision making: A methodological guide. *Journal of Biomedical Informatics, 38*(2), 154–171. doi:10.1016/j.jbi.2005.02.001.

Aronow, D.B., Cooley, J.R., & Soderland, S. (1995). Automated identification of episodes of asthma exacerbation for quality measurement in a computer-based medical record. *Proceedings of the Annual Symposium on Computer Applications in Medical Care*, 309–313.

Aronow, D., Feng, F., & Croft, W. B. (1999). Ad hoc classification of radiology reports. *Journal of the American Medical Informatics Association: JAMIA, 6*(5), 343–411.

Aronson, A.R. (2001). Effective mapping of biomedical text to the UMLS metathesaurus: the MetaMap program. *Proceedings of AMIA Symposium*, 17–21.

Aronson, A. R., & Lang, F. M. (2010). An overview of MetaMap: Historical perspective and recent advances. *Journal of the American Medical Informatics Association: JAMIA, 17*, 229–236.

Aronson, A., Mork, J., Gay, C., Humphrey, S.M., & Rogers, W. (2004). The NLM indexing initiative's medical text indexer. MEDINFO 2004. In *Proceedings of the Eleventh World Congress on Medical Informatics, San Francisco* (pp. 268–272). Retrieved from http://ii.nlm.nih.gov/resources/aronson-medinfo04.wheader.pdf

Aronson, A.R., Mork, J.G., Neveol, V., Shooshan, S.E., & Demner-Fushman, D. (2008). Methodology for creating UMLS content views appropriate for biomedical natural language processing. *AMIA Annual Symposium Proceedings*, 21–25.

Ash, J. S., Gorman, P. N., Lavelle, M., Payne, T. H., Massaro, T. A., Frantz, G. L., & Lyman, J. A. (2003a). A cross-site qualitative study of physician order entry. *Journal of the American Medical Informatics Association: JAMIA, 10*(2), 188–200. doi:10.1197/jamia.M770

Ash, J. S., Stavri, P. Z., & Kuperman, G. J. (2003b). A consensus statement on considerations for a successful CPOE implementation. *Journal of the American Medical Informatics Association: JAMIA, 10*(3), 229–234.

Ash, J. S., Berg, M., & Coiera, E. (2004). Some unintended consequences of information technology in health care: The nature of patient care information system-related errors. *Journal of the American Medical Informatics Association: JAMIA, 11*(2), 104–112.

Ash, J. S., Sittig, D. F., Poon, E. G., Guappone, K., Campbell, E., & Dykstra, R. H. (2007). The extent and importance of unintended consequences related to computerized provider order entry. *Journal of the American Medical Informatics Association: JAMIA, 14*(4), 415–423.

Ash, J. S., Anderson, N. R., & Tarczy-Hornoch, P. (2008). People and organizational issues in research systems implementation. *Journal of the American Medical Informatics Association: JAMIA, 15*(3), 283–289.

Ash, J. S., Sittig, D. F., Dykstra, R. H., Campbell, E., & Guappone, K. (2009). The unintended consequences of computerized provider order entry: Results of a mixed methods exploration. *International Journal of Medical Informatics, 78*(Supplement 1), S69–S76.

Ashburner, J., & Friston, K. J. (1997). Multimodal image coregistration and partitioning – a unified framework. *NeuroImage, 6*(3), 209–217.

Ashburner, M., Ball, C. A., Blake, J. A., et al. (2000). Gene ontology: Tool for the unification of biology. The gene ontology consortium. *Nature Genetics, 25*, 25–29.

Ashley, E. A., Butte, A. J., Wheeler, M. T., et al. (2010). Clinical assessment incorporating a personal genome. *The Lancet, 375*, 1525–1535.

Ashworth, M., & Millett, C. (2008). Quality improvement in uk primary care: The role of financial incentives. *The Journal of Ambulatory Care Management, 31*(3), 220–225.

Aspden, P., & Institute of Medicine (U.S.). Committee on Data Standards for Patient Safety. (2004). *Patient safety: Achieving a new standard for care*. Washington, D.C.: National Academies Press.

Association of American Medical Colleges (1984). Physicians for the twenty-first centry (Report of the Project Panel on the General Professional Education of the Physician and Collge Preparation for Medicine). J Med Educ 59(11):(Part 2)1-208.

Assimacopoulos, A., Alam, R., Arbo, M., et al. (2008). A brief retrospective review of medical records comparing outcomes for inpatients treated via telehealth versus in-person protocols: Is telehealth equally effective as in-person visits for treating neutropenic fever, bacterial pneumonia, and infected bacterial wounds. *Telemedicine Journal of E-Health, 14*, 762–768.

Atkinson, R. C., & Shiffrin, R. M. (1968). Human memory: A proposed system and its control processes. In K. W. Spence & J. T. Spence (Eds.), *The psychology of learning and motivation* (Vol. 2, pp. 89–195). New York: Academic Press.

Atkinson, A. J., Colburn, W. A., DeGruttola, V. G., et al. (2001). Biomarkers and surrogate endpoints: Preferred definitions and conceptual framework*. *Clinical Pharmacology and Therapeutics, 69*, 89–95.

Atkinson, N. L., Massett, H. A., Mylks, C., McCormack, L. A., Kish-Doto, J., Hesse, B. W., et al. (2011). Assessing the impact of user-centered research on a clinical trial eHealth tool via counterbalanced research design. *Journal of the American Medical Informatics Association: JAMIA, 18*(1), 24–31.

Atreya, R. V., Smith, J. C., McCoy, A. B., Malin, B., & Miller, R. A. (2013). Reducing patient re-identification risk for laboratory results within research datasets. *Journal of the American Medical Informatics Association: JAMIA, 20,* 95–101.

Avancha, S., Baxi, A., & Kotz, D. (2011). Privacy in mobile technology for personal healthcare. *ACM Computing Surveys, 45*(1), 3:1–3:54, to appear.

Avni. (2009). Addressing the ImageClef 2009 Challenge Using a Patch-based Visual Words Representation %U http://www.clef-campaign.org/2009/working_notes/avni-paperCLEF2009.pdf. Working Notes CLEF2009.

Baader, F. E., McGuinness, D. E., et al. (Eds.). (2003). *The description logic handbook: Theory, implementation and applications.* New York: Cambridge University Press.

Baars, M. J. H., Henneman, L., & Ten Kate, L. P. (2005). Deficiency of knowledge of genetics and genetic tests among general practitioners, gynecologists, and pediatricians: A global problem. *Genetics in Medicine, 7*(9), 605.

Babior, B. M., & Matzner, Y. (1997). The familial Mediterranean fever gene—cloned at last. *The New England Journal of Medicine, 337*(21), 1548–1549.

Bada, M., & Hunter, L. (2011). Desiderata for ontologies to be used in semantic annotation of biomedical documents. *Journal of Biomedical Informatics, 44*(1), 94–101.

Bai, C., & Elledge, S. J. (1997). Gene identification using the yeast two-hybrid system. *Methods in Enzymology, 283,* 141–156.

Baker, J. A., Kornguth, P. J., et al. (1995). Breast cancer: Prediction with artificial neural network based on BI-RADS standardized lexicon. *Radiology, 196*(3), 817–822.

Balas, E. A., & Boren, S. A. (2000). Managing clinical knowledge for health care improvement. In *Yearbook of medical informatics 2000: Patient-centered systems* (pp. 65–70). Stuttgart: Schattauer.

Baldi, P., & Brunak, S. (2001). *Bioinformatics: The machine learning approach.* Cambridge, MA: MIT Press.

Baldi, P., & Hatfield, G. W. (2002). *DNA microarrays and gene expression.* Cambridge: Cambridge University Press.

Ball, M., & Gold, J. (2006). Banking on health: Personal records and information exchange. *Journal of Healthcare Information Management, 20*(2), 71–83.

Bandura, A. (1977). Self-efficacy: Toward a unifying theory of behavioral change. *Psychological Review, 84,* 191–215.

Bandura, A. (1989). Social cognitive theory. In R. Vasta (Ed.), *Annals of child development* (Six theories of child development, Vol. 6, pp. 1–60). Greenwich: JAI Press.

Barabasi, A. L., Gulbahce, N., & Loscalzo, J. (2011). Network medicine: A network-based approach to human disease. *Nature Reviews Genetics, 12,* 56–68.

Barnett, G. O. (1968). Computers in patient care. *The New England Journal of Medicine, 279,* 1321–1327.

Barnett, G. O. (1984). The application of computer-based medical-record systems in ambulatory practice. *The New England Journal of Medicine, 310*(25), 1643–1650.

Barnett, G. O., Winickoff, R., Dorsey, J. L., Morgan, M. M., & Lurie, R. S. (1978). Quality assurance through automated monitoring and concurrent feedback using a computer-based medical information system. *Medical Care, 16*(11), 962–970.

Barnett, G. O., Justice, N. S., Somand, M. E., et al. (1979). COSTAR – a computer-based medical information system for ambulatory care. *Proceedings of the Institute of Electrical and Electronics Engineers (IEEE), 67,* 1226–1237.

Barnett, G. O., Cimino, J. J., Hurp, J. A., Hopper, E. P. (1987). DXplain: An evolving diagnostic decision-support system. *Journal of the American Medical Association, 258(1),* 67–74.

Baron, R. J. (2010). What's keeping us so busy in primary care? A snapshot from one practice. *The New England Journal of Medicine, 362*(17), 1632–1636.

Barrows, R. C., Jr., & Clayton, P. D. (1996). Privacy, confidentiality, and electronic medical records. *Journal of the American Medical Informatics Association: JAMIA, 3*(2), 139–148.

Bartlett, J., & Toms, E. (2005). Developing a protocol for bioinformatics analysis: An integrated information and behavior task analysis approach. *Journal of the American Society for Information Science and Technology, 56,* 469–482.

Bartolomeo, P. (2008). The neural correlates of visual mental imagery: An ongoing debate. *Cortex, 44*(2), 107–108. S0010-9452(07)00016-0 [pii].

Bashshur, R., Sanders, J., & Shannon, G. (1997). Telemedicine: Theory and Practice Charles C. Thomas, Springfield, IL.

Bashshur, R. L., Shannon, G. W., Krupinski, E. A., Grigsby, J., Kvedar, J. C., Weinstein, R. S., Sanders, J. H., Rheuban, K. S., Nesbitt, T. S., Alverson, D. C., Merrell, R. C., Linkous, J. D., Ferguson, A. S., Waters, R. J., Stachura, M. E., Ellis, D. G., Antoniotti, N. M., Johnston, B., Doarn, C. R., Yellowlees, P., Normandin, S., & Tracy, J. (2009). National telemedicine initiatives: Essential to healthcare reform. *Telemedicine and e-Health, 15,* 600–610.

Bates, D. W. (2000). Using information technology to reduce rates of medication errors in hospitals. *BMJ, 320,* 788–791.

Bates, D. W. (2006). Invited commentary: The road to implementation of the electronic health record. *Proceedings (Baylor University. Medical Center), 19*(4), 311–312.

Bates, D. W. (2009). The effects of health information technology on inpatient care. *Archives of Internal Medicine, 169*(2), 105–107.

Bates, D. W., & Bitton, A. (2010). The future of health information technology in the patient-centered medical home. *Health Affairs (Millwood), 29*(4), 614–621.

Bates, D. W., & Gawande, A. A. (2003). Improving safety with information technology. *The New England Journal of Medicine, 348*(25), 2526–2534.

Bates, D. W., Spell, N., Cullen, D. J., et al. (1997). The costs of adverse drug events in hospitalized patients. *Journal of the American Medical Association, 277*(4), 307–311.

Bates, D. W., Leape, L. L., Cullen, D. J., et al. (1998). Effect of computerized physician order entry and a team intervention on prevention of serious medication errors. *JAMA : The Journal of the American Medical Association, 280*(15), 1311–1316.

Bates, D. W., Ebell, M., Gotlieb, E., Zapp, J., & Mullins, H. C. (2003a). A proposal for electronic medical records in U.S. primary care. *Journal of the American Medical Informatics Association: JAMIA, 10*(1), 1–10.

Bates, D. W., Evans, R. S., Murff, H., et al. (2003b). Detecting adverse events using information technology. *Journal of the American Medical Informatics Association: JAMIA, 10*(2), 115–128.

Baud, R., Rassinoux, A. M., & Sherrer, J. R. (1992). Natural language processing and semantical representation of medical texts. *Methods of Information in Medicine, 31*, 117–125.

Baud, R., Lovis, C., Rassinoux, A. M., Michel, P. A., & Scherrer, J. R. (1998). Automatic extraction of linguistic knowledge from an international classification. *Studies in Health Technology and Informatics, 52*(Pt 1), 581–585.

Bauer, D. T., Guerlain, S., & Brown, P. J. (2010). The design and evaluation of a graphical display for laboratory data. *Journal of the American Medical Informatics Association: JAMIA, 17*(4), 416–424.

Baum, W. M. (2011). What is radical behaviorism? A review of Jay Moore's conceptual foundations of radical behaviorism. *Journal of the Experimental Analysis of Behavior, 95*(1), 119–126. doi:10.1901/jeab.2011.95-119.

Baumann, B., Gotzinger, E., et al. (2010). Segmentation and quantification of retinal lesions in age-related macular degeneration using polarization-sensitive optical coherence tomography. *Journal of Biomedical Optics, 15*(6), 061704.

Beccaro, M. A. D., Jeffries, H. E., Eisenberg, M. A., & Harry, E. D. (2006). Computerized provider order entry implementation: no association with increased mortality rates in an intensive care unit. *Pediatrics, 118*(1), 290–295.

Bechhofer, S., van Harmelen, F., et al. (2004). *OWL Web Ontology Language reference* (Technical Report REC-owl-ref-20040210). The WorldWideWeb Consortium. Available from http://www.w3.org/TR/2004/REC-owl-ref-20040210/

Bechtel, W., Abrahamsen, A., & Graham, G. (1998). Part I: The life of cognitive science. In W. Bechtel & G. Graham (Eds.), *A companion to cognitive science Blackwell companions to philosophy* (Vol. 13, pp. 2–104). Malden: Blackwell.

Becich, M. J. (2000). The role of the pathologist as tissue refiner and data miner: The impact of functional genomics on the modern pathology laboratory and the critical roles of pathology informatics and bioinformatics. *Molecular Diagnosis, 5*(4), 287–299.

Beck, J. R., & Pauker, S. G. (1983). The Markov process in medical prognosis. *Medical Decision Making, 3*(4), 419–458.

Beck, K., Beedle, M., et al. (2001). *Manifesto for Agile software development*. From www.agilemanifesto.org

Becker, K. G., Barnes, K. C., Bright, T. J., & Wang, S. A. (2004). The genetic association database. *Nature Genetics, 36*, 431–432.

Begun, J. W., Zimmerman, B., & Dooley, K. (2003). Health care organizations as complex adaptive systems. In S. M. Mick & M. Wyttenbach (Eds.), *Advances in health care organization theory* (pp. 253–288). San Francisco: Jossey-Bass.

Bela, K., & Hamel, D. (2010, October 26 2010). *Risky business: survey shows smartphone security concerns running high; yet 81% admit sneaking onto employer networks without permission*. From http://www.juniper.net/us/en/company/press-center/press-releases/2010/pr_2010_10_26-10_02.html

Benitez, K., & Malin, B. (2010). Evaluating re-identification risks with respect to the HIPAA privacy rule. *Journal of the American Medical Informatics Association: JAMIA, 17*, 169–177.

Benko, L.B. (2003, January 27). Back to the drawing board; Cedars-Sinai's physician order-entry system suspended. *Modern Healthcare, 12*.

Bennett, T. J., & Barry, C. J. (2009). Ophthalmic imaging today: An ophthalmic photographer's viewpoint – a review. *Clinical and Experimental Ophthalmology, 37*(1), 2–13.

Benson, D.A., Karsch-Mizrachi, I., Lipman, D.J., Ostell, J., Wheeler, D.L. (2003) GenBank. *Nucleic Acids Research, 31*(1):23–27. Available at http://www.ncbi.nlm.nih.gov

Berg, M. (1999). Patient care information systems and health care work: A sociotechnical approach. *International Journal of Medical Informatics, 55*(2), 87–101.

Berg, J. M., Tymoczko, J. L., & Stryer, L. (2010). *Biochemistry*. New York: W.H. Freeman.

Berners-Lee, T., Cailliau, R., Luotonen, A., Nielsen, H., & Secret, A. (1994). The world-wide web. *Communications of the ACM, 37*, 76–82.

Bernstam, E. V., Hersh, W. R., Johnson, S. B., et al. (2009). Synergies and distinctions between computational disciplines in biomedical research: Perspective from the Clinical and Translational Science Award programs. *Academic Medicine, 84*(7), 964–970.

Berstam, E. V., Smith, J. W., & Johnson, T. R. (2010). What is biomedical informatics? *Journal of Biomedical Informatics, 43*(1), 104–110.

Berwick, D. M. (2011). Launching accountable care organizations – the proposed rule for the Medicare shared savings program. *The New England Journal of Medicine, 364*, e32.

Besser, H. (2002). The next stage: moving from isolated digital collections to interoperable digital libraries. *First Monday, 7*(6). Retrieved from http://www.firstmonday.dk/issues/issue7_6/besser/

Beuscart-Zephir, M. C., Anceaux, F., Menu, H., Guerlinger, S., Watbled, L., & Evrard, F. (2005a).

User-centred, multidimensional assessment method of clinical information systems: a case-study in anaesthesiology. *International Journal of Medical Informatics, 74*(2–4), 179–189. S1386-5056(04)00167-4 [pii].

Beuscart-Zephir, M. C., Pelayo, S., Anceaux, F., Meaux, J. J., Degroisse, M., & Degoulet, P. (2005b). Impact of CPOE on doctor-nurse cooperation for the medication ordering and administration process. *International Journal of Medical Informatics, 74*(7–8), 629–641.

Beuscart-Zephir, M.C., Elkin, P., Pelayo, S., & Beuscart, R. (2007). The human factors engineering approach to biomedical informatics projects: state of the art, results, benefits and challenges. *Yearbook of Medical Informatics*, 109–127. me07010109 [pii].

Bickel, R. G. (1979). The TRIMIS concept. In *Proceedings of the 1979 annual symposium on Computer Applications in Medical Care* (pp. 839–842), Washington, D.C.

Bidgood, W. D., Jr., & Horii, S. C. (1992). Introduction to the ACR-NEMA DICOM standard. *Radiographics, 12*(2), 345–355.

Bird, K. T. (1972). Cardiopulmonary frontiers: quality health care via interactive television. *Chest, 61,* 204–205.

Bird, A. (2002). DNA methylation patterns and epigenetic memory. *Genes & Development, 16*(1), 6–21.

Bishop, C. M. (1995). *Neural networks for pattern recognition*. New York: Oxford University Press.

Bishop, C. (2007). *Pattern recognition and machine learning*. New York: Springer.

Biswal, S., Resnick, D. L., et al. (2007). Molecular imaging: integration of molecular imaging into the musculoskeletal imaging practice. *Radiology, 244*(3), 651–671.

Bittorf, A., & Bauer, J., et al. (1997). Web-based training modules in dermatology. *MD Comput, 14*(5): 371–376, 381.

Björk, B., Welling, P., Laakso, M., Majlender, P., Hedlund, T., & Guðnason, C. (2010). Open access to the scientific journal literature: situation 2009. *PLoS ONE, 5*(6), e11273. Retrieved from http://www.plosone.org/article/info%3Adoi%2F10.1371%2Fjournal.pone.0011273

Blake JA, Richardson JE, Bult CJ, Kadin JA, Eppig JT, & the members of the Mouse Genome Database Group. (2003). MGD: The mouse genome database. *Nucleic Acids Research,* 31, 193–195. Available at http://www.informatics.jax.org/

Bleich, H. (1972). Computer-based consultation: Electrolyte and acid–base disorders. *American Journal of Medicine, 53,* 285–291.

Blois, M. S., (1984). Information and Medicine: *The Nature of Medical Descriptions*. Berkeley: University of California Press.

Bloom, F. E., & Young, W. G. (1993). *Brain browser*. New York: Academic Press.

Bloomrosen, M., Starren, J., Lorenzi, N. M., Ash, J. S., Patel, V. L., & Shortliffe, E. H. (2011). Anticipating and addressing the unintended consequences of health IT and policy: A report from the AMIA 2009 Health Policy Meeting. *Journal of the American Medical Informatics Association: JAMIA, 18*(1), 82–90.

Bloxham, A. (2008, August 10). £13 Billion NHS computer system failures affecting patient care. *The Telegraph.*

Blum, B.I. (1986b). Clinical Information Systems: A review. Western Journal of Medicine, 145(6):791–797.

Blum, J. M., & Tremper, K. K. (2010). Alarms in the intensive care unit: too much of a good thing is dangerous: Is it time to add some intelligence to alarms? *Critical Care Medicine, 33,* 702–703. PMID 20083933.

Blumenthal, D. (2009). Stimulating the adoption of health information technology. *The New England Journal of Medicine, 360*(15), 1477–1479.

Blumenthal, D. (2010). Launching HITECH. *The New England Journal of Medicine, 362*(5), 382–385.

Blumenthal, D., & Glaser, J. P. (2007). Information technology comes to medicine. *The New England Journal of Medicine, 356*(24), 2527–2534.

Blumenthal, D., & Tavenner, M. (2010). The "meaningful use" regulation for electronic health records. *The New England Journal of Medicine, 363*(6), 501–504.

Bodenreider, O. (2004). The unified medical language system (UMLS): integrating biomedical terminology. *Nucleic Acids Research, 32,* D267–D270.

Bodenreider, O. (2008). Biomedical ontologies in action: role in knowledge management, data integration and decision support. Yearbook of Medical Informatics, 67–79.

Boeckmann, B., Bairoch, A., Apweiler, R., Blatter, M.C., Estreicher, A., Gasteiger, E., Martin, M.J., Michoud, K., O'Donovan, C., Phan, I., Pilbout, S., & Schneider, M. (2003). The SWISS-PROT protein knowledgebase and its supplement TrEMBL. *Nucleic Acids Research. 31,* 365–370. Available at http://us.expasy.org/sprot/

Bogun, F., Anh, D., Kalahasty, G., Wissner, E., Cou Serhal, C., Bazzi, R., Weaver, W. D., & Schuger, C. (2004). Misdiagnosis of atrial fibrillation and its clinical consequences. *American Journal of Medicine, 117,* 636–642. PMID 15501200.

Booth, R. (2000). *Project failures costly, TechRepublic/Gartner study finds*. Retrieved July 12, 2011, from http://www.techrepublic.com/article/it-project-failures-costly-techrepublicgartner-study-finds/1062043

Borgman, C. (1999). What are digital libraries? Competing visions. *Information Processing and Management, 35,* 227–244.

Bosch, A., Munoz, X., et al. (2006). Modeling and classifying breast tissue density in mammograms. *Computer Vision and Pattern Recognition, IEEE Computer Society Conference, 2,* 1552–1558.

Bosworth, K., Gustafson, D. H., Hawkins, R. P., Chewning, B., & Day, T. (1983). Adolescents, health education, and computers: The Body Awareness Resource Network (BARN). *Health Education, 14*(6), 58–60.

Bowden, D. M., & Martin, R. F. (1995). Neuronames brain hierarchy. *NeuroImage, 2,* 63–83.

Bowie, J., & Barnett, G. O. (1976). MUMPS: An economical and efficient time-sharing system for information management. *Computer Programs in Biomedicine, 6*, 11–22.

Bowker, G. C., & Starr, S. L. (2000). *Sorting things out: Classification and its consequences*. Cambridge: MIT Press.

Boyd, L. B., Hunicke-Smith, S. P., Stafford, G. A., et al. (2011). The caBIG life science business architecture model. *Bioinformatics, 27*(10), 1429–1435.

Boynton, J, Glanville, J, et al. (1998). Identifying systematic reviews in MEDLINE: developing an objective approach to search strategy design. *Journal of Information Science. 24*, 137–157.

Bradley, W. G., Golding, S. G., Herold, C. J., et al. (2011, August 27–29). Globalization of P4 medicine: Predictive, personalized, preemptive, and participatory–summary of the proceedings of the Eighth International Symposium of the International Society for Strategic Studies in Radiology. *Radiology, 258*, 571–582.

Bradshaw, K. E., Gardner, R. M., Clemmer, T. P., Orme, J. F., Thomas, F., & West, B. J. (1984). Physician decision-making: Evaluation of data used in a computerized ICU. *International Journal of Clinical Monitoring and Computing, 1*(2), 81–91.

Bradshaw, K. E., Sittig, D. F., Gardner, R. M., Pryor, T. A., & Budd, M. (1989). Computer-based data entry for nurses in the ICU. *MD Computing, 6*(5), 274–280. PMID 2486506.

Brain Innovation, B.V. (2001). *BrainVoyager*. From http://www.BrainVoyager.de/

'Brain' to store medical data. (1956, October 24). *The New York Times.*

Brannan, S. O., Dewar, C., Taggerty, L., & Clark, S. (2011). The effect of short messaging service text on non-attendance in a general ophthalmology clinic. *Scottish Medical Journal, 56*(3), 148–150.

Bransford, J., Brown, A. L., Cocking, R. R., & National Research Council (U.S.). Committee on Developments in the Science of Learning. (1999). *How people learn: Brain, mind, experience, and school*. Washington, D.C.: National Academy Press.

Bransford, J. D., Brown, A. L., & Cocking, R. R. (2000). *How people learn: Brain, mind, experience and school*. Washington, D.C.: The National Academies Press.

Braunwald, E. (1988). Evolution of the management of acute myocardial infarction: A 20th century saga. *The Lancet, 352*, 1771–1774. PMID 9848369.

Brechner, R. J., Cowie, C. C., Howie, L. J., Herman, W. H., Will, J. C., & Harris, M. I. (1993). Ophthalmic examination among adults with diagnosed diabetes mellitus. *JAMA : The Journal of the American Medical Association, 270*, 1714–1718.

Brender, J. (2005). *Handbook of evaluation methods for health informatics*. Burlington: Academic Press.

Brennan, P.F., Downs, S., Casper, G., & Kenron, D. (2007). Project HealthDesign: stimulating the next generation of personal health records. *AMIA Annual Symposium Proceedings*, 70–74.

Breslow, M. J. (2007). Remote ICU care programs: Current status. *Journal of Critical Care, 22*(1), 66–76.

Briggs, B. (2002). Clinical trials getting a hand. *Health Data Management, 10*(2), 56–60, 62.

Bright, R. A., & Brown, S. L. (2007). *Medical device epidemiology medical device epidemiology and surveillance* (pp. 21–42). Hoboken: Wiley.

Bright, T. J., Wong, A., Dhurjati, R., Bristow, E., Bastian, L., Coeytaux, R. R., Samsa, G., Hasselblad, V., Williams, J. W., Musty, M. D., Wing, L., Kendrick, A. S., Sanders, G. D., & Lobach, D. (2012). Effect of clinical decision-support systems: A systematic review. *Annals of Internal Medicine, 157*(1), 29–43.

Brin, S., & Page, L. (1998). The anatomy of a large-scale hypertextual Web search engine. *Computer Networks and ISDN Systems, 30*, 107–117. Retrieved from http://infolab.stanford.edu/pub/papers/google.pdf

Brinkley, J. F. (1985). Knowledge-driven ultrasonic three-dimensional organ modelling. *Patiernanalysis and Machine Intelligence, PAMI-7*(4), 431–441.

Brinkley, J. F. (1992). Hierarchical geometric constraint networks as a representation for spatial structural knowledge. *Proceedings of the 16th Annual Symposium on Computer Applications in Medical Care*, 140–144.

Brinkley, J. F. (1993a). A flexible, generic model for anatomic shape: Application to interactive two-dimensional medical image segmentation and matching. *Computers and Biomedical Research, 26*, 121–142.

Brinkley, J. F. (1993b). The potential for three-dimensional ultrasound. In F. A. Chervenak, G. C. Isaacson, & S. Campbell (Eds.), *Ultrasound in obstetrics and gynecology*. Boston: Little, Brown and Company.

Brinkley, J. F., Bradley, S. W., et al. (1997). The digital anatomist information system and its use in the generation and delivery of Web-based anatomy atlases. *Computers and Biomedical Research, 30*, 472–503.

Brinkley, J. F., Wong, B. A., et al. (1999). Design of an anatomy information system. *Computer Graphics and Applications, 19*(3), 38–48.

Brinkman, R. R., Courtot, M., Derom, D., et al. (2010). Modeling biomedical experimental processes with OBI. *Journal of Biomedical Semantics, 1*(Suppl 1), S7.

Brody, B. A. (1989). The ethics of using ICU scoring systems in individual patient management. *Problems in Critical Care, 3*, 662–670.

Brown, E. G., Wood, L., & Wood, S. (1999). The medical dictionary for regulatory activities (MedDRA). *Drug Safety, 20*, 109–117.

Brown, S. H., Lincoln, M. J., Groen, P. J., et al. (2003). VistA–U.S. Department of veterans affairs national-scale HIS. *International Journal of Medical Informatics, 69*(2–3), 135–156.

Brown, S.H., Fischietti, L.F., Graham, G., Bates, J., et al. (2007). Use of electronic health records in disaster response: The experience of department of veterans affairs after hurricane katrina. *American Journal of Public Health, 97*, S136–S141.

Brown, D.B., Gould, J.E., et al. (2009). Transcatheter Therapy for Hepatic Malignancy: Standardization of Terminology and Reporting Criteria. *Journal of*

Vascular and Interventional Radiology 20(7): S425–S434. (Reprinted from *Journal of Vascular and Interventional Radiology, 18*, 1469–1478, 2007)

Brownstein, J. S., Sordo, M., Kohane, I. S., & Mandl, K. D. (2007). The tell-tale heart: Population-based surveillance reveals an associaton f rofecoxib and celecoxib with myocardial infarction. *PLoS One, 2*(9), e840.

Bruer, J. T. (1993). *Schools for thought: A science of learning in the classroom*. Cambridge: MIT Press.

Bruls, T., & Weissenbach, J. (2011). The human metagenome: Our other genome? *Human Molecular Genetics, 20*(R2), R142–R148.

Buchanan, B. G., & Shortliffe, E. H. (1984). *Rule-based expert systems: The MYCIN experiments of the Stanford heuristic programming project*. Reading: Addison-Wesley.

Buetow, K. H. (2009). An infrastructure for interconnecting research institutions. *Drug Discovery Today, 14*(11–12), 605–610.

Buetow, K. H., & Niederhuber, J. (2009). Infrastructure for a learning health care system: CaBIG. *Health Affairs (Project Hope), 28*(3), 923–924; author reply 924–925.

Bug, W. J., Ascoli, G. A., et al. (2008). The NIFSTD and BIRNLex vocabularies: Building comprehensive ontologies for neuroscience. *Neuroinformatics, 6*(3), 175–194.

Buntin, M. B., Jain, S. H., & Blumenthal, D. (2010). Health information technology: Laying the infrastructure for national health reform. *Health Affairs (Millwood), 29*(6), 1214–1219.

Buntin, M. B., Burke, M. F., Hoaglin, M. C., & Blumenthal, D. (2011). The benefits of health information technology: A review of the recent literature shows predominantly positive results. *Health Affairs (Millwood), 30*(3), 464–471.

Burley, S. K., & Bonanno, J. B. (2002). Structuring the universe of proteins. *Annual Review of Genomics and Human Genetics, 3*, 243–262.

Burley, L., Scheepers, H., & Owen, L. (2009). *User involvement in the design and appropriation of a mobile clinical information system: Reflections on organisational learning*. New York: Springer.

Burnside, E., Rubin, D., et al. (2000). A Bayesian network for mammography. *Proceedings of the AMIA Symposium*, 106–110.

Burnside, E. S., Rubin, D. L., et al. (2004a). Using a Bayesian network to predict the probability and type of breast cancer represented by microcalcifications on mammography. *Studies in Health Technology and Informatics, 107*(Pt 1), 13–17.

Burnside, E. S., Rubin, D. L., et al. (2004b). A probabilistic expert system that provides automated mammographic-histologic correlation: Initial experience. *AJR. American Journal of Roentgenology, 182*(2), 481–488.

Burnside, E. S., Rubin, D. L., Fine, J. P., et al. (2006). Bayesian network to predict breast cancer risk of mammographic microcalcifications and reduce number of benign biopsy results: Initial experience. *Radiology, 240*(3), 666–673.

Burnside, E. S., Ochsner, J. E., et al. (2007). Use of microcalcification descriptors in BI-RADS 4th edition to stratify risk of malignancy. *Radiology, 242*(2), 388–395.

Burnside, E. S., Davis, J., et al. (2009). Probabilistic computer model developed from clinical data in national mammography database format to classify mammographic findings. *Radiology, 251*(3), 663–672.

Burykin, A., Peck, T., & Buchman, T. G. (2011). Using "off-the-shelf" tools for a terabyte-scale waveform recording in intensive care: Computer system design, database description and lessons learned. *Computer Methods and Programs in Biomedicine, 103*, 151–160. PMID 21093093.

Butler, D. (2001). Data, data, everywhere. *Nature, 414*(6866), 840–841.

Butte, A. J. (2008a). Medicine. The ultimate model organism. *Science, 320*(5874), 325–327.

Butte, A. J. (2008b). Translational bioinformatics: Coming of age. *Journal of the American Medical Informatics Association: JAMIA, 15*, 709–714.

Butte, A. (2009). Bioinformatic and computational analysis for genomic medicine. In G. S. Ginsburg & H. F. Willard (Eds.), *Essentials of genomic and personalized medicine*. Burlington: Elsevier.

Butte, A.J., & Chen, R. (2006). Finding disease-related genomic experiments within an international repository: first steps in translational bioinformatics. *AMIA Annual Symposium Proceedings*, 106–110.

Butte, A.J., Weinstein, D.A., & Kohane, I.S. (2000). Enrolling patients into clinical trials faster using RealTime Recuiting. *Proceedings of the AMIA Symposium*, 111–115.

Buxton, R. B. (2009). *Introduction to functional magnetic resonance imaging: Principles and techniques*. Cambridge/New York: Cambridge University Press.

Cabrera Fernandez, D., Salinas, H. M., et al. (2005). Automated detection of retinal layer structures on optical coherence tomography images. *Optics Express, 13*(25), 10200–10216.

Cairncross, F. (2001). *The death of distance: how the communications revolution is changing our lives (completely* (newth ed.). Boston: Harvard Business School Press.

California Health Care Foundation. (2005). *National Consumer Health Privacy Survey*. Available at: http://www.chcf.org/publications/2005/11/national-consumer-health-privacy-survey-2005. Accessed 12 Aug 2011.

Callen, J., Georgiou, A., Li, J., & Westbrook, J. I. (2011). The safety implications of missed test results for hospitalized patients: A systematic review. *BMJ Quality & Safety, 20*, 194–199. PMID 21300992.

Camon, E., Magrane, M., Barrell, D., et al. (2003). The gene ontology annotation (GOA) project: Implementation of GO in SWISS-PROT, TrEMBL, and InterPro. *Genome Research, 13*, 662–672.

Campbell, D. T., & Stanley, J. C. (1963). *Experimental and quasi experimental designs for research.* Boston: Houghton Mifflin, reprinted often since.

Campbell, K.E., Tuttle, M.S., Spackman, & K.A. (1998). A "lexically-suggested logical closure" metric for medical terminology maturity. In *Proceedings of the 1998 AMIA Annual Fall Symposium* (pp. 785–789), Orlando.

Campbell, M., Fitzpatrick, R., Haines, A., Kinmonth, A. L., Sandercock, P., Spiegelhalter, D., & Tyrer, P. (2000). Framework for design and evaluation of complex interventions to improve health. *BMJ, 321*(7262), 694–696.

Campbell, E. M., Sittig, D. F., Ash, J. S., Guappone, K. P., & Dykstra, R. H. (2006). Types of unintended consequences related to computerized provider order entry. *Journal of the American Medical Informatics Association: JAMIA, 13*(5), 547–556.

Campillos, M., Kuhn, M., Gavin, A. C., et al. (2008). Drug target identification using side-effect similarity. *Science, 321*, 263–266.

Campion, T. R., Jr., May, A. K., Waitman, L. R., Ozdas, A., Lorenzi, N. M., & Gadd, C. S. (2011). Characteristics and effects of nurse dosing overrides on computer-based intensive insulin therapy protocol performance. *Journal of the American Medical Informatics Association: JAMIA, 18*(3), 251–258.

Cao, Y., Liu, F., Simpson, P., Antieau, L., Bennett, A., Cimino, J. J., Ely, J., & Yu, H. (2011). AskHERMES: An online question answering system for complex clinical questions. *Journal of Biomedical Informatics, 44*(2), 277–288.

Caporaso, J. G., Deshpande, N., Fink, J. L., Bourne, P. E., Cohen, K. B., & Hunter, L. (2008). Intrinsic evaluation of text mining tools may not predict performance on realistic tasks. *Proceedings of the Pacific Symposium Biocomputing, 13*, 640–651.

Caputo, B., Tornmasi, T., et al. (2008). Discriminative cue integration for medical image annotation. *Pattern Recognition Letters, 29*(15), 1996–2002.

Carayon, P. (Ed.). (2007). *Handbook of human factors and ergonomics in health care and patient safety.* Mahwah: Lawrence Erlbaum Associates.

Carayon, P., Cartmill, R., Blosky, M. A., Brown, R., Hackenberg, M., Hoonakker, P., Hundt, A. S., Norfolk, E., Wetterneck, T. B., & Walker, J. M. (2011). ICU nurses' acceptance of electronic health records. *Journal of the American Medical Informatics Association: JAMIA, 18*(6), 812–819. PMID 21697291.

Card, S. K., Moran, T. P., & Newell, A. (1983). *The psychology of human-computer interaction.* Hillsdale: L. Erlbaum Associates.

Card, S. K., Mackinlay, J. D., & Shneiderman, B. (1999). *Readings in information visualization: Using vision to think.* San Francisco: Morgan Kaufmann Publishers.

Carneiro, G., Chan, A. B., et al. (2007). Supervised learning of semantic classes for image annotation and retrieval. *IEEE Transactions on Pattern Analysis and Machine Intelligence, 29*(3), 394–410.

Carpenter, A. E., Jones, T. R., et al. (2006). CellProfiler: Image analysis software for identifying and quantifying cell phenotypes. *Genome Biology, 7*(10), R100.

Carroll, J. M. (1997). Human-computer interaction: Psychology as a science of design [Literature review/research review]. *Annual Review of Psychology, 48*(1), 61–83.

Carroll, J. M. (2003). *HCI models, theories, and frameworks: Toward a multidisciplinary science.* San Francisco: Morgan Kaufmann.

Carroll, D. L., Dykes, P. C., & Hurley, A. C. (2010). Patients' perspectives of falling while in an acute care hospital and suggestions for prevention. *Applied Nursing Research, 23*(4), 238–241.

Carroll, A. E., Biondich, P. G., Anand, V., Dugan, T. M., Sheley, M. E., Xu, S. Z., & Downs, S. M. (2011). Targeted screening for pediatric conditions with the CHICA system. *Journal of the American Medical Informatics Association: JAMIA, 18*(4), 485–490.

Castro, D. (2007). *Improving health care: why a dose of IT may be just what the doctor ordered. Information Technology and Innovation Foundation.* Available at http://www.itif.org/publications/improving-healthcare-why-dose-it-may-be-just-what-doctor-ordered. Accessed 17 Dec 2012.

Cavalleranno, A. A., Cavallerano, J. D., Katalinic, P., Blake, B., Conlin, P. R., Hock, K., Tolson, A. M., Aiello, L. P., & Aiello, L. M. (2005). Joslin vision network research team. *American Journal of Ophthalmology, 139*, 597–604.

Caviness, V. S., Meyer, J., et al. (1996). MRI-based topographic parcellation of human neocortex: An anatomically specified method with estimate of reliability. *Journal of Cognitive Neuroscience, 8*(6), 566–587.

Cech, T. R. (2000). Structural biology. The ribosome is a ribozyme. *Science, 289*(5481), 878–879.

Cedar, H. (1988). DNA methylation and gene activity. *Cell, 53*, 3–4.

Celi, L. A., Hassan, E., Marquardt, C., Breslow, M., & Rosenfeld, B. (2001). The eICU: it's not just telemedicine. *Critical Care Medicine, 29*(8 Suppl), N183–N189. PMID 11496041.

Cella, D., Riley, W., Stone, A., et al. (2010). The patient-reported outcomes measurement information system (promis) developed and tested its first wave of adult self-reported health outcome item banks: 2005–2008. *Journal of Clinical Epidemiology, 63*(11), 1179–1194.

Centers for Disease Control and Prevention. (2011). *Public Health Information Network (PHIN) strategic plan: strategies to facilitate standards-based public health information exchange* (2011–2016). Atlanta, GA.

Chambrin, M. C. (2001). Alarms in the intensive care unit: how can the number of false alarms be reduced? *Critical Care, 5*, 184–188. PMID 11511330.

Chan, I. S., & Ginsburg, G. S. (2011). Personalized medicine: Progress and promise. *Annual Review of Genomics and Human Genetics, 12*, 217–244.

Chan, C. V., & Kaufman, D. R. (2011). A framework for characterizing eHealth literacy demands and barriers. *Journal of Medical Internet Research, 13*(4), e94. 0.2196/jmir.1750.

Chan, A. S., Coleman, R. W., Martins, S. B., Advani, A., Musen, M. A., Bosworth, H. B., Oddone, E. Z., Shilpak, M. G., Hoffman, B. B., & Goldstein, M. K. (2004). Evaluating provider adherence in a trial of a guideline-based decision support system for hypertension. *Studies in Health Technology and Informatics, 107*(Pt 1), 125–129.

Chan, E. Y., Qian, W. J., Diamond, D. L., et al. (2007). Quantitative analysis of human immunodeficiency virus type 1-infected CD4+ cell proteome: Dysregulated cell cycle progression and nuclear transport coincide with robust virus production. *Journal of Virology, 81*, 7571–7583.

Chan, K. S., Fowles, J. B., & Weiner, J. P. (2010). Review: Electronic health records and the reliability and validity of quality measures: A review of the literature. *Medical Care Research and Review, 67*(5), 503–527.

Chan, J., Shojania, K. G., Easty, A. C., & Etchells, E. E. (2011). Does user-centred design affect the efficiency, usability and safety of CPOE order sets? *Journal of the American Medical Informatics Association: JAMIA, 18*(3), 276–281.

Chandler, P., & Sweller, J. (1991). Cognitive load theory and the format of instruction. *Cognition and Instruction, 8*(4).

Channin, D. S., Mongkolwat, P., et al. (2009a). Computing human image annotation. *Conference of the Proceeding IEEE Engineering in Medicine and Biology Society, 1*, 7065–7068.

Channin, D. S., Mongkolwat, P., et al. (2009b). The caBIG annotation and image markup project. *Journal of Digital Imaging, 23*(2), 217–225.

Chapanis, A. (1996). *Human factors in systems engineering*. New York: Wiley.

Chapman, W. C., Dowling, J. N., & Wagner, M. M. (2004). Fever detection from free-text clinical records for biosurveillance. *Journal of Biomedical Informatics, 37*(2), 120–127.

Chapman, W. W., Bridewell, W., Hanbury, P., Cooper, G. F., & Buchanan, B. G. (2001). A simple algorithm for identifying negated findings and diseases in discharge summaries. *Journal of Biomedical Informatics, 34*(5), 301–310.

Charen, T. (1976). *MEDLARS indexing manual, part I: Bibliographic principles and descriptive indexing, 1977*. Springfield: National Technical Information Service.

Charen, T. (1983). *MEDLARS indexing manual, part II*. Springfield: National Technical Information Service.

Chase, W. G., & Simon, H. A. (1973). Perception in chess. *Cognitive Psychology, 4*(1), 55–81.

Chaudhry, B., Wang, J., Wu, S., Maglione, M., Mojica, W., Roth, E., Morton, S. C., et al. (2006). Systematic review: Impact of health information technology on quality, efficiency, and costs of medical care. *Annals of Internal Medicine, 144*(10), 742–752.

Chen, E. S., Zhou, L., Kashyap, V., Schaeffer, M., Dykes, P. C., & Goldberg, H. S. (2008). Early experiences in evolving an enterprise-wide information model for laboratory and clinical observations. *AMIA Annual Symposium Proceedings, 2008*, 106–110.

Chen, T., Clifford, G. D., & Mark, R. G. (2009). *Computers in Cardiology, 36*, 197–200. PMC2926988.

Cheung, N. T., Fung, K. W., Wong, K. C., et al. (2001). Medical informatics – the state of the art in the hospital authority. *International Journal of Medical Informatics, 62*, 113–119.

Chi, M. T. H., & Glaser, R. (1981). Categorization and representation of physics problems by experts and novices. *Cognitive Science, 5*, 121–152.

Chi, M. T. H., Glaser, R., & Farr, M. J. (1988). *The nature of expertise*. Hillsdale: L. Erlbaum Associates.

Chin, T. (2003). Doctors pull plug on paperless system. *American Medical News*.

Choi, H. S., Haynor, D. R., et al. (1991). Partial volume tissue classification of multichannel magnetic resonance images – a mixel model. *IEEE Transactions on Medical Imaging, 10*(3), 395–407.

Choi, M., Scholl, U. I., Ji, W., et al. (2009). Genetic diagnosis by whole exome capture and massively parallel DNA sequencing. *Proceedings of the National Academy of Sciences of the United States of America, 106*, 19096–19101.

Chopra, A., Park, T., & Levin, P.L. (2010). '*Blue Button*' provides access to downloadable personal health data. Available at http://www.whitehouse.gov/blog/2010/10/07/blue-button-provides-access-downloadable-personal-health-data. Accessed 17 Dec 2012.

Christensen, L., Haug, P., & Fiszman, P. (2002). MPLUS: a probabilistic medical language understanding system. *Proceedings of the ACL BioNLP*, 29–36.

Christensen, C. M., Grossman, J. H., & Hwang, J. (2009). *The innovator's prescription: A disruptive solution for health care*. New York: McGraw-Hill.

Chuang, J.H., Friedman, C., & Hripcsak, G. (2002). A comparison of the charlson comorbidities derived from medical language processing and administrative data. *Proceedings of the AMIA Symposium*, 160–164.

Chui, M., Loffler, M., & Roberts, R. (2010). *The internet of things*. McKinsey Quarterly, 2, 1–9.

Chung, T. K., Kukafka, R., & Johnson, S. B. (2006). Reengineering clinical research with informatics. *Journal of Neurocytology, 54*(6), 327–333.

Church, G., Heeney, C., Hawkins, N., et al. (2009). Public access to genome-wide data: Five views on balancing research with privacy and protection. *PLoS Genetics, 5*, e1000665.

Church, G. M., Gao, Y., & Kosuri, S. (2012). Next-generation digital information storage in DNA. *Science, 337*, 1628.

Chused, A. E., Kuperman, G. J., & Stetson, P. D. (2008). Alert override reasons: A failure to communicate. *Proceeding of the AMIA Annual Symposium*, 111–115.

Chute, C. G. (2000). Clinical classification and terminology: Some history and current observations. *Journal of the American Medical Informatics Association: JAMIA, 7*(3), 298–303.

Cimino, J. J. (1996). Review paper: Coding systems in health care. *Methods of Information in Medicine, 35*(4–5), 273–284.

Cimino, J. J. (1998). Desiderata for controlled medical vocabularies in the twenty-first century. *Methods of Information in Medicine, 37*(4–5), 394–403.

Cimino, J., & delFiol, G. (2007). Infobuttons and point of care access to knowledge. In R. Greenes (Ed.), *Clinical decision support: The road ahead* (pp. 345–371). Amsterdam: Elsevier.

Cimino, J.J., Sengupta, S., Clayton, P.D., Patel, V.L., Kushniruk, A., & Huang, X. (1998). Architecture for a Web-based clinical information system that keeps the design open and the access closed. [Research Support, U.S. Gov't, P.H.S.]. *Proceedings/AMIA ... Annual Symposium. AMIA Symposium,* 121–125.

Cimino, J.J., Li, J., Mendonca, E.A., Sengupta, S., Patel, V.L., & Kushniruk, A.W. (2000). An evaluation of patient access to their electronic medical records via the World Wide Web. *Proceeding of AMIA Symposium,* 151–155. D200410 [pii]

Cimino, J.J., Li, J., Bakken, S., & Patel, V. (2002a). Theoretical, empirical and practical approaches to resolving unmet information needs of clinical information system users. *Proceeding of the AMIA Annual Symposium,* 170–174.

Cimino, J. J., Patel, V. L., & Kushniruk, A. W. (2002b). The patient clinical information system (PatCIS): technical solutions for and experience with giving patients access to their electronic medical records. [Research Support, U.S. Gov't, P.H.S.]. *International Journal of Medical Informatics, 68*(1–3), 113–127.

Cirulli, E. T., & Goldstein, D. B. (2010). Uncovering the roles of rare variants in common disease through whole-genome sequencing. *Nature Reviews Genetics, 11,* 415–425.

Clancey, W. J., & Shortliffe, E. H. (1984). *Readings in medical artificial intelligence: The first decade.* Reading: Addison-Wesley.

Clancey, W. J. (1984). The epistemology of a rule-based system: A framework for explanation. *Artificial Intelligence, 20,* 215–251.

Clancy, C. M., Anderson, K. M., & White, P. J. (2009). Investing in health information infrastructure: can it help achieve health reform? *Health Affairs, 28*(2), 478–482.

Clark, R. C., & Mayer, R. E. (2011). *e-Learning and the science of instruction: Proven guidelines for consumers and designers of multimedia learning* (3rd ed.). San Francisco: Pfeiffer.

Clark, O., Clark, L., & Djulbegovic, B. (2001). Is clinical research still too haphazard? *The Lancet, 358*(9293), 1648.

Clark, A. P., Giuliano, K., & Chen, H. M. (2006). Pulse oximetry revisited "but His O2 was normal". *Clinical Nurssing Specialist CNS, 20,* 268–272. PMID 17149014.

Clark, E. N., Sejersten, M., Clemmensen, P., & MacFarland, P. W. (2010). Automated electrocardiogram interpretation programs versus cardiologists' triage decision making based on teletransmitted data in patients with suspected acute coronary syndrome. *The American Journal of Cardiology, 106,* 1696–1702. PMID 21126612.

Clarysse, P., Friboulet, D., et al. (1997). Tracking geometrical descriptors on 3-D deformable surfaces: Application to the left-ventricular surface of the heart. *IEEE Transactions on Medical Imaging, 16*(4), 392–404.

Classen, D. C., Pestotnik, S. L., Evans, R. S., & Burke, J. P. (1991). Computerized surveillance of adverse drug events in hospital patients. *JAMA : The Journal of the American Medical Association, 266,* 2847–2851. PMID 194452.

Classen, D. C., Pestotnik, S. L., Evans, R. S., Lloyd, J. F., & Burke, J. P. (1997). Adverse drug events in hospitalized patients. Excess length of stay, extra costs, and attributable mortality. *Journal of the American Medical Association, 277*(4), 301–306.

Classen, D. C., Avery, A. J., & Bates, D. W. (2007). Evaluation and certification of computerized provider order entry systems. *Journal of the American Medical Informatics Association: JAMIA, 14*(1), 48–55.

Clemmer, T. P. (2004). Computers in the ICU: Where we started and where we are now. *Journal of Critical Care, 19,* 204–207. PMID 15648035.

Clemmer, T. P., Spuhler, V. J., Berwick, D. M., & Nolan, T. W. (1998). Cooperation: The foundation of improvement. *Annals of Internal Medicine, 128*(12 Pt 1), 1004–1009. PMID 9625663.

CMS P4P. Retrieved July 17, 2011, from https://www.cms.gov/MedicaidCHIPQualPrac/

Cobb, J. P., Suffredini, A. F., & Danner, R. L. (2008). The fourth national institutes of health symposium on the functional genomics of critical injury: Surviving stress from organ systems and molecules. *Critical Care Medicine, 36,* 2905–2911. PMID 18828200.

Coenen, A., McNeil, B., Bakken, S., Bickford, C., Warren, J. J., & American Nurses Association Committee on Nursing Practice Information Infrastructure. (2001). Toward comparable nursing data: American Nurses Association criteria for data sets, classification systems, and nomenclatures. *Computers in Nursing, 19*(6), 240–246.

Coffey, R. (1979). *How medical information systems affect costs: the El Camino experience.* Washington, D.C.: Public Health Service. Publication DHEW-PHS-80-3626.

Cohen, J.D. (2001). *FisWidgets.* From http://neurocog.lrdc.pitt.edu/fiswidgets/

Cohen, A., Stavri, P., & Hersh, W. (2004). A categorization and analysis of the criticisms of evidence-based medicine. *International Journal of Medical Informatics, 73,* 35–43.

Cole, M., & Engestroem, Y. (1997). A cultural-historical approach to distributed cognition. In G. Salomon (Ed.), *Distributed cognition* (pp. 1–47). New York: Cambridge University Press.

Coletti, M., & Bleich, H. (2001). Medical subject headings used to search the biomedical literature. *Journal of the American Medical Informatics Association: JAMIA, 8,* 317–323.

College of American Pathologists. (1971). *Systematized nomenclature of pathology.* Chicago: The College of American Pathologists.

Collen, M. F. (1969). Value of multiphasic health check-ups. *The New England Journal of Medicine, 280*(19), 1072–1073.

Collen, M. F. (1995). *A history of medical informatics in the United States, 1950 to 1990.* Bethesda: American Medical Informatics Association.

Collen, M. F., Rubin, L., Neyman, J., Dantzig, G. B., Baer, R. M., & Siegelaub, A. B. (1964). Automated multiphasic screening and diagnosis. *American Journal of Public Health and the Nations Health, 54,* 741–750.

Collins, F. S. (2011). Reengineering translational science: The time is right. *Science Translational Medicine, 3*(90), 90cm17.

Collins, D. L., Neelin, P., et al. (1994). Automatic 3-D intersubject registration of MR volumetric data in standardized Talairach space. *Journal of Computer Assisted Tomography, 18*(2), 192–205.

Collins, D. L., Holmes, D. J., et al. (1995). Automatic 3-D model-based neuroanatomical segmentation. *Human Brain Mapping, 3,* 190–208.

Collins, S. A., Bakken, S., Vawdrey, D. K., Coiera, E., & Currie, L. (2011a). Model development for EHR interdisciplinary information exchange of ICU common goals. *International Journal of Medical Informatics, 80*(8), 141–149.

Collins, S. A., Bakken, S., Vawdrey, D. K., Coiera, E., & Currie, L. M. (2011b). Agreement between common goals discussed and documented in the ICU. *Journal of the American Medical Informatics Association: JAMIA, 18*(1), 45–50.

Collins, S. A., Bakken, S., Vawdrey, D. K., Coiera, E., & Currie, L. (2011c). Clinical preferences for verbal communication compared to EHR documentation in the ICU. *Journal of Applied Clinical Informatics, 2,* 190–201.

Colombet, I., Bura-Rivière, A., Chatila, R., Chatellier, G., Durieux, P., & PHRC-OAT study group. (2004). Personalized versus non-personalized computerized decision support system to increase therapeutic quality control of oral anticoagulant therapy: An alternating time series analysis. *BMC Health Services Research, 4*(1), 27.

Comaniciu, D., & Meer, P. (2002). Mean shift: A robust approach toward feature space analysis. *IEEE Transactions on Pattern Analysis and Machine Intelligence, 24*(5), 603–619.

Commission on Professional and Hospital Activities. (1978). *International classification of diseases, ninth revision, with clinical modifications (ICD-9-CM).* Ann Arbor: American Hospital Association.

Committee on Data Standards for Patient Safety. (2004). *Patient safety: Achieving a new standard for care. A report of the institute of medicine.* Washington, DC: The National Academies Press.

Committee on Quality of Health Care in America. (2001). *Crossing the quality chasm: A new health system for the 21st century. A report of the institute of medicine.* Washington, DC: National Academy Press.

Committee on the Robert Wood Johnson Foundation Initiative on the Future of Nursing at the Institute of Medicine. (2010). *The future of nursing: Leading change, advancing health.* Washington, DC: Institute of Medicine of the National Academies, The National Academies Press.

Concato, J., Shah, N., & Horwitz, R. I. (2000). Randomized, controlled trials, observational studies, and the hierarchy of research designs. *The New England Journal of Medicine, 342*(25), 1887–1892.

Congressional Budget Office. (2008). *Evidence on the costs and benefits of health information technology.* Washington, D.C.: CBO Paper.

Conn, J., & Lubell, J. (2006). Boosting personal records. Blues, AHIP offer model health record for patient use. *Modern Healthcare, 36*(50), 10.

Consortium, E. P. (2004). The ENCODE (ENCyclopedia of DNA elements) project. *Science, 306,* 636–640.

Corina, D.P., Poliakov, A.V., et al. (2000). Correspondences between language cortex identified by cortical stimulation mapping and fMRI. *Neuroimage (Human Brain Mapping Annual Meeting, June 12–16), 11*(5), S295.

Corn, M. (2009). Archiving the phenome: Clinical records deserve long-term preservation. *Journal of the American Medical Informatics Association: JAMIA, 16*(1), 1–6.

Côté, R. A., & Rothwell, D. J. (1993). *The systematised nomenclature of human and veterinary medicine, 1993.* Northfield: College of American Pathologits.

Coulet, A., Shah, N. H., Garten, Y., et al. (2010). Using text to build semantic networks for pharmacogenomics. *Journal of Biomedical Informatics, 43,* 1009–1019.

Courtney, P. K. (2011). Data liquidity in health information systems. *Cancer Journal, 17*(4), 219–221.

Covell, D., Uman, G., & Manning, P. (1985). Information needs in office practice: are they being met? *Annals of Internal Medicine, 103,* 596–599.

Cox, J., Jr. (1972). Digital analysis of the electroencephalogram, the blood pressure wave, and the electrocardiogram. *Proceedings of the IEEE, 60,* 1137.

Cox, R. W. (1996). AFNI: Software for analysis and visualization of functional magnetic resonance neuroimages. *Computers and Biomedical Research, 29,* 162–173.

Cresswell, K., & Sheikh, A. (2009). The nhs care record service (nhs crs): recommendations from the literature on successful implementation and adoption. *Informatics in Primary Care, 17*(3), 153–160.

Crick, F. (1970). Central dogma of molecular biology. *Nature, 227,* 561–563.

Cronenwett, L., Sherwood, G., & Gelmon, S. B. (2009). Improving quality and safety education: The QSEN Learning Collaborative. *Nursing Outlook, 57*(6), 304–312.

Crossley, G. H., Poole, J. E., Rozner, M. A., et al. (2011). The Heart Rhythm Society (HRS)/American Society of Anesthesiologists (ASA) Expert Consensus Statement on the Perioperative management Arrhythmia Monitors. *Heart Rhythm, 8,* 1114–1154. PMID 21722856.

Crowley, R. S., Naus, G. J., Stewart, J., 3rd, & Friedman, C. P. (2003). Development of visual diagnostic expertise in pathology – an information-processing study. *Journal of the American Medical Informatics Association: JAMIA, 10*(1), 39–51.

Crowley, R. S., Legowski, E., Medvedeva, O. M., Tseytlin, E., Roh, E., & Jukic, D. (2007). Evaluation of an intelligent tutoring system in pathology: Effects of external representation on performance gains, metacognition, and acceptance. *Journal of the American Medical Informatics Association: JAMIA, 14*(2), 182–190.

Cuadros, J., & Bresnick, G. (2009). EyePACS: An adaptable telemedicine system for diabetic retinopathy screening. *Journal of Diabetes Science and Technology, 3*, 509–516.

Cundick, R. M., Jr., & Gardner, R. M. (1980). Clinical comparison of pressure-pulse and indicator-dilution cardiac output determination. *Circulation, 62*, 371–376. PMID 6994922.

Curran, W. J., Stearns, B., & Kaplan, H. (1969). Privacy, confidentiality, and other legal considerations in the establishment of a centralized health-data system. *The New England Journal of Medicine, 281*, 241–248.

Cusack, C. M., Pan, E., Hook, J. M., Vincent, A., Kaelber, D. C., & Middleton, B. (2008). The value proposition in the widespread use of telehealth. *Journal of Telemedicine and Telecare, 14*(4), 167–168.

Cushing, H. (1903). On routine determination of arterial tension in operating room and clinic. *Boston Medical Surgical Journal, 148*:250.Dalto 1997

Cushman, R., Froomkin, M. A., Cava, A., Abril, P., & Goodman, K. W. (2010). Ethical, legal and social issues for personal health records and applications. *Journal of Biomedical Informatics, 43*, S51–S55.

D'Orsi, C. J., & Newell, M. S. (2007). BI-RADS decoded: Detailed guidance on potentially confusing issues. *Radiologic Clinics of North America, 45*(5), 751–763. v.

Da Vinci Surgery. Available at: http://www.davincisurgery.com. Accessed 28 June 2011.

Dale, A. M., Fischl, B., et al. (1999). Cortical surface-based analysis. I. Segmentation and surface reconstruction. *NeuroImage, 9*(2), 179–194.

Dalto, J. S., Johnson, K. V., Gardner, R. M., Spuhler, V. J., & Egbert, L. (1997). Medical information bus usage for automated IV pump data acquisition: Evaluation of use and nurse attitudes. *International Journal of Clinical Monitoring and Computing, 14*, 151–154. PMID 9387004.

Dameron, O., Roques E., et al. (2006). Grading lung tumors using OWL-DL based reasoning. *9th International Protégé Conference*. Stanford.

Damiani, G., Pinnarelli, L., Colosimo, S. C., Almiento, R., Sicuro, L., Galasso, R., Sommello, L., & Ricciardi, W. (2010). The effectiveness of computerized clinical guidelines in the process of care: A systematic review. *BMC Health Services Research, 10*, 2.

Damush, T. M., Weinberger, M., Clark, D. O., Tierney, W. M., Rao, J. K., Perkins, S. M., & Verel, K. (2002). Acute low back pain self management intervention for urban primary care patients: Rationale, design, and predictors of participation. *Arthritis and Rheumatism, 47*, 372–379.

Dansky, K. H., Palmer, L., Shea, D., & Bowles, K. H. (2001). Cost analysis of telehomecare. *Telemedicine Journal of E-Health, 7*(3), 225–232. doi:10.1089/153056201316970920.

Darmoni, S., Leroy, J., Baudic, F., Douyere, M., Piot, J., & Thirion, B. (2000). CISMeF: A structured health resource guide. *Methods of Information in Medicine, 9*, 30–35.

Datta, R., Joshi, D., et al. (2008). Image retrieval: ideas, influences, and trends of the new age. *ACM Computing Surveys, 40*(2), Article 5:1–60.

Davatzikos, C., & Bryan, R. N. (1996). Using a deformable surface model to obtain a shape representation of the cortex. *IEEE Transactions on Medical Imaging, 15*(6), 785–795.

David, J. M., Krivine, J. P., & Simmons, R. (Eds.). (1993). *Second generation expert systems*. Berlin: Springer.

Davies, K. (2008). Keeping score of your sequence. *BioIT World, 7*, 16–21.

Davies, K. (2010). Physicians and their use of information: A survey comparison between the United States, Canada, and the United Kingdom. *Journal of the Medical Library Association, 99*, 88–91.

Davis, L. S., Collen, M. F., Rubin, F. L., & Van Brunt, E. E. (1968). Computer stored medical record. *Computer Biomedical Research, 1*, 452–469.

Davis, R., Buchanan, B., & Shortliffe, E. H. (1977). Production rules as a representation for a knowledge-based consultation system. *Artificial Intelligence, 8*, 15–45.

Dayhoff, M. O. (1974). Computer analysis of protein sequences. *Federal Proceedings, 33*(12), 2314–2316.

de Dombal, F. T. (1987). Ethical considerations concerning computers in medicine in the 1980s. *Journal of Medical Ethics, 13*, 179–184.

de Dombal, F. T., Leaper, D. J., Staniland, J. R., McCann, A. P., & Horrocks, J. C. (1972). Computer-aided diagnosis of acute abdominal pain. *British Medical Journal, 1*, 376–380.

de Figueiredo, E. H., Borgonovi, A. F., et al. (2011). Basic concepts of MR imaging, diffusion MR imaging, and diffusion tensor imaging. *Magnetic Resonance Imaging Clinics of North America, 19*(1), 1–22.

Dean, J., & Ghemawat, S. (2008). MapReduce: Simplified data processing on large clusters. *Communications of the ACM, 51*(1), 107–113.

DeAngelis, C., Drazen, J., Frizelle, F., Haug, C., Hoey, J., Horton, R., & VanDerWeyden, M. (2005). Is this clinical trial fully registered? A statement from the International Committee of Medical Journal Editors. *Journal of the American Medical Association, 293*, 2927–2929.

DeBakey, M. (1991). The national library of medicine: Evolution of a premier information center. *Journal of the American Medical Association, 266*, 1252–1258.

Deci, E. L., & Ryan, R. M. (1985). *Intrinsic motivation and self-determination in human behavior.* New York: Plenum.

Decker, S. L., Jamoom, E. W., & Sisk, J. E. (2012). Physicians in nonprimary care and small practices and those age 55 and older lag in adopting electronic health record systems. *Health Affairs, 31*(5), 1108–1114.

DeClerq, P. A., Blom, J. A., Korsten, H. H., & Hasman, A. (2004). Approaches for creating computer-interpretable guidelines that facilitate decision support. *Artificial Intelligence in Medicine, 31*(1), 1–27.

Deflandre, E., Bonhomme, V., & Hans, P. (2008). Delta down compared with delta pulse pressure as an indicator of volaemia during intracranial surgery. *British Journal of Anaesthesia, 100*, 245–250. PMID 18083787.

DeGroot, A. T. (1965). *Thought and choice in chess.* The Hague: Mouton.

Del Fiol, G., Huser, V., Strasberg, H. R., et al. (2012). Implementations of the HL7 context-aware knowledge retrieval ("infobutton") standard: Challenges, strengths, limitations, and uptake. *Journal of Biomedical Informatics, 45*(4), 726–735.

Deleger, L., Merkel, M., & Zweigenbaum, P. (2009). Translating medical terminologies through word alignment in parallel text corpora. *Journal of Biomedical Informatics, 42*(4), 692–701.

Demiris, G., Speedie, S., & Finkelstein, S. (2000). A questionnaire for the assessment of patients' impressions of the risks and benefits of home telecare. *Journal of Telemedicine and Telecare, 6*(5), 278–284.

Demner-Fushman, D., & Lin, J. (2007). Answering clinical questions with knowledge-based and statistical techniques. *Computational Linguistics, 33*(1), 63–103.

Dempster, A. P., Laird, N. M., et al. (1977). Maximum likelihood from incomplete data via the EM algorithm. *Journal of the Royal Statistical Society Series B, 39*, 1–38.

Denny, J. C., Ritchie, M. D., Basford, M. A., et al. (2010). PheWAS: Demonstrating the feasibility of a phenome-wide scan to discover gene-disease associations. *Bioinformatics, 26*, 1205–1210.

Department of Health and Human Services. (1994). Essential public health functions. *Public Health in America.* Accessed 2005 at: http://www.health.gov/phfunctions/public.htm

Department of Health and Human Services. (2003) *Building the national health information infrastructure.* Available at http://aspe.hhs.gov/sp/nhii/. Accessed 12 Aug 2011.

Department of Health and Human Services. (2010). *Healthy people 2020.* Washington, DC: US Department of Health and Human Services. Available at http://healthypeople.gov/2020/topicsobjectives2020/objectiveslist.aspx?topicid=23. Accessed 29 Nov 2012.

Department of Health and Human Services. (2011). *Childhood overweight and obesity prevention initiative.* Washington, DC: National Academies Press.

Deselaers, T., Hegerath, A., et al. (2006). Sparse patch-histograms for object classification in cluttered images. In *DAGM 2006, Pattern Recognition, 27th DAGM Symposium, Lecture Notes in Computer Science* (pp. 202–211).

Deselaers, T., Muller, H., et al. (2007). The CLEF 2005 automatic medical image annotation task. *International Journal of Computer Vision, 74*(1), 51–58.

Deserno, T. M., Antani, S., et al. (2009). Ontology of gaps in content-based image retrieval. *Journal of Digital Imaging, 22*(2), 202–215.

DesRoches, C. M., et al. (2008). Electronic health records in ambulatory care – a national survey of physicians. *The New England Journal of Medicine, 359*, 50–60.

DesRoches, C. M., Worzala, C., Joshi, M. S., Kralovec, P. D., & Jha, A. K. (2012). Small, nonteaching, and rural hospitals continue to be slow in adopting electronic health record systems. *Health Affairs, 31*(5), 1092–1099.

Detmer, D. E. (2003). Building the national health information infrastructure for personal health, health care services, public health, and research. *BMC Medical Informatics and Decision Making, 3*, 1.

Dewey, F. E., Chen, R., Cordero, S. P., et al. (2011). Phased whole-genome genetic risk in a family quartet using a major allele reference sequence. *PLoS Genetics, 7*, e1002280.

Dexter, P. R., Perkins, S., Overhage, J. M., et al. (2001). A computerized reminder system to increase the use of preventive care for hospitalized patients. *The New England Journal of Medicine, 345*(13), 965–970.

Dexter, P. R., Perkins, S. M., Maharry, K. S., Jones, K., & McDonald, C. J. (2004). Inpatient computer-based standing orders vs. physician reminders to increase influenza and pneumococcal vaccination rates. *Journal of the American Medical Association, 292*(19), 2366–2371.

Dhenain, M., Ruffins, S. W., et al. (2001). Three-dimensional digital mouse atlas using high-resolution MRI. *Developmental Biology, 232*(2), 458–470.

Diamond, G., & Kaul, S. (2008). The disconnect between practice guidelines and clinical practice – stressed out. *Journal of the American Medical Association, 300*, 1817–1819.

DiCenso, A., Bayley, L., & Haynes, R. (2009). ACP Journal Club. Editorial: Accessing preappraised evidence: Fine-tuning the 5S model into a 6S model. *Annals of Internal Medicine, 151*(6), JC3-2. JC3-3.

Dick, R., & Steen, E. (Eds.) (1991). *The Computer-Based Patient Record: An Essential Technology for Health Care* (Rev. 1997). Washington, D.C.: Institute of Medicine, National Academy Press.

Diepgen, T. L., & Eysenbach, G. (1998). Digital images in dermatology and the Dermatology Online Atlas on the World Wide Web. *The Journal of Dermatology, 25*(12), 782–787.

Do, N. V., Barnhill, R., Heermann-Do, K. A., Salzman, K. L., & Gimbel, R. W. (2011). The military health system's personal health record pilot with Microsoft HealthVault and Google health. *Journal of the American Medical Informatics Association: JAMIA, 18*(2), 118–124.

Dodd, B. (1997, October). An independent "health information bank" could solve health data security issues. *British Journal of Healthcare Computing and Information Management, 14*(8), 2.

Doi, K. (2007). Computer-aided diagnosis in medical imaging: Historical review, current status and future potential. *Computerized Medical Imaging and Graphics, 31*(4–5), 198–211.

Doig, A. K., Drews, F. A., & Keefe, M. R. (2011). Informing the design of hemodynamic monitoring displays. *Computers, Informatics, Nursing, 29*(12), 706–713. PMID 21412150.

Doing-Harris, K. M., & Zeng-Treitler, Q. (2011). Computer-assisted update of a consumer health vocabulary through mining of social network data. *Journal of Medical Internet Research, 13*(2), e37.

Dolin, R.H., Giannone, G., & Schadow, G. (2007). Enabling Joint Commission medication reconciliation objectives with the HL7/ASTM Continuity of Care Document Standard. In *Proceedings of the 2007 AMIA Annual Symposium,* 186–190.

Donley, G., Hull, S. C., & Berkman, B. E. (2012). Prenatal whole genome sequencing. *The Hastings Center Report, 42,* 28–40.

Donovan, T., & Manning, D. J. (2007). The radiology task: Bayesian theory and perception. *The British Journal of Radiology, 80*(954), 389–391.

Doolan, D. F., Bates, D. W., & James, B. C. (2003). The use of computers for clinical care: A case series of advanced U.S. Sites. *Journal of the American Medical Informatics Association: JAMIA, 10*(1), 94–107.

Dossia Consortium. (2006). http://www.dossia.org. Accessed 17 Dec 2012.

Downs, S. M., Biondich, P. G., Anand, V., Zore, M., & Carroll, A. E. (2006). Using Arden syntax and adaptive turnaround documents to evaluate clinical guidelines. *AMIA Annual Symposium Proceedings, 2006,* 214–218.

Drazen, J., & Curfman, G. (2004). Public access to biomedical research. *The New England Journal of Medicine, 351,* 1343.

Drew, B. J., & Funk, M. (2006). Practice standards for ECG monitoring in hospital setting: Executive summary and guide for implementation. *Critical Care Nursing Clinics of North America, 18*(2), 157–168. PMID 16728301.

Drews, F. A., Musters, A., & Samore, M. H. (2008). Error producing conditions in intensive care unit. In *Advances in patient safety: New directions and alternative approaches* (Performance and tools, Vol. 3). Rockville: AHRQ. PMID 21249947.

Drucker, P. F. (1959). Long-range planning. *Management Science, 5*(3), 238–249.

Drury, H. A., & Van Essen, D. C. (1997). Analysis of functional specialization in human cerebral cortex using the visible man surface based atlas. *Human Brain Mapping, 5,* 233–237.

Du, X., Callister, S. J., Manes, N. P., et al. (2008). A computational strategy to analyze label-free temporal bottom-up proteomics data. *Journal of Proteome Research, 7,* 2595–2604.

Duch, W., Oentaryo, R.J., & Pasquier, M. (2008). *Cognitive architectures: Where do we go from here?* Paper presented at the proceeding of the 2008 conference on Artificial General Intelligence 2008: Proceedings of the First AGI Conference. Memphis, TN.

Duda, R. O., & Shortliffe, E. H. (1983). Expert systems research. *Science, 220,* 261–268.

Duda, R. O., Hart, P. E., et al. (2001). *Pattern classification.* New York: Wiley.

Dugas-Phocion, G., Ballester, M. A. G., et al. (2004). "Improved EM-based tissue segmentation and partial volume effect quantification in multi-sequence brain MRI." Medical Image Computing and Computer-Assisted Intervention – Miccai 2004, Pt 1. *Proceedings, 3216,* 26–33.

Duncan, R. G., Saperia, D., Dulbandzhyan, R., et al. (2001). Integrated web-based viewing and secure remote access to a clinical data repository and diverse clinical systems. *Proceedings of the AMIA Fall Symposium, 2001,* 149–153.

Dunham, I., Kundaje, A., Aldred, S. F., et al. (2012). An integrated encyclopedia of DNA elements in the human genome. *Nature, 489*(7414), 57–74.

Dupuits, F. M. (1994). The use of the Arden syntax for MLMs in HIOS+, a decision support system for general practitioners in The Netherlands. *Computers in Biology and Medicine, 24*(5), 405–410.

Durbin, R., Eddy, S. R., Krogh, A., & Mitchison, G. (1998). *Biological sequence analysis: Probabilistic models of proteins and nucleic acids.* Cambridge: Cambridge University Press.

Durfy, S. J. (1993). Ethics and the human genome project. *Archives of Pathology & Laboratory Medicine, 117*(5), 466–469.

Dykes, P. C., Carroll, D. L., Hurley, A. C., Benoit, A., & Middleton, B. (2009). Why do patients in acute care hospitals fall? Can falls be prevented? *The Journal of Nursing Administration, 39*(6), 299–304.

Dykes, P. C., Carroll, D. L., Hurley, A., Lipsitz, S., Benoit, A., Chang, F., et al. (2010). Fall prevention in acute care hospitals: A randomized trial. *Journal of the American Medical Association, 304*(17), 1912–1918.

Dyson, E. (2005, September). *Personal health information: data comes alive! Release* 1.0 24,1.

Earle, K. (2011). In people with poorly controlled hypertension, self-management including telemonitoring is more effective than usual care for reducing systolic blood pressure at 6 and 12 months. *Evidence-Based Medicine, 16*(1), 17–18.

East, T. D., Bohm, S. H., Wallace, C. J., Clemmer, T. P., Weaver, L. K., Orme, J. F., Jr., & Morris, A. H. (1992). A successful computerized protocol for clinical management of pressure control inverse ration ventilation. *Chest, 101*(3), 697–710. Edworthy 2006.

Ebbert J. O., Dupras D. M., Erwin P. J. (2003). Searching the medical literature using PubMed: a tutorial. *Mayo Clin Proc. 78(1)*, 87–91.

Eddy, D. M. (1992). *A manual for assessing health practices and designing practice policies: The explicit approach.* Philadelphia: American College of Physicians.

Edgar, E.P. (2009). *Physician retention in Army Medical Department. Strategic Research Project, U.S. Army War College, Carlisle Barracks PA* 17013–5050. Available at: http://handle.dtic.mil/100.2/ADA499087

Edgar, R., Domrachev, M., & Lash, A. E. (2002). Gene expression omnibus: NCBI gene expression and hybridization array data repository. *Nucleic Acids Research, 30*, 207–210.

Edworthy, J., & Hellier, E. (2006). Alarms and human behavior: Implications for medical alarms. *British Journal of Anaesthesia, 97*, 12–17. PMID 16698858.

Egan, D., Remde, J., Gomez, L., Landauer, T., Eberhardt, J., & Lochbaum, C. (1989). Formative design-evaluation of superbook. *ACM Transactions on Information Systems, 7*, 30–57.

EHI Primary Care. (2007). *NHS London orders data transfer review.*

Elhadad, N. (2006). Comprehending technical texts: predicting and defining unfamiliar terms. *Proceedings AMIA Symposium*, 239–243.

Elhadad, N., Kan, M. Y., Klavans, J. L., & McKeown, K. R. (2005). Customization in a unified framework for summarizing medical literature. *Artificial Intelligence in Medicine, 33*(2), 179–198.

Eliot CR, Woolf BP. (1996). A Simulation-Based Tutor that Reasons about Multiple Agents, Proceedings of the 13th National Conference on Artificial Intelligence (AAAI-96), Cambridge, MA: AAAI/MIT Press, pp. 409-415.

Elkin, P. L., Sorensen, B., De Palo, D., Poland, G., Bailey, K. R., Wood, D. L., & LaRusso, N. F. (2002). Optimization of a research web environment for academic internal medicine faculty. *Journal of the American Medical Informatics Association: JAMIA, 9*(5), 472–478.

Elstein, K. A., Shulman, L. S., & Sprafka, S. A. (1978). *Medical problem solving: An analysis of clinical reasoning.* Cambridge, MA: Harvard University Press.

Elter, M., & Horsch, A. (2009). CADx of mammographic masses and clustered microcalcifications: A review. *Medical Physics, 36*(6), 2052–2068.

Elwyn, G., Edwards, A., & Kinnersley, P. (1999). Shared decision-making in primary care: The neglected second half of the consultation. *The British Journal of General Practice, 49*(443), 477–482.

Ely, J., Osheroff, J., Ebell, M., Bergus, G., Levy, B., Chambliss, M., & Evans, E. (1999). Analysis of questions asked by family doctors regarding patient care. *British Medical Journal, 319*, 358–361.

Ely, J., Osheroff, J., Ebell, M., Chambliss, M., Vinson, D., Stevermer, J., & Pifer, E. (2002). Obstacles to answering doctors' questions about patient care with evidence: Qualitative study. *British Medical Journal, 324*, 710–713.

Embi, P. J., & Payne, P. R. (2009). Clinical research informatics: Challenges, opportunities and definition for an emerging domain. *Journal of the American Medical Informatics Association: JAMIA, 16*(3), 316–327.

Embi, P. J., Jain, A., Clark, J., Bizjack, S., Hornung, R., & Harris, C. M. (2005). Effect of a clinical trial alert system on physician participation in trial recruitment. *Archives of Internal Medicine, 165*(19), 2272–2277.

Eminovic, N., Wyatt, J. C., Tarpey, A. M., Murray, G., & Ingrams, G. J. (2004, June 02). First evaluation of the NHS direct online clinical enquiry service: A nurse-led Web chat triage service for the public. *Journal of Medical Internet Research, 6*(2), E17.

Engel, G. L. (1977). The need for a new medical model: A challenge for biomedicine. *Science, 196*, 129–136.

Erickson, B. (2011). Experience with importation of electronic images into the medical record from physical media. *Journal of Digital Imaging, 24*(4), 694–699.

Erickson, B., & Hangiandreou, N. (1998). The evolution of electronic imaging in the medical environment. *Journal of Digital Imaging, 11*(3 suppl 1), 71–74.

Erickson, B., Ryan, W., Gehring, D., & Pynadath, A. (2007, Summer). Top 10 features clinicians require in an image viewer. *SIIM News.*

Ericsson, K. A. (2006). *The Cambridge handbook of expertise and expert performance.* Cambridge/New York: Cambridge University Press.

Ericsson, K. A., & Simon, H. A. (1993). *Protocol analysis: Verbal reports as data (Rev. ed.).* Cambridge, MA: MIT Press.

Ericsson, K. A., & Smith, J. (1991). *Toward a general theory of expertise: Prospects and limits.* New York: Cambridge University Press.

Estes, W. K. (1975). The state of the field: General problems and issues of theory and metatheory. In W. K. Estes (Ed.), *Handbook of learning and cognitive processes* (Vol. 1). Hillsdale/New York: L. Erlbaum Associates.

Etheredge, L. M. (2007). A rapid-learning health system. *Health Affairs (Millwood), 26*(2), w107–w118.

Evans, D. (2002). Database searches for qualitative research. *Journal of the Medical Library Association, 90*(3), 290–293.

Evans, B. J. (2011). Much ado about data ownership. *Harvard Journal of Law & Technology, 25*(1), 70–130.

Evans, D. A., & Gadd, C. S. (1989). Managing coherence and context in medical problem-solving discourse. In D. A. Evans & V. L. Patel (Eds.), *Cognitive science in medicine: Biomedical modeling* (pp. 211–255). Cambridge, MA: MIT Press.

Evans, D. A., & Patel, V. L. (1989). *Cognitive science in medicine.* Cambridge, MA: MIT Press.

Evans, D. A., Cimino, J. J., Hersh, J. J., Huff, S. M., & Bell, D. S. (1994). Toward a medical-concept representation language. The Canon Group. *Journal of the American Medical Informatics Association: JAMIA, 1*(3), 207–217.

Evans, R. S., Pestotnik, S. L., Classen, D. C., Clemmer, T. P., Weaver, L. K., Orme, J. F., Lloyd, J. F., & Burke, J. P. (1998). A computer-assisted management program for antibiotics and other antinfective agents. *The New England Journal of Medicine, 338*(4), 232–238.

Evans, R. S., Carlson, R., Johnson, K. V., Palmer, B. K., & Lloyd, J. F. (2010). Enhanced notification of infusion pump programming errors. *Studies in Health Technology and Informatics, 160*(Pt 1), 734–738. PMID 20841783.

Evans, R.S., Johnson, K.V., Flint, V.B., Kinder, T., Lyon, C.R., Hawley, W.L., Vawdrey, D.K., Thomsen, G.E. (2005). Enhanced notification of critical ventilator events. *J Am Med Inform Assoc* 12, 589–95. PMID 16049226.

Eveillard, P. (2000). Bibliographic databases. Medline via PubMed. *La Revue du Praticien, 50*(16 Suppl), 1–34.

Executive Office of the President: President's Council of Advisors on Science and Technology. (2010). *Report to the President Realizing the Full Potential of Health Information Technology To Improve Healthcare For Americans: The Path Forward*. Washington, DC: Executive Office of the President of the United States.

Eysenbach, G. (2006). Citation advantage of open access articles. *PLoS Biology, 4*(5), e157.

Eysenbach, G. (2008). Medicine 2.0: Social networking, collaboration, participation, apomediation, and openness. *Journal of Medical Internet Research, 10*(3), e22.

Eysenbach, G., & Kohler, C. (2004). Health-related searches on the internet. *Journal of the American Medical Association, 291*, 2946.

Eysenbach, G., & Till, J. E. (2001). Ethical issues in qualitative research on internet communities. *BMJ, 323*(7321), 1103–1105.

Eysenbach, G., & Wyatt, J. (2002). Using the internet for surveys and health research. *Journal of Medical Internet Research, 4*(2), E13.

Eysenbach, G., Bauer, J., et al. (1998). An international dermatological image atlas on the WWW: Practical use for undergraduate and continuing medical education, patient education and epidemiological research. *Studies in Health Technology and Informatics, 52*(Pt 2), 788–792.

Eysenbach, G., Su, E., & Diepgen, T. (1999). Shopping around the internet today and tomorrow: Towards the millennium of cybermedicine. *British Medical Journal, 319*, 1294–1298.

Eysenbach, G., Tuische, J., & Diepgen, T. L. (2001). Evaluation of the usefulness of internet searches to identify unpublished clinical trials for systematic reviews. *Medical Informatics and the Internet in Medicine, 26*(3), 203–218.

Eysenbach, G., Powell, J., Kuss, O., & Sa, E.-R. (2002). Empirical studies assessing the quality of health information for consumers on the world wide web: A systematic review. *Journal of the American Medical Association, 287*, 2691–2700.

Eysenbach, G., Powell, J., Englesakis, M., Rizo, C., & Stern, A. (2004). Health related virtual communities and electronic support groups: Systematic review of the effects of online peer to peer interactions. *British Medical Journal, 328*(7449), 1166.

Fabienne, C., Olson, K. L., & Mandl, K. D. (2010). Health care reform- patients treated at multiple acute health care facilities: Quantifying information fragmentation. *Archives of Internal Medicine, 170*(22), 1989–1995.

Fafchamps, D., Young, C. Y., & Tang, P. C. (1991). Modelling work practices: Input to the design of a physician's workstation. In *Proceedings of the 15th annual symposium on Computer Applications in Medical Care* (pp. 788–792). Washington, D.C.: CAMC.

Fargher, E. A., Eddy, C., Newman, W., Qasim, F., Tricker, K., Elliott, R. A., & Payne, K. (2007). Patients" and healthcare professionals" views on pharmacogenetic testing and its future delivery in the NHS. *Pharmacogenomics, 8*(11), 1511–1519.

Fazi, P., Grifoni, P., Luzi, D., Ricci, F. L., & Vignetti, M. (2000). Is workflow technology suitable to represent and manage clinical trials? *Studies in Health Technology and Informatics, 77*, 302–306.

Fazi, P., Luzi, D., Manco, M., Ricci, F.L., Toffoli, G., & Vignetti, M. (2002). WITH: a system to write clinical trials using XML and RDBMS. *Proceedings of the AMIA Symposium, 240–244.

FDA (U.S. Food and Drug Administration). (2011). *Infusion pump software safety research at FDA*. Retrieval 1 Aug 2012: http://www.fda.gov/MedicalDevices/ProductsandMedicalProcedures/GeneralHospitalDevicesandSupplies/InfusionPumps/ucm202511.htm

Federative Committee on Anatomical Terminology. (1998). *Terminologia anatomica*. Stuttgart: Thieme.

Feero, W. G., Guttmacher, A. E., & Collins, F. S. (2010). Genomic medicine–an updated primer [Review]. *The New England Journal of Medicine, 362*(21), 2001–2011.

Fei-Fei, L., & Perona, P. (2005). A Bayesian hierarchical model for learning natural scene categories. In *Proceedings of IEEE Computer Vision and Pattern Recognition* (pp. 524–531), San Diego.

Feltovich, P. J., Johnson, P. E., Moller, J. H., & Swanson, D. B. (1984). The role and development of medical knowledge in diagnostic expertise. In W. J. Clancey & E. H. Shortliffe (Eds.), *Readings in medical artificial intelligence: The first decade* (pp. 275–319). Reading: Addison Wesley.

Ferguson, T. (1996). *Health Online: how to find health informaiton, support groups, and self help communities in cyberspace. The Millenium Whole Earth Catalogue*. Da Capo Press. Boston, MA.

Ferguson, T. (1997). Health care in cyberspace: Patients lead a revolution. *Futurist, 31*(6), 29–34.

Ferguson, T. (2002). From patients to end users: Quality of online patient networks needs more attention than quality of online health information. *British Medical Journal, 324*, 555–556.

Ferguson, G., Quinn, J., Horwitz, C., Swift, M., Allen, J., & Galescu, L. (2010). Towards a personal health management assistant. *Journal of Biomedical Informatics, 43*(5 Suppl), S13–S16.

Ferranti, J. M., Musser, R. C., Kawamoto, K., & Hammond, W. E. (2006). The clinical document architecture and the continuity of care record: A critical analysis. *Journal of the American Medical Informatics Association: JAMIA, 13*(3), 245–252.

Ferrucci, D., Brown, E., Chu-Carroll, J., et al. (2010). Building Watson: an overview of the DeepQA Project. *AI Magazine, 31*(3), 59–79. Retrieved from http://www.aaai.org/ojs/index.php/aimagazine/article/view/2303

Fiala, J. C., & Harris, K. M. (2001). Extending unbiased stereology of brain ultrastructure to three-dimensional volumes. *Journal of the American Medical Informatics Association: JAMIA, 8*(1), 1–16.

Ficarra, V., Novara, G., Fracalanza, S., et al. (2009). A prospective, non-randomized trial comparing robot-assisted laparoscopic and retropubic radical prostatectomy in one European institution. *BJU International, 104*, 534–539.

Fielding, N. G., & Lee, R. M. (1991). *Using computers in qualitative research*. Newbury Park: Sage Press.

Figurska, M., Robaszkiewicz, J., et al. (2010). Optical coherence tomography in imaging of macular diseases. *Klinika Oczna, 112*(4–6), 138–146.

Fiks, A. G., Alessandrini, E. A., Forrest, C. B., Khan, S., Localio, A. R., Gerber, A., et al. (2011). Electronic medical record use in pediatric primary care. *Journal of the American Medical Informatics Association: JAMIA, 18*(1), 38–44.

Final Rule: Centers for Medicare and Medicaid Services (CMS), HHS. Medicare and Medicaid Programs; Electronic Health Record Incentive Program—Stage 2, 77(171) Fed. Reg. 53968 (Sept. 4, 2012) (amending 42 C.F.R. § 412, 413, and 495).

Final Rule: Office of the National Coordinator (ONC) for Health Information Technology, Department of Health and Human Services. Health Information Technology: Standards, Implementation Specifications, and Certification Criteria for Electronic Health Record Technology, 2014 Edition; Revisions to the Permanent Certification Program for Health Information Technology, 77(171) Fed. Reg. 54163 (Sept. 4, 2012) (amending 45 C.F.R. § 170).

Fine, A. M., Nizet, V., & Mandl, K. D. (2011). Improved diagnostic accuracy of group a streptococcal pharyngitis with use of real-time biosurveillance. *Annals of Internal Medicine, 155*(6), 345–352.

Finkel, A. (ed.) (1977). CPT4: Physician's Current Procedural Terminology (4th ed.). Chicago: American Medical Association.

Fischer, B. A., & Zigmond, M. J. (2010). The essential nature of sharing in science. *Science and Engineering Ethics, 16*(4), 783–799.

Fischl, B., Sereno, M. I., et al. (1999). Cortical surface-based analysis. II: Inflation, flattening, and a surface-based coordinate system. *NeuroImage, 9*(2), 195–207.

Fisk, A. D., Rogers, W. A., Charness, N., Czaja, S. J., & Sharit, J. (2009). *Designing for older adults: Principles and creative human factors approaches*. Boca Raton: CRC Press.

Fiszman, M., Rindflesch, T., & Kilicoglu, H. (2004). Summarization of an online medical encyclopedia. MEDINFO 2004. In *Proceedings of the Eleventh World Congress on Medical Informatics* (pp. 506–510). San Francisco.

Fitzmaurice, J. M., Adams, K., & Eisenberg, J. M. (2002). Three decades of research on computer applications in health care: Medical informatics support at the agency for healthcare research and quality. *Journal of the American Medical Informatics Association: JAMIA, 9*(2), 144–160.

Fleurant, M., Kell, R., Love, J., Jenter, C., Volk, L. A., Zhang, F., Bates, D. W., & Simon, S. R. (2011). Massachusetts e-Health Project increased physicians' ability to use registries, and signals progress toward better care. *Health Affairs (Millwood), 30*(7), 1256–1264.

Flexner, A. (1910). *Medical education in the united states and Canada: A report to the Carnegie foundation for the advancement of teaching*. New York: The Carnegie Foundation for the Advancement of Teaching. OCLC 9795002.

Flin, R., & Patey, R. (2009). Improving patient safety through training in non-technical skills. *British Medical Journal, 339*, B3595. doi:10.1136/Bmj.B3595.

FMRIDB Image Analysis Group. (2001). *FSL – The FMRIB Software Libarary*. From http://www.fmrib.ox.ac.uk/fsl/index.html

Foley, D.D., Van Dam, A., Feiner, S.K., Hughes, J.F. (1990). *Computer Graphics: Principles and Practice. Reading*, MA: Addison-Wesley.

Forsythe, D.E. (1992). Using ethnography to build a working system: rethinking basic design assumptions. *Proceedings Annual Symposium Computer Applications in Medical Care*, 505–509.

Forsythe, D. E., Buchanan, B. G., Osheroff, J. A., & Miller, R. A. (1992). Expanding the concept of medical information: An observational study of physicians' information needs. *Computers and Biomedical Research, 25*, 181–200.

Foster, K.R. (2010, Spring). Telehealth in Sub-Saharan Africa. In *IEEE Technology and Society Magazine* (pp. 42–49).

Fougerousse, F., Bullen, P., et al. (2000). Human-mouse differences in the embryonic expression of developmental control genes and disease genes. *Human Molecular Genetics, 9*(2), 165–173.

Foulonneau, M., & Riley, J. (2008). *Metadata for digital resources: Implementation, systems design and interoperability*. New York: Neal-Schuman Publishers.

Fowler, F. J., Levin, C. A., & Sepucha, K. R. (2011). Informing and involving patients to improve the quality of medical decisions. *Health Affairs (Millwood), 30*(4), 699–706.

Fox, C. (1992). Lexical analysis and stop lists. In W. Frakes & R. Baeza-Yates (Eds.), *Information retrieval: Data structures and algorithms* (pp. 102–130). Englewood Cliffs: Prentice-Hall.

Fox, J. (1993). Decision support systems as safety-critical components: Towards a safety culture for medical informatics. *Methods of Information in Medicine, 32*, 345–348.

Fox, P. T. (Ed.) (2001). *Human brain mapping*. New York: Wiley.

Fox, S. (2011). *Health topics*. Washington, D.C.: Pew Internet & American Life Project. Retrieved from http://www.pewinternet.org/~/media//Files/Reports/2011/PIP_HealthTopics.pdf

Frackowiak, R. S. J., Friston, K. J., et al. (Eds.). (1997). *Human brain function*. New York: Academic Press.

Frakes, W. (1992). Stemming algorithms. In W. Frankes & R. Baeza-Yates (Eds.), *Information retrieval: Data structures and algorithms* (pp. 131–160). Englewood Cliffs: Prentice-Hall.

Frank, S.J. (1988). What AI practitioners should know about the law. *AI Magazine*. Part One 9:63–75; Part Two 9:109–114.

Franken, E. A., Jr., Berbaum, K. S., Marley, S. M., Smith, W. L., Sato, K., Kao, S. C., & Milam, S. G. (1992). Evaluation of a digital workstation for interpreting neonatal examinations. A receiver operating characteristic study. *Investigative Radiology, 27*, 732–737.

Franklin, K. B. J., & Paxinos, G. (1997). *The mouse brain in stereotactic coordinates*. San Diego: Academic Press.

Fred, M., Vawdrey, D., et al. (2009). *Enhancing a commercial electronic health record with a novel patient handoff application*. In Society of Hospital Medicine (SHM) Annual Meeting, Chicago, IL.

Frederiksen, C. H. (1975). Representing logical and semantic structure of knowledge acquired from discourse. *Cognitive Psychology, 7*(3), 371–458.

Frenk, J. (2010). The global health system: Strengthening national health systems as the next step for global progress. *PLoS Medicine, 7*(1), e1000089.

Frenk, J., Chen, L., Bhutta, Z. A., Cohen, J., Crisp, N., Evans, T., Fineberg, H., et al. (2010). Health professionals for a new century: Transforming education to strengthen health systems in an interdependent world. *The Lancet, 376*(9756), 1923–1958.

Freton A, Finger P. T. (2012). Spectral domain-optical coherence tomography analysis of choroidal osteoma. *The British Journal of Ophthalmology, 96(2)*, 224–8.

Friede, A., & O'Carroll, P. W. (1998). Public health informatics. In R. B. Wallace (Ed.), *Public health and preventive medicine* (14th ed., pp. 59–65). Stamford: Appleton & Lange.

Friede, A., McDonald, M. C., & Blum, H. (1995). Public health informatics: How information-age technology can strengthen public health. *Annual Review of Public Health, 16*, 239–252.

Friedman, C. P. (1994). The research we should be doing. *Academic Medicine, 69*(6), 455–457.

Friedman, C. P. (1995). Where's the science in medical informatics? *Journal of the American Medical Informatics Association: JAMIA, 2*(1), 65–67.

Friedman, T.L. (2007). *The world is flat: a brief history of the twenty-first century* (1st further updated and expanded hardcover ed.). New York: Farrar, Straus and Giroux.

Friedman, C. P. (2009). A "fundamental theorem" of biomedical informatics. *Journal of the American Medical Informatics Association: JAMIA, 16*(2), 169–170.

Friedman, C. P., & Abbas, U. L. (2003, March). Is medical informatics a mature science? A review of measurement practice in outcome studies of clinical systems. *International Journal of Medical Informatics, 69*(2–3), 261–272.

Friedman, B., & Dieterle, M. (1987). The impact of the installation of a local area network on physicians and the laboratory information system in a large teaching hospital. In *Proceedings of the 11th annual symposium on Computer Applications in Medical Care* (pp. 783–788), Washington, D.C.

Friedman, C., & Hripcsak, G. (1998). Evaluating natural language processors in the clinical domain. *Methods Inf Med, 37(4–5)*, 334–44.

Friedman, C. P., & Wyatt, J. C. (2005). *Evaluation methods in biomedical informatics* (2nd ed.). New York: Springer-Publishing, p. 386. ISBN 0-387-25889-2.

Friedman, C., Hripcsak, G., Johnson, S. B., Cimino, J. J., & Clayton, P. D. (1990). A generalized relational schema for an integrated clinical patient database. In R. A. Miller (Ed.), *Proceedings of the 14th annual SCAMC* (pp. 335–339). Los Alamitos: IEEE Computer Soc. Press.

Friedman, C., Alderson, P. O., Austin, J., Cimino, J. J., & Johnson, S. B. (1994). A general natural language text processor for clinical radiology. *Journal of the American Medical Informatics Association: JAMIA, 1*(2), 161–174.

Friedman, C., Huff, S. M., Hersh, W. R., Pattison-Gordon, E., & Cimino, J. J. (1995). The canon group's effort: Working toward a merged model. *Journal of the American Medical Informatics Association: JAMIA, 2*(1), 4–18.

Friedman, C., Kra, P., Krauthammer, M., Yu, H., & Rzhetsky, A. (2001). GENIES: A natural-langauge processing system for the extraction of molecular pathways from journal articles. *Bioinformatics, 17*(suppl), S74–S82.

Friedman, C., Shagina, L., Lussier, Y., & Hripcsak, G. (2004). Automated encoding of clinical documents based on natural language processing. *Journal of the American Medical Informatics Association: JAMIA, 11*(5), 392–402.

Friedman, C. P., Wong, A. K., & Blumenthal, D. (2010). Achieving a nationwide learning health system. *Science Translational Medicine, 2*(57), 57cm29.

Friefeld, O., Greenspan, H., et al. (2009). Multiple sclerosis lesion detection using constrained GMM and curve evolution. *Journal of Biomedical Imaging, 2009*, 1–13.

Fries, J. F. (1974). Alternatives in medical record formats. *Medical Care, 12*(10), 871–881.

Frisse, M. E., King, J. K., Rice, W. B., et al. (2008). A regional health information exchange: Architecture and implementation. *American Medical Informatics Association Annual Symposium Proceedings, 2008*, 212–216.

Frisse, M. E., Johnson, K., Nian, H., et al. (2011). The financial impact of health information exchange on emergency department care. *Journal of the American Medical Informatics Association: JAMIA, 19*(3), 328–333.

Friston, K. J., Holmes, A. P., et al. (1995). Statical parametric maps in functional imaging: A general linear approach. *Human Brain Mapping, 2*, 189–210.

Frost, J. H., & Massagli, M. P. (2008). Social uses of personal health information within PatientsLikeMe, an online patient community: What can happen when patients have access to one another's data. *Journal of Medical Internet Research, 10*(3), e15.

Frueh, F. W., & Gurwitz, D. (2004). From pharmacogenetics to personalized medicine: A vital need for educating health professionals and the community. *Pharmacogenomics, 5*, 571–579.

Fuchs, V. R., & Milstein, A. (2011). The $640 billion question–why does cost-effective care diffuse so slowly? *The New England Journal of Medicine, 364*(21), 1985–1987.

Fukuda, K., Tamura, A., Tsunoda, T., & Takagi, T. (1998). Toward information extraction: identifying protein names from biological papers. *Proceedings of the Pacific Symposium on Biocomputing*, 707–718.

Fung, K. W., Xu, J., Rosenbloom, S. T., et al. (2011). Testing three problem list terminologies in a simulated data entry environment. *American Medical Informatics Association Annual Symposium Proceeds, 2011*, 445–454.

Funk, M., & Reid, C. (1983). Indexing consistency in MEDLINE. *Bulletin of the Medical Library Association, 71*, 176–183.

Funk, M., Winkler, C. G., May, J. L., Stephens, K., Fennie, K. P., Rose, L. L., Turkman, Y. E., & Drew, B. J. (2010). Unnecessary arrhythmia monitoring and underutilization of ischemia and QT interval monitoring in current clinical practice: Baseline results of the practice Use of the latest standards for electrocardiography trial. *Journal of Electrocardiology, 43*, 542–547. PMID 20832819.

Gaba, D. M. (2004). The future vision of simulation in health care. *Quality & Safety in Health Care, 13*(Suppl 1), i2–i10.

Gabril, M. Y., & Yousef, G. M. (2010). Informatics for practicing anatomical pathologists: Marking a new era in pathology practice. *Modern Pathology, 23*(3), 349–358.

Galbraith, D. W. (2006). The daunting process of MIAME. *Nature, 444*(7115), 31.

Galperin, M., & Cochrane, G. (2011). The 2011 nucleic acids research database issue and the online molecular biology database collection. *Nucleic Acids Research, 39*(suppl1), D1–D6.

Gamazon, E. R., Huang, R. S., Cox, N. J., & Dolan, M. E. (2010). Chemotherapeutic drug susceptibility associated SNPs are enriched in expression quantitative trait loci. *Proceedings of the National Academy of Sciences of the United States of America, 107*, 9287–9292.

Garcia-Molina, H., Ullman, J. D., & Widom, J. D. (2002). *Database systems: The complete book.* Englewood Cliffs: Prentice-Hall.

Garcia-Molina, H., Ullman, J. D., & Widom, J. D. (2008). *Database systems: The complete book* (2nd ed.). Englewood Cliffs: Prentice-Hall.

Gardner, H. (1985). *The mind's new science: A history of the cognitive revolution.* New York: Basic Books.

Gardner, R. M. (1996). Accuracy and reliability of disposable pressure transducers coupled with modern pressure monitors. *Critical Care Medicine, 24*, 879–882. PMID 8706469.

Gardner, R. M. (2004). Computerized clinical decision-support in respiratory care. *Respiratory Care, 49*, 378–386. PMID 15030611.

Gardner, R.M. (2009). Clinical decision support systems: the fascination with closed-loop c control. *IMIA Yearbook of Medical Informatics*, 12–21. PMID 19855866.

Gardner, R. M., & Beale, R. J. (2009). Pressure to perform: Is cardiac output estimation from arterial waveforms good enough for routine use? *Critical Care Medicine, 37*, 337–338. EDITORIAL PMID 19112291.

Gardner, R. M., & Lundsgaarde, H. P. (1994). Evaluation of user acceptance of a clinical expert system. *Journal of the American Medical Informatics Association: JAMIA, 1*(6), 428–438.

Gardner, R. M., & Shabot, M. M. (2001). Computer-based patient-record systems. In E. H. Shortliffe & L. E. Perreault (Eds.), *Patient-monitoring systems* (2nd ed., pp. 443–485). New York: Springer Verlag.

Gardner, R. M., Warner, H. R., Toronto, A. F., & Gaisford, W. D. (1970). Cather-flush system for continuous monitoring of central arterial pulse waveform. *Journal of Applied Physiology, 29*, 911–913. PMID 5485368.

Gardner, R. M., Tariq, H., Hawley, W. L., & East, T. D. (1989). Medical information bus: The key to future integrated monitoring. *International Journal of Clinical Monitoring and Computing, 6*, 197–204. PMID 2628508.

Gardner, R. M., Hawley, W. H., East, T. D., Oniki, T., & Young, H. F. W. (1991). Real time data acquisition: Experience with the medical information bus (MIB). *Proceedings of the Annual Symposium on Computer Applications in Medical Care, 15*, 813–817. PMID 1807719.

Gardner, R. M., Pryor, T. A., & Warner, H. R. (1999). The HELP system: Update 1998. *International Journal of Medical Informatics, 54*, 169–182. PMID 10405877.

Gardner, R. M., Overhage, J. M., Steen, E., Holmes, J. H., Williamson, J. J., Detmer, D. E., & AMIA Board of Directors. (2009). Core content for the subspecialty of clinical informatics. *Journal of the American Medical Informatics Association: JAMIA, 16*, 153–157. PMID 19074296.

Garg, A. X., Adhikari, N. K. J., McDonald, H., et al. (2005). Effects of computerized clinical decision support systems on practitioner performance and patient outcomes: A systematic review. *Journal of the American Medical Association, 293*(10), 1223–1238.

Garten, Y., & Altman, R. B. (2009). Pharmspresso: A text mining tool for extraction of pharmacogenomic concepts and relationships from full text. *BMC Bioinformatics, 10*(Suppl 2), S6.

Garten, Y., Coulet, A., & Altman, R. B. (2010). Recent progress in automatically extracting information from the pharmacogenomic literature. *Pharmacogenomics, 11*, 1467–1489.

Gaschnig, J., Klahr, P., Pople, H., Shortliffe, E., & Terry, A. (1983). Evaluation of expert systems: Issues and case studies. In F. Hayes-Roth, D. A. Waterman, & D.

Lenat (Eds.), *Building expert systems*. Reading: Addison Wesley.

Gawande, A. (2009). *The checklist manifesto: How to get things right*. New York: Metropolitan Books.

Ge, D., Ruzzo, E. K., Shianna, K. V., et al. (2011). SVA: Software for annotating and visualizing sequenced human genomes. *Bioinformatics, 27*, 1998–2000.

Geissbuhler, A. J., & Miller, R. A. (1997). Desiderata for product labeling of medical expert systems. *International Journal of Medical Informatics, 47*(3), 153–163.

Gennari, J.H., Musen, M.A., Fergerson, R.W., Grosso, W.E., Crubézy, M., Eriksson, H., Noy, N.F., & Tu, S.W. (2003). The evolution of Protégé: an environment for knowledge-based systems development. *International Journal of Human–Computer Studies, 58*(1):89–123.

George, J. S., Aine, C. J., et al. (1995). Mapping function in human brain with magnetoencephalography, anatomical magnetic resonance imaging, and functional magnetic resonance imaging. *Journal of Clinical Neurophysiology, 12*(5), 406–431.

Gerstner, E. R., & Sorensen, A. G. (2011). Diffusion and diffusion tensor imaging in brain cancer. *Seminars in Radiation Oncology, 21*(2), 141–146.

Ghazvinian, A., Noy, N. F., & Musen, M. A. (2009). Creating mappings for ontologies in biomedicine: Simple methods work. *AMIA Annual Symposium Proceedings, 2009*, 198–202.

Ghazvinian, A., Noy, N. F., & Musen, M. A. (2011). How orthogonal are the OBO foundry ontologies? *Journal of Biomedical Semantics, 2*(Suppl 2), S2.

Gibson, K., & Scheraga, H. (1967). Minimization of polypeptide energy. I. Preliminary structures of bovine pancreatic ribonuclease S-peptide. *Proceedings of the National Academy of Sciences, 58*(2), 420–427.

Giger, M., & MacMahon, H. (1996). Image processing and computer-aided diagnosis. *Radiologic Clinics of North America, 34*(3), 565–596.

Giles, J. (2005). Internet encyclopaedias go head to head. *Nature, 438*, 900–901. Retrieved from http://www.nature.com/nature/journal/v438/n7070/full/438900a.html

Gillan, D. J., & Schvaneveldt, R. W. (1999). Applying cognitive psychology: Bridging the gulf between basic research and cognitive artifacts. In F. T. Durso, R. Nickerson, R. Schvaneveldt, S. Dumais, M. Chi, & S. Lindsay (Eds.), *Handbook of applied cognition* (pp. 3–31). Chichester/New York: Wiley.

Ginsburg, G. S., & Willard, H. F. (2009). Genomic and personalized medicine: Foundations and applications. *Translational Research, 154*, 277–287.

Giuse, D. A., & Mickish, A. (1996). Increasing the availability of the computerized patient record. *Proceedings of the AMIA Annual Fall Symposium, 1996*, 633–637.

Glaser, R. (Ed.). (2000). *Advances in instructional psychology: Education design and cognitive science* (Vol. 5). Mahwah: Lawrence Erlbaum and Associates.

Glaser, J. (2010). HITECH lays the foundation for more ambitious outcomes-based reimbursement. *The American Journal of Managed Care, 16*(12), SP19–SP23.

Goddard, K., Roudsari, A., & Wyatt, J. C. (2012). Automation bias: A systematic review of frequency, effect mediators, and mitigators. *Journal of the American Medical Informatics Association: JAMIA, 19*, 121–127.

Goetz, T. (2010). Sergey Brin's search for a Parkinson's cure. *Wired*, June 22

Goffman, E. (1959). *The presentation of self in everyday life*. Garden City: Doubleday.

Goh, K. I., Cusick, M. E., Valle, D., et al. (2007). The human disease network. *Proceedings of the National Academy of Sciences of the United States of America, 104*, 8685–8690.

Gold, J. D., & Ball, M. J. (2007). The health record banking imperative: A conceptual model. *IBM Systems Journal, 46*(1), 43–55.

Gold, M. R., Siegel, J. E., Russell, L. B., & Weinstein, M. C. (Eds.). (1996). *Cost effectiveness in health and medicine*. New York: Oxford University Press.

Goldberg, A. D., Allis, C. D., et al. (2007). Epigenetics: A landscape takes shape. *Cell, 128*(4), 635–638.

Goldberg, S. N., Grassi, C. J., et al. (2009). Image-guided tumor ablation: Standardization of terminology and reporting criteria. *Journal of Vascular and Interventional Radiology, 20*(7 Suppl), S377–S390.

Goldstein, M.K., Hoffman, B.B., Coleman, R.W., Musen, M.A., Tu, S.W., Advani, A., Shankar, R.D., O'Connor, M. (2000). Implementing clinical practice guidelines while taking account of evidence: ATHENA, an easily modifiable decision-support system for management of hypertension in primary care. In *Proceedings of the Annual AMIA Fall Symposium* (pp. 300–304). Philadelphia: Hanley & Belfus.

Goldzweig, C. L., Towfigh, A., Maglione, M., & Shekelle, P. G. (2009). Costs and benefits of health information technology: new trends from the literature. *Health Affairs (Millwood), 28*(2), w282–w293.

Gombas, P., Skepper, J. N., et al. (2004). Past, present and future of digital pathology. *Orvosi Hetilap, 145*(8), 433–443.

Gonzalez, R. C., Woods, R. E., et al. (2009). *Digital image processing using MATLAB*. S.I., Gatesmark Publishing. Natick, MA.

Gooch, P., & Roudsari, A. (2011). Computerization of workflows, guidelines, and care pathways: A review of implementation challenges for process-oriented health information systems. *Journal of the American Medical Informatics Association: JAMIA, 18*, 738–748.

Goodman, K. W. (1996). Ethics, genomics and information retrieval. *Computers in Biology and Medicine, 26*, 223–229.

Goodman, K. W. (1998a). Bioethics and health informatics: An introduction. In K. W. Goodman (Ed.), *Ethics, computing, and medicine: Informatics and the transformation of health care* (pp. 1–31). Cambridge: Cambridge University Press.

Goodman, K. W. (1998b). Outcomes, futility, and health policy research. In K. W. Goodman (Ed.), *Ethics, computing, and medicine: Informatics and the transformation of health care* (pp. 116–138). Cambridge: Cambridge University Press.

Goodman, K. W. (2000). Using the web as a research tool. *MD Computing, 17*(5), 13–14.

Goodman, K. W., & Cava, A. (2008). Bioethics, business ethics, and science: Bioinformatics and the future of healthcare. *Cambridge Quarterly of Healthcare Ethics, 17*(4), 361–372.

Goodman, K. W., Berner, E. S., Dente, M. A., Kaplan, B., Koppel, R., Rucker, D., Sands, D. Z., & Winkelstein, P. (2010). Challenges in ethics, safety, best practices, and oversight regarding HIT vendors, their customers, and patients. *Journal of the American Medical Informatics Association: JAMIA, 18*(1), 77–81.

Goodwin, J. O., & Edwards, B. S. (1975). Developing a computer program to assist the nursing process: Phase I – from systems analysis to an expandable program. *Nursing Research, 24*, 299–305.

Gorges, M., Markewitz, B. A., & Westenskow, D. R. (2009). Improving alarm performance in the medical intensive care unit using delays and clinical context. *Anesthesia and Analgesia, 108*, 1546–1552. PMID19372334.

Gorman, P., & Helfand, M. (1995). Information seeking in primary care: how physicians choose which clinical questions to pursue and which to leave unanswered. *Medical Decision Making, 15*, 113–119.

Goroll, A. H., Simon, S. R., Tripathi, M., Ascenzo, C., & Bates, D. W. (2009). Community-wide implementation of health information technology: The Massachusetts eHealth collaborative experience. *Journal of the American Medical Informatics Association: JAMIA, 16*(1), 132–139.

Gorry, G. A., & Barnett, G. O. (1968). Sequential diagnosis by computer. *JAMA : The Journal of the American Medical Association, 205*(12), 849–854.

Gottschalk, A., & Flocke, S. A. (2005). Time spent in face-to-face patient care and work outside the examination room. *Annals of Family Medicine, 3*(6), 488–493.

Granger, R. (2004). *The National Programme for Information Technology (NPfIT). Given at MEDINFO 2004 (San Francisco, CA).* Available at http://www.nhiiadvisors.com/slides/GrangerMedinfo 2004.ppt. Accessed 17 Dec 2012.

Grant, R. W., Wald, J. S., Poon, E. G., Schnipper, J. L., Gandhi, T. K., Volk, L. A., et al. (2006). Design and implementation of a web-based patient portal linked to an ambulatory care electronic health record: Patient gateway for diabetes collaborative care. *Diabetes Technology & Therapeutics, 8*(5), 576–586.

Grau, B., Horrocks, I., et al. (2008). Chapter 3: Description logics. In B. Porter, V. Lifschitz, & F. Van Harmelen (Eds.), *Handbook of knowledge representation* (Vol. 28, p. 1005). Amsterdam/Boston: Elsevier.

Gray Southon, F. C., Sauer, C., & Grant, C. N. (2004). Information technology in complex health services: Organizational impediments to successful technology transfer and diffusion. *Journal of the American Medical Informatics Association: JAMIA, 11*(2), 104–112.

Gray, J. E., Safran, C., Davis, R. B., Pompilio-Weitzner, G., Stewart, J. E., Zaccagnini, L., & Pursley, D. (2000). Baby CareLink: Using the internet and telemedicine to improve care for high-risk infants. *Pediatrics, 106*, 1318–1324.

Green, E. D., & Guyer, M. S. (2011). Charting a course for genomic medicine from base pairs to bedside. *Nature, 470*(7333), 204–213.

Green, B. B., Cook, A. J., Ralston, J. D., et al. (2008). Effectiveness of home blood pressure monitoring, web communication, and pharmacist care on hypertension control: A randomized controlled trial. *Journal of the American Medical Association, 299*(24), 2857–2867.

Green, R. C., Roberts, J. S., Cupples, L. A., et al. (2009). Disclosure of APOE genotype for risk of Alzheimer's disease. *The New England Journal of Medicine, 361*, 245–254.

Greenberg, M. D., Ridgely, M. S., & Hillestad, R. J. (2009). Crossed wires: how yesterday's privacy rules might undercut tomorrow's nationwide health information network. *Health Affairs (Millwood), 28*(2), 450–452.

Greenes, R. (1989, June). The radiologist as clinical activist: A time to focus outward. *Paper presented at the Proc First Internat Conf on Image Management and Communication in Patient Care: Implementation and Impact (IMAC 89),* Los Alamitos, CA.

Greenes, R. A. (Ed.). (2007). *Clinical decision support: The road ahead.* Burlington: Elsevier Inc.

Greenes, R. A., & Brinkley, J. F. (2001). Computer-based patient-record systems. In E. H. Shortliffe & L. E. Perreault (Eds.), *Patient-monitoring systems* (2nd ed., pp. 485–538). New York: Springer.

Greenes, R. A., & Shortliffe, E. H. (1990). Medical informatics: An emerging academic discipline and institutional priority. *Journal of the American Medical Association, 263*(8), 1114–1120.

Greenes, R. A., Barnett, G. O., Klein, S. W., Robbins, A., & Prior, R. E. (1970). Recording, retrieval, and review of medical data by physician-computer interaction. *The New England Journal of Medicine, 282*(6), 307–315.

Greenhalgh, T., Stramer, K., Bratan, T., Byrne, E., Russell, J., & Potts, H. W. W. (2010). Adoption and non-adoption of a shared electronic summary record in England: A mixed-method case study. *BMJ, 340*, c3111.

Greeno, J. G., & Simon, H. A. (1988). Problem solving and reasoning. In R. C. Atkinson & R. J. Herrnstein (Eds.), *Stevens' handbook of experimental psychology Vol 1: Perception and motivation; Vol 2: Learning and cognition* (2nd ed., Vol. 1, pp. 589–672). New York: Wiley.

Greenspan, H., & Pinhas, A. T. (2007). Medical image categorization and retrieval for PACS using the GMM-KL framework. *IEEE Transactions on Information Technology in Biomedicine, 11*(2), 190–202.

Greenspan, H., Ruf, A., et al. (2006). Constrained Gaussian mixture model framework for automatic segmentation of MR brain images. *IEEE Transactions on Medical Imaging, 25*(9), 1233–1245.

Greenspan, H., Avni, U., et al. (2011). X-ray categorization and retrieval on the organ and pathology level, using patch-based visual words. *IEEE Transactions on Medical Imaging, 30*(3), 733–746.

Gregg, R. E., Zhou, S. H., Lindauer, J. M., Helfendbein, E. D., & Giuliano, K. K. (2008). What is inside the electrocardiograph? *Journal of Electrocardiology, 41*, 8–14. PMID 1819652.

Gregory, S. (2011). Personal communication.

Grimm, R. H., Shimoni, K., Harlan, W. R., & Estes, E. H. J. (1975). Evaluation of patient-care protocol use by various providers. *The New England Journal of Medicine, 282*(10), 507–511.

Grishman, R., & Kittredge, R. (Eds.). (1986). *Analyzing language in restricted domains: Sublanguage description and processing.* Hillsdale: Erlbaum Associates.

Grishman, R., & Sundheim, B. (1996). Message Understanding Conference-6: A Brief History. In COLING, *96*, 466–471.

Grishman, R., Sager, N., Raze, C., & Bookchin, B. (1973). The linguistic string parser. *Proceedings of the National Computer Conference, 42*, 427–434.

Grosz, B., Joshi, A., & Weinstein, S. (1995). Centering: A framework for modeling the local coherence of discourse. *Computational Linguistics, 2*(21), 203–225.

Groves, R. H., Jr., Holcomb, B. W., Jr., & Smith, M. L. (2008). Intensive care telemedicine: Evaluating a model for proactive remote monitoring and intervention in the critical care setting. *Studies in Health Technology and Informatics, 131*, 131–146. PMID 18305328.

Grunfeld, A., & Ho, K. (1997). An internet primer, part II: Tools of the internet. *The Journal of Emergency Medicine, 15*(3), 401–404.

Grunfeld, A., Ho, K., & Walls, R. (1996). The internet: What's all the fuss about? *The Journal of Emergency Medicine, 14*(6), 769–770.

Guglin ME, Thatai D. Common errors in computer electrocardiogram interpretation. Int J Cardiol 2006; 106: 232–7. PMID 16321696.

Guide to Community Preventive Services. (2010). *Universally recommended vaccinations: immunization information systems.* Atlanta: Guide to Community Preventive Services. Available at http://www.thecommunityguide.org/vaccines/universally/imminfosystems.html. Accessed 29 Nov 2012.

Gur, D., & Sumkin, J. (2006). CAD in screening mammography. *AJR. American Journal of Roentgenology, 187*, 1474. 10.2214.

Gurses, A. P., & Xiao, Y. (2006). A systematic review of the literature on multidisciplinary rounds to design information systems. *Journal of the American Medical Informatics Association: JAMIA, 13*, 267–278. PMID 16501176.

Gusfield, D. (1997). *Algorithms on strings, trees and sequences: Computer science and computational biology.* Cambridge: Cambridge University Press.

Haddow, G., Bruce, A., Sathanandam, S., & Wyatt, J. C. (2011). 'Nothing is really safe': A focus group study on the processes of anonymizing and sharing of health data for research purposes. *Journal of Evaluation in Clinical Practice, 17*, 1140–1146.

Hagen, P. T., Turner, D., Daniels, L., & Joyce, D. (1998). Very large-scale distributed scanning solution for automated entry of patient information. *TEPR Proceedings (Toward an ElectronicPatient Record), 1*, 228–232.

Hagglund, M., Chen, R., & Koch, S. (2011). Modeling shared care plans using CONTsys and openEHR to support shared homecare of the elderly. *Journal of the American Medical Informatics Association: JAMIA, 18*(1), 66–69.

Hahn, U., Romacker, M., & Schulz, S. (1999). Discourse structures in medical reports – watch out! the generation of referentially coherent and valid text knowledge bases in the MEDSYNDIKATE system. *International Journal of Medical Informatics, 53*(1), 1–28.

Hahn, U., Romacker, M., & Schulz, S. (2002). MEDSYNDIKATE: A natural language system for the extraction of medical information from finding reports. *International Journal of Medical Informatics, 67*(1/3), 63–74.

Haislmaier, E.F. (2006). *Health care information technology: getting the policy right.* Available at http://www.heritage.org/Research/Reports/2006/06/Health-Care-Information-Technology-Getting-the-Policy-Right. Accessed 17 Dec 2012.

Halamka, J. D. (2010). Making the most of federal health information technology regulations. *Health Affairs (Millwood), 29*(4), 596–600.

Halamka, J. D., & Safran, C. (1998). CareWeb: A web-based medical record for an integrated healthcare delivery system. *Proceedings of Medinfo 1998, Part 1*, 36–39.

Halamka, J. D., Mandl, K. D., & Tang, P. C. (2008). Early experiences with personal health records. *Journal of the American Medical Informatics Association: JAMIA, 15*(1), 1–7.

Hamburg, M. A., & Collins, F. S. (2010). The path to personalized medicine. *The New England Journal of Medicine, 363*(4), 301–304.

Han, Y. Y., Carcillo, J. A., Venkataraman, S. T., Clark, R. S. B., Watson, R. S., Nguyen, T. C., Bayir, H., & Orr, R. A. (2005). Unexpected increased mortality after implementation of a commercially sold computerized physician order entry system. *Pediatrics, 116*(6), 1506–1512.

Hansell, D. M., Bankier, A. A., et al. (2008). Fleischner society: Glossary of terms for thoracic imaging. *Radiology, 246*(3), 697–722.

Hansen, L. K., Nielsen, F. A., et al. (1999). Lyngby – modeler's Matlab toolbox for spatio-temporal analysis of functional neuroimages. *NeuroImage, 9*(6), S241.

Hansen, N. T., Brunak, S., & Altman, R. B. (2009). Generating genome-scale candidate gene lists for pharmacogenomics. *Clinical Pharmacology and Therapeutics, 86*, 183–189.

Haralick, R. M. (1988). *Mathematical morphology.* Seattle: University of Washington.

Haralick, R. M., & Shapiro, L. G. (1992). *Computer and robot vision.* Reading: Addison-Wesley.

Harkema, H., Dowling, J. N., Thornblad, T., & Chapman, W. W. (2009). ConText: An algorithm for determining negation, experiencer, and temporal status from clinical reports. *Journal of Biomedical Informatics, 42*(5), 839–851.

Harmonizing State Privacy Law Collaborative. (2009). *Harmonizing state privacy law. Office of the National Coordinator of Health Information Technology.* Washington, DC.

Harney, A. S., & Meade, T. J. (2010). Molecular imaging of in vivo gene expression. *Future Medicinal Chemistry, 2*(3), 503–519.

Harris, Z. 1982. A grammar of English on mathematical principles. Wiley New York.

Harris, M. A. et al., for the Gene Ontology Consortium. (2004). The Gene Ontology (GO) database and informatics resource. *Nucleic Acids Research, 32* (Database issue) D258-6.

Harris, Z. (1991). *A theory of language and information – a mathematical approach.* New York: Oxford University Press.

Harris Interactive. (2007). *Many U.S. adults are satisfied with use of their personal health records.* Available at: http://www.harrisinteractive.com/vault/Harris-Interactive-Poll-Research-Health-Privacy-2007-03.pdf. Accessed 17 Dec 2012.

Harris, Z., Gottfried, M., Ryckman, T., Mattick, P., Daladier, A., Harris, T., & Harris, S. (1989). *The form of information in science – analysis of an immunology sublanguage.* Dordrecht: Kluwer Academic.

Harris, T.W., Lee, R., Schwarz, E., et al. (2003) WormBase: a cross-species database for comparative genomics. *Nucleic Acids Research, 31*:133–137. Available at http://www.wormbase.org

Harris, P. A., Taylor, R., Thielke, R., Payne, J., Gonzalez, N., & Conde, J. G. (2009). Research electronic data capture (REDCap)–a metadata-driven methodology and workflow process for providing translational research informatics support. *Journal of Biomedical Informatics, 42*(2), 377–381.

Harrison, M. I., Koppel, R., & Bar-Lev, S. (2007). Unintended consequences of information technologies in health care–an interactive sociotechnical analysis. *Journal of the American Medical Informatics Association: JAMIA, 14*(5), 542–549.

Hart, J., McBride, A., Blunt, D., Gishen, P., & Strickland, N. (2010). Immediate and sustained benefits of a "total" implementation of speech recognition reporting. *The British Journal of Radiology, 83*(989), 424–427.

Harter, S. (1992). Psychological relevance and information science. *Journal of the American Society for Information Science, 43*, 602–615.

Hartung, C., Anokwa, Y., Brunette, W., Lerer, A., Tseng, C., & Borriello, G. (2010). Open data kit: Tools to build information services for developing regions. *International Conference on Information and Communication Technologies and Development (ICTD2010) Proceedings.* http://www.gg.rhul.ac.uk/ict4d/ictd2010/papers/ICTD2010%20Hartung%20et%20al.pdf. Accessed 2 Jan 2012.

Hartzband, P., & Groopman, J. (2008). Off the record—avoiding the pitfalls of going electronic. *The New England Journal of Medicine, 358*(16), 1656–1658.

Hasan, K. M., Walimuni, I. S., et al. (2010). A review of diffusion tensor magnetic resonance imaging computational methods and software tools. *Computers in Biology and Medicine, 41*(12), 1062–1072.

Hassan, E., Badawi, O., Weber, R. J., & Cohen, H. (2010). Using technology to prevent adverse drug events in the intensive care unit. *Critical Care Medicine, 38*(6 Suppl), S97–S105. PMID 20502181.

Hassol, A., Walker, J. M., Kidder, D., Rokita, K., Young, D., Pierdon, S., et al. (2004). Patient experiences and attitudes about access to a patient electronic health care record and linked web messaging. *Journal of the American Medical Informatics Association: JAMIA, 11*(6), 505–513.

Hastie, T., Tibshirani, R., et al. (2009). *The elements of statistical learning: Data mining, inference, and prediction.* New York: Springer.

Haug, P. J., Ranum, D. L., & Frederick, P. R. (1990). Computerized extraction of coded findings from free-text radiology reports. *Radiology, 174*, 543–548.

Haug, P., Koehler, S., Lau, L.M., Wang, P., Rocha, R., & Huff, S. (1994). A natural language understanding system combining syntactic and semantic techniques. *Proceedings of the Annual Symposium on Computer Applications in Medical Care*, 247–251.

Haupt, M. T., Bekes, C. E., Brilli, R. J., Carl, L. C., Gray, A. W., Jastremski, M. S., Naylor, D. F., & Wedel, S. K. (2003). Guidelines on critical care services and personnel: Recommendations based on a system of categorization of thee levels of care. *Critical Care Medicine, 31*, 2877–2883. PMID 14805541.

Haynes, R. B. (2002). What kind of evidence is it that Evidence-Based Medicine advocates want health care providers and consumers to pay attention to? BMC Health Services Research. 2:3. http://www.biomedcentral.com/1472-6963/2/3.

Haynes, R.B. (Ed.) (2011). Computerized clinical decision support systems: how effective are they? [article collection] *Implementation Science, 6*, 87–108. Articles available at: http://www.implementationscience.com/series/CCDSS. Accessed 2 Jan 2012.

Haynes, R., McKibbon, K., Walker, C., Ryan, N., Fitzgerald, D., & Ramsden, M. (1990). Online access to MEDLINE in clinical settings. *Annals of Internal Medicine, 112*, 78–84.

Haynes, R., Wilczynski, N., McKibbon, K., Walker, C., & Sinclair, J. (1994). Developing optimal search strategies for detecting clinically sound studies in MEDLINE. *Journal of the American Medical Informatics Association: JAMIA, 1*, 447–458.

Haynes, R. B., Wilczynski, N. L., & Computerized Clinical Decision Support System (CCDSS) Systematic Review Team. (2010). Effects of computerized clinical decision support systems on practitioner performance and patient outcomes: Methods of a decision-maker-researcher partnership systematic review. *Implementation Science: IS, 5*, 12.

Hazlehurst, B., McMullen, C., Gorman, P., & Sittig, D. (2003). How the ICU follows orders: Care delivery as a complex activity system. *AMIA Annual Symposium Proceedings, 2003*, 284–288. D030003599 [pii].

Hazlehurst, B., McMullen, C. K., & Gorman, P. N. (2007). Distributed cognition in the heart room: how situation awareness arises from coordinated communications during cardiac surgery. *Journal of Biomedical Informatics, 40*(5), 539–551. doi:10.1016/j.jbi.2007.02.001. S1532-0464(07)00008-1 [pii].

Health Information Technology for Economic and Clinical Health (HITECH) Act, Title XIII of Division A and Title IV of Division B of the American Recovery and Reinvestment Act of 2009 (ARRA).(2009).

Health IT Standards Committee. (2011). *Recommendations to ONC on the assignment of code sets to clinical concepts [data elements] for use in quality measures. [Letter]*. Retrieved from http://www.healthit.gov/sites/default/files/standards-certification/HITSC_CQMWG_VTF_Transmit_090911.pdf. Accessed 3 Jan 2012.

Health Record Banking Alliance. (2006). http://www.healthbanking.org. Accessed 17 Dec 2012.

Health Record Banking Alliance. (2008). *Principles and fact sheet*. Available at http://www.healthbanking.org/docs/HRBAPrinciples & Fact Sheet 2008 FINAL.pdf. Accessed 17 Dec 2012.

Health Record Banking Alliance. (2012). *Health record banking: a foundation for myriad health information sharing models*. Available at http://www.healthbanking.org/docs/HRBABusiness Model White Paper Dec 2012.pdf. Accessed 17 Dec 2012.

Health Record Banking Alliance [2013]. A Proposed National Infrastructure for HIE Using Personally Controlled Records. Available at http://www.healthbanking.org/docs/HRBA%20Architecture%20White%20Paper%20Jan%202013.pdf. Accessed 7 Sep 2013.

Heath, B., Salerno, R., Hopkins, A., et al. (2009). Pediatric critical care telemedicine in rural underserved emergency departments. *Pediatric Critical Care Medicine, 10*, 588–591.

Heckerman, D., & Horvitz, E. (1986). The myth of modularity in rule-based systems for reasoning with uncertainty. In J. Lemmer & L. Kanal (Eds.), *Uncertainty in artificial intelligence 2*. Amersterdam: North Holland.

Heikamp, K., & Bajorath, J. (2011). Large-scale similarity search profiling of ChEMBL compound data sets. *Journal of Chemical Information and Modeling, 51*, 1831–1839.

Heiss, W. D., & Phelps, M. E. (Eds.). (1983). *Positron emission tomography of the brain*. Berlin/New York: Springer.

Held, K., Rota Kops, E., et al. (1997). Markov random field segmentation of brain MR images. *IEEE Transactions on Medical Imaging, 16*(6), 878–886.

Hellmich, M., Abrams, K. R., & Sutton, A. J. (1999). Bayesian approaches to meta-analysis of ROC curves. *Medical Decision Making, 19*, 252–264.

Henchley, A. (2003). Understanding Version 3. *A primer on the HL7 Versison 3 Communication Standard*. Munich:

Alexander Moench Publishing Co. Easily readable overview of HL7 Version 3 messaging standard.

Henderson, M. (2003). *HL7 messaging*. Silver Spring: OTech Inc.

Hennessy, J. L., & Patterson, D. A. (1996). *Computer architecture: A quantitative approach* (2nd ed.). San Francisco: Morgan Kaufmann.

Henriksen, K. (2008). *Understanding adverse events: A human factors framework. In H. R.G. (Ed.), patient safety and quality: An evidence-based handbook for nurses* (pp. 84–101). Rockville: Agency for Healthcare Research and Quality.

Henriksen, K. (2010). Partial truths in the pursuit of patient safety. *BMJ Quality & Safety Health Care, 19*(3), i3–i7.

Henry (Bakken), S. B., & Mead, C. N. (1997). Nursing classification systems: Necessary but not sufficient for representing "what nurses do" for inclusion in computer-based patient record systems. *Journal of the American Medical Informatics Association: JAMIA, 4*(3), 222–232.

Herasevich, V., Yilmaz, M., Khan, H., Hubmayr, R. D., & Gajic, O. (2009). Validation of an electronic surveillance system for acute lung injury. *Intensive Care Medicine, 35*, 1018–1023. PMID 19280175.

Herasevich, V., Pickering, B. W., Dong, Y., Peters, S. G., & Gajic, O. (2010). Informatics infrastructure for syndromic surveillance, decision support, reporting, and modeling of critical illness. *Mayo Clinic Proceedings, 85*, 247–254. PMID 21194152.

Herasevich, V., Afessa, B., & Pickering, B. W. (2011). Sepsis in critically ill patients with trauma. *Critical Care Medicine, 39*, 876–879. PMID 21613830.

Hersh, W. (1994). Relevance and retrieval evaluation: Perspectives from medicine. *Journal of the American Society for Information Science, 45*, 201–206.

Hersh, W. (1999). "A world of knowledge at your fingertips": the promise, reality, and future directions of on-line information retrieval. *Academic Medicine, 74*, 240–243.

Hersh, W. (2001). Interactivity at the text retrieval conference (TREC). *Information Processing and Management, 37*, 365–366.

Hersh, W. (2004). Healthcare information technology: Progress and barriers. *JAMA : The Journal of the American Medical Association, 292*, 2273–2274.

Hersh, W. (2009). *Information retrieval: A health and biomedical perspective* (3rd ed.). New York: Springer.

Hersh, W., & Hickam, D. (1995). An evaluation of interactive Boolean and natural language searching with an on-line medical textbook. *Journal of the American Society for Information Science, 46*, 478–489.

Hersh, W., & Hickam, D. (1998). How well do physicians use electronic information retrieval systems? A framework for investigation and review of the literature. *Journal of the American Medical Association, 280*, 1347–1352.

Hersh, W., & Rindfleisch, T. (2000). Electronic publishing of scholarly communication in the biomedical sciences. *Journal of the American Medical Informatics Association: JAMIA, 7*, 324–325.

Hersh, W., & Voorhees, E. (2009). TREC genomics special issue overview. *Information Retrieval, 12*, 1–15.

Hersh, W., Pentecost, J., & Hickam, D. (1996). A task-oriented approach to information retrieval evaluation. *Journal of the American Society for Information Science, 47*, 50–56.

Hersh, W., Crabtree, M., Hickam, D., et al. (2002). Factors associated with success for searching MEDLINE and applying evidence to answer clinical questions. *Journal of the American Medical Informatics Association: JAMIA, 9*, 283–293.

Hersh, W., Bhupatiraju, R., Ross, L., Johnson, P., Cohen, A., & Kraemer, D. (2006). Enhancing access to the bibliome: the TREC 2004 Genomics Track. *Journal of Biomedical Discovery and Collaboration, 1, 3*. Retrieved from http://www.j-biomed-discovery.com/content/1/1/3

Hersh, W., Muller, H., et al. (2009). The ImageCLEFmed medical image retrieval task test collection. *Journal of Digital Imaging, 22*(6), 648–655.

Hey, T., Tansley, S., & Tolle, K. (Eds.). (2009). *The fourth paradigm: Data-intensive scientific discovery*. Redmond: Microsoft Research.

Hickam, D. H., Shortliffe, E. H., Bischoff, M. B., Scott, A. C., Jacobs, C. D. (1985). The treatment advice of a computer-based cancer chemotherapy protocol advisor. *Annals of Internal Medicine, 103*(6 Pt 1), 928–936.

Hilgard, E. R., & Bower, G. H. (1975). *Theories of learning* (4th ed.). Englewood Cliffs: Prentice-Hall.

Hillestad, R., Bigelow, J., Bower, A., Girosi, F., Meili, R., Scoville, R., & Taylor, R. (2005). Can electronic medical record systems transform health care? Potential health benefits, savings, and costs. *Health Affairs, 24*, 1103–1117.

Himmelstein, D. U., & Woolhandler, S. (2010). Obama's reform: no cure for what ails us. *BMJ, 340*, c1778.

Hinshaw, K. P., Poliakov, A. V., et al. (2002). Shape-based cortical surface segmentation for visualization brain mapping. *NeuroImage, 16*(2), 295–316.

Hirschman, L., Yeh, A., Blaschke, C., & Valencia, A. (2005). Overview of BioCreAtIvE: Critical assessement of information extraction for biology. *BMC Bioinformatics, 6*(Suppl 1), S1.

Hirschorn, D., & Dreyer, K. (2006, April 27–30). *Comparison of consumer grade displays to medical grade displays for the primary interpretation of radiography*. Paper presented at the Society for Computer Applications in Radiology, Austin.

Hobbs, J. R., Appelt, D. E., Bear, J., Israel, D., Kameyama, M., Stickel, M., et al. (1996). FASTUS: A cascaded finite-state transducer for extracting information from natural-language text. In *Finite state devices for natural language processing*. Cambridge, MA: MIT Press.

Hoffman, R. R. (Ed.). (1992). *The psychology of expertise: Cognitive research and empirical AI*. Mahwah: Lawrence Erlbaum Associates.

Hoffman, M. A. (2007). The genome-enabled electronic medical record. *Journal of Biomedical Informatics, 40*, 44–46.

Hoffman, J. M., & Gambhir, S. S. (2007). Molecular imaging: The vision and opportunity for radiology in the future. *Radiology, 244*(1), 39–47.

Hoffman, M. A., & Williams, M. S. (2011). Electronic medical records and personalized medicine. *Human Genetics, 130*(1), 33–39.

Hoffman, R. R., Shadbolt, N. R., Burton, A. M., & Klein, G. (1995). Eliciting knowledge from experts – a methodological analysis. *Organizational Behavior and Human Decision Processes, 62*(2), 129–158.

Hohne, K., Bomans, M., et al. (1990). 3-D visualization of tomographic volume data using the generalized voxel model. *The Visual Computer, 6*(1), 28–36.

Hohne, K.H., Bomans, M., et al. (1992). A volume-based anatomical atlas. *IEEE Computer Graphics and Applications*, 72–78.

Hohne, K. H., Pflesser, B., et al. (1995). A new representation of knowledge concerning human anatomy and function. *Nature Medicine, 1*(6), 506–510.

Holden, R. J., & Karsh, B. (2007). A review of medical error reporting system design considerations and a proposed cross-level systems research framework. *Human Factors, 49*, 257–276.

Holford, N. H., Kimko, H. C., Monteleone, J. P., & Peck, C. C. (2000). Simulation of clinical trials. *Annual Review of Pharmacology and Toxicology, 40*, 209–234.

Hollingsworth, J. C., Chisholm, C. D., Giles, B. K., Cordell, W. H., & Nelson, D. R. (1998). How do physicians and nurses spend their time in the emergency department? *Annals of Emergency Medicine, 31*, 87–91.

Holroyd-Leduc, J. M., Lorenzetti, D., Straus, S. E., Sykes, L., & Quan, H. (2011). The impact of the electronic medical record on structure, process and outcomes within primary care: A systematic review of the evidence. *Journal of the American Medical Informatics Association: JAMIA, 18*, 732–737.

Homer, N., Szelinger, S., Redman, M., et al.(2008). Resolving individuals contributing trace amounts of DNA to highly complex mixtures using high-density SNP genotyping microarrays. *PLoS Genetics, 4*(8), e1000167.

Homerova, D., Sprusansky, O., Kutejova, E., & Kormanec, J. (2002). Some features of DNA-binding proteins involved in the regulation of the Streptomyces aureofaciens gap gene, encoding glyceraldehyde-3-phosphate dehydrogenase. *Folia Microbiologica (Praha), 47*, 311–317.

Hood, L., & Friend, S. H. (2011). Predictive, personalized, preventive, participatory (P4) cancer medicine. *Nature Reviews. Clinical Oncology, 8*, 184–187.

Horii, S.C. (1996). *Image acquisition: Sites, technologies and approaches*. In Greenes, R.A. and Bauman,

R.A. (eds.) Imaging and information management: computer systems for a changing health care environment. *The Radiology Clinics of North America, 34*(3):469-494.

Horrigan, J. B., Rainie, L., & Fox, S. (2001). *Online communities: Networks that nurture long-distance relationships and local ties*. Washington, D.C: Pew Internet & American Life Project.

Horsky, J., Kaufman, D. R., & Patel, V. L. (2003a). The cognitive complexity of a provider order entry interface. *AMIA Annual Symposium Proceedings*, 294–298. doi:D030003723 [pii].

Horsky, J., Kaufman, D. R., Oppenheim, M. I., & Patel, V. L. (2003b). A framework for analyzing the cognitive complexity of computer-assisted clinical ordering. *Journal of Biomedical Informatics, 36*(1-2), 4–22.

Horsky, J., Kuperman, G. J., & Patel, V. L. (2005). Comprehensive analysis of a medication dosing error related to CPOE. *Journal of the American Medical Informatics Association: JAMIA, 12*(4), 377–382. doi:10.1197/jamia.M1740. M1740 [pii].

House, E. (1980). *Evaluating with validity*. San Francisco: Sage.

Hoy, J. D., & Hyslop, A. Q. (1995). Care planning as a strategy to manage variation in practice: From care planning to integrated person-based record. *Journal of the American Medical Informatics Association: JAMIA, 2*(4), 260–266.

Hripcsak, G., & Wilcox, A. (2002). Reference standards, judges, and comparison subjects: Roles for experts in evaluating system performance. *Journal of the American Medical Informatics Association: JAMIA, 9*(1), 1–15.

Hripcsak, G., Ludemann, P., Pryor, T. A., Wigertz, O. B., & Clayton, P. D. (1994). Rationale for the Arden syntax. *Computers and Biomedical Research, 27*, 291–324.

Hripcsak, G., Friedman, C., Alderson, P. O., DuMouchel, W., Johnson, S. B., & Clayton, P. D. (1995). Unlocking data from narrative reports: A study of natural language processing. *Annals of Internal Medicine, 122*(9), 681–688.

Hripcsak, G., Kuperman, G. J., et al. (1998). Extracting findings from narrative reports: Software transferability and sources of physician disagreement. *Methods of Information in Medicine, 37*(1), 1–7.

Hripcsak, G., Cimino, J. J., & Sengupta, S. (1999). WebCIS: Large scale deployment of a web-based clinical information system. *Proceedings of the Annual AMIA Symposium, 1999*, 804–808.

Hripcsak, G., Vawdrey, D., Fred, M., & Bostwick, S. (2011). Use of electronic clinical documentation: Time spent and team interactions. *Journal of the American Medical Informatics Association: JAMIA, 18*(1), 112–117.

Hripcsak, G., Soulakis, ND., Li, L., Morrison, FP., Lai, AM., Friedman, C., Calman, NS., Mostashari, F. (2009) Syndromic surveillance using ambulatory electronic health records. *Journal of the American Medical Informatics Association: JAMIA, 16*(3):354–61. doi: 10.1197/jamia.M2922. Epub 2009 Mar 4.

Hsi-Yang Fritz, M., Leinonen, R., Cochrane, G., & Birney, E. (2011). Efficient storage of high throughput DNA sequencing data using reference-based compression. *Genome Research, 21*, 734–740. http://healthit.hhs.gov/portal/server.pt/gateway/PTARGS_0_12811_955546_0_0_18/HITSC_CQMWG_VTF_Transmit_090911.pdf

Hu, Z., Abramoff, M. D., et al. (2010a). Automated segmentation of neural canal opening and optic cup in 3D spectral optical coherence tomography volumes of the optic nerve head. *Investigative Ophthalmology and Visual Science, 51*(11), 5708–5717.

Hu, Z., Niemeijer, M., et al. (2010b). Automated segmentation of 3-D spectral OCT retinal blood vessels by neural canal opening false positive suppression. *Medical Image Computing and Computer Assisted Intervention, 13*(Pt 3), 33–40.

Hudson, D. L., & Cohen, M. E. (2009). Multidimensional medical decision making. *Conference Proceedings – IEEE Engineering in Medicine and Biology Society, 1*, 3405–3408.

Hudson, H. E., & Parker, E. B. (1973). Medical communication in Alaska by satellite. *The New England Journal of Medicine, 289*, 1351–1356.

Hudson, K. L., Holohan, M. K., & Collins, F. S. (2008). Keeping pace with the times–the Genetic Information Nondiscrimination Act of 2008. *The New England Journal of Medicine, 358*, 2661–2663.

Humphreys, B. L. (Ed.). (1990). *UMLS knowledge sources – first experimental edition documentation*. Bethesda: National Library of Medicine.

Humphreys, B., Lindberg, D., Schoolman, H., & Barnett, G. (1998). The unified medical language system: An informatics research collaboration. *Journal of the American Medical Informatics Association: JAMIA, 5*, 1–11.

Humphreys, K., Demetriou, G., & Gaizauskas, R. (2000). Two applications of information extraction to biological science journal articles: enzyme interactions and protein structures. *Proceedings of the Pacific Symposium on Biocomputing*, 505–516.

Hunt, D. L., Haynes, R. B., et al. (1998). Effects of computer-based clinical decision support systems on physician performance and patient outcomes: A systematic review. *JAMA : The Journal of the American Medical Association, 280*(15), 1339–1346.

Hutchins, E. (1995). *Cognition in the wild*. Cambridge, MA: MIT Press.

Iezzoni, L. I. (1990). Using administrative diagnostics data to assess the quality of hospital care: Pitfalls and potential of ICD-9-CM. *International Journal of Technology Assessment in Health Care, 6*(2), 272–281.

Imai, K., Kricka, L. J., & Fortina, P. (2011). Concordance study of 3 direct-to-consumer genetic-testing services. *Clinical Chemistry, 57*(3), 518–521.

Imhoff, M., & Kuhls, S. (2006). Alarm algorithms in critical care monitoring. *Anesthesia and Analgesia, 102*, 1525–1537. PMID 16632837.

Institute of Medicine. (1988). *The future of public health*. Washington, DC: National Academy Press.

Institute of Medicine. (1991). *The computer-based patient record: An essential technology for patient care.* Washington, DC: National Academy Press.

Institute of Medicine. (1999). *Committee on quality of health care in America. To Err is human: Building a safer health care system.* Washington, DC: National Academy Press.

Institute of Medicine. (2003). *Patient safety: Achieving a new standard for care.* Washington, D.C.: National Academy Press.

Institute of Medicine. (2007). *The learning healthcare system: Workshop summary.* Washington, DC: National Academies Press.

Institute of Medicine. (2011a). *Engineering a learning healthcare system: A look at the future.* Washington, DC: National Academies Press.

Institute of Medicine. (2011b). *Health IT and patient safety: Building safer systems for better care.* Washington: The National Academies Press.

Institute of Medicine. (2011c). *Digital infrastructure for the learning health system: The foundation for continuous improvement in health and healthcare* (Workshop series summary). Washington: The National Academies Press.

Institute of Medicine. (2012). *Best care at lower cost: The path to continuously learning health care in America.* Washington, DC: National Academies Press.

Institute of Medicine (IOM) Committee on Improving the Patient Record. (1997). *The Computer-Based Patient Record: An essential technology for healthcare* (revised edition) Dick, R.S., Steen E.B., & Detmer, D.E. (Eds.), Washington: National Academy Press. Available at: http://www.iom.edu/Reports/1997/The-Computer-Based-Patient-Record-An-Essential-Technology-for-Health-Care-Revised-Edition.aspx. Accessed 2 Jan 2012.

Institute of Medicine (IOM) Committee on Improving the Patient Record. (2001). *Crossing the Quality Chasm: A New Health System for the 21st Century.* Washington, D.C.: National Academy Press. Available at: http://www.iom.edu/Reports/2001/Crossing-the-Quality-Chasm-A-New-Health-System-for-the-21st-Century.aspx. Accessed 2 Jan 2012.

International Anatomical Nomenclature Committee. (1989). *Nomina anatomica.* Edinburgh: Churchill Livingstone.

International Classification of Primary Care. (1998). Singapore: World Organization of National Colleges, Academies and Academic Associations of General Practitioners/Family Physicians.

International Health Terminology Standards Development Organization. (2011). *SNOMED CT (Systematized Nomenclature of Medicine-Clinical Terms).* Retrieved August 31, 2011, from http://www.ihtsdo.org/

International Standards Organization 1087. (2000). *Terminology work – Vocabulary.* (ISO 1087-1:2000): International Standards Organization. Geneva, Switzerland.

International Standards Organization. (1987). *Information processing systems-Concepts and terminology for the conceptual schema and the information base.* (ISO TR 9007:1987): International Standards Organization. Geneva, Switzerland.

InTouch Health. Available at: http://www.intouchhealth.com. Accessed 6 May 2011.

Irwin, J. J., & Shoichet, B. K. (2005). ZINC–a free database of commercially available compounds for virtual screening. *Journal of Chemical Information and Modeling, 45,* 177–182.

Isaac, T., Weissman, J., Davis, R., Massagli, M., Cyrulik, A., Sands, D., & Weingart, S. (2009). Overrides of medication alerts in ambulatory care. *Archives of Internal Medicine, 169*(3), 305.

Issel-Tarver, L., Christie, K.R., Dolinski, K., Andrada, R., Balakrishnan, R., Ball, C.A., Binkley, G., Dong, S., Dwight, S.S., Fisk, D.G., Harris, M., Schroeder, M., Sethuraman, A., Tse, K., Weng, S., Botstein, D., & Cherry, J.M. (2001). Saccharomyces genome database. *Methods Enzymol, 350,* 329–346. Available at http://www.yeastgenome.org/

Ivers, M.T., Timson, G.F., von Blankensee, H., Whitfield, G., Keltz, P.D., & Pfeil, C.N. (1983). Large scale implementation of compatible hospital computer systems within the Veterans Administration. *Proceedings of the Sixth Annual Symposium on Computer Applications in Medical Care,* 53–56.

Jadad, A. (1999). Promoting partnerships: Challenges for the internet age. *British Medical Journal, 319,* 761–764.

James, B. C., & Savitz, L. A. (2011). How intermountain trimmed health care costs through robust quality improvement efforts. *Health Affairs (Millwood), 30*(6), 1185–1191.

Janamanchi, B., Katsamakas, E., Raghupathi, W., & Gao, W. (2009). The state and profile of open source software projects in health and medical informatics. *International Journal of Medical Informatics, 78*(2009), 457–472.

Jaspers, M. W. (2009). A comparison of usability methods for testing interactive health technologies: Methodological aspects and empirical evidence. *International Journal of Medical Informatics, 78*(5), 340–353.

Jaspers, M. W., Smeulers, M., Vermeulen, H., & Peute, L. W. (2011). Effects of clinical decision-support systems on practitioner performance and patient outcomes: A synthesis of high-quality systematic review findings. *Journal of the American Medical Informatics Association: JAMIA, 18*(3), 327–334.

Jenders, R. A. (2008). Suitability of the Arden syntax for representation of quality indicators. *AMIA Annual Symposium Proceedings, 6,* 991.

Jenders, R.A., & Shah, A. (2001). Challenges in using the Arden Syntax for computer-based nosocomial infection surveillance. *Proceedings of the AMIA Symposium,* 289–293.

Jenssen, T.K., & Vinterbo, S. (2000). A set-covering approach to specific search for literature about human genes. *Proceedings of the AMIA Symposium,* 384–388.

Jewett, A. I., Huang, C. C., & Ferrin, T. E. (2003). MINRMS: An efficient algorithm for determining protein structure similarity using root-mean-squared-distance. *Bioinformatics, 19*(5), 625–634.

Jha, A. K., Doolan, D., Grandt, D., Scott, T., & Bates, D. W. (2008). The use of health information technology in seven nations. *International Journal of Medical Informatics, 77*(12), 848–854.

Jha, A. K., DesRoches, C. M., Campbell, E. G., Donelan, K., Rap, S. R., Ferris, T. G., Shields, A., Rosenbaum, S., & Blumenthal, D. (2009). Use of electronic health records in U.S. Hospitals. *The New England Journal of Medicine, 360*, 1628–1638. PMID 19321858.

Jha, A. K., Prasopa-Plaizier, N., Larizgoitia, I., & Bates, D. W. (2010). Patient safety research: An overview of the global evidence. *Quality & Safety in Health Care, 19*(1), 42–47. doi:10.1136/qshc.2008.029165.

Jiang, Y.-G., Ngo C.-W, et al. (2007). Towards optimal bag-of-features for object categorization and semantic video retrieval. In *Proceedings of the 6th ACM international conference on Image and video retrieval* (pp. 494–501), Amsterdam: ACM.

Jimison, H. B., Pavel, M., Larimer, N., & Mullen, P. (2007) A general architecture for computer based health coaching. In *Proceedings of the International Conference on Technology & Aging*, Toronto.

Johnson, S. B. (2000). Natural language processing in biomedicine. In J. D. Bronzino (Ed.), *The handbook of biomedical engineering* (p. 188-1-6). Boca Raton: CRC Press.

Johnson, K.A., & Becker, J.A. (2001). *The whole brain atlas.* From http://www.med.harvard.edu/AANLIB/home.html

Johnson, S.B., Friedman, C., Cimino, J.J., Clark, T., Hripcsak, G., & Clayton, P.D. (1991). Conceptual data model for a central patient database. *Proceedings of the Symposium on Computer Applications in Medical Care*, 381–385.

Johnson, P.D., Tu, S.W., Musen, M.A., & Purves, I. (2001a). A virtual medical record for guideline-based decision support. In *Proceedings of the AMIA Annual Symposium*, 294–298, Washington, DC.

Johnson, K. B., Ravert, R. D., & Everton, A. (2001c). Hopkins teen central: Assessment of an internet-based support system for children with cystic fibrosis. *Pediatrics, 107*(2), E24.

Johnson, S. B., Bakken, S., Dine, D., Hyun, S., Mendonca, E., Morrison, F., et al. (2008). An electronic health record based on structured narrative. *Journal of the American Medical Informatics Association: JAMIA, 15*(1), 54–64.

Johnston, D., Pan, E., Walker, J., Bates, D. W., & Middleton, B. (2003). *The value of computerized provider order entry in ambulatory settings.* Boston: Center for Information Technology Leadership, Partners Healthcare.

Jollis, J. G., Ancukiewicz, M., DeLong, E. R., Pryor, D. B., Muhlbaier, L. H., & Mark, D. B. (1993). Discordance of databases designed for claims payment versus clinical information systems. Implications for outcomes research. *Annals of Internal Medicine, 119*(8), 844–850.

Jones, S. S., Heaton, P. S., Rudin, R. S., & Schneider, E. C. (2012). Unraveling the IT productivity paradox — lessons for health care. *The New England Journal of Medicine, 366*(24), 2243–2245.

Jonquet, C., Musen, M. A., & Shah, N. H. (2010). Building a biomedical ontology recommender web service. *Journal of Biomedical Semantics, 1*(Suppl 1), S1.

Jonquet, C., LePendu, P., Falconer, S., Coulet, A., Noy, N. F., Musen, M. A., & Shah, N. H. (2011). NCBO resource index: Ontology-based search and mining of biomedical resources. *Journal of Web Semantics: Science, Services and Agents on the World Wide Web, 9*(3), 316–324.

Jordan, D. A., McKeown, K. R., Concepcion, K. J., Feiner, S. K., & Hatzivassiloglou, V. (2001). Generation and evaluation of intraoperative inferences for automated health care briefings on patient status after bypass surgery. *Journal of the American Medical Informatics Association: JAMIA, 8*(3), 267–280.

Joshi-Tope, G., Gillespie, M., Vastrik, I., et al. (2005). Reactome: A knowledgebase of biological pathways. *Nucleic Acids Research, 33*, D428–D432.

Joyce, V. R., Barnett, P. G., Bayoumi, A. M., Griffin, S. C., Kyriakides, T. C., Yu, W., Sundaram, V., Holodniy, M., Brown, S. T., Cameron, W., Youle, M., Sculpher, M., Anis, A. H., & Owens, D. K. (2009). Health-related quality of life in a randomized trial of antiretroviral therapy for advanced HIV disease. *Journal of the Acquired Immunodeficiency Syndrome, 50*, 27–36.

Joyce, V. R., Barnett, P. G., Chow, A., Bayoumi, A. M., Griffin, S. C., Sun, H., Holodniy, M., Brown, S. T., Cameron, D. W., Youle, M., Sculpher, M., Anis, A. H., & Owens, D. K. (2012). Effect of treatment interruption and intensification of antiretroviral therapy on health-related quality of life in patients with advanced HIV: A randomized controlled trial. *Medical Decision Making, 32*, 70–82.

Juni, P., Altman, D. G., & Egger, M. (2001). Systematic reviews in health care: Assessing the quality of controlled clinical trials. *British Medical Journal, 323*(7303), 42–46.

Jurafsky, D., & Martin, J. H. (2009). *Speech and language processing. An introduction to natural language processing, computational linguistics and speech recognition.* Upper Saddle River: Prentice Hall.

Jurie, F., & Triggs, B. (2005). *Creating efficient codebooks for visual recognition.* Proceedings of the tenth IEEE international conference on Computer Vision (ICCV'05) Volume 1 – Volume 01, IEEE Computer Society: 604–610 %@ 600-7695-2334-X-7601.

Kaelber, D., & Pan, E.C. (2008). The value of personal health record (phr) systems. *AMIA Annual Symposium Proceedings*, 343–347.

Kaelber, D. C., et al. (2008). *The value of personal health records. Center for information technology leadership, partners healthcare (Boston)* (p. 52). Chicago: Health Information Management and Systems Society.

Kahn, J. M. (2011a). The use and misuse of ICU telemedicine. *Editorial JAMA, 305*, 2176–2183. PMID 21576623.

Kahn, S. D. (2011b). On the future of genomic data. *Science, 331*(6018), 728–729.

Kahn, C. E., & Rubin, D. L. (2009). Automated semantic indexing of figure captions to improve radiology image retrieval. *Journal of the American Medical Informatics Association: JAMIA, 16*(3), 380–386.

Kahn, C. E., Roberts, L. M., Shaffer, K. A., & Haddawy, P. (1997). Construction of a Bayesian network for mammographic diagnosis of breast cancer. *Computers in Biology and Medicine, 27,* 19–29.

Kahn, C. E., Jr., Langlotz, C. P., et al. (2009). Toward best practices in radiology reporting. *Radiology, 252*(3), 852–856.

Kane, B., & Sands, D. Z. (1998). Guidelines for the clinical use of electronic mail with patients. *Journal of the American Medical Informatics Association: JAMIA, 5,* 104–111.

Kang, J. H., & Chung, J. K. (2008). Molecular-genetic imaging based on reporter gene expression. *Journal of Nuclear Medicine, 49*(Suppl 2), 164S–179S.

Kang, M. J., Lee, C. G., Cho, S. J., et al. (2006). IFN-gamma-dependent DNA injury and/or apoptosis are critical in cigarette smoke-induced murine emphysema. *Proceedings of the American Thoracic Society, 3,* 517–518.

Kaplan, B., & Harris-Salamone, K. D. (2009). Health IT success and failure: Recommendations from literature and an AMIA workshop. *Journal of the American Medical Informatics Association: JAMIA, 16,* 291–299.

Kapur, T., Grimson, W. E., et al. (1996). Segmentation of brain tissue from magnetic resonance images. *Medical Image Analysis, 1*(2), 109–127.

Karat, J. (1994). Workplace applications – tools for motivation and tools for control. *Information Processing '94, Vol Iii, 53,* 382–387.

Karplus, M., & Weaver, D. L. (1976). Protein-folding dynamics. *Nature, 260*(5550), 404–406.

Karr, J. R., Sanghvi, J. C., et al. (2012). A whole-cell computational model predicts phenotype from genotype. *Cell, 150*(2), 389–401.

Karsh, B.-T., Weinger, M. B., Abbott, P. A., & Wears, R. L. (2010). Health information technology: Fallacies and sober realities. *Journal of the American Medical Informatics Association: JAMIA, 17*(6), 617–623.

Kass, B. (2001). *Reducing and preventing adverse drug events to decrease hospital costs.* Research in Action, Issue 1. AHRQ Publication Number 01–0020. Available at http://www.ahrq.gov/qual/aderia/aderia.htm. Accessed 12 Aug 2011.

Kass, M., Witkin, A., et al. (1987). Snakes: Active contour models. *International Journal of Computer Vision, 1*(4), 321–331.

Kassirer, J.P., & Gorry, G.A. (1978). Clinical problem solving: A behavioral analysis. *Anns Int Med, 89*(2):245–255.

Kastor, J. (2001). *Mergers of teaching hospitals in Boston, New York, and Northern California.* Ann Arbor: University of Michigan Press.

Kato, P. M., & Beale, I. L. (2006). Factors affecting acceptability to young cancer patients of a psychoeducational video game about cancer. *Journal of Pediatric Oncology Nursing, 23*(5), 269–275.

Kaufman, D. R., Patel, V. L., & Magder, S. (1996). The explanatory role of spontaneously generated analogies in a reasoning about physiological concepts. *International Journal of Science Education, 18,* 369–386.

Kaufmann, A., Meltzer, M., & Schmid, G. (1997). The economic impact of a bioterrorist attack: Are prevention and post-attack intervention programs justifiable? *Emerging Infectious Diseases, 3*(2), 83–94.

Kaufman, D. R., Patel, V. L., Hilliman, C., Morin, P. C., Pevzner, J., Weinstock, R. S., Starren, J. (2003). Usability in the real world: assessing medical information technologies in patients' homes. *J Biomed Inform, 36*(1-2), 45–60.

Kaufman, D. R., Pevzner, J., Rodriguez, M., Cimino, J. J., Ebner, S., Fields, L., & Starren, J. (2009). Understanding workflow in telehealth video visits: Observations from the IDEATel project. *Journal of Biomedical Informatics, 42*(4), 581–592.

Kaushal, R., Shojania, K. G., & Bates, D. W. (2003). Effects of computerized physician order entry and clinical decision support systems on medication safety: A systematic review. *Archives of Internal Medicine, 163*(12), 1409–1416.

Kawamoto, K., Del Fiol, G., Strasberg, H.R., et al. (2010). Multi-national, multi-institutional analysis of clinical decision support data needs to inform development of the HL7 Virtual Medical Record standard. *AMIA Annual Symposium Proceedings*, 377–381.

Keiser, M. J., Setola, V., Irwin, J. J., et al. (2009). Predicting new molecular targets for known drugs. *Nature, 462,* 175–181.

Kelley, M. A., Angus, D., Chalfin, D. B., Crandall, E. D., Ingbar, D., Johanson, W., Medina, J., Sessler, C. N., & Vender, J. S. (2004). The critical care crisis in the united states: A report from the profession. *Chest, 125,* 1514–1517. PMID 15078767.

Kemper, A. R., Trotter, T. L., Lloyd-Puryear, M. A., Kyler, P., Feero, W. G., & Howell, R. R. (2010). A blueprint for maternal and child health primary care physician education in medical genetics and genomic medicine: Recommendations of the United States secretary for health and human services advisory committee on heritable disorders in newborns and children [Research Support, U.S. Gov't, P.H.S.]. *Genetics in Medicine: Official Journal of the American College of Medical Genetics, 12*(2), 77–80.

Kendall, D. B. (2009). Protecting patient privacy through health record trusts. *Health Affairs, 28*(2), 444–446.

Kennedy, D. (2001). *Internet brain segmentation repository.* From http://neuro-www.mgh.harvard.edu/cma/ibsr

Kennelly, R. J., & Gardner, R. M. (1997). Perspectives on development of IEEE 1073: The medical information bus (MIB) standard. *International Journal of Clinical Monitoring and Computing, 14*(3), 143–149.

Kent, H. (2001). Hands across the ocean for the world's first trans-Atlantic surgery. *CMAJ: Canadian Medical Association Journal, 13,* 1374.

Kent, W. J. (2003). BLAT – the BLAST-like alignment tool. *Genome Research, 12*(4), 656–664.

Keren, H., Burkhoff, D., & Squara, P. (2007). Evaluation of a non-invasive continuous cardiac output monitoring system based on thoracic bioreactance. *American Journal of Physiology - Heart and Circulatory Physiology, 293*, H583–H589. PMID 17384132.

Kershaw, A. (2003). Patient use of the internet to obtain health information. *Nursing Times, 99*(36), 30–32.

Keselman, A., Tse, T., Crowell, J., Browne, A., Ngo, L., & Zeng, Q. (2007). Assessing consumer health vocabulary familiarity: An exploratory study. *Journal of Medical Internet Research, 9*(1), e5.

Kevles, B. (1997). *Naked to the bone: Medical imaging in the twentieth century*. New Brunswick: Rutgers University Press.

Khajouei, R., & Jaspers, M. W. (2010). The impact of CPOE medication systems' design aspects on usability, workflow and medication orders: A systematic review. *Methods of Information in Medicine, 49*(1), 3–19.

Khatri, P., & Draghici, S. (2005). Ontological analysis of gene expression data: Current tools, limitations, and open problems. *Bioinformatics, 21*, 3587–3595.

Kho, A. N., Pacheco, J. A., Peissig, P. L., et al. (2011). Electronic medical records for genetic research: Results of the eMERGE consortium. *Science Translational Medicine, 3*, 79re71.

Kidd, M. R. (2008). Personal electronic health records: MySpace or HealthSpace? *British Medical Journal, 336*, 1029–1030.

Kilo, C. M., & Wasson, J. H. (2010). Practice redesign and the patient-centered medical home: History, promises, and challenges. *Health Affairs (Millwood), 29*(5), 773–778.

Kim, M., & Johnson, K. (2004). Patient entry of information: Evaluation of user interfaces [Comparative study]. *Journal of Medical Internet Research, 6*(2), e13.

Kim, J. H., Kohane, I. S., & Ohno-Machado, L. (2002). Visualiztion and evaluation of clusters for exploratory analysis of gene expression data. *Journal of Biomedical Informatics, 35*, 25–36.

Kim, J. D., Ohta, T., Tateisi, Y., & Tsujii, J. (2003). GENIA corpus – semantically annotated corpus for biotextmining. *Bioinformatics, 19*(suppl 1), i180–i182.

Kim, H., Dykes, P. C., Thomas, D., Winfield, L. A., & Rocha, R. A. (2011). A closer look at nursing documentation on paper forms: Preparation for computerizing a nursing documentation system. *Computational Biology in Medicine, 41*(4), 182–189.

Kimborg, D.Y., & Aguirre, G.K. (2002). *A flexible architecture for neuroimaging data analysis and presentation*. From http://www.nimh.nih.gov/neuroinformatics/kimberg.cfm

King, W., Proffitt, J., et al. (2000). The role of fluorescence in situ hybridization technologies in molecular diagnostics and disease management. *Molecular Diagnosis, 5*(4), 309–319.

Kinnings, S. L., Liu, N., Buchmeier, N., et al. (2009). Drug discovery using chemical systems biology: Repositioning the safe medicine Comtan to treat multi-drug and extensively drug resistant tuberculosis. *PLoS Computational Biology, 5*, e1000423.

Kintsch, W. (1998). *Comprehension: A paradigm for cognition*. Cambridge/New York: Cambridge University Press.

Kirkpatrick, D. L. (1994). *Evaluating training programs*. San Francisco: Berrett-Koehler.

Kittredge, R., & Lehrberger, J. (Eds.). (1982). *Sublanguage – studies of language in restricted semantic domains*. New York: De Gruyter.

Kleinke, J. D. (2005). Dot-gov: Market failure and the creation of a national health information technology system. *Health Affairs (Millwood), 24*(5), 1246–1262.

Kleinmuntz, B. (1968). Formal Representation of Human Judgment (Vol. 3). New York: Wiley.

Kleinmuntz, D. N., & Schkade, D. A. (1993). Information displays and decision-processes. *Psychological Science, 4*(4), 221–227.

Kleinmuntz, D. N., & Schkade, D. A. (1993). Information displays and decision-processes. *Psychological Science, 4*(4), 221–227.

Knaus, W. A., Wagner, D. P., & Lynn, J. (1991). Short-term mortality predictions for critically ill hospitalized adults: Science and ethics. *Science, 254*, 389–394.

Knox, C., Law, V., Jewison, T., et al. (2011). DrugBank 3.0: A comprehensive resource for 'omics' research on drugs. *Nucleic Acids Research, 39*, D1035–D1041.

Kohane, I. S. (2011). Using electronic health records to drive discovery in disease genomics. *Nature Reviews Genetics, 12*(6), 417–428.

Kohane, I. S., & Altman, R. B. (2005). Health-information altruists–a potentially critical resource. *The New England Journal of Medicine, 353*(19), 2074–2077.

Kohane, I., & Mandl, K. (2011). *SHARP research area three: substitutable medical apps, reusable technologies. Strategic Health IT Advanced Research Projects (SHARP) Program*. 2012, from http://healthit.hhs.gov/portal/server.pt/community/sharp:_area_3/3127/home/20707

Kohane, I. S., Churchill, S. E., & Murphy, S. N. (2011b). A translational engine at the national scale: Informatics for integrating biology and the bedside. *Journal of the American Medical Informatics Association: JAMIA, 19*(2), 181–185.

Kohn, L. T., Corrigan, J., & Donaldson, M. S. (2000). *To err is human: Building a safer health system*. Washington, D.C.: National Academy Press.

Kohn, L., Corrigan, J., & Donaldson, M. (Eds.). (2002). *To err is human: Building a safer health system. Institute of medicine*. Washington: National Academy Press.

Kolodner, R., & Douglas, J. V. (1997). *Computerizing large integrated health networks: The VA success*. New York: Springer.

Komaroff, A., Black, W., & Flatley, M. (1974). Protocols for physician assistants: Management of diabetes and hypertension. *The New England Journal of Medicine, 290*, 307–312.

Kong, Y. M., Dahlke, X., Xiang, Q., Qian, Y., Karp, D., & Scheuermann, R. H. (2011). Toward an ontology-based framework for clinical research databases. *Journal of Biomedical Informatics, 44*(1), 48–58.

Koppel, R., & Kreda, D. (2009). Health care information technology vendors' "hold harmless" clause: Implications for patients and clinicians. *Journal of the American Medical Association, 301*, 1276–1278.

Koppel, R., Metlay, J. P., Cohen, A., Abaluck, B., Localio, A. R., Kimmel, S. E., & Strom, B. L. (2005). Role of computerized physician order entry systems in facilitating medication errors. *JAMA : The Journal of the American Medical Association, 293*(10), 1197–1203.

Koreen, S., Gelman, R., Martinez-Perez, M. E., et al. (2007). *Ophthalmology, 114*, e59–e67.

Korner, M., Weber, C. H., et al. (2007). Advances in digital radiography: Physical principles and system overview. *Radiographics, 27*(3), 675–686.

Kosara, R., & Miksch, S. (2002). Visualization methods for data analysis and planning in medical applications. *International Journal of Medical Informatics, 68*(1–3), 141–153.

Koshy, S., Feustel, P. J., Hong, M., & Kogan, B. A. (2010). Scribes in an ambulatory urology practice: Patient and physician satisfaction. *Journal of Urology, 184*(1), 258–262.

Koslow, S. H., & Huerta, M. F. (Eds.). (1997). *Neuroinformatics: An overview of the human brain project.* Mahwah: Lawrence Erlbaum.

Kostyack, P. (2002). The emergence of the healthcare information trust. *Matrix: Journal of Law-Medicine, 12*(293), 339–447.

Kouwenhoven, W. B., Jude, J. R., & Knickerbocker, G. G. (1960). Closed-chest cardiac massage. *JAMA : The Journal of the American Medical Association, 173*, 1064–1067. PMID 14411374.

Kowalczyk, L. (2011). *Patient alarms often unheard, unheeded.* Boston Globe.

Kraus, V. B., Burnett, B., Coindreau, J., et al. (2011). Application of biomarkers in the development of drugs intended for the treatment of osteoarthritis. *Osteoarthritis and Cartilage, 19*, 515–542.

Kremkau, F. W. (2006). *Diagnostic ultrasound principles and instruments.* St. Louis: Saunders Elsevier.

Krishnaral, A., Lee, J., Laws, S., & Crawford, T. (2010). Voice recognition software: Effect on radiology report turnaround time at an academic medical center. *AJR. American Journal of Roentgenology, 195*(1), 194–197.

Krist, A., Woolf, S., & Rothemich, S. (2010). *Improving care through AHRQ health IT tools.* Retrieved July10, 2011, from http://www.ahrq.gov/about/annualconf10/krist_rosenthal/krist.HTM.

Krist, A. H., & Woolf, S. H. (2011). A vision for patient-centered health information systems. *JAMA : The Journal of the American Medical Association, 305*(3), 300–301.

Kuchenbecker, J., Dick, H. B., Schmitz, K., & Behrens-Baumann, W. (2001). Use of internet technologies for data acquisition in large clinical trials. *Telemedicine Journal of E-Health, 7*(1), 73–76.

Kuchinke, W., Aerts, J., Semler, S. C., & Ohmann, C. (2009). CDISC standard-based electronic archiving of clinical trials. *Medical Informatics and the Internet in Medicine, 48*(5), 408–413.

Kuhn, I.M., Wiederhold, G., Rodnick, J.E., et al. (1984). Automated ambulatory medical record systems in the U.S. In Blum, B. (Ed.), *Information Systems for Patient Care* (pp.199–217), New York: Springer. Original 1982 report available at: http://infolab.stanford.edu/TR/CS-TR-82-928.html. Accessed 2 Jan 2012.

Kuhn, M., Campillos, M., Letunic, I., Jensen, L. J., & Bork, P. (2010). A side effect resource to capture phenotypic effects of drugs. *Molecular Systems Biology, 6*, 343.

Kulikowski, C. A. (1997). Medical imaging informatics: Challenges of definition and integration. *Journal of the American Medical Informatics Association: JAMIA, 4*(3), 252–253.

Kulikowski, C. A., Shortliffe, E. H., et al. (2012) AMIA Board white paper: Definition of biomedical informatics and specification of core competencies for graduate education in the discipline. *Journal of the American Medical Informatics Association, 19*(6), 931–938.

Kulkarni, A., Aziz, B., Shams, I., & Busse, J. (2009). Comparisons of citations in web of science, Scopus, and Google scholar for articles published in general medical journals. *Journal of the American Medical Association, 302*, 1092–1096.

Kullo, I. J., Fan, J., Pathak, J., Savova, G. K., Ali, Z., & Chute, C. G. (2010). Leveraging informatics for genetic studies: use of the electronic medical record to enable a genome-wide association study of peripheral arterial disease. *Journal of the American Medical Informatics Association: JAMIA, 17*(5), 568–574.

Kuperman, G. J., & Gibson, R. F. (2003). Computer physician order entry: Benefits, costs, and issues. *Annals of Internal Medicine, 139*(1), 31–39.

Kuperman, G. J., Gardner, R. M., & Pryor, T. A. (1991). *HELP: A dynamic hospital information system.* New York: Springer.

Kurtzke, J. F. (1979). ICD-9: A regression. *American Journal of Epidemiology, 108*(4), 383–393.

Kush, R. D., Helton, E., Rockhold, F. W., & Hardison, C. D. (2008). Electronic health records, medical research, and the tower of Babel. *The New England Journal of Medicine, 358*(16), 1738–1740.

Kushniruk, A. W., Kaufman, D. R., Patel, V. L., Levesque, Y., & Lottin, P. (1996). Assessment of a computerized patient record system: A cognitive approach to evaluating medical technology. *MD Computing, 13*(5), 406–415.

Kushniruk, A. W., Triola, M. M., Borycki, E. M., Stein, B., & Kannry, J. L. (2005). Technology induced error and usability: The relationship between usability problems and prescription errors when using a handheld application. *International*

Journal of Medical Informatics, 74(7–8), 519–526. doi:10.1016/j.ijmedinf.2005.01.003. S1386-5056(05)00011-0 [pii].

Labkoff, S. E., & Yasnoff, W. A. (2007). A framework for systematic evaluation of health information infrastructure progress in communities. *Journal of Biomedical Informatics, 40*(2), 100–105.

Laine, C., Horton, R., DeAngelis, C., Drazen, J., Frizelle, F., Godlee, F., & Verheugt, F. (2007). Clinical trial registration: Looking back and moving ahead. *Journal of the American Medical Association, 298,* 93–94.

Lamb, A. (1955). *The Presbyterian Hospital and the Columbia-Presbyterian Medical Center, 1868–1943: A history of a great medical adventure.* New York: Columbia University Press.

Lamb, J. (2007). The connectivity map: A new tool for biomedical research. *Nature Reviews Cancer, 7*(1), 54–60.

Lamb, J., Crawford, E. D., Peck, D., et al. (2006). The connectivity map: Using gene-expression signatures to connect small molecules, genes, and disease. *Science, 313,* 1929–1935.

Lancet (1879). Practice by telephone. *Lancet, 114*(2985), 819.

Lander, E. S., Linton, L. M., Birren, B., et al. (2001). Initial sequencing and analysis of the human genome. *Nature, 409,* 860–921.

Landrigan, P. J., Trasande, L., Thorpe, L. E., et al. (2006). The National Children's Study: A 21-year prospective study of 100,000 American children. *Pediatrics, 118,* 2173–2186.

Lane, W. A. (1936, November). What the mouth reveals. *New Health, 11,* 34–35.

Langer, S. (2002). Impact of speech recognition on radiologist productivity. *Journal of Digital Imaging, 15*(4), 203–209.

Langer, S., Fetterly, K., Mandrekar, J., Harmsen, S., Bartholmai, B., Patton, C., et al. (2006). ROC study of four LCD displays under typical medical center lighting conditions. *Journal of Digital Imaging, 19*(1), 30–40.

Langheier, J. M., & Snyderman, R. (2004). Prospective medicine: The role for genomics in personalized health planning. *Pharmacogenomics, 5*(1), 1–8.

Langley, P., Laird, J. E., & Rogers, S. (2009). Cognitive architectures: Research issues and challenges. *Cognitive Systems Research, 10*(2), 141–160. doi: 10.1016/j.cogsys.2006.07.004.

Langlotz, C. P. (2006). RadLex: A new method for indexing online educational materials. *Radiographics, 26*(6), 1595–1597.

Langridge, R. (1974). Interactive three-dimensional computer graphics in molecular biology. *Federation Proceedings, 33*(12), 2332–2335.

Lapsia, V., Lamb, K., & Yasnoff, W. A. (2012). Where should electronic records for patients be stored? *International Journal of Medical Informatics, 81*(12), 821–827.

Larabell, C. A., & Nugent, K. A. (2010). Imaging cellular architecture with X-rays. *Current Opinion in Structural Biology, 20*(5), 623–631.

Larkin, J. H., & Simon, H. A. (1987). Why a diagram is (sometimes) worth 10000 words. *Cognitive Science, 11*(1), 65–99.

Larkin, J., McDermott, J., Simon, D. P., & Simon, H. A. (1980). Expert and novice performance in solving physics problems. *Science, 208*(4450), 1335–1342.

Larsen, R. A., Evans, R. S., Burke, J. P., Pestotnik, S. L., Gardner, R. M., & Classen, D. C. (1989). Improved perioperative antibiotic Use and reduced surgical wound infections through use of computer decision analysis. *Infection Control and Hospital Epidemiology, 10*(7), 316–320.

Lashkari, D. A., DeRisi, J. L., McCusker, J. H., Namath, A. F., Gentile, C., Hwang, S. Y., Brown, P. O., & Davis, R. W. (1997). Yeast microarrays for genome wide parallel genetic and gene expression analysis. *Proceedings of the National Academy of Sciences, 94*(24), 13057–13062.

Lau, F., Kuziemsky, C., Price, M., & Gardner, J. (2010). A review on systematic reviews of health information system studies. *Journal of the American Medical Informatics Association: JAMIA, 17*(6), 637–645.

Lauer, M. S., & Collins, F. S. (2010). Using science to improve the nation's health system: NIH's Commitment to comparative effectiveness research. *JAMA: The Journal of the American Medical Association, 303*(21), 2182–2183.

Laurent, M., & Vickers, T. (2009). Seeking health information online: Does Wikipedia matter? *Journal of the American Medical Informatics Association: JAMIA, 16,* 471–479.

Lawrence, S. (2001). Free online availability substantially increases a paper's impact. *Nature, 411,* 521.

Le Bihan, D., Mangin, J. F., et al. (2001). Diffusion tensor imaging: Concepts and applications. *Journal of Magnetic Resonance Imaging, 13*(4), 534–546.

Leape, L. L. (1994). Error in medicine. *JAMA: The Journal of the American Medical Association, 272*(23), 1851–1857. doi:10.1001/jama.1994.03520230061039.

Leape, L. L., Brennan, T. A., Laird, N., Lawthers, A. G., Localio, A. R., Barnes, B. A., & Hiatt, H. (1991). The nature of adverse events in hospitalized patients. *The New England Journal of Medicine, 324*(6), 377–384. doi:10.1056/NEJM199102073240605.

Leatherman, S., Berwick, D., Iles, D., et al. (2003). The business case for quality: Case studies and an analysis. *Health Affairs, 22*(2), 17–30.

Leavitt, M., & Gallagher, L. (2006). The EHR seal of approval: CCHIT introduces product certification to spur EHR adoption. *Journal of AHIMA, 77*(5), 26–30; quiz 33–24.

Ledley R. (1965) Use fo Computers in Biology and Medicine. New Yord: McGraw-Hill.

Ledley, R. S., & Lusted, L. B. (1959). Probability, logic and medical diagnosis. *Science, 130*(3380), 892–930.

Ledley, R. S., & Lusted, L. B. (1991). Reasoning foundations of medical diagnosis. *MD Computing, 8*(5), 300–315.

Lee, D. H. (2003). Magnetic resonance angiography. *Advances in Neurology, 92,* 43–52.

Lee, J. K. T. (2006). *Computed body tomography with MRI correlation*. Philadelphia: Lippincott Williams & Wilkins.

Lee, J., & Mark, R. G. (2010). An investigation of patterns in hemodynamic data indicative of impending hypotension in intensive care. *Biomedical Engineering, 9*, 62. PMID 20973998.

Lee, T., & Mongan, J. (2009). *Chaos and organization in healthcare*. Cambridge, MA: The MIT Press.

Lee, Y., Kim, N., et al. (2009). Bayesian classifier for predicting malignant renal cysts on MDCT: Early clinical experience. *AJR. American Journal of Roentgenology, 193*(2), W106–W111.

Lee, J. Y., Du, Y. E., Coki, O., Flynn, J. T., Starren, J., & Chiang, M. F. (2010). Parental perceptions toward digital imaging and telemedicine for retinopathy of prematurity management. *Graefe's Archive for Clinical and Experimental Ophthalmology, 248*, 141–147.

Leeflang, M. M. G., Deeks, J. J., & Gatsonis, C. (2008). Bossuyt PMM on behalf of the Cochrane diagnostic test accuracy working group. Systematic reviews of diagnostic tests. *Annals of Internal Medicine, 149*, 889–897.

Lehmann, T. M., Guld, M. O., et al. (2004). Content-based image retrieval in medical applications. *Methods of Information in Medicine, 43*(4), 354–361.

Leiner, F., & Haux, R. (1996). Systematic planning of clinical documentation. *Methods of Information in Medicine, 35*, 25–34.

Lenert, L. A., Michelson, D., Flowers, C., & Bergen, M. R. (1995). *IMPACT: An object-oriented graphical environment for construction of multimedia patient interviewing software* (pp. 319–323). Washington, D.C.: Proceedings of the Annual Symposium of Computer Applications in Medical Care.

Lenfant, C. (2003). Shattuck lecture – clinical research to clinical practice – lost in translation? *The New England Journal of Medicine, 349*, 868–874.

Leong, F. J., & Leong, A. S. (2003). Digital imaging applications in anatomic pathology. *Advances in Anatomic Pathology, 10*(2), 88–95.

Leong, K. C., Chen, W. S., Leong, K. W., Mastura, I., Mimi, O., Sheikh, M. A., et al. (2006). The use of text messaging to improve attendance in primary care: A randomized controlled trial. *Family Practice, 23*(6), 699–705.

Lependu, P., Musen, M. A., & Shah, N. H. (2011a). Enabling enrichment analysis with the human disease ontology. *Journal of Biomedical Informatics, 44*(Suppl 1), S31–S38.

LePendu, P., Racunas, S,A., Iyer, S., et al. (2011b). *Annotation analysis for testing drug safety signals*. The 14th Bio-Ontologies SIG meeting at ISMB 2011, Vienna, Austria.

Lesgold, A. (1984). Human skill in a computerized society: Complex skills and their acquisition. *Behavior Research Methods, 16*(2), 79–87. doi:10.3758/bf03202363.

Lesgold, A., Rubinson, H., Feltovich, P., Glaser, R., Klopfer, D., & Wang, Y. (1988). Expertise in a complex skill: Diagnosing x-ray pictures. In M. T. H. Chi, R. Glaser, et al. (Eds.), *The nature of expertise* (pp. 311–342). Hillsdale: Lawrence Erlbaum Associates.

Lesk, M. (2005). *Understanding digital libraries* (2nd ed.). San Francisco: Morgan Kaufmann.

Lester, R. T., Ritvo, P., Mills, E. J., Kariri, A., Karanja, S., Chung, M. H., Jack, W., Habyarimana, J., Sadatsafavi, M., Najafzadeh, M., Marra, C. A., Estambale, B., Ngugi, E., Ball, T. B., Thabane, L., Gelmon, L. J., Kimani, J., Ackers, M., & Plummer, F. A. (2010). Effects of a mobile phone short message service on antiretroviral treatment adherence in Kenya (WelTel Kenya1): a randomised trial. *The Lancet, 376*(9755), 1838–1845.

Leu, M. G., Cheung, M., Webster, T. R., Curry, L., Bradley, E. H., Fifield, J., et al. (2008). Centers speak up: The clinical context for health information technology in the ambulatory care setting. *Journal of General Internal Medicine, 23*(4), 372–378.

Levine (1999), "Telestroke": The Application of Telemedicine for Stroke. Steven R. Levine and Mark Gorman. Stroke. *30*, 464-469, doi:10.1161/01.STR.30.2.464.

Levine, S. R., & Gorman, M. (2009). "Telestroke": the application of telemedicine for stroke. *Stroke, 30*, 464–469.

Levitt, M. (1983). Molecular dynamics of native protein. I. Computer simulation of trajectories. *Journal of Molecular Biology, 168*(3), 595–617.

Levy, M. A., & Rubin, D. L. (2008). Tool support to enable evaluation of the clinical response to treatment. *AMIA Annual Symposium Proceedings, 2008*, 399–403.

Levy, M. A., & Rubin, D. L. (2011). Current and future trends in imaging informatics for oncology. *Cancer Journal, 17*(4), 203–210.

Levy, M. A., O'Connor, M. J., et al. (2009). Semantic reasoning with image annotations for tumor assessment. *AMIA Annual Symposium Proceedings, 2009*, 359–363.

Lexe, G., Monaco, J., et al. (2009). Towards improved cancer diagnosis and prognosis using analysis of gene expression data and computer aided imaging. *Experimental Biology and Medicine (Maywood, N.J.), 234*(8), 860–879.

Li, Q., Mark, R. G., & Clifford, G. D. (2009). Artificial arterial blood pressure artifact models and an evaluation of a robust blood pressure and heart rate estimator. *Biomedical Engineering Online, 8*, 13. PMID 19586547.

Libicki, M. C. (1995). *Information technology standards: Quest for the common byte*. Boston: Digital Press.

Lichtenbelt, B., Crane, R., et al. (1998). *Introduction to volume rendering*. Upper Saddle River: Prentice Hall.

Lieberman, M. A. (1988). The role of self-help groups in helping patients and families cope with cancer. *CA: A Cancer Journal for Clinicians, 38*(3), 162–168.

Lieberman, D. A. (2001). Management of chronic pediatric diseases with interactive health games: Theory and research findings. *The Journal of Ambulatory Care Management, 24*(1), 26–38.

Lilly, C. M., Cody, S., Zhao, H., et al. (2011). Hospital mortality, length of stay, and preventable complications among critically Ill patients before and after Tele-ICU reengineering of critical care processes. *JAMA: The Journal of the American Medical Association, 305*, 2175–2183. doi: 10.1001/jama.2011.697. Epub 2011 May 16. PubMed PMID: 21576622.

Lin, J., & Dyer, C. (2010). *Data-intensive text processing with MapReduce*. San Rafael: Morgan & Claypool Publishers.

Lin, L., Isla, R., Doniz, K., Harkness, H., Vicente, K. J., & Doyle, D. J. (1998). Applying human factors to the design of medical equipment: Patient-controlled analgesia. *Journal of Clinical Monitoring and Computing, 14*(4), 253–263.

Lin, N.D., Martins, S.B., Chan, A.S., Coleman, R.W., Bosworth, H.B., Oddone, E.Z., Shankar, R.D., Musen, M.A., Hoffman, B.B., & Goldstein, M.K. (2006). Identifying barriers to hypertension guideline adherence using clinician feedback at the point of care. *AMIA Annual Symposium Proceedings*, 494–498.

Lindberg, D.A.B. (1965). *Collection, evaluation, and transmission of hospital laboratory data. Presented at the Seventh IBM Medical Symposium*, Poughkeepsie, NY.

Lindberg, D. (1967). Collection, evaluation, and transmission of hospital laboratory data. *Methods of Information in Medicine, 6*(3), 97–107.

Lindberg, D., & Humphreys, B. (2005). 2015 – The future of medical libraries. *The New England Journal of Medicine, 352*, 1067–1070.

Lindberg, D. A. B., Humphreys, B. L., & McCray, A. T. (1993). The unified medical language system. *Methods of Information in Medicine, 32*, 281–291.

Linder, J. A., Ma, J., Bates, D. W., Middleton, B., & Stafford, R. S. (2007). Electronic health record use and the quality of ambulatory care in the united states. *Archives of Internal Medicine, 167*(13), 1400–1405.

Lindgren, H. (2008). Decision support system supporting clinical reasoning process – an evaluation study in dementia care. *Studies in Health Technology and Informatics, 136*, 315–320.

Lindhurst, M. J., Sapp, J. C., Teer, J. K., et al. (2011). A mosaic activating mutation in AKT1 associated with the Proteus syndrome. *The New England Journal of Medicine, 365*(7), 611–619.

Lipton, E., & Johnson, K. (2001, December 26). The anthrax trail; tracking bioterror's tangled course. *New York Times*, Section A, p. 1

Littlejohns, P., Wyatt, J. C., & Garvican, L. (2003, April 19). Evaluating computerised health information systems: Hard lessons still to be learnt. *BMJ, 326*(7394), 860–863.

Liu, J. L. Y., & Wyatt, J. C. (2011). The case for randomized controlled trials to assess the impact of clinical information systems. *Journal of the American Medical Informatics Association: JAMIA, 18*(2), 173–180.

Liu, T., Lin, Y., Wen, X., Jorissen, R. N., & Gilson, M. K. (2007). BindingDB: A web-accessible database of experimentally determined protein-ligand binding affinities. *Nucleic Acids Research, 35*, D198–D201.

Liu, Y. I., Kamaya, A., et al. (2009). A controlled vocabulary to represent sonographic features of the thyroid and its application in a Bayesian network to predict thyroid nodule malignancy. *Summit on Translational Bioinformatics, 2009*, 68–72.

Liu, Y. I., Kamaya, A., et al. (2011). A Bayesian network for differentiating benign from malignant thyroid nodules using sonographic and demographic features. *AJR. American Journal of Roentgenology, 196*(5), W598–W605.

Lorensen, W. E., & Cline, H. E. (1987). Marching cubes: A high resolution 3-D surface construction algorithm. *ACM SIGGRAPH Computer Graphics, 21*(4), 163–169.

Lowe, D. (1999). Object recognition from local scale invariant features. In *Proceedings of the International Conference on Computer Vision* (pp. 1150–1157), Greece.

Lowe, H.J., Antipov, I., et al. (1998). Towards knowledge-based retrieval of medical images. The role of semantic indexing, image content representation and knowledge-based retrieval. *Proceedings of the AMIA Symposium*, 882–886.

Lown, B., Amarasingham, R., & Neuman, J. (1962). New method for terminating cardiac arrhythmias. Use of synchronous capacitor discharge. *JAMA: The Journal of the American Medical Association, 182*, 548–555. PMID 12921298.

Lu, Z. (2011). PubMed and beyond: A survey of Web tools for searching biomedical literature. *Database (Oxford), 2011*, baq036.

Luce, R. E. (2008). A New Value Equation Challenge: The Emergence of eResearch and Roles for Research Libraries. In Council on Library and Information Resources (Ed.), *No Brief Candle: Reconceiving Research Libraries for the 21st Century* (pp. 42–50). Washington, D.C: Council on Library and Information Resources.

Lundsgaarde, H. P. (1987). Evaluating medical expert systems. *Social Science & Medicine, 24*, 805–819.

Lunshof, J. E., Bobe, J., Aach, J., et al. (2010). Personal genomes in progress: From the human genome project to the personal genome project. *Dialogues in Clinical Neuroscience, 12*, 47–60.

Lupski, J. R., Reid, J. G., et al. (2010). Whole-genome sequencing in a patient with Charcot–Marie–tooth neuropathy. *The New England Journal of Medicine, 362*(13), 1181–1191.

Lussier, Y., Shagina, L., & Friedman, C. (2001). Automating SNOMED coding using medical language understanding: a feasibility study. *Proceedins of the AMIA Symposium*, 418–422.

Lusted, L. B. (1960). Logical analysis in roentgen diagnosis. *Radiology, 74*, 178–193.

Lutz, S., & Henkind, S. J. (2000). Recruiting for clinical trials on the web. *Healthplan, 41*(5), 36–43.

MacDonald, D. (1993). *Register, McConnel Brain Imaging Center*. Montreal: Neurological Institute. Montreal, Canada.

MacDonald, D., Kabani, N., et al. (2000). Automated 3-D extraction of inner and outer surfaces of cerebral cortex from MRI. *NeuroImage, 12*(3), 340–356.

Mackinnon, A. D., Billington, R. A., Adam, E. J., Dundas, D. D., & Patel, U. (2008). Picture archiving and communication systems lead to sustained improvements in reporting times and productivity: Results of a 5-year audit. *Clinical Radiology, 63*, 796–804.

Macklin, R. (1992). Privacy and control of genetic information. In G. J. Annas & S. Elias (Eds.), *Gene mapping: Using law and ethics as guides* (pp. 157–172). New York: Oxford University Press.

Mailman, M. D., Feolo, M., Jin, Y., et al. (2007). The NCBI dbGaP database of genotypes and phenotypes. *Nature Genetics, 39*, 1181–1186.

Majchrowski, B. (2010). Medical software's increasing impact on healthcare and technology management. *Biomedical Instrumentation and Technology, 44*(1), 70–74.

Major, K., Shabot, M. M., & Cunneen, S. (2002). Wireless clinical alerts and patient outcomes in the surgical intensive care unit. *American Surgery, 68*, 1057–1060.

Malcolm, S., & Goodship, J. (Eds.). (2007). *Genotype to phenotype* (2nd ed.). Oxford: BIOS Scientific Publishers.

Malin, B., & Sweeney, L. (2004). How (not) to protect genomic data privacy in a distributed network: Using trail re-identification to evaluate and design anonymity protection systems. *Journal of Biomedical Informatics, 37*, 179–192.

Malin, B., Loukides, G., Benitez, K., & Clayton, E. W. (2011). Identifiability in biobanks: Models, measures, and mitigation strategies. *Human Genetics, 130*, 383–392.

Mandl, K. D., & Kohane, I. S. (2008). Tectonic shifts in the health information economy. *The New England Journal of Medicine, 358*(16), 1732–1737.

Mandl, K. D., & Kohane, I. S. (2009). No small change for the health information economy. *The New England Journal of Medicine, 360*(13), 1278–1281.

Mandl, K. D., & Kohane, I. S. (2012). Escaping the EHR trap — the future of health IT. *The New England Journal of Medicine, 366*, 2240–2242.

Mandl, K. D., Simons, W. W., Crawford, W. C., & Abbett, J. M. (2007). Indivo: A personally controlled health record for health information exchange and communication. *BMC Medical Informatics and Decision Making, 7*, 25. Research Support, N.I.H., Extramural.

Mani, I. (2001). *Automatic summarization*. Amsterdam: John Benjamins.

Manning, C., & Schütze, H. (1999). *Foundations of statistical natural language processing*. Cambridge, MA: MIT Press.

Manolio, T. A., Collins, F. S., Cox, N. J., et al. (2009). Finding the missing heritability of complex diseases. *Nature, 461*, 747–753.

Mant, J., & Hicks, N. (1995). Detecting differences in quality of care: The sensitivity of measures of process and outcome in treating acute myocardial infarction. *BMJ, 311*, 793–796.

Marcetich, J., Rappaport, M., & Kotzin, S. (2004). *Indexing consistency in MEDLINE*. MLA 04 Abstracts (pp. 10–11). Washington, DC.

Marcin, J. P., Nesbitt, T. S., Kallas, H. J., et al. (2004). *Journal of Pediatrics, 144*, 375–380.

Marcus, M., Santorini, B., & Marcinkiewicz, M. (1993). Building a large annotated corpus of English: The Penn Treebank. *Computational Linguistics, 19*, 313–330.

Margolis, D. J., Hoffman, J. M., et al. (2007). Molecular imaging techniques in body imaging. *Radiology, 245*(2), 333–356.

Markle Foundation. (2006). *The connecting for health common framework*. Retrieved October 1, 2011. From http://www.connectingforhealth.org/health

Markle Foundation, C.f.H.A.P.-P.C. (2004). *The personal health working group: Final report*. New York: Markle Foundation.

Marks, L., & Power, E. (2002). Using technology to address recruitment issues in the clinical trial process. *Trends in Biotechnology, 20*(3), 105–109.

Marks, R. G., Conlon, M., & Ruberg, S. J. (2001). Paradigm shifts in clinical trials enabled by information technology. *Statistics in Medicine, 20*(17–18), 2683–2696.

Maroto, M., Reshef, R., Munsterberg, A. E., Koester, S., Goulding, M., & Lassar, A. B. (1997). Ectopic Pax-3 activates MyoD and Myf-5 expression in embryonic mesoderm and neural tissue. *Cell, 89*, 139–148.

Marquet, G., Dameron, O., et al. (2007). Grading glioma tumors using OWL-DL and NCI Thesaurus. AMIA Annual Symposium Proceedings, 508–512.

Marroquin, J. L., Vemuri, B. C., et al. (2002). An accurate and efficient Bayesian method for automatic segmentation of brain MRI. *IEEE Transactions on Medical Imaging, 21*(8), 934–945.

Martin, R. F., & Bowden, D. M. (2001). *Primate brain maps: Structure of the macaque brain*. New York: Elsevier Science.

Martin, R.F., Mejino, J.L.V., et al. (2001). Foundational model of neuroanatomy: implications for the Human Brain Project. *Proceedings of the AMIA Annual Fall Symposium*, 438–442. Washington, D.C.

Marwede, D., Schulz, T., et al. (2008). Indexing thoracic CT reports using a preliminary version of a standardized radiological lexicon (RadLex). *Journal of Digital Imaging, 21*(4), 363–370.

Massaro, T. A. (1993). Introducing physician order entry at a major academic medical center. *Academic Medicine, 68*, 20–30.

Massoud, T. F., & Gambhir, S. S. (2003). Molecular imaging in living subjects: Seeing fundamental biological processes in a new light. *Genes & Development, 17*, 545–580.

Masys, D. R. (2002). Effects of current and future information technologies on the health care workforce. *Health Affairs, 21*(5), 33–41.

Masys, D. R., Jarvik, G. P., Abernethy, N. F., Anderson, N. R., Papanicolaou, G. J., Paltoo, D. N., Hoffman, M. A., Kohane, I. S., & Levy, H. P. (2012). Technical desiderata for the integration of genomic data into electronic health records. *Journal of Biomedical Informatics, 45*(3), 419–422.

Mathews, S. C., & Pronovost, P. J. (2011). The need for systems integration in health care. *JAMA: The Journal of the American Medical Association, 305*, 934–935. PMID 21364143.

Mattern, C., Erickson, B., King, B., & Okryznski, T. (1999). Impact of electronic imaging on clinician behavior in the urgent care setting. *Journal of Digital Imaging, 12*(2 Suppl 1), 148–151.

Mayes, T.J., Draper, S.W., McGregor, A.M., & Koatley, K. (1988). *Information flow in a user interface: The effect of experience and context on the recall ofMac-Write screens.* Paper presented at the Conference on People and Computers IV, Cambridge.

McCarty, C. A., Chisholm, R. L., et al. (2011). The eMERGE Network: A consortium of biorepositories linked to electronic medical records data for conducting genomic studies. *BMC Medical Genomics, 4*, 13.

McClellan, M., McKethan, A. N., Lewis, J. L., Roski, J., & Fisher, E. S. (2010). A national strategy to put accountable care into practice. *Health Affairs (Millwood), 29*(5), 982–990.

McConnell, S. (1996). *Rapid development: Taming wild software schedules/Steve McConnell.* Redmond: Microsoft Press.

McCullough, J. S., Casey, M., Moscovice, I., & Prasad, S. (2010). The effect of health information technology on quality in U.S. Hospitals. *Health Affairs (Millwood), 29*(4), 647–654.

McDonald, C. J. (1976). Protocol-based computer reminders, the quality of care and the nonperfectibility of man. *The New England Journal of Medicine, 295*(24), 1351–1355.

McDonald, C. J. (1981). *Action-oriented decisions in ambulatory medicine.* Philadelphia: Mosby.

McDonald, C. J. (Ed.). (1987a). *Images, signals, and devices* (M.D. Computing: Benchmark Papers). New York: Springer.

McDonald, C. J. (Ed.). (1987b). *Tutorials* (M.D. Computing: Benchmark Papers). New York: Springer.

McDonald, C. J. (1997). The barriers to electronic medical record systems and how to overcome them. *Journal of the American Medical Informatics Association: JAMIA, 4*(3), 213–221.

McDonald, C. J., & Abhyankar, S. (2011). Clinical decision support and rich clinical repositories: A symbiotic relationship. Invited commentary. *Archives of Internal Medicine, 171*(10), 903–905.

McDonald, M. H., & McDonald, C. J. (2012). Electronic medical records and preserving primary care physicians' time: Comment on "electronic health record-based messages to primary care providers". *Archives of Internal Medicine, 172*(3), 285–287.

McDonald, C.J., Bhargava, B., Jeris, D.W. (1975). *A clinical information system (CIS) for ambulatory care.* Proceedings AFIPS National Computing Conference, Anaheim.

McDonald, C.J., Wiederhold, G., Simborg, D., Hammond, W.E., Jelovsek, F., Schneider, K. (1984a). A discussion of the draft proposal for data exchange standards for clinical laboratory results. *Proceedings of the 8th Annual Symposium on Computer Applications in Medical Care*, 406–413.

McDonald, C. J., Hui, S. L., Smith, D. M., et al. (1984b). Reminders to physicians from an introspective computer medical record. A two year randomized trial. *Annals of Internal Medicine, 100*(1), 130–138.

McDonald, C. J., Overhage, J. M., Dexter, P., Takesue, B. Y., & Dwyer, D. M. (1997). A framework for capturing clinical data sets from computerized sources. *Annals of Internal Medicine, 127*(8), 675–682.

McDonald, C. J., Overhage, J. M., Tierney, W. M., et al. (1999). The regenstrief medical record system: A quarter century experience. *International Journal of Medical Informatics, 54*(3), 225–253.

McDonald, C. J., Huff, S. M., Suico, J. G., et al. (2003). LOINC, a universal standard for identifying laboratory observations: A 5-year update. *Clinical Chemistry, 49*(4), 624–633.

McDonald, C. J., Overhage, J. M., Barnes, M., Schadow, G., Blevins, L., Dexter, P. R., & Mamlin, B. W. (2005). The Indiana network for patient care: A working local health information infrastructure (LHII). *Health Affairs (Millwood)., 24*(5), 1214–1220.

McGettigan, P., & Henry, D. (2006). Cardiovascular risk and inhibition of cyclooxygenase: A systematic review of the observational studies of selective and nonselective inhibitors of cyclooxygenase 2. *JAMA: The Journal of the American Medical Association, 296*(13), 1633–1644.

McGlynn, E. A., Asch, S. M., Adams, J., et al. (2003). The quality of health care delivered to adults in the United States. *The New England Journal of Medicine, 348*, 2635–2645.

McInerney, T., & Terzopoulos, D. (1997). Medical image segmentation using topologically adaptable surfaces. Cvrmed-Mrcas'97. *Lecture Notes in Computer Science, 1205*, 23–32.

McKibbon, K., & Fridsma, D. (2006). Effectiveness of clinician-selected electronic information resources for answering primary care physicians' information needs. *Journal of the American Medical Informatics Association: JAMIA, 13*, 653–659.

McKibbon, K., Haynes, R., Dilks, C. W., Ramsden, M., Ryan, N., Baker, L., & Fitzgerald, D. (1990). How good are clinical MEDLINE searches? A comparative study of clinical end-user and librarian searches. *Computers and Biomedical Research, 23*(6), 583–593.

McLachlan, G. J., & Peel, D. (2000). *Finite mixture models.* New York: Wiley.

McManus, J., & Wood-Harper, T. (Understanding the sources of information systems project failure). *Management Services, 51*, 38–43.

McNeer, J. F., Wallace, A. G., Wagner, G. S., Starmer, C. F., & Rosati, R. A. (1975). The course of acute myocardial infarction: Feasibility of early discharge of the uncomplicated patient. *Circulation, 51*, 410–413.

McPhee, S. J., Bird, J. A., Fordham, D., Rodnick, J. E., & Osborn, E. H. (1991). Promoting cancer prevention activities by primary care physicians: Results of a randomized, controlled trial. *Journal of the American Medical Association, 266*(4), 538–544.

Mead, N., & Bower, P. (2000). Patient-centredness: A conceptual framework and review of the empirical literature. *Social Science & Medicine, 51*(7), 1087–1110.

Mechouche, A., Golbreich, C., et al. (2008). Ontology-based annotation of brain MRI images. *AMIA Annual Symposium Proceedings*, 460–464.

Meckley, L. M., & Neumann, P. J. (2010). Personalized medicine: Factors influencing reimbursement. *Health Policy, 94*, 91–100.

Mehta, T. S., Raza, S., et al. (2000). Use of Doppler ultrasound in the evaluation of breast carcinoma. *Seminars in Ultrasound, CT, and MR, 21*(4), 297–307.

Meigs, J., Barry, M., Oesterling, J., & Jacobsen, S. (1996). Interpreting results of prostate-specific antigen testing for early detection of prostate cancer. *Journal of General Internal Medicine, 11*(9), 505–512.

Mell, P., & Grance, T. (2011). *The NIST Definition of Cloud Computing*. NIST Special Publication 800–145, National Institute of Standards and Technology. Gathersburg, MD.

Melton, L. J., 3rd. (1996). History of the Rochester epidemiology project. *Mayo Clinic Proceedings, 71*, 266–274.

Menachemi, N., Powers, T. L., & Brooks, R. G. (2011). Physician and practice characteristics associated with longitudinal increases in electronic health records adoption. *Journal of Healthcare Management, 56*(3), 183–198.

Mervis, J. (2012). U.S. Science policy: Agencies rally to tackle big data. *Science, 336*, 22.

Merzweiler, A., Knaup, P., Weber, R., Ehlerding, H., Haux, R., & Wiedemann, T. (2001). Recording clinical data–from a general set of record items to case report forms (CRF) for clinics. *Medinfo, 10*(Pt 1), 653–657.

Meyer, B. C., Raman, R., Hemmen, T., et al. (2008). Efficacy of site-independent telemedicine in the STRokEDOC trial: A randomized, blinded, prospective trial. *Lancet Neurology, 7*, 787–795.

Michaelis, J., Wellek, S., & Willems, J. L. (1990). Reference standards for software evaluation. *Methods of Information in Medicine, 29*, 289–297.

Michel, A., Zorb, L., Dudeck, J. (1996). Designing a low-cost bedside workstation for intensive care units. In *Proceedings of the 1996 AMIA Annual Fall Symposium* (pp. 777–781), Washington, DC.

Microsoft. (2012). Microsoft HealthVault Ecosystem Overview. http://www.healthvault.com/Industry/ecosystem/application-providers/index.aspx. Accessed 17 Dec 2012.

Microsoft. (2012). http://msdn.microsoft.com/en-us/healthvault/hh922966. Accessed 17 December 2012.

Middleton, B. (2009). The clinical decision support consortium. *Studies in Health Technology and Informatics, 150*, 26–30.

Miles, W. (1982). *A history of the national library of medicine: The Nation's treasury of medical knowledge*. Bethesda: U.S. Department of Health and Human Services.

Miller, R. A. (1989). Legal issues related to medical decision support systems. *International Journal of Clinical Monitoring and Computing, 6*, 75–80.

Miller, R. A. (1990). Why the standard view is standard: People, not machines, understand patients' problems. *The Journal of Medicine and Philosophy, 15*, 581–591.

Miller, R. A., Massarie, F. (1990). The demise of the Greek oracle model for medical diagnosis systems. *Methods of Information in Medicine, 29*, 1–2.

Miller, R. A. (1997). Predictive models for primary caregivers: Risky business? *Annals of Internal Medicine, 127*(7), 565–567.

Miller, G. C., & Britt, H. (1995). A new drug classification for computer systems: The ATC extension code. *International Journal of Bio-Medical Computing, 40*, 121–124.

Miller, R. A., & Gardner, R. M. (1997a). Summary recommendations for the responsible monitoring and regulation of clinical software systems. *Annals of Internal Medicine, 127*(9), 842–845.

Miller, R. A., & Gardner, R. M. (1997b). Recommendations for responsible monitoring and regulation of clinical software systems. *Journal of the American Medical Informatics Association: JAMIA, 4*, 442–457.

Miller, R. A., & Goodman, K. W. (1998). Ethical challenges in the use of decision-support software in clinical practice. In K. W. Goodman (Ed.), *Ethics, computing, and medicine: Informatics and the transformation of health care* (pp. 102–115). Cambridge: Cambridge University Press.

Miller, R. A., & Miller, S. M. (2007). Legal and regulatory issues related to the use of clinical software in health care delivery. In R. A. Greenes (Ed.), *Clinical decision support: The road ahead* (pp. 423–444). Boston: Elsevier.

Miller, A. R., & Tucker, C. (2009). Privacy protection and technology diffusion: The case of electronic medical records. *Management Science, 55*, 1077–1093.

Miller, R. A., Schaffner, K. F., & Meisel, A. (1985). Ethical and legal issues related to the use of computer programs in clinical medicine. *Annals of Internal Medicine, 102*, 529–536.

Miller, R. A., Gardner, R. M., Johnson, K. B., & Hripcsak, G. (2005a). Clinical decision support and electronic prescribing systems: A time for responsible thought and action. *Journal of the American Medical Informatics Association: JAMIA, 12*(4), 403–409.

Miller, R. A., Waitman, L. R., Chen, S., & Rosenbloom, S. T. (2005b). The anatomy of decision support during inpatient care provider order entry (CPOE): empirical observations from a decade of CPOE experience at Vanderbilt. *Journal of Biomedical Informatics, 38*(6), 469–485.

Miller, H., Yasnoff, W., & Burde, H. (2009). *Personal health records: The essential missing element in twenty-first century healthcare*. Chicago: Health Information and Management Systems Society.

Min, J.J., & Gambhir, S.S. (2008). Molecular imaging of PET reporter gene expression. *Handbook of Experimental Pharmacology*, (185 Pt 2), 277–303.

Minsky, M. (1975). A framework for representing knowledge. In P. H. Wintson (Ed.), *The psychology of computer vision*. New York: McGraw-Hill.

Mittal, M. K., Dhuper, S., Siva, C., Fresen, J. L., Petruc, M., & Velazquez, C. R. (2010). Assessment of email communication skills of rheumatology fellows: A pilot study. *Journal of the American Medical Informatics Association: JAMIA, 17*(6), 702–706.

Modayur, B., Prothero, J., et al. (1997). Visualization-based mapping of language function in the brain. *NeuroImage, 6,* 245–258.

Modi, P., Rodriguez, E., & Chitwood, W. R., Jr. (2009). Robot-assisted cardiac surgery. *Interactive Cardiovascular and Thoracic Surgery, 9,* 500–505.

Moed, H. (2007). The effect of open access on citation impact: An analysis of ArXiv's condensed matter section. *Journal of the American Society for Information Science and Technology, 58,* 2047–2054.

Morel, G., Amalberti, R., & Chauvin, C. (2008). Articulating the differences between safety and resilience: The decision-making process of professional sea-fishing skippers. *Human Factors, 50*(1), 1–16.

Mork, J. G., Bodenreider, O., Demner-Fushman, D., et al. (2010). Extracting Rx information from clinical narrative. *Journal of the American Medical Informatics Association: JAMIA, 17,* 536–539.

Morris, A. H. (2000). Developing and implementing computerized protocols for standardization of clinical decisions. *Annals of Internal Medicine, 132,* 373–383. PMID 10691588.

Morris, A. H. (2001). Rational use of computerized protocols in the intensive care unit. *Critical Care, 5,* 249–254. PMID 11737899.

Morris, A. H. (2003). Treatment algorithms and protocolized care. *Current Opinion in Critical Care, 9,* 236–240. PMID 12771677.

Morrison JL, Cai Q, Davis N, Yan Y, Berbaum ML, Ries M, Solomon G. (2010) Clinical and economic outcomes of the electronic intensive care unit: results from two community hospitals. *Crit Care Med, 38(1),* 2–8. doi: 10.1097/CCM.0b013e3181b78fa8. PubMed PMID: 19730249.

Morrison, J. L., Cai, Q., Davis, N., et al. (2010). Clinical and economic outcomes of the electronic intensive care unit: Results from two community hospitals. *Critical Care Medicine, 38,* 2–8.

Mort, M., Evani, U. S., Krishnan, V. G., et al. (2010). In silico functional profiling of human disease-associated and polymorphic amino acid substitutions. *Human Mutation, 31,* 335–346.

Moses, L. E., Littenberg, B., & Shapiro, D. (1993). Combining independent studies of a diagnostic test into a summary ROC curve: Data-analytic approaches and some additional considerations. *Statistics in Medicine, 12*(4), 1293–1316.

Mostashari, F. (2011). Moving forward on meaningful use. The ONC's Farzad Mostashari, MD, offers his perspectives on the road ahead. Interview by Mark Hagland. *Healthcare Informatics, 28*(3), 51–52.

Motik, B., Grau, B. C., et al. (2008). OWL 2: The next step for OWL. *Journal of Web Semantics, 6*(4), 309–322.

Motik, B., Shearer, R., et al. (2009). Hypertableau reasoning for description logics. *Journal of Artificial Intelligence Research, 36,* 165–228.

Muller, H., Michoux, N., et al. (2004). A review of content-based image retrieval systems in medical applications-clinical benefits and future directions. *International Journal of Medical Informatics, 73*(1), 1–23.

Mullett, C. J., Evans, R. S., Christenson, J. C., & Dean, J. M. (2001). Development and impact of a computerized pediatric antiinfective decision support program. *Pediatrics, 108,* 1–7. PMID 11581483.

Multiple authors. (2010). Special issue on translational bioinformatics. *Journal of Biomedical Informatics, 43*(3), 355–357.

Multiple authors. (2011a). JAMIA special issue on natural language processing. *Journal of the American Medical Informatics Association: JAMIA, 18*(5), 539–667.

Multiple authors. (2011b). Special issue: Dealing with data [Series]. *Science, 331*(6018), 639–806.

Munasinghe, R. L., Arsene, C., Abraham, T. K., Zidan, M., & Siddique, M. (2011). Improving the utilization of admission order sets in a computerized physician order entry system by integrating modular disease specific order subsets into a general medicine admission order set. *Journal of the American Medical Informatics Association: JAMIA, 18*(3), 322–326.

Murphy, R. L. H., Block, P., Bird, K. T., & Yurchak, P. (1973). Accuracy of cardiac auscultation by microwave. *Chest, 63,* 578–581.

Murphy, S.N., Mendis, M.E., Berkowitz, D.A., Kohane, I. S., & Chueh, H.C. (2006). *Integration of clinical and genetic data in the i2b2 architecture.* Paper presented at the AMIA annual symposium. Washington, DC.

Murphy, S. N., Dubey, A., Embi, P. J., et al. (2012). Current state of information technologies for the clinical research enterprise across academic medical centers. *Clinical and Translational Science, 5*(3), 281–284.

Murray, M. D., Harris, L. E., Overhage, J. M., Zhou, X. H., Eckert, G. J., Smith, F. E., Buchanan, N. N., Wolinsky, F. D., McDonald, C. J., & Tierney, W. M. (2004, March). Failure of computerized treatment suggestions to improve health outcomes of outpatients with uncomplicated hypertension: Results of a randomized controlled trial. *Pharmacotherapy, 24*(3), 324–337.

Musen, M. A. (1997). Modeling for decision support. In J. van Bemmel & M. Musen (Eds.), *Handbook of medical informatics* (pp. 431–448). Heidelberg: Springer.

Musen, M. A. (1998). Domain ontologies in software engineering: Use of PROTÉGÉ with the EON architecture. *Methods of Information in Medicine, 37*(4–5), 540–550.

Musen, M. A., Tu, S. W., Das, A. K., & Shahar, Y. (1996). EON: A component-based approach to automation of protocol-directed therapy. *Journal of the American Medical Informatics Association: JAMIA, 3*(6), 367–388.

Musen, M. A., Noy, N. F., Shah, N. H., et al. (2011). The national center for biomedical ontology. *Journal of the American Medical Informatics Association: JAMIA, 18*(4), 441–448.

Mutalik, P. G., Deshpande, A., & Nadkarni, P. M. (2001). Use of general-purpose negation detection to augment concept indexing of medical documents: A quantitative study using the UMLS. *Journal of the American Medical Informatics Association: JAMIA, 8*(6), 598–609.

Mynatt, B., Leventhal, L., Instone, K., Farhat, J., & Rohlman, D. (1992). Hypertext or book: Which is better for answering questions? *Proceedings of Computer-Human Interface, 92,* 19–25.

Nadkarni, P., Chen, R., & Brandt, C. (2001). UMLS concept indexing for production databases: A feasibility study. *Journal of the American Medical Informatics Association: JAMIA, 8*(1), 80–91.

Nadkarni, P. M., Ohno-Machado, L., & Chapman, W. W. (2011). Natural language processing: An introduction. *Journal of the American Medical Informatics Association: JAMIA, 18*(5), 544–551.

Nahn, V. D., Barnhill, R., Heermann-Do, K., Salzman, K. L., & Gimbel, R. W. (2011). The military health system's personal health record pilot with Microsoft HealthVault and Google Health. *Journal of the American Medical Informatics Association: JAMIA, 18*(1), 118–124.

Nambisan, P. (2011). Information seeking and social support in online health communities: Impact on patients' perceived empathy. *Journal of the American Medical Informatics Association: JAMIA, 18*(3), 298–304.

Napel, S. A., Beaulieu, C. F., et al. (2010). Automated retrieval of CT images of liver lesions on the basis of image similarity: Method and preliminary results. *Radiology, 256*(1), 243–252.

National Committee on Vital and Health Statistics. (2001) Information for health: A strategy for building the National Health Information Infrastructure. Report and Recommendations from the National Committee on Vital and Health Statistics. Available at http://www.ncvhs.hhs.gov/nhiilayo.pdf. Accessed 17 Dec 2012.

National Council for Prescription Drug Programs. (1994). *Data dictionary.* Scottsdale, AZ: National Council for Prescription Drug Programs.

National e-Health Transition Authority (NEHTA). (2011). *NEHTA strategic plan* 2011–2012. Available at http://www.nehta.gov.au/component/docman/doc_download/1338-nehta-strategic-plan-20112012. Accessed 25 Aug 2011.

National High Blood Pressure Education Program. (2004). *The Seventh Report of the Joint National Committee on Prevention, Detection, Evaluation, and Treatment of High Blood Pressure.* National Heart, Lung, and Blood Institute, National Insitutes of Health.

National Institutes of Standards and Technology (NIST). (2005). *Guidelines for the selection and use of transport layer security (TLS) implementations* (NIST Special Publication 800–52). Gaithersburg: U.S. Department of Commerce. http://csrc.nist.gov/publications/nistpubs/800-52/SP800-52.pdf

National Library of Medicine. (1999). *Medical subject headings – Annotated alphabetic list.* Bethesda: U.S. Department of Health and Human Services, Public Health Service.

National Library of Medicine. (1999). *Next generation internet phase I awards.* Retrieved June 17, 2007, from http://www.nlm.nih.gov/research/ngisumphase1.html

National Library of Medicine. (2003). *Scaleable information infrastructure awards.* Retrieved June 30, 2007, from http://www.nlm.nih.gov/research/siiawards.html

National Research Council. (1997). *For the record: Protecting electronic health information.* Washington, D.C.: National Academy Press.

National Research Council. (2001). Computer science and telecommunications board. *Networking health: Prescriptions for the internet.* Washington, DC: National Academy Press.

National Research Council (U.S.). Committee on Enhancing the Internet for Health and Biomedical Applications: Technical Requirements and Implementation Strategies. (2000). *Networking health: Prescriptions for the internet.* Washington, D.C.: National Academy Press.

National Research Council (US) Committee on Engaging the Computer Science Research Community in Health Care Informatics, Stead, W. W., & Lin, H. S. (2009). *Computational technology for effective health care: Immediate steps and strategic directions. The national academies collection: Reports funded by National Institutes of Health.* Washington (DC): National Academies Press (US).

National Research Council of the National Academies. (2011). *Health Care Comes Home.* Washington (DC): National Academies Press (US). Washington, DC.

National Science and Technology Council (U.S.). Interagency Working Group on Digital Data. (2009). *Harnessing the power of digital data for science and society: Report of the Interagency Working Group on Digital Data to the Committee on Science of the National Science and Technology Council.* Washington, D.C.: Interagency Working Group on Digital Data.

National Science Foundation (U.S.), & Cyberinfrastructure Council (National Science Foundation). (2007). *Cyberinfrastructure vision for 21st century discovery* (pp. iii, 58 p.). Retrieved from http://www.nsf.gov/pubs/2007/nsf0728/index.jsp

Nazi, K. M., Woods, S. S., & Woods, S. S. (2008). MyHealtheVet PHR: a description of users and patient portal use. *AMIA … Annual Symposium proceedings/AMIA Symposium. AMIA Symposium,* 1182.

Nease, R. F., Jr., & Owens, D. K. (1994). A method for estimating the cost-effectiveness of incorporating patient preferences into practice guidelines. *Medical Decision Making, 14*(4), 382–392.

Nease, R. F., Jr., & Owens, D. K. (1997). Use of influence diagrams to structure medical decisions. *Medical Decision Making, 17*(13), 263–275.

Nease, R. F., Jr., Kneeland, T., O'Connor, G. T., Sumner, W., Lumpkins, C., Shaw, L., Pryor, D., & Sox, H. C. (1995). Variation in patient utilities for the outcomes of the management of chronic stable angina. Implications for clinical practice guidelines. *Journal of the American Medical Association, 273*(15), 1185–1190.

Needleman, S. B., & Wunsch, C. D. (1970). A general method applicable to the search for similarities in the amino acid sequence of two proteins. *Journal of Molecular Biology, 48*(3), 443–453.

NEHI and Massachusetts Technology Collaborative (2010, December). *Critical care, critical choices: the care for tele-ICU in intensive care.*

Nelson, S.J., Brown, S.H., Erlbaum, M.S., Olson, N., Powell, T., Carlsen, B., Carter, J., Tuttle, M.S., & Hole, W.T. (2002). A semantic normal form for clinical drugs in the UMLS: Early experience with the VANDF. *Proceedings of the AMIA Fall Symposium, 557–561.*

Nelson, N. C., Evans, R. S., Samore, M. H., & Gardner, R. M. (2005). Detection and prevention of medication errors using real-time nurse charting. *Journal of the American Medical Informatics Association: JAMIA, 12,* 390–397. PMID 15802486.

Nelson, S. J., Zeng, K., Kilbourne, J., Powell, T., & Moore, R. (2011). Normalized names for clinical drugs: RxNorm at 6 years. *Journal of the American Medical Informatics Association: JAMIA, 18,* 441–448.

Neville, A. J. (2009). Problem-based learning and medical education forty years on. A review of its effects on knowledge and clinical performance. *Medical Principles and Practice, 18,* 1–9.

New York Academy of Medicine (1961). *Standard nomenclature of diseases and operations.* (5th ed.). New York: McGraw-Hill.

Newell, A. (1990). *Unified theories of cognition.* Cambridge, MA: Harvard University Press.

Newell, A., & Simon, H. A. (1972). *Human problem solving.* Englewood Cliffs: Prentice-Hall.

Ng, A. Y., M. Jordan, et al. (2001). On spectral clustering: analysis and an algorithm. In *Advances in Neural Information Processing Systems* (*NIPS* 13).

Ng, S. B., Buckingham, K. J., Lee, C., et al. (2010). Exome sequencing identifies the cause of a mendelian disorder. *Nature Genetics, 42,* 30–35.

NHS Centre for Coding and Classification. (1994). *Read Codes* (Version 3). (April ed.). London: NHS Management Executive, Department of Health.

Nicholson, D. (2006). *An evaluation of the quality of consumer health information on Wikipedia.* Portland: Capstone, Oregon Health & Science University. Retrieved from http://www.ohsu.edu/dmice/people/students/theses/2006/upload/Nicholson_CapstoneFinal06.pdf

Nicolae, D. L., Gamazon, E., Zhang, W., et al. (2010). Trait-associated SNPs are more likely to be eQTLs: Annotation to enhance discovery from GWAS. *PLoS Genetics, 6,* e1000888.

Nielsen, J. (1993). *Usability engineering.* Boston: Academic Press.

Nielsen, J. (1994). *Usability inspection methods.* Paper presented at the conference companion on human factors in computing systems, Boston.

Nielsen, J., & Landauer, T.K. (1993, April 24–29). A mathematical model of the finding of usability problems. In *Proceedings of the ACM INTERCHI'93 Conference* (pp. 206–13), Amsterdam.

Nielsen, B., Albregtsen, F., et al. (2008). Statistical nuclear texture analysis in cancer research: A review of methods and applications. *Critical Reviews in Oncogenesis, 14*(2–3), 89–164.

Nissenbaum, H. F. (2010). *Privacy in context: Technology, policy, and the integrity of social life.* Stanford: Stanford Law Books.

Noble, M., Bruening, W., Uhl, S., & Schoelles, K. (2009). Computer-aided detection mammography for breast cancer screening: Systematic review and meta-analysis. *Archives of Gynecology and Obstetrics, 279*(6), 881–890.

Nolte, E., & McKee, C. M. (2008). Measuring the health of nations: Updating an earlier analysis. *Health Affairs (Millwood), 27*(1), 58–71.

Norman, D. A. (1986). Cognitive engineering. In D. A. Norman & S. W. Draper (Eds.), *User centered system design: New perspectives on human-computer interaction* (pp. 31–61). Hillsdale: Lawrence Erlbaum Associates.

Norman, D. A. (1988). *The psychology of everyday things.* New York: Basic Books.

Norman, D. A. (1993). *Things that make us smart: Defending human attributes in the age of the machine.* Reading: Addison-Wesley Pub. Co.

Novack, D. H., Plumer, R., Smith, R. L., et al. (1979). Changes in physicians' attitudes toward telling the cancer patient. *JAMA: The Journal of the American Medical Association, 241,* 897–900.

Nowak, E., Jurie, F., et al. (2006). "Sampling strategies for bag-of-features image classification." computer vision – Eccv 2006, Pt 4. *Proceedings, 3954,* 490–503.

NSF-NIH Interagency Initiative. (2012). Core techniques and technologies for advancing big data science and engineering (BIGDATA). http://grants.nih.gov/grants/guide/notice-files/NOT-GM-12-109.html. Accessed 24 Nov 2012 and http://www.nsf.gov/funding/pgm_summ.jsp?pims_id=504767. Accessed 24 Nov 2012.

O'Carroll, P. W., Yasnoff, W. A., Ward, M. E., Ripp, L. H., & Martin, E. L. (Eds.). (2003). Public health informatics and information systems. New York: Springer..

O'Connell, E.M., Teich, J.M., Pedraza, L.A., Thomas, D. (1996). A comprehensive inpatient discharge system. *Proceedings of the 1996 AMIA Annual Fall Symposium, 699–703.*

O'Connor, A. M., Rostom, A., Fiset, V., Tetroe, J., Entwistle, V., Llewellyn-Thomas, H., et al. (1999). Decision aids for patients facing health treatment or screening decisions: Systematic review. *BMJ, 319*(7212), 731–734.

O'Connor, A.M., Bennett, C.L., Stacey, D., Barry, M., Col, N.F., Eden, K.B., et al. (2009). Decision aids for people facing health treatment or screening decisions. *Cochrane Database of Systematic Reviews,* (3), CD001431.

Obeid, J., Gabriel, D., & Sanderson, I. (2010). A biomedical research permissions ontology: Cognitive and knowledge representation considerations. In *Proceedings of the 2010 workshop on Governance of Technology, Information and Policies* (pp. 9–13). Austin: ACM.

Ohmann, C., & Kuchinke, W. (2009). Future developments of medical informatics from the viewpoint of networked clinical research: Interoperability and integration. *Methods of Information in Medicine, 48*(1), 45–54.

Ohno-Machado, L. (2012). Big science, big data, and a big role for biomedical informatics. *Journal of the American Medical Informatics Association: JAMIA, 19*, e1.

Ohno-Machado, L., Wang, S.J., et al. (1999). Decision support for clinical trial eligibility determination in breast cancer. *Proceedings of the AMIA Symposium*, 340–344.

Olsen, L., Grossman, C., & McGinnis, J. M. (Eds.). (2011). *Learning what works: Infrastructure required for comparative effectiveness research*. Washington: The National Academics Press.

Olson, S. (2007, July/August). Who's your daddy? *The Atlantic*.

Omenn, G. S. (2006). Grand challenges and great opportunities in science, technology, and public policy. *Science, 314*, 1696–1704.

Ong, K. (2011). *Medical informatics: An executive primer, second edition*. Chicago: Healthcare and Management Information Systems Society.

Ong, M. S., & Coiera, E. (2011, June). A systematic review of failures in handoff communication during intrahospital transfers. *Joint Commission Journal on Quality and Patient Safety, 37*(6), 274–284.

Oniki, T. A., Clemmer, T. P., & Pryor, T. A. (2003). The effect of computer-generated reminders on charting deficiencies in the ICU. *Journal of the American Medical Informatics Association: JAMIA, 10*, 177–187.

Openchowski, M. W. (1925). The effect of the unit record system and improved organization on hospital economy and efficiency. *Archives of Surgery, 10*(3), 925–934.

Organization for Human Brain Mapping. (2001). *Annual Conference on Human Brain Mapping*. Brighton.

Ormond, K. E., Wheeler, M. T., Hudgins, L., et al. (2010). Challenges in the clinical application of whole-genome sequencing. *Lancet, 375*, 1749–1751.

Ornstein, C. (2003, January 22). Hospital heeds doctors, suspends use of software. *Los Angeles Times*.

Osborn, C. Y., Mayberry, L. S., Mulvaney, S. A., & Hess, R. (2010). Patient web portals to improve diabetes outcomes: A systematic review. *Current Diabetes Reports, 10*(6), 422–435.

Osborn, C. Y., Rosenbloom, S. T., Stenner, S. P., Anders, S., Muse, S., Johnson, K. B., et al. (2011). MyHealthAtVanderbilt: Policies and procedures governing patient portal functionality. *Journal of the American Medical Informatics Association : JAMIA, 18*(Suppl 1), i18–i23.

Osheroff, J., Pifer, E., Sittig, D., & Jenders, R. (2004). *Clinical decision support implementers' workbook*. Chicago: HIMSS.

Osheroff, J. A., Teich, J. M., Middleton, B., Steen, E. B., Wright, A., & Detmer, D. E. (2007). A roadmap for national action on clinical decision support. *Journal of the American Medical Informatics Association: JAMIA, 14*(2), 141–145.

Oster, S., Langella, S., Hastings, S., et al. (2008). CaGrid 1.0: An enterprise grid infrastructure for biomedical research. *Journal of the American Medical Informatics Association: JAMIA, 15*(2), 138–149.

Overby, C. L., Tarczy-Hornoch, P., Hoath, J. I., Kalet, I. J., & Veenstra, D. L. (2010). Feasibility of incorporating genomic knowledge into electronic medical records for pharmacogenomic clinical decision support. *BMC Bioinformatics, 11*(Suppl 9), S10.

Overhage, J. M., Suico, J., & McDonald, C. J. (2001). Electronic laboratory reporting: Barriers, solutions and findings. *Journal of Public Health Management and Practice, 7*(6), 60–66.

Overhage, J. M., Grannis, S., & McDonald, C. J. (2008). A comparison of the completeness and timeliness of automated electronic laboratory reporting and spontaneous reporting of notifiable conditions. *American Journal of Public Health, 98*(2), 344–350.

Overington, J. (2009). ChEMBL. An interview with John Overington, team leader, chemogenomics at the European Bioinformatics Institute Outstation of the European Molecular Biology Laboratory (EMBL-EBI). Interview by Wendy A. Warr. *Journal of Computer-Aided Molecular Design, 23*, 195–198.

Owens, D. K. (1998). Patient preferences and the development of practice guidelines. *Spine, 23*(9), 1073–1079.

Owens, D. K., & Nease, R. F., Jr. (1993). Development of outcome-based practice guidelines: A method for structuring problems and synthesizing evidence. *The Joint Commission Journal on Quality Improvement, 19*(7), 248–263.

Owens, D. K., & Nease, R. F., Jr. (1997). A normative analytic framework for development of practice guidelines for specific clinical populations. *Medical Decision Making, 17*(4), 409–426.

Owens, D., Harris, R., Scott, P., & Nease, R. F., Jr. (1995). Screening surgeons for HIV infection: A cost-effectiveness analysis. *Annals of Internal Medicine, 122*(9), 641–652.

Owens, D. K., Holodniy, M., Garber, A. M., Scott, J., Sonnad, S., Moses, L., Kinosian, B., & Schwartz, J. S. (1996a). The polymerase chain reaction for the diagnosis of HIV infection in adults: A meta-analysis with recommendations for clinical practice and study design. *Annals of Internal Medicine, 124*(9), 803–815.

Owens, D. K., Holodniy, M., McDonald, T. W., Scott, J., & Sonnad, S. (1996b). A meta-analytic evaluation of the polymerase chain reaction (PCR) for diagnosis of human immunodeficiency virus (HIV) infection in infants. *Journal of the American Medical Association, 275*(17), 1342–1348.

Owens, D. K., Shachter, R. D., & Nease, R. F., Jr. (1997). Representation and analysis of medical decision problems with influence diagrams. *Medical Decision Making, 17*(3), 241–262.

Ozbolt, J. (2000). Terminology standards for nursing: Collaboration at the summit. *Journal of the American Medical Informatics Association: JAMIA, 7*, 517–522.

Ozbolt, J. (2003). Reference terminology for therapeutic goals: A new approach. *Proceedings of the AMIA Fall Symposium, Journal of the American Medical*

Informatics Association, Symposium Supplement, 2003, 504–508.

Ozbolt, J. G., Schultz, S., Swain, M. A. P., Abraham, I. L., & Stein, K. F. (1984). Developing expert systems for nursing practice. In G. S. Cohen (Ed.), *Proceedings of the eighth annual symposium on computer applications in medical care* (pp. 654–657). Silver Spring: IEEE Computer Society.

Ozbolt, J., Brennan, G., & Hatcher, I. (2001). PathworX: An informatics tool for quality improvement. *Proceedings of the AMIA Fall Symposium, Journal of the American Medical Informatics Association, Symposium Supplement, 2001*, 518–522.

Özdas, A., Speroff, T., Waitman, L. R., Ozbolt, J., Butler, J., & Miller, R. A. (2006). Integrating "best of care" protocols into clinicians' workflow via care provider order entry: Impact on quality of care indicators for acute myocardial infarction. *Journal of the American Medical Informatics Association: JAMIA, 13*(2), 188–196.

Ozdas, A., Miller, R. A., & Waitman, L. R. (2008). Care Provider Order Entry (CPOE): A perspective on factors leading to success or to failure. *Yearbook of Medical Informatics, 2007*, 128–137. Review. Erratum in: Yearbook of Medical Informatics. 2008:19.

Ozkaynak, M., Brennan, P. F., Hanauer, D. A., Johnson, S., Aarts, J., Zheng, K., & Haque, S. N. (2013, March 28). Patient-centered care requires a patient-oriented workflow model. *Journal of the American Medical Informatics Association: JAMIA, 20*(e1), e14–e16.

Paddock, S. W. (1994). To boldly glow. Applications of laser scanning confocal microscopy in developmental biology. *BioEssays, 16*(5), 357–365.

Padkin, A., Rowan, K., & Black, N. (2001). Using high quality clinical databases to complement the results of randomised controlled trials: The case of recombinant human activated protein C. *BMJ, 323*(7318), 923–926.

Pagliari, C., Detmer, D., & Singleton, P. (2007). Potential of electronic personal health records. *BMJ, 335*(7615), 330–333.

Palda, V. A., & Detsky, A. S. (1997). Perioperative assessment and management of risk from coronary artery disease. *Annals of Internal Medicine, 127*(4), 313–328.

Palfrey, J., Gasser, U. (2010). Born digital: Understanding the first generation of digital natives. New York: Basic Books; Robertson, J. (2011). *Insulin pumps, monitors vulnerable to hacking*. Retrieval 15 Aug 2011: http://www.ap.org/

Palmer, M., Gildea, D., & Kingsbury, P. (2005). The proposition bank: An annotated corpus of semantic roles. *Computational Linguistics, 31*(1), 71–105.

Palotie, A., Widen, E., & Ripatti, S. (2013). From genetic discovery to future personalized health research. *New Biotechnology, 30*(3), 291–295.

Park, T. (2011). Opening access to high-value data sets. In L. A. Olsen, R. S. Saunders, & J. M. McGinnis (Eds.), *Patients charting the course: Citizen engagement and the learning health system* (pp. 74–87). Washington: National Academies Press.

Park, J. C., Kim, H. S., & Kim, J. J. (2001). Bidirectional incremental parsing for automatic pathway identification with combinatory categorial grammar. *Proceedings of the Pacific Symposium on Biocomputing, 6*, 396–407.

Parrish, F., Do, N., Bouhaddou, O., & Warnekar, P. (2006). Implementation of RxNorm as a terminology mediation standard for exchanging pharmacy medication between federal agencies. *AMIA Annual Symposium Proceedings*, 1057.

Paskin, N. (2006). The DOI handbook. Oxford: International DOI Foundation. Retrieved from http://www.doi.org/handbook_2000/DOIHandbook-v4-4.pdf

Patel, V. L., & Cohen, T. (2008). New perspectives on error in critical care. *Current Opinion in Critical Care, 14*(4), 456–459.

Patel, V. L., & Groen, G. J. (1986). Knowledge based solution strategies in medical reasoning. *Cognitive Science, 10*(1), 91–116.

Patel, V. L., & Groen, G. J. (1991a). Developmental accounts of the transition from medical student to doctor: Some problems and suggestions. *Medical Education, 25*(6), 527–535.

Patel, V. L., & Groen, G. J. (1991b). The general and specific nature of medical expertise: A critical look. In K. A. Ericsson & J. Smith (Eds.), *Toward a general theory of expertise: Prospects and limits* (pp. 93–125). New York: Cambridge University Press.

Patel, V. L., & Kaufman, D. R. (1998). Medical informatics and the science of cognition. *Journal of the American Medical Informatics Association: JAMIA, 5*(6), 493–502.

Patel, V. L., & Zhang, J. (2007). Cognition and patient safety in healthcare. In F. T. Durso, R. S. Nickerson, S. Dumais, S. Lewandowsky, & T. Perfect (Eds.), *Handbook of applied cognition* (2nd ed., pp. 307–331). New York: Wiley.

Patel, V. L., Groen, G. J., & Frederiksen, C. H. (1986). Differences between students and physicians in memory for clinical cases. *Medical Education, 20*, 3–9.

Patel, V. L., Groen, G. J., & Arocha, J. F. (1990). Medical expertise as a function of task-difficulty. *Memory and Cognition, 18*(4), 394–406.

Patel, V.L., Arocha, J.F., & Kaufman, D.R. (1994). Diagnostic reasoning and medical expertise. In Medin, D.L. (Ed.), The psychology of learning and motivation: Advances in research and theory, Vol. 31 (Vol. 19970101, pp. 187–252 ix, 366pp.). San Diego: Academic Press, Inc.

Patel, V. L., Ramoni, M. F., et al. (1997). Cognitive models of directional inference in expert medical reasoning. In P. J. Feltovich & K. M. Ford (Eds.), *Expertise in context: Human and machine* (pp. 67–99). Cambridge: The MIT Press.

Patel, V. L., Kushniruk, A. W., Yang, S., & Yale, J. F. (2000). Impact of a computer-based patient record system on data collection, knowledge organization, and reasoning. *Journal of the American Medical Informatics Association*, 7(6), 569–585.

Patel, V. L., Arocha, J. F., & Kaufman, D. R. (2001). Review? A primer on aspects of cognition for medical informatics. *Journal of the American Medical Informatics Association: JAMIA*, 8(4), 324–343.

Patel, V. L., Branch, T., & Arocha, J. F. (2002a). Errors in interpreting quantities as procedures: The case of pharmaceutical labels. *International Journal of Medical Informatics*, 65(3), 193–211.

Patel, V. L., Kaufman, D. R., & Arocha, J. F. (2002b). Emerging paradigms of cognition in medical decision-making. *Journal of Biomedical Informatics*, 35(1), 52–75.

Patel, V. L., Arocha, J. F., & Zhang, J. (2005). Thinking and reasoning in medicine. In K. J. Holyoak (Ed.), *Cambridge handbook of thinking and reasoning* (pp. 727–750). Cambridge: Cambridge University Press.

Patel, A., Schieble, T., Davidson, M., Tran, M. C., Schoenberg, C., Delphin, E., et al. (2006). Distraction with a hand-held video game reduces pediatric preoperative anxiety. *Paediatric Anaesthesia*, 16(10), 1019–1027.

Patel, V. L., Zhang, J., Yoskowitz, N. A., Green, R., & Sayan, O. R. (2008). Translational cognition for decision support in critical care environments: A review. *Journal of Biomedical Informatics*, 41, 413–431.

Patel, V. L., Yoskowitz, N. A., Arocha, J. F., & Shortliffe, E. H. (2009). Cognitive and earning sciences in biomedical and health instructional design: A review with lessons for biomedical informatics education. *Journal of Biomedical Informatics*, 42, 176–197.

Patel, V. L., Arocha, J. F., & Zhang, J. (2010). Medical reasoning and thinking. In K. J. Holyoak & R. G. Morrison (Eds.), *Oxford handbook of thinking and reasoning*. Oxford: Oxford University Press.

Patel, V. L., Cohen, T., Murarka, T., et al. (2011). Recovery at the edge of error: Debunking the myth of the infallible expert. *Journal of Biomedical Informatics*, 44(3), 413–424.

Patient Centered Medical Home 2011. Retrieved July 17, 2011, from http://www.ncqa.org/.

Patient Centered Medical Homes Resource Center. Retrieved July 17, 2011, from http://www.pcmh.ahrq.gov/portal/server.pt/community/pcmh_home/1483.

Patton, M. Q. (1999, December). Enhancing the quality and credibility of qualitative analysis. *Health Services Research*, 34(5 Pt 2), 1189–1208.

Pauker, S.G., Gorry, G.A., Kassirer, J.P., & Schwartz, W.B. (1976). Towards the simulation of clinical cognition: Taking a present illness by computer. *Amer J Med*, 60(7):981–996.

Pauker, S. G., & Kassirer, J. P. (1980). The threshold approach to clinical decision making. *The New England Journal of Medicine*, 34(5 Pt 2), 1189–1208.

Pauker, S. G., & Kassirer, J. P. (1981). Clinical decision analysis by computer. *Archives of Internal Medicine*, 141(13), 1831–1837.

Pavel, M., Jimison, H., Hayes, T., Larimer, N., Hagler, S., Vimegnon, Y., et al. (2010). Optimizing medication reminders using a decision-theoretic framework. *Studies in Health Technology and Informatics*, 160(Pt 2), 791–795.

Pawson, R., & Tilley, N. (1997). *Realistic evaluation*. London: Sage Press.

Paxinos, G., & Watson, C. (1986). *The rat brain in stereotaxic coordinates*. San Diego: Acedemic Press.

Payne, S. J. (2003). Users' mental models: The very ideas. In J. M. Carroll (Ed.), *HCI models, theories, and frameworks: Toward a multidisciplinary science* (1st ed., pp. 135–156). San Francisco: Morgan Kaufmann.

Payne, P. R., Johnson, S. B., Starren, J. B., Tilson, H. H., & Dowdy, D. (2005). Breaking the translational barriers: The value of integrating biomedical informatics and translational research. *Journal of Investigative Medicine*, 53(4), 192–200.

Payne, P. R., Embi, P. J., & Sen, C. K. (2009). Translational informatics: Enabling high-throughput research paradigms. *Physiological Genomics*, 39(3), 131–140.

Payne, P. R., Embi, P. J., & Niland, J. (2010). Foundational biomedical informatics research in the clinical and translational science era: A call to action. *Journal of the American Medical Informatics Association: JAMIA*, 17(6), 615–616.

Payton, F., Pare, G., LeRouge, C., & Madhu, R. (2011). Health care IT: Process, people, patients and interdisciplinary considerations. *Journal of the Association for Information Systems*, 12(2/3), 1–13.

Peabody, G. (1922). The physician and the laboratory. *Boston Medical Surgery Journal*, 187, 324.

Pearce, C., Arnold, M., Phillips, C., Trumble, S., & Dwan, K. (2011). The patient and the computer in the primary care consultation. *Journal of the American Medical Informatics Association: JAMIA*, 18(2), 138–142.

Peleg, M., Tu, S., Bury, J., Ciccarese, P., Fox, J., Greenes, R. A., Hall, R., Johnson, P. D., Jones, N., Kumar, A., Miksch, S., Quaglini, S., Seyfang, A., Shortliffe, E. H., & Stefanelli, M. (2003). Comparing computer-interpretable guideline models: A case-study approach. *Journal of the American Medical Informatics Association: JAMIA*, 10, 52–68.

Pencina, M. J., D'Agostino, R. B., Sr., D'Agostino, R. B., Jr., & Vasan, R. S. (2008). Evaluating the added predictive ability of a new marker: From area under the ROC curve to reclassification and beyond. *Statistics in Medicine*, 27, 157–172; discussion 207–112.

Perkins, D. N., Schwartz, S., & Simmons, R. (1990). A view from programming. In M. Smith (Ed.), *Toward a unified theory of problem solving: Views from content domains* (pp. 45–67). Hillsdale: Lawrence Erlbaum Associates.

Perkins, G., Renken, C., et al. (1997). Electron tomography of neuronal mitochondria: Three-dimensional structure and organization of cristae and menbrane contacts. *Journal of Structural Biology*, 119(3), 260–272.

Perreault, L. E., & Metzger, J. B. (1999). A pragmatic framework for understanding clinical decision support. *Heathcare Information Management*, 13(2), 5–21.

Perry, M. (2003). Distributed cognition. In J. M. Carroll (Ed.), *HCI models, theories, and frameworks: Toward a multidisciplinary science* (pp. 193–223). San Francisco: Morgan Kaufmann Publishers.

Pestian, J. P., & Matykiewicz, P. (2008). Classification of suicide notes using natural language processing. *Proceedings of the ACL BioNLP*, 96–97.

Pestian, J. P., Brew, C., Matykiewicz, P., Hovermale, D. J., Johnson, N., Cohen, K. B., & Duch, W. (2007). A shared task involving multi-label classification of clinical free text. *Proceedings of the Workshop on BioNLP*, Association for Computational Linguistics Stroudsburg, PA: 97–104.

Pestotnik, S. L. (2005). Expert clinical decision support systems to enhance antimicrobial stewardship programs: Insights from the Society of Infectious Diseases Pharmacists. *Pharmacotherapy, 25*(8), 1116–1125.

Peterson, W., Birdsall, T. (1953). The Theory of Signal Detectability. (Technical Report No. 13.): Electronic Defense Group, University of Michigan, Ann Arbor.

Petratos, G. N., Kim, Y., Evans, R. S., & Gardner, R. M. (2010). Comparing the effectiveness of computerized adverse drug event monitoring systems to enhance clinical decision support for hospitalized patients. *Applied Clinical Informatics, 1*, 293–303.

Peute, L. W., Aarts, J., Bakker, P. J., & Jaspers, M. W. (2009). Anatomy of a failure: A sociotechnical evaluation of a laboratory physician order entry system implementation. *International Journal of Medical Informatics, 79*(4), e58–e70.

Pevsner, P. (2009). *Bioinformatics and functional genomics*. Hoboken, NJ: Wiley.

Pew Internet and American Life Project. Health Topics. (2011). http://pewinternet.org/Reports/2011/HealthTopics.aspx. Accessed 21 Nov 2011.

Pew Internet and American Life Project. Peer-to-peer Healthcare. (2011). http://pewinternet.org/Presentations/2011/Aug/NIH-Mind-the-Gap.aspx. Accessed 21 Nov 2011.

Pham, D. L., Xu, C. Y., et al. (2000). Current methods in medical image segmentation. *Annual Review of Biomedical Engineering, 2*, 315.

Pham, H. H., Schrag, D., O'Malley, A. S., Wu, B., & Bach, P. B. (2007). Care patterns in medicare and their implications for pay for performance. *The New England Journal of Medicine, 356*(11), 1130–1139.

Phansalkar, S., Desai, A. A., Bell, D., et al. (2012a). High-priority drug-drug interactions for use in electronic health records. *Journal of the American Medical Informatics Association: JAMIA, 19*(5), 735–743.

Phansalkar, S., van der Sijs, H., Tucker, A. D., et al. (2012b). Drug-drug interactions that should be non-interruptive in order to reduce alert fatigue in electronic health records. *Journal of the American Medical Informatics Association: JAMIA, 20*(3), 489–493.

Pickering, B. W., Herasevich, V., & Gajic, A. A. (2010). Novel representation of clinical information in the ICU – developing user interfaces which reduce information overload. *Applied Clinical Informatics, 1*, 116–131. PMID – NONE [Patent applied for!!].

Pinsky, P. F., Miller, A., Kramer, B. S., Church, T., Reding, D., Prorok, P., Gelmann, E., Schoen, R. E., Buys, S., Hayes, R. B., & Berg, C. D. (2007, April 15). Evidence of a healthy volunteer effect in the prostate, lung, colorectal, and ovarian cancer screening trial. *American Journal of Epidemiology, 165*(8), 874–881.

Plunkett, R. J., (1952). Standard Nomenclature of Diseases and Operations – 4th ed., American Medical Association. New York: McGraw-Hill

Pluye, P., & Grad, R. (2004). How information retrieval technology may impact on physician practice: An organizational case study in family medicine. *Journal of Evaluation in Clinical Practice, 10*, 413–430.

Polifka, J. E., & Friedman, J. M. (2002). Teratogen update: Azathioprine and 6-mercaptopurine. *Teratology, 65*(5), 240–261.

Pollack, A. (2011, July 29). Ruling upholds gene patent in cancer test. *The New York Times*. New York City: The New York Times Company.

Polson, P. G., Lewis, C., Rieman, J., & Wharton, C. (1992). Cognitive walkthroughs – a method for theory-based evaluation of user interfaces. *International Journal of Man–machine Studies, 36*(5), 741–773.

Poon, K. B. (2005). *Fusing multiple heart rate signals to reduce alarms in adult intensive care unit*. Master of Science Thesis from Department of Medical Informatics, University of Utah. Salt Lake City, UT.

Poon, E. G., Kuperman, G. J., Fiskio, J., & Bates, D. W. (2002). Real-time notification of laboratory data requested by users through alphanumeric pagers. *Journal of the American Medical Informatics Association: JAMIA, 9*, 217–222.

Poon, E. G., Keohane, C. A., Yoon, C. S., Ditmore, M., Bane, A., Levtzion-Korach, O., et al. (2010). Effect of bar-code technology on the safety of medication administration. *The New England Journal of Medicine, 362*(18), 1698–1707.

Pople, H. (1982). Heuristic methods for imposing structure on ill-structured problems: The structuring of medical diagnosis. In Szolovits P. (ed.), Artificial Intelligence in Medicine. Boulder, CO: Westview Press.

Porter, M., & Teisberg, E. (2006). *Redefining healthcare: Creating value-based competition on results*. Cambridge, MA: Harvard Business School Press.

Pouratian, N., Sheth, S. A., et al. (2003). Shedding light on brain mapping: Advances in human optical imaging. *Trends in Neurosciences, 26*(5), 277–282.

Prastawa, M., Gilmore, J., et al. (2004). Automatic segmentation of neonatal brain MRI. Medical Image Computing and Computer-Assisted Intervention – Miccai 2004, Pt 1. *Proceedings, 3216*, 10–17.

Preece, J., Rogers, Y., & Sharp, H. (2007). *Interaction design: Beyond human-computer interaction* (2nd ed.). West Sussex: Wiley.

President's Council of Advisors on Science and Technology. (2010). *Realizing the full potential of health information technology to improve healthcare for Americans: The path forward* (p. 40). Washington, DC: Executive Office of the President. Available at http://www.whitehouse.gov/sites/default/files/microsites/ostp/pcast-health-it-report.pdf. Accessed 12 Aug 2011.

President's Information Technology Advisory Committee. (2001, February). Panel on Transforming Health Care. *Transforming health care through information technology*. Available at http://www.itrd.gov/pubs/pitac/pitac-hc-9feb01.pdf. Accessed 17 Dec 2012.

Pressler, T. R., Yen, P. Y., Ding, J., Liu, J., Embi, P. J., & Payne, P. R. (2012). Computational challenges and human factors influencing the design and use of clinical research participant eligibility pre-screening tools. *BMC Medical Informatics and Decision Making, 12*, 47.

Prochaska, J. O., & DiClemente, C. C. (2005). The transtheoretical approach. In J. C. Norcross & M. R. Goldfried (Eds.), *Handbook of psychotherapy integration* (2nd ed., pp. 147–171). New York: Oxford University Press. http://en.wikipedia.org/wiki/Special:BookSources/0195165799. ISBN 0195165799.

Prothero, J. S., & Prothero, J. W. (1986). Three-dimensional reconstruction from serial sections IV. The reassembly problem. *Computers and Biomedical Research, 19*(4), 3610373.

Pruitt, K.D., Maglott, D.R. (2001). RefSeq and LocusLink: NCBI gene-centered resources. *Nucleic Acids Research, 29*(1), 137–140. Available at http://www.ncbi.nlm.nih.gov/LocusLink/

Pryor, T. A. (1988). The HELP medical record system. *MD Computing, 5*(5), 22–33.

Pryor, T. A. (1989). Computerized nurse charting. *International Joural of Clinical Monitoring and Computing, 6*, 173–179. PMID 2592844.

Pryor, T. A., & Hripcsak, G. (1993). The Arden syntax for medical logic modules. *International Journal of Clinical Monitoring and Computing, 10*(4), 215–224.

Pryor, T. A., Gardner, R. M., Clayton, P. D., & Warner, H. R. (1983). The HELP system. *Journal of Medical Informatics, 7*(2), 87–102.

Public Health Informatics Institute. (2011). *Collaborative requirements development methodology*. Decatur: Public Health Informatics Institute.

Pysz, M. A., Gambhir, S. S., et al. (2010). Molecular imaging: Current status and emerging strategies. *Clinical Radiology, 65*(7), 500–516.

Qin, J., Li, R., et al. (2010). A human gut microbial gene catalogue established by metagenomic sequencing. *Nature, 464*(7285), 59–65.

Qiu, G. (2002). Indexing chromatic and achromatic patterns for content-based colour image retrieval. *Pattern Recognition, 35*(8), 1675–1686.

Quake, S. (2011). Personal communication.

Rahimi, B., Vimarlund, V., & Timpka, T. (2009). Health information system implementation: A qualitative meta-analysis. *Journal of Medical Systems, 33*(5), 359–368.

Rahmani, R., Goldman, S. A., et al. (2008). Localized content-based image retrieval. *IEEE Transactions on Pattern Analysis and Machine Intelligence, 30*(11), 1902–1912.

Ralston, J. D., Carrell, D., Reid, R., Anderson, M., et al. (2007). Patient web services integrated with a shared medical record: Patient use and satisfaction. *Journal of the American Medical Informatics Association: JAMIA, 14*(6), 798.

Ralston, J. D., Carrell, D., Reid, R., Anderson, M., Moran, M., & Hereford, J. (2007). Patient web services integrated with a shared medical record: Patient use and satisfaction. *Journal of the American Medical Informatics Association, 14*(6), 798–806. Epub 2007 Aug 21. Erratum in: Journal of the American Medical Informatics Association. 2008;15(2):265.

Ramnarayan, P., Kapoor, R. R., Coren, M., Nanduri, V., Tomlinson, A. L., Taylor, P. M., Wyatt, J. C., & Britto, J. F. (2003, November–December). Measuring the impact of diagnostic decision support on the quality of clinical decision making: Development of a reliable and valid composite score. *Journal of the American Medical Informatics Association: JAMIA, 10*(6), 563–572.

Ramsaroop, P., & Ball, M. (2000). The "bank of health": a model for more useful patient health records. *MD Computing, 17*, 45–48.

Ransohoff, D. F., & Feinstein, A. R. (1978). Problems of spectrum and bias in evaluating the efficacy of diagnostic tests. *The New England Journal of Medicine, 299*(17), 926–930.

Rausch, T., & Jackson, J. (2007). *Using clinical workflows to improve medical device/system development*. Paper presented at the Joint Workshop on High-Confidence Medical Devices, Software, and Systems and Medical Device Plug-and-Play Interoperability. Cambridge, MA.

Ray, P. (2011). Multimodality molecular imaging of disease progression in living subjects. *Journal of Biosciences, 36*(3), 499–504.

Ray, P., & Gambhir, S. S. (2007). Noninvasive imaging of molecular events with bioluminescent reporter genes in living subjects. *Methods in Molecular Biology, 411*, 131–144.

Read, J. D. (1990). Computerizing medical language. In H. DeGlanville & J. Roberts (Eds.), *Current perspectives in health computing HC90* (pp. 203–208). Computing: British Journal of Health Care.

Read, J. D., & Benson, T. J. (1986). Comprehensive coding. *British Journal of Health Care Computing, 3*, 622–625.

Reason, J. T. (1990). *Human error*. Cambridge/New York: Cambridge University Press.

Rector, A. L., Nowlan, W. A., et al. (1993). Goals for concept representation in the GALEN project. In C. Safran (Ed.), *Proceedings of the 17th annual symposium on Computer Applications in Medical Care (SCAMC 93)* (pp. 414–418). New York: McGraw Hill.

Rector, A. L., Glowinski, A. J., Nowlan, W. A., & Rossi-Mori, A. (1995). Medical-concept models and medical records: An approach based on GALEN and PEN & PAD. *Journal of the American Medical Informatics Association: JAMIA, 2*(1), 19–35.

Redd, W. H., Jacobsen, P. B., Die-Trill, M., Dermatis, H., McEvoy, M., & Holland, J. C. (1987). Cognitive/attentional distraction in the control of conditioned nausea in pediatric cancer patients receiving chemotherapy. *Journal of Consulting and Clinical Psychology, 55*(3), 391–395.

Reiner, B. I., Siegel, E. L., & Hooper, F. J. (2002). Accuracy of interpretation of CT scans: Comparing PACS monitor displays and hard-copy images. *AJR. American Journal of Roentgenology, 179*, 1407–1410.

Reiser, S. (1991). The clinical record in medicine. Part 1: Learning from cases. *Annals of Internal Medicine, 114*(10), 902–907.

Research Support, U.S. Gov't, P.H.S. (2006). *Journal of the American Medical Informatics Association: JAMIA, 13*(1), 91–95.

Research Support, U.S. Gov't, P.H.S. (2007). *BMC medical informatics and decision making, 7*, 25.

Research Support, U.S. Gov't, P.H.S. (2008). *The New England Journal of Medicine, 358*(16), 1732–1737.

Research Support, U.S. Gov't, P.H.S. (2010). *Journal of medical Internet research, 12*(2), e14.

Research Support, U.S. Gov't, P.H.S. (2011). *PloS one, 6*(4), e19256.

Rhee, S. Y., Wood, V., Dolinski, K., & Draghici, S. (2008). Use and misuse of the gene ontology annotations. *Nature Reviews Genetics, 9*, 509–515.

Ribaric, S., Todorovski, L., et al. (2001). Presentation of dermatological images on the internet. *Computer Methods and Programs in Biomedicine, 65*(2), 111–121.

Ricci, M. A., Caputo, M., Amour, J., et al. (2003). Telemedinicine reduces discrepancies in rural trauma care. *Telemedicine Journal and E-Health, 9*, 3–11.

Ricci, F., Rokach, L., Shapira, B., & Kantor, P. B. (Eds.). (2011). *Recommender systems handbook*. New York/London: Springer.

Richardson, J. S. (1981). The anatomy and taxonomy of protein structure. *Advances in Protein Chemistry, 34*, 167–339.

Richesson, R. L., & Krischer, J. (2007, November–December). Data standards in clinical research: Gaps, overlaps, challenges and future directions. *Journal of the American Medical Informatics Association: JAMIA, 14*(6), 687–696.

Richter, G. M., Williams, S. L., Starren, J., Flynn, J. T., & Chiang, M. F. (2009). Telemedicine for retinopathy of prematurity diagnosis: Evaluation and challenges. *Survey of Ophthalmology, 54*, 671–685.

Rigby, M., Forsström, J., Ruth, R., & Wyatt, J. (2001). Verifying quality and safety in health informatics services. *BMJ, 323*, 552–556.

Rimoldi, H. J. (1961). The test of diagnostic skills. *Journal of Medical Education, 36*, 73–79.

Rindflesch, T.C., Tanabe, L., Weinstein, J.N., & Hunter, L. (2000). EDGAR: extraction of drugs, genes and relations from the biomedical literature. *Proceedings of the Pacific Symposium Biocomputing*, 517–528.

Ritchie, C. J., Edwards, W. S., et al. (1996). Three-dimensional ultrasonic angiography using power-mode Doppler. *Ultrasound in Medicine and Biology, 22*(3), 277–286.

Ritchie, M. D., Denny, J. C., Crawford, D. C., et al. (2010). Robust replication of genotype-phenotype associations across multiple diseases in an electronic medical record. *American Journal of Human Genetics, 86*, 560–572.

Riva, A., Mandl, K. D., Oh, D. H., Nigrin, D. J., Butte, A., Szolovits, P., et al. (2001). The personal internetworked notary and guardian. *International Journal of Medical Informatics, 62*(1), 27–40.

Robertson, J. (2011, August 4). Insulin pumps, monitors vulnerable to hacking. Associated Press via various media, e.g., *The Washington Times*. Retrieval 1 Aug 2012: http://www.washingtontimes.com/news/2011/aug/4/insulin-pumps-monitors-vulnerable-to-hacking/?page=all

Robinson, P. J. (1997). Radiology's Achilles' heel: Error and variation in the interpretation of the Rontgen image. *The British Journal of Radiology, 70*(839), 1085–1098.

Robinson, A., & Thomson, R. (2001). Variability in patient preferences for participating in medical decision making: Implication for the use of decision support tools. *Quality in Health Care: QHC, 10*(Suppl 1), i34–i38.

Rocca-Serra, P., Brandizi, M., Maguire, E., et al. (2010). ISA software suite: Supporting standards-compliant experimental annotation and enabling curation at the community level. *Bioinformatics, 26*, 2354–2356.

Roden, D. M., Pulley, J. M., Basford, M. A., Bernard, G. R., Clayton, E. W., Balser, J. R., & Masys, D. R. (2008, September). Development of a large-scale de-identified DNA biobank to enable personalized medicine. *Clinical Pharmacology and Therapeutics, 84*(3), 362–369.

Rodríguez-Campos, L. (2012, November). Advances in collaborative evaluation. *Evaluation and Program Planning, 35*(4), 523–528.

Rogers, Y. (2004). New theoretical approaches for HCI. *Annual Review of Information Science and Technology, 38*, 87–143.

Rogers, W. J., Canto, J. G., Lambrew, C. T., Tiefenbrunn, A. J., Kinkaid, B., Shoultz, D. A., Frederick, P. D., & Every, N. (2000). Temporal trends in the treatment of over 1.5 million patients with myocardial infarction in the US from 1990 thru 1999: The National Registry of Myocardial Infarction 1, 2 and 3. *Journal of the American College of Cardiology, 36*, 2056–2063. PMID 11127441.

Rohlfing, T., & Maurer, C. R., Jr. (2003). Nonrigid image registration in shared-memory multiprocessor environments with application to brains, breasts, and bees. *IEEE Transactions on Information Technology in Biomedicine, 7*(1), 16–25.

Romano, M. J., & Stafford, R. S. (2011). Electronic health records and clinical decision support systems: Impact on national ambulatory care quality. *Archives of Internal Medicine, 171*(10), 897–903.

Rose, M. T. (1989). *The open book: A practical perspective on OSI*. Upper Saddle River: Prentice Hall.

Rosen, G. (1993). *History of public health*. Baltimore: Johns Hopkins University Press.

Rosen, G.D., Williams, A.G., et al. (2000). The mouse brain library @ www.mbl.org. *International Mouse Genome Conference, 14*, 166.

Rosenbloom, S. T., Geissbuhler, A. J., Dupont, W. D., Giuse, D. A., Talbert, D. A., Tierney, W. M., Plummer, W. D., Stead, W. W., & Miller, R. A. (2005). *Effect of CPOE User Interface Design on User-Initiated Access* to Educational and Patient Information during Clinical Care Journal of the American Medical Informatics Association: JAMIA, 12(4), 458–473.

Rosencrance, L. (2006, November 13). Problems abound for Kaiser e-health records management system. Computerworld, 40(46), 1–3.

Rosenfeld, B. A., Dorman, T., Breslow, M. J., et al. (2000). Intensive care unit telemedicine: Alternate paradigm for providing continuous intensivist care. Critical Care Medicine, 28, 3925–3931.

Ross, B., & Bluml, S. (2001). Magnetic resonance spectroscopy of the human brain. Anatomical Record (New Anat), 265(2), 54–84.

Ross, D. T., Scherf, U., Eisen, M. B., et al. (2000). Systematic variation in gene expression patterns in human cancer cell lines. Nature Genetics, 24, 227–235.

Rosse, C. (2000). Terminologia anatomica; considered from the perspective of next-generation knowledge sources. Clinical Anatomy, 14, 120–133.

Rosse, C., & Mejino, J. L. V. (2003). A reference ontology for bioinformatics: The foundational model of anatomy. Journal of Bioinformatics, 36(6), 478–500.

Rosse, C., Mejino, J. L., et al. (1998a). Motivation and organizational principles for anatomical knowledge representation: The digital anatomist symbolic knowledge base. Journal of the American Medical Informatics Association: JAMIA, 5(1), 17–40.

Rosse, C., Shapiro, L.G., et al. (1998b). The Digital Anatomist foundational model: principles for defining and structuring its concept domain. Proceedings, American Medical Informatics Association Fall Symposium (pp. 820–824), Orlando.

Roth, E. M., Patterson, E. S., & Mumaw, R. J. (2002). Cognitive engineering: Issues in user-centered system design. In J. J. Marciniak (Ed.), Encyclopedia of software engineering. New York: Wiley.

Rothenberg, J. (1999). Ensuring the longevity of digital information, from http://www.clir.org/pubs/archives/ensuring.pdf

Rotman, B. L., Sullivan, A. N., McDonald, T. W., Brown, B. W., DeSmedt, P., Goodnature, D., Higgins, M. C., Suermondt, H. J., Young, C., & Owens, D. K. (1996). A randomized controlled trial of a computer-based physician workstation in an outpatient setting: Implementation barriers to outcome evaluation. Journal of the American Medical Informatics Association: JAMIA, 3(5), 340–8. PMID: 8880681 [PubMed - indexed for MEDLINE].

Rozenblum, R., Jang, Y., Zimlichman, E., Salzberg, C., Tamblyn, M., Buckeridge, D., Forster, A., Bates, D. W., & Tamblyn, R. (2011). A qualitative study of canada's experience with the implementation of electronic health information technology. CMAJ: Canadian Medical Association journal, 183(5), E281–E288.

RSNA. (2009). RSNA to create image sharing network with NIBIB grant. Retrieved June 24, 2011, from http://www.rsna.org/Publications/rsnanews/November-2009/1109_announcements.cfm. Accessed 27 Jan 13.

Rubin, D. L. (2008). Creating and curating a terminology for radiology: Ontology modeling and analysis. Journal of Digital Imaging, 21(4), 355–362.

Rubin, D. L. (2011, October). Measuring and improving quality in radiology: Meeting the challenge with informatics. Radiographics, 31(6), 1511–1527.

Rubin, D. L., & Napel, S. (2010). Imaging informatics: toward capturing and processing semantic information in radiology images. Yearbook of Medical Informatics, 34–42.

Rubin, D.L., Gennari, J., & Musen, M.A. (2000). Knowledge representation and tool support for critiquing clinical trial protocols. Proceedings of the AMIA Symposium, 724–728.

Rubin, D. L., Bashir, Y., et al. (2004). Linking ontologies with three-dimensional models of anatomy to predict the effects of penetrating injuries. Conference Proceedings: IEEE Engineering in Medicine and Biology Society, 5, 3128–3131.

Rubin, D. L., Bashir, Y., et al. (2005). Using an ontology of human anatomy to inform reasoning with geometric models. Studies in Health Technology and Informatics, 111, 429–435.

Rubin, D.L., Grossman, D., et al. (2006a). Ontology-based representation of simulation models of physiology. AMIA Annual Symposium Proceedings, 664–668.

Rubin, D. L., Dameron, O., et al. (2006b). Using ontologies linked with geometric models to reason about penetrating injuries. Artificial Intelligence in Medicine, 37(3), 167–176.

Rubin, D.L., Rodriguez, C., et al. (2008). iPad: Semantic annotation and markup of radiological images. AMIA Annual Symposium Proceedings, 626–630.

Rubin, D. L., Talos, I. F., et al. (2009a). Computational neuroanatomy: Ontology-based representation of neural components and connectivity. BMC Bioinformatics, 10(Suppl 2), S3.

Rubin, D. L., Supekar, K., et al. (2009b). Annotation and Image Markup: Accessing and Interoperating with the Semantic Content in Medical Imaging. IEEE Intelligent Systems, 24(1), 57–65.

Rubin, D. L., Flanders, A., et al. (2011). Ontology-assisted analysis of Web queries to determine the knowledge radiologists seek. Journal of Digital Imaging, 24(1), 160–164.

Rudin, R. S. (2010). The litmus test for health information exchange success: Will small practices participate?: comment on "health information exchange". Archives of Internal Medicine, 170(7), 629–630.

Rudin, R. S., Salzberg, C. A., Szolovits, P., Volk, L. A., Simon, S. R., & Bates, D. W. (2011). Care transitions as opportunities for clinicians to use data exchange services: how often do they occur? Journal of the American Medical Informatics Association: JAMIA, 18(6), 853–858.

Ruiz, M.E. (2006). Combining image features, case descriptions and UMLS concepts to improve retrieval of medical images. AMIA Annual Symposium Proceedings, 674–678.

Rusk, N. (2010). Expanding HapMap. *Nature Methods, 7*, 780–781.

Saccavini, C., & Greco, F. (2004). *Health Current Account Project*. Presented at EuroPAC MIR (Session 7.19).

Saeed, M., Lieu, C., Raber, G., & Mark, R. G. (2002). MIMIC II: A massive temporal ICU patient database to support research in intelligent patient monitoring. *Computers in Cardiology, 29*, 641–644.

Saeed, M., Villarroel, M., Reisner, A. T., Clifford, G., Lethman, L. W., Moody, G., Heldt, T., Kyaw TH Moody, B., & Mark, R. G. (2011). Multiparameter intelligent monitoring in intensive care II: A public-access intensive care unit database. *Critical Care Medicine, 39*, 952–960. PMID 21283005.

Saffle, J. R., Edelman, L., Theurer, L., et al. (2009). Telemedicine evaluation of acute burns is accurate and cost-effective. *The Journal of Trauma, 67*, 358–365.

Safran, C., Porter, D., Lightfoot, J., Rury, C. D., Underhill, L. H., Bleich, H. L., & Slack, W. V. (1989). ClinQuery: A system for online searching of data in a teaching hospital. *Annals of Internal Medicine, 111*(9), 751–756.

Safran, C., Rury, C., Rind, D., & Taylor, W. C. (1991). A computer-based outpatient medical record for a teaching hospital. *MD Computing, 8*, 291–299.

Safran, C., Shabot, M. M., Munger, B. S., Holmes, J. H., Steen, E. B., Lumpkin, J. R., & Detmer, D. E. (2009, March–April). AMIA board of directors. Program requirements for fellowship education in the subspecialty of clinical informatics. *Journal of the American Medical Informatics Association: JAMIA, 16*, 158–166. PMID 19074295.

Sager, N. (1972). Syntactic formatting of science information. *Proceedings of the AFIPS* (pp. 791–800). In Kittredge, R., &Lehrberger, J., (Eds.), Reprinted in Sublanguage: Studies of language in restricted semantic domains (pp. 9–26). Berlin (1982): Walter de Gruyter.

Sager, N. (1978). Natural language information formatting: The automatic conversion of texts to a structured data base. In M. C. Yovits (Ed.), *Advances in computers* (Vol. 17, pp. 89–162). New York: Academic Press.

Sager, N. (1981). *Natural language information processing: A computer grammer of english and its applications*. Reading: Addison-Wesley.

Sager, N., Friedman, C., & Lyman, M. (1987). *Medical language processing – computer management of narrative data*. Reading: Addison-Wesley.

Saleem, J. J., Russ, A. L., Justice, C. F., Hagg, H., Ebright, P. R., Woodbridge, P. A., & Doebbeling, B. N. (2009a). Exploring the persistence of paper with the electronic health record. *International Journal of Medical Informatics, 78*(9), 618–628.

Saleem, J., Russ, A., Sanderson, P., Johnson, T., Zhang, J., & Sittig, D. (2009b). Current challenges and opportunities for better integration of human factors research with development of clinical information systems. *Yearbook of Medical Informatics, 2009*, 48–58.

Saleem, J. J., Russ, A. L., Neddo, A., Blades, P. T., Doebbeling, B. N., & Foresman, B. H. (2011). Paper persistence, workarounds, and communication breakdowns in computerized consultation management. *International Journal of Medical Informatics, 80*(7), 466–479.

Salomon, G., Perkins, D. N., & Globerson, T. (1991). Partners in cognition: Extending human intelligence with intelligent technologies. *Educational Researcher, 20*(3), 2–9. doi:10.3102/0013189x020003002.

Salpeter, S. R., Sanders, G. D., Salpeter, E. E., & Owens, D. K. (1997). Monitored isoniazid prophylaxis for low-risk tuberculin reactors older than 35 years of age: A risk-benefit and cost-effectiveness analysis. *Annals of Internal Medicine, 127*(12), 1051–1061.

Salton, G. (1991). Developments in automatic text retrieval. *Science, 253*, 974–980.

Salton, G., & McGill, M. (1983). *Introduction to modern information retrieval*. New York: McGraw-Hill.

Salton, G., Fox, E., & Wu, H. (1983). Extended Boolean information retrieval. *Communications of the ACM, 26*, 1022–1036.

Saltz, J., Hastings, S., Langella, S., Oster, S., Kurc, T., Payne, P., & Chue Hong, N. (2008). A roadmap for caGrid, an enterprise grid architecture for biomedical research. *Studies in Health Technology and Informatics, 138*, 224–237.

Samantaray, R., Njoku, V. O., Brunner, J. W., Raghavan, V., Kendall, M. L., & Shih, S. C. (2011). Promoting electronic health record adoption among small independent primary care practices. *The American Journal of Managed Care, 17*(5), 353–358.

Sander, C. (2000). Genomic medicine and the future of health care. *Science, 287*(5460), 1977–1978.

Sanders, G. D., Hagerty, C. G., Sonnenberg, F. A., Hlatky, M. A., & Owens, D. K. (1999). Distributed dynamic decision support using a web-based interface for prevention of sudden cardiac death. *Medical Decision Making, 19*(2), 157–166.

Sanders, G. D., Hlatky, M. A., & Owens, D. K. (2005). Cost effectiveness of the implantable cardioverter defibrillator (ICD) in primary prevention of sudden death. *The New England Journal of Medicine, 353*, 1471–1478.

Sandor, S., & Leahy, R. (1997). Surface-based labeling of cortical anatomy using a deformable atlas. *IEEE Transactions on Medical Imaging, 16*(1), 41–54.

Sansone, S. A., Fan, T., et al. (2007). The metabolomics standards initiative. *Nature Biotechnology, 25*(8), 846–848.

Sansone, S. A., Rocca-Serra, P., et al. (2008). The first RSBI (ISA-TAB) workshop: "can a simple format work for complex studies?". *OMICS A Journal of Integrative Biology, 12*(2), 143–149.

Saria, S., Rajani, A. K., Gould, J., Koller, D., & Penn, A. A. (2010). Integration of early physiological responses predicts later illness severity in preterm infants. *Science Translational Medicine, 2*(48), 48ra65.

Sarkar, I. N., & Payne, P. R. (2011). The joint summits on translational science: Crossing the translational chasm. *Journal of Biomedical Informatics, 44*(Suppl 1), S1–S2.

Sarkar, I. N., & Starren, J. (2002). Desiderata for personal electronic communications in clinical systems. *Journal of the American Medical Informatics Association: JAMIA, 9,* 209–216.

Sarkar, I. N., Butte, A. J., Lussier, Y. A., et al. (2011a). Translational bioinformatics: Linking knowledge across biological and clinical realms. *Journal of the American Medical Informatics Association: JAMIA, 18,* 354–357.

Sarkar, U., Karter, A. J., Liu, J. Y., Adler, N. E., Nguyen, R., Lopez, A., et al. (2011b). Social disparities in internet patient portal use in diabetes: Evidence that the digital divide extends beyond access. *Journal of the American Medical Informatics Association: JAMIA, 18*(3), 318–321.

Satava, R. M. (2007). The future of sugical simulation and surgical robotics. *Bulletin of the American College of Surgeons, 92*(3), 13–19.

Saunders, C. J., Miller, N. A., Soden, S. E., et al. (2012). Rapid whole-genome sequencing for genetic disease diagnosis in neonatal intensive care units. *Science Translational Medicine, 4*(154), 154ra135.

Sayers, E., Barrett, T., Benson, D., Bolton, E., Bryant, S., Canese, K., & DiCuccio, M. (2011). Database resources of the national center for biotechnology information. *Nucleic Acids Research, 39*(suppl1), D38–D51.

Scaife, M., & Rogers, Y. (1996). External cognition: How do graphical representations work? *International Journal of Human Computer Studies, 45*(2), 185–213.

Scalbert, A., Brennan, L., et al. (2009). Mass-spectrometry-based metabolomics: Limitations and recommendations for future progress with particular focus on nutrition research. *Metabolomics, 5*(4), 435–458.

Schadt, E. E. (2012). The changing privacy landscape in the era of big data. *Molecular Systems Biology, 8,* 612.

Schaefer, C. F., Anthony, K., Krupa, S., et al. (2009). PID: The pathway interaction database. *Nucleic Acids Research, 37,* D674–D679.

Schaltenbrand, G., & Warren, W. (1977). *Atlas for stereotaxy of the human brain.* Stuttgart: Thieme.

Schedlbauer, A., Prasad, V., Mulvaney, C., Phansalkar, S., Stanton, W., Bates, D. W., & Avery, A. J. (2009). What evidence supports the use of computerized alerts and prompts to improve clinicians' prescribing behavior? *Journal of the American Medical Informatics Association: JAMIA, 16*(4), 531–538.

Scheuner, M. T., Sieverding, P., & Shekelle, P. G. (2008). Delivery of genomic medicine for common chronic adult diseases: A systematic review. *JAMA: The Journal of the American Medical Association, 299*(11), 1320–1334.

Schimel, A. M., Fisher, Y. L., et al. (2011). Optical coherence tomography in the diagnosis and management of diabetic macular edema: Time-domain versus spectral-domain. *Ophthalmic Surgery, Lasers & Imaging, 42*(4), S41–S55.

Schmidt, H. G., & Rikers, R. M. (2007). How expertise develops in medicine: Knowledge encapsulation and illness script formation. *Medical Education, 41*(12), 1133–1139. doi:10.1111/j.1365-2923.2007.02915.x. MED2915 [pii].

Schnall, R., Gordon, P., Camhi, E., & Bakken, S. (2011a). Perceptions of factors influencing use of an electronic record for case management of persons living with HIV. *AIDS Care, 23*(3), 357–365.

Schnall, R., Cimino, J. J., Currie, L. M., & Bakken, S. (2011b). Information needs of case managers caring for persons living with HIV. *Journal of the American Medical Informatics Association: JAMIA, 18*(3), 305–308.

Schnipper, J. L., Gandhi, T. K., Wald, J. S., Grant, R. W., Poon, E. G., Volk, L. A., et al. (2008a). Design and implementation of a web-based patient portal linked to an electronic health record designed to improve medication safety: The Patient Gateway medications module. *Informatics in Primary Care, 16*(2), 147–155.

Schnipper, J. L., Linder, J. A., Palchuk, M. B., Einbinder, J. S., Li, Q., Postilnik, A., & Middleton, B. (2008b). "Smart forms" in an electronic medical record: Documentation-based clinical decision support to improve disease management. *Journal of the American Medical Informatics Association: JAMIA, 15*(4), 513–523.

Schultz, J. R., Cantrill, S. V., & Morgan, K. G. (1971). *AFIPS Conference Proceedings, 38,* 239–264.

Schultz, E. B., Price, C., et al. (1997). Symbolic anatomic knowledge representation in the read codes version 3: Structure and application. *Journal of the American Medical Informatics Association: JAMIA, 4,* 38–48.

Schwamm, L. H., Holloway, R. G., Amarenco, P., Audebert, H. J., Bakas, T., Chumbler, N. R., Handschu, R., Jausch, E. C., Knight, W. A., 4th, Levine, S. R., Mayberg, M., Meyer, B. C., Meyers, P. M., Skalabrin, E., & Wechsler, L. R. (2009). American heart association stroke council; interdisciplinary council on peripheral vascular disease. *Stroke, 40,* 2616–2634.

Schwartz, W. B. (1970). Medicine and the computer: The promise and problems of change. *The New England Journal of Medicine, 283*(23), 1257–1264.

Schwartz, D., & Collins, F. (2007). Medicine. Environmental biology and human disease. *Science, 316,* 695–696.

Schwartz, R. J., Weiss, K. M., & Buchanan, A. V. (1985). Error control in medical data. *MD Computing, 2*(2), 19–25.

Scott, G. P., Shah, P., Wyatt, J. C., Makubate, B., & Cross, F. W. (2011, August 11). Making electronic prescribing alerts more effective: Scenario-based experimental study in junior doctors. *Journal of the American Medical Informatics Association: JAMIA, 18*(6), 789–798.

Seal, R. L., Gordon, S. M., Lush, M. J., et al. (2011). Genenames.org: The HGNC resources in 2011. *Nucleic Acids Research, 39,* D514–D519.

Seidenari, S., Pellacani, G., et al. (2003). Computer description of colours in dermoscopic melanocytic lesion images reproducing clinical assessment. *British Journal of Dermatology, 149*(3), 523–529.

Sekimizu, T., Park, H. S., & Tsujii, J. (1998). Identifying the interaction between genes and gene products based on frequently seen verbs in Medline abstracts. *Genome Informatics Ser Workshop on Genome Informatics, 9*, 62–71.

Senathirajah, Y., & Bakken, S. (2009). Architectural and usability considerations in the development of a Web 2.0-Based EHR. *Student Health Technology Informatics, 143*, 315–321.

Sensor Systems Inc. (2001). *MedEx.* from http://medx.sensor.com/products/medx/index.html

Shabo, A. (2005). The implications of electronic health record for personalized medicine. *Biomedical papers of the Medical Faculty of the University Palacký, Olomouc, Czechoslovakia, 149*(2), suppl 251–8.

Shabo, A. (2006). A global socio-economic-medico-legal model for the sustainability of longitudinal health records. *Methods of Information in Medicine, 45*, 240–245 (Part 1), 498–505 (Part 2).

Shabot, M. M. (1995). Computers in the intensive care unit: Was pogo correct? *Journal of Intensive Care Medicine, 10*, 211–212.

Shabot, M. M., & Gardner, R. M. (Eds.). (1994). *Decision support systems in critical care.* Boston: Springer.

Shah, N. H., & Musen, M.A. (2008). UMLS-Query: a perl module for querying the UMLS. *AMIA Annual Symposium Proceedings*, Washington, DC: 652–656.

Shah, N. R., Seger, A. C., Seger, D. L., Fiskio, J. M., Kuperman, G. J., Blumenfeld, B., Recklet, E. G., et al. (2006). Improving acceptance of computerized prescribing alerts in ambulatory care. *Journal of the American Medical Informatics Association: JAMIA, 13*(1), 5–11.

Shah, N. H., Rubin, D. L., Espinosa, I., et al. (2007). Annotation and query of tissue microarray data using the NCI thesaurus. *BMC Bioinformatics, 8*, 296.

Shah, N. H., Jonquet, C., Chiang, A. P., et al. (2009a). Ontology-driven indexing of public datasets for translational bioinformatics. *BMC Bioinformatics, 10*(Suppl 2), S1.

Shah, S. H., Crosslin, D.R., Nelson, S., et al. (2009b). Metabolomic profiles are associated with baseline insulin resistance and improvement in insulin resistance with weight loss in the WLM trial. *Ciculation.*

Shahar, Y., & Musen, M. A. (1996). Knowledge-based temporal abstractions in clinical domains. *Artificial Intelligence in Medicine, 8*(3), 267–298.

Shapiro, L. G., & Stockman, G. C. (2001). *Computer vision.* Upper Saddle River: Prentice Hall.

Shea, S., Starren, J., Weinstock, R. S., et al. (2002). Columbia University's informatics for diabetes education and telemedicine (IDEATel) project: Rationale and design. *Journal of the American Medical Informatics Association: JAMIA, 9*(1), 49–62.

Shea, S., Weinstock, R. S., Teresi, J. A., et al. (2009). A randomized trial comparing telemedicine case management with usual care in older, ethnically diverse, medically underserved patients with diabetes mellitus: 5 Year results of the IDEATel study. *Journal of the*

American Medical Informatics Association: JAMIA, 16(4), 446–456.

Shekelle, P.G., Morton, S.C., et al. (2006). Costs and benefits of health information technology. *Evidence Reports Technology Assessesment (Full Report),* (132), 1–71.

Shekelle, P. G., Pronovost, P. J., Wachter, R. S., et al. (2011). Advancing the science of patient safety. *Annals of Internal Medicine, 154*(10), 693–696.

Sherifali, D., Greb, J. L., Amirthavasar, G., Hunt, D., Haynes, R. B., Harper, W., Holbrook, A., Capes, S., Goeree, R., O'Reilly, D., Pullenayegum, E., & Gerstein, H. C. (2011). Effect of computer-generated tailored feedback on glycemic control in people with diabetes in the community: A randomized controlled trial. *Diabetes Care, 34*(8), 1794–1798.

Sherry, S. T., Ward, M. H., Kholodov, M., Baker, J., Phan, L., Smigielski, E. M., & Sirotkin, K. (2001). DbSNP: The NCBI database of genetic variation. *Nucleic Acids Research, 29*, 308–311.

Shi, J. B., & Malik, J. (2000). Normalized cuts and image segmentation. *IEEE Transactions on Pattern Analysis and Machine Intelligence, 22*(8), 888–905.

Shiffman, R. N., Karras, B. T., Agrawal, A., Chen, R., Marenco, L., & Nath, S. (2000). GEM: A proposal for a more comprehensive guideline document model using XML. *Journal of the American Medical Informatics Association: JAMIA, 7*(5), 488–498.

Shih, S. C., McCullough, C. M., Wang, J. J., Singer, J., & Parsons, A. S. (2011). Health information systems in small practices. Improving the delivery of clinical preventive services. *Am J Prev Med, 41*(6), 603–609. doi:10.1016/j.amepre.2011.07.024.

Shim, E.-J., Lee, K.-S., Park, J.-H., & Park, J.-H. (2011). Comprehensive needs assessment tool in cancer (CNAT): the development and validation. *Supportive Care in Cancer, 19*(12), 1957–1968.

Shirky, C. (2010). *Cognitive surplus: Creativity and generosity in a connected age.* New York: Penguin Press.

Shneiderman, B. (1998). *Designing the user interface: Strategies for effective human-computer-interaction* (3rd ed.). Reading: Addison Wesley Longman.

Shortell, S. M., Gillies, R. R., Anderson, D. A., et al. (2000). *Remaking healthcare in America: The evolution of organized delivery* (2nd ed.). San Francisco: Jossey-Bass.

Shortliffe, E. H., Buchanan, B. G. (1975). A model of inexact reasoning in medicine. *Mathematical Biosciences, 23*(3), 351–379.

Shortliffe, E. H. (1976). *Computer-based medical consultations: MYCIN.* New York: Elsevier/North Holland.

Shortliffe, E. H. (1993). Doctors, patients, and computers: Will information technology dehumanize health-care delivery? *Proceedings of the American Philosophical Society, 137*(3), 390–398.

Shortliffe, E. H. (1994). Dehumanization of patient care. Are computers the problem or the solution? *Journal of the American Medical Informatics Association: JAMIA, 1*, 76–78.

Shortliffe, E.H. (1998a). The Next Generation Internet and health care: A civics lesson for the informatics community. *Proceedings of the AMIA Annual Fall Symposium* (pp. 8–14), Orlando.

Shortliffe, E. H. (1998b). *The evolution of health-care records in the era of the Internet, Proceedings of Medinfo 98*. Seoul/Amsterdam: IOS Press.

Shortliffe, E. H. (2000). Networking health: Learning from others, taking the lead. *Health Affairs, 19*(6), 9–22.

Shortliffe, E. H. (2005). Strategic action in health information technology: Why the obvious has taken so long. *Health Affairs, 24*, 1222–1233.

Shortliffe, E. H. (2010). Biomedical informatics in the education of physicians. *Journal of the American Medical Association, 304*(11), 1227–1228.

Shortliffe, T., (2012). *The Future of Biomedical Informatics: A Perspective from Academia.* Keynote Presentation, Medical Informatics Europe 2012, Pisa, Italy.

Shortliffe, E. H., & Blois, M. S. (2001). The computer meets medicine and biology: Emergence of a discipline. In E. H. Shortliffe & L. E. Perreault (Eds.), *Medical informatics: Computer applications in health care and biomedicine* (2nd ed., pp. 3–40). New York: Springer.

Shortliffe, E.H., Sondik, E. (2004). *The informatics infrastructure: Anticipating its role in cancer surveillance.* Proceedings of the C-Change Summit on Cancer Surveillance and Information: The Next Decade, Phoenix

Shortliffe, E. H., Buchanan, B. G., & Feigenbaum, E. (1979). Knowledge engineering for medical decision making; a review of computer-based clinical decision aids. *Proceedings of the IEEE, 67*, 1207–1224.

Shortliffe, E. H., Califano, A., & Hunter, L. (2009). New JBI emphasis on translational bioinformatics. *Journal of Biomedical Informatics, 42*, 199–200.

Shubin, H., & Weil, M. H. (1966). Efficient monitoring with a digital computer of cardiovascular function in seriously ill patients. *Annals of Internal Medicine, 65*(3), 453–460.

Shuldiner, A. R., O'Connell, J. R., Bliden, K. P., et al. (2009). Association of cytochrome P450 2C19 genotype with the antiplatelet effect and clinical efficacy of clopidogrel therapy. *JAMA: The Journal of the American Medical Association, 302*, 849–857.

Siebert, U., Alagoz, O., Bayoumi, A. M., Jahn, B., Owens, D. K., Cohen, D., et al. (2012). State-transition modeling: A report of the ISPOR-SMDM modeling good research practices task force-3. *Medical Decision Making, 32*, 690–700.

Siebig, S., Kuhls, S., Imhoff, M., Gather, U., Scholmerich, J., & Wrede, C. E. (2010). Intensive care unit alarms – how many do we need? *Critical Care Medicine, 38*, 451–456. PMID 20016379.

Siegler, E. L. (2010). The evolving medical record. *Annals of Internal Medicine, 153*(10), 671–677.

Siek, K. A., Khan, D. U., Ross, S. E., Haverhals, L. M., Meyers, J., & Cali, S. R. (2011). Designing a personal health application for older adults to manage medications: A comprehensive case study. *Journal of Medical Systems, 35*(5), 1099–1121.

Silberg, W., Lundberg, G., & Musacchio, R. (1997). Assessing, controlling, and assuring the quality of medical information on the internet: Caveat lector et viewor – let the reader and viewer beware. *Journal of the American Medical Association, 277*, 1244–1245.

Simborg, D. W., Chadwick, M., Whiting-O'Keefe, Q. E., Tolchin, S. G., Kahn, S. A., & Bergan, E. S. (1983). Local area networks and the hospital. *Computers and Biomedical Research, 16*(3), 247–259.

Simon, H. A. (1980). The behavioral and social sciences. *Science, 209*(4452), 72–78.

Simon, D. P., & Simon, H. A. (1978). Individual differences in solving physics problems. In R. S. Siegler (Ed.), *Children's thinking: What develops?* (Vol. 11, pp. 325–348). Hillsdale: Lawrence Erlbaum Associates.

Simon, R., Brennecke, R., Hess, O., Meier, B., Reiber, H., & Zeelenberg, C. (1994). Report of the ESC task force on digital imaging in cardiology. Recommendations for digital imaging in angiocardiography. *European Heart Journal, 15*, 1332–1334.

Simonaitis, L., Belsito, A., Warvel, J., Hui, S., & McDonald, C. J. (2006). Extensible stylesheet language formatting objects (XSL-FO): a tool to transform patient data into attractive clinical reports. *AMIA Annual Symposium Proceedings, 2006*, 719–723.

Singer, E. (2011). A family learns the secrets of its genomes. *MIT Technology Review.*

Singh, A., Massoud, T. F., et al. (2008). Molecular imaging of reporter gene expression in prostate cancer: An overview. *Seminars in Nuclear Medicine, 38*(1), 9–19.

Sirota, M., Dudley, J. T., Kim, J., et al. (2011). Discovery and preclinical validation of drug indications using compendia of public gene expression data. *Science Translational Medicine, 3*, 96ra77.

Sistrom, C., Dang, P., Weilburg, J., Dreyer, K., Rosenthal, D., & Thrall, J. (2009). Effect of computerized order entry with integrated decision support on the growth of outpatient procedure volumes: Seven-year time series analysis. *Radiology, 251*, 147–155.

Sittig, D. F. (1994). Grand challenges in medical informatics? *Journal of the American Medical Informatics Association: JAMIA, 1*(5), 412–413.

Sittig, D., & Singh, H. (2009). Eight rights of safe electronic health record use. *JAMA: The Journal of the American Medical Association, 302*(10), 1111–1113.

Sittig, D. F., & Singh, H. (2011). Defining health information technology-related errors: new developments since to err is human. *Archives of Internal Medicine, 171*(14), 1281–1284.

Sittig, D. F., Krall, M., Kaalaas-Sittig, J., & Ash, J. S. (2005). Emotional aspects of computer-based provider order entry: A qualitative study. *Journal of the American Medical Informatics Association: JAMIA, 12*(5), 561–567.

Sittig, D. F., Wright, A., Osheroff, J. A., et al. (2008). Grand challenges in clinical decision support. *Journal of Biomedical Informatics, 41*(2), 387–392.

Sittig, D. F., Wright, A., Meltzer, S., Simonaitis, L., Evans, R. S., Nichol, W. P., Ash, J. S., & Middleton, B.

(2011). Comparison of clinical knowledge management capabilities of commercially-available and leading internally-developed electronic health records. *BMC Medical Informatics and Decision Making, 11,* 13. PMID 21329520.

Sivic, J., & Zisserman, A. (2003). Video Google: A text retrieval approach to object matching in videos. *Proceedings of the International Conference on Computer Vision, 2,* 1470–1477.

Skinner, B. F. (1938). *The behavior of organisms.* New York: Appleton-Century-Crofts.

Slack, W. V., & Bleich, H. L. (1999). The CCC system in two teaching hospitals: A progress report. *International Journal of Medical Informatics, 54*(3), 183–196.

Slack, W. V., Hicks, G. P., Reed, C. E., & Van Cura, L. J. (1966). A computer-based medical-history system. *The New England Journal of Medicine, 274*(4), 194–198. PubMed PMID: 5902618.

Slack, W. V., Peckham, B. M., Van Cura, L. J., & Carr, W. F. (1967). A computer-based physical examination system. *JAMA: The Journal of the American Medical Association, 200*(3), 224–228.

Slagle, J. M., Gordon, J. S., Harris, C. E., Davison, C. L., Culpepper, D. K., Scott, P., et al. (2010). MyMediHealth – designing a next generation system for child-centered medication management. *Journal of Biomedical Informatics, 43*(5 Suppl), S27–S31.

Sloboda, J. (1991). Musical expertise. In K. A. Ericsson & J. Smith (Eds.), *Toward a general theory of expertise: Prospects and limits* (pp. 153–171). New York: Cambridge University Press.

Slutsky, J. R., & Clancy, C. M. (2010). Patient-centered comparative effectiveness research: Essential for high-quality care. *Archives of Internal Medicine, 170*(5), 403–404.

Smelcer, J., Miller-Jacobs, H., et al. (2009). Usability of electronic medical records. *Journal of Usability Studies, 4*(2), 70–84.

Smeulders, A. W. M., Worring, M., et al. (2000). Content-based image retrieval at the end of the early years. *IEEE Transactions on Pattern Analysis and Machine Intelligence, 22*(12), 1349–1380.

Smith, L. (1985). Medicine as an art. In J. Wyngaarden & L. Smith (Eds.), *Cecil textbook of medicine.* Philadelphia: W. B. Saunders.

Smith, A. (2011, July). *Smartphone adoption and usage.* Washington, D.C: Pew Internet and American Life Project.

Smith, T., & Waterman, M. (1981). Identification of common molecular subsequences. *Journal of Molecular Biology, 147*(1), 195–197.

Smith, M.K., Welty, C., et al. (2004). *OWL web ontology language guide,* http://www.w3.org/TR/owl-guide/

Smith, P. C., Araya-Guerra, R., Bublitz, C., Parnes, B., Dickinson, L. M., Vorst, R. V., Westfall, J. M., & Pace, W. D. (2005). Missing clinical information during primary care visits. *JAMA: The Journal of the American Medical Association, 293*(5), 565–571.

Smith, B., Ashburner, M., Rosse, C., et al. (2007). The OBO foundry: Coordinated evolution of ontologies to support biomedical data integration. *Nature Biotechnology, 25,* 1251–1255.

Smith, M. Q., Staley, C. A., et al. (2009). Multiplexed fluorescence imaging of tumor biomarkers in gene expression and protein levels for personalized and predictive medicine. *Current Molecular Medicine, 9*(8), 1017–1023.

Sobradillo, P., Pozo, F., & Agusti, A. (2011). P4 medicine: The future around the corner. *Archivos de Bronconeumología, 47,* 35–40.

Sohrab, M. A., Smith, R. T., et al. (2011). Imaging characteristics of dry age-related macular degeneration. *Seminars in Ophthalmology, 26*(3), 156–166.

Sollins, K., & Masinter, L. (1994). *Functional requirements for uniform resource names: Internet Engineering Task Force.* Retrieved from http://www.w3.org/Addressing/rfc1737.txt

Solomon, M., Liu, Y., et al. (2011). Optical imaging in cancer research: Basic principles, tumor detection, and therapeutic monitoring. *Medical Principles and Practice, 20*(5), 397–415.

Sommerville, I. (2002). Software engineering. *Reading.* MA: Addison Wesley.

Sonnenberg, F. A., & Beck, J. R. (1993). Markov models in medical decision making: A practical guide. *Medical Decision Making, 13*(4), 322–338.

Sordo, M., Boxwala, A. A., Ogunyemi, O., & Greenes, R. A. (2004). Description and status update on GELLO: A proposed standardized object-oriented expression language for clinical decision support. *Studies in Health Technology and Informatics, 107,* 164–168.

Soto, G. E., Young, S. J., et al. (1994). Serial section electron tomography: A method for three-dimensional reconstruction of large structures. *NeuroImage, 1,* 230–243.

Southon, F. C., Sauer, C., & Grant, C. N. (1997). Information technology in complex health services: Organizational impediments to successful technology transfer and diffusion. *Journal of the American Medical Informatics Association: JAMIA, 4*(2), 112–24. PMID: 9067877 [PubMed - indexed for MEDLINE].

Sox, H. (2009). Medical journal editing: who shall pay? *Annals of Internal Medicine, 151,* 68–69.

Sox, H. C., Blatt, M. A., Higgins, M. C., & Marton, K. I. (1988). *Medical decision making.* Boston: Butterworth Publisher.

Spackman, K. A. (2000). SNOMED RT and SNOMEDCT. Promise of an international clinical terminology. *MD Computing, 17*(6), 29.

Spackman, K. A. (2004). SNOMED CT milestones: Endorsements are added to already-impressive standards credentials. *Healthcare Informatics, 21*(54), 56.

Spackman, K.A., Campbell, K.E., & Cote, R.A. (1997a). SNOMED RT: a reference terminology for health care. *Proceedings of the AMIA Annual Fall Symposium,* 640–644.

Spackman, K. A., Campbell, K. E., et al. (1997b). SNOMED-RT: A reference terminology for health care. In D. R. Masys (Ed.), *Proceedings, AMIA annual fall symposium* (pp. 640–644). Philadelphia: Hanley and Belfus.

Spiegelhalter, D. J. (1983). Evaluation of medical decision-aids, with an application to a system for dyspepsia. *Statistics in Medicine, 2,* 207–216.

Spilker, B. (1991). *Guide to clinical trials.* New York: Raven Press.

Spitzer, V. M., & Whitlock, D. G. (1998). The visible human dataset: The anatomical platform for human simulation. *Anatomical Record, 253*(2), 49–57.

Spyns, P. (1996). Natural language processing in medicine: An overview. *Methods of Information in Medicine, 35,* 285–301.

Srinivasan, P., Rindflesch, T. (2002). Exploring text mining from MEDLINE. *Proceedings of the AMIA Symposium,* pp. 722–726.

Sriram, K. B., Larsen, J. E., Yang, I. A., Bowman, R. V., & Fong, K. M. (2011). Genomic medicine in non-small cell lung cancer: Paving the path to personalized care. *Respirology (Carlton, Vic.), 16*(2), 257–263.

Staffa, J. A., Chang, J., & Green, L. (2002). Cerivastatin and reports of fatal rhabdomyolysis [Letter]. *The New England Journal of Medicine, 346*(7), 539–540.

Stallings, W. (1987a). *The open systems interconnection (OSI) model and OSI-related standards* (Vol. 1). New York: Macmillian.

Stallings, W. (1987b). *Handbook of computer-communications standards.* New York: Macmillan.

Stallings, W. (1997). *Data and computer communications.* Englewood Cliffs: Prentice-Hall.

Stanfill, M., Williams, M., Fenton, S., Jenders, R., & Hersh, W. (2010). A systematic literature review of automated clinical coding and classification systems. *Journal of the American Medical Informatics Association: JAMIA, 17,* 646–651.

Starr, P. (1982). The Social Transformation of American Medicine. New York: Basic Books.

Starr, P. (1983). The Social Transformation of American Medicine. *Basic Books.*

Starren, J., & Johnson, S. B. (2000). An object-oriented taxonomy of medical data presentations. *Journal of the American Medical Informatics Association: JAMIA, 7*(1), 1–20.

Starren, J., Hripcsak, G., Sengupta, S., Abbruscato, C. R., Knudson, P. E., Weinstock, R. S., & Shea, S. (2002). Columbia University's informatics for diabetes education and telemedicine (IDEATel) project: Technical implementation. *Journal of the American Medical Informatics Association: JAMIA, 9*(1), 25–36.

State of Washington Health Care Authority. (2006). *Washington State health information infrastructure: Final report and roadmap for state action.* Available at http://www.hca.wa.gov/documents/legreports/finalreport.pdf. Accessed 21 Jul 2013.

Stead, W. W. (2010). Electronic health records. *Studies in Health Technology and Informatics, 153,* 119–143.

Stead, W. W., & Hammond, W. E. (1988). Computer-based medical records: The centerpiece of TMR. *MD Computing, 5*(5), 48–62.

Stead, W. W., & Lin, H. S. (Eds.). (2009). *Computational technology for effective health care: Intermediate*

steps and strategic directions. Washington, DC: National Academies Press.

Stead, W. W., & Lorenzi, N. M. (1999). Health informatics: Linking investment to value. *Journal of the American Medical Informatics Association: JAMIA, 6,* 341–348.

Stead, W., Haynes, R. B., Fuller, S., et al. (1994). Designing medical informatics research and library projects to increase what is learned. *Journal of theAmerican Medical Informatics Association, 1,* 28–34.

Stead, W. W., Borden, R., Bourne, J., Giuse, D., Giuse, N., Harris, T. R., Miller, R. A., & Olsen, A. J. (1996). The Vanderbilt University fast track to IAIMS: From planning to implementation. *Journal of the American Medical Informatics Association: JAMIA, 3,* 308–317.

Stead, W. W., Patel, N. R., & Starmer, J. M. (2008). Closing the loop in practice to assure the desired performance. *Transactions of the American Clinical and Climatological Association, 119,* 185–194; discussion 194–185.

Stead, W. W., Searle, J. R., Fessler, H. E., Smith, J. W., & Shortliffe, E. H. (2011). Biomedical informatics: Changing what physicians need to know and how they learn. *Academic Medicine: Journal of the Association of American Medical Colleges, 86*(4), 429–434.

Stearns, M. Q., Price, C., Spackman, K. A., & Wang, A. Y. (2001). SNOMED clinical terms: Overview of the development process and project status. *Proceedings of the AMIA Symposium,* 662–666.

Stein, L. D. (2010). The case for cloud computing in genome informatics. *Genome Biology, 11,* 207.

Stein, P. D., Fowler, S. E., Goodman, L. R., Gottschalk, A., Hales, C. A., et al. (2006). Multidetector computed tomography for acute pulmonary embolism. *The New England Journal of Medicine, 354,* 2317–2327.

Stein, D.M., Vawdrey, D.K., Stetson, P.D., & Bakken, S. (2010). An analysis of team checklists in physician signout notes. *American Medical Informatics Association Annual Symposium Proceedings,* 767–771.

Steinbrook, R. (2008). Personally controlled online health data – the next big thing in medical care? *New England Journal of Medicine, 358*(16), 1653–1656.

Steinbrook, R. (2009). Health care and the American Recovery and Reinvestment Act. *The New England Journal of Medicine, 360*(11), 1057–1060.

Stensaas, S. S., & Millhouse, O.E. (2001). *Atlases of the brain.* From http://medstat.med.utah.edu/kw/brain_atlas/credits.htm

Stenson, P. D., Mort, M., Ball, E. V., et al. (2009). The human gene mutation database: 2008 update. *Genome Medicine, 1,* 13.

Sternberg, R. J., & Horvath, J. A. (Eds.). (1999). *Tacit knowledge in professional practice: Researcher and practitioner.* Mahwah: Lawrence Erlbaum Associates.

Stevens, R. H., Lopo, A. C., & Wang, P. (1996). Artificial neural networks can distinguish novice and expert strategies during complex problem solving. *Journal of the American Medical Informatics Association: JAMIA, 3,* 131–138.

Steyerberg, E. W., Pencina, M. J., Lingsma, H. F., et al. (2011). Assessing the incremental value of diagnostic and prognostic markers: A review and illustration. *European Journal of Clinical Investigation, 42*(2), 216–228.

Storey, J. D., & Tibshirani, R. (2003). Statistical significance for genomewide studies. *Proceedings of the National Academy of Sciences of the United States of America, 100*(16), 9440–9445.

Strahan, R., & Schneider-Kolsky, M. (2010). Voice recognition versus transcriptionist: Error rates and productivity in MRI reporting. *Journal of Medical Imaging and Radiation Oncology, 54*(5), 411–414.

Straus, S., Richardson, W., Glasziou, P., & Haynes, R. (2005). *Evidence based medicine: How to practice and teach EBM* (3rd ed.). New York: Churchill Livingstone.

Stremikis, D. (2009, January). *Health information technology: Key lever in health system transformation.* From the President, pp. 1–5.

Strom, B. L. (2006). How the US drug safety system should be changed. *JAMA: The Journal of the American Medical Association, 295*(17), 2072–2075.

Strom, B. L., Schinnar, R., Aberra, F., Bilker, W., Hennessy, S., Leonard, C. E., & Pifer, E. (2010). Unintended effects of a computerized physician order entry nearly hard-stop alert to prevent a drug interaction: A randomized controlled trial. *Archives of Internal Medicine, 170*(17), 1578–1583.

Subramaniam, B., Hennessey, J. G., et al. (1997). Software and methods for quantitative imaging in neuroscience: The Kennedy Krieger Institute Human Brain Project. In S. H. Koslow & M. F. Huerta (Eds.), *Neuroinformatics: An overview of the human brain project* (pp. 335–360). Mahwah: Lawrence Erlbaum.

Subramanian, A., Tamayo, P., Mootha, V. K., et al. (2005). Gene set enrichment analysis: A knowledge-based approach for interpreting genome-wide expression profiles. *Proceedings of the National Academy of Sciences of the United States of America, 102*, 15545–15550.

Suchman, L. A. (1987). Understanding computers and cognition – a new foundation for esign – Winograd, T., Flores, F. *Artificial Intelligence, 31*(2), 227–232.

Sumner, W., Nease Jr., R.F., Littenberg, B. (1991). U-titer: A utility assessment tool. In *Proceedings of the 15th annual symposium on Computer Applications in Medical Care* (pp. 701–705), Washington, DC.

Sun, J. X., Reisner, A. T., Saeed, M., Heldt, T., & Mark, R. G. (2009). The cardiac output from pressure algorithms trial. *Critical Care Medicine, 37*, 72–80. PMID 19112280.

Sundsten, J.W., Conley, D.M., et al. (2000). Digital Anatomist web-based interactive atlases. From http://www9.biostr.washington.edu/da.html

Sung, N. S., Crowley, W. F., Jr., Genel, M., et al. (2003). Central challenges facing the national clinical research enterprise. *JAMA: The Journal of the American Medical Association, 289*(10), 1278–1287.

Sussman, S. Y. (2001). *Handbook of program development for health behavior research & practice.* Thousand Oaks: Sage.

Swanson, D. (1988). Historical note: Information retrieval and the future of an illusion. *Journal of the American Society for Information Science, 39*, 92–98.

Swanson, L. W. (1992). *Brain maps: Structure of the rat brain.* Amsterdam/New York: Elsevier.

Swanson, L. W. (1999). *Brain maps: Structure of the rat brain.* New York: Elsevier Science.

Sweeney, L. (1997). Weaving technology and policy together to maintain confidentiality. *The Journal of Law, Medicine & Ethics, 25*, 98–110.

Swets, J. A. (1973). The relative operating characteristic in psychology. *Science, 182*, 990.

Szczepura, A., & Kankaanpaa, J. (1996). *Assessment of health care technologies.* London: Wiley.

Szolovits, P., & Pauker, S. G. (1979). Computers and clinical decision making: Whether, how much, and for whom? *Proceedings of the IEEE, 67*, 1224–1226.

Szolovits, P., Doyle, J., Long, W.J., Kohane, I., Pauker, S.G. (1994). *Guardian angel: Patient-Centered Health Information Systems* (Technical Report MIT/LCS/TR-604), Boston: Massachusetts Institute of Technology Laboratory for Computer Science.

Tai, B. C., & Seldrup, J. (2000). A review of software for data management, design and analysis of clinical trials. *Annals of the Academy of Medicine, Singapore, 29*(5), 576–581.

Talairach, J., & Tournoux, P. (1988). *Co-planar stereotaxic atlas of the human brain.* New York: Thieme Medical Publishers.

Talmon, J., Ammenwerth, E., Brender, J., de Keizer, N., Nykänen, P., & Rigby, M. (2009). STARE-HI—statement on reporting of evaluation studies in health informatics. *International Journal of Medical Informatics, 7*, 1–9.

Talos, I. F., Rubin, D. L., et al. (2008). A prototype symbolic model of canonical functional neuroanatomy of the motor system. *Journal of Biomedical Informatics, 41*(2), 251–263.

Tamersoy, A., Loukides, G., Nergiz, M. E., Saygin, Y., & Malin, B. (2012). Anonymization of longitudinal electronic medical records. *IEEE Transactions on Information Technology in Biomedicine, 16*, 413–423.

Tanenbaum, A. S. (1987). *Computer networks* (2nd ed.). Englewood Cliffs: Prentice Hall.

Tanenbaum, A. (1996). *Computer networks* (3rd ed.). Englewood Cliffs: Prentice-Hall.

Tang, P.C. (2003). *Key Capabilities of an Electronic Health Record System* (Letter Report). Committee on Data Standards for Patient Safety. Board on Health Care Services, Institute of Medicine.

Tang, P. C., & McDonald, C. J. (2001). Computer-based patient-record systems. In E. H. Shortliffe & L. E. Perreault (Eds.), *Medical informatics: Computer applications in health care and biomedicine* (2nd ed., pp. 327–358). New York: Springer.

Tang, P. C., & Patel, V. L. (1994). Major issues in user interface design for health professional workstations: Summary and recommendations. *International Journal of Biomedical Computing, 34*(104), 130–148.

Tang, P. C., Annevelink, J., Suermondt, H. J., & Young, C. Y. (1994a). Semantic integration in a physician's workstation. *International Journal of Bio-Medical Computing, 35*(1), 47–60.

Tang, P.C., Fafchamps, D., Shortliffe, E.H. (1994b). Traditional medical records as a source of clinical data in the outpatient setting. *Proceedings of the Annual Symposium Computer Applications in Medical Care,* 575–579.

Tang, P.C., Jaworski, M.A., Fellencer, C.A., Kreider, N., LaRosa, M.P., & Marquardt, W.C. (1996). Clinician information activities in diverse ambulatory care practices. *Proceedings: a conference of the American Medical Informatics Association / … AMIA Annual Fall Symposium. AMIA Fall Symposium,* 12–16.

Tang, P., Newcomb, C., Gorden, S., & Kreider, N. (1997). Meeting the information needs of patients: results from a patient focus group. *Proceedings of the 1997 AMIA Annual Fall Symposium* (pp. 672–676), Nashville.

Tang, P. C., LaRosa, M. P., & Gorden, S. M. (1999a). Use of computer-based records, completeness of documentation, and appropriateness of documented clinical decisions. *Journal of the American Medical Informatics Association: JAMIA, 6*(3), 245–251.

Tang, P. C., Marquardt, W. C., Boggs, B., et al. (1999b). NetReach: Building a clinical infrastructure for the enterprise. In J. M. Overhage (Ed.), *Fourth annual proceedings of the Davies CPR recognition symposium* (pp. 25–68). Chicago: McGraw-Hill.

Tang, P. C., Ash, J. S., Bates, D. W., Overhage, J. M., & Sands, D. Z. (2006). Personal health records: Definitions, benefits, and strategies for overcoming barriers to adoption. *Journal of the American Medical Informatics Association: JAMIA, 13*(2), 121–126.

Tang, P. C., Ralston, M., Arrigotti, M. F., Qureshi, L., & Graham, J. (2007). Comparison of methodologies for calculating quality measures based on administrative data versus clinical data from an electronic health record system: Implications for performance measures. *Journal of the American Medical Informatics Association: JAMIA, 14,* 10–15.

Tarczy-Hornoch, P., Markey, M. K., Smith, J. A., & Hiruki, T. (2007). Bio*medical informatics and genomic medicine: Research and training. *Journal of Biomedical Informatics, 40,* 1–4.

Tate, K.E., Gardner, R.M., & Scherting, K. (1995). Nurses, pagers, and patient-specific criteria: Three keys to improved critical value reporting. *Proceedings of the Annual Symposium on Computer Applications in Medical Care,* 154–8. PMID 8563258.

Tatonetti, N. P., Fernald, G. H., & Altman, R. B. (2011a). A novel signal detection algorithm for identifying hidden drug-drug interactions in adverse event reports. *Journal of the American Medical Informatics Association: JAMIA, 19*(1), 79–85.

Tatonetti, N. P., Denny, J. C., Murphy, S. N., et al. (2011b). Detecting drug interactions from adverse-event reports: Interaction between paroxetine and pravastatin increases blood glucose levels. *Clinical Pharmacology and Therapeutics, 90,* 133–142.

Taylor, H. (2010). *"Cyberchondriacs" on the rise? Those who go online for healthcare information continues to increase.* Rochester: Harris Interactive. Retrieved from http://www.harrisinteractive.com/vault/HI-Harris-Poll-Cyberchondriacs-2010-08-04.pdf

Taylor, C. F., Field, D., Sansone, S. A., Aerts, J., et al. (2008). Promoting coherent minimum reporting guidelines for biological and biomedical investigations: The MIBBI project. *Nature Biotechnology, 26,* 889–896.

Teich, J. M., Kuperman, G. J., & Bates, D. W. (1997). Clinical decision support: Making the transition from the hospital to the community network. *Healthcare Information Management, 11*(4), 27–37.

Teich, J. M., Glaser, J. P., Beckley, R. F., et al. (1999). The Brigham integrated computing system (BICS): Advanced clinical systems in an academic hospital environment. *International Journal of Medical Informatics, 54*(3), 197–208.

Teich, J. M., Merchia, P. R., Schmiz, J. L., et al. (2000). Effects of computerized physician order entry on prescribing practices. *Archives of Internal Medicine, 160*(18), 2741–2747.

Tenenbaum, J., James, A., & Paulyson-Nuñez, K. (2012). An altered treatment plan based on direct to consumer (DTC) genetic testing: Personalized medicine from the patient/pin-cushion perspective. *Journal of Personalized Medicine, 2*(4), 192–200.

The FlyBase Consortium. (2003). The FlyBase database of the Drosophila genome projects and community literature. *Nucleic Acids Research, 31,* 172–175. Available at http://flybase.org/

The Gene Ontology Consortium. (2003). Gene ontology: tool for the unification of biology. *Nature Genetics, 25,* 25–29. Available at http://www.geneontology.org/

Thomas, E. J., Lucke, J. F., Wueste, L., Weavind, L., & Patel, B. (2009). *JAMA: The Journal of the American Medical Association, 302,* 2671–2678.

Thompson, C. B., Snyder-Halpern, R., & Staggers, N. (1999). Clinical informatics case studies: Analysis, processes, and techniques. *Computers in Nursing, 17*(5), 203–206.

Thompson, E. T., & Hayden, A. C. (1961). Standard Nomenclature of Diseases and Operations, 5th ed., American Medical Association. New York: McGraw-Hill.

Thompson, J. P., & Mahajan, R. P. (2006). Monitoring the monitors – beyond risk management. *British Journal of Anaesthesia, 97,* 1–3. PMID 16769701.

Thorisson, G. A., Smith, A. V., Krishnan, L., & Stein, L. D. (2005). The international HapMap project web site. *Genome Research, 15,* 1592–1593.

Tierney, W. M., Miller, M. E., Overhage, J. M., & McDonald, C. J. (1993). Physician inpatient order writing on microcomputer workstations: Effects on resource utilization. *Journal of the American Medical Association, 269*(3), 379–383.

Toga, A. W. (2001). UCLA Laboratory for Neuro Imaging (LONI). From http://www.loni.ucla.edu/

Toga, A. W., Ambach, K. L., et al. (1994). High-resolution anatomy from in situ human brain. *NeuroImage, 1*(4), 334–344.

Toga, A. W., Santori, E. M., et al. (1995). A 3-D digital map of rat brain. *Brain Research Bulletin, 38*(1), 77–85.

Toga, A. W., Frackowiak, R. S. J., et al. (Eds.). (2001). *Neuroimage: A journal of brain function.* New York: Academic Press.

Tommasi, T., Caputo, B., et al. (2010). Overview of the CLEF 2009 medical image annotation track. In *Proceedings of the 10th international conference on cross-language evaluation forum: Multimedia experiments* (pp. 85–93). Corfu: Springer.

Toomre, D., & Bewersdorf, J. (2010). A new wave of cellular imaging. *Annual Review of Cell and Developmental Biology, 26,* 285–314.

Torda, P., Han, E. S., & Scholle, S. H. (2010). Easing the adoption and use of electronic health records in small practices. *Health Affairs (Millwood), 29*(4), 668–675.

Torrance, G. W., & Feeny, D. (1989). Utilities and quality-adjusted life years. *International Journal of Technology Assessment in Health Care, 5*(4), 559–575.

Trafton, J., Martins, S., Michel, M., Lewis, E., Wang, D., Combs, A., Scates, N., Tu, S., & Goldstein, M. K. (2010). Evaluation of the acceptability and usability of a decision support system to encourage safe and effective use of opioid therapy for chronic, noncancer pain by primary care providers. *Pain Medicine, 11*(4), 575–585.

Trotti, A., Colevas, A. D., & Setser, A. (2003). CTCAE v3.0: Development of a comprehensive grading system for the adverse effects of cancer treatement. *Seminars in Radiation Oncology, 13*(3), 176–181.

Trusheim, M. R., Berndt, E. R., & Douglas, F. L. (2007). Stratified medicine: Strategic and economic implications of combining drugs and clinical biomarkers. *Nature Reviews Drug Discovery, 6,* 287–293.

Tsarkov, D., & Horrocks, I. (2006). FaCT++ description logic reasoner: System description. *Automated Reasoning, Proceedings, 4130,* 292–297.

Tu, H. T., & Cohen, G. R. (2008). Striking jump in consumers seeking health care information. *Tracking Report*, (20), 1–8.

Tufte, E. (2006). *Beautiful evidence.* Cheshire: Graphics Press. ISBN 978-0-9613921-7-8.

Tversky, A., & Kahneman, D. (1974). Judgment under uncertainty: Heuristics and biases. *Science, 185,* 1124–1131.

Tysyer, D.A. (1997). Database legal protection. *Bitlaw.* Retrieval 1 Aug 2012: http://www.bitlaw.com/copyright/database.html

Ullman-Cullere, M. H., & Mathew, J. P. (2011). Emerging landscape of genomics in the electronic health record for personalized medicine. *Human Mutation, 32*(5), 512–516. doi:10.1002/humu.21456.

Uzuner, O. (2009). Recognizing obesity and comorbidities in sparse data. *Journal of the American Medical Informatics Association: JAMIA, 16*(4), 561–570.

Uzuner, O., Goldstein, I., Luo, Y., & Kohane, I. (2008). Identifying patient smoking status from medical discharge records. *Journal of the American Medical Informatics Association: JAMIA, 15*(1), 14–24.

Uzuner, O., Solti, I., & Cadag, E. (2010). Extracting medication information from clinical text. *Journal of the American Medical Informatics Association: JAMIA, 17*(5), 514–518.

Uzuner, O., South, B. R., Shen, S., & Duvall, S. L. (2011). 2010 i2b2/VA challenge on concepts, assertions, and relations in clinical text. *Journal of the American Medical Informatics Association: JAMIA, 18*(5), 552–556.

Valdes, I. (2008). *Free and open source software in healthcare 1.0. American Medical Informatics Association Open Source Working Group White Paper.* Available at: http://www.scribd.com/doc/14109414/AMIA-Free-and-Open-Source-Software-in-Healthcare-10. Accessed 2 Jan 2012.

van Bemmel, J. H. (1997). A changing world of grand challenges. *International Journal of Medical Informatics, 44*(1), 53–55.

van der Lei, J., Musen, M. A., van der Does, E., Man in 't Veld, A. J., & vanr Bemmel, J. H. (1991). Comparison of computer-aided and human review of general practitioners' management of hypertension. *The Lancet, 338*(8781), 1504–1508.

van der Sijs, H., Aarts, J., Vulto, A., & Berg, M. (2006). Overriding of drug safety alerts in computerized physician order entry. *Journal of the American Medical Informatics Association: JAMIA, 13*(2), 138–147.

Van Essen, D. C., & Drury, H. A. (1997). Structural and functional analysis of human cerebral cortex using a surface-basec atlas. *Journal of Neuroscience, 17*(18), 7079–7102.

Van Essen, D. C., Drury, H. A., et al. (2001). An integrated software suite for surface-based analysis of cerebral cortex. *Journal of American Medical Association, 8*(5), 443–459.

van Gennip, E. M., & Talmon, J. L. (Eds.). (1995). *Assessment and evaluation of information technologies in medicine.* Amsterdam: IOS Press.

Van Leemput, K., Maes, F., et al. (1999). Automated model-based tissue classification of MR images of the brain. *IEEE Transactions on Medical Imaging, 18*(10), 897–908.

Van Noorden, S. (2002). Advances in immunocytochemistry. *Folia Histochemica et Cytobiologica, 40*(2), 121–124.

van Walraven, C., Taljaard, M., Bell, C. M., Etchells, E., Zarnke, K. B., Stiell, I. G., & Forster, A. J. (2008). Information exchange among physicians caring for the same patient in the community. *Canadian Medical Association Journal, 179*(10), 1013–1018.

Van Way, C. W., Murphy, J. R., Dunn, E. L., & Elerding, S. C. (1982). A feasibility study of computer-aided diagnosis in appendicitis. *Surgery Gynecol & Obstet, 155,* 685–688.

Van't Veer, L. J., Dai, H., van de Vijver, M. J., et al. (2002). Gene expression profiling predicts clinical outcome of breast cancer. *Nature, 415*(6871), 484–485.

Vandemheen, K. L., Aaron, S. D., Poirier, C., Tullis, E., & O'Connor, A. (2010). Development of a decision aid for adult cystic fibrosis patients considering referral for lung transplantation. *Progress in Transplantation, 20*(1), 81–87.

van Rijsbergen, C. (1979). *Information retrieval.* London: Butterworth.

Vapnik, V. N. (2000). *The nature of statistical learning theory*. New York: Springer.

Varma, M., & Zisserman, A. (2003). Texture classification: Are filter banks necessary? In *Proceedings of the IEEE Conference on Computer Vision and Pattern Recognition, Madison, Wisconsin, 2*, (pp. 691–698).

Vawdrey, D. K., Gardner, R. M., Evans, R. S., Orme, J. F., Jr., Clemmer, T. P., Greenway, L., & Drews, F. A. (2007). Assessing the data quality in manual data entry of ventilator settings. *Journal of the American Medical Informatics Association: JAMIA, 14*, 295–303. PMID 17329731.

Vawdrey, D., Wilcox, L., Collins, S., Bakken, S., Feiner, S., & Boyer, A. (2011, October 22–26). A tablet computer application for patients to participate in their hospital care. *Proceedings of the 2011 AMIA Annual Fall Symposium*, 1428–1435.

Venter, J. C., Adams, M. D., Myers, E. W., et al. (2001). The sequence of the human genome. *Science, 291*, 1304–1351.

Via, M., Gignoux, C., & Burchard, E. G. (2010). The 1000 genomes project: new opportunities for research and social challenges. *Genome Medicine, 2*, 3.

Vicente, K. J. (1999). *Cognitive work analysis: Toward safe, productive & healthy computer-based work*. Mahwah: Lawrence Erlbaum Associates Publishers.

Vigoda, M. M., & Lubarsky, D. A. (2006). Failure to recognize loss of incoming data in an anesthesia record-keeping system may have increased medical liability. *Anesthesia and Analgesia, 102*, 1798–1802.

Vincze, V., Szarvas, G., Farkas, R., Mora, G., & Csirik, J. (2008). The BioScope corpus: Biomedical texts annotated for uncertainty, negation, and their scopes. *BMC Bioinformatics, 9*(S11), S9.

Vogel, L. H. (2003). Finding value from information technology investments: Exploring the elusive ROI in healthcare. *Journal for Health Information Management, 17*(4), 20–28.

Vogel, L. H. (2006, September 1) Everyone gets to play. *CIO*.

von Dijk, T. A., & Kintsch, W. (1983). *Strategies of discourse comprehension*. New York: Academic Press.

Voorhees, E., & Harman, D. (Eds.). (2005). *TREC: Experiment and evaluation in information retrieval*. Cambridge, MA: MIT Press.

Voorhees, E., & Hersh, W. (2012). Overview of the TREC 2012 Medical Records Track. *The Twenty-First Text REtrieval Conference proceedings* (*TREC* 2012). Gaithersburg: National Institute for Standards and Technology.

Voorhees, E., & Tong, R. (2011). Overview of the TREC 2011 Medical Records Track. *The Twentieth Text REtrieval Conference proceedings* (*TREC* 2011). Gaithersburg: National Institute for Standards and Technology. Gaithersburg, MD.

Vreeman, D. J., McDonald, C. J., & Huff, S. M. (2010). Representing patient assessments in LOINC®. *American Medical Informatics Association Annual Symposium Proceedings, 2010*, 832–836.

Wachter, S. B., Agutter, J., Syroid, N., Drews, F., Weinger, M. B., & Westenskow, D. (2003). The employment of an iterative design process to develop a pulmonary graphical display. *Journal of the American Medical Informatics Association: JAMIA, 10*(4), 363–372.

Wadman, M. (2007). Experts call for active surveillance of drug safety. *Nature, 446*(7134), 358–359.

Wagner, M. M., Dato, V., Dowling, J. N., & Allswede, M. (2003). Representative threats for research in public health surveillance. *Journal of Biomedical Informatics, 36*(3), 177–188.

Wald, J.S., Grant, R.W., Schnipper, J.L., Gandhi, T.K., Poon, E.G., Businger, A.C., et al. (2009). Survey analysis of patient experience using a practice-linked PHR for type 2 diabetes mellitus. *Proceedings of the 2009 AMIA Annual Symposium*, 678–682.

Walker, J., Pan, E., Johnston, D., Adler-Milstein, J., Bates, D. W., & Middleton, B. (2004). *The value of healthcare information exchange and Interoperability*. Boston: Center for Information Technology Leadership, Partners Healthcare.

Walker, J., Pan, E., Johnston, D., Adler-Milstein, J., Bates, D. W., and Middleton, B. (2005). The value of health care information exchange and interoperability. *Health Aff (Millwood)*, Suppl Web Exclusives: W5–10–W5–18.

Wang, J. Z., Wiederhold, G., et al. (1997). Content-based image indexing and searching using Daubechies' wavelets. *International Journal on Digital Libraries, 1*(4), 311–328.

Wang, S. J., Middleton, B., Prosser, L. A., Bardon, C. G., Spurr, C. D., Carchidi, P. J., Kittler, A. F., Goldszer, R. C., Fairchild, D. G., Sussman, A. J., Kuperman, G. J., & Bates, D. W. (2003). A cost-benefit analysis of electronic medical records in primary care. *American Journal of Medicine, 114*(5), 397–403.

Wang, X., Hripcsak, G., Markatou, M., & Friedman, C. (2009a). Active computerized pharmacovigilance using natural language processing, statistics, and electronic health records: A feasibility study. *Journal of the American Medical Informatics Association: JAMIA, 16*(3), 328–337.

Wang, Y., Xiao, J., Suzek, T. O., et al. (2009b). PubChem: A public information system for analyzing bioactivities of small molecules. *Nucleic Acids Research, 37*, W623–W633.

Wang, Y., Bolton, E., Dracheva, S., Karapetyan, K., Shoemaker, B. A., Suzek, T. O., Wang, J., Xiao, J., Zhang, J., & Bryant, S. H. (2010). An overview of the PubChem BioAssay resource. *Nucleic Acids Research, 38*, D255–D266.

Ward, J. R., & Clarkson, P. J. (2007). Human factors engineering and the design of medical devices. In P. Carayon (Ed.), *Handbook of human factors and ergonomics in health care and patient safety* (pp. 367–382). Mahwah: Lawrence Erlbaum Associates.

Ware, C. (2003). Design as applied perception. In J. M. Carroll (Ed.), *HCI models, theories, and frameworks:*

Toward a multidisciplinary science (pp. 11–26). San Francisco: Morgan Kaufmann Publishers.

Warner, H. R. (1972). A computer-based patient information system for patient care. In G. A. Bekey & M. D. Schwartz (Eds.), *Hospital information systems* (pp. 293–332). New York: Marcel Dekker.

Warner, H. R. (1979). *Computer-assisted medical decision-making*. New York: Academic Press.

Warner, H. R., Swan, H. J., Connolly, D. C., Tompkins, R. G., & Wood, E. H. (1953). Quantitation of beat-to-beat changes in stroke volume from the aortic pulse contour in man. *Journal of Applied Physiology, 5*, 495–507. PMID 13034677.

Warner, H. R., Toronto, A. F., & Veasy, L. (1964). Experience with Bayes' theorem for computer diagnosis of congenital heart disease. *Annals of the New York Academy of Science, 115*, 2–16.

Warner, H. R., Gardner, R. M., & Toronto, A. F. (1968). Computer-based monitoring of cardiovascular function in postoperative patients. *Circulation, 37* (4 Suppl), II68–II74.

Wasson, J. H., Sox, H. C., Neff, R. K., & Goldman, L. (1985). Clinical prediction rules: Applications and methodological standards. *The New England Journal of Medicine, 313*, 793–799.

Weeber, M., Mork, J., & Aronson, A. (2001). Developing a test collection for biomedical word sense disambiguation. *Proceedings of the AMIA Symposium*, 746–750.

Weed, L. L. (1968). Medical records that guide and teach. *The New England Journal of Medicine, 278*(12), 652–657.

Weed, L. L. (1975). *Your health care and how you can manage it*. Burlington: PROMIS Laboratory, University of Vermont.

Wei, L., Altman, R.B. (1998). Recognizing protein binding sites using statistical descriptions of their 3D environments. *Proceedings of the pacific symposium on Biocomputing '98* (pp. 497–508), Singapore.

Weibel, S., & Koch, T. (2000). *The Dublin Core Metadata Initiative: mission, current activities, and future directions*. D-Lib Magazine, 6. Retrieved from http://www.dlib.org/dlib/december00/weibel/12weibel.html

Weil, T. P. (2001). *Health networks: Can they be the solution?* Ann Arbor: University of Michigan Press.

Weill, P., & Ross, J. W. (2004). *IT governance: How top performers manage IT decision rights for superior performance*. Boston: Harvard Business School Press.

Weinfurt, P. T. (1990). Electrocardiographic monitoring: An overview. *Journal of Clinical Monitoring, 6*(2), 132–138.

Weingart, S. N., Toth, M., Sands, D. Z., Aronson, M. D., Davis, R. B., & Phillips, R. S. (2003). Physicians' decisions to override computerized drug alerts in primary care. *Archives of Internal Medicine, 163*(21), 2625–2631.

Weingart, S. N., Rind, D., Tofias, Z., & Sands, D. Z. (2006). Who uses the patient internet portal? The PatientSite experience. *J Am Med Inform Assoc, 13*, (1), 91–95.

Weinger, M.B., & Slagle, J. (2001). Human factors research in anesthesia patient safety. *Proceedings of the AMIA Symposium*, 756–760. doi:D010001242 [pii].

Weinstein, M. C., & Fineberg, H. (1980). *Clinical decision analysis*. Philadelphia: W. B. Saunders.

Weinstock, R. S., Izquierdo, R., Goland, R., Palmas, W., Teresi, J. A., Eimicke, J. P., & Consortium, I. D. (2010). Lipid treatment in ethnically diverse underserved older adults with diabetes mellitus: Statin use, goal attainment, and health disparities in the informatics for diabetes education and telemedicine project. *Journal of American Geriatrics Society, 58*(2), 401–402.

Weir, C. R., Hammond, K. W., Embi, P. J., et al. (2011). An exploration of the impact of computerized patient documentation on clinical collaboration. *International Journal of Medical Informatics, 80*(8), e62–e71.

Weiser, M. (1993a). Some computer science issues in ubiquitous computing. *Communications of the ACM, 36*(7), 75–84.

Weiser, M. (1993b). Ubiquitous computing. *Computer, 26*(10), 71–72.

Weissleder, R., & Mahmood, U. (2001). Molecular imaging. *Radiology, 219*, 316–333.

Weitzman, E. R., Kaci, L., & Mandl, K. D. (2010). Sharing medical data for health research: The early personal health record experience. *J Med Internet Res, 12*(2), e14.

Weitzman, E. R., Adida, B., Kelemen, S., & Mandl, K. D. (2011a). Sharing data for public health research by members of an international online diabetes social network. *PLoS One, 6*(4), e19256.

Weitzman, E. R., Cole, E., Kaci, L., & Mandl, K. D. (2011b). Social but safe? Quality and safety of diabetes-related online social networks [Research Support, N.I.H., Extramural]. *Journal of the American Medical Informatics Association: JAMIA, 18*(3), 292–297.

Weizenbaum, J. (1966). A computer program for the study of natural language communication between man and machine. *Communications of the ACM, 9*(1), 36–45.

Wellcome Department of Cognitive Neurology. (2001). Statistical parametric mapping. From http://www.fil.ion.ucl.ac.uk/spm/

Wennberg, J. (2010). *Tracking medicine: A Researcher's quest to understand health care*. Oxford: Oxford University Press.

Wennberg, J., & Gittelsohn, A. (1973). Small area variations in health care delivery. *Science, 182*(117), 1102–1108.

Were, M. C., Shen, C., Tierney, W. M., Mamlin, J. J., Biondich, P. G., Li, X., Kimaiyo, S., & Mamlin, B. W. (2011). Evaluation of computer-generated reminders to improve CD4 laboratory monitoring in sub-Saharan Africa: A prospective comparative study. *Journal of the American Medical Informatics Association: JAMIA, 18*(2), 150–155.

Wessels, J. T., Yamauchi, K., et al. (2010). Advances in cellular, subcellular, and nanoscale imaging in vitro and in vivo. *Cytometry. Part A, 77*(7), 667–676.

Westbrook, J., Coiera, E., & Gosling, A. (2005). Do online information retrieval systems help experienced clinicians answer clinical questions? *Journal of the American Medical Informatics Association: JAMIA, 12*, 315–321.

Weston, A. D., & Hood, L. (2004). Systems biology, proteomics, and the future of health care: Toward predictive, preventative, and personalized medicine. *Journal of Proteome Research, 3*, 179–196.

Whelan, T., Levine, M., Willan, A., Gafni, A., Sanders, K., Mirsky, D., et al. (2004). Effect of a decision aid on knowledge and treatment decision making for breast cancer surgery: A randomized trial. *JAMA: The Journal of the American Medical Association, 292*(4), 435–441.

White, B.Y., & Frederiksen, J.R. (1990). Causal model progressions as a foundation for intelligent learning environments. In W.J. Clancey & E. Soloway (Eds.), *Artificial intelligence and learning environments Special issues of "Artificial Intelligence": An International Journal"* (pp. 99–157).

Whiting-O'Keefe, Q. E., Simborg, D. W., Epstein, W. V., & Warger, A. (1985). A computerized summary medical record system can provide more information than the standard medical record. *Journal of the American Medical Association, 254*(9), 1185–1192.

Wickland, E. (2011, August 18). *Australia taps Accenture, Oracle, Orion Health for national PHR project. Health Information Technology News.* Available at http://www.healthcareitnews.com/news/australia-taps-accenture-oracle-orion-health-national-phr-project. Accessed 25 Aug 2011.

Wicks, P., Vaughan, T. E., Massagli, M. P., & Heywood, J. (2011). Accelerated clinical discovery using self-reported patient data collected online and a patient-matching algorithm. *Nature Biotechnology, 29*(5), 411–414.

Wiederhold, G. (1981). *Databases for health care.* New York: Springer.

Wiederhold, G., & Clayton, P. D. (1985). Processing biological data in real time. *M.D. Computing, 2*(6), 16–25.

Wild, D. J. (2009). Grand challenges for cheminformatics. *Journal of Cheminformatics, 1*, 1.

Wildemuth, B., deBliek, R., Friedman, C., & File, D. (1995). Medical students' personal knowledge, searching proficiency, and database use in problem solving. *Journal of the American Society for Information Science, 46*, 590–607.

Willmann, J. K., van Bruggen, N., et al. (2008). Molecular imaging in drug development. *Nature Reviews Drug Discovery, 7*(7), 591–607.

Willson, D. (1994). Survey of nurse perception regarding the utilization of bedside computers. *Proceedings of the Annual Symposium on Computer Applications in Medical Care*, 553–557. PMID 7949989.

Willson, D., Nelson, N. C., Rosebrock, B. J., Hujcs, M. T., Wilner, D. G., & Buxton, R. B. (1994). Using an integrated point of care system: A nursing perspective. *Topics in Health Information Management, 14*, 24–29. PMID 19134757.

Wilson, T. (1990). *Confocal microscopy.* San Diego: Academic Press Ltd.

Wing, J. M., & Barr, V. (2011). Jeannette M. Wing @ PCAST; Barbara Liskov keynote. *Communications of the ACM, 54*(9), 10–11.

Winograd, T. (1972). Understanding natural language. *Cognitive Psychology, 3*(1), 1–191.

Wishart, D. S. (2008). Metabolomics: A complementary tool in renal transplantation. *Contributions to Nephrology, 160*, 76–87.

Wishart, D. S. (2011). Advances in metabolite identification. *Bioanalysis, 3*, 1769–1782.

Wong, B.A., Rosse, C., et al. (1999). Semi-automatic scene generation using the Digital Anatomist Foundational Model. *Proceedings, American Medical Informatics Association Fall Symposium* (pp. 637–641), Washington, D.C.

Woods, W. (1973). Progress in NLU – an application to lunar geology. *Proceeding of AFIPS, 42*, 441–450.

Woods, C. R., & Kemper, K. J. (2009). Curriculum resource use and relationships with educational outcomes in an online curriculum. *Academic Medicine, 84*(9), 1250–1258.

Woods, R. P., Cherry, S. R., et al. (1992). Rapid automated algorithm for aligning and reslicing PET images. *Journal of Computer Assisted Tomography, 16*, 620–633.

Woods, R. P., Mazziotta, J. C., et al. (1993). MRI-PET registration with automated algorithm. *Journal of Computer Assisted Tomography, 17*, 536–546.

Woods, D. D., Patterson, E. S., & Cook, R. I. (2007). Behind human error: Taming complexity to improve patient safety. In P. Carayon (Ed.), *Handbook of human factors and ergonomics in health care and patient safety* (pp. 459–476). Mahwah: Lawrence Erlbaum Associates.

Wootton R, (Ed.). (2009). *Telehealth in the developing world.* London: Royal Society of Medicine Press. Available at: http://web.idrc.ca/openebooks/396-6/. Accessed 6 Oct 2011.

World Health Organization. (1992). *International classification of diseases index. Tenth revision. Volume* (Tabular list, Vol. 1). Geneva: The World Health Organization.

WorldWideWeb Consortium. (W3C Recommendation 10 Feb 2004). *OWLWeb Ontology Language Reference.* Cambridge, MA.

Worthey, E. A., Mayer, A. N., Syverson, G. D., et al. (2011). Making a definitive diagnosis: Successful clinical application of whole exome sequencing in a child with intractable inflammatory bowel disease. *Genetics in Medicine, 13*(3), 255–262.

Wrenn, J. O., Stein, D. M., Bakken, S., & Stetson, P. D. (2010). Quantifying clinical narrative redundancy in an electronic health record. *Journal of the American Medical Informatics Association: JAMIA, 17*(1), 49–53.

Wright, P. C., Fields, R. E., & Harrison, M. D. (2000). Analyzing human-computer interaction as distributed cognition: The resources model. *Human Computer Interaction, 15*(1), 1–41.

Wright, A., Sittig, D. F., Ash, J. S., Sharma, S., Pang, J. E., & Middleton, B. (2009). Clinical decision support capabilities of commercially-available clinical information systems. *Journal of the American Medical Informatics Association: JAMIA, 16*(5), 637–644.

Wright, A., Sittig, D. F., Ash, J. S., Feblowitz, J., et al. (2011). Development and evaluation of comprehensive clinical decision support taxonomy: Comparison of front-end tools in commercial and internally developed electronic health records. *Journal of the American Medical Informatics Association: JAMIA, 18*, 232–242. PMID 21415065.

WTCCC. (2007). Genome-wide association study of 14,000 cases of seven common diseases and 3,000 shared controls. *Nature, 447*, 661–678.

Wubbelt, P., Fernandez, G., & Heymer, J. (2000). Clinical trial management and remote data entry on the internet based on XML case report forms. *Studies in Health Technology and Informatics, 77*, 333–337.

Wyatt, J., & Spiegelhalter, D. (1990). Evaluating medical expert systems: What to test and how? *Medical Informatics (Lond), 15*, 205–217.

Wyatt, J., & Wyatt, S. (2003). When and how to evaluate clinical information systems ? *International Journal of Medical Informatics, 69*, 251–259.

Wyatt, J. C., Batley, R. P., & Keen, J. (2010, October). GP preferences for information systems: Conjoint analysis of speed, reliability, access and users. *Journal of Evaluation in Clinical Practice, 16*(5), 911–915.

Yakushiji, A., Tateisi, Y., Miyao, Y., & Tsujii, J. (2001). Event extraction from biomedical papers using a full parser. *Proceedings of the Pacific Symposium Biocomputing, 6*, 408–419.

Yamin, C. K., Emani, S., Williams, D. H., Lipsitz, S. R., Karson, A. S., Wald, J. S., & Bates, D. W. (2011). The digital divide in adoption and use of a personal health record. *Archives of Internal Medicine, 171*(6), 568–574.

Yan, J., & Gu, W. (2009). Gene expression microarrays. In Y. Lu & R. I. Mahato (Eds.), *Cancer research pharmaceutical perspectives of cancer therapeutics* (pp. 645–672). New York: Springer.

Yasnoff, W.A. (2006). Health record banking: A practical approach to the national health information infrastructure. Available at http://williamyasnoff.com/?p=26. Accessed 17 Dec 2012.

Yasnoff, W. A., & Miller, P. L. (2003). Decision support and expert systems in public health. In P. W. O'Carroll, W. A. Yasnoff, M. E. Ward, L. H. Ripp, & E. L. Martin (Eds.), *Public health informatics and information systems* (pp. 494–512). New York: Springer.

Yasnoff, W. A., O'Carroll, P. W., Koo, D., Linkins, R. W., & Kilbourne, E. M. (2000). Public health informatics: Improving and transforming public health in the information age. *Journal of Public Health Management and Practice, 6*(6), 67–75.

Yasnoff, W. A., Humphreys, B. L., Overhage, J. M., Detmer, D. E., Brennan, P. F., Morris, R. W., Middleton, B., Bates, D. W., & Fanning, J. P. (2004). A consensus action agenda for achieving the national health information infrastructure. *Journal of the American Medical Informatics Association: JAMIA, 11*(4), 332–338.

Yasnoff, W. A., Sweeney, L., & Shortliffe, E. H. (2013). Putting health IT on the path to success. *Journal of the American Medical Association, 309*(10), 989–990.

Yildirim, M. A., Goh, K. I., Cusick, M. E., et al. (2007). Drug-target network. *Nature Biotechnology, 25*, 1119–1126.

Yoo, T. S. (2004). *Insight into images: Principles and practice for segmentation, registration, and image analysis.* Wellesley: A K Peters.

Youngner, S. J. (1988). Who defines futility? *Journal of the American Medical Association, 260*, 2094–2095.

Yu, F., & Ip, H. H. (2008). Semantic content analysis and annotation of histological images. *Computers in Biology and Medicine, 38*(6), 635–649.

Yu, V. L., Buchanan, B. G., Shortliffe, E. H., Wraith, S. M., Davis, R., Scott, A. C., & Cohen, S. N. (1979a). Evaluating the performance of a computer-based consultant. *Computer Programs in Biomedicine, 9*(1), 95–102.

Yu, V. L., Fagan, L. M., Wraith, S. M., Clancey, W. J., Scott, A. C., Hannigan, J., Blum, R. L., Buchanan, B. G., & Cohen, S. N. (1979b). Antimicrobial selection by a computer. A blinded evaluation by infectious disease experts. *Journal of the American Medical Association, 242*(12), 1279–1282.

Zalis, M. E., Barish, M. A., et al. (2005). CT colonography reporting and data system: A consensus proposal. *Radiology, 236*(1), 3–9.

Zarin, D. A. (2011). Letter: The ClinicalTrials.gov results database. *The New England Journal of Medicine, 364*(22), 2170.

Zarin, D., Tse, T., Williams, R., Califf, R., & Ide, N. (2011). The ClinicalTrials.gov results database-update and key issues. *The New England Journal of Medicine, 364*, 852–860.

Zerhouni, E. A. (2006). Clinical research at a crossroads: The NIH roadmap. *Journal of Investigative Medicine, 54*, 171–173.

Zhang, J. (1997). The nature of external representations in problem solving. *Cognitive Science, 21*(2), 179–217.

Zhang, J. J., & Norman, D. A. (1994). Representations in distributed cognitive tasks. *Cognitive Science, 18*(1), 87–122.

Zhang, Y., & Szolovitz, P. (2008). Patient-specific learning in real time for adaptive monitoring in critical care. *Journal of Biomedical Informatics, 41*, 452–460. PMID 18463000.

Zhang, J., & Walji, M. F. (2011). TURF: Toward a unified framework of EHR usability. *Journal of Biomedical Informatics, 44*(6), 1056–1067.

Zhang, Y. Y., Brady, M., et al. (2001). Segmentation of brain MR images through a hidden Markov random field model and the expectation-maximization algorithm. *IEEE Transactions on Medical Imaging, 20*(1), 45–57.

Zhang, J., Patel, V. L., Johnson, K. A., & Malin, J. (2002). Designing human-centered distributed information systems. *IEEE Intelligent Systems, 17*(5), 42–47.

Zhang, J., Patel, V.L., Johnson, T.R., & Shortliffe, E.H. (2004). A cognitive taxonomy of medical errors. *Journal of Biomedical Informatics*, 37(3), 193–204.

Zhang, J., Johnson, T. R., Patel, V. L., Paige, D. L., & Kubose, T. (2003). Using usability heuristics to evaluate patient safety of medical devices. *Journal of Biomedical Informatics, 36*(1–2), 23–30. S1532046403000601 [pii].

Zhang, J., Patel, V. L., Johnson, T. R., & Shortliffe, E. H. (2004). A cognitive taxonomy of medical errors. *Journal of Biomedical Informatics, 37*(3), 193–204.

Zhang, H., Fiszman, M., Shin, D., Miller, C. M., Rosemblat, G., & Rindflesch, T. C. (2011). Degree centrality for semantic abstraction summarization of therapeutic studies. *Journal of Biomedical Informatics, 44*(5), 830–838.

Zheng, B., Sumkin, J., Good, W., Maitz, G., Chang, Y., & Gur, D. (2000). Applying computer-assisted detection schemes to digitized mammograms after JPEG data compression: An assessment. *Academic Radiology, 7*(8), 595–602.

Zhenyu, H., Yanjie, Z., et al. (2009). *Combining text retrieval and content-based image retrieval for searching a large-scale medical image database in an integrated RIS/PACS environment*, SPIE. Bellingham, WA.

Zhou, L., Soran, C. S., Jenter, C. A., Volk, L. A., Orav, E. J., Bates, D. W., et al. (2009). The relationship between electronic health record use and quality of care over time. *Journal of the American Medical Informatics Association: JAMIA, 16*(4), 457–464.

Zhu, J., Zhang, B., & Schadt, E. E. (2008). A systems biology approach to drug discovery. *Advances in Genetics, 60*, 603–635.

Zhu, V. J., Overhage, M. J., Egg, J., Downs, S. M., & Grannis, S. J. (2009). An empiric modification to the probabilistic record linkage algorithm using frequency-based weight scaling. *Journal of the American Medical Informatics Association: JAMIA, 16*(5), 738–745.

Zhu, Q., Ge, D., Maia, J. M., et al. (2011). A genome-wide comparison of the functional properties of rare and common genetic variants in humans. *American Journal of Human Genetics, 88*, 458–468.

Zielstorff, R. D., Hudgings, C. L., & Grobe, S. J. (1993). *Next-generation nursing information systems: Essential characteristics for professional practice.* Washington, DC: American Nurses Publishing.

Zijdenbos, A. P., Evans, A. C., et al. (1996). Automatic quantification of multiple sclerosis lesion volume using stereotactic space. Proc. In *4th International conference on visualization in biomedical computing. Hamburg* (pp. 439–448).

Zoll, P. M., Linethal, A. J., Gibson, W., Paul, M. H., & Norman, L. R. (1956). Termination of ventricular fibrillation in man by externally applied countershock. *The New England Journal of Medicine, 254*, 727–732. PMID 13309666.

Zong, W., Moody, G. B., & Mark, R. G. (2004). Reduction of false arterial blood pressure alarms using signal quality assessment and relationship between the electrocardiogram and arterial blood pressure. *Medical & Biological Engineering & Computing, 42*, 698–706. PMID 15503972.

Zuriff, G. E. (1985). *Behaviorism: A conceptual reconstruction.* New York: Columbia University Press.

Zweigenbaum, P. (1994). MENELAS: An access system for medical records using natural language. *Computer Methods and Programs in Biomedicine, 45*(1–2), 117–120.

Zweigenbaum, P., & Courtois, P. (1998). Acquisition of lexical resources from SNOMED for medical language processing. *Proceedings of Medinfo, 9*(Pt 1), 586–590.

Ledley R. (1965) Use of Computers in Biology and Medicine. New York: McGraw-Hill.

Association of American Medical Colleges (1984). Physicians for the twenty-first century (Report of the Project Panel on the General Professional Education of the Physician and College Preparation for Medicine). J Med Educ 59(11):(Part 2) 1–208.

Name Index

A

Aanestad, M., 440
Abbey, L., 252
Abernathy, N., 753
Aboukhalil, A., 575
Adams, I., 649
Adams, K., 478, 483, 500
Adler-Milstein, J., 427, 439, 440, 516, 528, 790, 795
Advani, A., 666
Afrin, J., 551
Agrawal, M., 318
Aguirre, G., 289
Ahern, D., 478, 500
Ahmed, A., 579, 586–588
Aine, C., 289
Ajzen, I., 530
Akerkar, R., 627, 628
Akin, O., 115
Alberini, J., 289, 294
Albert, K., 617
Aldrich, C., 689
Alecu, I., 739
Allard, F., 122
Allemann, P., 555
Alpert, S., 338
Altman, R., 35, 695, 701, 718, 721, 740, 753, 805, 806
Altschul, S., 705
Altschuler, D., 745
Amarasingham, R., 784
Amernco, P., 559
Ammenwerth, E., 783
Ancker, J., 140
Anderson, J., 114, 117, 119, 335, 357, 381
Anderson, N., 753, 777
Andrews, J., 252
Andrews, R., 577
André, B., 312
Angrist, M., 746, 747, 749, 753
Aristotle, 32
Armstrong, R., 297
Arocha, J., 65, 118, 135, 141, 148
Aronow, D., 272
Aronson, A., 257, 272, 628, 731
Ash, J., 129, 136, 367, 375, 484, 493, 496, 648, 671, 673, 756, 777
Ashburner, J., 319, 732

Ashley, E., 747
Assimacopoulos, A., 554
Atkinson, R., 113, 498
Atreya, R., 339
Audebert, H., 559
Austin, G., 113
Avancha, S., 798, 809
Avni, Z., 311
Aydin, C., 335, 381

B

Baars, M., 648
Babbage, C., 22
Babior, B., 699
Bada, M., 802
Baeza-Yates, R., 641
Bai, C., 696
Bailey, N., 36
Bajorath, J., 743
Bakas, T., 559
Baker, J., 301
Bakken, S., 475, 489. *See also* Henry, S.B.
Balas, A., 26, 27, 425
Baldi, P., 718
Ball, M., 435
Bandura, A., 530
Barabasi, A., 735, 737
Barnard, F., 287
Barnett, G.O., 23, 30, 39, 394, 420, 649, 658
Barr, V., 807
Barrows Jr., R., 419
Barry, C., 297
Bartholmai, B., 604
Bartlett, J., 616
Bartolomeo, P., 119
Bashshur, R., 542, 559
Bastian, L., 672
Bates, D., 195, 412, 419, 420, 424, 440, 456, 495, 516, 648, 673, 762, 781, 785, 790, 792, 794, 795
Baud, R., 257
Bauer, D., 411
Baum, W.M., 112
Baumann, B., 297
Bayes, T., 64
Bayir, H., 195

Beale, I., 521
Beale, R., 570
Bechhofer, S., 323
Bechtel, W., 111, 112
Becich, M., 296
Beck, J., 97
Beck, K., 196
Becker, J., 305
Bedenreider, O., 301, 731, 739
Beedle, M., 196
Begun, J., 16
Bela, K., 536
Bell, A., 543
Benitez, K., 339
Benko, L., 129
Bennett, T., 297
Benoit, A., 500
Benson, D., 230, 265, 282
Benson, T., 252
Berg, J., 718
Berg, M., 143, 785
Berner, E., 353, 420
Berners-Lee, T., 615
Bernstam, E., 58, 65, 761
Berwick, D., 783, 786
Besser, H., 639
Beuscart-Zephir, M., 133, 136
Bewersdorf, J., 296
Bickel, R., 487
Bidgood, W., 299
Bieber, E., 420
Bigelow, J., 515, 795
Billings, J., 614
Bird, A., 703
Bird, K., 543
Bishop, M., 258, 311, 315
Biswal, S., 294, 296
Bitton, A., 792, 794
Bittorf, A., 297
Blake, J., 273, 277, 282
Bleich, H., 394, 464, 624, 657
Blois, M.S., 3, 32, 109, 110
Bloom, F., 300, 305
Bloomrosen, M., 138, 648, 785, 793
Bloxham, A., 494
Blum, B., 58
Blum, H., 515
Blum, J., 574
Blumenthal, D., 192, 647, 648, 789, 790, 800
Bluml, S., 289
Bodenreider, O., 626
Boeckmann, B., 282
Bogun, F., 568
Bonanno, J., 714
Boone, K., 252
Booth, R., 494
Boren, S., 26, 27, 425
Borgman, C., 615, 638
Bosch, A., 312

Bosworth, K., 520, 521
Bowden, M., 300, 305
Bower, A., 515, 795
Bower, G., 112
Bower, P., 518
Bowie, J., 30
Boyd, S., 768
Boynton, J., 633
Bradshaw, K., 576, 577, 581
Branch, T., 141
Brand, W., 503
Brannan, S., 534
Bransford, J., 120, 677, 692
Branstetter, B., 610
Braunwald, E., 567
Brechner, R., 548
Brender, J., 357, 381
Brennan, P., 440, 516, 533
Breslow, M., 554, 585, 808
Bresnick, G., 548
Briggs, A., 96, 105
Briggs, B., 762
Bright, R., 136
Bright, T., 648, 672
Brin, S., 630
Brinkley, J., 142, 285, 304, 305, 311, 314, 326, 593
Brinkman, R., 731
Bristow, E., 672
Britt, H., 739
Brody, W., 343
Bromberg, Y., 753
Brown, A., 692
Brown, D., 302
Brown, E., 739, 770
Brown, S., 136, 208, 394
Brownstein, J., 416
Bruer, J., 115
Bruls, T., 752
Brunak, S., 718
Bruner, J., 113
Bryan, R., 314, 315
Buchanan, B., 655, 659
Buetow, K., 767, 770, 773
Bug, W., 300
Buntin, M., 419, 425, 430, 783, 800
Burke, J., 195, 399
Burley, S., 495, 714
Burnside, E., 301, 321, 808
Burykin, A., 569, 572, 575
Bush, G.W., 782
Butler, D., 762
Butte, A., 722, 724, 754, 756, 765
Buxton, R., 292

C
Cabrera Fernandez, D., 297
Cairncross, F., 798
Callan, J., 581

Campbell, D., 367
Campbell, E., 484, 496, 673
Campbell, K., 230
Campbell, M., 381
Campillos, M., 743
Campion, T., 497
Cao, Y., 260
Caporaso, J., 277
Capriotti, E., 753
Caputo, B., 313
Carayon, P., 111, 133, 134, 148, 578
Carcillo, J.A., 195
Card, S., 113, 130, 139, 141, 142
Carneiro, G., 303
Caro, J., 103, 105
Carpenter, A., 296
Carroll, D., 500
Carroll, J., 116, 128–130, 148, 406
Carter, J., 208
Castro, D., 440
Cava, A., 339, 353
Cavalleranno, A., 548
Caviness, V., 307
Cech, T., 700
Cedar, H., 722
Celi, L., 585, 586
Chambrin, M., 572
Chan, A., 303, 661
Chan, G., 129, 496
Chan, I., 648, 750, 752, 799, 809
Chan, K., 786, 795
Chandler, P., 117
Chang, F., 500
Channin, D., 301–303
Chapanis, A., 133, 134
Chapman, K., 258, 272
Charen, T., 627
Chase, W., 122
Chaudhry, B., 196, 589
Chaudry, B., 666, 783
Chen, E., 492
Chen, R., 570, 724
Cheung, N., 394
Chi, M., 121, 122, 128
Chiang, M.F., 541, 549, 559
Chin, T., 495
Choi, H., 314
Chomsky, N., 113
Chopra, A., 429, 534
Christensen, C., 473, 527, 528, 808, 810
Christensen, L., 257
Chuang, J., 279
Chui, M., 798, 810
Chumbler, N., 559
Chung, J., 295
Chung, T., 756, 766, 772, 777
Church, G., 55, 745–747
Chused, A., 671
Chute, C., 252

Cimino, J.J., 47, 129, 211, 252, 301, 481, 526, 527, 559, 616, 656, 755, 759
Cirulli, E., 728
Clancey, W., 115, 659, 661
Clancy, C., 647, 774
Clark, E., 568, 570
Clark, O., 762
Clark, R.C., 688
Clark, R.S.B., 195
Clarkson, P., 136
Clarysse, P., 310
Classen, D., 195, 351, 399, 419, 583
Clayton, P., 161, 184, 419
Clemmer, T.P., 195, 561, 567, 578, 587, 588, 590
Cline, H., 314
Cobb, J., 589
Cochrane, G., 622
Cocking, R., 692
Coenen, A., 232
Coeytaux, R., 672
Coffey, R., 394
Cohen, A., 619
Cohen, G., 522
Cohen, J., 289
Cohen, M., 320
Cohen, P., 381
Cohen, T., 136, 579
Cole, M., 143
Coletti, M., 624
Collen, M., 22, 23, 35, 394, 420, 487, 520
Collins, D., 314, 318, 577
Collins, F., 752, 774, 799, 806
Collins, S., 486, 497
Colombet, I., 648
Conn, J., 526
Cook, D., 691, 692
Cook-Deegan, R., 750
Coreira, E., 35, 378
Corina, D., 289
Corn, M., 799
Corrigan, J., 478, 483, 500
Coté, R., 57, 230
Coulet, A., 742
Council, N., 184
Courtney, P., 524
Courtois, P., 257
Covell, D., 400, 616, 646
Cox, J., 567
Cresswell, K., 790
Crick, F., 696, 723
Critchfield, A., 551
Croft, W., 641
Cronenwett, L., 489
Crossley, G., 569
Crowley, R., 128, 684, 692
Crowley, W., 777
Cuadros, J., 548
Cullen, D., 195
Cundick, R., 569

Curgman, G., 617
Curran, W., 349
Cusack, C., 785
Cushing, H., 564
Cushman, R., 329, 346, 353

D
D'Orsi, C., 302
Daladier, A., 283
Dale, A., 314, 315
Dalto, J., 571, 578, 587
Dameron, O., 325
Damiani, G., 397
Damush, T., 415
Dansky, K., 129
Darmoni, S., 627
Datta, R., 320
Davatzikos, C., 314, 315
David, J., 659
Davies, K., 615, 702, 753
Davis, L., 394
Davis, R., 120, 559
Day, H., 140
Dayhoff, M., 704
DeAngelis, C., 623
DeBakey, M., 614
DeClerq, P., 661
DeGroot, A., 121
Dean, J., 630
Deci, E., 518
Decker, S., 647
Deflandre, E., 570
Del Fiol, G., 400
Deleger, L., 260
Demiris, G., 370, 383
Demner-Fushman, D., 259, 260
Dempster, A., 315
Dente, M., 353
DesRoches, C., 429, 647
Deselaers, R., 313, 320
Deserno, T., 320, 326
Detmer, D., 440, 516
Detmer, W., 518, 613
Detsky, A., 74
Dev, P., 675, 678, 679
Dewey, F., 702, 747
Dewey, M., 32
Dexter, P., 399
Dhenian, M., 306
Dhurjati, R., 672
DiCenso, A., 619
Diamond, G., 616
Dick, R., 4, 6
Diepgen, T., 297
Dieterle, M., 466
Dodd, B., 435
Doig, K., 571
Doing-Harris, K., 491

Dolin, R., 491
Donaldson, M., 500
Donley, G., 748
Donovan, T., 321
Doolan, D., 488, 495
Douglas, J., 465
Dowdy, D., 777
Downs, S.M., 406
Draghici, S., 732
Draper, S., 143
Drazen, E., 617
Drew, B., 569
Drews, F., 570, 571
Dreyer, K., 602, 610
Drucker, P., 797, 801, 802
Drury, H., 307
Du, X., 752
Duch, W., 116
Duda, R., 311, 315, 331
Dugas-Phocion, G., 316
Duncan, R., 394
Dunham, I., 745
Dunker, A., 718
Dupuits, F., 204
Durbin, R., 718
Durfy, S., 698
Dyer, C., 630
Dykes, P., 475, 492, 494, 500
Dyson, E., 435

E
Earle, K., 401
East, T., 577, 581, 588
Ebbert, J., 762
Eddy, D., 104
Eddy, S., 718
Edgar, E., 406
Edwards, B., 476
Edworthy, J., 573
Egan, D., 636
Einthoven, W., 565
Elhadad, N., 255, 260
Eliot, C., 683
Elkin, P., 129
Elledge, S., 696
Elstein, A., 29, 35, 60, 62, 64, 105, 115, 125, 126
Elter, M., 604
Ely, J., 616
Embi, P.J., 753, 755–757, 762, 774, 775, 777
Eminovic, N., 358
Engel, G., 647
Engestrom, Y., 143
Erickson, B., 593, 602, 608
Ericsson, K., 114, 122
Estes, W., 113
Etheredge, L., 805
Evans, B., 809
Evans, D., 120, 128, 148, 282, 762

Evans, R., 195, 398, 399, 561, 581–583
Eveillard, P., 762
Eysenbach, G., 276, 297, 522, 526, 616–618, 762

F
Fafchamps, D., 411, 413
Fanning, J., 440, 516
Fargher, E., 648
Fazi, P., 765
Feeny, D., 94
Feero, W., 806
Fei-Fei, L., 312
Feltovich, P., 125
Fenwick, E., 105
Ferguson, T., 522, 533, 618
Ferrucci, D., 638
Fiala, J., 318
Ficarra, V., 555
Fielding, N., 378
Fields, R., 146
Figurska, M., 297
Fiks, A., 499
Fine, A., 806
Fineberg, H., 658
Finger, P., 297
Fink, A., 381
Finkel, A., 58
Finley, S., 500
Fischer, B., 712
Fischl, B., 315
Fisk, A.D., 116
Fiszman, M., 638
Fitzmaurice, M., 394
Fitzpatrick, J., 327
Fleurant, M., 404
Flexner, A., 393, 647, 675
Flin, R., 133
Flocke, S., 405
Florence, V., 797
Floyer, J., 564
Flynn, T., 559
Foley, D., 310
Forsythe, D., 367, 374
Foster, I.T., 149
Foster, K., 558
Fougerousse, F., 305
Foulonneau, M., 614
Fowler, F., 792, 795
Fox, C., 615, 616, 629
Fox, J., 356
Fox, P., 289
Fox, S., 539
Frackowiak, R., 289
Frakes, W., 629, 641
Franken, E., 548
Franklin, K., 300
Fred, M., 204
Frederiksen, C., 118

Frederiksen, J., 119
Freeman, H., 381
Frenk, J., 675, 676, 805
Freton, A., 297
Fridsma, D., 637
Friede, A., 503, 505, 506, 515
Friedman, B., 466
Friedman, C., 255, 257, 262, 266, 272, 275, 282,
     283, 285
Friedman, C.P., 35, 128, 331, 355–357, 367, 369, 370,
     375, 381, 384, 490–492, 495, 691, 692, 773, 808
Friedman, J., 753, 806
Friedman, T., 808, 810
Friefeld, O., 316, 317
Friend, S., 744
Fries, J., 413
Frisse, M.E., 404, 797, 801
Friston, K., 289, 314, 319
Froomkin, M., 353
Frost, J., 525
Frueh, F., 750
Fukuda, K., 257
Fung, K., 406
Funk, M., 569, 628

G
Gaba, D., 681, 692
Gabril, M., 296, 808
Gadd, C., 120
Galbraith, D., 711
Galilei, G., 564
Gallagher, L., 192
Gallin, J., 759, 777
Galperin, M., 622
Gamazon, E., 740
Gambhir, S., 294–296
Garcia-Molina, H., 171, 184
Gardner, R.M., 113, 142, 335, 339, 351, 352, 399, 418,
     420, 561, 569–571, 575–578, 580, 586–590
Garg, A., 398
Garten, Y., 742
Gaschnig, J., 357
Gasser, U., 336
Gauld, R., 420
Gawande, A., 456, 648, 654
Ge, D., 746
Geissbuhler, A., 348
Genel, M., 777
Gennari, J., 664
Geoff, D., 610
George, J., 290
Gerstner, E., 293
Ghazvinian, A., 732
Ghemawat, S., 630
Gibson, K., 146, 704
Gibson, R., 331
Giger, M., 297
Gilder, D., 283

Giles, J., 622
Gillan, D., 110, 116
Ginsburg, G., 647, 648, 725, 750, 752, 799, 809
Girosi, F., 515, 795
Gittelsohn, A., 522
Giuse, D., 394
Glaser, J., 340, 648
Glaser, R., 121, 128
Glasziou, P., 105, 641
Goddard, K., 385
Goetz, T., 728
Goffman, E., 518
Goh, K., 735, 736
Gold, J., 435
Gold, M., 95, 105
Goldberg, A., 703
Goldberg, S., 302
Goldfinch, S., 420
Goldstein, D., 728
Goldstein, M., 661, 662
Goldzweig, C., 456
Gollschalk, A., 405
Gombas, P., 296
Gonzalez, R., 308, 327
Gooch, P., 807
Goodman, K., 329, 335, 339, 341, 343, 344,
        353, 765
Goodnow, J., 113
Goodship, J., 718
Goodwin, J., 476
Gorges, M., 569, 574
Gorman, M., 554
Gorman, P., 615, 616
Gorroll, A., 394
Gorry, G.A., 60, 658
Gottfried, M., 283
Gould, J., 87
Grad, R., 637
Grance, T., 182, 184
Granger, R., 431
Grannis, S., 515
Grant, R., 492
Gray, J., 553, 559
Greco, F., 435
Green, B., 401
Green, E., 798, 810
Green, R., 750
Greenberg, M., 794
Greenes, R., 5, 15, 30, 142, 285, 590, 593,
        598, 643, 672
Greenhalgh, T., 791
Greeno, J., 113–115
Greenspan, H., 285, 313, 317, 320
Gregg, R., 568
Gregory, S., 728
Grigsby, J., 559
Grimm, R., 657
Grishman, R., 257, 258, 262, 274
Grobe, S., 478, 481
Groen, G., 29, 118, 122, 123, 126

Groen, P., 208
Groopman, J., 351
Grossman, J., 473, 810
Grosz, B., 274
Groves, R., 565
Grunfeld, A., 522
Gu, W., 707
Guba, E., 381
Guglin, M., 568
Gur, D., 604
Gurses, A., 579
Gurwitz, D., 750
Gusfield, D., 705, 718
Gustafson, D., 520–522
Guyer, M., 798, 810

H
Haddow, G., 377
Hagglund, M., 491
Hahn, U., 257, 275
Haislmeier, E., 435
Halamka, J., 394, 527, 528, 791
Hallestad, R., 515
Hamburg, M., 806
Hamel, D., 536
Hammond, W.E., 211, 394
Han, Y.Y., 195
Hangiandreou, N., 602
Hansen, L., 289
Hansen, N., 743
Haralick, R., 311, 313, 314
Hardison, C., 777
Harkema, H., 272
Harman, D., 635
Harney, A., 295
Harris, K., 318
Harris, M., 234
Harris, P., 765
Harris, S., 283
Harris, T., 282, 283
Harris, Z., 257, 264, 283
Harris-Salamone, K., 331, 495
Harrison, M., 146, 484, 648, 671
Hart, J., 603
Harter, S., 635, 636
Hartung, C., 409
Hartzband, P., 351
Hasan, K., 293
Hassan, E., 583
Hasselblad, V., 672
Hassol, A., 492
Hastie, T., 709, 753
Hatfield, G., 718
Haug, P., 257, 653
Haupt, M., 565
Haux, R., 494
Haynes, R., 195, 397, 618, 633, 636, 648
Hazlehurst, B., 147
Heaton, P., 795

Heckerman, D., 661
Heikamp, K., 743
Heiss, W., 289
Held, K., 317
Helfand, M., 615, 616
Hellier, E., 573
Hellmich, M., 81
Helton, E., 777
Henchley, A., 252
Henderson, M., 252
Henkind, S., 765
Hennessey, J., 184
Henriksen, K., 133, 134, 148
Henry, D., 805
Henry, S.B., 232. *See also* Bakken, S.
Herasevich, V., 584
Herbranson, E., 680
Hersh, W.R., 311, 320, 613, 614, 616, 619, 625, 626,
     633, 635–639, 641
Hey, T., 798
Hickam, D., 633, 636, 673
Hicks, N., 385
Higgins, M., 105, 494
Hilgard, E., 112
Hillestad, R., 425, 785, 795
Himmelstein, D., 456
Hinman, A., 515
Hinshaw, K., 314, 315
Hirschorn, D., 602
Hirshman, L., 282
Ho, K., 522
Hobbs, J., 273
Hoffman, J., 294, 296
Hoffman, M., 648, 727, 752, 753
Hoffman, R., 122
Hohne, K., 305, 307
Holden, R., 136
Holford, N., 762
Hollingsworth, J., 405
Holloway, R., 559
Holroyd-Leduc, J., 331
Hood, L., 725, 744
Horii, S., 291, 299
Horrigan, J., 525
Horrocks, J., 323
Horsch, A., 604
Horsky, J., 137, 146
Horvath, J., 122
Horvitz, E., 661
House, E., 366
Houston, T., 500
Hoy, J., 493
Hoyt, R., 36
Hripcsak, G., 194, 204, 257, 258, 275, 391, 394, 496,
     577, 586
Hsi-Yang Fritz, M., 726
Hu, Z., 297
Hudgings, C., 479, 481
Hudson, D., 320
Hudson, L., 543

Huerta, M., 287
Huff, S.M., 211, 232
Humphreys, B., 58, 234, 257, 440, 516, 613,
     625, 638, 641
Hunink, M., 105
Hunt, D., 195, 399
Hunter, L., 718, 802
Hurley, A., 500
Hutchins, E., 143, 146, 147
Hwang, J., 473, 810
Hyslop, A., 493

I
Iezzoni, L., 769
Imai, K., 748
Imhoff, M., 573
Ip, H., 303
Irwin, J., 738
Isaac, T., 671
Issel-Tarver, L., 282
Ivers, M., 487

J
Jackson, J., 493
Jadad, A., 617
Jaffe, C., 211
Jagadish, H., 184
Jain, R., 381
James, A., 159
James, B., 456, 495
Janamanchi, B., 410
Jarvik, G., 753
Jaspers, M., 128, 133, 397, 496
Jenders, R., 204
Jensen, T., 440
Jenssen, T., 257
Jewett, A., 706
Jha, A., 136, 440, 572, 790
Jiang, Y., 312
Jihong, W., 610
Jimison, H., 517, 526, 533, 534
Johnson, K., 305, 425, 517, 525, 529, 533
Johnson, P., 125, 661
Johnson, R., 537
Johnson, S., 141, 142, 394, 411, 413, 488, 777
Johnson, T., 65, 135
Johnston, D., 425, 515, 795
Jollis, J., 212
Jones, S., 795
Jonquet, C., 732
Jordan, D., 260
Joshi-Tope, G., 741
Joyce, V., 95
Jukic, D., 692
Juni, P., 691
Jurafsky, D., 261, 263, 264, 267, 270–273, 283
Jurie, F., 311

K

Kaelber, D., 437, 784, 785
Kahn, C., 302, 658
Kahn, M., 585, 753, 799
Kahneman, D., 72, 105
Kalet, I., 36
Kane, B., 545
Kang, J., 295
Kang, M., 744
Kankaanpaa, J., 357
Kann, M., 753
Kaplan, B., 331, 353, 495
Kapur, T., 316
Karat, C., 128
Karnon, J., 105
Karplus, M., 704
Karr, J., 703
Karsh, B., 136, 589, 671
Kass, M., 314, 424
Kassirer, J., 60, 98, 99, 658
Kastor, J., 444
Kato, P., 521
Kaufman, D., 65, 109, 110, 117, 119, 129, 133, 140,
    146–148
Kaufmann, A., 425
Kaul, S., 616
Kaushal, R., 462
Kawamoto, K., 660, 667
Keiser, M., 743
Kelley, M., 565
Kemper, K., 804, 806
Kendall, D., 435
Kendrick, A., 672
Kennedy, D., 314
Kennelly, R., 571, 578
Kent, H., 555
Kent, W., 705
Keren, H., 570
Kershaw, A., 522
Keselman, A., 260
Kevles, B., 290
Khajouei, R., 397
Khatri, P., 732
Kho, A., 734, 806
Kidd, M., 435
Kilbourne, E., 516
Kilo, C., 792
Kim, H., 492
Kim, J., 258, 282, 762
Kim, M., 529
Kimborg, D., 289
King, W., 296
Kinning, S., 742
Kintsch, W., 114, 117, 118
Kirkpatrick, D., 692
Kittredge, R., 258, 262
Klasnja, P., 65
Klein, T., 718
Kleinke, J., 790, 795
Kleinmuntz, B., 125, 139

Knaus, W., 341, 659
Knox, C., 738
Koatley, K., 143
Koch, T., 627
Kohane, I.S., 35, 208, 416, 435, 529, 535, 538, 669, 753,
    797, 798, 803, 805, 806, 810
Kohler, C., 616
Kohn, L., 482, 500, 523, 646, 676
Kolodner, R., 465
Komaroff, A., 657
Kong, Y., 769
Koo, D., 515, 516
Koppel, R., 128, 129, 138, 148, 341, 353, 358, 380,
    484, 493
Koreen, S., 558
Korner, M., 291
Korotkoff, N., 564
Kosara, R., 141
Koslow, S., 287
Kouwenhoven, W., 565
Kowalczyk, L., 572
Kraus, V., 728
Kreda, D., 341
Kremkau, F., 292
Krischer, J., 777
Krishnaral, A., 603
Krist, A., 435, 440, 476, 492
Krogh, A., 718
Krupinski, E., 559
Kubler, S., 283
Kuchenbecker, J., 765
Kuchinke, W., 768
Kuhls, S., 572
Kuhn, I., 394, 406
Kukafka, R., 777
Kulikowski, C., 22, 286
Kulkarni, A., 623
Kullo, I., 802
Kuntz, K., 105
Kuperman, G., 136, 194, 331, 420, 487, 576, 577, 590,
    649, 652
Kurtzke, J., 226
Kuruchitthan, P., 503
Kush, R., 777
Kushniruk, A., 120, 132, 137, 144, 146
Kvedar, J., 559

L

LaVenture, M., 503, 509, 515
Labkoff, S., 439
Laennec, R., 564
Laine, C., 623
Lamb, A., 394
Lamb, J., 730, 740
Lander, E., 696, 723
Landrigan, P., 752
Lang, F., 731
Langer, S., 602, 603
Langheier, J., 648

Langley, P., 116
Langlotz, C., 301
Langridge, R., 704
Lapsia, V., 434
Larabell, C., 296
Larkin, J., 117, 122, 126, 139, 141
Larsen, R., 399
Lashkari, D., 696
Lau, F., 419
Lauer, M., 774
Laurent, M., 622
Lawrence, S., 616
Le Bihan, D., 293
LePendu, P., 733, 734
Leahy, R., 314
Leape, L., 134, 195, 646
Leatherman, S., 456
Leavitt, M., 192
Ledley, R., ix, 125, 321, 649, 673
Lee, D., 293
Lee, J., 291, 558, 584
Lee, R., 378
Lee, T., 473
Lee, Y., 321
Leeflang, M., 81
Legowski, E., 692
Lehmann, T., 320
Lehrberger, J., 262
Leiner, F., 494
Lenert, L., 95
Lenfant, C., 724
Leong, A., 296
Leong, F., 296
Leong, K., 534
Lesgold, A., 121, 123, 128
Lesk, M., 640
Lester, R., 361, 364, 365
Leu, M., 495
Levick, D., 420
Levine, S., 554
Levinson, A., 681
Levitt, M., 701, 704
Levy, H., 753
Levy, M., 304, 326
Lewitter, F., 753
Lexe, G., 295
Li, Q., 569
Libicki, M., 215
Lichtenbelt, B., 310
Lieberman, M., 519, 521
Lighthowler, M., 500
Lightstone, S., 184
Lilly, C., 555, 585, 587, 588
Lin, H., 209, 483, 492, 500, 800, 810
Lin, J., 259, 260, 630
Lin, L., 110, 128, 136, 137, 142
Lin, N., 661
Lincoln, M., 208
Lincoln, Y., 381
Lindberg, D., 234, 265, 300, 394, 487, 613, 638, 641

Linder, J., 783
Lindgren, H., 648
Lindhurst, M., 745
Linkins, R., 516
Lipsey, M., 381
Lipsits, S., 500
Lipton, E., 425
Littlejohns, P., 357
Liu, J., 372
Liu, T., 740
Liu, Y., 290, 321, 610
Lloyd, J., 195
Lobach, D., 672
Loffler, M., 810
Lorensen, W., 314
Lowe, D., 297, 311
Lown, B., 565
Lu, Z., 799
Lubarsky, D., 411
Lubell, J., 526
Luce, R., 799
Lundsgaarde, H., 356, 577
Lunshof, J., 746, 747
Lupski, J., 716
Lussier, Y., 754
Lusted, L., 125, 320, 649, 673
Lutz, S., 765

M
MacDonald, D., 314, 315, 319
MacMahon, H., 297
Mackinnon, A., 548
Macklin, R., 339
Magder, S., 119
Maglione, M., 196
Maglott, D., 282
Magrabi, F., 35
Mahajan, R., 573
Mahmood, U., 290, 294
Mahon, B., 416
Mailman, M., 740, 770
Majchrowski, B., 349
Major, K., 401
Malcolm, S., 718
Malik, J., 316
Malin, B., 339
Mandl, K.D., 208, 435, 517, 528, 529, 535, 538, 539, 669, 797, 798
Manning, C., 258, 283
Manning, D., 321
Mant, J., 385
Marcetich, J., 899
Marcin, J., 554
Marcus, M., 258, 262
Margolis, D., 294, 296
Mark, R.G., 561, 584
Marks, L., 762, 765
Marks, R., 762, 765
Maroto, M., 258

Marquet, G., 325
Marroquin, J., 317
Martin, E., 515
Martin, J., 261, 263, 264, 267, 270–273, 283
Martin, R., 300, 305
Marwede, D., 302
Masarie, F., 654
Masinter, L., 639
Massagli, M., 525
Massaro, T., 484
Massoud, T., 294
Masys, D., 55, 424, 697, 753
Mathew, J., 648
Mathews, S., 571, 578
Mattern, C., 603
Mattick Jr.P., 283
Matykiewicz, P., 260
Matzner, Y., 699
Maurer, C., 317
Mayer, R., 688
Mayes, R., 143
McCarthy, J., 182
McCarty, C., 697
McClellan, M., 786
McConnell, S., 196, 208
McCormick, K., 35
McCullough, J., 456
McDonald, C., 142, 232, 391, 394, 398, 399, 404, 406,
    411, 414, 426, 465, 487, 515, 654, 762
McDonald, M., 406, 515
McDonald, R., 283
McGettigan, P., 805
McGill, M., 631, 635
McGlynn, E., 424, 616, 786
McGregor, A., 143
McInerny, T., 317
McKee, C., 786
McKibbon, K., 636, 637
McLachlan, G., 315
McManus, J., 494
McNeer, J., 33
McPhee, S., 399
Mead, C., 232
Mead, N., 518
Meade, T., 295
Mechouche, A., 303
Meckley, L., 753
Medvedeva, O., 692
Meer, P., 315
Mehta, T., 288
Meigs, J., 86
Meili, R., 515, 795
Meisel, A., 353
Mejino, J., 300
Mell, P., 182, 184
Melton III, L., 393
Mervis, J., 55
Merzweiler, A., 765
Metzger, J., 462
Metzler, D., 641

Meyer, B., 554
Michaelis, J., 370
Michel, A., 493
Mickish, A., 394
Middleton, B., 440, 516, 643, 670, 673, 795
Miksch, S., 141
Miles, W., 614, 641
Miller, A., 794
Miller, B.S., 440
Miller, G., 113, 739
Miller, H., 435, 514
Miller, K., 753
Miller, P., 35
Miller, R.A., 329–333, 335, 339, 342–344, 347–349,
    351–353, 397, 398, 400, 418, 654, 793
Miller, R.H., 440
Miller, S., 349
Miller-Jacobs, H., 195
Millhouse, O., 305
Milstein, A., 786, 787
Min, J., 295
Minsky, M., 272
Mitchison, G., 718
Mittal, M., 498
Modayur, B., 314
Moed, H., 616
Mohr, D., 74
Mojica, W., 196
Moller, J., 125
Mongan, J., 473
Mooney, S., 695
Moore, G., 25, 417
Morel, G., 135
Morgenstern, D., 94
Mork, J., 731
Morris, A., 577, 584, 588, 590
Morris, R., 440, 516
Morrison, J., 554, 555
Mort, M., 733
Morton, S.C., 194, 196
Moses, L., 81
Mostashari, F., 192
Motik, B., 323
Muller, H., 320
Mullett, C., 582
Mulley, A., 522
Munasinghe, R., 496
Murphy, R., 543
Murphy, S., 770, 772
Musen, M., 105, 643, 649, 659, 661, 662, 731, 732
Musty, M., 672
Mutalik, P., 272
Mynatt, B., 636

N
Nadeau, T., 184
Nadkarni, P., 272
Nahn, V., 499
Nambisan, P., 498

Napel, S., 286, 287, 304, 320, 808
Narus, S.P., 185
Naus, G., 128
Nazi, K., 527
Nease Jr., R., 94, 95, 101, 104, 105
Needleman, S., 704
Nehrt, N., 753
Nelson, S., 576, 577, 587
Nesbitt, T.S., 541
Neumann, P., 753
Neville, A., 676
Newell, A., 113, 114, 116
Newell, M., 302
Ng, G., 316
Ng, S., 702, 745
Nguyen, T.C., 195
Nicholson, D., 622
Nicolae, D., 740
Niederhuber, J., 770
Nielsen, B., 297
Nielsen, J., 128, 129, 132, 358, 383
Nissenbaum, H., 798, 800, 809
Nivre, J., 283
Noble, M., 808
Nolte, E., 786
Norman, D., 117, 128, 130–132, 139, 140, 146, 148
Novack, D., 749
Nowak, E., 311, 312
Nugent, K., 296

O

O'Carroll, P., 503, 505, 506, 515, 516
O'Connell, E., 493
O'Connor, A., 531, 785
Obeid, J., 726
Ognibene, F., 759, 777
Ohmann, C., 768
Ohno-Machado, L., 55, 65, 204, 754
Olsen, L., 799, 805
Olson, S., 749
Omenn, G., 801
Ong, K., 473
Ong, M., 378
Oniki, T., 576, 577
Openshowski, M., 393
Ormond, K., 747, 749, 750
Orne, J., 195
Ornstein, C., 494, 495
Orr, R.A., 195
Osborn, C., 527
Osheroff, J., 420, 643, 670, 673
Oster, S., 773
Overby, C., 648
Overhage, M., 425, 440, 509, 515, 516
Owens, D., 67, 68, 81, 95, 97, 101, 102, 104, 105
Ozbolt, J.M., 35, 475–477, 491, 494
Ozdas, A., 398, 494
Ozkaynak, M., 17

P

Paddock, S., 296
Padkin, A., 762
Page, L., 630
Pagliari, C., 528
Palda, V., 74
Palfrey, J., 336
Palmas, W., 559
Palmer, M., 283
Palmer, S., 258
Palotie, A., 55
Paltiel, A., 105
Paltoo, D., 753
Pan, E., 516, 784, 785, 795
Papanicoloaou, G., 753
Park, J., 143, 257
Park, T., 801
Parker, E., 543
Parrish, F., 738
Paskin, N., 639
Patel, V.L., 29, 65, 109, 110, 117–120, 122, 123, 126–128, 134–136, 141, 143–146, 148, 411, 412, 418, 521, 579, 671
Patey, R., 133
Patterson, D., 184
Patton, M., 387
Pauker, S., 62, 97–99, 330, 658
Pavel, M., 533
Pawson, R., 386
Paxinos, G., 300
Payne, P., 753, 755–757, 762, 766, 772, 774, 775, 777
Payne, S., 119
Payton, F., 476
Peabody, G., 68
Pearce, C., 499
Peel, D., 315
Perkins, D., 122
Perkins, G., 296
Perona, P., 312
Perreault, L., 443, 462
Perry, M., 143
Pestian, J., 260, 282
Pestonik, S., 195, 398, 399
Petratos, G., 583
Peute, L., 492
Pevsner, P., 718
Pham, H., 316, 327, 784
Phansalkar, S., 397
Phelps, M., 289
Pickering, B., 577, 579, 586, 587
Pinhas, A., 320
Pinsky, P., 371
Pliskin, J., 105
Plummer, H., 393
Pluye, P., 637
Polifka, J., 806
Polson, P., 131
Pompilio-Weitzner, G., 559
Poon, A., 488, 575
Poon, E., 401

Pople, H., 62, 64
Porter, M., 473
Potchen, E., 327
Pouratian, N., 290
Power, E., 762, 765
Prastawa, M., 317
Pratt, W., 65
Preece, J., 115, 128, 148
Pressler, T., 765
Price, R., 156
Prince, J., 327
Prochaska, J., 530
Pronovost, P., 571, 578
Prothero, J.S., 318
Prothero, J.W., 318
Pruitt, K., 282
Pryor, T., 203, 394, 420, 576, 577, 590
Pysz, M., 294, 296

Q
Qin, J., 702
Quake, S., 747
Qui, G., 320

R
Raghavan, P., 283
Rahimi, B., 492, 495
Rahmani, R., 320
Raiffa, H., 105
Rall, M., 692
Ralston, J., 492, 527
Ramnarayan, P., 370
Ramsaroop, P., 435
Rausch, T., 493
Ravert, R., 521, 525
Ray, P., 290, 294, 296
Read, J., 230
Reason, J., 135
Rector, A., 232, 300
Redd, W., 521
Reid, C., 628
Reiner, B., 548
Rhee, S., 732
Ribaric, S., 297
Ribeiro-Neto, B., 641
Ricci, F., 553, 803
Richards, F., 420
Richardson, J., 704
Richesson, R., 252, 777
Richter, G., 548, 559
Rigby, M., 358
Rikers, R., 128
Riley, J., 614
Rimoldi, H., 125
Rindfleisch, T., 257, 616
Ripp, L., 515
Ritchie, C., 292
Ritchie, M., 734

Riva, A., 526, 528
Riva-Rocci, S., 564
Robb, R., 327
Roberts, R., 810
Robertson, J., 335, 349
Robinson, P., 319
Rocca-Serra, P., 712
Rockhold, F., 777
Roden, D., 416
Rodriguez-Campos, L., 387
Roentgen, W., 290
Rogers, W., 567
Rogers, Y., 109, 110, 130, 139, 146, 148
Roh, E., 692
Rohlfing, T., 317
Rohn, J., 45, 47, 51
Romano, M., 419
Rose, M., 237
Rosen, G., 305, 515
Rosenbloom, S.T., 398
Rosencrance, L., 494
Rosenfeld, B., 554, 585
Ross, B., 289, 515, 603
Ross, D., 740
Ross, J., 459
Ross, S., 533
Rosse, C., 300, 326
Rossi, P., 381
Roth, E., 130, 196
Rothemich, S., 492
Rothenberg, J., 640
Rothwell, D., 57, 230
Rotman, B., 494
Roudsari, A., 807
Rozenblum, R., 791
Rubin, D., 285–287, 301–304, 322, 325, 326
Rubin, R., 765, 808
Rucker, D., 353
Rudin, R., 781, 784, 791, 795
Ruiz, M., 320
Rusk, N., 740
Russell, L., 105
Ryan, S., 518
Ryckmann, T., 283

S
Saccavini, C., 435
Saeed, M., 282, 569, 572, 575
Saffle, J., 553
Safran, C., 394, 464, 559, 590
Sager, N., 257, 258, 264, 266, 283
Salber, P., 777
Saleem, J., 495, 792
Salomón, G., 144, 146
Salpeter, S., 97
Salton, G., 629, 631, 635
Saltz, J., 773
Samantaray, R., 419
Samsa, G., 672

Sanders, G., 97, 104, 672
Sandor, S., 314
Sands, D., 353, 545
Sandy, L., 777
Sansone, S., 711
Santorii, S., 564
Saria, S., 658
Sarkar, I., 498, 545, 722, 753, 754, 774
Satava, R., 805
Saunders, C., 748
Savitz, L., 456
Sayers, E., 622
Scablert, A., 711
Scaife, M., 139
Schacter, R., 105
Schadt, E., 753
Schaefer, C., 741
Schaffner, K., 353
Schaltenbrand, G., 307
Schedlbauer, A., 397, 648
Scheraga, H., 704
Schimel, A., 297
Schkade, D., 139
Schleyer, T.K.L., 675
Schmidt, H., 124, 128
Schnall, R., 491, 496
Schneider, E., 795
Schneider-Kolsky, M., 603
Schnipper, J., 492, 666
Schultz, E., 300
Schultz, J., 394
Schutze, H., 258, 283
Schvaneveldt, R., 110, 116
Schwamm, L., 554, 559
Schwartz, D., 752
Schwartz, W., 25, 672
Scott, G., 357, 364, 365
Scoville, R., 515, 795
Sculpher, M., 105
Seibig, S., 574
Sekimizu, T., 257
Seldrup, J., 765
Senathirajah, Y., 489
Senders, J., 133
Shabot, M., 142, 581, 588, 590
Shah, A., 204
Shah, N.H., 65, 721, 727, 731, 734
Shah, N.R., 671
Shahar, Y., 643, 649
Shannon, G., 559
Shapiro, L., 311, 313, 314, 327
Sharp, H., 148
Shea, S., 133, 559
Sheikh, A., 790
Shekelle, P., 194, 793
Sherifali, D., 401
Sherry, S., 745
Sherwood, L., 777
Shi, J., 316
Shiffman, R., 668

Shiffrin, R., 113
Shih, S., 331
Shirky, C., 800
Shneiderman, B., 128
Shoichet, B., 738
Shortell, S., 444
Shortliffe, E.H., 3, 5, 10, 11, 15, 18, 26, 29, 35, 36, 39, 60, 109, 110, 115, 135, 148, 185, 331, 344, 643, 649, 650, 655, 659, 724, 788
Shubin, H., 567
Shuldiner, A., 741
Shulman, L., 35, 125, 126
Siebert, U., 97, 105
Siegel, J., 105
Siegler, E., 488
Siek, K., 533
Silberg, W., 618
Silverstein, J.C., 149
Simborg, D., 23, 213
Simon, D., 122
Simon, H.A., 112–115, 122, 139, 141
Simon, R., 608
Simonaitis, L., 412, 415
Singer, E., 747
Singh, A., 295
Singh, H., 671
Sintchenko, V., 97, 105
Sirota, M., 730
Sistrom, C., 607
Sittig, D., 330, 588, 671, 673, 801
Skinner, B.F., 112, 518
Slack, W., 394, 464, 520
Slagle, J., 110, 112, 534
Sloboda, F., 122
Slutsky, J., 774
Smelcer, J., 195
Smeulders, A., 320
Smith, A., 538
Smith, J., 122
Smith, J.W., 66
Smith, L., 69
Smith, M., 290
Smith, P., 784
Smith, T., 704
Snyder-Halpern, R., 195
Snyderman, R., 648
Sobradillo, P., 749
Sollins, K., 639
Solomon, M., 290
Somerville, I., 357, 363
Sondik, E., 11
Sonka, M., 327
Sonnenberg, F., 97
Sordo, M., 660
Sorenson, A., 293
Soto, G., 318
Southon, F., 494
Sox, H., 67, 86, 94, 99, 105, 616, 617, 658
Spackman, K., 230, 300, 739
Spiegelhalter, D., 355, 357

Spilker, B., 760, 761
Spitzer, V., 318
Spock, B., 333
Sprafka, S., 35, 125, 126
Spyns, P., 257
Srinivasan, P., 257
Staffa, J., 805
Stafford, R., 419
Staggers, N., 195
Stallings, W., 237, 252
Stanfill, M., 638
Stanley, J., 367
Starkes, J., 122
Starren, J., 133, 141, 142, 411, 413, 541, 545,
    549, 559, 777
Stavri, P., 136, 613
Stead, W., 209, 380, 394, 483, 489, 492, 500, 800,
    803, 807, 810
Stearns, M., 58
Steen, E., 4, 6
Stein, D., 403, 726
Steinbrook, R., 435, 440
Stensaas, S., 305
Stenson, P., 740
Stephenson, R., v
Sternberg, R., 122
Stevens, R., 680
Stewart, J., 128, 559
Stockman, G., 314, 327
Storey, J., 710
Stormo, G., 35
Strahan, R., 603
Straus, S., 618, 641
Strohman, T., 641
Strom, B., 393, 671, 805
Stryer, L., 718
Subramaniam, A., 733
Subramaniam, B., 314
Suchman, S., 143
Sumkin, J., 604
Sumner, W., 95
Sun, J., 570
Sundheim, B., 274
Sundsten, J., 304
Sung, N., 756, 777
Sussman, S., 112
Swanson, D., 125, 635
Swanson, L., 300, 305
Sweeney, L., 339
Sweller, J., 117
Szczepaniak, M., 35
Szczepura, A., 357
Szolovits, P., 330, 435, 526, 575

T
Tai, B., 765
Talairach, J., 306
Talmon, J., 357, 380
Talos, I., 325
Tamersoy, A., 339

Tanenbaum, A., 184, 237
Tang, P., 142, 209, 391, 404, 411–413, 417, 418, 618,
    781, 784, 786, 792
Taonetti, N., 740, 742, 743
Tarczy-Hornoch, P., 29, 723, 754, 777
Tate, K., 581, 588
Taube, L., 564
Tavenner, M., 192, 647
Taylor, C., 711
Taylor, H., 615, 616
Taylor, R., 515
Teich, J., 394, 399, 420, 462, 673
Teisberg, E., 473
Tenenbaum, J., 695, 721, 747
Teorey, T., 184
Teresi, J., 559
Terzopoulos, D., 314, 317
Thomas, E., 555
Thompson, C.B., 195
Thompson, J., 573
Thorisson, G., 734
Tibshirani, R., 710, 753
Tierney, W., 394, 419
Till, J., 276
Tilley, N., 386
Tilson, H., 777
Toga, A., 289, 305, 306
Tommasi, T., 313
Toms, E., 616
Tong, R., 635
Toomre, D., 296
Torda, P., 792
Toronto, A., v
Torrance, G., 94
Tournoux, P., 306
Trafton, J., 664
Tremper, K., 574
Triggs, B., 311
Trotti, A., 770
Trushkeim, M., 725
Tsarkov, D., 323
Tseytlin, E., 692
Tu, S., 522
Tuck, D., 36
Tucker, C., 794
Tufte, E., 411
Tversky, A., 72, 105
Tymoczko, J., 718
Tysyer, D., 350

U
Ullman, J., 184
Ullman-Cullere, M., 648
Uzuner, O., 282

V
Valdes, I., 419
van Bemmel, J., 801
van Dijk, T., 114, 117

van Essen, D., 307, 314, 315
van Gennip, E., 357
van Leemput, K., 317
van Noorden, S., 296
van Rijsbergen, C., 629
van Walsaven, C., 784
van Way, C., 371
van der Lei, J., 656, 673
van der Sijs, H., 671
van't Veer, L., 708
Vandemheen, K., 531
Vapnik, V., 312
Varma, M., 312
Vawdrey, D., 185, 204, 488, 571, 575, 578, 581, 587
Veasey, L., v
Venkataraman, S.T., 195
Vester, C., 723, 746
Via, M., 740
Vicente, K., 115
Vickers, T., 622
Vigoda, M., 411
Vincze, V., 282
Vinterbo, S., 257
Vogel, L., 443, 451, 455, 459
Volker, N., 748
von Neumann, J., 94, 150
Voorhees, E., 635
Vreeman, D., 396

W
Wachter, S., 129
Wadman, M., 805
Wagner, M., 425
Wald, J., 492
Walji, M., 671
Walker, J., 420, 785, 795
Wang, J., 196, 320
Wang, S., 204, 420, 785
Wang, X., 258, 738
Ward, J.R., 136
Ward, M., 515
Ware, C., 141
Warner, H., v, vi, 23, 394, 569, 575, 649
Warren, W., 307
Wasson, J., 371, 792
Waterman, M., 704
Watson, C., 300
Watson, J., 696, 749
Watson, R.S., 195
Waxman, A., 745
Weaver, D., 704
Weaver, L., 195
Weeber, M., 282
Weed, L., 394, 420, 487
Weeks, J., 105
Wei, L., 701
Weibel, S., 627
Weil, M., 567
Weil, T., 444
Weill, P., 459

Weiner, J., 795
Weinfurt, P., 568
Weingart, S., 526
Weinger, M., 110, 112
Weinstein, M., 105, 658
Weinstein, R., 559
Weinstock, R., 133, 559
Weir, C., 409
Weiser, M., 537, 797
Weissenbach, J., 752
Weissleder, R., 290, 294
Weitzman, E., 498, 526, 535, 806
Weizenbaum, J., 257
Wennberg, J., 616
Wennenberg, J., 522
Were, M., 410
Wessels, J., 296
Westbrook, J., 637
Weston, A., 725
Wetherall, D., 184
Whelan, T., 531
White, B., 119
Whiting-O'Keefe, Q., 394
Whitlock, D., 318
Wicks, P., 806
Wiederhold, G., 23, 161, 171, 184, 185, 465
Wilcox, A., 185, 275
Wild, D., 801
Wildemuth, B., 636
Willard, H., 647, 725
Williams, J., 672
Williams, M., 648
Williams, S., 559
Williamson, J., 35
Willman, J., 294, 296
Willson, D., 577
Wilson, T., 296
Wing, J., 807
Wing, L., 672
Winkelstein, P., 353
Winkler, H., 723
Winograd, T., 257
Wishart, D., 703, 752
Witkin, A., 314
Wolfgang, B., 610
Wong, A., 672
Wong, B., 305
Wood-Harper, T., 494
Woods, C., 804
Woods, D., 133, 134, 136
Woods, R., 318, 319, 327
Woods, S., 500
Woods, W., 257
Woolf, S., 435, 440, 476, 492
Woolhandler, S., 456
Wootton, R., 558
Worthey, E., 748
Wrenn, J., 409
Wright, A., 351, 673
Wright, P., 146, 588
Wu, S., 196

Wubbelt, P., 765
Wunsch, C., 704
Wyatt, J., 355, 356, 362, 372, 373, 381, 384, 762, 808
Wyatt, S., 372

X
Xiao, Y., 579
Xu, C., 327
Xue, N., 283

Y
Yakushiji, A., 257
Yamin, C., 784
Yan, J., 707
Yasnoff, W., 8, 423, 427, 434, 439, 440, 503, 505,
    506, 514–516
Yildrim, M., 736, 737
Yoo, T., 308, 327
Yoshihashi, A., 36
Yoskowitz, N., 148
Young, W., 300, 305
Youngner, S., 343
Yousef, G., 296, 808
Yu, F., 303

Z
Zaccagnini, L., 559
Zalis, M., 302
Zarin, D., 623, 771, 772
Zeng-Treitler, Q., 491
Zerhouni, E., 724
Zhang, H., 317
Zhang, J., 116, 128, 134–137, 139, 260,
    575, 671
Zhenyu, H., 320
Zhou, L., 489
Zhu, J., 735
Zhu, Q., 744
Zhu, V., 395
Zielstorff, R., 479, 481, 501
Zigmond, M., 712
Zijdenbos, A., 314
Zimmerman, B., 16
Zimmerman, J., 252
Zisserman, A., 312
Zoll, P., 565
Zong, W., 575
Zuriff, G., 112
Zweigenbaum, P., 257

Subject Index

A

AAFP. *See* American Academy of Family
    Physicians (AAFP)
AAMC. *See* American Association of Medical
    Colleges (AAMC)
AAMSI. *See* American Association for Medical Systems
    and Informatics (AAMSI)
Abstraction, 225
Academic Medicine (journal), 691
Access, 639, 640
Accountable care organizations (ACO), 213, 340, 444,
    450, 485, 486, 783, 786
Accountability, 176
Accredited canvass, 221
Accredited Standards Organization (ASC), 219
    ASC X12, 213, 219, 221, 245ff
ACC. *See* American College of Cardiology (ACC)
Accuracy, 142
Action, model of, 130, 131
Active failure, 135
Active storage, 153
ACO. *See* Accountable care organizations (ACO)
ACR/NEMA. *See* American College of Radiology/
    National Electrical Manufacturers
    Association (ACR/NEMA)
Ad hoc standards development, 215
ADA. *See* American Dental Association *and* American
    Diabetes Association (ADA)
Ada, 165
Address, 153
ADE. *See* Adverse drug event (ADE)
AdEERS. *See* Adverse Event Expedited Reported
    System (AdEERS)
ADL. *See* Archetype Definition Language (ADL)
ADMD. *See* Administration Management Domain
    (ADMD)
Administration Management Domain (ADMD), 163
Admission-discharge-transfer (ATD), 212, 460
Adoption of information technology, 4
Advanced Distributed Learning, 689
Advanced Informatics in Medicine (AIM), 232
Advanced Research Projects Agency (ARPA), 10
Adverse drug event (ADE), 582, 583
Adverse Event Expedited Reported System
    (AdEERS), 772
Affordable Care Act of 2010, 485, 486

Agency for Health Care Research and Quality (AHRQ),
    24, 400, 483, 530, 620, 621, 687, 774
Agile software development model, 196
Aggregated content, 623–4
AHA. *See* American Heart Association (AHA)
AHIMA. *See* American Health Information Management
    Association (AHIMA)
AHRQ. *See* Agency for Health Care Research and
    Quality (AHRQ)
AIM. *See* Advanced Informatics in Medicine (AIM)
Alaska Satellite Biomedical Demonstration
    project, 543
Alarms, 567, 572ff
Alerts, 41, 188, 190, 564, 765
Algorithms, 22, 315
    Smith-Waterman. *See* Smith-Waterman Algorithm
Allscripts, Inc., 403
Alphanumeric sequence, 629
AMA. *See* American Medical Association (AMA)
Ambulatory medical record systems, 445, 478. *See also*
    Electronic health records
American Academy of Family Physicians (AAFP), 240
American Academy of Pediatrics, 240
American Association for Medical Systems and
    Informatics (AAMSI), 235
American Association of Medical Colleges
    (AAMC), 685–7
  Group on Educational Affairs, 688
American Cancer Society, 519
American College of Cardiology, 664
American College of Critical Care Medicine, 565
American College of Physicians (ACP)
American College of Radiology/National Electrical
    Manufacturers Association (ACR/NEMA), 213,
    235, 238, 600
American Dental Association (ADA), 246
American Diabetes Association (ADA), 687
American Health Information Management Association
    (AHIMA), 218, 350, 622
American Heart Association (AHA), 444, 519, 568,
    664, 687
American Immunization Registry Association
    (AIRA), 510
American Medical Association (AMA), 229, 557
American Medical Association Medical Information
    Network. *See* AMA/NET

American Medical Informatics Association (AMIA), 21,
    350, 489, 495, 590, 685, 723, 724, 774
  Nursing Informatics Special Interest Group, 232
  10x10 programs, 685, 775
  Summit on Translational Science, 724, 774
American National Standards Institute (ANSI), 212, 218,
    219, 221, 241, 247, 660, 667, 689, 690
  Committee on Dental Informatics, 689
American Nurses Association, 350
American Psychiatric Association, 230
American Recovery and reinvestment Act of 2009
    (ARRA), 17, 470, 647
American Society for Testing and Materials. See ASTM
American Society of Anesthesiologists, 565
American Standard Code for Information Interchange.
    See ASCII
American Stroke Association, 554
American Telemedicine Association (ATA), 552, 557
AMIA. See American Medical Informatics Association
    (AMIA)
Analog signal, 43, 159
Analog-to-digital conversion, 159–61
Anatomical-Therapeutic-Chemical classification
    (ATC), 233
Anatomy, 299
Anchoring and adjustment, 73
Ancillary services, 460
Android, 529
Angiography
Anonymization, 339
Annotated corpora (or content), 282, 622, 623
Annotation schema, 282
ANSI. See American National Standards Institute (ANSI)
ANSI X12. See ASC X12 under Accredited Standards
    Organization
Antibiograms, 581
Antibiotic Assistant program, 564, 581, 582
Apache, 208
APACHE III Critical Care Series, 480, 555, 581
API (Application Programming Interface), 167, 168, 206
Apple Computer, 350
Applets, 174, 207
Application Level, 172
Application Programming Interface. See API
Application research, 26
Appropriate use, 330
  and educational standards, 332
Archetype Definition Language (ADL), 224
Archival storage, 153
Arden Syntax, 203, 240, 652, 660, 661, 667
Aries system, 619
Arguments
ARPA. See Advanced Research Projects Agency (US
    Department of Defense)
ARPAnet, 10, 173
ARRA. See American Recovery and reinvestment Act of
    2009 (ARRA)
Artificial intelligence (AI), 33
Artificial neural networks (ANNs), 681
ASC. See Accredited Standards Organization (ASC)

ASCII, 152, 211, 268
Assembly language, 164
Association of Academic Health Center Libraries, 350
ASTM (American Society for Testing Materials), 213,
    219, 221, 240
  ASTM E31 committee, 221, 222, 235
  ASTM standard 1238, 235, 239, 1241
  ASTM Standard E1460, 240
Asynchronous communication, 544
Asynchronous transfer mode (ATM), 157
ATA. See American Telemedicine Association (ATA)
ATC. See Anatomic Therapeutic Chemical Classification
    (ATC)
ATHENA system, 228, 661, 662
Atlases, 304
ATM. See Asynchronous transfer mode (ATM)
Attribute list address, 163
Audit trails, 176, 178
Auditing, 766
Australian Royal Flying Doctor Service (RFDS), 543
Authentication, 176
Authorization, 176
Availability, 176
Availability heuristic, 73

B
Backbone links, 162
Backbone networks, 10
Background question, 618
Backward chaining, 651
Bag-of-words approach (natural language processing),
    257
Bandwidth, 158, 543
Barcode scanner, 577
BARN. See Body Awareness Resource Network (BARN)
Base 2 numbering system, 151
BLAST. See Basic Linear Alignment and Search
    Technique (BLAST)
Basic Linear Alignment and Search Technique (BLAST),
    705
Basic research, 26
Basic sciences, 26
Baby CareLink, 553
Bayes' theorem, 64, 81ff, 99, 321, 649, 650
  cautions in application, 87
  derivation of, 107
  implications of, 85
  odds-ratio form, 83
Bayesian diagnosis programs, 657ff
Baylor College of Medicine, 748
Bedside monitor, 565, 567, 572
Bedside terminals, 577
Behavioral research, 756
Behavior management, 530
Behaviorism, 111, 676
Beth Israel-Deaconess Medical Center, 394, 464, 526
Belief networks, 101, 658
Best-of-breed systems, 197, 198, 213, 445
Bibliographic content, 619

Bibliographic database, 620, 762
BICS. *See* Brigham Integrated Computing System (BICS)
Big data, 4, 55, 251, 538, 807, 808
Billing systems, 212
Binary digit. *See* Bit
Biobanks, 726
Biocomputation, 20
    and medical practice
    progress in, 695ff, 721ff
BioCreAtIvE challenges, 282
Bioinformatics, 28, 695ff, 721ff
    ethical issues, 339, 746, 749
Biological models, 803
Biomarkers, 725, 727ff
Biomed Central (BMC), 617
Biomedical computing. *See* Biocomputation
Biomedical engineering, 31
Biomedical informatics, 15, 18ff
    and biomedical engineering, 31
    and biomedical science and medical practice, 25ff
    and cognitive science, 30
    and computer science, 30
    component sciences, 30ff
    definition, 21
    history, 22ff
Biomedical information retrieval. *See* Information
    retrieval
Biomedical Information Science and Technology
    Initiative (BISTI), 20
Biomedical Research Integrated Domain Group
    (BRIDG), 247, 768
Biomedical science
Biometric identifier
Biomolecular imaging, 29, 597
BioScope, 282
Biosurveillance, 258
BI-RADS, 302
BISTI. *See* Biomedical Information Science and
    Technology Initiative (BISTI)
Bit, 151
Bit depth, 155
Bit rate, 157
Blackberry alphanumeric pager, 581
Blinding, 758
Blog, 622
Blood pressure monitoring, 569
Blue Button, 534
Blue Cross. *See* Insurance
Blue Shield. *See* Insurance
BMC. *See* Biomed Central (BMC)
BMJ. *See* British Medical Journal (BMJ)
Body Awareness Resource Network (BARN), 520ff
Body of knowledge (BOK), 622
Bonferroni method, 709
Boolean operators, 630
Boolean searching, 630
Bootstrap, 153
Bottom up parsing, 271
Bound morphemes, 261
Branching logic, 657

BRIDG. *See* Biomedical Research Integrated Domain
    Group (BRIDG)
Bridges, 157
Brigham and Women's Hospital, 488, 492, 493
Brigham Integrated Computing System (BICS), 464, 493
BrighamRad, 622
British Medical Journal (BMJ), 621
Broadband, 158, 558
    "medical grade" 544
Browsing, 174
Business-logic layer, 469
Buttons, 174

C
C (programming language), 165
C++ 165
caBIG. *See* Cancer Biomedical Informatics Grid (caBIG)
Cancer Biomedical Informatics Grid (caBIG), 303, 767ff
    Clinical Trials Management Workspace, 767–8
Cancer Therapy Evaluation Program (CTEP), 770, 772
Canon Group, 282
Canonical form, 624
CAP. *See* College of American Pathologists (CAP)
Capitation, 35
Cardiac output, 569
Cardiac imaging, 607
CareVue, 575
Case (letters), 268, 269
Case-based learning, 679ff
Case coordinator, 478
Case manager, 478
Case sensitivity, 163
Catalogue et Index et Sites Médicaux Francophones
    (CISMeF), 627
Cataloging, 615
Causal networks, 735
CCD. *See* Continuity of Care Document or charge
    coupled device (CCD)
CCHIT. *See* Certification Commission for Health
    Information Technology (CCHIT)
CCOW. *See* Clinical Context Object Workgroup (CCOW)
CCR. *See* Continuity of Care Record (CCR)
CD Plus. *See* Ovid
CDA. *See* Clinical Document Architecture (CDA)
CDC. *See* Centers for Disease Control and
    Prevention (CDC)
CDER. *See* Center for Drug Evaluation and
    Research (CDER)
CDEs. *See* Common Data Elements (CDEs)
CDISC. *See* Clinical Data Interchange Standards
    Consortium (CDISC)
CDL. *See* Constraint Definition Language (CDL)
CDR. *See* Clinical data repository (CDR)
CDSS. *See* Clinical decision-support system (CDSS)
CDW. *See* Clinical data warehouse (CDW)
Cedars-Sinai Medical Center, 129, 581
Cellular imaging, 296
CEN. *See* Comité Européen de Normalisation (CEN)
Center for Clinical Computing, 464

Center for Drug Evaluation and Research (CDER), 772
Center for Healthcare Information Management, 350
Centers for Disease Control and Prevention (CDC), 56, 250, 400, 506ff, 621, 687
Centers for Medicare and Medicaid Services (CMS), 17, 213, 483, 485, 486, 552, 557, 685, 753, 773
Central processing unit (CPU), 24, 150, 151ff
Certification Commission for Health Information Technology (CCHIT), 192, 217
Certification process, 217
Challenge evaluations, 635
Chat rooms, 689
Cellular phones, 558. *See also* Smart phones
Centering theory, 274, 275
Change of shift, 579
Character sets, 268
Chart parsing, 271
Check tags, 625
Chemical Abstracts, 233
CHESS. *See* Comprehensive Health Evaluation and Social Support System (CHESS)
CHI. *See* Consumer health informatics (CHI)
Children's Hospital of Philadelphia, 748
Children's Mercy Hospital and Clinics, 748
CHIN. *See* Community Health Information Networks (CHIN)
Chunking, 122, 270
CIMI. *See* Clinical Information Modeling Initiative (CIMI)
CINAHL (Cumulative Index to Nursing and Allied Health Literature), 620
    Subject Headings, 625
CISMeF. *See* Catalogue et Index et Sites Médicaux Francophones (CISMeF)
Citation database, 622, 623
Citrix, 198
Class, 264
Classification, 225, 615
Client-server interaction, 175
Clinical algorithm, 663. *See also* Algorithm
Clinical and Translational Science Awards (CTSAs), 722, 724, 773, 782
Clinical Context Object Workgroup (CCOW), 199, 248
Clinical Data Interchange Standards Consortium (CDISC), 219, 225, 248, 768, 770
Clinical data repository (CDR), 277, 467, 468
Clinical data warehouse (CDW), 9, 277, 762, 763
Clinical decisions. *See* Decision making; decision support
Clinical decision-support system (CDSS), 496–7, 564, 586ff, 643ff, 646, 762. *See also* Decision support systems
Clinical Document Architecture (CDA), 241ff, 277
Clinical documentation, 461
Clinical Element Models, 225
Clinical evidence, 623
Clinical Genomics Workgroup (HL7), 726
Clinical guidelines, 7, 13, 105, 423, 584, 585, 764
Clinical informatics, 26, 697, 715
Clinical Information Modeling Initiative (CIMI), 225
Clinical information systems, 445

Clinical models, 222ff
Clinical pathways, 7, 461
Clinical practice guidelines. *See* Clinical guidelines
Clinical prediction rules, 73
Clinical research, 6, 13, 50, 53, 338, 415, 756–62, 778, 779, 802
Clinical research informatics (CRI), 755ff
Clinical research management systems (CRMS), 765ff
Clinical trial management system (CTMS), 763, 765
Clinical trials, 6, 9, 722
    active phase, 761
    enrollment phase, 761
    Phase I, 722, 760
    Phase II, 760
    Phase III, 760
    Phase IV, 760
    Preparatory phase
    randomized, 50, 758ff
Clinically relevant population, 73
ClinicalTrials.gov, 623, 770, 772, 773
ClinQuery, 464
CLOCKSS, 640
Closed-loop therapy, 461, 488, 589
Cloud computing, 34, 182, 183, 485, 610, 763
Clustering algorithm, 315
CMS. *See* Centers for Medicare and Medicaid Services (CMS)
Coaching, 683
Coagulation meter, 547
COBOL, 165, 211
Cochrane Database of Systematic Reviews, 623
Cocke-Younger-Kasami (CYK) parsing, 271
Coded terminologies, 222ff
Cognition architecture, 115
Cognitive artifacts, 110
Cognitive engineering, 130
Cognitive heuristics, 72
Cognitive resources, 127
Cognitive science, 19, 30, 109ff, 676
    explanatory framework, 112
Cognitive task analysis, 131, 137
Cognitive walkthrough, 132, 147
Cohort discovery, 764
Collaboration, 517
Collaborative practices, 518
Collaborative workspaces, 129
College of American Pathologists (CAP), 230
Color resolution, 155
Columbia University, 394, 402, 509, 526, 527, 552, 652
Comité Européen de Normalisation (CEN; European Committee for Standardization), 213, 245
    Technical Committee 251 (TC251), 213, 218ff, 232
Commercial off-the-shelf software (COTS), 193, 198
Commodity Internet, 547
Common Data Elements (CDEs), 769
Common Object Request Broker Architecture (CORBA)
Common Terminology Criteria for Adverse Events (CTCAE), 770, 771
Communications. *See* Data communications
Community-based research, 756

Community Health Information Networks (CHINs), 426
Compactness, 142
Comparative effectiveness research, 256
Comparative studies, 372
Complexity, 517
Comprehensibility, 178
Comprehensive Health Evaluation and Social Support
    System (CHESS)
Computational biology. *See* Bioinformatics
Computed radiography (CR), 600
Computed tomography (CT), 35, 291, 594
Computer-aided diagnosis (CAD), 604. *See also*
    Decision-support systems
Computer architectures, 149, 150
Computer-assisted learning, 520
    didactic, 679
    drill and practice, 677, 678
    exploration vs structured interaction, 678
    feedback and guidance, 683
Computer instructions, 153
Computer literacy, 35
Computer memory, 150, 153
Computer science, 30
Computer-based monitoring, 561ff
    intensive care unit, 567
Computer-Based Patient Record Institute (CPRI),
    350, 426
Computer-based patient records (CPRs). *See* Electronic
    health records
Computer-Stored Ambulatory Record (COSTAR), 487
Computerized provider order-entry (CPOE), 13, 138,
    397, 425, 452, 461, 462, 493, 495ff, 607, 785
Computerized Unified Patient Interaction Device
    (CUPID), 488
Computers and Biomedical Research (journal), 20, 21
Concept, 225, 624
Concept Unique Identifier (CUI), 265, 626
Conceptual graph based semantics, 264, 272
Conceptual knowledge, 119
Conceptual operators, 137
Concordance, 77
Conditional independence, 72ff, 87
Confidentiality, 8, 175, 335, 349, 454
Consensus standards development, 215
Consent, 435
Constraint Definition Language (CDL), 224, 225
Constructivism, 676–7
Consumer decision making, 518, 520, 530
Consumer engagement, 518, 523
Consumer-facing software, 522, 523
Consumer health informatics (CHI), 29, 344, 517ff, 542
Consumer-to-consumer communication, 519
Content standardization, 492
Context, 630
Contingency tables, 76
Continuity of Care Record (CCR), 240ff
Continuity of Care Document (CCD), 241ff, 491, 666
Continuum of care, 48, 486
Contract management, 463
Contrast radiography, 296

Contrast resolution, 155, 156, 295
Control, 178
Control intervention, 758
Controlled terminologies, 624ff, 662
Copyright, 350
Coreference chains, 267
Coreference resolution, 274
Corpora, 282, 283
Correctional telehealth, 542, 543, 551
Cost-benefit tradeoffs, 419, 455, 648
Cost control, 35, 785
COSTAR (Computer-Stored Ambulatory Record), 394
COTS. *See* Commercial off-the-shelf software (COTS)
COURSEWRITER III
CPOE. *See* Computerized provider order entry (CPOE)
CPR. *See* Computer-based patient record (CPR)
CPT. *See* Current Procedural Terminology (CPT)
Creative Commons, 350
Credentialing, 535
CRI. *See* Clinical research informatics (CRI)
CRMS. *See* Clinical research management systems
    (CRMS)
Cryptographic encoding, 177
CT imaging. *See* Computed tomography (CT)
CTCAE. *See* Common Terminology Criteria for Adverse
    Events (CTCAE)
CTEP. *See* Cancer Therapy Evaluation Program (CTEP)
CTMS. *See* Clinical trial management system (CTMS)
CTSA. *See* Clinical and Translational Science
    Awards (CTSA)
CUI. *See* Concept Unique Identifier (CUI)
Culture change, 457
Cumulative Index to Nursing and Allied Health
    Literature. *See* CINAHL
CUPID. *See* Computerized Unified Patient
    Interaction Device
Curly braces problem, 660
Current Procedural Terminology (CPT), 58, 229, 249
Curriculum Inventory Portal, 686
CURRMIT, 686
Cursors, 154

D
Dana Farber Cancer Institute, 492
DARPA. *See* Advanced Research Projects Agency (US
    Department of Defense)
Dashboard, 499, 606, 644, 803
Data, 39ff, 58
    access, 5
    acquisition, 5, 43, 159ff, 188ff, 479, 480, 586,
        587, 655
    capture, 404
    display, 189, 410
    entry, 64
    exchange, 790
    genetic, 339, 699ff
    independence, 170
    integration, 450
    layer, 467

Data, 39ff (*cont.*)
  liquidity, 524, 534
  management, 9, 167, 646
  medical (*see* Medical data)
  mining, 733, 742
  presentation, 480
  processing, 480
  quality, 586
  recording, 43
  reuse, 250, 256, 481
  sharing, 335, 712
  sponge, 239
  standards, 802
  storage, 188ff, 480, 726
  summarization, 189, 638
  timeliness, 587
  transformation, 480
  validation, 410, 655
Data buses, 150
Data communications, 157
  Internet (*see* Internet)
Data Encryption Standard (DES), 177
Data interchange standards, 235ff
Data layer, 467
Data Link Level, 172
Data-driven reasoning, 126, 671
Database, 59, 154, 169
  citation, 622
  EBM (evidence-based medicine),
    622, 623
  genomics, 29, 622
  phenotypic, 29
  regional, 13
Database management systems, 169ff, 622
Database of Genome and Phenome. *See* dbGAP
Datum
dbGAP (Database of Genome and Phenome), 770
DCI. *See* Dossier of Clinical Information (DCI)
DCMI. *See* Dublin Core Metadata Initiative (DCMI)
de facto standards development, 215
Debuggers, 169
Decentralized Hospital Computer Program
  (DHCP), 487
Decision analysis, 90ff, 658
Decision making, 39, 644, 656ff, 803, 804
Decision nodes, 91
Decision science, 30, 67ff
Decision support systems, 4, 8, 14, 188, 190, 333, 397,
  423, 456, 461, 643ff
  data-driven, 580
  human-computer interaction, 110
  in the intensive care unit, 579ff
Decision tree, 89
deCode Genetics, 748
De-duplication, 514
De-identified data, 425
Demand for trainees, 15, 18
Dental informatics, 26
Dermatologic imaging, 297
Department of Defense, 224, 499
Department of Health and Human Services, 241

Department of Veterans Affairs. *See* Veterans Health
  Administration
Departmental systems, 23, 465
Dependency grammar, 264
Dependent variables, 368
Derivational morphemes, 261
DermIS, 622
DES. *See* Data Encryption Standard (DES)
Description logic, 323
Descriptive studies, 372
Design validation, 362
Diagnosis, 29, 67, 319ff, 333, 594, 603, 644
Diagnosis-Related Groups (DRG), 226, 227, 229, 430,
  462, 684
Diagnostic and Statistical Manual of Mental Disorders
  (DSM), 230
Diagrams, 141
DICOM. *See* Digital Imaging and Communications in
  Medicine (DICOM)
Dictionary, 225
Differential diagnosis, 60, 594
Digital Anatomist Dynamic Scene Generator, 305
Digital Anatomist Interactive Atlases, 304
Digital certificates, 178
Digital computers, 159
Digital image, 593. *See also* Image
Digital Imaging and Communications in Medicine
  (DICOM), 213, 220, 238–40, 299, 395,
  548, 600, 606
Digital lectures, 677
Digital libraries, 613–41, 638
  intellectual property, 640
  preservation, 640, 809
Digital Mammography Imaging Screening Trial.
  See DMIST
Digital Object Identifier (DOI), 639
Digital radiography, 600
Digital signal processing (DSP), 161
Digital Subscriber Line (DSL), 157
Digital subtraction angiography, 309
Direct Project, 534, 791
Directionality of reasoning, 122
Disambiguation, 272, 282
Discordance, 77
Discourse, 260, 266, 274ff
Discrete-event simulation models, 103
Discussion rooms, 689
Distributed cognition, 139, 142ff
Distributed databases, 181
Distributed Hospital Computer Program
  (DHCP), 465
Distributed systems, 178ff, 465
  programming, 180
DNA, 698
DNS. *See* Domain Name System (DNS)
Doctoral dissertations, 30
DOI. *See* Digital Object Identifier (DOI)
Domain expert, 122
Domain Name System (DNS), 162, 404
Domains, 279
Dossier of Clinical Information (DCI), 144, 145

Double-blinded, randomized, placebo-controlled
    trial, 759
Double blinding, 54, 758, 759
Draft standard for trial use (DTSU), 217
Drawings in patient records, 44
DRG. *See* Diagnosis-Related Groups (DRG)
Drug codes, 232–4
Drug repurposing, 730
DSL. *See* Digital Subscriber Line (DSL)
DSM. *See* Diagnostic and Statistical Manual of Mental
    Disorders (DSM)
DSP. *See* Digital signal processing (DSP)
DTSU. *See* Draft standard for trial use (DTSU)
Dublin Core Metadata Initiative (DCMI), 627, 628
DXplain system, 623, 649
Dynamic programming, 705
Dynamic simulation, 681
Dynamic transition models, 103

E
E-mail, 10, 173, 174
E-prescribing, 405, 790
Early parsing method, 271
EBCDIC, 211
EBM. *See* Evidence-based medicine (EBM)
ECG. *See* Electrocardiogram (ECG)
ECOCYC project, 715
eCRFs. *See* Electronic case report forms (eCRFs)
ED (emergency department) *See* Emergency room
EDC. *See* Electronic data capture (EDC)
EDIFACT. *See* Electronic Data Interchange for
    Administration, Commerce, and Transport
    (EDIFACT)
Education, 15, 29, 595, 675ff, 802
    computers in. (*see* Computer-assisted learning)
    consumer health education, 686, 687, 804
EHRs. *See* Electronic health records
eHuman, 684
EKG. *See* Electrocardiogram (EKG)
El Camino Hospital, 23, 394, 464
electrocardiogram (ECG or EKG), 159–61, 547, 565ff
    automated analysis of, 568
Electrocardiographic Society, 568
Electroencephalography, 290
Electromagnetic interference, 159
Electronic case report forms (eCRFs), 766
Electronic data capture (EDC), 763, 765, 766
Electronic data interchange (EDI), 462
Electronic Data Interchange for Administration,
    Commerce, and Transport, 213, 235, 247, 248
Electronic health records (EHRs), 4, 41, 186, 189, 198,
    199, 250, 251, 340, 391ff, 425ff, 489, 495ff, 513,
    550, 575, 616, 623, 646, 687, 733, 758, 762, 763,
    774, 782ff, 799, 806
    clinician order entry (*see* CPOE)
    certification, 217
    distributed cognition, 142ff
Electronic-long, paper-short. *See* ELPS (electronic-long,
    paper-short)
Electronic mail. *See* E-mail

Electronic medical records, 47. *See also* Electronic
    health records
Electronic support groups, 525
Eligibility criteria, 663
Eliza, 257
ELPS (electronic-long, paper-short), 621
EMBASE, 620
    ETREE, 625
EMERGE Research Network, 697, 734
Emergency department. *See* Emergency room
Emergency room (ER), 561
Emergency telemedicine, 552–4
Emotion detection, 260
Emory University, 509
EMRs (Electronic Medical Records). *See* Electronic
    Health Records
EN13606
ENCODE (Encyclopaedia of DNA Elements), 745
Encryption, 12, 174
ENIAC computer, 22
Enrichment analysis, 732
Enrollment, 761
Enterprise information warehouse, 468
Entrez system, 622, 701, 710
Entry term, 624
ePad, 304
Epic Systems, 416
Epidemiology, 22, 506, 756
Epigenetics, 703, 723
Epistemologic framework, 120, 121
ER. *See* Emergency room (ER)
Erlang, 165
Error, 135, 482
Error analysis, 276
Error checking, 12
Extreme programming, 197
Ethernet, 601
Ethics, 276, 329ff, 746ff, 749ff
Ethnography, 374
ETL. *See* Extraction-transformation-load (ETL)
EudraCT (European Union Drug Regulating Authorities
    Clinical Trials), 772
European Committee for Standardization Technical
    Committee. *See* Comité Européen de
    Normalisation
European Union Drug Regulating Authorities Clinical
    Trials. *See* EudraCT
Evaluation, 355ff, 439
    data analysis, 376ff
    data collection, 376ff
    communicating results, 378ff
    contract, 359
    extrinsic, 275
    informatics, 689
    information retrieval, 634
    intrinsic, 275
    negotiation phase, 359
    study types, 364
    summative, 689
    system oriented, 634
    user oriented, 635–6

Event-condition-action (ECA) rules, 653
Event monitors, 462
Evidence-based guidelines, 7. *See also* Clinical
    guidelines
Evidence-based medicine (EBM), 7, 340, 618, 633, 637
Exabyte, 153
Exact-match retrieval, 630
Expected-value decision making, 87ff
Exomes, 716
Experimental intervention, 758
Experimental science, 26
Expert, 122
Expert systems, 330
expertise, 122
Expressiveness, 278
Extended Binary Coded Decimal Interchange Code.
    See EBCDIC
eXtensible Markup Language. *See* XML
External representations, 138, 139
External validity, 761
Extraction-transformation-load (ETL), 181, 766
Extreme programming, 197
Extrinisic evaluation, 275

F
F measure, 276
Facebook, 525
Facts (program), 532
Factual knowledge, 120
Falls prevention, 493
Falls risk assessment, 493
False alarms, 575
False negatives, 76ff, 276
False positives, 76ff, 276
False-negative rate, 77ff
False-positive rate, 77ff
Fast Health care Interoperability Resources (FHIR),
    242–3, 251
FDA. *See* Food and Drug Administration (FDA)
FDAAA. *See* Food and Drug Administration
    Amendments Act of 2007 (FDAAA)
FDDI. *See* Fiber Distributed Data Interface (FDDI)
Feasibility analysis, 762
Federal Children's Bureau, 519
Federal Trade Commission, 349
Federated database system, 179
Federated queries, 179, 181
Fee-for-service, 450
Feedback. *See* Haptic feedback
Fellowship. *See* National Library of Medicine
    postdoctoral fellowship
Fiber Distributed Data Interface, 239, 601
Fiberoptic cable, 158
Fields, 169
File Transfer Protocol (FTP), 173, 174
File, 170
File servers, 158
File system, 154
Firewall, 177

Filtering algorithms, 161
Financial savings, 648. *See also* Cost-benefit tradeoffs
Finite state automata, 261
    cascading, 271
FHIR. *See* Fast Health care Interoperability Resources
    (FHIR)
Flexner report, 393
Flexnerian learning, 675
Flybase, 282
FM. *See* Frequency modulation (FM)
Food and Drug Administration (FDA), 233, 349–51, 456,
    583, 610, 741, 761, 768, 770
Food and Drug Administration Amendments Act of 2007
    (FDAAA), 772
Foreground question, 618
Force feedback. *See* Haptic feedback
Form factor, 470
Formative evaluation, 689
FORTRAN, 165
Forward chaining, 651
Foundational Model of Anatomy, 300, 301, 304
Fourier transform, 161
Frame based semantics, 264
Frame relay, 157
Frames, 272
Free morphemes, 261
Frequency, 160
Frequency modulation, 161
Front-end applications, 170
FTP. *See* File Transfer Protocol (FTP)
Full-text content, 620ff
Functional imaging, 288, 597
Functional magnetic resonance imaging (fMRI), 289
Functional mapping, 597
Future of EHRs, 10

G
GALEN, 232, 300
GALEN Representation and Integration Language
    (GRAIL), 232
Gateways, 158
GELLO, 660, 668
GENBANK, 265, 282, 700, 704, 708, 712, 717
Gene expression data, 696, 701, 707
Gene Expression Omnibus (GEO), 700
Gene Ontology (GO), 234, 282, 717
General Electric Corporation, 225, 570
General purpose graphical processing unit
    (CPGPU), 154
Genetic Information Nondiscrimination Act (GINA),
    350, 698, 746
GENIA corpus, 282
Genome, 698, 723
    analysis, 702
    databases, 712
Genome-wide association studies (GWAS), 726, 741
Genomic medicine, 725
Genomics, 696
    in critical care, 589

Genotype, 698
Geographic information systems (GIS), 503, 507
Georgetown Home Health Care Classification
	(HHCC), 232
Gestalt psychology, 141
Gigabytes, 153
GINA. *See* Genetic Information Nondiscrimination Act
	(GINA)
GIS. *See* Geographic information systems (GIS)
GLIF. *See* GuideLine Interchange Format (GLIF)
Global processing, 309
Globus Online, 174
GO. *See* Gene Ontology (GO)
Goals, Operators Methods and Selection Rules
	(GOMS), 130
Google, 630, 633, 807
Google Health, 498, 499, 534, 538
Google Scholar, 623
Gopher, 521
Governance, 432, 458, 513
Government roles, 13, 215, 506
GPU. *See* Graphical processing unit (GPU)
GPGPU. *See* General purpose graphical processing unit
	(GPGPU)
GRAIL. *See* GALEN Representation and Integration
	Language (GRAIL)
Grammar, 262
	context-free, 263, 266
	probabilistic, 262–4, 266
Grammar rule, 266
Grand challenges, 801ff
Granularity, 630
Graphical processing unit (GPU), 150, 154
Graphical user interface, 169
Graphs, 735
Grid computing, 182
Group Health Cooperative, 492, 527
Growth charts, 49
GS1, 219
Guardian Angel Manifesto (Proposal), 526
Guideline Element Model (GEM), 668
GuideLine Interchange Format (GLIF), 668
Guidelines. *See* Clinical guidelines
Gulf of evaluation, 131
Gulf of execution, 131

H
Hadoop, 181
Handovers, 577, 579
Haptic feedback, 154, 555, 595, 682
Harmonic mean, 276
Harrison's Online, 623
Harvard Medical Practice Study, 134
Harvard University, 208, 747
HCFA (Health Care Financing Administration) former
	name for Centers for Medicare and Medicaid
	Services (CMS)
HCI. *See* Human-computer interaction (HCI)
Head word, 262

Health Care Financing Administration (HCFA) former
	name for Centers for Medicare and Medicaid
	Services (CMS)
Health Desk, 532
Health Evaluation Logical Processing system. *See* HELP
	System
Health Industry Business Communications Council
	(HIBCC), 247
Health informatics education, 685
Health information exchange (HIE), 207, 404, 425,
	790, 801
Health information infrastructure (HII), 17, 404, 423ff,
	503, 514, 523
Health Information Management Systems Society
	(HIMSS), 240
Health information and communications technology
	(HICT), 542. *See also* Health information
	technology
Health information technology. *See* EHRs, CPOE,
	departmental systems, HIE
Health Information Technology for Economic and
	Clinical Health Act of 2009 (HITECH), 17, 331,
	341, 349, 405, 415, 427, 470, 478, 483, 534, 535,
	647, 788ff, 800
Health information technology policy, 781ff
Health Insurance Portability and Accountability Act of
	1976 (HIPAA), 12, 245, 276, 338, 349, 392, 418,
	428, 454, 486, 550, 610
Health Level 7 (HL7), 12, 204, 216, 218–20, 235, 237,
	241, 242, 396, 445, 575, 607, 656, 660, 722, 770
	Clinical Document Architecture (CDA), 224,
	277, 770
	Clinical Genomics Workgroup, 726
	Individual Case Safety Reports, 772
	Reference Information Model (RIM), 224, 241, 243,
	248, 251
	Terminfo, 224
Health literacy, 111
Health maintenance organizations (HMOs), 213, 447
Health on the Net Foundation (HON), 522, 535, 618
	HON Select, 620
Health promotion, 13
Health Record Banking Alliance (HRBA), 433, 435
Health record banks (HRBs), 434ff
Health services research, 756
Health Wise, 532
Healthcare financing, 34. *See also* Insurance
Healthcare informatics. *See* Biomedical informatics
Healthcare information systems (HCIS), 443ff
Healthcare organizations (HCOs), 443ff
Healthcare team, 43
Healthfinder, 620
HealthGate Data Corporation, 532
HealthVault. *See* Microsoft HealthVault
HELP (Health Evaluation Logical Processing) System,
	304, 487, 563, 576, 578, 580ff, 649, 652ff, 660
Helpers, 174
Heritage Foundation, 435
Heuristic evaluation, 132, 137
Heuristics, 59. *See also* Cognitive heuristics

HGNC. *See* HUGO Gene Nomenclature Committee (HGNC)

HHCC. *See* Home Health Care Classification (HHCC)

HIBCC. *See* Health Industry Business Communications Council (HIBCC)

HICT. *See* health information and communications technology (HICT)

HIE. *See* Health information exchange (HIE)

Hierarchy, 624

Highwire Press, 616, 634

HII. *See* Health information infrastructure (HII)

HIMSS. *See* Health Information Management Systems Society (HIMSS)

Hindsight bias, 135

HIPAA. *See* Health Insurance Portability and Accountability Act (HIPAA)

HIS. *See* Hospital information systems (HIS)

Historical control, 758

HIT. *See* Health information technology (HIT)

HITECH. *See* Health Information Technology for Economic and Clinical Health Act (HITECH)

HL7. *See* Health Level 7 (HL7)

HMOs. *See* Health maintenance organizations

Home computing, 537

Home Health Care Classification (HHCC), 232

Home telehealth, 542, 551–3
  monitoring, 558

Home telemedicine unit, 549, 551, 553

HON. *See* Health on the Net Foundation (HON)

Hopkins Teen Central, 521, 525

Hospital-acquired infections. *See* Nosocomial infections

Hospital information systems, 22, 189, 212, 216, 444

HTML (HyperText Markup Language), 173, 174, 267, 627

HTTP. *See* HyperText Transfer Protocol (HTTP)

HUGO Gene Nomenclature Committee (HGNC), 234

Human Brain Project, 306

Human Disease Network, 736

Human factors, 110, 133ff. *See also* Usability

Human Gene Mutation Database, 698

Human Genome Project, 55, 251, 696, 711, 723

Human-computer interaction, 110, 128ff. *See also* Usability

Hypertext, 174

HyperText Markup Language. *See* HTML (HyperText Markup Language)

HyperText Transfer Protocol (HTTP), 173, 206

Hypothesis generation, 60, 63, 256

Hypothesis-driven reasoning, 126

Hypothetico-deductive approach, 60, 70, 125

I

I2b2 (Informatics for Integrating Bench and Bedside), 282, 770

IAIMS. *See* Integrated Academic Information Management Systems (IAIMS)

ICANN. *See* Internet Corporation for Assigned Names and Numbers (ICANN)

ICD-10. *See* International Classification of Diseases, Tenth Revision (ICD-10)

ICD-10-CM. *See* International Classification of Diseases, Tenth Revision-Clinical Modifications (ICD-10-CM)

ICD-9. *See* International Classification of Diseases, Ninth Revision

ICD-9-CM. *See* International Classification of Diseases, Ninth Revision-Clinical Modifications

ICMP. *See* Internet Control Message Protocol (ICMP)

Icons

ICNP. *See* International Classification of Nursing Practice (ICNP)

ICPC. *See* International Classification of Primary Care (ICPC)

ICHPPC. *See* International Classification of Health Problems in Primary Care (ICHPPC)

IDEATel. *See* Informatics for Diabetes Education and Telemedicine (IDEATel)

IDF. *See* Inverse document frequency (IDF)

IDF*TF weighting. *See* TF*IDF weighting

IDNs. *See* Integrated delivery networks (IDNs)

IEEE. *See* Institute of Electrical and Electronics Engineers (IEEE)

IHE. *See* Integrating the Healthcare Enterprise (IHE)

IHTSDO. *See* International Health Terminology Standards Development Organization (IHTSDO)

Image
  acquisition, 286ff, 600
  biomolecular, 597
  compression, 544
  content representation, 297
  database, 622
  enhancement, 309
  exchange, 609
  interpretation, 286, 319ff, 599
  link-based, 630
  metadata, 299
  patches, 311
  quality, 295ff
  quantitation, 310, 321
  registration, 317ff
  rendering, 309
  retrieval, 319
  segmentation, 313ff

Image-guided procedures, 595

Image processing, 286, 307ff

Imaging informatics, 28, 285ff, 593

Imaging systems, 593ff

iMDSoft, 575

IMIA. *See* International Medical Informatics Association (IMIA)

Immersive simulated environments, 129, 682

Immunization
  registries, 510
  informatics issues, 511ff
  information systems (IIS), 595

Implementation science, 759

IMS Global Learning Consortium, 689

Incentive Programs for Electronic Health Records rule, 483, 484
Independent variables, 72, 369
Index, 259
Index Medicus, 614, 704
Indexing, 614, 624ff
  automated, 624, 628ff
  controlled terminologies, 624ff
  manual, 624, 626ff
Indirect care, 479
Individualized medicine. *See* Personalized medicine
Infectious disease monitoring, 581
Inference, 320
Inflectional morphemes, 261
Influence diagrams, 101ff, 658
Infobutton, 400, 402, 481, 644, 656, 687
InfoPOEMS, 623
InfoRAD, 601
Informatics for Diabetes Education and Telemedicine (IDEATel), 140, 549, 552
Informatics for Integrating Bench and Bedside. *See* i2b2
Information, 19, 58
  extraction, 258, 638
  management, 443ff
  model, 303
  need, 615
  nature of, 32ff
  needs, 646
  requirements, 448
  resources, 356
  science, 19, 30
  structure, 26
  theory, 20
Information retrieval (IR), 110, 259, 613ff, 762
  evaluation, 634
  exact-match, 630, 631
  partial-match, 631, 632
  retrieval systems, 632ff
Ink-jet printers, 155
Input devices, 154
Institute of Electrical and Electronics Engineers (IEEE), 213, 218, 219, 235, 245
  Learning technology Standards Committee, 689
Institute of Medicine (IOM), 14, 419, 482, 483, 488, 504, 523, 524, 805
Institutional Review Boards (IRBs), 178, 339, 761
Insurance, 444
  Blue Cross, 444
  Blue Shield, 444
  Medicaid, 444
  Medicare, 444
Integrated Academic Information Management Systems (IAIMS), 489
Integrated circuits, 567
Integrated delivery networks (IDNs), 157, 338, 443ff, 484, 486
Integrated Services Digital Network (ISDN), 239, 550, 552
Integrating the Healthcare Enterprise (IHE), 219–21
Integration, 8, 450, 607, 695

Intelihealth, 622
Intellectual property, 350, 640
Intelligent tutoring systems, 683, 684
Intensive care unit (ICU), 561ff
  neonatal (NICU), 553, 561
  surgical (SICU), 565
Interactions, 735
Interactive television, 518
Interactive video, 522
Interdisciplinary care, 478, 479
Interface Definition Language (IDL), 180
Interface engine, 445
Interface technology, 405
Intermediate effect, 123
Intermountain Healthcare, 398, 571, 576, 580, 581
Internal representations, 138
Internal Revenue Service, 214, 225
Internal validity, 761
International Classification of Diseases 56, 226, 249, 655, 769
  Ninth Revision (ICD-9), 226–8, 734
  Ninth Edition-Clinical Modification (ICD-9-CM), 226, 227, 277, 282, 464, 769, 771
  Tenth Revision (ICD-10), 57, 226, 228
  Tenth Edition-Clinical Modification (ICD-10-CM), 226, 228
International Classification of Health Problems in Primary Care (ICHPPC), 228
International Classification of Nursing Practice (ICNP), 232
International Classification of Primary Care (ICPC), 228
International Council of Nurses, 232
International Health Terminology Standards Development Organization (IHTSDO), 219, 221, 230, 491
International Medical Informatics Association (IMIA), 495
International Standards Organization (ISO), 212, 245, 627
  Technical Committee 215 (Health Informatics) (TC215), 213, 218, 219
  ISO/CEN 13606, 224
  ISO Standard 1087, 225
Internet, 162, 239
  addresses, 162
  development of, 10
  service providers (ISP), 163
  support group (ISG), 522, 525
Internet Corporation for Assigned Names and Numbers (ICANN), 162
Internet Control Message Protocol (ICMP), 173
Interstate Nurse Licensure Compact, 557
Interoperability, 8, 250, 276, 472, 639, 640, 670, 764
Interpreter, 165
Intervention, 758
Interventional radiology, 598
Interviews, 377
Intravenous (IV) pump, 563, 583, 584
Intrinsic evaluation, 275
Inverse document frequency (IDF), 629

IOM. *See* Institute of Medicine (IOM)
iPhone, 529, 587
IPA. *See* Individual practice associations
iPad, 587
IR. *See* Information retrieval (IR)
ISDN. *See* Integrated Services Digital Network (ISDN)
ISG. *See* Internet support group (ISG)
ISO. *See* International Standards Organization (ISO)
ISP. *See* Internet service provider (ISP)
IV pump. *See* Intravenous (IV) pump

J

JAMIA. *See Journal of the American Medical*
        Informatics Association
Java, 165
JavaScript, 165
JavaScript Object Notation (JSON), 180
JBI. *See Journal Biomedical Informatics*
JCAHO. *See* Joint Commission, The
JIC. *See* Joint Initiative Council (JIC)
Jobs, 168. *See also* Training
Joint Commission, The (TJC; formerly, Joint
        Commission for Accreditation of Health Care
        Organizations; JCAHO), 250, 449, 485
Joint Initiative Council (JIC), 219
Johns Hopkins University, 690
Journal of Biomedical Informatics (JBI), 21, 29,
        724, 774
Journal of Educational Research, 692
Journal of the American Medical Informatics
        Association, 724, 774
JSON. *See* JavaScript Object Notation
Judgment. *See* Clinical judgment
"Just in time" information model, 522, 531, 553,
        687, 691

K

Kaiser Health System, 23, 430, 520, 527, 532
KEGG. *See* Kyoto Encyclopaedia of Genes and
        Genomes (KEGG)
Kernel, 167, 169
Key fields, 170
Key performance indicators (KPIs), 606
Keyboards, 154
Keyword approach (natural language processing), 257
KF. *See* Knowledge Finder (KF)
Kilobytes, 153
Knowledge, 58
    acquisition, 651
    compilation, 120
    discovery, 638
    evidence-based, 19
    organization of, 117
    procedural, 119
    representation, 298ff
Knowledge base, 65, 659, 664, 717
    conceptual, 119
    reasoning, 322

Knowledge based systems, 659. *See also* Expert systems
Knowledge Finder (KF), 637
Kyoto Encyclopaedia of Genes and Genomes (KEGG)

L

Labor and delivery suites, 561
Laboratory information system (LIS), 190, 197
LANs. *See* Local-area networks (LANs)
Laser printers, 155
Latency, 142, 555
Latent conditions, 135
Latent failure, 135
Law of proximity, 141, 142
Law of symmetry, 141, 142
LCD. *See* Liquid crystal display (LCD)
LDS Hospital, 23, 394, 399, 576ff, 581, 652
LEAN, 458
Learning assessment, 687
Learning health system, 14, 17, 672, 773, 805
Learning through design, 681
Legal issues, 50, 347ff, 513. *See also* Regulation
Library, 638
Licensure, 557
Leadership
Leapfrog Group
Learning center, 687, 688
LED. *See* Light-emitting diode (LED)
Leeds abdominal pain system, 649
Legacy systems, 488
Lexemes, 261
Lexical-statistical retrieval, 631
Lexicography
Lexicon, 261, 262, 606
Liability under tort law, 347
Library of Congress, 640
Light-emitting diode (LED), 154
Likelihood ratios, 83
LingPipe, 283
Linguistic knowledge, 260
Linguistic String Project, 257
Linux, 208
Liquid crystal display (LCD), 154
LIS. *See* Laboratory information system (LIS)
LISP, 165
List servers, 173
Literature reference databases, 519, 619
Local-area networks, 4, 157ff, 239, 465, 601
        protocols, 158
Lockheed Corporation, 23, 464
LOCKSS project (National Digital Information
        Infrastructure Preservation Program), 640
LocusLink, 282
Logan International Airport, 543
Logic-based semantics, 264
Logical Observations, Identifiers, Names, and Codes
        (LOINC), 232–4, 249, 282
Logical Record Architecture, 225
LOINC. *See* Logical Observations, Identifiers, Names,
        and Codes (LOINC)

Long-term memory, 117
Long-term storage, 153, 154
Lossless compression, 602
Lossy compression, 602
Lots of Copies Keep Stuff Safe. *See* LOCKSS project
Low-level processes
Low-resource environments, 558
LUNAR, 257

M

M (computer language). *See* MUMPS
Machine language, 164
Machine learning, 260, 584, 708, 709, 802
Machine translation, 260
Macros, 164
Magnetic media, 150
Magnetic-resonance imaging (MRI), 35, 289, 293, 595
Magnetic-resonance spectroscopy, 289
Magnetoencephalography, 290
Mainframe computers, 463
Malpractice, 348
Managed care, 34
Managed competition
Management of uncertainty, 67ff
Management science, 30
MAP. *See* Mean average precision (MAP)
MapReduce, 181
Markle Foundation, 527
Markov models, 96, 261
Marshfield Clinic, 550, 558
Massachusetts General Hospital (MGH), 23, 30, 492, 520, 543
Massachusetts General Hospital Utility Multiprogramming System. *See* MUMPS
Massachusetts Institute of Technology (MIT), 678
Massachusetts Medical Society (MMS), 240
Mayo Clinic, 393, 491, 577, 579, 584, 587
Mayo Health Advisor, 532
Master patient index (MPI), 459
McMaster University, 680
MDConsult, 621, 623, 627
Mean average precision (MAP), 635
Meaningful use (of electronic health records), 13, 17, 192, 200, 241, 396, 454, 509, 545, 646, 773, 782ff. *See also* HITECH
Means-ends analysis, 113
Measurement, 369
Medbiquitous standards, 686, 690
MedEd PORTAL, 685, 687
Mediators, 181
Medicaid. *See* Centers for Medicaid and Medicare Services (CMS); Insurance
Medical cognition, 110, 121ff
Medical College of Wisconsin, 748
Medical computer science, 19
Medical Data Interchange Standards, 235
Medical devices, 31, 793
Medical Dictionary of Regulatory Affairs (MedRA), 249, 282, 770, 771

Medical entities dictionary, 469
Medical errors, 111
Medical expertise, 125
Medical informatics, 26. *See also* Biomedical informatics
Medical Information Bus (MIB), 245, 571, 578, 587
Medical Knowledge Self-Assessment Program
Medical library, 687
Medical Library Association, 350
Medical Literature Analysis and Retrieval System (MEDLARS), 614, 627
Medical logic modules (MLMs), 204, 240, 652, 660, 661
Medical home. *See* Patient centered medical home
Medical history taking, 520
Medical record committees, 339
Medical records. *See* Electronic health records
Medical Subject Headings (MeSH), 234, 282, 301, 614, 624, 625, 627, 739
Medicare. *See* Centers for Medicaid and Medicare Services (CMS); Insurance
MEDINET project, 23
MEDITECH, 467
MEDLARS. *See* Medical Literature Analysis and Retrieval System (MEDLARS)
MEDLARS Online. *See* MEDLINE
MedLEE, 257
MEDLINE, 282, 464, 480, 614, 619, 626ff, 631ff, 636, 637
MEDLINEplus, 400, 623, 687, 739, 807
Medscape, 687
MEDSYNDIKATE, 257
MedRA. *See* Medical Dictionary of Regulatory Affairs (MedRA)
MedWISE, 489
Megabits, 157
Megabytes, 153
Memorandum of understanding, 376
Memory (human), 116, 117
Memory sticks, 472
Mental images, 119
Mental models, 119
Mental representations, 115
Mentoring, 683, 684
Merck Medicus, 623
MERLOT, 689, 690
MeSH. *See* Medical Subject Headings (MeSH)
Messaging, 214, 245
Meta-analysis, 81
Meta-tools
Metabolomics, 711, 727
Metadata, 170, 614, 726, 763
Metagenomics, 702, 752
Metathesaurus (UMLS), 234, 281, 6256
MetaVision, 575
MGH. *See* Massachusetts General Hospital (MGH)
MGH Utility Multi-Programming System. *See* MUMPS
mHealth. *See* Mobile health
MHS. *See* Military Health System (MHS)
MIAME. *See* Minimum Information About a Microarray Experiment (MIAME)
MiCare, 499

Microarray chips, 696. *See also* Gene expression data, MIAME

Microcomputers, 24

Micromedex, 400, 480

Microprocessor, 24, 567

Microsimulation models, 103

Microsoft HealthVault, 431, 499, 529

Microsoft, Inc., 350, 431

Microsoft Bing, 630, 633

MIF. *See* Model Interchange Format (MIF)

Military Health System (MHS), 498

MIME. *See* Multipurpose Internet Mail Extensions (MIME)

MIMIC-II (Multiparameter Intelligent Monitoring in Intensive Care), 276, 584

Minicomputers, 444, 567

Minimum Information About a Microarray Experiment (MIAME), 711, 717

Misspellings, 277, 278

Mistakes, 135

MIT. *See* Massachusetts Institute of Technology (MIT)

Mixed-initiative dialog, 655

MKSAP. *See* Medical Knowledge Self-Assessment Program (MKSAP)

MLMs. *See* Medical logic modules (MLMs)

MMS. *See* Massachusetts Medical Society

Mobile phones, 558, 587. *See also* Smart phones

Mock-ups, 193

Model Interchange Format (MIF), 224

Model organisms databases, 282, 624

Modifiers, 259

Molecular biology, 696

Molecular Biology Database Collection, 622

Molecular imaging, 294

Monotonicity, 123

Moore's Law, 25, 417, 717

Morbidity and Mortality Weekly Report (MMWR), 507

Morphemes, 260, 261, 268

Morphological knowledge, 261, 265

Morphology, 260, 261, 630

Morphometrics, 597

Mosaic, 207

Motion artifacts, 544

Mouse, 154

Mouse Genome Informatics, 282, 624

MPI. *See* Master patient index (MPI)

MPLS. *See* Multiprotocol label switching (MPLS)

MRI. *See* Magnetic resonance imaging (MRI)

Multi-axial terminology, 230

Multidisciplinary Epidemiology and Translational Research in Intensive Care Data Mart, 584

Multimodal interfaces, 129

Multiparameter Intelligent Monitoring in Intensive Care database. *See* MIMIC-II

Multiphasic screening, 394

Multiprocessing, 168

Multiprogramming, 168

Multiprotocol label switching (MPLS), 544

Multipurpose Internet Mail Extensions (MIME), 173

Multiuser systems, 168

MUMPS, 165, 445, 464

MyChart, 526

MYCIN, 649ff, 659, 661

MyHealtheVet, 527

MyMediHealth, 533

N

NAHIT. *See* National Alliance for Health Information Technology (NAHIT)

Naïve Bayes, 657

Name, 225

Name authority, 469

Name-servers, 162

Named entity normalization, 259

Named-entity recognition, 259

NANDA. *See* North American Nursing Diagnosis Association (NANDA)

NAR. *See* Nucleic Acids Research (NAR) database

NASA. *See* National Aeronautics and Space Administration (NASA)

Narrative data, 303

National Academy of Sciences, 482–3

National Aeronautics and Space Administration (NASA), 543

National Alliance for Health Information Technology

National Cancer Institute (NCI), 621, 745, 767, 769, 770

National Center for Biomedical Computing, 770

National Center for Biomedical Ontology (NCBO), 732

National Center for Biotechnology Information (NCBI), 234, 619, 710, 713, 770

 NCBI Bookshelf, 621

National Center for Microscopy and Imaging Research, 318

National Committee for Quality Assurance

National Committee on Vital and Health Statistics (NCVHS), 426

National Council of State Boards of Nursing, 557

National Council for Prescription Drug Programs (NCPDP), 213, 219, 235, 245

National Digital Information Infrastructure Preservation Program (NDIIPP), 640

National Drug Codes (NDC), 234

National Electronic Disease Surveillance System

National Guidelines Clearinghouse (NGC), 620

National Health and Nutrition Examination (NHANES), 508

National health goals, 783

National Health Information Infrastructure (NHII). *See* Health information infrastructure

National Health Information Network (NHIN), 483, 486

 NHIN Connect, 483

 NHIN Direct, 483

National Health Service (UK) (NHS), 224, 230, 545

 NHS Direct, 545

National Heart, Lung and Blood Institute, 522

National Human Genome Research Institute (NHGRI), 702, 745

National Information Standards Organization (NISO), 627

National Institute for Standards and Technology (NIST), 181, 219, 635
National Institutes of Health (NIH), 24, 616, 623, 686, 687, 724, 756, 770, 774
    NIH Reporter, 623
    Pain Consortium, 769
National Library of Medicine (NLM), 24, 25, 233, 234, 282, 400, 411, 542, 614, 620, 621, 624, 628, 632, 634, 687, 731, 739, 772
    NLM Gateway, 634
    postdoctoral fellowship, 774
National Provider Identifier (NPI), 213
National Quality Forum (NQF), 220, 250
National Research Council, 338, 426, 482, 483, 489
National Science Foundation (NSF), 10, 538, 617
Nationwide Health Information Network (NwHIN), 404
Natural history study, 758, 759
Natural language, 251
Natural language processing (NLP), 251ff, 405, 656, 733
Natural language query, 631
Naturalistic studies, 375
NCBI. See National Center for Biotechnology Information (NCBI)
NCBO. See National Center for Biomedical Ontology (NCBO)
NCPDP. See National Council for Prescription Drug Programs (NCPDP)
NCI. See National Cancer Institute (NCI)
NCVHS. See National Committee on Vital and Health Statistics (NCVHS)
NDC. See National Drug Codes (NDC)
NDIIPP. See National Digital Information Infrastructure Preservation Program (NDIIPP)
Nebraska Psychiatric Institute, 543
NEDSS. See National Electronic Disease Surveillance System (NEDSS)
Needs assessment, 362, 689
Negation, 278
Negative dictionary, 629
Negative predictive value, 84
Negligence theory, 347
Nested structures, 263
Net reclassification improvement (NRI), 730
Netter Interactive 3D, 684
NetWellness, 622
Network access providers, 157, 158, 163
Network analysis, 735
Network Level, 172
Network operations center (NOC), 434
Network stack, 171, 172
Network topology, 172
Neuroinformatics, 287, 317
NeuroNames, 300
New York Presbyterian Hospital (NYPH), 393, 552
New York State Psychiatric Institute (NYSPI), 551
NGC. See National Guidelines Clearinghouse (NGC)
NHII. See National Health Information Infrastructure (NHII)
NHIN. See National Health Information Network (NHIN)
NHS. See National Health Service (UK)

NIC. See Nursing Interventions Classification (NIC)
NICU. See Neonatal intensive care unit (NICU)
NISO. See National Information Standards Organization (NISO)
NIST. See National Institute for Standards and Technology (NIST)
NLP. See Natural language processing (NLP)
NLTK (Natural Language Tool Kit), 283
NOC. See Nursing Outcomes Classification (NOC)
Noise, 161
Nomenclature, 55, 222ff
North American Nursing Diagnosis Association (NANDA), 232
Nosocomial infections, 563
NPI. See National Provider Identifier (NPI)
NSF. See National Science Foundation (NSF)
Nuclear magnetic resonance (NMR), 293
Nuclear medicine imaging, 293
Nucleic Acids Research (NAR) database, 622
Nursing care, 477
Nursing informatics, 26
Nursing terminologies, 232
Nursing Interventions Classification (NIC), 232
Nursing Outcomes Classification (NOC), 232
Nutritionist, 478
Nyquist frequency, 161
NYPH. See New York Presbyterian Hospital (NYPH)
NYSPI. See New York State Psychiatric Institute (NYSPI)

O

Object Management Group (OMG), 668
Objectivist studies, 367
OBI. See Ontology for Biomedical Investigations
Object, 225
Observational cohort study, 759
Occupational therapist, 478
Odds, 82
Odds ratio, 82
Office of Civil Rights, 349
Office of the National Coordinator for Health Information Technology (ONC; formerly ONCHIT), 17, 192, 217, 404, 483, 671, 773, 782ff
OLAP. See On line analytic processing
OLTP. See On line transaction processing
Omaha System, 232
    omics data, 722
    omics technologies, 707
Omnibus Budget Reconciliation Act 1981
Omnibus Budget Reconciliation Act 1989
On line analytic processing (OLAP), 171
On line transaction processing (OLTP), 171
ONC (formerly; ONCHIT). See Office of the National Coordinator for Health Information Technology
Online Mendelian Inheritance in Man (OMIM) database, 621, 622, 715, 736, 738
Online Registry of Biomedical Informatics Tools (ORBIT), 283

Ontologies, 222ff, 272, 278, 323, 661, 730
Ontology for Biomedical Investigations (OBI), 769
Open access, 617
Open CL, 154
Open Course Ware movement, 678
Open data interface (ODI), 404
Open Directory, 620, 627, 628
Open standards development policy, 217
Open Standards Interconnect (OSI) protocol, 236, 237
Open source, 207, 419
OpenEHR Foundation, 220, 224, 491
OpenGALEN, 232
OpenMRS, 409
OpenNLP, 283
Operating characteristics (of tests), 75
Operating rooms, 561
Operating systems, 167ff
Ophthalmologic imaging, 297
Optical character recognition, 410
Optical coherence tomography, 297
Optical disks, 150
ORBIT. *See* Online Registry of Biomedical Informatics
    Tools (ORBIT)
Order-entry systems. *See* Computerized provider order
    entry (CPOE)
Order sets, 7
Organizational change, 16
Oscilloscope, 567
OSI. *See* Open Standards Interconnect protocol (OSI)
Osirix, 684
Outcome
    data, 342, 786
    variables, 368
Outcomes research, 756
Output devices, 154–5
Overload, 190
OVID (formerly, CD Plus), 619, 621, 637, 686, 762
OWL (Web Ontology Language), 224, 323
Oximeter. *See* Pulse oximeter

P

Packets, 158
PACS. *See* Picture archiving and communications
    systems (PACS)
PageRank algorithm, 630
Pages, 168
Palo Alto Research Center (PARC), 797
Paper records, 4ff, 50ff, 392ff
PaperChase, 464
Parallel computing, 181
Parallel database management system, 181
Parallel processing, 151, 181
Parse tree, 269
Part of speech, 261, 263, 269
    tagging, 270
Partial-match searching, 631
Partial parsing. *See* Shallow parsing
Partners Health Care, 401, 492, 494, 748
Participant recruitment, 764

Participant registration, 766
Participant screening, 766
Pascal, 165
PatCIS. *See* Patient Clinical Information
    System (PatCIS)
Patents, 350
Pathognomonic tests, 62
Pathology Education Instruction Resource (PEIR), 622
Patient
    identifiers, 213, 214
    engagement, 518
    tracking, 460
    triage, 463
Patient care information management, 475ff
Patient care information systems, 480
Patient-centered care, 17, 476ff
Patient-centered communication, 523
Patient centered systems, 14, 485, 495
Patient centered medical home, 478, 792
Patient Centered Outcomes Research Institute
    (PCORI), 774
Patient Clinical Information System (PatCIS), 526, 527
Patient Gateway, 492
Patient identifiers, 794
Patient monitoring, 561ff
    intensive care units, 561, 564
Patient portals, 517, 526ff, 545
Patient safety, 111, 133ff, 357, 793
Patient-care systems, 475ff
Patient simulator, 682
Patient tracking, 460
Patients Like Me, 525
PatientSite, 526
Pattern recognition, 802
Pay for performance, 450, 457, 485, 486
PCAST. *See* President's Council of Advisors on Science
    and Technology (PCAST)
PCHR. *See* Personally controlled health record (PCHR)
PCORI. *See* Patient Centered Outomes Research Institute
    (PCORI)
PCPs. *See* Primary care physicians (PCPs)
PDAs. *See* Personal digital assistants (PDAs)
PDF. *See* Portable Document Format (PDF)
PEM. *See* Privacy-Enhanced Mail (PEM)
Perimeter definition, 175
Performance indicators. *See* Key performance indicators
Perl, 165
Personal computers (PCs), 4, 24
Personal electronic communications, 545
Personal Genome Project (PGP), 698, 746
Personal health applications, 517
Personal health information (PHI), 803
Personal health records (PHR), 345, 417, 498, 499,
    517ff, 526ff, 610, 784, 792, 805, 806
    tethered, 492
Personalized medicine, 55, 647, 721, 724, 806
Personally controlled health record (PCHR), 529
PET scan. *See* Positron emission tomography (PET)
Petabyte, 153
Pharmacogenomics, 29, 737ff

Pharmacogenomics Knowledge Base (PharmGKB), 698, 739, 740
Pharmacovigilence, 256
Phenome-wide association scan (PheWAS), 734
Phenotype, 256, 610, 698
PHI. *See* Personal health information (PHI)
Phillips Corporation, 570
PHIN. *See* Public Health Information Network (PHIN)
PHRs. *See* Personal health records (PHRs)
Physical Transport Level, 172
Physical therapist, 478
Physicians' Information and Education Resource (PIER), 623
Picture-archiving and communication systems (PACS), 197, 296, 308, 548, 601
PIER. *See* Physicians' Information and Education Resource (PIER)
PITAC. *See* President's Information Technology Advisory Committee (PITAC)
Pittsburgh Note Repository, 282
Pixels, 155, 298
PL/1, 165
Placebo, 758, 759
Placebo-controlled trial, 759
Planning, 325
Plug-ins, 174
PLoS. *See* Public Library of Science (PLoS)
Podcast, 678
Pointing devices, 154
Policy, 513, 808. *See also* HIT policy
Polysemy, 280, 630
Portable Document Format (PDF), 630
Portico, 640
Positive predictive value, 84
Positron-emission tomography (PET), 289
Post-test probability, 71
Postcoordination, 223, 229
Postdoctoral fellowship. *See* National Library of Medicine postdoctoral fellowship
Postgenomic databases, 725
POTS (plain old telephone system). *See* Telephone
PPO. *See* Preferred provider organizations (PPO)
Practice management systems, 445
Practice redesign, 792
Pragmatics, 260, 266
Precision, 276, 634
Precision medicine, 610. *See also* Personalized medicine
Precoordination, 223, 229
Predicate calculus, 118
Predicate logic, 257, 271
Prediction of function, 707, 742
Predictive biomarkers. *See* Biomarkers
Predictive value, 63
    negative, 84
    positive, 63, 84
Preferred provider organizations, 213
President's Council of Advisors on Science and Technology (PCAST), 427, 439, 806
President's Information Technology Committee (PITAC), 426

Pretest probability, 70
Prevalence, 63
Prevention (of disease), 11, 13
Primal pictures, 684
Primary knowledge-based information, 615
Prior probability. *See* Pretest probability
Privacy, 8, 175, 198, 249, 276, 335, 349, 419, 427, 793, 809
Privacy-Enhanced Mail (PEM), 173
Private Management Domain (PRMD), 163
PRMD. *See* Private Management Domain (PRMD)
Probabilistic approach (natural language processing), 258
Probabilistic systems, 657
Probability, 64, 67ff
    subjective assessment, 71
    threshold, 98
Problem-based learning, 675, 767, 679ff
Problem solving, 645. *See also* Decision making
Problem space, 113
Problem-Oriented Medical Information System (PROMIS), 487
Procedural knowledge, 119, 120
Process integration, 451
Process reengineering, 16, 457
Production rules, 120
Productivity, 455
Professional Standards Review Organizations (PSROs), 485
Professional-patient relationship, 334, 344
Prognostic scoring system, 341
Programming languages, 164ff
Project HealthDesign Initiative, 345, 529, 533, 537
PROMIS. *See* Problem-Oriented Medical Information System (PROMIS)
PROSPECT. *See* Prospective Outcome Systems using Patient-specific Electronic Data to Compare Tests and Therapies (PROSPECT)
Prospective Outcome Systems using Patient-specific Electronic Data to Compare Tests and Therapies (PROSPECT), 484
Prospective studies, 53, 416
Protected memory, 168
Protégé system, 665
Protein Data Bank (PDB), 700, 704, 714
Proteomics, 696
Protocol (clinical), 7, 584, 585
Protocol analysis, 113
Protocol authoring, 765
Protocol management, 766
Provider communications, 46
Provider-profiling systems, 462
Pseudo-identifiers, 507
PSRO. *See* Professional Standards Review Organizations (PSRO)
Public health, 339, 504ff, 645
    informatics, 28, 503ff
Public Health Information Network (PHIN), 509, 515
Public-key cryptography, 177, 404
Public Library of Science (PLoS), 617

Public policy. *See* Policy
PubMed, 276, 400, 619, 621ff, 631ff, 704, 762, 799
PubMed Central (PMC), 276
Pulse oximeter, 570
Punctuation, 268
Python, 165

Q

QALYs. *See* Quality-adjusted life years (QALYs)
QOS. *See* Quality of service (QOS)
QRS wave, 160
QSEN. *See* Quality and Safety Education for Nurses
    (QSEN)
Quality-adjusted life years, 91, 96
Quality and Safety Education for Nurses (QSEN), 489
Quality
    assurance, 666
    control, 12
    management, 455, 486
    measurement, 785ff
    reporting, 415
Quality of service (QOS), 544
Quasi-experiement, 758, 759
Query, 614
Query and reporting tools, 766
Query language, 170
Query-response cycle, 433
Question answering, 259, 638
Question understanding, 256

R

Radiology, 593ff
Radiology systems, 593ff
    information systems, 603ff
Radiology Society of North America (RSNA), 220,
    234, 600
RadLex, 234, 301ff, 325, 606
RAM (random access memory), 153
Randomized clinical trials (RCTs), 50, 373, 758, 759
RCRIM. *See* Regulated Clinical Research Information
    Management (RCRIM)
RCTs. *See* Randomized clinical trials (RCTs)
RDF. *See* Resource Description Framework (RDF)
RSS. *See* Really Simple Syndication (RSS)
Read Clinical Codes, 57, 230, 231, 300
Read-only memory. *See* ROM (read-only memory)
Real-time data acquisition, 159
Real-time monitoring, 568, 569
Really Simple Syndication (RSS), 268, 620
Recall, 276, 634
Receiver, 235
Receiver-operating characteristic (ROC) curve, 78, 79,
    81, 729
Records, 170. *See also* Medical records
Reference Information Model. *See* Health Level Seven
    Reference Information Model
Reference resolution, 259
Reference standards, 275

Referential expression, 267, 274, 275
Referral bias, 73, 80
Regenstrief Institute, 407, 413, 415, 654
Regenstrief Medical Record System (RMRS), 394, 487
Regional extension centers, 427
Regional Health Information Organizations (RHIOs), 427
Regional network, 162
Registers, 151, 153
Registries, 14
Regular expression, 261, 262, 265
Regulated Clinical Research Information Management
    (RCRIM), 768
Regulation, 341, 347ff, 750, 793
Relationships (natural language processing), 259
Relative recall, 634, 635
Relevance judgement, 635
Relevance ranking, 630
Reminders, 188, 190, 414, 654
Remote consultation. *See* Teleconsultation
Remote intensive care, 542, 554, 555
Remote interpretation, 545, 547
Remote monitoring, 472, 545–7, 559
Remote presence healthcare. *See* Telemedicine
Report generation, 170
Representation, 225
Representational state, 147
Representational State Transfer (REST), 180
Representativeness, 72
Research monitoring tools, 766
Research planning, 763
REST. *See* Representational State Transfer (REST)
Resource Description Framework (RDF), 627–8
Results reporting, 461
RESUME system
Retrieval, 614, 630ff
Retrospective chart review, 53
Retrospective research study, 50, 416, 758, 759
Return on investment (ROI), 648
Review of systems (ROS), 61
RFDS. *See* Australian Royal Flying Doctor Service
    (RFDS)
RHIO. *See* Regional Health Information Organization
    (RHIO)
Rich Site Summary. *See* Really Simple Syndication
Rich Text Format (RTF), 267
Risk attitude, 94
Risk-neutral, 94
RIM. *See* Health Level Seven Reference Information
    Model (RIM)
RNA, 698
Roadmap for Medical Research (NIH), 724
Robert Wood Johnson Foundation, 345, 486, 530, 537
Robotic surgery, 555
ROC curve. *See* Receiver-operating characteristic
    (ROC) curve
Role-limited access, 178
ROM (read-only memory), 153
Rounds report, 579, 580, 587
Routers, 158
    external, 162

RS-232, 571
RSNA. *See* Radiology Society of North
America (RSNA)
RSS. *See* Really Simple Syndication (RSS)
RTF. *See* Rich text Format (RTF)
Rule-based approach (natural language
processing), 258
Rule-based systems, 659. *See also* MYCIN
RxNorm, 233, 234, 282, 396, 731, 734, 738

S

Saccharomyces Database, 282
Safe, Timely, Effective, Efficient, Equitable, Patient-
centered (STEEP) care, 524
Safety. *See* Patient safety
Sampling, 160, 370
Sandia National Laboratory, 659
Satellite, 11, 543, 558
Scenario-based learning, 679ff
Schema, 118, 170
Science Citation Index (SCI), 622
Scientific American Medicine, 636
SCO. *See* Standard Development Organizations Charter
Committee (SCO)
SCOPUS, 623
SCORM. *See* Sharable Content Object Reference Model
(SCORM)
Screening tools, 765
SCRIPT, 245
Script, 166
SDLC. *See* Software development lifecycle (SDLC)
SDOs. *See* Standards development organizations (SDOs)
Search. *See* Information retrieval
Secondary knowledge-based information, 615
Secondary use of data. *See* Data reuse
Secret-key cryptography, 177
Secure FTP (SFTP), 174
Secure Shell (SSH), 173
Secure Sockets Layer (SSL), 174
Security, 8, 175, 198, 214, 419, 454, 766, 809
Self care, 518
Self-help, 520
Semantic analysis, 272
Semantic grammar, 265
Semantic Network (UMLS), 281, 626
Semantic patterns, 264
Semantic sense, 264
Semantic types, 264
Semantic web, 627
Semantics, 260, 264, 272ff
Sender, 235
Sensitivity, 62, 67ff
Sensitivity analysis, 95ff
Sensors, 800
Sentences, 268
Sentiment analysis, 260
Sequence, 700
alignment, 705
databases, 712

Sequencing, 702, 703, 744
next generation, 702, 745
Service-oriented architecture (SOA), 205, 206, 243, 470,
668, 763
Set-based searching, 630
Set-top boxes, 11
Setting-specific factors (SSF), 669
SFTP. *See* Secure FTP (SFTP)
Shallow parsing, 270
Sharable Content Object Reference Model
(SCORM), 690
SHARE models, 225
Shared decision making, 518
SHARP Program. *See* Strategic Health IT Research
Projects
Shielding, 161
Short Message Service (SMS), 558
Short-term memory, 117
SHRDLU, 257
SICU. *See* Intensive care unit, surgical
Side effects, 743
Signal processing, 159ff
Simple Mail Transport Protocol (SMTP), 173, 534
Simple Object Access Protocol (SOAP), 206
Simulated patients, 685
Simulation, 681ff, 691, 762
Simulation center, 685, 688
Single nucleotide polymorphisms, 697, 740, 741
Single photon emission computed tomography
(SPECT), 294
Single-signon, 199
Single user systems, 168
Six Sigma, 458
Skype, 526
SlideShare, 678
SlideTutor, 684
Slips, 135
Slots, 272
Smalltalk, 165
SMArt (Substitutable Medial Applications, reusable
technologies), 208, 225, 529, 530
Smart phones, 4, 45, 461, 558
Smith Waterman algorithm, 704, 706
SMK. *See* Structured Meta Knowledge (SMK)
SMS. *See* Short Message Service (SMS)
SMTP. *See* Simple Mail Transport Protocol (SMTP)
SNOMED-CT (Systematized Nomenclature of
Medicine-Clinical Terms), 57, 221–3, 230, 232,
234, 249, 277, 282, 300, 301, 396, 464, 491, 655,
731, 734, 770, 771
SNOP (Standardized Nomenclature of
Pathology), 57
SNP. *See* Single nucleotide polymorphism (SNP)
SOA. *See* Service-oriented architecture (SOA)
SOAP. *See* Simple Object Access Protocol (SOAP)
Social networking, 4, 517, 525
Social Science Citation Index (SSCI), 622
Societal change, 472
Software, 164ff, 186ff
certification, 351

Software development, 191ff, 196, 197
  analysis, 191, 192
  evaluation, 195, 196
  implementation phase, 194
  integration, 202
  lifecycle (SDLC), 191ff
  integration, 194
  planning, 191, 192
  testing, 193
Software oversight committees, 351
Software psychology, 130
Solid state drives, 150
Spamming, 173
Spatial resolution, 155, 156, 295
Specialist Lexicon (UMLS), 281, 626
Specificity, 63, 67ff
SPECT. *See* Single photon emission computed
  tomography (SPECT)
Spectrum bias, 80
Speech recognition, 162, 406, 603
Spirometer, 547
SPRUS, 257
SQL. *See* Structured Query Language (SQL)
SSCI. *See* Social Science Citation Index (SSCI)
SSH. *See* Secure Shell (SSH)
SSL. *See* Secure Sockets Layer (SSL)
ST segment, 162
STEEP. *See* Safe, Timely, Effective, Efficient, Equitable,
  Patient-centered (STEEP) care
Standard of care, 334
Standard development organizations, 215, 218ff
Standard Development Organizations Charter Committee
  (SCO), 220
Standard Guidelines for the Design of Educational
  Software, 689
Standard ML, 165
Standards, 8, 211ff, 418, 436, 670
  data in clinical research, 764, 767ff
  data definitions, 12
  data transmission and sharing, 12
  development process, 215ff
Standards and Certification Criteria for Electronic Health
  Records rule, 483
Standards development organizations (SDO), 214, 491
Stanford University, 23, 615, 739, 747
Stat! Ref, 621
Static simulation, 681
Stem cells, 744
Stemming, 629
Stimulus Bill. *See* American Reinvestment and Recovery
  Act (ARRA)
Stop words, 629
STOR, 394
Storage, 34
  active, 153
  archival, 153
  long-term, 153, 1544
Store and forward, 544, 545, 549
Strategic Health IT Research Projects (SHARP
  program), 483, 491

Stratified medicine. *See* Genomic medicine
Strict product liability, 347
Structural alignment, 705
Structural analysis, 703
Structural imaging, 288
Structural informatics, 28. *See also* Imaging informatics
Structure validation, 363
Structured data entry, 656
Structured Meta Knowledge (SMK), 232
Structured Query Language (SQL), 170
Study arm, 758
Subdomains, 279
Subheadings, 625
Subjectivist studies, 374
Sublanguage, 262
Substitutable Medial Applications, reusable technologies.
  See Substitutable Medial Applications, reusable
  technologies (SMArt)
Summative evaluation, 689
Supervised learning, 658, 728
Support vector machine (SVM), 312, 709. *See also*
  Machine learning
Surescripts, 397
Surgical intensive care unit. *See* Intensive care unit,
  surgical
Surveillance, 11, 191, 425, 505
  syndromic, 337, 584
Sustainability, 513
Switches, 158
Symbolic-programming languages, 164
Synchronous communication, 544
Syndromic software integration, 256
Syndromic surveillance. *See* Surveillance, syndromic
Synonymy, 280, 624, 630
Syntactic knowledge, 262ff
Syntactic parse, 269
Syntax, 260, 261, 269ff
Systematic review, 618
System learnability, 110
Systematized Nomenclature of Medicine–Clinical Terms.
  See Systematized Nomenclature of Medicine–
  Clinical Terms (SNOMED-CT)
Systematized Nomenclature of Pathology. *See* SNOP
  (Standardized Nomenclature of Pathology)
Systems biology, 699, 703
Systems programs, 169

T
Tablet computers, 45, 461
Tabulating machines, 23
Tactile feedback. *See* Haptic feedback
Tailored information, 799
Tales from the Heart, 680
TATRC. *See* Telemedicine and Advanced Technology
  Resource Center (TATRC)
TBI. *See* Translational bioinformatics (TBI)
TCP/IP. *See* Transmission Control Protocol/Internet
  Protocol (TCP/IP)
Technical Advisory Group, 220

Technicon Data Systems (TDS), 23
Technicon Medical Information System, 464
Telecardiology, 547
Telecommunications, 11
Teleconsultation, 543, 550
Teledermatology, 547
Telegraphic language, 262
Telehealth, 535, 541ff, 784, 792
    licensure and economics, 557
    networks, 543
    video-based, 550, 552
Telehome care. See Home telehealth
Tele-ICU, 554, 555, 585, 586
Telemedicine, 5, 15, 344, 541, 542
Telemedicine and Advanced Technology Resource
        Center (TATRC), 538
Teleophthalmology, 542, 547
Telepathology, 547, 548
Telephone, 545, 549ff
    cellular, 558
Telepresence, 344, 542, 544, 545, 555, 556, 595
Telepsychiatry, 542, 551
Teleradiology, 15, 542, 543, 547, 548, 557, 606
Telerobotics, 555, 556
Telestroke, 554
Telesurgery, 542, 555
Temporal resolution, 295
Terabyte, 153
Term, 225, 624
Term frequency
Term weighting, 629
Terminals
Terminologies, 8, 225, 226
    for clinical research, 768ff
Terminology authority, 469
Terminology services, 469
Test collection, 635
Test-interpretation, 62, 79ff
Test-referral bias, 80
Tests. See Diagnostic tests
Text comprehension, 113
Text generation, 260
Text mining, 638, 742, 762
Text processing, 267
Text REtrieval Conference (TREC), 635
Text readability assessment, 260
Text simplification, 260
Text summarization, 260, 638
TF. See Term frequency (TF)
TF*IDF weighting, 629
The Medical Record (TMR), 394, 487
Therapeutic targeting, 728
Thesaurus, 624
Thick clients, 198
Thin clients, 198
Think-aloud protocols, 113
Thomson-Reuters, 623
Threads, 166
Three-dimensional environment, 691
Time-shared computers, 23

Time-sharing networks, 614
Tissue imaging, 296TJC. See Joint Commission, The
TMIS. See Technicon Medical Information System
        (TMIS)
TMR. See The Medical Record (TMR)
Tokens, 261, 268
Tokenization, 267, 268
Tolven, 224
Top down parsing, 271
Tooth Atlas, 679
Tort law, 347
Touchscreen, 154
Tower of Hanoi, 113, 114
Track pad, 154
Training, 15, 595, 750
Transaction sets, 235
Transcription, 406
Transducer, 569
Transition matrix, 270
Transition probabilities, 97
Translating Research into Practice (TRIP), 620
Translational bioinformatics, 717, 721ff
Translational medicine, 721. See also CTSAs
Translational research, 759
Transmission Control Protocol/Internet Protocol (TCP/
        IP), 162, 172, 173, 239, 466, 600
Transport level, 172
Transport level security (TLS), 174, 410
TREC. See Text REtrieval Conference (TREC)
Tree. See Decision tree
Tri-Service Medical Information System (TRIMIS), 487
Triage, 463
Trigger event, 238, 583
TRIMIS. See Tri-Service Medical Information (TRIMIS)
TRIP. See Translating Research into Practice (TRIP)
True negatives, 76ff
True positives, 76ff
True-negative rate, 77ff
True-positive rate, 77ff
Twenty-three and Me (23andMe), 748, 751
Twisted-pair wires, 158
Type checking, 165
Type I errors, 709
Typographical errors, 277, 278

U
Ubiquitous computing, 129
UCC. See Uniform Code Council (UCC)
UCUM, 396
UDP. See User Datagram Protocol (UDP)
Ultrasound, 292
UMIA, 283
UML. See Unified Modeling Language (UML)
UMLS. See Unified Medical Language System (UMLS)
Unicode, 152, 268
Unified Medical Language System (UMLS), 58, 234ff,
        265, 281, 282, 301, 469, 625, 626, 731, 739
Unified Modeling Language UML), 224, 225, 272, 768
Uniform Code Council (UCC), 247

Uniform Resource Identifier (URI), 639
Uniform Resource Name (URN), 639
Unique health identifier (UHI), 794
Unintended consequences, 136ff, 493, 496
United Nations, 235
Universal Product Number Repository, 247
Uniform Resource Locator (URL), 174, 639
Universal System Bus (USB), 571
University Hospital of Giessen, 493
University of Colorado, 345
University of Columbia Missouri, 487
University of Leeds, 649
University of Michigan, 466
University of Pennsylvania, 289
University of Pittsburgh, 289
University of California Los Angeles, 306
University of California San Francisco, 465
University of California Santa Cruz
University of Washington, 301, 306, 409
University of Wisconsin, 520
Up-To-Date, 400, 480, 623, 687
URAC (Utilization Reviewed Acredditation,
    Commission (518)
URI. *See* Uniform Resource Identifier (URI)
URL. *See* Universal Resource Locator (URL)
URN. *See* Uniform Resource Name (URN)
Usability testing, 133, 363, 418, 493
USB. *See* Universal System Bus (USB)
User authentication, 198
User Datagram Protocol (UDP), 172
User interfaces, 128, 803
User-interface layer, 469
Utility, 89, 94, 658, 671

V
Validation, 195
Validity, 761
Value theory, 89ff
Vanderbilt University, 493, 494
Vector mathematics, 631
Vector-space model, 631
Vendors (of clinical systems), 340
Ventilator alarms, 581
Verification, 195
Vertical integration, 446
Veterans Health Administration, 208, 224, 232, 332, 392,
    395, 430, 465, 527, 534, 548, 665
    National Drug File (VANDF), 234
Veterinary informatics, 26
Video-based Telehealth, 548
Videoconferencing, 544, 545
Video display terminals (VDTs), 463
View(s), 170
View schemas, 170
Virginia Commonwealth University, 492
Virtual address, 169
Virtual Patient, 685
Virtual reality, 683

Virtual memory, 168, 169
Virtual Private Networks (VPNs), 177, 609
Virtual reality, 129
Viruses, 176
Visible Body, 684
Visible Human Project, 622
VistA system, 208, 332, 395, 661, 665
Visual analog scales, 94
Visual diagnosis, 127
VisualDX, 622
Visualization, 605, 684, 762
Vital signs, 564, 565
Vocabulary, 55, 198, 225, 226, 624
Volatile memory, 153
Volume rendering, 310
Volunteer effect, 371
Von Neuman machines, 150, 151
Voxel, 289, 291, 317
Voxelman, 305
VPNs. *See* Virtual Private Networks (VPNs)

W
WANs. *See* Wide-area networks (WANs)
Washington DC Principles for free access to science, 617
Washington Heights/Inwood Informatics Infrastructure
    for Comparative Effectiveness Research
    (WICER), 484
Waterfall software development model, 196, 197
Wearable computers, 798
Web-based Clinical Information System (WebCIS), 552
Web browsers, 174
Web catalog, 620
Web of Science, 622, 623
Web Ontology Language. *See* OWL
Web services, 180
Web Services Description Language (WSDL), 180, 206
WebCIS. *See* Web-based Clinical Information System
    (WebCIS)
Webinar, 678
Weblog. *See* Blog
WebMD, 687
WebPath, 622
WebTV, 525
WEDI. *See* Workgroup for Electronic Data Interchange
Weight Watchers Online, 531
White space, 268
WHO. *See* World Health Organization (WHO)
WHO Drug Dictionary
WHO-ART. *See* World Health Organization Adverse
    Reactions Terminology
Whole slide digitization, 609
WICER. *See* Washington Heights/Inwood Informatics
    Infrastructure for Comparative Effectiveness
    Research
Wide-area networks (WAN), 157, 163, 238
WIPO. *See* World Intellectual Property Organization
    (WIPO)
Wireless networking, 4

WIRM. *See* Web Interfacing Repository Manager (WIRM)
Wishard Memorial Hospital, 394
WizOrder, 400
WONCA. *See* World Organization of National Colleges, Academies and Academic Associations of General Practitioners/Family Physicians (WONCA)
Word(s), 153, 268
Word sense, 264, 272, 282
Word sense disambiguation (WSD), 272, 282
Workflow management, 606, 669
Workflow modelling, 492, 493, 764
Workforce training, 763
Workgroup for Electronic Data Interchange (WEDI), 220
Working memory. *See* Short-term memory
Workstations, 45
World Health Organization (WHO), 56, 226, 582
WHO Drug Dictionary, 232
World Intellectual Property Organization (WIPO), 640
World Organization of National Colleges, Academies and Academic Associations of General Practitioners/Family Physicians (WONCA), 228
World Wide Web (WWW), 174, 175, 521, 614

Worm(s), 176
WormBase Database, 282
WSD. *See* Word sense disambiguation
WSDL. *See* Web Services Description Language
WWW. *See* World Wide Web (WWW)

X
X.25, 239
X-rays
Xerox PARC. *See* Palo Alto Research Center
XML (Extensible Mark-up Language), 175, 206, 216, 235, 240, 242, 267, 303, 471, 628, 666, 772

Y
Y2K problem, 40
Yale University, 226
YouTube, 678

Z
Z39.84, 639
Zynx, 623

CPSIA information can be obtained
at www.ICGtesting.com
Printed in the USA
LVHW06*1328210818
587645LV00002B/5/P